PRINCIPLES OF MOLECULAR CARDIOLOGY

CONTEMPORARY CARDIOLOGY

CHRISTOPHER P. CANNON, MD
SERIES EDITOR

PRINCIPLES
OF MOLECULAR CARDIOLOGY

Edited by

MARSCHALL S. RUNGE, MD, PhD

Department of Medicine
UNC School of Medicine, Chapel Hill, NC

CAM PATTERSON, MD

Carolina Cardiovascular Biology Center
Chapel Hill, NC

Foreword by

JAMES T. WILLERSON, MD

University of Texas Medical School
Houston, TX

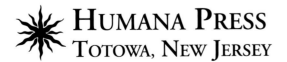

HUMANA PRESS
TOTOWA, NEW JERSEY

Cover illustrations: Figure 2, Chapter 6, by M. Ashe and D. Bader; Fig. 2, Chapter 11, by M. W. Majesky; Fig. 8, Chapter 14, by D. D. Miller and S. C. Herrmann; Fig. 3, Chapter 12, by G. A. Stouffer.

Cover design by Patricia F. Cleary.

This publication is printed on acid-free paper. ∞
ANSI Z39.48-1984 (American National Standards Institute) Permanence of Paper for Printed Library Materials.

Printed in the United States of America. 10 9 8 7 6 5 4 3 2 1

Library of Congress Cataloging-in-Publication Data
Principles of molecular cardiology / edited by Marschall S. Runge and Cam Patterson ; foreword by James T. Willerson.
        p. ; cm. — (Contemporary cardiology)
    Includes bibliographical references and index.
    ISBN 1-58829-201-0 (hardcover : alk. paper) eISBN 1-59259-878-1
    1. Heart—Diseases—Molecular aspects.
    [DNLM: 1. Cardiovascular Diseases—genetics. 2. Cardiovascular Diseases—physiopathology. WG 120 P957 2005] I. Runge, Marschall Stevens, 1954- II. Patterson, Cam. III. Series: Contemporary cardiology (Totowa, N.J.: Unnumbered)

C682.9.P754 2005   616.1'2042—dc22
2004014202

FOREWORD

Principles of Molecular Cardiology provides a broad and up-to-date treatment of the molecular biology of cardiovascular diseases. This is a timely volume given the impact of cardiovascular diseases in our society and the numerous advances in understanding cardiovascular disease that have followed the molecular and genomic revolutions. This book begins with a broad historical overview of the major themes in molecular cardiology: cardiovascular genetics, the molecular biology of the cardiovascular system, genomics, gene therapy, and stems cells and progenitor cells in cardiovascular disease. These chapters provide concise information about how these areas can be used to understand and develop treatments for cardiovascular diseases.

This overview is followed by a discussion of cardiac function and dysfunction. Subjects covered include the molecular and structural events in heart development; the molecular biology of inherited myocardial diseases with a specific focus on hypertrophic cardiomyopathies and muscular dystrophies that affect the heart; the molecular regulation of inotropic function and the events that occur in cardiomyocytes that contribute to progressive systolic dysfunction; the process of inflammation within the heart with emphasis on how adhesion molecules affect this process; and common cardiac defects and the molecular basis for these defects.

The third section of this book focuses on the important topic of coronary artery disease. This section includes excellent chapters addressing the differentiation of the coronary arteries; the evolution of coronary vascular lesions with emphasis on the effects of platelets, smooth muscle cells, and inflammatory cells in this process; the molecular pathways that activate platelets and the pharmacologic actions of antiplatelet drugs; pathophysiologic events that result in myocardial infarction; the development of arterial disease after cardiac transplantation; the scientific basis for thrombolytic therapy; and the molecular basis for restenosis following percutaneous coronary interventions and recently developed new treatment modalities, including radiation therapy.

The section on cardiac arrhythmias is timely given recent progress in understanding the molecular basis and genetics of arrhythmias and sudden death. Topics covered in this section include the molecular biology of the development of the cardiac conduction system, the electrical events that cause sudden death and the development of arrhythmias, emerging new therapies for arrhythmias based on the molecular understanding, and the genetic basis for arrhythmias.

The section on vascular diseases includes state-of-the-art chapters discussing the molecular events that regulate angiogenesis and the potential for angiogenic therapy, the molecular basis for the metabolism and actions of nitric oxide, the role of inflammation in vascular disease, the pathophysiology of pulmonary hypertension and the genetics that influence its development, the molecular and genetic events that cause malformations of the vascular system, and the molecular events involved in thrombosis.

The book concludes with a section on risk factors for cardiovascular disease. These chapters succinctly summarize the molecular basis for lipid metabolism, the molecular biology of aging and its impact on the cardiovascular system, the role of oxidative species in atherosclerosis, the molecular consequences of diabetes on the cardiovascular system, and the molecular determinants of inflammation and its amelioration with proper risk factor modification.

An understanding of these topics is critically important to anyone who wishes to conduct serious research in any of these areas or teach others about them. Moreover, new therapies that develop in these areas will be based on an understanding of the molecular biology and genetics of these cardiovascular problems.

I believe *Principles of Molecular Cardiology* is an outstanding book. Anyone interested in the development, genetics, and pathologies that affect the cardiovascular system will want to have this book available for ready reference.

James T. Willerson, MD

Texas Heart Institute
The University of Texas Health Science Center at Houston
Houston, TX

PREFACE

In recent years, molecular studies have had a major impact on cardiovascular clinical practice and outcomes. The rationale for drug therapies for treating cardiovascular diseases such as heart failure has been based primarily on data derived from basic science investigations. The Human Genome Project has implications for biology and mankind that are unparalleled, in part because having such an abundance of information on the inner workings of humans is unprecedented. Our understanding of genetic links to cardiovascular diseases has increased dramatically, helping redefine the etiology and diagnostic criteria for numerous conditions and leading to new, individualized treatments.

Principles of Molecular Cardiology was undertaken to explore the latest developments in molecular cardiology research. In this text, we review the complex process of heart development, explain the molecular bases of cardiovascular diseases, describe the application of research advances in clinical treatment, and provide a historical perspective for important areas within this discipline. This book is intended for researchers, clinicians, students, and healthcare professionals who want to keep abreast of current findings in molecular cardiology research. The authors, all leading specialists, provide a unique perspective of what the future in molecular research holds for their respective fields.

Genetics research and advances in gene therapy are recurring themes throughout this text. Certain genetic mutations are clearly associated with severe cardiovascular disease, and new disease-causing mutations are being identified with increasing frequency. Some researchers estimate that there are probably only 200–300 genes that provide susceptibility for the 20 diseases that account for 80% of all deaths globally. Given the genetic and physical maps of the human genome and the technology of high-throughput nucleotide sequencing, it is conceivable that all human genes that contribute to the genetic risk of major cardiovascular diseases will be known within the next decade.

In the field of vascular biology, the number of genes that have been cloned and linked to vascular wall disease is growing exponentially. Because of their association with cardiovascular function, genes encoding the proteins endothelin-1—a potent vasoactive hormone—and the angiotensin receptor have proven to be attractive sites for pharmacologic intervention, but it is clear that the genes identified today will be the therapeutic targets of tomorrow. In addition, gain-of-function and loss-of-function mice, created through genetic manipulations, have provided enormous insights into such processes as lipid metabolism and the function of cardiac- and vascular wall-specific genes.

Although studies using mouse models have been a major tool to push the field of molecular cardiology forward, advances in human genetics have contributed significantly to the understanding of inherited cardiac diseases such as long QT syndrome and hypertrophic obstructive cardiomyopathy. Although advances have been made in understanding the pathophysiologic and genetic bases of cardiac arrhythmias, current treatment options are still inadequate, prompting a search for genetic strategies to treat these conditions.

Research in the complex area of atherosclerosis continues. Despite the great strides made in recent years, many of the processes involved in atherosclerosis remain poorly characterized. Studies of atherosclerosis in humans are limited by the complexity of the cellular and molecular mechanisms that contribute to the process and the long time course of disease development. There is also significant variability seen in pathogenetic mechanisms. In this text, the authors discuss the latest developments in understanding the pathogenesis of atherosclerosis—its manifestations (coronary artery disease, acute coronary syndromes) and its underlying mechanisms (oxidative stress and inflammation).

Platelets play a central role in the pathogenesis of atherosclerosis. Therefore, platelet inhibition has proven to be a logical therapeutic strategy for acute and chronic treatment of atherosclerosis and its clinical sequelae. The need for efficient inhibition of platelet function is even more evident in the situation of a vascular injury associated with angioplasty. Strategies for inhibiting platelet function are discussed in this text. There are many different potential ways to inhibit platelet activation, and several receptors are considered promising therapeutic targets, including the thrombin receptor and the TXA_2 receptor.

Restenosis following percutaneous coronary interventions remains a serious problem. Because of the number of molecular targets available for targeting the cell cycle in antirestenosis therapy, gene therapy is a second clinical approach for inhibiting small muscle cell proliferation. Although results from antirestenotic gene therapy trials in humans have not been published, results from animal models are promising. A second antirestenotic gene therapy that affects the cell cycle makes use of the overexpression of cell cycle inhibitory molecules. Experimental data support the use of gene therapy as a cell cycle inhibitor; however, the application of gene therapy to clinical medicine will depend not only on the ability of cell cycle arrest to block restenosis in clinical settings, but also on the demonstration of acceptable safety profiles.

The field of developmental biology of the cardiovascular system has also accelerated during the past decade. New developments in the study of blood vessel development and a strong clinical interest in therapeutic angiogenesis have led to greater understanding of the molecular biology of the assembly of cardiovascular structures, and many of these ideas are being translated to clinical practice to treat obstructive vascular disease.

Despite these advances and promising new discoveries, cardiovascular disease remains the leading cause of death in the United States. The aging of the population will undoubtedly be a factor in the increasing incidence of coronary artery disease, heart failure, and stroke. Of the more than 64 million Americans with one or more types of cardiovascular disease, more than 25 million are estimated to be age 65 and older (*Heart Disease and Stroke Statistics—2004 Update*, American Heart Association). For reasons not entirely clear, there is also an increased prevalence of obesity and type 2 diabetes—the major cardiovascular risk factors—in this country. Related complications—hypertension, hyperlipidemia, and atherosclerotic vascular disease—also have increased.

In the next decade, new tools will be applied to the study of cardiovascular disease and function. These instruments will include DNA microarrays, proteomic approaches, comparative DNA analysis, and markers of human genetic variation. The innovative use of these new and powerful tools hold promise to accelerate the pace of discovery in cardiovascular medicine.

There is an untapped potential for molecular and cellular biology to lead to substantial new discoveries in the near future. These discoveries will only be achieved with intensive and focused research. We hope this text will provide a foundation of knowledge and inspiration for investigators to continue the progress in this crucial field of research. As clinicians and scientists, the advancements in molecular cardiology over the preceding decade have inspired the editors in the laboratory and at the bedside, and we are grateful to our colleagues for moving the field so rapidly during this time.

We would like to thank the many individuals who contributed to the success of this book. We especially commend all our authors for devoting their time, energy, and scholarship to preparing these chapters—we asked for the best from our contributors, and we got it. We also thank the following editors who assisted in preparation of the text. Rebecca Bartow, PhD, was primary manuscript editor, and Jennifer King, PhD, also edited and reviewed many chapters; their contributions to this project can be appreciated whenever consistency and cogency are detected in this book. Angela Rego, BBA, coordinated manuscripts, handled correspondence between physician editors and authors, and served as adjutant general for all aspects of this project. Rebecca Teaff, MA, coordinated the editing process and reviewed manuscripts, for which the editors extend their gratitude. Carolyn Kruse, BS, DC, served as a manuscript editor. Kakky Baugher, BA, Erin Allingham, BA, Elizabeth Schramm, BA, and Kelly Scarlett assisted in manuscript review and formatting, as well as verifying references. Katie O'Brien, MA, and Angela Rego, BBA, assisted in preparation of graphics for the text. We would also like to thank Craig Adams of Humana Press for his enthusiastic support in ushering this book through the publication process.

We also extend our appreciation to our colleagues, collaborators, trainees, and laboratory members, including Nageswara Madamanchi, Yaxu Wu, and Holly McDonough, who inspired our desire to tackle this project. We dedicate this book to the memory of Edgar Haber. Dr. Haber trained many of the contributors to this project and influenced all of them. His family—his wife Carol, his sons Eben, Justin, and Graham, and his sister Ruth—shared him with us, for which we are grateful.

Cam Patterson, MD
Marschall S. Runge, MD, PhD

CONTENTS

CONTRIBUTORS

EINARI AAVIK, MS • *Transplantation Laboratory, Haartman Institute, Rational Drug Design Programme, Biomedicum Helsinki, University of Helsinki, Helsinki, Finland*

JULIUS AITSEBAOMO, MD • *Carolina Cardiovascular Biology Center, University of North Carolina at Chapel Hill, Chapel Hill, NC*

STEPHEN L. ARCHER, MD • *Department of Medicine, University of Alberta Hospital, Edmonton, AL, Canada*

MABELLE ASHE • *Department of Medicine, Vanderbilt University, Nashville, TN*

DAVID BADER, PhD • *Department of Medicine, Vanderbilt University, Nashville, TN*

LIZA BARKI-HARRINGTON, PhD • *Department of Medicine, Duke University Medical Center, Durham, NC*

ALLAN R. BRASIER, MD • *Departments of Internal Medicine and Human Biological Chemistry and Genetics, The University of Texas Medical Branch at Galveston, Galveston, TX*

W. VIRGIL BROWN, MD • *Department of Medicine, Emory University School of Medicine, Atlanta, GA*

RAMON BRUGADA, MD • *Masonic Medical Research Laboratory, Utica, NY*

WAYNE E. CASCIO, MD • *Department of Medicine, University of North Carolina at Chapel Hill, Chapel Hill, NC*

YI CHU, PhD • *Department of Internal Medicine, University of Iowa College of Medicine, Iowa City, IA*

DAVID R. CLEMMONS, MD • *Department of Medicine, University of North Carolina at Chapel Hill, Chapel Hill, NC*

MARSHALL A. CORSON, MD • *Department of Medicine, University of Washington School of Medicine, Seattle, WA*

J. KEVIN DONAHUE, MD • *Institute of Molecular Cardiobiology, Johns Hopkins University School of Medicine, Baltimore, MD*

DANIEL DU TOIT • *Department of Surgery, Stellenbosch University, Cape Town, South Africa*

MOHSEN S. ELEDRISI, MD • *Department of Internal Medicine, King Abdulaziz National Guard Medical Center, Saudi Arabia*

RONALD J. FALK, MD • *Departments of Medicine and Pathology and Laboratory Medicine, University of North Carolina at Chapel Hill, Chapel Hill, NC*

VIDU GARG, MD • *Department of Pediatrics, The University of Texas Southwestern Medical Center, Dallas, TX*

ROBERT G. GOURDIE, PhD • *Department of Cell Biology and Anatomy, Medical University of South Carolina, Charleston, SC*

PEKKA HÄYRY, MD, PhD • *Transplantation Laboratory, Haartman Institute, Rational Drug Design Programme, Biomedicum Helsinki, Univerity of Helsinki, Helsinki, Finland and Juvantia Pharma Ltd, Turku, Finland*

DONALD D. HEISTAD, MD • *Department of Internal Medicine, University of Iowa College of Medicine, Iowa City, IA*

STEVEN C. HERRMANN, MD, PhD • *Department of Internal Medicine, St. Louis University, St. Louis, MO*

KUI HONG, MD, PhD • *Masonic Medical Research Laboratory, Utica, NY*

TATSURO ISHIDA, MD, PhD • *Department of Medicine, Stanford University School of Medicine, Stanford, CA*

J. CHARLES JENNETTE, MD • *Departments of Medicine and Pathology and Laboratory Medicine, University of North Carolina at Chapel Hill, Chapel Hill, NC*

NOBUYUKI KANZAWA, PhD • *Department of Cell Biology, Cornell University Medical College, New York, NY*

EDWARD G. LAKATTA, MD • *National Institute on Aging, National Institutes of Health, Baltimore, MD*

NGOC-ANH LE, PhD • *Department of Medicine, Emory University School of Medicine, Atlanta, GA*

PHILIPPE LE CORVOISIER, MD • *Department of Medicine, Duke University Medical Center, Durham, NC*

NAGESWARA R. MADAMANCHI, PhD • *Carolina Cardiovascular Biology Center, University of North Carolina at Chapel Hill, Chapel Hill, NC*

MARK W. MAJESKY, PhD • *Departments of Medicine and Genetics, Carolina Cardiovascular Biology Center, University of North Carolina at Chapel Hill, Chapel Hill, NC*

DOUGLAS L. MANN, MD • *Winters Center for Heart Failure Research, Baylor College of Medicine, Houston, TX*

EDUARDO MARBÁN, MD, PhD • *Institute of Molecular Cardiobiology, Johns Hopkins University School of Medicine, Baltimore, MD*

KEITH L. MARCH, MD, PhD • *Departments of Medicine and Cellular and Integrative Physiology, Indiana University School of Medicine, Indianapolis, IN*

DOUGLAS A. MARCHUK, PhD • *Department of Genetics, Duke University Medical Center, Durham, NC*

ELIZABETH M. MCNALLY, MD, PhD • *Departments of Medicine and Human Genetics, The University of Chicago, Chicago, IL*

EVANGELOS D. MICHELAKIS, MD • *Department of Medicine, University of Alberta Hospital, Edmonton, AL, Canada*

TAKASHI MIKAWA, PhD • *Department of Cell Biology, Cornell University Medical College, New York, NY*

D. DOUGLAS MILLER, MD • *Department of Internal Medicine, St. Louis University, St. Louis, MO*

STEPHAN MOLL, MD • *Department of Medicine, University of North Carolina at Chapel Hill, Chapel Hill, NC*

MARTIN MOSER, MD • *Carolina Cardiovascular Biology Center, University of North Carolina at Chapel Hill, Chapel Hill, NC*

SAMER S. NAJJAR, MD • *National Institute on Aging, National Institutes of Health, Baltimore, MD*

CAM PATTERSON, MD • *Carolina Cardiovascular Biology Center, University of North Carolina at Chapel Hill, Chapel Hill, NC*

DAVID J. PENNISI, PhD • *Department of Cell Biology, Cornell University Medical College, New York, NY*

KARLHEINZ PETER, MD • *Department of Cardiology and Angiology, University of Freiburg, Freiburg, Germany*

CLIFTON P. POMA, BSc • *Department of Cell Biology, Cornell University Medical College, New York, NY*

THOMAS QUERTERMOUS, MD • *Department of Medicine, Stanford University School of Medicine, Stanford, CA*

ADRIAN RECINOS III, PhD • *Department of Internal Medicine, The University of Texas Medical Branch at Galveston, Galveston, TX*

GUY L. REED III, MD • *Department of Genetics and Complex Diseases, Harvard School of Public Health, Boston, MA*

JALEES REHMAN, MD • *Krannert Institute of Cardiology, Indiana University School of Medicine, Indianapolis, IN*

ROBERT ROBERTS, MD • *Departments of Medicine and Cell Biology, Baylor College of Medicine, Houston, TX*

HOWARD A. ROCKMAN, MD • *Departments of Medicine, Cell Biology, and Genetics, Duke University Medical Center , Durham, NC*

ROGER D. ROSSEN, MD • *Department of Immunology, Baylor College of Medicine, Houston, TX*

MARSCHALL S. RUNGE, MD, PhD • *Carolina Cardiovascular Biology Center, and Department of Medicine, University of North Carolina at Chapel Hill, Chapel Hill, NC*

MINNIE SARWAL, MD, PhD • *Department of Pediatrics, Stanford University Medical Center, Stanford, CA*

CHRISTINE SEIDMAN, MD • *Departments of Medicine and Genetics, Harvard Medical School, Boston, MA*

CHRISTOPHER SEMSARIAN, MB, BS, PhD • *Molecular Cardiology Group, Centenary Institute, Newtown, NSW, Australia*

MAXIM SHULIMOVICH, BSc • *Department of Cell Biology, Cornell University Medical College, New York, NY*

JAI PAL SINGH, PhD • *Cardiovascular Research Division, Eli Lilly and Company, Indianapolis, IN*

SUSAN SMYTH, MD, PhD • *Carolina Cardiovascular Biology Center, University of North Carolina at Chapel Hill, Chapel Hill, NC*

DEEPAK SRIVASTAVA, MD • *Departments of Pediatrics and Molecular Biology, The University of Texas Southwestern Medical Center, Dallas, TX*

GEORGE A. STOUFFER, MD • *Department of Medicine, University of North Carolina at Chapel Hill, Chapel Hill, NC*

SHAYELA SUVARNA, PhD • *Department of Medicine, Duke University Medical Center, Durham, NC*

MIWAKO SUZUKI, MD, PhD • *Department of Medicine, Duke University Medical Center, Durham, NC*

RAYMOND TABIBIAZAR, MD • *Department of Medicine, Stanford University School of Medicine, Stanford, CA*

KIMIKO TAKEBAYASHI-SUZUKI. PhD • *Department of Cell Biology, Cornell University Medical College, New York, NY*

TONY TRAN, MD • *Department of Medicine, Baylor College of Medicine, Houston, TX*

JOANNIS VAMVAKOPOULOS, MS, PhD • *Transplantation Laboratory, Haartman Institute, Rational Drug Design Programme, Biomedicum Helsinki, Univerity of Helsinki, Helsinki, Finland*

J. ANTHONY WARE, MD • *Cardiovascular Research Division, Eli Lilly and Company, Indianapolis, IN*

SCOTT M. WASSERMAN, MD • *Department of Medicine, Stanford University School of Medicine, Stanford, CA*

NEAL L. WEINTRAUB, MD • *Department of Internal Medicine, University of Iowa College of Medicine, Iowa City, IA*

GILBERT C. WHITE II, MD • *Departments of Medicine and Pharmacology, University of North Carolina at Chapel Hill, Chapel Hill, NC*

JAMES T. WILLERSON, MD • *Texas Heart Institute, The University of Texas Health Science Center at Houston, Houston, TX*

EUGENE YANG, MD • *Department of Medicine, Stanford University School of Medicine, Stanford, CA*

I OVERVIEW

1

Cardiovascular Genetics

Christopher Semsarian, MBBS, PhD and Christine Seidman, MD

CONTENTS

INTRODUCTION
GENETIC BASIS OF CARDIOVASCULAR DISORDERS
IMPACT OF CARDIOVASCULAR GENETICS ON RESEARCH
IMPACT OF CARDIOVASCULAR GENETICS ON CLINICAL MEDICINE
FUTURE STUDIES
REFERENCES

INTRODUCTION

When the double helical structure of DNA was first proposed in 1953 by Watson and Crick in a two-page *Nature* article *(1)*, no one could have predicted the tremendous impact this discovery would have in establishing the study of human genetic diseases. This discovery was an important landmark in the development of the field of cardiovascular genetics. In the last 30 years, several technological advances have fueled a surge in cardiovascular genetic research. Such advances include the understanding of biochemical components of DNA, the development of cloning techniques and DNA sequencing, the amplification of DNA by polymerase chain reaction (PCR), the identification of restriction enzymes (the molecular biologist's "scalpel") for handling small pieces of DNA, and the undertaking of the Human Genome Project *(2)*. Today, cardiovascular genetics is characterized by the integration of high-technology laboratory studies and clinical medicine. Within the last decade, cardiovascular genetics has redefined the etiology and diagnostic criteria for numerous diseases and has led to the development of new, individualized treatment for cardiovascular diseases.

GENETIC BASIS OF CARDIOVASCULAR DISORDERS

A genetic basis has been identified for many cardiovascular disorders (Table 1). Hypertrophic cardiomyopathy, an autosomal dominant disorder, was the first primary cardiomyopathy identified as having a genetic basis and, therefore, has served as a paradigm for the study of genetic cardiovascular disorders. After initial genetic studies in 1989 mapped the gene for familial hypertrophic cardiomyopathy to chromosome 14q1 *(3)*, mutations in the β-myosin heavy chain gene were identified as the cause of hypertrophic cardiomyopathy (Fig. 1A). In the last 10 years, more than 200 mutations in only 10 genes have been identified as causing hypertrophic cardiomyopathy *(5,6)*. Because all 10 genes encode sarcomeric proteins, hypertrophic cardiomyopathy has been redefined as a "disease of the sarcomere." Over the last 5 years, mutations in several genes have been identified as contributing to other cardiovascular diseases (Table 1), including dilated cardiomyopathy *(7–9)*, cardiomyopathies of the right ventricle such as arrhythmogenic right ventricular dysplasia *(10)*, and mitochondrial myopathies *(11)*. In addition, genetic mutations have been linked to arrhythmogenic disorders such as the autosomal dominant (Romano–Ward syndrome) and recessive (Jervell and Lange-Nielsen syndrome) forms of long QT syndrome, and the Brugada syndrome *(12–14)*. These arrhythmogenic disorders have been called "ion channelopathies," because the mutations lie in genes encoding sodium or potassium channel proteins.

Cardiovascular genetics has had an impact on the study of congenital heart diseases and vascular disorders. For example, mutations in the transcription factor TBX5 gene cause Holt–Oram syndrome *(15)*, whereas genetic

From: *Contemporary Cardiology: Principles of Molecular Cardiology*
Edited by: M. S. Runge and C. Patterson © Humana Press Inc., Totowa, NJ

3

Table 1
The Genetics of Cardiovascular Disorders

Type of disorder	Pattern of inheritance	Locus	Gene product
Arrhythmias			
ARVD	Dominant	1q42	Ryanodine receptor
		2q32	Unknown
		3p23	Unknown
		10p14	Unknown
		14q23-24	Unknown
Brugada syndrome	Dominant	3p21-24	Sodium channel SCN5A
Long QT syndrome	Dominant	3p21-24	Sodium channel SCN5A
		4q25-27	Unknown
		7q35-36	Potassium channel HERG
		11p15.5	Potassium channel KVLQT1
Naxos (ARVD + palmarplantas keratoderma)	Recessive	6p24	Desmoplakin
		17q21	Plakoglobin
Stress-induced ventricular tachycardia	Dominant	1q42	Ryanodine receptor
Cardiomyopathies			
Barth syndrome	X-linked	Xq28	Tafazzin
Dilated	Dominant	1q3	Cardiac troponin T
		2q31	Titin
		14q12	Cardiac β myosin
		15q2	α tropomyosin
		15q14	Cardiac actin
Dilated + conduction disease	Dominant	1p1-q21	Lamin A and C splice variant
		3q22-p25	Unknown
Dilated + muscular dystrophy	Dominant	2q35	Desmin
		6q23	Unknown
	X-lined	Xp21	Dystrophin
Hypertrophic	Dominant	1q3	Cardiac troponin T
		2q31	Titin
		3p	Regulatory light chain
		11p13-q13	Myosin binding protein-C
		12q2	Essential light chain
		14q12	Cardiac β myosin
		15q2	α tropomyosin
		15q14	Cardiac actin
		19q13	Cardiac troponin I
Hypertrophic + conduction disease	Dominant	7q3	γ2 regulatory subunit AMP-activated protein kinase
Congenital			
Alagille syndrome		20q12	Jagged-1 (Notch receptor ligand)
Anomalous pulmonary venous return	Dominant	4q13-q12	Unknown
ASD + atrial aneurysm	Dominant	5p	Unknown
ASD + AV block	Dominant	5q35	Transcription factor NKX2.5

(Continued)

Table 1 Continued

Type of disorder	Pattern of inheritance	Locus	Gene product
Carney complex (myxomas)	Dominant	17q2	Protein kinase A regulatory subunit 1α
		2	Unknown
Char syndrome (patent ductus arteriosus)	Dominant	6p12-p21	Neural crest transcription factor TFAP2B
Heterotaxy + structural malformations	X-linked	Xq26.2	ZIC3
Holt-Oram syndrome (ASD, VSD)	Dominant	12q2	T-box transcription factor TBX5
Velocranial facial syndrome (Tetralogy of Fallot)	Dominant	22q11.21-q11.23	T-box transcription factor TBX1
Metabolic			
Amyloidosis (iron storage)	Dominant	18q11.2-q12.1	Transthyretin
Familial hypercholesterolemia	Dominant	19p13.2	LDL receptor
(↑LDL-cholesterol)	Recessive	1p35	Adaptor protein
Familial hypoapolipoproteinemia	Dominant	11q23	Apolipoprotein A-1
(↓HDL-C)		9q22-q31	ATP-binding cassette transporter-1
Hemochromatosis	Recessive	6p21.3	HFE (HLA-H)
Homocystinuria	Recessive	21q22	Cystathionine beta-synthase
Hypobetalipoproteinemia (↓LDL)	Dominant	2p24	Apolipoprotein (apoB)
↑ Lipoprotein (a)	Dominant	6q26-q27	Lp(a) lipoprotein
Pseudoxanthoma elasticum	Recessive	16p13	ATP-binding cassette transporter-C
	Dominant		(ABCC6)
Sitosterolemia + hypercholesterolemia	Recessive	2p21	ATP-binding cassette transporters (ABCG8, ABCG5)
Tangier disease	Recessive	9q22-q31	ATP-binding cassette transporter-1
Vascular			
Ehlers-Danlos syndrome	Dominant	2q14-q21	Type III procollagen
Familial aortic aneurysm	Dominant	2q14-q21	Type III procollagen
		11p23-24	Unknown
		5q12-14	Unknown
Marfan's syndrome	Dominant	15q21	Fibrillin
Osler Webb Rendu syndrome	Dominant	9q	Endoglin
Supravascular aortic stenosis	Dominant	7q11.2	Elastin

ARVD, arrhythmogenic right ventricular dysplasia; ASD, atrial septal defect; AV, atrioventricular; HDL, high-density lipoprotein; HLA-H, human leukocyte antigen-H; LDL, low-density lipoprotein.

defects in another transcription factor gene, NKX2.5, cause familial atrial septal defects with conduction disease (16). In addition, genetic defects have been identified in vascular disorders characterized by a cardiac phenotype. Marfan's syndrome, an autosomal dominant disorder characterized by multisystem clinical features including cardiac, ocular, and skeletal malformations, is caused by mutations in the gene for fibrillin, a major component of the microfibrils that function in adhesion of connective tissue structures (17). Furthermore, lipid disorders, hypertension, and other vasculopathies have been associated with genetic mutations (18–20). Over the next 10 years,

A

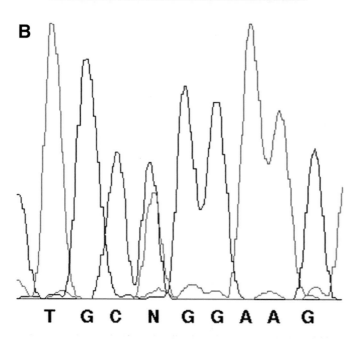

B

T G C N G G A A G

Fig. 1. Molecular genetics of hypertrophic cardiomyopathy. **(A)** Pathologic specimen showing classic anatomical features of hypertrophic cardiomyopathy caused by a missense mutation in the β myosin heavy chain gene. Note marked biventricular hypertrophy (bar = 25 mm) of the free wall and the interventricular septum and enlargement of the left atrium. Chronic atrial fibrillation may have contributed to the development of mural thrombus (arrowhead) present within each atrium. **(B)** DNA sequence analysis showing a missense mutation in the β myosin heavy chain gene that causes hypertrophic cardiomyopathy. Genomic DNA extracted from peripheral blood was amplified by PCR, and the β myosin heavy chain gene was sequenced. The sequence trace

the molecular genetics of other cardiovascular diseases will be outlined. The identification of the genetic nature of diseases will be accelerated by information obtained from the sequencing of the human genome and by the study of cardiac development in animal models and the identification of homologous genes in humans.

IMPACT OF CARDIOVASCULAR GENETICS ON RESEARCH

The identification of genes that cause cardiac diseases has had multiple implications for basic science research and clinical medicine. Although many more disease-causing genes will be identified, the major focus of future research involves understanding the function of such genes. How does a single basepair substitution in a gene lead to a complex cardiac disorder? In the case of hypertrophic cardiomyopathy, a basepair change (Fig. 1B) in one of 3.2 billion basepairs can result in a clinical disorder with a wide gamut of symptoms. The spectrum ranges from a patient with no symptoms and a normal life expectancy to a patient with severe symptoms and risk of sudden death *(21,22)*. What signaling steps are involved in the pathogenesis of genetic cardiovascular disorders? What factors can modify the phenotypic expression of the mutated gene? Are environmental factors or secondary gene–gene interactions involved in the phenotypic expression? This latter question is illustrated by the different clinical presentations in siblings carrying the same genetic mutation *(23)*. To address these fundamental issues, significant research efforts have focused on the development of animal models of human disease. The animal model used most often for the study of cardiovascular genetics is the mouse genome *(24–26)*. The molecular basis of disease is studied by conducting experiments of gene transfer into cultured cardiac myocytes *(27,28)*, by creating transgenic animals via gene transfer into germ line cells *(29,30)*, or by ablating genes via homologous recombination to produce gene knockout models. In some mouse models, a single point mutation is introduced in, or knocked in, to one allele of the mouse genome, mimicking the heterozygotic situation in humans in which the gene of interest is under normal regulatory mechanisms *(26)*. The Arg403Gln mouse model of hypertrophic cardiomyopathy illustrates how an animal model can be used to understand the

Fig. 1. *(Continued)* indicates an ambiguous nucleotide (N) because one β cardiac myosin heavy chain gene contains a mutation. The substitution of one nucleotide alters the amino acid residue encoded at position 719, substituting glutamine for arginine.

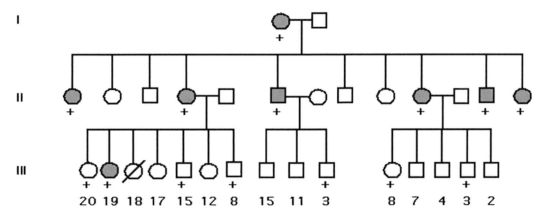

Fig. 2. Genotype versus phenotype in familial hypertrophic cardiomyopathy. Autosomal dominant transmission of clinical disease (filled symbols) and a missense mutation in a β cardiac myosin heavy chain gene (+) is evident in generations I and II. Young children in generation III who carry the mutation do not exhibit cardiac hypertrophy (open symbols), a finding that is consistent with age-dependent penetrance of phenotype in hypertrophic cardiomyopathy. Squares, males; circles, females; and slash, deceased.

functional and physiological effects of a disease gene in humans *(26)*. In the Arg403Gln model, mice develop the features of the hypertrophic cardiomyopathy in humans, including cardiac hypertrophy, myofibrillar disarray, fibrosis, diastolic dysfunction, and, in some cases, sudden death *(26,31)*. This model has provided information on how the mutation affects sarcomere function *(32)* and alters Ca^{2+} handling *(33)*, and how the phenotype can be modified by genetic background *(34)*. Such animal models are invaluable for understanding disease pathogenesis, assessing pharmacological therapies, and identifying new molecular targets for therapy.

IMPACT OF CARDIOVASCULAR GENETICS ON CLINICAL MEDICINE

The effects of cardiovascular genetics on clinical medicine are numerous. Identification of disease-causing genetic defects has led to more rapid and accurate diagnoses. For example, in families in which the genetic mutation for hypertrophic cardiomypathy is known, family members can be screened early for identification of the defective gene (Fig. 2), and the diagnosis can be made before symptoms or clinical features develop. The disease-causing mutation has been identified in many individuals in whom cardiac hypertrophy has not developed; these patients, previously classified as unaffected, are now identified as genotype positive/phenotype negative with this preclinical diagnosis. The most important goal of a preclinical diagnosis in the absence of cardiac hypertrophy is the prevention of cardiac events. Although preclinical diagnosis may have deleterious psychosocial implications, identifying these patients allows for the

early initiation of treatment and the possible prevention of clinical features. In addition, genetic diagnosis has led to the recognition that certain gene mutations cause late-onset disease. For example in hypertrophic cardiomyopathy, defects in the gene encoding myosin-binding protein C usually produce hypertrophy in the fourth and fifth decades of life, whereas mutations in the β-myosin heavy chain gene cause hypertrophy by the age of 20 years in more than 90% of individuals with the mutation *(4,5,23,35)*. Thus, the absence of hypertrophy does not exclude an individual in a family with known hypertrophic cardiomyopathy from carrying the genetic defect.

A second, often overlooked, impact of molecular diagnosis in genetic cardiovascular disorders is the "negative result." The identification of the mutation in one family member allows for the screening of any member of the family. Thus, testing children can preempt longitudinal clinical evaluations. If a child does not inherit the mutation, annual clinical screening is not necessary, the child can participate in school sports and extracurricular activities, and parents find relief from worry.

Making a genetic diagnosis in a medical disease has numerous advantages. A genetic diagnosis can help resolve ambiguous diagnoses, such as those in patients with a borderline or modest increase in left ventricular wall thickness that can occur in some trained athletes with hypertrophy. Genetic testing can aid in the diagnosis of patients with systemic hypertension and suspected hypertrophic cardiomyopathy and patients with hypertrophy in less common sites such as apical hypertrophic cardiomyopathy, where diagnosis can be difficult. Furthermore, antenatal diagnoses can be made in families in which a mutation is known. Although associated with many ethical issues, prenatal diagnosis may be warranted in a family with a clearly documented "malignant" phenotype.

Limitations in the availability of laboratory equipment and the labor-intensive nature of genetic techniques preclude the routine use of genetic diagnosis in patients with suspected cardiovascular diseases. Patients with a family history of disease are the most likely ones to undergo genetic testing. Alternative genetic techniques, such as linkage analysis, can be used to identify which gene is involved; therefore, an accurate family history, the cornerstone of management of patients with genetic disease, is of utmost importance in all inherited medical disorders. Of particular importance in obtaining an accurate family history, the ages at death and the causes of death may give an estimation of the risk of death within a family. Patients with a family history of a genetic disorder are at much greater risk of disease or death than the general population, and clinical screening of such patients is justified. However, within the next decade, the development of molecular technology such as DNA chips or mass spectrometry will allow researchers to assess thousands of mutations within hours, thereby enabling more widespread screening of familial and sporadic cases of genetic cardiovascular disorders.

Molecular studies have contributed significantly to clinical medicine by identifying potential sites of intervention and by allowing targeting of treatment. Certain genetic mutations (malignant mutations) are clearly associated with severe cardiovascular disease *(4,23,35)*. Identification of malignant mutations, which put patients at high risk of sudden cardiac death, allows clinicians to consider preventive measures, such as implantation of a cardioverter-defibrillator to prevent sudden death. Future interventions in cardiovascular genetic disorders may involve correcting the underlying genetic defects. Furthermore, with an increased understanding of genetic mechanisms, target therapy may be developed to mitigate the genetic defect or to correct the molecular abnormality, thereby curing the disease.

FUTURE STUDIES

During the last 10 years, our knowledge of genetic cardiovascular diseases has increased remarkably. With the recent completion of the Human Genome Project, the next decade should bring an unprecedented escalation in our identification and understanding of genetic cardiovascular diseases. Furthermore, new disease-causing genes are being identified with increasing frequency. The challenge that lies ahead is determining what these genes do, how they function, how they interact with other genes, how they activate signal pathways to cause disease, and how environmental factors affect the development of disease. More investigation is required to maximize the potential of molecular genetics for improving clinical medicine. We must analyze the effect of genotype on disease expression and therapeutic response to understand fully how genetic studies can be used to enhance health care in the 21st century. Answering such questions will require collaborative efforts between clinicians and basic scientists. An improved understanding of disease pathogenesis and the development of individualized therapeutic regimens based on a patient's genetic profile will have a substantial impact on the diagnosis and treatment of cardiovascular diseases. Proper integration of genetic technologies and clinical medicine will eventually reduce human disease and suffering and prolong human life.

REFERENCES

1. Watson JD, Crick FH. Molecular structure of nucleic acids: a structure of deoxyribose nucleic acid. Nature 1953;171:737–738.
2. Macilwain C. World leaders heap praise on human genome landmark. Nature 2000;405:983–984.
3. Jarcho JA, McKenna WJ, Pare JAP, et al. Mapping a gene for familial hypertrophic cardiomyopathy to chromosome 14q1. N Engl J Med 1989;321:1372.
4. Genomics of Cardiovascular Development, Adaptation, and Remodeling. NHLBI Program for Genomic Applications, Beth Israel Deaconess Medical Center. Available at: http://genetics.med.harvard.edu/~seidman/cg3/. Accessed January 10, 2003.
5. Seidman CE, Seidman JG. The genetic basis for cardiomyopathy: from mutation identification to mechanistic paradigms. Cell 2001;104:557–567.
6. Semsarian C, Seidman CE. Molecular medicine in the 21st century. Intern Med J 2001;31:53–59.
7. Fatkin D, MacRae C, Sasaki T, et al. Missense mutations in the rod domain of the lamin A/C gene as causes of dilated cardiomyopathy and conduction-system disease. N Engl J Med 1999;341:1715–1724.
8. Olson TM, Michels VV, Thibodeau SN, Tai YS, Keating MT. Actin mutations in dilated cardiomyopathy, a heritable form of heart failure. Science 1998;280:750–752.
9. Li D, Tapscott T, Gonzalez O, et al. Desmin mutations responsible for idiopathic dilated cardiomyopathy. Circulation 1999;100:461–464.
10. Tiso N, Stephan DA, Nava A, et al. Identification of mutations in the cardiac ryanodine receptor gene in families affected with arrhythmogenic right ventricular cardiomyopathy type 2 (ARVD2). Hum Mol Genet 2001;10:189–194.
11. Wallace DC. Mitochondrial defects in cardiomyopathy and neuromuscular disease. Am Heart J 2000;139:70–85.
12. Wang Q, Shen J, Splawski I, et al. SCN5A mutations associated with an inherited cardiac arrhythmia, long QT syndrome. Cell 1995;80:805–811.
13. Curran ME, Splawski I, Timothy KW, et al. A molecular basis for cardiac arrhythmia: HERG mutations cause long QT syndrome. Cell 1995;80:795–803.
14. Vatta M, Li H, Towbin JA. Molecular biology of arrhythmic syndromes. Curr Opin Cardiol 2000;15:12–22.

15. Basson CT, Bachinsky DR, Lin RC, et al. Mutations in human TBX5 cause limb and cardiac malformation in Holt-Oram syndrome. Nat Genet 1997;15:30–35.

16. Schott JJ, Benson DW, Basson CT, et al. Congenital heart disease caused by mutations in the transcription factor NKX2-5. Science 1998;281:108–111.

17. Milewicz DM. Molecular genetics of Marfan syndrome and Ehlers-Danlos type IV. Curr Opin Cardiol 1998;13:198–204.

18. Lehrman MA, Goldstein JL, Brown MS, et al. Internalization-defective LDL receptors produced by genes with nonsense and frameshift mutations that truncate the cytoplasmic domain. Cell 1985;41:735–743.

19. Poch E, Gonzalez D, Giner V, et al. Molecular basis of salt sensitivity in human hypertension: evaluation of renin-angiotensin-aldosterone system gene polymorphisms. Hypertension 2001;38:1204–1209.

20. den Hollander AI, Heckenlively JR, van den Born LI, et al. Leber congenital amaurosis and retinitis pigmentosa with Coats-like exudative vasculopathy are associated with mutations in the crumbs homologue 1 (CRB1) gene. Am J Hum Genet 2001;69:198–203.

21. Maron BJ, Shirani J, Poliac LC, et al. Sudden death in young competitive athletes–clinical, demographic and pathological profiles. JAMA 1996;276:199–204.

22. Maron BJ, Epstein SC, Roberts WC. Hypertrophic cardiomyopathy: a common cause of sudden death in the young competitive athlete. Eur Heart J 1983;4:135–142.

23. Anan R, Greve G, Thierfelder L, et al. Prognostic implications of novel β-cardiac myosin heavy chain gene mutations that cause familial hypertrophic cardiomyopathy. J Clin Invest 1994;93:280–285.

24. Bruneau BG, Nemer G, Schmitt JP, et al. A murine model of Holt-Oram syndrome defines roles of the T-box transcription factor Tbx5 in cardiogenesis and disease. Cell 2001;106:709–721.

25. Tardiff JC, Hewett TE, Palmer BM, et al. Cardiac troponin T mutations result in allele-specific phenotypes in a mouse model for hypertrophic cardiomyopathy. J Clin Invest 1999;104:469–481.

26. Geisterfer-Lowrance AA, Christe M, Conner DA, et al. A mouse model of familial hypertrophic cardiomyopathy. Science 1996;272:731–734.

27. Marian AJ, Yu QT, Mann DL, Graham FL, Roberts R. Expression of a mutation causing hypertrophic cardiomyopathy in adult feline cardiocytes disrupts sarcomere assembly. Circ Res 1995;77:98–106.

28. Sweeney HL, Feng HS, Yang Z, Watkins H. Functional analyses of troponin T mutations that cause hypertrophic cardiomyopathy: insights into disease pathogenesis and troponin function. Proc Natl Acad Sci USA 1998;95:14406–14410.

29. Vikstrom KL, Factor SM, Leinwand LA. Mice expressing mutant myosin heavy chains are a model for familial hypertrophic cardiomyopathy. Mol Med Today 1996;2:556–567.

30. Oberst L, Zhao G, Park JT, et al. Dominant negative effect of a mutant cardiac troponin T on cardiac structure and function in transgenic mice. J Clin Invest 1998;102:1498–1505.

31. McConnell BK, Fatkin D, Semsarian C, et al. Comparison of two murine models of familial hypertrophic cardiomyopathy. Circ Res 2001;88:383–389.

32. Tyska MJ, Hayes E, Giewat M, et al. Single molecule mechanics of R403Q cardiac myosin isolated from the mouse model of familial hypertrophic cardiomyopathy. Circ Res 2000;86:737–744.

33. Fatkin D, McConnell BK, Semsarian C, et al. An abnormal Ca^{2+} response in mutant sarcomere protein–mediated familial hypertrophic cardiomyopathy. J Clin Invest 2000;106:1351–1359.

34. Semsarian C, Healy M, Fatkin D, et al. A polymorphic modifier gene alters the hypertrophic response in a murine model of familial hypertrophic cardiomyopathy. J Mol Cell Cardiol 2001;33:2055–2060.

35. Fananapazir L, Epstein ND. Genotype-phenotype correlations in hypertrophic cardiomyopathy. Insights provided by comparisons of kindreds with distinct and identical beta-myosin heavy chain gene mutations. Circulation 1994;89:22–32.

2

Molecular Biology Applications in Cardiovascular Medicine

Eugene Yang, MD, Scott M. Wasserman, MD, Tatsuro Ishida, MD, PhD, Raymond Tabibiazar, MD, and Thomas Quertermous, MD

CONTENTS

INTRODUCTION

Basic science research has made great contributions to the field of cardiovascular medicine. Scientific studies have had a major impact on clinical practices and outcomes. For example, the principles of cardiac contractile function and unique aspects of hemodynamic loading on the ventricles were defined in animal studies. These findings translated directly into pressure monitoring devices used for patients in the acute care setting. The rationale for drug therapies for treating cardiovascular diseases was based primarily on data derived from basic science investigations. For example, the treatment of heart failure and cardiac arrhythmias evolved from elegant pharmacologic and physiologic studies. A clear path has emerged from the basic science laboratory to the bedside.

During the past decade, scientists have supported the application of cellular and molecular biology to the study of cardiovascular disease and function. Endothelin-1, a potent vasoactive hormone, and angiotensin receptor were among the most heralded new genes to be cloned because of their association with cardiovascular function. The field of vascular biology has expanded rapidly; many endothelial cell genes have been cloned and linked to vascular wall disease. Gain-of-function and loss-of-function mice, created through genetic manipulations, have provided great insight into lipid metabolism and the function of cardiac- and vascular wall–specific genes. In addition, the field of developmental biology of the cardiovascular system has developed during this decade. Increased study of blood vessel development and a strong clinical interest in therapeutic angiogenesis led to great advances in the understanding of the molecular biology of the assembly of cardiovascular structures. Finally, human genetics studies have contributed significantly to the understanding of inherited cardiac diseases such as long QT syndrome and hypertrophic obstructive cardiomyopathy.

Unlike earlier scientific discoveries that successfully translated to clinical practice, the application of recent studies in cellular and molecular cardiovascular science has been slow. Although the identification of genes and their encoded proteins has generated optimism about

From: *Contemporary Cardiology: Principles of Molecular Cardiology*
Edited by: M. S. Runge and C. Patterson © Humana Press Inc., Totowa, NJ

finding new therapeutic targets, the path from target to drug development is a complex, arduous process; therefore, success has been limited in this era of cloning and molecular biology with the exception of plasminogen activator molecules. Furthermore, gene therapy has been viewed as a way to apply directly the findings of basic genetic research to patient treatment, but again this therapeutic approach has been slow to materialize. During this decade, therefore, the major advances in the treatment of cardiovascular disease have evolved not from basic science applications, but from the development of new technologies such as the angioplasty catheter and the coronary artery stent.

In the next decade, new tools will be applied to the study of cardiovascular disease and function. These instruments will include DNA microarrays, protein chips, and other proteomics methodologies, vast amounts DNA sequences from humans and other species, and markers of human genetic variation. The innovative use of these new and powerful tools may accelerate the pace of discovery. For example, DNA microarrays can provide quantitative information about differences in gene expression between two conditions for 20,000 genes simultaneously and can relate these changes to virtually all other genes in the transcriptome. Genes that have coordinate regulation across many manipulations would be expected to have similar functions or to be involved in the same, or related, signaling pathways.

The greatest promise of DNA microarrays and other new tools is that cardiovascular researchers will be able to evaluate the behavior of every gene involved in a specific disease process or biological pathway. We can now identify all genes that are differentially regulated in the blood vessel wall of patients with vascular disease by comparing their gene expression profile with those generated from the normal vessel wall of individuals with known risk factors (such as diabetes) and those without risk factors. Human genetic epidemiology studies can be used to evaluate the association of disease and the vascular wall genes whose expression is temporally linked to vascular disease and risk factor status. Identification of the pathways that underlie cardiovascular disease will accelerate the development of new therapeutic strategies.

We believe that the great, untapped potential of molecular and cellular biology and the emergence of new genomics and human genetics initiatives will lead to substantial new discoveries in cardiovascular disease. However, these discoveries will not be achieved without intensively focused research. In this chapter, we provide a brief overview of basic molecular biology

techniques and applications useful to a cardiovascular researcher.

OVERVIEW OF RECOMBINANT DNA TECHNOLOGY

The study of the human genome, which encompasses approximately 3 billion nucleotides, is a daunting task that has been made possible by recombinant DNA technology. In its basic form, recombinant DNA technology is the process of combining DNA from two or more sources. This technology is based on several common techniques of molecular biology, including the use of restriction endonucleases to cleave DNA into manageable segments, sequence analysis of purified DNA to confirm the identity of a particular fragment, DNA cloning strategies to produce large amounts of identical DNA sequence(s), and hybridization methodologies to identify particular nucleic acid sequences. Improvements in reagents and techniques have allowed for the recent, large-scale sequencing of the human genome.

In general terms, cloning is the process of isolating and amplifying a particular DNA sequence. A clone, which is defined as a large number of exact copies of a unique DNA sequence, can exist as a double-stranded DNA fragment in solution or in a vector (e.g., plasmid, bacteriophage, or plasmid–bacteriophage hybrid). Polymerase chain reaction (PCR)-based or cell-based techniques can be used for cloning. In PCR-based cloning, a target sequence is exponentially amplified by adding oligonucleotide primers designed for the sequence of interest and a DNA template to a PCR reaction mixture. This amplicon can then be used for various purposes, such as creating a probe for *in situ* hybridization or for ligating into a vector for cell-based cloning. Although fast, this PCR-based technique has several problems associated with in vitro enzymatic reaction systems, including failed PCR reactions, decreased efficiency of cloning lengthy sequences (>2 kb DNA segments), limited production of and random mutations in the amplicon, a need for *a priori* knowledge of sequence information for primer design, and high costs. Innovations in the field, such as the use of enzymes such as *Pfu*, with its proofreading feature, have resolved some of these issues. Cell-based cloning, however, remains the most versatile and widely used method for cloning.

Cell-based cloning involves inserting a foreign DNA sequence into a vector and introducing this vector into a host cell that reproduces the foreign DNA in large quantities. The genetic material of interest can be obtained directly from cells or tissues by a PCR-based approach that uses oligonucleotide primers to generate an amplicon. In addition, DNA can be obtained from a complementary DNA (cDNA) library, which is a collection of distinct DNA sequences generated by converting cellular mRNA into cDNA, or by fragmentation of genomic DNA. The isolated DNA sequence is packaged into a vector, which is then introduced into host cells (i.e., bacteria or yeast) in a process known as transformation. Once inside the host, the vector does not incorporate into the host genome and therefore reproduces itself independent of the host cell. This process generates large amounts of the unique DNA sequence. After the host cells have been transformed, the clones are plated onto agar at a density that permits the isolation of individual clones. These clones multiply and become colonies (for plasmid cloning vectors) or plaques (phage cloning vectors). Each colony or plaque represents one clone comprising a group of host cells with a unique, genetically identical recombinant DNA sequence. The colony or plaque with the DNA element of interest is picked through a screening process and further expanded in liquid media. The target DNA is isolated by using standard biochemical protocols for further analyses such as sequencing or screening a library.

Cloned DNA fragments isolated from the vector sequence can be used for several purposes, including Northern blotting and *in situ* hybridization studies to evaluate mRNA expression levels of a specific gene. When the cloned DNA fragment encodes a cDNA, protein expression can be used for a more detailed analysis. In expression cloning, the expressed protein rather than the DNA sequence can be identified after transfection of the target sequence into a cell or tissue. Expression and purification of proteins derived from cloned cDNAs can be used in protein function studies, such as receptor–ligand binding assays and other functional assays (e.g., ion flux and phosphorylation). Finally, expressed nucleic acid sequences can be used for *in situ* hybridization or for functional analysis with antisense strategies.

GENETIC TOOLS

Restriction Enzymes

Restriction endonucleases are bacterial enzymes that protect the host bacteria by degrading foreign double-stranded DNA. The endonucleases act as molecular scissors by cutting double-stranded DNA at unique nucleotide recognition sequences. Bacteria can protect these particular sites from enzymatic degradation by methylating certain nucleotide residues (i.e., adenine and cytosine).

Because of their ability to recognize and cut specific sequence motifs, restriction endonucleases can be used by molecular biologists to cut large pieces of DNA into more manageable fragments. These smaller fragments can be cloned, sequenced, and even used to decipher the primary structure of the larger sequence. Several hundred enzymes have been isolated, characterized, and named based on the bacteria from which they were isolated. For example, *Eco*R1 originates from *Escheria coli*, *Sma*I from *Serratia marcescens*, and *Pst*I from *Providencia stuartii (1)*.

Each restriction enzyme recognizes and cuts a particular 4–8 basepair sequence. Enzymes that recognize the same sequence are called isoschizimers. Based on the probability of finding a 4–8 nucleotide recognition site composed of any combination of bases, an 8-base cutter, such as *Pac*I, should cut human genomic DNA every 1×10^6 basepairs, whereas a 4-base cutter, such as *Hae*II, should cut every 250 nucleotides *(2)*. This calculation assumes that each nucleotide is equally represented in the genome, which is not completely true. Furthermore, endonuclease restriction sites are not evenly and randomly placed in the genome. Enzymes that have CpG in their recognition sequence more frequently in regions of the genome that are rich in C and G nucleotides. Recognition sites are often palindromic, and most have a twofold axis of symmetry with the nucleic acid sequence for each strand being the same when read in the 5' to 3' direction.

After binding to its recognition site, the restriction endonuclease hydrolyzes a phosphodiester bond at the same point in each 5' to 3' sequence. This cleavage can occur symmetrically or asymmetrically. Restriction fragments produced by restriction endonucleases that cut symmetrically have blunt-ends, whereas enzymes that cut asymmetrically yield fragments with 5' or 3' overhangs. These asymmetric overhangs are often called cohesive termini, or sticky ends, because the overhanging ends are complementary and can associate with themselves by hydrogen bonds to yield a circular molecule or with each other to form linear or circular concatamers. The fragments with either blunt or sticky ends can be ligated into a plasmid cloning vector that has been linearized (i.e., cut with a restriction enzyme). These intramolecular and intermolecular associations of restriction fragment ends depend on the DNA concentration and whether the fragment and cloning vector ends are blunt or have compatible overhangs.

High DNA concentrations favor concatamerization, whereas low DNA concentrations favor intramolecular cyclization *(3)*. When ligating or joining by enzymatic reaction the DNA fragment of interest with a linearized vector, the concentrations of the DNA insert and vector are optimized to ensure ligation of one DNA insert copy per vector. Several techniques can be used to improve the efficiency of cloning the fragment into a vector, such as the use of two restriction enzymes that do not produce complementary ends or the use of vector dephosphorylation.

Restriction enzyme digestion of DNA, either genomic or cDNA, produces fragments of different lengths. A digest reaction can be complete or partial. In a complete restriction digest, all of the recognition sites for that restriction endonuclease are cleaved. Partial digests, which occur when the amount of enzyme is limited or when the time for digestion is decreased, result in a random cleavage of only a fraction of the available restriction sites. Complete digestion of the target DNA is usually desired. Restriction fragments can be separated by gel electrophoresis, and their sizes can be calculated by comparing the fragments to DNA standards of known molecular weights. This DNA fingerprint can be compared to fingerprints generated from digests with other restriction enzymes to yield a restriction map. These restriction maps, which provide useful information for other molecular biological tools, are linear or circular maps that document the relative positions of various restriction sites for a specific segment of DNA.

Cloning Vectors

A cloning vector is a vehicle for the delivery of foreign DNA into a host cell and the replication of that DNA independent of the host cell cycle. Foreign DNA is first inserted into the vector in vitro. This hybrid molecule is transferred to a host cell where it uses the host's cellular machinery to generate multiple copies of itself without incorporating into the host's genome. The most commonly used cloning vectors are plasmids and bacteriophages. Both of these naturally occurring species have been genetically engineered to replicate in a foreign host, to transform the host efficiently, and to allow the recovery of vector with its target DNA. Several new hybrid vectors, such as cosmids, yeast artifical chromosomes (YACs), and bacterial artificial chromosomes (BACs), have been constructed to clone larger pieces of DNA. In addition, cloning vectors can be engineered to produce nucleic acid sequences or proteins (4). These vectors, called expression vectors, have special sequences that direct the transcription of nucleic acids and the translation of amino acids independent of the host cell cycle. The generated nucleic acid and protein sequences can be used in several assays such as in situ hybridization, and the amino acid sequences can be assessed for function or antibody binding.

PLASMIDS

Plasmids are naturally occurring, circular molecules of extra-chromosomal, double-stranded DNA that can self-replicate. Plasmids carry genes that can confer unique properties on their host, such as drug resistance, sexual fertility, and the ability to synthesize a rare amino acid. Found in the cytoplasm of many prokaryotes and eukaryotes, such as bacteria, yeast, and mammalian cells, plasmids can be transferred to neighboring cells through bacterial conjugation or to daughter cells through host cell division. Because of their innate ability to carry genes and their compatibility with various cell types, these natural structures have been genetically engineered for use as cloning vectors.

Plasmid vectors have various unique properties based on their intended use; however, they all have three basic characteristics. First, plasmid vectors must have the means to self-replicate; thus, plasmids contain an origin of replication site and other genes required for replication. Second, plasmid vectors need a polylinker, a 50–150 nucleotide sequence comprising multiple, distinct recognition sites for restriction endonucleases, that allows the simple insertion and removal of foreign DNA sequence in and out of the vector. The third feature is the need for selectable markers that will differentiate host cells with no vector, empty vector, or vector with foreign DNA. These markers usually bestow properties on the transformed cell that it normally does not possess. For example, bacteria transformed with a plasmid that encodes an antibiotic resistance gene will no longer die in the presence of that antibiotic.

Several genes have been used as selectable markers, including genes that encode resistance to ampicillin (β-lactamase), chloramphenicol (chloramphenicol acetyltransferase), kanamycin (kanamycin phosphotransferase), and tetracycline (3). Bacteria transformed with plasmids encoding these genes will survive when grown on agar implanted with the appropriate antibiotic.

In addition, markers can be used to determine whether a plasmid vector contains foreign DNA sequence. To achieve this goal, β-galactosidase can be inserted into the polylinker site. When foreign DNA is cloned into the polylinker, the marker gene is interrupted, resulting in insertional inactivation. Thus, cells transformed with empty vector turn blue when grown on X-gal impregnated agar, whereas those cells transformed with plasmid containing the insert will be colorless. Furthermore, this technique of insertional inactivation can be used with antibiotic resistance genes. In this case, two antibiotic resistance genes are used; one is placed within the polylinker and the other is outside of the polylinker. Transformed bacteria are grown in duplicate on agar plates containing both antibiotics. Colonies that are sensitive to the antibiotic resistance gene in the polylinker, but resistant to the antibiotic gene outside of the polylinker, contain the plasmid with the foreign DNA. Colonies that are resistant to both antibiotics contain empty vector.

Foreign DNA can be ligated into plasmid vectors with DNA ligase in vitro. Plasmid vectors are ideal for the cloning of cDNAs because most mRNA transcripts are smaller than 5 kb. Bacteria are transformed with the plasmid and grown on an agar plate impregnated with the appropriate selectable marker(s). Colonies with the insert are expanded in large volumes of media. Several plasmid purification kits are available for isolating pure plasmid DNA from the bacterial host. Because of their ease of use and widespread availability, plasmids are a fundamental tool in molecular cloning. The major limitations with plasmids are that the foreign DNA insert must be smaller than 5–10 kb and the inefficiency of bacterial transformation (1). Plasmid vectors are commercially available from several vendors. These products range from the straightforward plasmids used for cloning restriction fragments to more advanced vectors designed to produce functional proteins.

BACTERIOPHAGE

Bacteriophage λ, a bacterial virus engineered for cloning, can transform bacteria more efficiently than plasmids and can accept inserts up to 23 kb in size. The wild-type bacteriophage λ virion comprises a protein coat that holds nearly 50 kb of linear double-stranded DNA. A temperate virus, bacteriophage λ can exist in a lytic or lysogenic growth state once it has infected a host. In the lytic cycle, the virus makes multiple copies of its genome and coat proteins. The viral genome is then packaged into new phage particles that are released when the host cell lyses. The neighboring cells are infected by the phage and the cycle of replication and release continues. In the lysogenic cycle, the viral genome is integrated into the host chromosome and replicates along with the host chromosome.

The bacteriophage and its lytic growth cycle, when used in recombinant DNA technology, is an effective and efficient cloning vector. The middle portion of the bacteriophage λ genome encodes proteins that are not vital for lytic growth and can be excised so that foreign DNA can be ligated between the two "arms" of essential genetic sequence. This recombinant DNA, which must be 37–52 kb, is then packaged in vitro by coat proteins into infectious phage particles (1). The infectious virions are grown with bacteria. Bacteria infected by the bacteriophage λ undergo lysis, which leaves a "hole" known as a plaque on the bacterial lawn. Each plaque represents a single clone with a unique insert. Clones are picked and

expanded in a broth medium. Then, the phage are purified and DNA is isolated. Because they are easier to handle than cosmids, YACs, and BACs, bacteriophage are ideal for cloning midsized 10–20 kb segments (5).

COSMIDS

Cosmids are hybrids of plasmids and bacteriophage λ designed to hold 30–44 kb DNA fragments that efficiently transform bacteria (1). Cosmids contain a plasmid backbone composed of selection markers, an origin of replication, a polylinker, and a cos site from the bacteriophage λ. Cos sites are cohesive termini found at the 5′ ends of linear phage DNA that are ligated by the host cell, which produces a circular molecule capable of replication. For cloning, the cosmid vector is linearized and mixed with the DNA fragments to be cloned. DNA ligase joins cut vector and insert fragments into concatemeric molecules. These molecules are mixed with packaging extract containing proteins necessary to package naked phage DNA into phage heads. The infectious phage inject their DNA, which contains the insert into the host bacteria. The linear cosmid DNA recircularizes in the host and replicates as a plasmid. Bacterial colonies are chosen based on their selection markers. Although these hybrid molecules clone larger fragments than plasmids or phage, and transform bacteria as efficiently as phage, cosmids tend to rearrange and/or delete DNA insert segments.

YEAST ARTIFICIAL CHROMOSOMES

Yeast artificial chromosomes (YACs) are recombinant vectors generated to clone large fragments of genomic DNA by taking advantage of chromosomal replication during cell division (2,6,7). Recombinant DNA technology is used to place four sequences required for chromosomal replication in a plasmid backbone: an autonomous replication sequence, a centromere sequence (central region of chromosome), and two telomere sequences (chromosome ends). This plasmid backbone contains cloning sites and selectable markers. A YAC plasmid vector is linearized and then cut into two fragments. Foreign DNA 0.2–2.0 million bases (Mb) in length is ligated between these two arms, creating an artificial chromosome with two telomeres capping the chromosome ends and a central centromere. The cell walls of the yeast *Saccharomyces cerevisiae* are removed (thereby producing spheroplasts) and embedded in agar for support and stability. The yeast are transformed with the artificial chromosomes, which have a low transformation efficiency. More starting DNA is required to ensure complete representation of the genome when this strategy is used to generate a recombinant genomic library. The yeast grow in their selective environment and regenerate their walls. Selection markers allow only YAC-containing yeast to be propagated. The foreign DNA is replicated during cell division, resulting in a single copy per cell. The low yields, creation of inserts composed of two or more noncontiguous genomic fragments, and a complicated DNA isolation process are drawbacks to this technique. Furthermore, generation of recombinant YACs is time consuming and technically difficult. Only a few universities and national laboratories support YAC cloning. Nonetheless, YACs are important tools for generating physical genome maps over multiple megabases and have permitted the cloning of regions with repetitive sequences common to eukaryotes.

BACTERIOPHAGE P1 VECTORS AND ARTIFICIAL CHROMOSOMES

Cloning of eukaryotic genomes has been complicated by the large size of the genome and by the presence of structurally unstable repetitive sequence elements. YACs have been engineered to alleviate these problems but are technically challenging; therefore, several alternative vectors have been created. Bacteriophage P1 is a plasmid–bacteriophage hybrid vector engineered to accommodate 70–100 kb of foreign DNA *(8,9)*. Target DNA sandwiched between two plasmid arms is packaged in P1 phage in vitro. These infectious virions inject their DNA into a host where it circularizes into a plasmid and replicates. P1 artificial chromosomes are a combination of the *Escherichia coli* fertility factor (F-factor) plasmid and bacteriophage P1 *(10)*. BACs based on the F factor plasmid were created as an alternative to YAC cloning *(11)*. The F factor plasmid is a low copy number plasmid (one or two copies per cell), which reduces the potential for genetic recombination events, and the F factor plasmid can accept DNA fragments up to 300 kb. *E. coli* are transformed by electroporation, which is 10–100 times more efficient than yeast spheroplast transformation. Therefore, less starting material is required to create a comprehensive genomic library. Conventional colony lift and hybridization techniques are used in BAC screening. DNA isolation is easier and chimeric DNA inserts are formed less frequently with BACs than with YACs.

Expression Vectors and Systems

Expression vectors are cloning vectors designed to express or produce substantial quantities of a gene or its protein. For example, an mRNA product of an expression vector can be used as a probe for *in situ* hybridization or as an antisense RNA for functional–therapeutic assessment. The expressed gene products or recombinant proteins can be used as molecular reagents such as restriction endonucleases, as therapeutic proteins such as erythropoietin, or as reagents for structural analyses, functional assays,

antibody production, or drug screening. These expression vectors have many features of cloning vectors, such as the polylinker cloning sites and selectable markers. In addition, expression vectors have specific sequences that target the cloned cDNA for transcription and translation in the host cell. Some vectors have molecular switches called inducible promoters that can turn the transcription of a gene on and off through the addition of an inert reagent. The inducible promoter protects the host from potentially toxic effects of the recombinant protein or its production. The most commonly used expression vectors are plasmids with bacteriophage sequence elements and viral vectors. Host systems range from bacteria to mammalian cell lines. The vector choice is usually based on the application of the expressed gene or recombinant protein.

E. COLI RECOMBINANT PROTEIN EXPRESSION SYSTEM

E. coli transformed with plasmid/bacteriophage-based expression vectors generate recombinant proteins for antibody screening, functional studies, and structural determination. This system is best suited for generating small, intracellular proteins because large polypeptides cannot be properly folded, and post-translational modifications are minimal or nonexistent in the *E. coli* system. Eukaryotic proteins are usually not very stable in bacteria. Producing a fusion protein by inserting the foreign cDNA downstream of a sequence that encodes a highly expressed host cell gene can increase protein stability and expression. For example, a cDNA of interest can be inserted into the *E. coli lacZ* gene, which results in a fusion protein consisting of the cloned gene product at the carboxy-terminus and β-galactosidase at the amino-terminus. Amino-terminal tags, glutathione-*S*-transferase and polyhistidine, can be added to the cloned gene product to facilitate protein purification *(2)*. To ensure that expression of the target protein is not harmful to the host, expression vectors often have an inducible promoter that turns on the production of the cloned gene product in the presence of a reagent, such as isopropyl-β-d-thiogalactopyranoside. The *E. coli* recombinant protein system is inexpensive and simple, and most molecular biologists are familiar with the techniques and reagents. However, recombinant protein stability and solubility are problems in this system. Despite efforts to create a "bacterial" fusion gene product, these proteins still degrade easily. The use of *E. coli* strains deficient in proteases has met with limited success. High levels of protein expression can result in the formation of inclusion bodies, which are dense aggregates of insoluble recombinant protein *(3)*. Although they may improve protein purification, the aggregates can cause the protein to be incorrectly folded and inactive. The level of expression, temperature, and the bacterial strain can be varied to mitigate this problem *(3,12)*.

BACULOVIRUS-INSECT RECOMBINANT PROTEIN EXPRESSION SYSTEM

Large quantities of recombinant protein can be produced with the baculovirus expression system in insect cells. Baculoviruses are large, enveloped arthropod viruses containing double-stranded DNA. Like other bacteriophage vectors, the sizable 130 kb baculovirus genome contains significant amounts of genetic material that can be discarded without hindering its ability to replicate and infect a host. Therefore, this viral vector system can support large segments of foreign DNA.

The baculovirus vector is prepared through homologous recombination. Target DNA is ligated into a transfer plasmid flanked by the polyhedrin promoter and viral-specific sequences. The polyhedrin protein is a protective viral coat protein that is produced in substantial quantities but is not critical for viral replication or infection. Insect cells lacking polyhedrin cannot form occlusion bodies and thus have unique plaque morphologies. A small transfer plasmid with the foreign DNA fragment and wild-type baculovirus DNA must be applied together and transform *Spodoptera frugiperda* (Sf9)–cultured insect cells. The cloned gene is incorporated into the baculovirus DNA by replacing the polyhedrin gene inside the cell through an inefficient process called homologous recombination. Proper recombination is confirmed by PCR or nucleic acid hybridization. The viral mixture composed of wild-type and recombinant baculovirus is plated onto Sf9 cells, and plaques with recombinant virus are chosen and expanded for protein purification. A substantial quantity of soluble recombinant protein is generated with relative ease. However, this process requires a high level of expertise and is time consuming. Insect cells can be infected with more than one recombinant virus, which permits the expression of more than one protein or protein subunit per cell. Because the baculovirus system is eukaryotic, the recombinant protein often assumes the proper cellular location and can undergo some post-translation modification. However, excessive recombinant protein production can distort the cellular compartmentalization. This recombinant protein strategy is confined to insect cells because baculovirus does not infect vertebrates, and its promoters do not function in mammalian cells.

RECOMBINANT PROTEIN EXPRESSION IN MAMMALIAN CELLS

Mammalian cell expression of recombinant proteins is essential for the proper synthesis, processing, and folding of complex polypeptides. Recombinant proteins have successfully been expressed in mammalian cells with multiple techniques, including transient transfection, stable transfection, viral transduction of cultured cells, transgenic animals, and cell lines derived from transgenic animals. In transient transfection, plasmid-based vectors drive the expression of recombinant proteins for a brief period of time (i.e., days to weeks). Several methods, such as DEAE-dextran, electroporation, and liposome formulations, can be used to transfect the host cell with the plasmid vector carrying the foreign DNA. Although it varies with the technique and cell type, the transfection efficiency is low, with approximately 5–50% of the cell population expressing the recombinant protein. This technique is useful for getting quick information about subcellular localization or cellular function, but it is not useful for producing protein for biochemical characterization.

Strategies have been developed to increase the production of recombinant protein by transiently transfecting eukaryotic cells. These methods use COS cells, a simian kidney cell line with a stably integrated, replication origin-defective SV40 genome *(13)*. COS cells transfected with a plasmid vector containing foreign DNA and a SV40 origin of replication produce high levels of target protein expression. This target protein is processed and appropriately secreted or targeted to its subcellular location. Thus, the COS cell expression system is a good transient transfection strategy to determine receptor–ligand interactions and to reliably produce sufficient amounts of recombinant protein in mammalian cells.

The use of viruses is another method for expressing recombinant protein in mammalian cells both in vitro and in vivo. Vaccinia viruses, adenoviruses, and retroviruses have been used to insert foreign DNA into mammalian cells. The gene of interest is usually expressed under the control of viral expression elements. After infecting mammalian cells, the virus uses the host cell translational machinery to produce large amounts of the protein of interest, which can be purified for further analyses. The in vivo application of viral-mediated gene delivery, known as gene therapy, is beyond the scope of this chapter, but will be discussed elsewhere in this book.

Stable integration of a foreign gene into a host cell chromosome through transfection or generation of transgenic animals results in the reliable production of large amounts of recombinant protein. An expression plasmid can be integrated into the cellular genome of cultured cells by selection for stable expression of a drug resistance gene such as the neomycin resistance gene. With these methods, identical stable cell lines can be developed and selected for high level expression of recombinant protein.

The use of engineered Chinese hamster ovary cells in combination with plasmid vectors carrying specific drug resistance genes allows for the production of cell lines with high levels of protein expression. Transgenic animals are produced to accept an expression construct in the germ line through manipulation of fertilized eggs or embryonic cells in culture. In one clever application of this technique, transcriptional regulatory sequences in the expression construct direct expression of the protein in milk-producing cells so that the recombinant protein can be extracted from milk. Alternatively, stable cell lines can be adapted from the transgenic animal for the in vitro production of recombinant protein.

RECOMBINANT LIBRARIES

A DNA library is a compendium of DNA clones isolated from a particular type of cell, tissue, or organism. The goal of developing such a library is to obtain the genetic information that determines a particular species of animal or plant, to examine the expressed genetic information that characterizes a specific cell or tissue, and to observe how a cell or tissue responds to certain environmental stimuli. Cloning and sequence characterization of numerous genomes together with identifying expressed sequence tags (EST) from large numbers of cells and tissues has provided many physical clones that can be obtained directly. Access to these clones has decreased the need for generating and screening libraries. All genes will eventually exist as a catalogued collection of well-characterized clones that can be rapidly obtained for a small fee.

Genomic libraries are constructed from the high-molecular-weight DNA that is contained in the nuclei of eukaryotic cells and transmitted during reproduction. This DNA, which contains all the organism's genetic information, directs the development, differentiation, and function of cells and specialized tissues. All cells of an organism contain the same genetic information, with the notable exceptions of T and B cells and some tumor cells. Of course, some degree of dissimilarity is seen between the genomes of same species members; these differences define our intraspecies variability. The obvious advantage of this type of library is that it contains all of the inherited genetic material for the species. In additional, the DNA sequences that regulate gene expression can be examined only by studying DNA obtained from genomic libraries. The major disadvantage of this approach, however, is the presence within a structural gene of large regions of untranslated sequence. Genomic libraries are usually screened by hybridization with DNA probes derived from cDNA clones.

Alternatively, high-throughput PCR can be used to screen arrayed genomic libraries where DNA is available for each clone. Screening of genomic libraries should decrease with the completion of the entire human genome sequence and the availability of cloned DNA fragments.

A cDNA library is constructed from mRNA that is expressed by a cell or tissue at a specific point in time. This library reflects not only the type of cell or tissue used in the study, but also the cell's response to various hormones, growth factors, and biophysical forces. cDNA does not exist in nature but is synthesized from mRNA, which specifies and directs assembly of protein sequences. Because mRNA cannot be cloned directly, the synthesis of cDNA allows for easy characterization of the coding portion of the structural gene and provides for rapid bioinformatics analysis of the conceptual protein. cDNA libraries offer several unique advantages. First, the coding region of a gene is usually much smaller than the genomic structural sequence that contains both intronic and regulatory sequences. Second, the cDNA can be used to direct synthesis of an mRNA that will encode the same protein as the original mRNA, allowing for rapid development of expression constructs for generating recombinant protein. This feature of cDNAs is used in the screening of expression libraries, where clones are evaluated on the basis of the proteins that they encode. Third, the numbers of genes that are expressed by a single cell or tissue are much smaller than the total number of genes in the genome, and thus the number of clones that need to be examined to identify a cDNA for a specific gene may be smaller. cDNA clones isolated from many cells and tissues have been identified through sequencing and made available to researchers. Availability of these EST clones and the development of PCR cloning is decreasing the need to screen cDNA libraries to obtain clones. However, cloning methodology will continue because of the need to identify genes that encode specific functions through expression cloning, or those that characterize a specific cellular process through subtraction cloning. cDNA libraries are usually screened with labeled DNA probes, but expression libraries can be screened with antibodies and other reagents that depend on protein function.

Obtaining a population of clones that represents the complete genome or all mRNA transcripts can be difficult. Mathematical models are used to ensure that the library is large enough to encompass the entire sequence repertoire (14). The number of independent clones that are formed by ligating the cloned DNA into a cloning vector is called the base of the library. A base of approximately 1 million clones is usually necessary for λ phage genomic libraries and cDNA libraries. The larger the base of the library, the more likely it is that the gene of interest will be found. To examine all of the clones of a library, a number of clones representing at least three times the base of the library should be screened. Although the availability of genomic DNA for the construction of genomic libraries is rarely a problem, cDNA must be biochemically synthesized and is often limiting. The use of high-efficiency bacteria for the generation of the clones in the primary plating of a library is important to capture as many recombinant molecules as possible. The quality, purity, and size of the DNA are crucial to the generation of a library. High-quality DNA ensures an accurate representation of the DNA because exogenous, contaminating genetic material can cause erroneous results. The creation of a DNA library is not a trivial undertaking. Well-characterized genomic and cDNA libraries are available from academic and commercial sources. Libraries that have been amplified several times by plating on bacteria should be used with care because the library quality declines with overamplification, which can result in loss of rare transcripts.

Genomic DNA Library

All nucleated cells of an organism have the same general genomic information. Genomic DNA comprise coding regions or exons and non-coding regions or introns. Within the non-coding regions are sequences that control the patterns of individual gene expression (i.e., transcriptional regulatory elements). Most of the genome of higher eukaryotes is non-coding DNA. A complete genomic DNA library contains at least one copy of each region of the genome being evaluated. A sub-genomic library can be generated that contains only a defined portion of the species genome. Such libraries can be based on fractionated chromosomes, a particular chromosome band, or genomic DNA fragments of specific molecular weight. Genomic DNA libraries have been used to determine structural information such as the location of introns, exons, and transcriptional regulatory elements. In addition, genomic libraries have been used to clone genes with homology to other known genes and genes with little information regarding cellular expression pattern.

Genomic DNA can be prepared from any type of cell or tissue. Accessible cells, such as semen or blood cells, are an excellent source of genomic DNA. In the human genome project, a genomic library for nucleotide sequencing of the human genome was created from the blood of five donors (15). To establish a genomic library, high-molecular-weight DNA is carefully isolated and then randomly digested by partial restriction enzyme digestion or sheared by physical forces. Either process yields overlapping DNA fragments of optimum size to clone into a vector. The fragments of genomic DNA are usually inserted into vectors with a large carrying capacity, such as bacteriophage, cosmids, YACs, or BACs. When the starting sequence material is represented by fewer clones, screening of the cloned sequences is more rapid and thorough. Finally, generating sufficient numbers of clones to represent the entire genome is important in establishing genomic DNA libraries. A genome equivalent, which is an estimate of the number of independent clones required to adequately represent the entire genome (2), can be calculated by dividing the genome size by the average insert size. For example, a genome equivalent for a human genomic DNA library (3×10^9 bases) composed of inserts of 30 kb would be 100,000 clones, creating a onefold library. A library of several genomic equivalents is usually needed to ensure representation of the entire genome. Vectors with high transformation efficiency and the ability to assimilate large DNA inserts minimize the complexity of the library (i.e., the number of independent genomic clones).

cDNA Library

mRNA is the genetic blueprint or coding sequence that dictates the primary amino acid sequence of the encoded protein. mRNA represents the combined sequences of the various exons that make up the structural gene, with intronic regions removed from an initial large RNA molecule by RNA splicing. The mRNA is only a small fraction of the total cellular RNA, which also includes ribosomal RNA (rRNA) and transfer RNA (tRNA). mRNA is a fragile, single-stranded molecule sensitive to RNase, a ubiquitous enzyme that degrades RNA. Single-stranded mRNA can be converted into cDNA in vitro by reverse transcriptase. The cDNA molecule can be used as a template to synthesize a second DNA strand, to produce double-stranded cDNA. cDNA is composed of sense and antisense strands; the sense strand has the same sequence as the mRNA. A cDNA library is a collection of different double-stranded molecules that represent the different mRNAs found in the cell or tissue being studied. The frequency of a single clone usually represents the relative abundance of the mRNA for that gene in the starting mRNA sample.

Isolation of mRNA is facilitated by its characteristeric poly-adenylated 3′ tail. These poly-A tails bind to oligo(dT) or poly(U) columns while the remaining RNA elutes off the column. Application of high-ionic-strength buffers to the column disrupts the non-covalent hydrogen bonds between nucleotides and permits the elution of purified mRNA. Total cellular RNA or mRNA is converted to double-stranded cDNA by reverse transcriptase in vitro. cDNA synthesis requires primers that can be either random, such as oligo(dT), or gene-specific to begin the reaction. The type of primer used in cDNA synthesis is based on the starting RNA material and the intended use of the cDNA. Double-stranded cDNA is first ligated into a cloning vector and then transformed in a host cell to generate colonies for plating and selection. Because most genes are less than 5 kb, plasmids and bacteriophage are the most commonly used vectors for cDNA library construction.

Like genomic libraries, a critical issue for cDNA libraries is the adequate representation of all mRNAs expressed by a cell or tissue. The abundance of mRNA transcripts varies and is a function of the number of transcripts generated and the rate at which they are degraded. Rare mRNAs may be difficult to detect, whereas other transcripts may not be expressed in a particular cell or tissue. For cDNA cloning, therefore, determining which tissue source will be most enriched for the genes of interest is critical.

RECOMBINANT LIBRARY SCREENING

Nucleic Acid Hybridization

Nucleic acid hybridization involves the non-covalent association of nucleic acids from two complementary single strands into a double-stranded molecule. In a typical hybridization reaction, DNA/RNA from a library or gel is transferred to a nitrocellulose or nylon membrane. The membrane-bound, denatured double-stranded DNA or single-stranded RNA is exposed to a labeled or tagged nucleic acid probe. The probe binds to complementary RNA/DNA on the membrane, which is washed at various stringencies to remove nonspecific probe. Binding of the nucleic acid probe to the membrane or blot is assessed by autoradiography or phosphoimaging. DNA or RNA that hybridizes to the probe contains either the exact or a highly homologous DNA/RNA sequence. Northern blotting is the technique of RNA nucleic acid hybridization, and Southern blotting is DNA nucleic acid hybridization.

The typical nucleic acid probe is 50–1000 bases long and can be generated by several techniques, including oligonucleotide synthesis, PCR, and expression cloning. Oligonucleotide probes are single-stranded, synthetic molecules 15–50 bases long and are usually custom designed and purchased from a commercial supplier. Because of their short length, oligonucleotide probes can be designed to detect specific protein motifs like zinc-finger or other conserved functional domains. PCR with sequence-specific primers, cell-based cloning, and expression cloning can be used to generate nucleic acid probes. Probes are usually labeled by incorporating a nucleotide

with a radioactively labeled phosphate (i.e., [P32]dCTP) into the probe synthesis reaction. Less common labeling methodologies include digoxigenin-labeled probes, which can be detected with an enzyme-linked assay, and biotinylated probes, which can be detected with avidin-based systems. Colonies, plaques, or DNA/RNA fragments that bind the labeled probe appear as distinct spots or bands on the membrane. This hybridization information is then correlated with the original plate or gel to isolate the sequence of interest.

Differential Screening, Subtraction Hybridization, and Subtraction Cloning

These methods have been developed to clone cDNAs that represent genes that are differentially expressed between different cell types or the same cell type that is undergoing stimulation. Subtraction cloning is a powerful technique that generates a cDNA library or subtraction library, enriched for genes that are different between two conditions. The construction of subtraction libraries is based on the assumption that cells with or without a stimulus will express the same genes except for those genes affected by the stimulus. mRNA is isolated from two cell populations to create a subtraction library. For example, mRNA can be isolated from endothelial cells grown in the presence or absence of the inflammatory cytokine, tumor necrosis factor-α (TNF-α). Single-stranded cDNA is synthesized from mRNA of one condition (e.g., endothelial cells exposed to TNF-α) and hybridized to an excess of mRNAs from the second condition (unstimulated endothelial cells). DNA–RNA hybrids form between genes that are common to both conditions, whereas genes expressed in only one condition remain single-stranded. These single-stranded cDNA are then converted to double-stranded cDNA and ligated into a cloning vector to produce a library of the differentially expressed genes. This classic approach, however, is tedious and technically challenging. More simple PCR-based methods have recently been developed to generate subtracted libraries enriched for low transcript messages. This technique, called suppression subtraction hybridization, has been used extensively in our laboratory to clone genes that are expressed by endothelial cells undergoing angiogenesis in vitro (16,17).

Differential screening is similar to subtraction hybridization but does not require the creation of a new library. A cDNA library is chosen that is expected to contain the genes that are expressed in the cell under stimulation. Labeled cDNA is made from mRNA isolated from cells or tissues to be compared. The labeled probes from each condition are hybridized separately to replicate membranes made by transfer of bacteriophage or plasmid library clones. Autoradiography of the hybridized filters is performed, and the spots on the replicate membranes are compared. Spots that differ between the two membranes correlate with genes that are differentially expressed between the two conditions. In this type of experiment, changes in gene expression are qualitative because the amount of cDNA per colony is not the same on the replicate blots. Furthermore, this type of analysis requires that the radioactive probes be comparable in specific activity and that the exposure times be modified to yield a similar intensity of hybridization. Although used successfully in the past, this technique is technically challenging, and genes that are differentially regulated at a modest level are often missed (18). Finally, finding a library that will fully represent the stimulated condition may be difficult.

Recombinant Protein Screening

One of the most powerful methods developed for molecular cloning is the ability to directly clone a molecule based on some feature of its encoded protein. The gene encoding the potent vasoactive factor endothelin-1 was cloned on the basis of its ability to induce the contraction of vascular tissue in a bioassay. Numerous cell-surface receptors have been cloned by transfecting cells able to adhere to a plastic dish coated with antibodies, interacting proteins, or radiolabeled ligands. Transcription factors have been cloned on the basis of their ability to bind specific DNA regulatory sequences. Although the importance of many forms of molecular cloning by library screening has decreased because of the wide availability of ESTs, expression cloning will continue to be essential for the identification of molecules that mediate a specific molecular function.

Expression cloning requires a cDNA library that is constructed from the cells or tissues known to express the protein or functional activity of interest. Because many of the screens have low efficiency rates and are laborious to perform, finding a cellular source that is enriched for the protein and mRNA to be cloned is imperative. The choice of vector is important; it must be capable of directing expression in either bacteria or eukaryotic cells. Inducible transcriptional systems improve specificity and prevent the loss of cells caused by protein toxicity. Expression libraries require a larger base than other cDNA libraries to ensure representation of all proteins expressed by the target cell or tissue. For each cDNA, only one in six clones will be expressed as a protein because the gene can insert itself in the 5'-3' or the 3'-5' direction or in any one of three reading frames. In recent methods, directional

insertion of the cDNA has reduced the frequency to one in three clones. Although the expression vector contains the machinery to direct transcription, the initiating ATG sequence must be provided by the cloned cDNA. Because of these technical demands, expression library construction is challenging and difficult.

Several cloning strategies have taken advantage of the availability of antibodies for proteins of interest. Such immunologic screening is based on the ability of an antibody to recognize and bind an antigen. The antibody can be either monoclonal (i.e., recognize one epitope) or polyclonal (i.e., recognize multiple epitopes). For screening purposes, a polyclonal antibody or a mixture of monoclonal antibodies is usually preferable because the antisera can bind many epitopes of an individual protein antigen. One early such strategy in bacteria took advantage of the expression of recombinant protein in the λ phage vector λgt11. Libraries created with this vector expressed a beta-galactosidase fusion protein, and nitrocellulose filters lifted from the library plates were evaluated by exposing them to antiserum labeled directly or identified by a second labeled antibody. Cloning was performed by picking areas of the bacteriophage lawn where spots were seen on autoradiograph. This process was repeated until clones were pure. The major problem with this screening strategy is that proteins expressed in bacteria do not undergo eukaryotic post-translation modifications and may not be folded correctly. Furthermore, a protein that adheres to a membrane is essentially denatured. As a result, the types of antibodies that can be used in antibody screening in bacteria are restricted. Similar methods have been used with plates of eukaryotic cells by using cDNA libraries in eukaryotic expression plasmids such as pCDNA3. Lawns of COS cells transfected with an expression library have been screened by incubating the antisera directly on the lawn of cells. The cells expressing the protein of interest can be identified with a chromogenic substrate reaction directed by an enzyme tag on the antibodies. Plasmid DNA isolated from these cells is amplified, transfected into COS cells again, and the process repeated until clones are pure.

Antibody-directed screening, a common method, was used to clone cell-surface receptors with expression libraries transfected into COS cells. High-level transient expression of the library clones in these eukaryotic cells produced large amounts of these receptors on the COS cell surface. Transfected cells were applied to plastic plates coated with a specific antibody, and cells containing the clone of interest were selected. Plasmid expression constructs were harvested back from the cells that adhered to the plates, and the process was repeated until a small number of plasmids were isolated. This technique has allowed for the cloning of many genes, such as T cell-surface genes for which large amounts of monoclonal antibodies are available.

An important advantage of screening with eukaryotic cell expression systems is that the recombinant proteins are folded and modified correctly. However, the antibody must be able to identify the protein in its native state. In addition, transfection and handling of eukaryotic cells is difficult.

Binding assays have been used in expression cloning strategies to clone important molecules. The most rapid and straightforward techniques parallel those used for antibody screening of expression libraries. For instance, bacteriophage expression libraries have been widely used to clone DNA binding proteins. In these experiments, a double-stranded DNA segment encoding a cognate DNA binding element recognized by a transcriptional regulatory protein is radiolabeled and incubated with filters containing recombinant proteins from the library plates. Spots identified on autoradiographs are used to guide "picking" regions of the phage lawn, and a pure clone that is responsible for the binding is obtained by serial screenings. In another approach analogous to antibody screening of plated eukaryotic cells, a radiolabeled ligand is applied directly to plates of COS cells expressing transfected libraries. These plates are either overlaid with photographic emulsion or exposed to film, and the area of cells generating a signal is identified. Plasmid DNA isolated from these cells is amplified and retransfected for several rounds until a single clone is obtained. This ligand screening technique was used for the cloning of the most sought after receptor in cardiovascular biology, the angiotensin receptor (19). A more labor-intensive strategy uses a radiolabeled ligand in solution that has been reacted with pools of transfected eukaryotic cells expressing a fraction of the expression library. These pools can be evaluated for radioligand binding as a group, yielding a subset of genes that includes the desired receptor. The pools are subdivided, and smaller pools of genes are evaluated in subsequent binding reactions. This process of reductionist cloning is repeated until a single clone remains for characterization. This technique has been used to clone numerous cell surface receptors (20,21). For these strategies to work, a high-affinity receptor must be selected whose binding properties are not altered by the radiolabeling process, and information about ligand concentrations must be available.

Additional strategies of reductionist cloning or screening of pools have been used with other creative assays to clone a wide variety of different functional classes of proteins. For instance, a bioassay of vascular contraction to screen for the physiological activity of vasoconstriction was used to clone endothelin-1. Other creative methods have used the in vitro generation of cRNA transcripts from pools of clones, which are then injected into a cell that can be functionally evaluated. Such techniques have paired expression screening of cRNA pools by microinjection into oocytes of *Xenopus laevis*. These RNAs are translated at high efficiency allowing for functional screening by patch clamp, for example, to look for new ion fluxes. These approaches have been used to clone new molecules that may contibute to cardiovascular development.

Finally, the most efficient expression cloning strategies take advantage of a biological selection process to enrich for those clones encoding the gene of interest. One good example is the use of a transformation assay to identify genes that confer the ability to grow in a transformed fashion on NIH 3T3 fibroblasts. Genes that have the ability to transform these cells are called oncogenes, and they are readily identified because they are the only genes that permit the transfected cells to grow in this selection process. Another example is the cloning of the Na^+/H^+ antiporter (22). A cell line lacking antiporter activity was developed and transfected with human DNA. These transfected cells were then subjected to selection conditions that permitted survival only of cells expressing the human gene for this antiporter protein.

Cloning with Synthetic Recombinant Expression Libraries

All of the cloning strategies discussed above are aimed at the cloning of naturally occurring genes. In some cases, the function of the gene is known, whereas in other cases the gene is identified only through its association with specific biological processes or functional activities. Robust strategies are available to clone sequences that do not necessarily exist in nature, but rather, are selected to fit a specific functional profile. These strategies are used extensively by the pharmaceutical industry when a specific molecular function is needed, but no known biological reagent has been identified or adapted for the desired purpose. In one such methodology, short DNA segments encoding random peptides are generated and screened for their ability to bind to the molecules, cells, or tissues of interest. Very large recombinant libraries can be made in bacteriophage vectors to express proteins on their surfaces. Recombinant clones encoding peptides that bind are selected by repeated interaction with a target protein. This technique has recently been used to characterize peptides that recognize endothelial cell-surface epitopes (23). These peptides may be used to define endothelial cell markers that mediate tumor metastasis and endothelial functions. Another application of the screening of synthetic DNA segments is to generate high-affinity recombinant monoclonal antibodies. "Random" DNA fragments can be inserted into cloning sites in an antibody framework at a position that codes for the hypervariable region of the antibody, thus simulating the biological process of antibody diversity. Large libraries of recombinant synthetic antibodies have been generated in this way and screened by repeated affinity purification of the antigen epitope to be targeted. This method allows for the rapid development of constructs that encode recombinant antibodies that can be expanded by using bacterial expression systems, thus eliminating the need for animal use.

ANALYSIS OF GENE EXPRESSION

Genetic information that is stored in the inherited genome must first be "turned on" or transcribed into mRNA and then translated into protein to affect biological processes. Regulation of these processes determines the phenotypic differences between hair cells, gut epithelial cells, and other cell types, and the ability of a cell to respond to stimuli such as the hormone estrogen. The most critical regulatory step probably occurs at the mRNA level, as determined by the concentration of an mRNA species for a gene of interest in a specific cell type. Steady-state mRNA levels reflect both synthesis and degradation. These levels can be determined with Northern blots and microarrays, which are usually called gene expression studies. Transcriptional regulation studies evaluate the rate of transcription and are usually directed at understanding the DNA and protein elements that mediate transcription. mRNA stability is rarely measured, but this aspect of gene expression is clearly a universal mechanism for transcriptional regulation. In this section, we will briefly review the various techniques used to analyze gene expression in a specific cell or tissue type.

Northern Blotting

Northern blotting is the most commonly used method to detect and quantify a particular mRNA in a mixture of RNAs isolated from cells or tissues. For this analysis, an RNA sample, often total RNA, is denatured by treatment with formaldehyde to prevent hydrogen bonding between basepairs. This step ensures that all of the RNA molecules have an unfolded, linear conformation. Individual RNAs are then separated according to size by gel electrophoresis and transferred to a nitrocellulose or nylon membrane. The membrane is exposed to a radiolabeled DNA or RNA probe, hybridized and washed, and then subjected to autoradiography.

The signal for a specific hybridization can vary because of differences in RNA concentrations; therefore, examining expression levels of "housekeeping genes," such as β-actin or cyclophilin, that do not change across experimental conditions is important. Because these genes may occasionally be regulated by a stimulus, more than one housekeeping gene should be used under these circumstances. The signals are quantified by densitometry measurements of autoradiographs or by a phosphoimager that calculates a ratio for the expression level of an experimental versus a control gene. By modifying the conditions of the hybridization and wash, such as salt concentration and temperature, a probe can be used to detect mRNA species that do not have an identical sequence. This "low stringency" hybridization technique enables the detection of mRNAs representing orthologs or paralogs of the probe sequence.

The probe used for Northern blotting can be either labeled RNA or DNA. Although radioactively labeled nucleotides have usually been used for incorporation during enzymatic amplification of the probe sequence, nonradioactive methods are rapidly gaining acceptance. The size of the labeled probe varies from 100 to 1000 basepairs but, recently, oligonucleotides comprising as few as 15 basepairs have been end-labeled and used as probes as long as hybridization and washing conditions are modified to account for the low affinity hybridization seen with such short sequences (24).

Ribonuclease Protection Assay

The ribonuclease protection assay (RPA) is an extremely sensitive technique used for the detection and quantification of mRNA and for analysis of mRNA structure (25,26). This assay is based on the principle that ribonucleases digest single-stranded but not double-stranded RNAs. For this assay, a labeled antisense RNA probe is synthesized that is complementary to part of the target RNA to be analyzed. Both radioactive and nonradioactive probes can be used. Antisense probe RNA is prepared by inserting the DNA region that encodes a particular RNA into one of the common transcription vectors that contains a T3, T7, or SP6 bacteriophage promoter. Highly specific RNA transcripts are generated by using the corresponding T3, T7, or SP6 RNA polymerases (27). The labeled probe is then mixed with the sample RNA and incubated under normal hybridization conditions. After hybridization, the mixture is treated with ribonuclease to degrade single-stranded, unhybridized probes, so that only labeled probes that hybridized to complementary RNA in the sample will be protected from ribonuclease digestion. Hybridized probe is then separated on a polyacrylamide gel and visualized by autoradiography. When the probe is present in molar excess over the target mRNA in the hybridization reaction, the intensity of the resulting band will be directly proportional to the amount of cRNA in the original mixture.

RPA is usually more sensitive than Northern blotting and can therefore be used to detect less abundant mRNAs. However, the higher sensitivity of this assay often results in a higher background signal. RPA has several important applications. For example, genes with multiple-splice variants can be identified with a single probe designed to hybridize to all variants of the gene (28). These hybridized fragments can be separated on a gel and variants can be verified by their relative sizes. An additional advantage of the RPA is that multiple probes for different target RNAs can be assessed in a single reaction.

Polymerase Chain Reaction

PCR is a powerful and sensitive technique for rapid enzymatic amplification of genes present in very low copy numbers. In addition to amplifying genomic DNA templates, PCR can be used to accurately measure mRNA levels by amplification of cDNA that is reverse-transcribed from RNA.

In a typical PCR reaction (29,30), the DNA sequence between two primers undergoes repeated doublings in an exponential fashion. In the first cycle, heating to 95°C melts the double-stranded DNA, and subsequent cooling to 42–68°C then allows for the primers to hybridize (anneal) to their complementary sequences on the target DNA. The thermostable *Taq* DNA polymerase is used to extend each primer sequence at 72°C in the 5′ to 3′ direction, generating newly synthesized DNA strands. In the second cycle, the original and newly made DNA strands are separated at 95°C; primers again anneal to their complementary sequence at 42–68°C; and each primer is again extended by *Taq* polymerase to the end of the other primer sequence. Thus, all DNA strands synthesized in the amplification cycles exactly equal the length of the region to be amplified, as determined by the sequence of the primers. In the third cycle, two double-stranded DNA molecules are generated that are equal to the sequence of the region to be amplified. These two are doubled in the fourth cycle and are doubled again with each successive cycle. In this way, after 25–40 cycles of PCR, the yield of target molecules will be 2^n, where n equals the number of cycles.

To measure mRNA levels by PCR, the mRNA must first be converted to cDNA, which then serves as a template for the polymerase reaction (31). Oligo (dT) primers, random decamers, or gene-specific antisense primers are used to synthesize single-stranded cDNA by reverse transcriptase.

Standard PCR is then performed after addition of the gene-specific sense and antisense primers. The PCR products are fractionated by size on agarose gels for visualization. In this assay, contaminating genomic DNA must be removed from the RNA samples before synthesizing cDNA because amplification from DNA will cause spuriously high estimates of mRNA concentrations. Because of its sensitivity, PCR is inherently non-quantitative. Thus, standard PCR, although excellent for rapid and easy detection of mRNA expression in an individual RNA sample, is not ideal for relative quantification.

Relative quantification of mRNA levels can be achieved by using reverse transcription coupled with PCR (RT-PCR) with primers for the gene of interest and control primers for a control amplification. The reaction is terminated and analyzed with both targets in the exponential phase of amplification (32). However, conditions under which both PCR reactions are simultaneously in the exponential phase can be difficult to determine because common control genes are usually expressed at much higher levels than the transcript of interest. Small variations among samples sometimes result in large differences in product yield. Competitive RT-PCR (33,34) is a more reliable method for accurate quantification.

In competitive PCR, a known amount of an exogenous standard (competitor) template is added to a target RNA sample, and RT-PCR with a common set of primers is performed to amplify simultaneously both target and standard templates, which are distinguished from each other by their size differences on gel electrophoresis. The abundance of the target is determined by comparing signals obtained for the competitor and target. For example, serial 10-fold dilutions of competitor RNA are added to reactions containing a constant amount of target RNA. RT-PCR is performed, followed by gel electrophoresis. Product yield is determined by measurements of radioactivity incorporated during amplification (31) or by analysis of gels stained with intercalating dyes such as ethidium bromide (35). Because the amount of competitor added to each reaction is known, the amount of endogenous target in the sample RNA can be determined by comparison. The ratio of products obtained from the endogenous and competitor targets at the end of amplification reflects the initial ratio of target to competitor RNA.

In recent years, more sophisticated techniques have been developed to quantify mRNA levels. Real-time RT-PCR (36) is a new, noncompetitive technology that can detect products while they are being formed. The accumulation of products is assessed with several probes, including fluorogenic 5′ nuclease probes and molecular beacons (37,38). In this assay, fluorescence measurements are made in real time during each cycle of PCR with a thermocycler connected to an optical excitation and detection device. During the exponential phase of PCR, the amount of amplified product synthesized in each cycle increases in a semigeometric fashion. The cycle during which the amount of released fluorescence exceeds a baseline threshold fluorescence is known as the threshold cycle (Ct). This Ct value is inversely proportional to the amount of starting target. Thus, high-copy number samples will have low Ct values, whereas low-copy number samples will have high values. For rigorous quantification of mRNAs, a standard curve is generated with in vitro transcribed RNA. A Ct value is determined for different concentrations of this control RNA. Ct values are then plotted against the RNA concentrations to generate a standard curve for quantifying the level of expression in unknown samples. Because fluorescence monitoring is highly sensitive and accurate with a linear dose response over a wide range of target concentrations, real-time PCR is superior to conventional PCR quantification, which only analyzes end-point products.

The yield of PCR products from real-time RT-PCR was initially estimated by the amount of fluorescence released by DNA-binding dyes such as ethidium bromide, SYBR Green I, or oxazole yellow derivatives. TaqMan PCR *(37)*, which uses an oligonucleotide labeled at its 5′ end with a fluorescent dye and a quenching dye at its 3′ end, was recently developed to increase the specificity of the amplified products. This probe anneals to an internal sequence within the amplified DNA fragment. PCR is performed with the labeled oligonucleotide and primer pairs to amplify the target sequence. When both the fluorescent and quenching dyes are present in close proximity on the intact hybridization probe, fluorescence emission from the dye is absorbed by the quenching dye. As the amount of target DNA increases during PCR, greater amounts of oligonucleotide probe hybridize to the denatured target DNA. However, during the extension phase of the PCR cycle, the 5′→3′ exonuclease activity of *Taq* polymerase cleaves the fluorophore from the probe. Because the fluorophore is no longer adjacent to the quencher, it begins to fluoresce. The intensity of fluorescence, therefore, is proportional to the amount of target PCR product. Real-time PCR is an excellent technique used not only to measure the abundance of DNA, but also to screen for mutations and single nucleotide polymorphisms.

In situ *Hybridization*

The *in situ* detection of mRNA on microscopic sections provides direct visualization of the spatial location of mRNA at the cellular level. Knowing the location of

mRNA is useful during early phases of study with a new gene because it helps in developing hypotheses about cellular function of the gene product. Furthermore, *in situ* data are often critical for understanding the molecular functions of well-characterized genes. For example, if a gene is thought to encode a cell-surface receptor that responds to locally secreted ligands, documentation of the spatial coordinate regulation of this receptor and its ligands at the cellular level is essential. The ability to examine gene expression at the cellular level is critical for complex tissues such as the kidney, brain, and even the blood vessel wall, where the expression of an individual gene might have different implications, depending on the cell type involved.

In situ hybridization can be used for analysis of cells or tissue sections mounted on slides, or for whole mount analysis of embryos or tissue fragments in suspension *(39)*. The tissues must be pretreated before beginning the assay to increase accessibility of the target RNA. In addition, a labeled nucleic acid probe must be generated for subsequent detection of the RNA. The strategy for making single-stranded labeled cRNA probes is similar to RNase protection assays. For tissue sections, both isotope probes and non-isotope probes with digoxigenin or biotin can be used *(40)*. Resolution is maximal with low-energy radioisotopes such as ^{35}S or ^{33}P. Labeled probes are incubated with cells or tissue specimens fixed on glass slides. For whole mount detection, nonradioactive probes must be used *(17)*. For example, in nonradioactive detection of target RNA, antibodies to digoxigenin are used that contain a tagged enzyme that catalyzes the conversion of a chromogenic substrate so the hybridization pattern can be seen. For radiolabeled probe detection, slides are covered with photographic emulsion for several weeks before the film is developed. These slides can be counterstained so that the normal cellular architecture is maintained, thereby permitting immunohistochemical analysis. Whole mount–stained specimens can be photographed and then embedded, sectioned, and examined under a microscope, with or without secondary counterstaining. The specificity of the signal depends on the stringency of washing and the extent of similarity between the probe and the intended target sequence. Although less sensitive and more difficult to optimize than radioactive detection, nonradioactive detection is much faster and can provide data in a few days rather than several weeks for radioactive labeling methods.

In situ hybridization is an excellent technique for locating sites of mRNA expression, but it is not ideal for quantification. The advantage of this technique is that only a small region of transcribed sequence is necessary to obtain extensive information about the cellular pattern of expression. It is possible to begin with an EST obtained by searching genomic databases and complete a quick survey of its expression in a matter of days. In some cases, *in situ* methods have been optimized to allow high-throughput screening of novel database sequences to identify those that are expressed in a tissue- or cell-specific pattern.

Nuclear Run-off Assay

Nuclear run-off assays measure the rate of gene transcription rather than steady state mRNA levels by quantifying newly transcribed RNA molecules in cells undergoing manipulation. This assay is the most sensitive tool for measuring specific gene transcription as a function of cell state. Cell nuclei contain RNA that is being transcribed. Transcription can be completed in a test tube by adding ribonucleotides. The newly synthesized RNA can be labeled to high specific activity in isolated nuclei by including a radiolabeled ribonucleotide in the reaction. Transcription cannot be initiated under these same conditions; therefore, the level of transcription occurring at the moment that the nuclei were collected can be measured. In contrast to Northern blotting, an unlabeled, specific probe is immobilized on a filter that is hybridized to a reaction mixture containing radiolabeled transcripts to detect specific RNA species. These radiolabeled mRNAs represent all of the mRNAs elongated during the in vitro reaction; therefore, levels of transcription for many different mRNAs can be simultaneously analyzed by blotting multiple probes on a single filter. This assay is useful for evaluating whether changes in mRNA levels reflect differences in gene transcription or rates of mRNA degradation and often precedes more detailed transcriptional regulation experiments.

Promoter Analysis

Gene expression in cells or organs is strictly regulated under physiological conditions by DNA regulatory sequences that are located within hundreds to thousands of basepairs from the transcribed regions of the gene. These regulatory elements can be either positive or negative regulators of transcription, and may determine tissue specificity, developmental patterns of expression, or cell-specific responses to a variety of stimuli. The complex methodology for the study of DNA and the proteins that mediate transcriptional regulation of eukaryotic genes is beyond the scope of this chapter. However, because of the availability of useful DNA constructs that have been made in many laboratories and the ability to transfect most cell types with liposome reagents, these studies can be an excellent complement to more traditional mRNA studies.

Unlike nuclear run-off studies that are technically demanding, basic promoter studies are a simpler method for assessing rates of transcription. The primary tool for evaluating transcription is the reporter gene transfection assay. Various segments of the structural gene under study are linked to a reporter gene that can be easily assessed in a simple cell lysate. The level of activity of the reporter gene indicates the relative rate of transcription, as determined by the activity of the regulatory sequences. The firefly luciferase gene is a common example of a reporter gene.

The primary transcriptional element for each gene is the promoter, which is usually a sequence immediately upstream of the transcription start site. Whether a TATA element is present or not, promoter sequences initiate the assembly of a complex milieu of proteins that mediate transcription. Careful experiments must map the site of initiation of transcription before studies can be performed with reporter constructs. Primer extension and RNAse protection assays are used in the mapping process. In addition, other proteins, binding to cognate DNA sequences within introns or further upstream or downstream, can regulate transcription through interaction with the basal apparatus. In reporter gene experiments, a portion of the native promoter region is used, with or without additional putative regulatory sequences.

Construction of reporter plasmids for analysis requires flanking and intronic genomic sequence, which are usually obtained by cloning and mapping the intron–exon organization of the gene. In humans, predicted organizational information in the human genome sequence is used for mapping. Promoter regions of varying lengths are initially used in different constructs to map the important upstream elements. These studies are complemented by mutagenesis analyses to define more accurately the regulatory sequences. Protein binding experiments with nuclear protein and radiolabeled DNA promoter fragments are useful in these studies. Such footprint assays and gel shift assays can define possible protein binding sequences, although functional verification is required. If the expression pattern of reporter genes containing only upstream sequence does not parallel the known expression pattern, then the intronic or flanking sequence is also included in the reporter construct *(41)*.

Finally, reporter assays are performed by transfecting the plasmid containing the promoter and reporter into appropriate cell types. For cell specificity studies, the plasmid must be transfected into cells that either express or do not express the gene under investigation. Transcriptional regulation of genes expressed in heart cells has been difficult to study in vitro, mainly because of the lack of a good cell culture model. In cases where in vitro models for transfection studies are lacking, or the in vitro studies do not provide the expected results, transgenic animals can be used for reporter gene experiments (42,43).

GENOMICS

Dramatic changes are currently reshaping the experimental approach to the study of cardiovascular disease. The advanced technologies necessary for these new approaches require focus on the details of experimental methodology and on the use of rigorous statistical tools. With this caveat, advances in the field of cardiovascular medicine will be made at a significant rate in the coming decade. These breakthroughs will result from studies of gene expression, protein production and regulation, and genetic markers associated with cardiovascular disease.

Human Genome Project

As recombinant DNA technologies emerged in the early 1980s, the rate of research into the genetic basis of human diseases accelerated because of our knowledge of the human genome. In 1990, a formal 15-year plan to sequence the entire human genome was initiated by the National Institutes of Health and the U.S. Department of Energy and was entitled the Human Genome Project. This large-scale international consortium, aided by advances in DNA sequencing technology and challenged by a privately funded initiative at Celera, announced in February 2001 that the initial working draft of the human genome was complete (44).

This working draft showed that the total size of the genome is approximately 3.2 gigabases, with an estimate of 30,000 to 35,000 human structural genes (44). Although 10% of the genome is not sequenced, the correct orientation of large fragments of DNA is incomplete, and the extent of the human transcriptome is not well defined, the wealth of information now available will have a dramatic impact on the study of human disease. In addition to the preliminary sequence information that was reported, more than 1.4 million single nucleotide polymorphisms (SNPs) were identified and mapped to the reference sequence. This figure will increase to over 3 million. The importance of this information is manifold; these single-base differences between genomes may confer individual susceptibility to or protection from all human diseases, including cardiovascular disease. Because the genetic basis of cardiovascular diseases such as atherosclerosis and hypertension are polygenic, identification of SNPs in disease-related genes will play a vital role in our understanding of their pathophysiological basis.

Microarrays

The basic principles of microarrays have evolved from traditional nucleic acid blots used by molecular biologists to analyze the expression levels of multiple mRNA or DNA sequences immobilized on nitrocellulose or nylon membranes. The microarray was directly adapted from the Northern blot, where multiple DNA samples are dot blotted on a membrane and then probed with radiolabeled cDNA made from the RNA of interest. Radiographic film is used to detect the amount of radioactivity for each DNA molecule on the membrane, and densitometry is used to quantify nucleic acid levels. This technique, however, is limited by problems with standardization of data and a narrow dynamic range for accurate quantification.

Microarrays or gene chips work similarly by hybridization of a labeled cDNA (or RNA) sample to DNA molecules fixed at specific locations on a suitable substrate. Because of recent technological developments, this type of analysis can be conducted in a high-throughput, automated fashion. A major breakthrough has been the identification of glass as an excellent substrate for DNA hybridization. In addition, DNA samples can be labeled with fluorescent dyes such as cy3 and cy5 instead of radioactivity, which increases the dynamic range for measurement of gene expression. These advances, in conjunction with new robotics technologies for synthesizing and depositing nucleic acids at very high densities, have allowed for the creation of microarrays containing tens of thousands of genes on a single microscope glass slide (45). Furthermore, sophisticated analytical tools have been developed to analyze the large amount of data generated from these array hybridization studies. As a result, expression levels for tens of thousands of genes can be simultaneously measured in an accurate and reproducible manner.

The complex technologies for the deposition or creation of specific DNA fragments on glass slides can be viewed most simply as variants of two platforms, one that uses synthetic chemical methods in situ to build an array of known oligonucleotide gene sequences one base at a time and the other that uses spotting of presynthesized DNA fragments of known or unknown sequence. Ed Southern of Oxford University first described the basic concepts for creation of DNA microarrays in the late 1980s. Affymetrix, a company that has provided high quality oligonucleotide arrays for scientific studies, adapted photolithography technology from the computer industry. The use of spotted cDNA fragments amplified by PCR to make arrays was developed in the laboratory of Patrick O. Brown at Stanford University, who, along with Dr. David Botstein, adapted this platform to study yeast biology and cancer genetics (46).

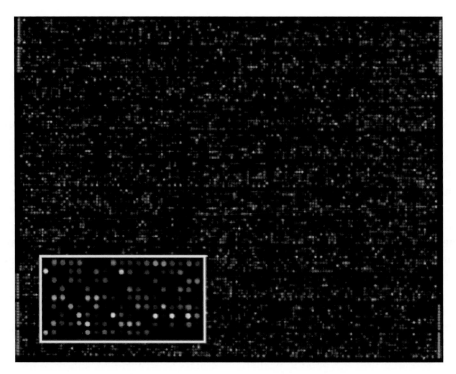

Fig. 1. Image of a high-density cDNA microarray printed on a glass slide. Inset shows a close-up view of array features or probes. Spots represent probes that have hybridized preferentially to cDNA labeled with a fluorescent dye.

Oligonucleotide arrays currently contain the highest density of "features" or probes, up to several hundred thousand elements per array. Up to 50,000 cDNA fragments can be printed onto a conventional microscope glass slide by using a bank of printing pens attached to a robotic arm. One difficulty with pen printing is the relative lack of uniformity of the spotted features. In a recent modification of the basic spotting methodology for array construction, pen spotting is used to deposit large presynthesized oligonucleotides instead of cDNAs. These oligos are typically 50–60 bases long, whereas oligos on the Affymetrix chips are 20–25 bases long. Sensitivity and specificity are better with longer oligos. These chips will likely become a dominant platform for DNA expression analysis when the entire human transcriptome is complete. Furthermore, Agilent Technologies has entered the microarray domain by applying its ink-jet technology to produce high quality *in situ* oligonucleotide arrays and spotted cDNA arrays (Fig. 1).

Both the oligonucleotide and spotted cDNA methods allow for the simultaneous examination of mRNA expression levels of thousands of genes; however, each has unique advantages and disadvantages. Because oligonucleotides can be generated from sequence information alone, probes can be customized to represent the most unique part of a given transcript, such as the

5′ untranslated region; therefore, splice variants or closely related genes can be more reliably detected *(47)*. However, hybridization kinetics are less specific with short 20–30-base pair oligos, and the costs of synthesizing oligos for custom arrays and purchasing commercially available products are high. Although cDNA microarrays are more difficult to produce because of the laborious steps necessary to generate cDNA probes for printing, they offer greater flexibility to customize specific probe sets. Furthermore, arrays comprising unsequenced clones and ESTs generated from cDNA libraries are powerful reagents for gene discovery *(47)*. Finally, whereas some oligonucleotide platforms, such as Affymetrix, compare fluorescent signals generated by hybridization of RNA samples from two tissues or cell types onto separate arrays, cDNA microarrays examine competitive hybridization of the two RNA samples labeled with different dyes to the same array. Instead of an indirect comparison of fluorescent signals on two separate arrays, a ratio for the intensity of the fluorescent signal from each channel can be calculated to determine the relative mRNA expression level for each gene on the array *(47)*.

Although it is in the early stages of development, microarray technology has already been used in many scientific studies to obtain useful information about human disease and basic biological processes. For example, microarray studies have led to a new paradigm for the molecular characterization of tumors. Alizadeh et al. *(48)* used cDNA microarrays to discover unique gene expression patterns to subclassify forms of diffuse large B-cell lymphoma (DLBCL). This approach not only identified distinct subtypes of DLBCL, but also predicted which patients had better survival rates based on molecular classification of their tumors *(48)*. In addition, subtypes based on gene expression profiles have been defined for breast cancer *(49,50)*. Recently, van't Veer et al. *(51)* used oligonucleotide arrays to identify a "poor prognosis" molecular pattern in breast tumors that correlated highly with clinical outcomes. This pattern was better than current consensus guidelines for predicting high-risk patients in need of adjuvant therapy while simultaneously reducing the number of patients receiving unnecessary treatment *(51)*. Furthermore, the use of microarrays has been successful in studying basic biological processes. For example, Spellman et al. *(52)* identified a comprehensive list of cell cycle–regulated genes in the yeast by using cDNA microarrays. They not only compiled a list of 800 genes whose transcript levels varied with the cell cycle, but also identified specific promoter elements within these genes that were predictive of cell cycle regulation.

Only a few basic studies have been conducted using this platform to study cardiovascular disease. Haley et al. *(53)* used a cDNA array to identify eotaxin, an eosinophil-attracting chemokine, as a potential new candidate gene associated with atherosclerosis. Stanton et al. *(54)* used microarrays to examine gene expression profiles in an animal model of myocardial infarction. They identified more than 700 genes with altered expression patterns in myocardial infarction, including many unknown genes. One group recently studied changes in gene expression associated with heart failure by using high-density oligonucleotide arrays to compare transcriptional profiles of normal and failing human hearts *(55)*. At the basic molecular level, several studies have used microarrays to identify novel pathways for endothelial cell signaling *(56–59)*. Finally, Adams et al. *(60)* defined the molecular phenotypes of arteries and veins by comparing their respective gene expression profiles on cDNA arrays.

In summary, microarrays are a powerful new technology for studying gene expression on a global scale. With the imminent completion of the entire human genome sequence, the transcriptional profile of all human genes can be examined. Some of the studies highlighted in this section not only testify to the power of these tools, but also provide a glimpse of their future application to study human disease. Microarrays may someday be used to diagnose different diseases, to determine the likelihood of an individual patient's response to a specific treatment, and to predict clinical outcomes, all based on gene expression profile studies.

Proteomics

Although high-throughput genomics tools such as microarrays have greatly increased our understanding of human disease, evidence indicates that mRNA levels correlate poorly with protein levels *(61)*. Furthermore, many proteins can arise from a single open reading frame because of post-transcriptional modifications such as alternative splicing and RNA editing and post-translational modifications, including glycosylation and phosphorylation *(61)*. In fact, three to six proteins may be produced per gene in humans *(62)*. Therefore, an analysis of the relative abundance of proteins and modifications to proteins is required to understand any physiological processes.

Unlike genomics, which has advanced rapidly with the development of tools such as microarrays, proteomics, or the study of the entire protein complement of the genome, has lagged behind because of many technical obstacles *(63)*. Dynamic changes in protein levels induced by specific physiological stimuli are often complemented by modifications of existing proteins, thereby producing an added layer of complexity to proteomic analysis. In addition to the high cost and labor-intensive nature of these studies, proper experimental design is daunting because of post-translational processing and the rapid changes in protein levels.

The basic techniques involved in proteomic studies are protein separation, protein identification, and classification of protein modifications *(63)*. The current mainstay of protein separation is two-dimensional gel electrophoresis (2-DE). Proteins are resolved first by their charge with isoelectric focusing (IEF) and second by their size with sodium dodecyl sulfate polyacrylamide gel electrophoresis. Large gels can separate up to 10,000 proteins *(64)*. These proteins are detected by staining the gel with silver or zinc, radiolabeling with ^{32}P or ^{35}S, or labeling with a fluorescent dye. The most sensitive method is radiolabeling, but the most commonly used technique is silver staining *(63)*. Specialized software analysis tools are used to identify proteins and calculate their relative expression levels from 2-DE images. Other protein separation methods, though not commonly used, include affinity chromatography, high-performance liquid chromatography, capillary IEF, and ion exchange.

Although protein separation methods have been perfected over the past 25 years, the most significant advance in proteomic analysis has been the development of mass spectrometry (MS) for protein identification *(63)*.

Peptide mass mapping is often used for MS protein identification. Proteins separated by 2-DE are digested with proteases such as trypsin or chemical reagents to produce smaller peptide sequences, which yield a set of distinct peptides specific to each protein (63). These peptides are then ionized by electrospray ionization from the liquid phase or matrix-assisted laser desorption ionization (MALDI) from the solid phase. A unique peptide mass fingerprint (PMF) is generated from the masses of peptides measured by MS (63,65). Finally, the protein is identified by comparing the peptide signature to PMFs for known, partial, or predicted protein sequences found in protein databases such as SWISS-PROT.

The most difficult task in proteomic analysis is the identification and characterization of post-translational modifications. Traditional biochemical methods such as periodic acid/Schiff staining to identify glycosylated proteins and ^{32}P radiolabeling to detect phosphorylated proteins are not readily amenable to high-throughput strategies. MS is emerging, however, as a potential solution to this problem. MS PMF data can be used to identify up to 22 different post-translational modifications and to predict possible modifications based on amino acid sequence homology (63). Furthermore, new technologies such as MALDI-time of flight-post source decay have greatly increased the ability to detect post-translational modifications by fragmenting proteins into very small peptides comprising only a few amino acids.

Most proteomic studies, like genomics studies, have been conducted in the area of cancer research. For example, Ostergaard et al. (66) used 2-DE to analyze protein expression patterns of squamous cell carcinomas of the bladder and to identify unique markers of tumor differentiation. Proteomic applications to cardiovascular disease have focused primarily on protein expression profiles in cardiomyopathies. Pleissner et al. (67) performed a proteomic analysis of heart tissue from patients with or without dilated cardiomyopathy and identified several proteins that are differentially expressed by myocardial tissue from cardiomyopathy patients, including cytoskeletal proteins and proteins associated with energy production and stress responses.

Proteomics is a promising complement to genomics-based strategies. However, until technical difficulties are solved, proteomics will not gain the same level of interest as genomics. Methods to detect low-abundance proteins and to identify post-translational modifications are still in early stages of development (65). Protein separation techniques are difficult to automate, and robust bioinformatics tools are lacking. Despite these limitations, proteomics will eventually become an essential platform to study biological processes and human disease.

Single Nucleotide Polymorphisms

Rare diseases such as Huntington's disease and cystic fibrosis are caused by mutation of a single gene. Classical linkage studies in families identified these highly penetrant alleles, which usually occur at a frequency of less than 1% of the population. In contrast, common diseases such as atherosclerosis are caused by a complex interaction between environmental risk factors and multiple genetic loci. These genetic variants are usually found at moderate to high frequency in the general population. Linkage analysis methods with classical markers do not have the power to discriminate common alleles that determine disease susceptibility. Instead, identification of a large set of markers dispersed throughout the genome is required. These markers can be used in an extensive genetic analysis to understand the hereditary basis of complex disorders such as atherosclerosis. The most attractive candidates for markers are SNPs.

SNPs are single base pair differences in a DNA sequence between individuals of a population. SNPs occur about every 1000 base pairs throughout the genome. The effects that SNPs will have on a specific phenotype depend on their location within the genome. Coding SNPs are found within the coding regions of genes and may alter the function or structure of encoded proteins resulting in a disease state. Most SNPs, however, are located within non-coding regions and probably have little effect on phenotype (68). Two main strategies are used for studying SNPs and complex diseases—candidate gene approach and linkage disequilibrium mapping.

The candidate gene approach is based on prior knowledge about the genes that are likely to contribute to the pathogenesis of a specific disease. SNPs are identified in the candidate genes, and association studies determine a link between the polymorphic variation and the disease. These studies are limited in scope, however, since a priori knowledge of the genes involved is required for any analysis.

The recent efforts by the Human Genome Project and others have led to the identification and mapping of more than 2 million SNPs. These high-density SNP maps may allow scientists to identify disease phenotypes by using linkage disequilibrium mapping. Linkage disequilibrium is defined as two alleles at different loci that occur in an individual at a frequency greater than would be predicted by random chance (69). The strength of linkage disequilibrium decreases with time, or successive generations, because of recombinatorial events between loci. Loci that are close to each other are more likely to be inherited together than those that are far apart. When specific haplotypes (i.e., combinations of segregating alleles at different loci) are in linkage disequilibrium and associated with a disease phenotype, a susceptibility gene can be mapped to a precise location in the genome *(68,70)*. New genetic variants associated with human disease may therefore be rapidly identified through large-scale genotyping of populations and linkage disequilibrium mapping studies.

The technological advances made in genomics and proteomics have improved high-throughput methods for identifying and genotyping SNPs. Although other methods for SNP identification exist, sequence-specific detection is the preferred method for large-scale genotyping and is based on four mechanisms for allelic discrimination: allele-specific hybridization, nucleotide primer extension, oligonucleotide ligation, and enzymatic cleavage *(68,71)*.

Hybridization methods are based on designing two allele-specific probes to hybridize to a target sequence when a perfect complementary sequence is present. Under optimal conditions, a one basepair mismatch is sufficiently destabilizing to prevent the probe from annealing to its target *(71)*. The most widely used allele-specific oligonucleotide (ASO) hybridization method to distinguish SNP alleles is real-time PCR in homogeneous, solution-phase hybridization reactions with fluorescence detection (TaqMan™ and Molecular Beacon assays). The major problem with this approach, which has hindered the development of high-throughput multiplex assays with this platform, is the difficulty in predicting optimal reaction conditions or a probe that will provide the greatest distinction between two alleles *(68)*. However, microarrays have recently been used for multiplex allele-specific probe hybridization reactions by spotting hundreds of ASO probes for each SNP on glass slides.

Primer extension protocols, which are very flexible, are excellent for allelic discrimination and require the smallest number of primers and probes for detection *(71)*. In this approach, a primer anneals to its target sequence immediately adjacent to the SNP and is extended by a DNA polymerase with a single nucleotide complementary to the oligonucleotide at the site of the SNP. This method is based on the high accuracy of nucleotide incorporation by DNA polymerases *(68)*. Assay design and optimization are minimal, which makes this approach the best suited for high-throughput genotype applications; therefore, many detection systems and platforms have been developed with primer extension protocols. Pyrosequencing, with the use of an enzyme-based luminometric detection of pyrophosphate; mass spectrometry, such as MALDI-time of flight mass spectrometry; enzyme-linked immunosorbent assays; and microarrays are platforms currently used for detection of SNPs.

Microarray-based strategies appear to be particularly tailored for large-scale SNP analysis *(68)*.

Ligation methods rely on the ability of DNA ligases to discriminate mismatches at the ligation site of adjacent oligonucleotides annealed to a DNA template *(68,71)*. Ligation occurs, therefore, only when oligonucleotides are exactly complementary to the template at the junction. Ligation methods have the highest level of specificity and are easy to optimize; however, they are the slowest reaction and require the greatest number of probes *(71)*. High-throughput strategies have been developed including microarray formats, multiplex detection with fluorescently labeled probes, and real time PCR assays.

The final allelic discrimination method is invasive cleavage of oligonucleotide probes. This approach is based on the use of two target-specific oligonucleotides, one with a 5′-region noncomplementary to the target sequence and the other an upstream complementary probe. When the probes are matched at the SNP, the three-dimensional structure formed at this site is cleaved by a 5′-endonuclease, or FLAP endonuclease. The enzyme releases the 5′-sequence of the signaling probe, which can be detected directly, or can be further amplified *(68)*. MS and fluorescence polarization methods are currently used for SNP detection. The invasive assays do not require a PCR amplification step and therefore are isothermal reactions. Unfortunately, these assays require a large amount of target DNA and extremely pure probes to ensure specificity of the reactions.

Genetic variants associated with cardiovascular disease have been studied extensively. In most of these studies, a candidate gene approach was used in which many of the genes analyzed are purported to play a role in the disease process. For example, increased plasminogen-activator inhibitor 1 (PAI-1) activity is commonly found in patients with coronary artery disease. In studies by Eriksson et al. *(72)* and Margaglione et al. *(73)*, the 4G/5G polymorphism in the PAI-1 promoter was associated with higher plasma PAI-1 activity, and the 4G allele was found more often in patients with a history of myocardial infarction. Inflammation contributes significantly to the progression of atherosclerosis. Cytokines that mediate inflammatory responses are good candidate genes for association studies. CX3CR1, a chemokine receptor expressed on monocytes, acts either as a chemotactic receptor or as an adhesion molecule, depending on the nature of its ligand, fractalkine. In a recent study, a common CX3CR1 genetic variant (I249) was an independent risk factor for coronary artery disease *(74)*. Finally, Ranade et al. *(75)* identified two polymorphisms (T-344C, Lys-173/Arg) in the aldosterone synthase gene that conferred increased susceptibility to insulin resistance and diabetes *(75)*. Although interesting, these findings from candidate gene studies need to be independently verified in additional cohorts.

In summary, SNPs are an important genetic determinant of complex human diseases. Classical candidate gene approaches have produced a vast amount of data linking genetic variants with human disease. These types of studies are limited in scope, however, because they require *a priori* knowledge of the disease-associated genes. Furthermore, such candidate gene association studies require large, carefully selected cohorts to obtain reproducible results. Full definition of the haplotype structure of the human genome, in concert with the refinement of high-throughput technologies for SNP detection and genotyping, will allow SNP-based association studies to make significant contributions to the study of the genetics of cardiovascular disease.

GENETIC ANIMAL MODELS FOR THE STUDY OF CARDIOVASCULAR DISEASE

Animal models, always important in biomedical research, have been used to study the pathophysiology of disease and to evaluate the beneficial and toxic effects of pharmacological therapies. With the advent of molecular biology and the development of techniques to manipulate the genome, the use of animal models has become even more important. In particular, the mouse has been used as a model to study human diseases such as hypertension, diabetes, insulin resistance, hyperlipidemia, and atherosclerosis. In this section, we briefly describe the tools required for genetic manipulation of the mouse and then examine in more detail how genetic mouse models have increased our understanding of atherosclerosis.

Genetic Manipulation of the Mouse
GENE TARGETING OR KNOCKOUT METHODS

The goal of gene targeting experiments is to analyze the phenotype of mice fractionally lacking a single gene. Many genes have been targeted in mice, and these analyses have provided significant information about the function of specific genes.

The first step in gene knockout or deletion studies is the assembly of a targeting construct that will introduce a desired mutation in the chosen gene when it integrates into one of the endogenous alleles. The targeting construct is designed to replace an essential portion of the structural gene. Targeting vectors typically contain genomic homology regions cloned on either side of genes for neomycin resistance and thymidine kinase *(76)*. Homologous recombination events within these homology regions result in the replacement of genomic DNA with the neomycin resistance gene and the concomitant loss of the thymidine kinase gene. Random integration of the construct, however, leads to genomic incorporation of the thymidine kinase gene. Positive selection with G418 selects for transfected cells that have incorporated the targeting construct, whereas negative selection with gancyclovir eliminates cells that have a functional thymidine kinase gene as a result of random integration. Despite this dual selection process, only a small percentage of G418 resistant cells contain the targeting construct; therefore, screening the individual G418 colonies by Southern blot with restriction digests and probes that map to the locus of interest is essential.

The next step in this process is to introduce the targeted deletion into the germline. For this step, the deletion is generated through homologous recombination in cultured pluripotent embryonic stem (ES) cells, and then these cells are implanted into chimeric mice. Only one allele is usually altered in the stem cells, and the mutation is established in the germline of heterozygous animals. Chimeric mice generated from injection of the targeted ES cells into blastocysts have patchy coat colors reflecting the beige color of the 129 line used to generate the ES cells and the black color of the C57Bl6 line used to produce the blastocysts. The chimeric mice are then bred back with wild-type animals. True chimeric mice will transmit the targeted allele to the F1 generation. These heterozygous animals usually develop normally and are fertile; therefore, mutations that otherwise would be lethal in the homozygous state can be maintained in the population. By cross-breeding this F1 generation, homozygous or knockout mice are generated that represent a loss of function model for the targeted gene. These mice are then assessed for Mendelian segregation of the targeted allele. If the targeted gene is not essential for embryonic development, homozygous animals will make up about one fourth of the offspring. Although this technique initially requires a high level of expertise, gene targeted deletions are done in many laboratories, and many institutions have core facilities that support the more difficult aspects of this process.

Information gained through gene-targeting experiments varies greatly. In cases where the gene serves an essential early function, the embryo often does not survive *(77–79)*. Although these studies provide helpful information about embryogenesis, they have often hindered the analysis of the functional role of these genes in the adult animal. In a few cases, loss of only one allele was lethal, implying that the amount of protein was critical for normal development, a situation called the "gene dosage" effect *(80,81)*. In contrast, targeted deletion studies of genes thought to be functionally important have frequently produced no discernible phenotypic abnormalities *(82)*. These results have been interpreted as evolutionary safeguards, or a functional redundancy, in molecular pathways of genes critical to survival of a species. However, careful scrutiny of animals with a normal phenotype under routine growth and maintenance conditions has shown abnormal responses to various environmental stimuli.

Among the numerous gene targeting studies, some of the most notable work has examined the functional importance of endothelial cell genes. Gene deletion studies of the vascular endothelial growth factor receptors, flk1 and flt1, angiopoietin receptor tek/tie2, and the orphan tie1 receptor have provided tremendous insight on the early developmental events associated with endothelial cell origin and/or proliferation such as vasculogenesis and angiogenesis *(77–79)*. Much has been learned about the function of vascular endothelial-cadherin and various selectins in targeting studies *(83,84)*.

DOUBLE KNOCKOUTS

Double gene knockout mice can be generated by breeding mice with different single-gene deletions and screening the progeny for both mutated genes. Alternatively, ES cells homozygous for one knockout can be targeted to a second locus with a construct that contains a different drug resistance gene *(85)*. Double knockout animals have been developed with ApoE deficient mice as a genetic background to evaluate whether a second gene can modify the development or progression of atherosclerosis. This approach has been used to analyze genes such as monocyte chemotactic protein-1 (MCP-1), E-selectin, and P-selectin. In addition, mice with multiply targeted genes have been used to determine the functional overlap of different genes and to unmask redundancies in specific signaling pathways. For example, the role of all three src-related genes (fyn, yes, and src) in cytoplasmic signaling was defined in combined targeting studies *(86)*.

CRE/LOXP REGULATED GENE TARGETING

Many gene knockouts result in embryonic lethality, indicating that the gene plays a critical role in the development of the embryo. Although characterizing the defective phenotype indicates the functional requirement for the gene and encoded protein in embryogenesis, loss of the mutant animal before birth obviates investigation of the gene within the pathophysiological context of adulthood. In addition, compensatory mechanisms during development can potentially mask important and relevant phenotypes, and residual effects that linger into adulthood may alter responses to disease stimuli. Confining the cell types where the gene is inactivated or regulating the time at which the gene deletion occurs may circumvent these limitations to gene targeting techniques.

DNA recombinases have been used to address these limitations. In the most extensively studied system in the mouse, the Cre recombinase is used because of its ability to manipulate DNA flanked by LoxP recognition sequences *(87,88)*. The first step in generating a regulated or conditional mutation is to use homologous recombination to insert two LoxP recognition sites on either side of the sequence to be deleted *(89,90)*. These sequences, when placed outside of the coding regions of the gene, do not appear to disturb transcription, RNA processing, or translation. The altered allele is then passed into the germline, as described above for generating knockout mice.

Recombination, which is achieved by breeding the LoxP mice to mice that express Cre in a temporal and/or cell-specific fashion, results in loss of the LoxP flanked sequence *(91–93)*. Cre recognizes and cleaves the LoxP sites and joins the chromosomal ends to yield an allele that contains only a single residual LoxP site. Several methods are used to introduce Cre in a cell- or tissue-specific fashion *(94)*. For example, cardiac- and endothelial cell–specific promoters have been used to drive restricted expression of Cre in these tissues *(95)*. Alternatively, the Cre protein can be introduced into a tissue by infecting it with an adenovirus that expresses the recombinase *(96)*. Finally, combining the Cre-LoxP system with an inducible gene expression system that exploits tetracycline regulatory elements can be used for cell-specific and inducible regulation of recombination *(97,98)*.

Transgenesis

Transgenesis is the introduction of exogenous DNA into the genome of an animal such that it becomes part of the animal's germline. The DNA that is to be integrated into the germline typically contains a gene (usually in the form of a cDNA), a promoter to drive expression of the cDNA, and an untranslated sequence to direct correct polyadenylation of the synthetic transcript. The main techniques for generation of transgenic mice involve either microinjecting the desired DNA into the pronucleus of a fertilized egg or introducing the transgene directly into ES cells. Methods of ES cell manipulation are similar to those described for gene knockouts, with the exception that integration does not have to occur at a specific locus. Tissue-specific promoters can be used to drive expression of the transgene in particular cell types.

Transgenic animals have been widely used in gain-of-function experiments to determine the effects that over-expression or changes in the temporal or spatial expression patterns have on the function of a targeted gene. For example, the keratin14 promoter has been used to express putative angiogenic factors in the skin, where vessel structure and function are easily observed in vivo *(99)*. Lipoprotein lipase (LPL) expression has been targeted to different tissues and evaluated in an LPL-deficient setting *(100,101)* so that local function of the enzyme in tissues where it is normally expressed can be evaluated. Finally, transgenic animals have been used to decipher DNA sequences that direct cell-specific and developmental patterns of gene expression. In this approach, various portions of a non-coding sequence are paired with the native or heterologous promoter sequence upstream of a reporter gene whose transcription can be easily assessed *(102)*.

A common problem seen in transgenic studies is that the level of transgene expression often depends on where it integrates in the genome. Although transgenes often integrate in large copy numbers, expression is low and variable because sufficient transcriptional regulatory elements are not included in the construct to direct site-independent expression. Variability in expression levels between different lines of mice is particularly frustrating when transgenic animals are used for in vivo mapping of cell-specific regulatory elements. The inclusion of introns into a construct increases the level of expression, and several constructs now contain introns from several highly expressed genes. Transgenic mice can be produced by microinjection of a large region of genomic DNA, often in the form of a BAC *(103)*. In addition to the exons encoding the gene of interest, regulatory regions of the gene are included, which significantly increase the likelihood of obtaining adequate levels of expression.

Several investigators now use homologous recombination in ES cells to eliminate variable expression levels caused by integration of the transgene into different genomic sites. In this approach, an endogenous locus is specifically targeted for incorporation of the transgene construct *(104)*. This approach results in not only a greater uniformity of expression between different lines of mice but also a higher level of expression. This method is more time consuming and requires more expertise than the usual technique of pronuclear injection. Currently under development is the use of homologous recombination in bacteria to genetically engineer large regions of DNA that can be microinjected into pronuclei for the rapid development of stable and highly expressed transgenes *(105)*.

Regulated Transgene Expression

To provide experimentally regulated expression of foreign genes in transgenic animals, drug-inducible tran-scriptional elements have been developed. The most widely used transcriptional element originates from the tetracycline response system *(106)*. In the classical approach, tetracycline (or the potent analog doxycycline), which inhibits transcription of the transgene, is continuously supplied in the animal's drinking water *(107)*. Gene expression is initiated, therefore, only upon removal of the drug. In this technique, two transcriptional units are used. The first contains a promoter that drives the expression of a regulatory protein that interacts with tetracycline, and when bound to the drug, does not allow it to bind and inhibit the transcription of a second promoter. This second promoter, under constant inhibition when tetracycline is present, drives the expression of the experimental gene. The most widely used method takes advantage of the ability of a cell-specific promoter to drive expression of the tetracycline operator protein, thus conferring both spatial and temporal regulation of gene expression. This paradigm, where presence of the drug inhibits transcription, is called a "tet-off" system. In a commonly used variant of this system, an operator protein, which can activate rather than inhibit transcription when bound to the drug, is used and forms the basis for a "tet-on" system. Both tet-on and tet-off approaches have drawbacks related to the leakiness of trangene expression in the repressed state. For both systems, each of the transcriptional units can be incorporated into individual lines of mice and then combined by breeding the mice, or both transcriptional units can be simultaneously injected with a single construct. These systems can be evaluated by breeding animals containing a regulatory transgene with a reporter mouse that has a tetracycline-regulated reporter gene. The expression of the reporter gene can then be measured in the presence or absence of the drug.

Animal Models of Atherosclerosis

HISTORICAL PERSPECTIVE

Although progress has been made in understanding the pathophysiology of atherosclerosis, the molecular mechanisms underlying atherosclerosis at its various stages are largely unknown, due in large part to the inaccessibility of human vascular diseased tissue to study. Mouse models of atherosclerosis provide access to the vessel wall during the progression of the disease process, and genetic manipulation of the mouse makes possible the study of interactions between the environment and the genetic factors that contribute to disease progression.

The mouse has traditionally been the species of choice for genetic manipulation and for the development of experimental disease models. Extensive early work on mouse reproduction and development and the advanced status of mouse genetics have contributed to the use of the mouse model. Rodents have been used for the study of atherosclerosis because of our knowledge of their physiology, the feasibility of genetic manipulation, low housing costs, and the ease of maintenance. Their relative resistance to atherosclerosis along with their excessive mortality on high-fat diets originally discouraged many researchers from using rodent models. In addition, the distinct lipid profiles of mice contributed to the initial lack of interest in rodent models of atherosclerosis. As molecular techniques for genetic manipulation in mice improved, a small number of insightful researchers began to alter mice genetically by perturbing their lipid metabolism (108–110). Well-formulated questions could clearly be addressed by using the mouse model. Highly characterized knockout mice and transgenic mice have contributed greatly to the understanding of lipoprotein and inflammatory pathways and their role in atherosclerosis. These studies have identified a limited set of candidate genes that modulate the disease process at its various stages (111–113).

INBRED MICE

Mice, with typical cholesterol levels of less than 100 mg/dL, are highly resistant to atherosclerosis. In the 1980s, several researchers tried to produce atherosclerosis in mice to identify possible candidate genes (114–116). On high-fat, high-cholesterol diets, several strains of inbred mice, such as C57Bl/6, developed increased cholesterol levels and several layers of foam cells reminiscent of early atherosclerotic lesions (113,117). In contrast, other strains such as C3H/HeJ mice did not develop such lesions. Although an atherogenic diet decreased high-density lipoprotein (HDL) levels in the B6 strain, C3H mice were resistant to these changes (109). Crosses between susceptible and resistant strains were used to identify potential loci for genetic susceptibility (118). One well-studied locus was Ath1, which encoded for the second most abundant HDL apolipoprotein (ApoA-II) (119–121). The use of inbred mice to study atherosclerosis raised several critical issues. The histology and vascular distribution of the lesions were different from those found in humans (122). Furthermore, the atherogenic diet used in the mice was nonphysiologic and caused a chronic inflammation in C57Bl/6 mice (113,123); therefore, the development of lesions in some inbred mice could be attributed to diet-induced inflammation rather than atherosclerosis. Recent studies, however, suggest that endothelial cells, not inflammatory cells or plasma lipid levels, may contribute to the differences in susceptibility to atherosclerosis (124–127).

GENETIC MANIPULATION: ROLE OF CANDIDATE GENES IN DISEASE

Mouse models of atherosclerosis have become the most powerful experimental approach to study the roles of candidate genes in vivo. In the early 1990s, two laboratories used gene knockout technology to generate atherosclerosis-prone ApoE deficient mice (110,128). As a result, the popularity of mouse models of atherosclerosis has dramatically increased (112,113). The ApoE knockout mouse, used either as a single knockout or as the genetic background for a second gene mutation, is one of the most widely used models of atherosclerosis. The delayed clearance of certain lipoproteins in ApoE mice increases cholesterol levels. On a normal diet, these mice can develop atherosclerotic lesions spontaneously, and a high-fat diet increases the lesion size and the rate of disease progression (110,128). The time course for the development of atherosclerotic lesions and the various stages of the lesions are well characterized (129). Although complex lesions do not occur, the histological changes and regions of susceptibility are similar to those seen in humans.

ATHEROGENIC AND ANTIATHEROGENIC GENES

Several well-characterized transgenic and gene knockout mouse models have contributed greatly to the understanding of critical pathways in atherosclerosis. Several genes have been identified that either promote or prevent the disease process in these mouse models (Tables 1 and 2) (111,112). Endothelial injury and subsequent endothelial dysfunction may be an initiating event during atherosclerosis. The role of oxidative stress at initial stages of disease has been studied in several mouse models. A reduction in atherosclerosis was reported in 15-lipoxygenase (15-LO)/ApoE double knockout mice, which suggests a proatherogenic role of 15-LO as an oxidant-generating enzyme (130). Similar findings have been described for iNOS/ApoE double knockout mice (131), confirming the potent oxidative properties of inducible NOS. These oxidant-generating pathways may modify low-density lipoprotein (LDL) to its oxidized and highly atherogenic form. Degradation of the biologically active lipids within oxidized LDL may potentially reduce disease susceptibility. The finding of increased lesion formation in mice deficient in paraxonase, which degrades oxidized phospholipids, supports this theory (132–134). Hypertension contributes to endothelial injury. A marked increase in atherosclerotic lesions is seen in hypertensive mice lacking eNOS and ApoE genes (135,136). In contrast, atherosclerosis was not accelerated in hypertensive mice without hyperlipidemia (137). Finally, diabetic and hyperinsulinemic mice may be at risk for atherosclerosis (138,139).

Table 1
Candidate Atherogenic Genes Involved in Atherosclerosis

Gene (Ref)	Genetic background	Mouse model	Degree of atherosclerosis	Pathway
C57Bl/6 (109)	Wild type	Control	↑	Wild type
iNOS (131,167)	ApoE−/−	DKO	↓	Endothelial function
12/15-LO (130)	ApoE−/−	DKO	↓	Lipid metabolism
12/15-LO (168)	LDLR−/−	TG	↑	Lipid metabolism
ApoAII (169)	Wild type	TG	↑	Lipid metabolism
ApoB48 (170)	ApoE−/−	TG/KO	↑	Lipid metabolism
ApoB48 (171)	LDLR−/−	TG/KO	↑	Lipid metabolism
ApoC1 (172)	Wild type	TG	↑	Lipid metabolism
CETP (164)	Wild type	TG	↑	Lipid metabolism
Lp(a) (173)	Wild type	TG	↑	Lipid metabolism
SR-A (149)	ApoE−/−	DKO	↓	Lipid metabolism
CCR2 (147,174)	ApoE−/−	DKO	↓	Inflammation
CD154 (175)	ApoE−/−	DKO	↓	Inflammation
CXCR2 (148)	LDLR−/−	DKO	↓	Inflammation
E selectin (144)	LDLR−/−	DKO	↓	Inflammation
P selectin (144)	LDLR−/−	DKO	↓	Inflammation
ICAM-1 (143)	ApoE−/−	DKO	↓	Inflammation
MCP-1 (145)	ApoB+	KO/TG	↓	Inflammation
MCP-1 (146)	LDLR−/−	DKO	↓	Inflammation
MCP-1 (176)	ApoE−/−	DKO	↓	Inflammation
MCSF (141)	ApoE−/−	DKO	↓	Inflammation
CD36 (150)	ApoE−/−	DKO	↓	Inflammation
PPARA (177)	ApoE−/−	DKO	↓	Insulin resistance

CCR2, chemokine (cc motif) receptor 2; CETP, cholesteryl ester transfer protein; DKO, double knockout; ICAM, intercellular adhesion molecule; iNOS, inducible nitric oxide synthase; KO, knockout; LDLR, low density lipoprotein receptor; LO, lipoxygenase; Lp(a), Lipoprotein (a); MCP, monocyte chemotactic protein; MCSF, macrophage colony-stimulating factor; PPARA, peroxisome proliferator activated receptor α (alpha); SR-A, scavenger receptor A; TG, transgenic.

Recruitment of monocytes, their differentiation into macrophages, and progressive accumulation of oxidized LDL leads to the development of atherosclerotic lesions. Mice that lack the gene for macrophage colony stimulating factor are extremely resistant to atherosclerosis when bred onto an ApoE-deficient background *(140,141)*, which confirms the critical role of macrophages in the development of disease. The recruitment of monocytes to the vascular wall is regulated by cell adhesion molecules that are expressed on endothelial cell surfaces. Several of these molecules may contribute to the progression of atherosclerosis. Monocyte recruitment to atherosclerotic lesions was significantly reduced in ApoE-deficient mice with an intracellular adhesion molecule-1 deficiency *(142,143)* or E or P selectin deficiency *(144)*. Other studies have described the important

role of monocyte migration into the arterial wall. The extent of atherosclerotic lesions is markedly reduced in mice that lack the genes for MCP-1 *(145,146)* or its receptor (CCR2) *(147)*. In addition, disruption of the CXCR2 gene for the IL-8 receptor significantly reduced disease burden *(148)*.

The production of foam cells with fatty streak formation is the hallmark of atherosclerotic lesions. Uptake of oxidized LDL by macrophages is mediated by several different molecules. Lesion development is reduced in scavenger receptor A (SR-A) and CD36 knockout mice bred to an ApoE-deficient background, suggesting that recognition of oxidized LDL by scavenger receptors is important in the disease process *(149,150)*.

The critical role of cholesterol efflux in the progression of atherosclerosis has been shown in several

Table 2
Candidate Antiatherogenic Genes Involved in Atherosclerosis

Gene (Ref)	Genetic background	Mouse model	Degree of atherosclerosis	Pathway
C3H/HeJ (109)	Wild type	Control	↓	
eNOS (135–137)	ApoE–/–	DKO	↓	Endothelial function
ABC A1 (178)	Wild type	KO	? ↑	Lipid metabolism
ABC A1 (179)	Wild type	TG	? ↓	Lipid metabolism
ApoAI (151)	ApoB+	KO/TG	↑	Lipid metabolism
ApoAI (180,181)	ApoE–/–	TG/KO	↓	Lipid metabolism
ApoAI (182)	LDLR–/–	TG/KO	↓	Lipid metabolism
ApoB 100 (170)	ApoE–/–	TG/KO	↓	Lipid metabolism
ApoE (110,128)	Wild type	KO	↑	Lipid metabolism
LDLR (183)	ApoE–/–	DKO	↑	Lipid metabolism
LDLR (108)	Wild type	KO	↓	Lipid metabolism
LIPC (184)	Wild type	KO	↑	Lipid metabolism
LPL (185)	Wild type	KO	? ↑	Lipid metabolism
PON1 (186,187)	ApoE–/–	DKO	↑	Lipid metabolism
SR-B1 (165)	LDLR–/–	DKO	↑	Lipid metabolism
SR-B1 (166)	LDLR–/–	TG/KO	↓	Lipid metabolism
IRS-1 (138)	Wild type	KO	? ↑	Insulin resistance
PPARG (188)	LDLR–/–	DKO	↑	Insulin resistance
IL-10 (189)	Wild type	KO	↑	Inflammation

ABC, ATP-binding cassette transporter; DKO, double knockout; eNOS, endothelial nitric oxide synthase; IL-10, interleukin-10; IRS-1, insulin receptor substrate-1; KO, knockout; LDLR, low density lipoprotein receptor; LIPC, hepatic lipase; LPL, lipoprotein lipase; PON1, paraxonase 1; PPARG, peroxisome proliferator activated receptor γ (gamma); SR-B1, scavenger receptor B1; TG, transgenic.

studies. HDL is important in "reverse cholesterol transport," thus explaining the inverse correlatation between HDL and the risk of atherosclerosis. Deletion of the ApoA-1 gene, which encodes for the major protein component of HDL, causes severe atherosclerosis in ApoB transgenic mice (151). Other molecules important in cholesterol transport modulate atherosclerosis, including ACAT-1 (152–154), ABC-1 (ATP binding cassette family of transporters) (155–160), lecithin-chol acyltransferase (161,162), cholesteryl ester transfer protein (163,164), and SR-B1 (HDL receptor in liver) (165,166). Studies in genetically manipulated mice have indicated that several other families of genes, such as the nuclear receptors PPAR-α and LXRs, and genes involved in cellular immunity such as interleukin-4, interleukin-10, and interferon-gamma, contribute to the progression of atherosclerotic lesions (112). Many new genes will likely be identified as important modulators of atherosclerosis in these same animal models.

POTENTIAL DISADVANTAGES OF MOUSE MODELS OF ATHEROSCLEROSIS

The mouse model for atherosclerosis has some disadvantages. Mice have different lipid profiles and cardiac physiology than humans, and vascular manipulation is often difficult because of their small size. In addition, atherosclerosis in mice is a relatively rapid process, whereas in humans, it is slow and progressive. Although increases in cholesterol are extremely high in most mouse models, the model best suited for studying atherosclerosis in humans has not been identified. Distal coronary disease and evidence of complications from ischemia are not usually seen in mice. Furthermore, thrombotic events that cause myocardial infarction are not usually found in the mouse model. Although the ApoE/eNOS double knockout mouse addresses some of these shortcomings (135,136), many other differences in the disease process between mice and humans cannot be resolved. The extent to which findings in the mouse model can be extrapolated to humans is unknown.

FUTURE DIRECTIONS

Recent advances in high-throughput genomics technology offer a novel, systematic approach to study the expression of thousands of genes simultaneously. This technology can be used to study differential gene expression in different strains of mice that are either resistant or susceptible to atherosclerosis. In addition, these methods can be used to determine genome-wide responses of cellular components of the vascular wall (i.e., smooth muscle cells, endothelial cells, and macrophages) to atherogenic stimuli or therapeutic interventions. Moreover, the different patterns of gene expression during various stages of development of the disease can be studied in a mouse model of cardiovascular disease, an approach that cannot be replicated in humans. New candidate genes may be identified from studies of temporal patterns of gene expression. The use of animal models in combination with emerging genomic and proteomic technologies should accelerate the pace of discovery for the molecular determinants of cardiovascular disease and offer direct benefits for humans in the future.

REFERENCES

1. Strachan T, Read AP. Human Molecular Genetics. 2nd ed. New York: John Wiley & Sons, 1999:576.
2. Grompe M, Johnson W, Jameson JL. Recombinant DNA and genetic techniques. In: Jameson JL, Collins FS, eds. Principles of Molecular Medicine. Totowa, NJ: Humana Press, 1998: 9–24.
3. Janssen K. Analysis of RNA by Northern and slot blot hybridization. In: Ausubel FM, Brent R, Kingston RE, et al., eds. Current Protocols in Molecular Biology. New York: Greene Publishing and John Wiley & Sons, 1994: 4.9.1–4.9.11.
4. Muyrers JP, Zhang Y, Stewart AF. Techniques: Recombinogenic engineering—new options for cloning and manipulating DNA. Trends Biochem Sci 2001;26:325–331.
5. Monaco AP, Larin Z. YACs, BACs, PACs and MACs: artificial chromosomes as research tools. Trends Biotechnol 1994; 12:280–286.
6. Burke DT, Carle GF, Olson MV. Cloning of large segments of exogenous DNA into yeast by means of artificial chromosome vectors. Science 1987;236:806–812.
7. Schlessinger D. Yeast artificial chromosomes: tools for mapping and analysis of complex genomes. Trends Genet 1990; 6:248,255–258.
8. Shepherd NS, Smoller D. The P1 vector system for the preparation and screening of genomic libraries. Genet Eng (N Y) 1994;16:213–228.
9. Sternberg NL. Cloning high molecular weight DNA fragments by the bacteriophage P1 system. Trends Genet 1992;8:11–16.
10. Ioannou PA, Amemiya CT, Garnes J, et al. A new bacteriophage P1-derived vector for the propagation of large human DNA fragments. Nat Genet 1994;6:84–89.
11. Shizuya H, Birren B, Kim UJ, et al. Cloning and stable maintenance of 300-kilobase-pair fragments of human DNA in Escherichia coli using an F-factor-based vector. Proc Natl Acad Sci USA 1992;89:8794–8797.
12. Schein CH. Optimizing protein folding to the native state in bacteria. Curr Opin Biotechnol 1991;2:746–750.
13. Gluzman Y. SV40-transformed simian cells support the replication of early SV40 mutants. Cell 1981;23:175–182.
14. Seed B, Parker RC, Davidson N. Representation of DNA sequences in recombinant DNA libraries prepared by restriction enzyme partial digestion. Gene 1982;19:201–209.
15. Venter JC, Adams MD, Myers EW, et al. The sequence of the human genome. Science 2001;291:1304–1351.
16. Hirata K, Dichek HL, Cioffi JA, et al. Cloning of a unique lipase from endothelial cells extends the lipase gene family. J Biol Chem 1999;274:14170–14175.
17. Hirata K, Ishida T, Penta K, et al. Cloning of an immunoglobulin family adhesion molecule selectively expressed by endothelial cells. J Biol Chem 2001;276:16223–16231.
18. Dogan Temizer PLH, Shi-Chung Ng, Quertermous T. Molecular cloning strategies. In: Fozzard HA, ed. The Heart and Cardiovascular System. New York: Raven Press, 1992:561–579.
19. Sasaki K, Yamano Y, Bardhan S, et al. Cloning and expression of a complementary DNA encoding a bovine adrenal angiotensin II type-1 receptor. Nature 1991;351:230–233.
20. Lin HY, Wang XF, Ng-Eaton E, Weinberg RA, Lodish HF. Expression cloning of the TGF-beta type II receptor, a functional transmembrane serine/threonine kinase. Cell 1992;68:775–785.
21. D'Andrea AD, Lodish HF, Wong GG. Expression cloning of the murine erythropoietin receptor. Cell 1989;57:277–285.
22. Franchi A, Perucca-Lostanlen D, Pouyssegur J. Functional expression of a human Na^+/H^+ antiporter gene transfected into antiporter-deficient mouse L cells. Proc Natl Acad Sci USA 1986;83:9388–9392.
23. Pasqualini R, Ruoslahti E. Organ targeting in vivo using phage display peptide libraries. Nature 1996;380:364–366.
24. Sambrook J, Russell DW. Preparation of radiolabeled DNA and RNA probes. Molecular cloning. A Laboratory Manual, vol. 2. New York: Cold Spring Harbor Laboratory Press, 2001:9.4-9.75.
25. Zinn K, DiMaio D, Maniatis T. Identification of two distinct regulatory regions adjacent to the human beta-interferon gene. Cell 1983;34:865–879.
26. Myers RM, Larin Z, Maniatis T. Detection of single base substitutions by ribonuclease cleavage at mismatches in RNA:DNA duplexes. Science 1985;230:1242–1246.
27. Melton DA, Krieg PA, Rebagliati MR, Maniatis T, Zinn K, Green MR. Efficient in vitro synthesis of biologically active RNA and RNA hybridization probes from plasmids containing a bacteriophage SP6 promoter. Nucleic Acids Res 1984;12:7035-56.
28. Calzone FJ, Britten RJ, Davidson EH. Mapping of gene transcripts by nuclease protection assays and cDNA primer extension. Methods Enzymol 1987;152:611–632.
29. Temizer D, Huang PL, Ng S-C, Quertermous T. Molecular cloning strategies. In: Fozzard HA, et al., eds. The Heart and Cardiovascular System. New York: Raven Press, 1992: 561–579.
30. Lodish H, Berk A, Zipursky SL, Matsudaira P, Baltimore D, Darnell J. Recombinant DNA and genomics. Molecular Cell Biology. New York: W. H. Freeman, 1999:207–253.
31. Sambrook J, Russell DW. In vitro amplification of DNA by polymerase chain reaction. Molecular cloning. A Laboratory Manual, vol. 2. New York: Cold Spring Harbor Laboratory Press, 2001:8.18–8.106.
32. Murphy LD, Herzog CE, Rudick JB, Fojo AT, Bates SE. Use of the polymerase chain reaction in the quantitation of mdr-1 gene expression. Biochemistry 1990;29:10351–10356.

33. Siebert PD, Larrick JW. Competitive PCR. Nature 1992; 359:557–558.

34. Gilliland G, Perrin S, Blanchard K, Bunn HF. Analysis of cytokine mRNA and DNA: detection and quantitation by competitive polymerase chain reaction. Proc Natl Acad Sci USA 1990;87:2725–2729.

35. Tsai SJ, Wiltbank MC. Quantification of mRNA using competitive RT-PCR with standard-curve methodology. Biotechniques 1996;21:862–866.

36. Heid CA, Stevens J, Livak KJ, Williams PM. Real time quantitative PCR. Genome Res 1996;6:986–994.

37. Holland PM, Abramson RD, Watson R, Gelfand DH. Detection of specific polymerase chain reaction product by utilizing the 5–3′ exonuclease activity of Thermus aquaticus DNA polymerase. Proc Natl Acad Sci USA 1991;88:7276–7280.

38. Tyagi S, Bratu DP, Kramer FR. Multicolor molecular beacons for allele discrimination. Nat Biotechnol 1998;16:49–53.

39. Wilkinson DG. The theory and practice of in situ hybridization. In: Wilkinson DG, ed. in situ Hybridization. A Practical Approach. New York: Oxford University Press, 1998.

40. Hidai C, Zupancic T, Penta K, et al. Cloning and characterization of developmental endothelial locus-1: an embryonic endothelial cell protein that binds the alphavbeta3 integrin receptor. Genes Dev 1998;12:21–33.

41. Kadonaga JT, Tjian R. Affinity purification of sequence-specific DNA binding proteins. Proc Natl Acad Sci USA 1986;83:5889–5893.

42. Schlaeger TM, Qin Y, Fujiwara Y, Magram J, Sato TN. Vascular endothelial cell lineage-specific promoter in transgenic mice. Development 1995;121:1089–1098.

43. Fadel BM, Boutet SC, Quertermous T. Octamer-dependent in vivo expression of the endothelial cell-specific TIE2 gene. J Biol Chem 1999;274:20376–20383.

44. Lander ES, Linton LM, Birren B, et al. Initial sequencing and analysis of the human genome. Nature 2001;409:860–921.

45. Lockhart DJ, Winzeler EA. Genomics, gene expression and DNA arrays. Nature 2000;405:827–836.

46. Schena M, Shalon D, Davis RW, Brown PO. Quantitative monitoring of gene expression patterns with a complementary DNA microarray. Science 1995;270:467–470.

47. Schulze A, Downward J. Navigating gene expression using microarrays—a technology review. Nat Cell Biol 2001; 3:E190–E195.

48. Alizadeh AA, Eisen MB, Davis RE, et al. Distinct types of diffuse large B-cell lymphoma identified by gene expression profiling. Nature 2000;403:503–511.

49. Perou CM, Sorlie T, Eisen MB, et al. Molecular portraits of human breast tumours. Nature 2000;406:747–752.

50. Sorlie T, Perou CM, Tibshirani R, et al. Gene expression patterns of breast carcinomas distinguish tumor subclasses with clinical implications. Proc Natl Acad Sci USA 2001;98:10869–10874.

51. van 't Veer LJ, Dai H, van de Vijver MJ, et al. Gene expression profiling predicts clinical outcome of breast cancer. Nature 2002;415:530–536.

52. Spellman PT, Sherlock G, Zhang MQ, et al. Comprehensive identification of cell cycle-regulated genes of the yeast Saccharomyces cerevisiae by microarray hybridization. Mol Biol Cell 1998;9:3273–3297.

53. Haley KJ, Lilly CM, Yang JH, et al. Overexpression of eotaxin and the CCR3 receptor in human atherosclerosis: using genomic technology to identify a potential novel pathway of vascular inflammation. Circulation 2000;102:2185–2189.

54. Stanton LW, Garrard LJ, Damm D, et al. Altered patterns of gene expression in response to myocardial infarction. Circ Res 2000;86:939–945.

55. Yang J, Moravec CS, Sussman MA, et al. Decreased SLIM1 expression and increased gelsolin expression in failing human hearts measured by high-density oligonucleotide arrays. Circulation 2000;102:3046–3052.

56. McCormick SM, Eskin SG, McIntire LV, et al. DNA microarray reveals changes in gene expression of shear stressed human umbilical vein endothelial cells. Proc Natl Acad Sci USA 2001;98:8955–8960.

57. Hossain MA, Bouton CM, Pevsner J, Laterra J. Induction of vascular endothelial growth factor in human astrocytes by lead. Involvement of a protein kinase C/activator protein-1 complex-dependent and hypoxia-inducible factor 1-independent signaling pathway. J Biol Chem 2000;275:27874–27882.

58. Zhang S, Day IN, Ye S. Microarray analysis of nicotine-induced changes in gene expression in endothelial cells. Physiol Genomics 2001;5:187–92.

59. Chen BP, Li YS, Zhao Y, et al. DNA microarray analysis of gene expression in endothelial cells in response to 24-h shear stress. Physiol Genomics 2001;7:55–63.

60. Adams LD, Geary RL, McManus B, Schwartz SM. A comparison of aorta and vena cava medial message expression by cDNA array analysis identifies a set of 68 consistently differentially expressed genes, all in aortic media. Circ Res 2000;87:623–631.

61. Dunn MJ. Studying heart disease using the proteomic approach. Drug Discov Today 2000;5:76–84.

62. Wilkins MR, Sanchez JC, Williams KL, Hochstrasser DF. Current challenges and future applications for protein maps and post-translational vector maps in proteome projects. Electrophoresis 1996;17:830–838.

63. Arrell DK, Neverova I, Van Eyk JE. Cardiovascular proteomics: evolution and potential. Circ Res 2001;88:763–773.

64. Klose J, Kobalz U. Two-dimensional electrophoresis of proteins: an updated protocol and implications for a functional analysis of the genome. Electrophoresis 1995;16:1034–1059.

65. Banks RE, Dunn MJ, Hochstrasser DF, et al. Proteomics: new perspectives, new biomedical opportunities. Lancet 2000; 356:1749–1756.

66. Ostergaard M, Rasmussen HH, Nielsen HV, et al. Proteome profiling of bladder squamous cell carcinomas: identification of markers that define their degree of differentiation. Cancer Res 1997;57:4111–4117.

67. Pleissner KP, Soding P, Sander S, et al. Dilated cardiomyopathy-associated proteins and their presentation in a WWW-accessible two-dimensional gel protein database. Electrophoresis 1997; 18:802–808.

68. Syvanen AC. Accessing genetic variation: genotyping single nucleotide polymorphisms. Nat Rev Genet 2001;2:930–942.

69. Risch NJ. Searching for genetic determinants in the new millennium. Nature 2000;405:847–856.

70. Roses AD. Pharmacogenetics and the practice of medicine. Nature 2000;405:857–865.

71. Kwok PY. Methods for genotyping single nucleotide polymorphisms. Annu Rev Genomics Hum Genet 2001;2:235–258.

72. Eriksson P, Kallin B, van 't Hooft FM, Bavenholm P, Hamsten A. Allele-specific increase in basal transcription of the plasminogen-activator inhibitor 1 gene is associated with myocardial infarction. Proc Natl Acad Sci USA 1995; 92:1851–1855.

73. Margaglione M, Cappucci G, Colaizzo D, et al. The PAI-1 gene locus 4G/5G polymorphism is associated with a family history of coronary artery disease. Arterioscler Thromb Vasc Biol 1998;18:152–156.

74. Moatti D, Faure S, Fumeron F, et al. Polymorphism in the fractalkine receptor CX3CR1 as a genetic risk factor for coronary artery disease. Blood 2001;97:1925–1928.

75. Ranade K, Wu KD, Risch N, et al. Genetic variation in aldosterone synthase predicts plasma glucose levels. Proc Natl Acad Sci USA 2001;98:13219–13224.

76. Ramirez-Solis R, Davis AC, Bradley A. Gene targeting in embryonic stem cells. In: Wassarman PM, DePamphilis ML, eds. Guide to Techniques in Mouse Development. San Diego: Academic Press, 1993:855–878.

77. Fong G, Rossant J, Breitman ML. Role of the Flt-1 receptor tyrosine kinase in regulating the assembly of vascular endothelium. Nature 1995;376:66–70.

78. Sato TN, Tozawa Y, Deutsch U, et al. Distinct roles of the receptor tyrosine kinases Tie-1 and Tie-2 in blood vessel formation. Nature 1995;376:70–74.

79. Shalaby F, Rossant J, Yamaguchi TP, et al. Failure of blood-island formation and vasculogenesis in Flk-1-deficient mice. Nature 1995;376:62–66.

80. Ferrara N, Carver-Moore K, Chen H, et al. Heterozygous embryonic lethality induced by targeted inactivation of the VEGF gene. Nature 1996;380:439–442.

81. Carmeliet C, Ferreira V, Brier G, et al. Abnormal blood vessel development and lethality in embryos lacking a single VEGF allele. Nature 1996;380:435–439.

82. Hynes RO. Targeted mutations in cell adhesion genes: what have we learned from them? Dev Biol 1996;180:402–412.

83. Carmeliet P, Lampugnani MG, Moons L, et al. Targeted deficiency or cytosolic truncation of the VE-cadherin gene in mice impairs VEGF-mediated endothelial survival and angiogenesis. Cell 1999;98:147–157.

84. Bischoff J. Cell adhesion and angiogenesis. J Clin Invest 1997;100:S37–S39.

85. te Riele H, Maandag ER, Clarke A, Hooper M, Berns A. Consecutive inactivation of both alleles of the pim-1 proto-oncogene by homologous recombination in embryonic stem cells. Nature 1990;348:649–651.

86. Klinghoffer RA, Sachsenmaier C, Cooper JA, Soriano P. Src family kinases are required for integrin but not PDGFR signal transduction. Embo J 1999;18:2459–2471.

87. Sauer B, Henderson N. Site-specific DNA recombination in mammalian cells by the Cre recombinase of bacteriophage P1. Proc Natl Acad Sci USA 1988;85:5166–5170.

88. Sauer B, Henderson N. Cre-stimulated recombination at loxP-containing DNA sequences placed into the mammalian genome. Nucleic Acids Res 1989;17:147–161.

89. Odell J, Caimi P, Sauer B, Russell S. Site-directed recombination in the genome of transgenic tobacco. Mol Gen Genet 1990;223:369–378.

90. Sauer B, Henderson N. Targeted insertion of exogenous DNA into the eukaryotic genome by the Cre recombinase. New Biol 1990;2:441–449.

91. Lewandoski M, Martin GR. Cre-mediated chromosome loss in mice. Nat Genet 1997;17:223–225.

92. Lewandoski M, Wassarman KM, Martin GR. Zp3-cre, a transgenic mouse line for the activation or inactivation of loxP-flanked target genes specifically in the female germ line. Curr Biol 1997;7:148–151.

93. Brocard J, Warot X, Wendling O, et al. Spatio-temporally controlled site-specific somatic mutagenesis in the mouse. Proc Natl Acad Sci USA 1997;94:14559–14563.

94. Jiang X, Rowitch DH, Soriano P, McMahon AP, Sucov HM. Fate of the mammalian cardiac neural crest. Development 2000;127:1607–1616.

95. Isermann B, Hendrickson SB, Zogg M, et al. Endothelium-specific loss of murine thrombomodulin disrupts the protein C anticoagulant pathway and causes juvenile-onset thrombosis. J Clin Invest 2001;108:537–546.

96. Rijnkels M, Rosen JM. Adenovirus-Cre-mediated recombination in mammary epithelial early progenitor cells. J Cell Sci 2001;114:3147–3153.

97. Sohal DS, Nghiem M, Crackower MA, et al. Temporally regulated and tissue-specific gene manipulations in the adult and embryonic heart using a tamoxifen-inducible Cre protein. Circ Res 2001;89:20–25.

98. St-Onge L, Furth PA, Gruss P. Temporal control of the Cre recombinase in transgenic mice by a tetracycline responsive promoter. Nucleic Acids Res 1996;24:3875–3877.

99. Suri C, McClain J, Thurston G, et al. Increased vascularization in mice overexpressing angiopoietin-1. Science 1998;282:468–471.

100. Levak-Frank S, Hofmann W, Weinstock PH, et al. Induced mutant mouse lines that express lipoprotein lipase in cardiac muscle, but not in skeletal muscle and adipose tissue, have normal plasma triglyceride and high-density lipoprotein-cholesterol levels. Proc Natl Acad Sci USA 1999;96:3165–3170.

101. Levak-Frank S, Weinstock PH, Hayek T, et al. Induced mutant mice expressing lipoprotein lipase exclusively in muscle have subnormal triglycerides yet reduced high density lipoprotein cholesterol levels in plasma. J Biol Chem 1997;272:17182–17190.

102. Boutet SC, Quertermous T, Fadel BM. Identification of an octamer element required for in vivo expression of the TIE1 gene in endothelial cells. Biochem J 2001;360:23–29.

103. Pennacchio LA, Olivier M, Hubacek JA, et al. An apolipoprotein influencing triglycerides in humans and mice revealed by comparative sequencing. Science 2001;294:169–173.

104. Guillot PV, Liu L, Kuivenhoven JA, Guan J, Rosenberg RD, Aird WC. Targeting of human eNOS promoter to the Hprt locus of mice leads to tissue-restricted transgene expression. Physiol Genomics 2000;2:77–83.

105. Copeland NG, Jenkins NA, Court DL. Recombineering: a powerful new tool for mouse functional genomics. Nat Rev Genet 2001;2:769–779.

106. St-Onge L, Furth PA, Gruss P. Temporal control of the Cre recombinase in transgenic mice by a tetracycline responsive promoter. Nucleic Acids Res 1996;24:3875–3877.

107. Freundlieb S, Baron U, Bonin AL, Gossen M, Bujard H. Use of tetracycline-controlled gene expression systems to study mammalian cell cycle. Methods Enzymol 1997;283:159–173.

108. Ishibashi S, Brown MS, Goldstein JL, Gerard RD, Hammer RE, Herz J. Hypercholesterolemia in low density lipoprotein receptor knockout mice and its reversal by adenovirus-mediated gene delivery. J Clin Invest 1993;92:883–893.

109. Ishida BY, Blanche PJ, Nichols AV, Yashar M, Paigen B. Effects of atherogenic diet consumption on lipoproteins in mouse strains C57BL/6 and C3H. J Lipid Res 1991;32:559–568.

110. Plump AS, Smith JD, Hayek T, et al. Severe hypercholesterolemia and atherosclerosis in apolipoprotein E-deficient mice created by homologous recombination in ES cells. Cell 1992;71:343–353.

111. Lusis AJ. Atherosclerosis. Nature 2000;407:233–241.
112. Glass CK, Witztum JL. Atherosclerosis. The road ahead. Cell 2001;104:503–516.
113. Breslow JL. Mouse models of atherosclerosis. Science 1996;272:685–688.
114. Paigen B, Morrow A, Brandon C, Mitchell D, Holmes P. Variation in susceptibility to atherosclerosis among inbred strains of mice. Atherosclerosis 1985;57:65–73.
115. Paigen B, Ishida BY, Verstuyft J, Winters RB, Albee D. Atherosclerosis susceptibility differences among progenitors of recombinant inbred strains of mice. Arteriosclerosis 1990;10:316–323.
116. Nishina PM, Wang J, Toyofuku W, Kuypers FA, Ishida BY, Paigen B. Atherosclerosis and plasma and liver lipids in nine inbred strains of mice. Lipids 1993;28:599–605.
117. Paigen B, Plump AS, Rubin EM. The mouse as a model for human cardiovascular disease and hyperlipidemia. Curr Opin Lipidol 1994;5:258–264.
118. Paigen B, Albee D, Holmes PA, Mitchell D. Genetic analysis of murine strains C57BL/6J and C3H/HeJ to confirm the map position of Ath-1, a gene determining atherosclerosis susceptibility. Biochem Genet 1987;25:501–511.
119. Paigen B, Mitchell D, Reue K, Morrow A, Lusis AJ, LeBoeuf RC. Ath-1, a gene determining atherosclerosis susceptibility and high density lipoprotein levels in mice. Proc Natl Acad Sci USA 1987;84:3763–3767.
120. Mehrabian M, Qiao JH, Hyman R, Ruddle D, Laughton C, Lusis AJ. Influence of the apoA-II gene locus on HDL levels and fatty streak development in mice. Arterioscler Thromb 1993;13:1–10.
121. LeBoeuf RC, Doolittle MH, Montcalm A, Martin DC, Reue K, Lusis AJ. Phenotypic characterization of the Ath-1 gene controlling high density lipoprotein levels and susceptibility to atherosclerosis. J Lipid Res 1990;31:91–101.
122. Paigen B, Morrow A, Holmes PA, Mitchell D, Williams RA. Quantitative assessment of atherosclerotic lesions in mice. Atherosclerosis 1987;68:231–240.
123. Plump A. Atherosclerosis and the mouse: a decade of experience. Ann Med 1997;29:193–198.
124. Shi W, Haberland ME, Jien ML, Shih DM, Lusis AJ. Endothelial responses to oxidized lipoproteins determine genetic susceptibility to atherosclerosis in mice. Circulation 2000;102:75–81.
125. Shi W, Wang NJ, Shih DM, Sun VZ, Wang X, Lusis AJ. Determinants of atherosclerosis susceptibility in the C3H and C57BL/6 mouse model: evidence for involvement of endothelial cells but not blood cells or cholesterol metabolism. Circ Res 2000;86:1078–1084.
126. Grimsditch DC, Penfold S, Latcham J, Vidgeon-Hart M, Groot PH, Benson GM. C3H apoE(−/−) mice have less atherosclerosis than C57BL apoE(−/−) mice despite having a more atherogenic serum lipid profile. Atherosclerosis 2000;151:389–397.
127. Van Lenten BJ, Prieve J, Navab M, Hama S, Lusis AJ, Fogelman AM. Lipid-induced changes in intracellular iron homeostasis in vitro and in vivo. J Clin Invest 1995;95:2104–2110.
128. Zhang SH, Reddick RL, Piedrahita JA, Maeda N. Spontaneous hypercholesterolemia and arterial lesions in mice lacking apolipoprotein E. Science 1992;258:468–471.
129. Napoli C, Palinski W, Di Minno G, D'Armiento FP. Determination of atherogenesis in apolipoprotein E-knockout mice. Nutr Metab Cardiovasc Dis 2000;10:209–215.
130. Cyrus T, Witztum JL, Rader DJ, et al. Disruption of the 12/15-lipoxygenase gene diminishes atherosclerosis in apo E-deficient mice. J Clin Invest 1999;103:1597–1604.
131. Kuhlencordt PJ, Chen J, Han F, Astern J, Huang PL. Genetic deficiency of inducible nitric oxide synthase reduces atherosclerosis and lowers plasma lipid peroxides in apolipoprotein E-knockout mice. Circulation 2001;103:3099–3104.
132. Shih DM, Gu L, Xia YR, et al. Mice lacking serum paraoxonase are susceptible to organophosphate toxicity and atherosclerosis. Nature 1998;394:284–287.
133. Shih DM, Xia YR, Wang XP, et al. Combined serum paraoxonase knockout/apolipoprotein E knockout mice exhibit increased lipoprotein oxidation and atherosclerosis. J Biol Chem 2000;275:17527–17535.
134. Costa LG, Li WF, Richter RJ, Shih DM, Lusis A, Furlong CE. The role of paraoxonase (PON1) in the detoxication of organophosphates and its human polymorphism. Chem Biol Interact 1999;119–120,429–438.
135. Knowles JW, Reddick RL, Jennette JC, Shesely EG, Smithies O, Maeda N. Enhanced atherosclerosis and kidney dysfunction in eNOS(−/−)Apoe(−/−) mice are ameliorated by enalapril treatment. J Clin Invest 2000;105:451–458.
136. Kuhlencordt PJ, Gyurko R, Han F, et al. Accelerated atherosclerosis, aortic aneurysm formation, and ischemic heart disease in apolipoprotein E/endothelial nitric oxide synthase double-knockout mice. Circulation 2001;104:448–454.
137. Shesely EG, Maeda N, Kim HS, et al. Elevated blood pressures in mice lacking endothelial nitric oxide synthase. Proc Natl Acad Sci USA 1996;93:13176–13181.
138. Abe H, Yamada N, Kamata K, et al. Hypertension, hypertriglyceridemia, and impaired endothelium-dependent vascular relaxation in mice lacking insulin receptor substrate-1. J Clin Invest 1998;101:1784–1788.
139. Schreyer SA, Wilson DL, LeBoeuf RC. C57BL/6 mice fed high fat diets as models for diabetes-accelerated atherosclerosis. Atherosclerosis 1998;136:17–24.
140. Smith HO, Anderson PS, Kuo DY, et al. The role of colony-stimulating factor 1 and its receptor in the etiopathogenesis of endometrial adenocarcinoma. Clin Cancer Res 1995;1:313–325.
141. Qiao JH, Tripathi J, Mishra NK, et al. Role of macrophage colony-stimulating factor in atherosclerosis: studies of osteopetrotic mice. Am J Pathol 1997;150:1687–1699.
142. Collins RG, Velji R, Guevara NV, Hicks MJ, Chan L, Beaudet AL. P-Selectin or intercellular adhesion molecule (ICAM)-1 deficiency substantially protects against atherosclerosis in apolipoprotein E-deficient mice. J Exp Med 2000;191:189–194.
143. Bourdillon MC, Poston RN, Covacho C, Chignier E, Bricca G, McGregor JL. ICAM-1 deficiency reduces atherosclerotic lesions in double-knockout mice (ApoE(−/−)/ICAM-1(−/−)) fed a fat or a chow diet. Arterioscler Thromb Vasc Biol 2000;20:2630–2635.
144. Dong ZM, Chapman SM, Brown AA, Frenette PS, Hynes RO, Wagner DD. The combined role of P- and E-selectins in atherosclerosis. J Clin Invest 1998;102:145–152.
145. Gosling J, Slaymaker S, Gu L, et al. MCP-1 deficiency reduces susceptibility to atherosclerosis in mice that overexpress human apolipoprotein B. J Clin Invest 1999;103:773–778.
146. Gu L, Okada Y, Clinton SK, et al. Absence of monocyte chemoattractant protein-1 reduces atherosclerosis in low density lipoprotein receptor-deficient mice. Mol Cell 1998;2:275–281.
147. Boring L, Gosling J, Cleary M, Charo IF. Decreased lesion formation in CCR2−/− mice reveals a role for chemokines in the initiation of atherosclerosis. Nature 1998;394:894–897.

148. Boisvert WA, Santiago R, Curtiss LK, Terkeltaub RA. A leukocyte homologue of the IL-8 receptor CXCR-2 mediates the accumulation of macrophages in atherosclerotic lesions of LDL receptor-deficient mice. J Clin Invest 1998;101:353–363.

149. Suzuki H, Kurihara Y, Takeya M, et al. A role for macrophage scavenger receptors in atherosclerosis and susceptibility to infection. Nature 1997;386:292–296.

150. Febbraio M, Podrez EA, Smith JD, et al. Targeted disruption of the class B scavenger receptor CD36 protects against atherosclerotic lesion development in mice. J Clin Invest 2000;105: 1049–1056.

151. Voyiaziakis E, Goldberg IJ, Plump AS, Rubin EM, Breslow JL, Huang LS. ApoA-I deficiency causes both hypertriglyceridemia and increased atherosclerosis in human apoB transgenic mice. J Lipid Res 1998;39:313–321.

152. Yagyu H, Kitamine T, Osuga J, et al. Absence of ACAT-1 attenuates atherosclerosis but causes dry eye and cutaneous xanthomatosis in mice with congenital hyperlipidemia. J Biol Chem 2000;275:21324–21330.

153. Buhman KF, Accad M, Farese RV. Mammalian acyl-CoA:cholesterol acyltransferases. Biochim Biophys Acta 2000;1529:142–154.

154. Accad M, Smith SJ, Newland DL, et al. Massive xanthomatosis and altered composition of atherosclerotic lesions in hyperlipidemic mice lacking acyl CoA:cholesterol acyltransferase 1. J Clin Invest 2000;105:711–719.

155. Rust S, Rosier M, Funke H, et al. Tangier disease is caused by mutations in the gene encoding ATP-binding cassette transporter 1. Nat Genet 1999;22:352–355.

156. Drobnik W, Lindenthal B, Lieser B, et al. ATP-binding cassette transporter A1 (ABCA1) affects total body sterol metabolism. Gastroenterology 2001;120:1203–1211.

157. Brooks-Wilson A, Marcil M, Clee SM, et al. Mutations in ABC1 in Tangier disease and familial high-density lipoprotein deficiency. Nat Genet 1999;22:336–345.

158. Bodzioch M, Orso E, Klucken J, et al. The gene encoding ATP-binding cassette transporter 1 is mutated in Tangier disease. Nat Genet 1999;22:347–351.

159. Lawn RM, Wade DP, Garvin MR, et al. The Tangier disease gene product ABC1 controls the cellular apolipoprotein-mediated lipid removal pathway. J Clin Invest 1999;104:R25–R31.

160. Marcil M, Brooks-Wilson A, Clee SM, et al. Mutations in the ABC1 gene in familial HDL deficiency with defective cholesterol efflux. Lancet 1999;354:1341–1346.

161. Ng DS, Francone OL, Forte TM, Zhang J, Haghpassand M, Rubin EM. Disruption of the murine lecithin:cholesterol acyltransferase gene causes impairment of adrenal lipid delivery and up-regulation of scavenger receptor class B type I. J Biol Chem 1997;272:15777–15781.

162. Lambert G, Sakai N, Vaisman BL, et al. Analysis of glomerulosclerosis and atherosclerosis in lecithin cholesterol acyltransferase-deficient mice. J Biol Chem 2001;276:15090–15098.

163. Plump AS, Masucci-Magoulas L, Bruce C, Bisgaier CL, Breslow JL, Tall AR. Increased atherosclerosis in ApoE and LDL receptor gene knock-out mice as a result of human cholesteryl ester transfer protein transgene expression. Arterioscler Thromb Vasc Biol 1999;19:1105–1110.

164. Marotti KR, Castle CK, Boyle TP, Lin AH, Murray RW, Melchior GW. Severe atherosclerosis in transgenic mice expressing simian cholesteryl ester transfer protein. Nature 1993; 364:73–75.

165. Huszar D, Varban ML, Rinninger F, et al. Increased LDL cholesterol and atherosclerosis in LDL receptor-deficient mice with attenuated expression of scavenger receptor B1. Arterioscler Thromb Vasc Biol 2000;20:1068–1073.

166. Kozarsky KF, Donahee MH, Glick JM, Krieger M, Rader DJ. Gene transfer and hepatic overexpression of the HDL receptor SR-BI reduces atherosclerosis in the cholesterol-fed LDL receptor-deficient mouse. Arterioscler Thromb Vasc Biol 2000;20:721–727.

167. Niu XL, Yang X, Hoshiai K, et al. Inducible nitric oxide synthase deficiency does not affect the susceptibility of mice to atherosclerosis but increases collagen content in lesions. Circulation 2001;103:1115–1120.

168. Harats D, Shaish A, George J, et al. Overexpression of 15-lipoxygenase in vascular endothelium accelerates early atherosclerosis in LDL receptor-deficient mice. Arterioscler Thromb Vasc Biol 2000;20:2100–2105.

169. Warden CH, Hedrick CC, Qiao JH, Castellani LW, Lusis AJ. Atherosclerosis in transgenic mice overexpressing apolipoprotein A-II. Science 1993;261:469–472.

170. Veniant MM, Pierotti V, Newland D, et al. Susceptibility to atherosclerosis in mice expressing exclusively apolipoprotein B48 or apolipoprotein B100. J Clin Invest 1997;100:180–188.

171. Farese RV, Jr., Veniant MM, Cham CM, et al. Phenotypic analysis of mice expressing exclusively apolipoprotein B48 or apolipoprotein B100. Proc Natl Acad Sci USA 1996; 93:6393–6398.

172. Shachter NS, Ebara T, Ramakrishnan R, et al. Combined hyperlipidemia in transgenic mice overexpressing human apolipoprotein Cl. J Clin Invest 1996;98:846–855.

173. Lawn RM, Wade DP, Hammer RE, Chiesa G, Verstuyft JG, Rubin EM. Atherogenesis in transgenic mice expressing human apolipoprotein(a). Nature 1992;360:670–672.

174. Dawson TC, Kuziel WA, Osahar TA, Maeda N. Absence of CC chemokine receptor-2 reduces atherosclerosis in apolipoprotein E-deficient mice. Atherosclerosis 1999;143:205–211.

175. Lutgens E, Gorelik L, Daemen MJ, et al. Requirement for CD154 in the progression of atherosclerosis. Nat Med 1999;5:1313–1316.

176. Aiello RJ, Bourassa PA, Lindsey S, et al. Monocyte chemoattractant protein-1 accelerates atherosclerosis in apolipoprotein E-deficient mice. Arterioscler Thromb Vasc Biol 1999;19: 1518–1525.

177. Tordjman K, Bernal-Mizrachi C, Zemany L, et al. PPARalpha deficiency reduces insulin resistance and atherosclerosis in apoE-null mice. J Clin Invest 2001;107:1025–1034.

178. Christiansen-Weber TA, Voland JR, Wu Y, et al. Functional loss of ABCA1 in mice causes severe placental malformation, aberrant lipid distribution, and kidney glomerulonephritis as well as high-density lipoprotein cholesterol deficiency. Am J Pathol 2000;157:1017–1029.

179. Singaraja RR, Bocher V, James ER, et al. Human ABCA1 BAC transgenic mice show increased high density lipoprotein cholesterol and ApoAI-dependent efflux stimulated by an internal promoter containing liver X receptor response elements in intron 1. J Biol Chem 2001;276:33969–33979.

180. Benoit P, Emmanuel F, Caillaud JM, et al. Somatic gene transfer of human ApoA-I inhibits atherosclerosis progression in mouse models. Circulation 1999;99:105–110.

181. Plump AS, Scott CJ, Breslow JL. Human apolipoprotein A-I gene expression increases high density lipoprotein and suppresses atherosclerosis in the apolipoprotein E-deficient mouse. Proc Natl Acad Sci USA 1994;91:9607–9611.

182. Tangirala RK, Tsukamoto K, Chun SH, Usher D, Pure E, Rader DJ. Regression of atherosclerosis induced by liver-directed gene transfer of apolipoprotein A-I in mice. Circulation 1999; 100:1816–1822.

183. Ishibashi S, Herz J, Maeda N, Goldstein JL, Brown MS. The two-receptor model of lipoprotein clearance: tests of the hypothesis in "knockout" mice lacking the low density lipoprotein receptor, apolipoprotein E, or both proteins. Proc Natl Acad Sci USA 1994;91:4431–4435.

184. Homanics GE, de Silva HV, Osada J, et al. Mild dyslipidemia in mice following targeted inactivation of the hepatic lipase gene. J Biol Chem 1995;270:2974–2980.

185. Weinstock PH, Bisgaier CL, Aalto-Setala K, et al. Severe hypertriglyceridemia, reduced high density lipoprotein, and neonatal death in lipoprotein lipase knockout mice. Mild hypertriglyceridemia with impaired very low density lipoprotein clearance in heterozygotes. J Clin Invest 1995;96:2555–2568.

186. Durrington PN, Mackness B, Mackness MI. Paraoxonase and atherosclerosis. Arterioscler Thromb Vasc Biol 2001;21:473–480.

187. Mackness B, Davies GK, Turkie W, et al. Paraoxonase status in coronary heart disease: are activity and concentration more important than genotype? Arterioscler Thromb Vasc Biol 2001;21:1451–1457.

188. Chawla A, Boisvert WA, Lee CH, et al. A PPAR gamma-LXR-ABCA1 pathway in macrophages is involved in cholesterol efflux and atherogenesis. Mol Cell 2001;7:161–171.

189. Pinderski Oslund LJ, Hedrick CC, Olvera T, et al. Interleukin-10 blocks atherosclerotic events in vitro and in vivo. Arterioscler Thromb Vasc Biol 1999;19:2847–2853.

3

Genomics and Its Application to Cardiovascular Disease

Robert Roberts, MD

Contents

INTRODUCTION

Genomics refers to the study or science of genomes, which contain all of the DNA that codes for an organism. Knowing the human genome has implications for biology and mankind that are unparalleled, in part because having such an abundance of information regarding the inner workings of humans is unprecedented. Because a genomic sequence is a blueprint of the biological activities of an organism, determining what regulates a genome has implications that stimulate the imagination. For example, there are probably only 200–300 genes that provide susceptibility for the 20 diseases that account for 80% of all deaths globally, and most of these genes will be identified in the next 5 years. The genomes and genes of the organisms *Haemophilus influenzae* and *Treponema pallidum* have been identified *(1)*. These genes and their end products provide novel targets for the development of antibiotics and vaccines. The cloning of growth factors that selec-tively modulate cardiac myocyte growth or inhibit fibrosis is to be expected.

In the 1940s, it was established that DNA—not proteins—passes on inherited characteristics. In humans, the genome consists of the DNA contained in the 23 pairs of chromosomes that are enclosed in the nucleus. Twenty-two of these chromosomes are paired with a homologous chromosome and are referred to as autosomes. The remaining two chromosomes are the sex chromosomes, of which females have two X chromosomes and males have an X and a Y chromosome. The X and Y chromosomes share only a small area of homology. Homologous chromosomes share the same set of genes, but because each set came from a different parent, there are minor differences between the DNA sequences. These differences may or may not alter gene function, although they are very important genetic markers and are frequently used for mapping and identifying genes.

Each chromosome is a single, long, linear molecule of DNA. The three-dimensional structure of DNA consists

From: *Contemporary Cardiology: Principles of Molecular Cardiology*
Edited by: M. S. Runge and C. Patterson © Humana Press Inc., Totowa, NJ

of two long helical strands coiled around a common axis, forming a double helix. Each strand of DNA is composed of four different monomers called nucleotides. The two strands of DNA are coiled antiparallel to each other and are held together by hydrogen bonds formed between the bases. A nucleotide consists of a phosphate group linked by a phosphodiester bond to a pentose (five-carbon sugar molecule) that in turn is linked to an organic base. In DNA, the pentose is deoxyribose; in RNA it is ribose. The number of organic bases found in DNA is limited to four: adenine (A), guanine (G), thymine (T), and cytosine (C). The same is true for RNA, except it contains uracil (U) instead of thymine. Thus, each chromosome is a macromolecule of repeat sequences of various combinations of the four bases—A, C, G, and T. DNA sequences are read from left to right, with the proximal sequence (left) referred to as the 5′ end and the distal sequence (right) as the 3′ end. The hydrogen bonds that hold the two strands of DNA together form between the organic bases in a precise and obligatory manner. Adenine can only pair with thymine, and it does so through two hydrogen bonds. Guanine can only pair with cytosine, and it does so through three hydrogen bonds. This complementary base pairing between the two strands contributes to the stability of the double helix and is also a unique feature of DNA. When DNA is denatured—for example, by increased temperature—the hydrogen bonds break and the helix separates into two single strands. Restoration of the lower temperature induces annealing, and the two DNA strands come together in the same precise order as prior to separation. Practically all DNA diagnostic tests capitalize upon DNA's ability to denature and reanneal.

STRUCTURE OF THE HUMAN GENOME

If joined head to tail, the 46 human chromosomes would span about 3 m. Yet the average cell only spans about 0.0015 cm, and the nucleus containing the chromosomes occupies less than 10% of the volume of the cell. The chromosomes, compacted to occupy very little space, are wound around proteins—primarily around histone proteins—in a specific structure that has important implications for gene regulation. The combination of DNA and protein is referred to as chromatin. The family of histones that comprise the bulk of chromatin are rich in lysine, a positively charged amino acid that binds to negatively charged phosphate groups in DNA. As viewed using an electron microscope, chromatin exhibits bead-like structures referred to as nucleosomes. Nucleosomes are about 30 nm in diameter and are the primary structural unit of chromatin. The DNA, wound around the surface of the protein core, makes slightly less than two turns for every 146 basepairs (bp) of DNA. DNA that is not undergoing transcription is more compact—and probably more tightly bound to histones—than DNA that is undergoing transcription. Acetylation and deacetylation of histone proteins is now recognized as fundamental to the regulation of gene expression (2). Histone acetyltransferases (HAT) acetylate the lysine groups on histones, which disrupts histone binding to DNA and results in relaxation of the chromatin and increased transcription. Histone deacetylases (HDAC) antagonize this action and repress transcription. There are 16 known HDACs in humans. Class II HDACs are known to repress transcription of myocyte enhancer factor (MEF-2), one of the pivotal transcription factors in myogenesis (3). When chromosomes are fully compacted, access of RNA polymerase and possibly other proteins required for transcription is blocked. Thus, chromatin compaction and decompaction determines whether a gene will be transcribed and expressed into its functional unit—the protein.

GENE STRUCTURE AND REGULATION

The total human genome has about 3 billion bp. The average chromosome has about 135 million bp. The longest chromosome (chromosome 1) has over 250 million bp, and the smallest chromosome (chromosome 21) has only 50 million. The hereditary characteristics of an individual are determined by the linear sequence of the four bases and are passed on by genes. A gene is a distinct unit of heredity whose transcript, or messenger RNA (mRNA), encodes a single polypeptide. Genes have a start and stop site, and they vary in size from 10,000 to 2 million bp. It is estimated that an average human gene is 20,000 bp long. Genes themselves do not participate in cellular function, but through their intermediary mRNA they code for a polypeptide with specific amino acids. The precise linear sequence of the amino acids in a polypeptide corresponds to the linearity of the codons, which are triplets of bases, in the gene. Each codon encodes a specific amino acid. It is estimated that the human genome has about 40,000 genes. Thus, genes represent only about 2% of human DNA (Table 1). About 20–30% of the DNA is transcribed into mRNA, but most of it is spliced out in the process of making mature mRNA that will exit the nucleus and serve as the polypeptide template. Those sequences that form mRNA for proteins

Table 1
Web Pages Related to Genome Searches

Find Exon in Genome

http://translate.google.com/translate?hl=en&sl=fr&u=http://gamay.univ-perp.fr./analyse_seq/
sim4&prev=/search%3Fq%3Dsim4%26hl%3Den%26dsafe%3Doff

Multi-Sequence Alignment

http://searchlauncher.bcm.tmc.edu/multi-align/multi-align.html

NCBI Sequence BLAST®

http://www.ncbi.nlm.nih.gov/BLAST/

NCBI Conserved Peptide Sequence Domain Search

http://www.ncbi.nlm.nih.gov/Structure/cdd/wrpsb.cgi

NCBI Pairwise Sequence Alignment

http://www.ncbi.nlm.nih.gov/blast/bl2seq/bl2.html

NCBI Human Genome Homepage, Including Unigene, SNP, LocusLink, Genome Search, etc.

http://www.ncbi.nlm.nih.gov/genome/guide/human/

NCBI Human Genome BLAST®

http://www.ncbi.nlm.nih.gov/genome/seq/page.cgi?F=HsBlast.html&&ORG=Hs

NCBI ORF Finder

http://www.ncbi.nlm.nih.gov/gorf/gorf.html

NCBI Human/Mouse Homology Map

http://www.ncbi.nlm.nih.gov/Homology

NCBI DART: Peptide Domain Architecture Retrieval Tool

http://www.ncbi.nlm.nih.gov/Structure/lexington/lexington.cgi?cmd=rps

or for transfer or ribosomal RNA are referred to as exons (exiting the nucleus), while the intervening sequences are referred to as introns (remain in the nucleus).

Because genes occupy such a small percentage of the whole genome, identifying them can be an extremely difficult and tedious task. While genes do have start and stop sites, these sites cannot be easily discerned from other genomic sequence. The start site of a gene does not have a specific universal sequence; instead, it has promoter elements proximal to its 5′ end to which transcription initiation factors bind. Promoters are proteins that increase transcription and are referred to as transcription factors or DNA binding proteins. Proteins that enhance or facilitate transcription are referred to as enhancers, and proteins which repress transcription are silencers (Fig. 1). The 3′ end of a gene has a sequence that is the signal for polyadenylation. Thus, a gene has interspersed coding and noncoding sequences. Important regulatory sequences are at the 5′ and 3′ ends.

The function of most human DNA remains unknown. It is estimated that 30–50% of the human genome consists of repeat sequences (4,5). The most common form of repeat sequences are the long interspersed elements (LINES) that are 6000–7000 bp in length and comprise 15% of the human genome. These elements are considered to be mobile units that move around the human genome. Short interspersed elements (SINES) are also common repeat sequences, and they are about 300 bp long and account for about 10% of the human genome. SINES are fairly well conserved and occur in about 1 million sites in the human genome, and because they can be digested by the restriction enzyme Alu, they have been collectively referred to as the Alu family. Another 4% of human DNA consists of repeat sequences that have been transposed into the human genome by retroviruses. The larger repeat sequences such as LINES and SINES are often referred to as satellite repeat DNA, while the smaller clusters of short sequences are referred to as minisatellite DNA. There are many other small repeat sequences of di-, tri-, or tetranucleotides that occur throughout the human genome and are referred to as microsatellites. While the functions of these repeat sequences remain to be determined, the microsatellite repeats are used as DNA markers for chromosomal mapping of genes. The intervening sequences offer structural stability and may contribute to survival. Mutations

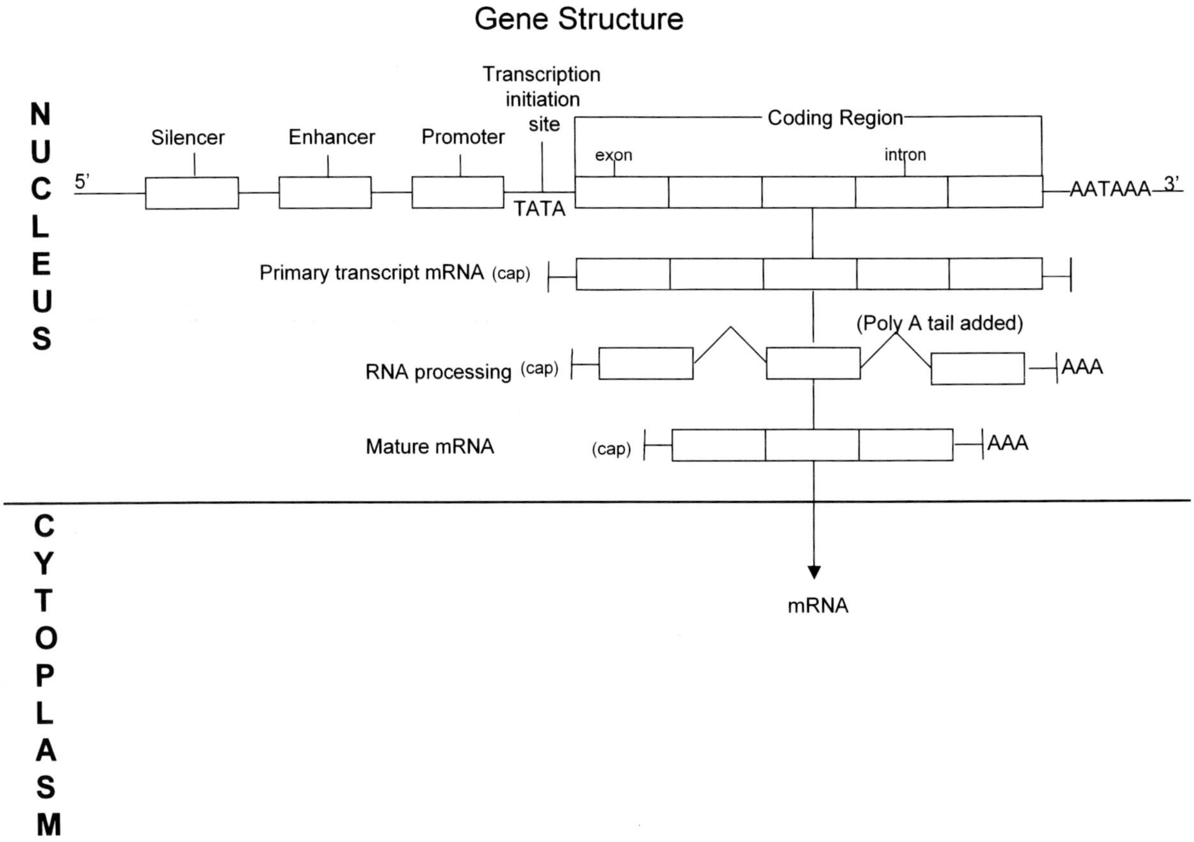

Gene Structure

Fig. 1. Gene structure. Transcription occurs in the nucleus, producing mRNA that is processed into mature mRNA and transported to the cytoplasm. In the cytoplasm, translation occurs. The mRNA codes for specific amino acids that will be linked together to form a polypeptide and ultimately a mature protein.

occur more commonly in introns, which account for more than 90% of DNA, but since introns are not expressed, the mutations unlikely affect protein function.

THE HUMAN GENOME PROJECT

The overall goal of the Human Genome Project (HGP) was to obtain a physical map of the human genome by determining the sequence of all the bases in each chromosome. It was the first international project devoted to understanding the biology of humans. When the project was initiated in 1990, it was expected to be completed in 2005. Currently there is a rough draft covering about 90% of the human sequence, and the draft is expected to be completed by the year 2003 *(6–9)*. The HGP has also developed genetic maps that mark the chromosomal locations of short DNA sequences. Chromosomal markers to map the human genome were available prior to the HGP, but they were limited in their distribution and provided minimal information. The new set of DNA markers was developed from repeat microsatellite sequences. These markers are repeats of di-, tri-, or tetranucleotides referred to as short tandem repeat polymorphisms (STRPs). Currently available genetic maps have thousands of markers that span the human genome at intervals of less than 1 million bp. These genetic markers made possible the widespread application of genetic linkage analysis. This is a computerized technique used to map the chromosomal location, or locus, of a defective gene of a familial disease and has led to the identification of several genes responsible for inherited cardiovascular disease.

The HGP also spurred the process of making a genetic map of markers that are expressed sequences. Expressed sequence tags (ESTs) are unique genomic sequences present only in genes *(10)*. ESTs are short sequences of 200 or 300 bp that can be used as a probe to identify the full genomic sequence of a gene. It may be surprising that one could obtain expressed sequences without knowing the gene. But because all genes are expressed through an mRNA intermediary, gene expression in a cell can be determined by extracting all of the mRNA from a cell. The mRNA sequence is then converted to cDNA by the enzyme reverse transcriptase, and the cDNA can in turn be amplified into multiple copies by using polymerase chain reaction (PCR). Hundreds of thousands of ESTs have been sequenced and entered into GenBank, an international database. These ESTs are cloned in vectors, some of which are bacterial, and multiple copies of the vectors can be obtained. Many ESTs have been mapped to their chromosomal location. The ultimate aim of the HGP is to have an EST accurately mark a chromosomal position at intervals less than 100,000 bp throughout the human genome. Identifying genetic markers and ESTs has markedly accelerated chromosomal mapping and identification of genes.

It must not be assumed that sequencing the human genome is the same as identifying human genes. Having human genomic sequences available will markedly facilitate gene identification, but it does not in itself provide a means to identify genes. Identifying most or all human genes remains a goal of the future. Given the genetic and physical maps of the human genome and the technology of high-throughput nucleotide sequencing, it is conceivable that all human genes will be identified in the next 5 years. Identifying the genes remains a major effort and will require closer collaboration of physicians and scientists. Improved identification of phenotypes due to Single-gene disorders is a major opportunity and a challenge for physicians. It will require increased awareness of genetics and improved clinical observations. The human genome will provide immense insight into how genes interact with environmental stimuli. There is a worldwide interest in the human genome, and those interests are scientifically, culturally, racially, medically, and commercially motivated. It is predicted that within 5–10 years personalized medicine will be a reality, and an individual's genetic profile will determine the types and doses of drugs that will be provided for treating diseases. The commercial spin-off and utilization of genomic technology is already evident from the large role biotechnology occupies in our everyday commercial world.

COMPUTERIZED DATABASES OF GENES, cDNAs, AND PROTEINS

Once the human genome project was underway, it became evident there was a need for a computerized network of gene databases (11). The computerized gene bank GenBank (accessible at http://www.ncbi.nlm.nih.gov) was established by the National Center for Biotechnology Information (NCBI). The NCBI is part of the International Nucleotide Sequence Database Collaboration, which also includes the European Molecular Biology Laboratory's

(EMBL's) nucleotide database from the European Bioinformatics Institute (EBI, Hinxton, United Kingdom) and the DNA Databank of Japan (DDBJ, Mishima, Japan). While data are entered at each center separately, the three centers communicate daily to make all of the data available to the world. GenBank is continually updated with human genome sequences and other relevant information. It is available at no cost to physicians and scientists throughout the world. It contains billions of DNA sequences from over 40,000 species and expands on a daily basis. GenBank, EMBL's database, and DDBJ are generated from direct submission of information from authors who do so either voluntarily or as part of the requirement for publication. Investigators are required to enter any newly discovered DNA, cDNA, or amino acid sequence into GenBank prior to publication. These databases contain nucleotide sequences of the human genome, other species' genomes, ESTs, and cDNAs. Known genes, ESTs, and available cDNA sequences are annotated to their approximate chromosomal region within the genome. The amino acid sequence of proteins and their known function are also included. These databases include programs for searching DNA sequences to identifying known and unknown genes, and similar programs are available to search for known cDNA and protein sequences. There are many commercial databases available—some contain both DNA and protein sequence information, while others are dedicated to either genomic, cDNA, or amino acid sequences. GenBank and its two partners, United Kingdom and Japan, provide sequence information obtained from investigators and are regarded as primary databases. These original data may be organized and modified to the interest of any commercial enterprise or investigator. Such derived databases are usually referred to as secondary databases. There are databases that are dedicated to the genes of a particular organism, organ, or functioning cellular network. Table 1 lists web sites of gene databases. Using these databases is a requisite for research in human molecular genetics and biology.

BIOINFORMATICS—PREDICTING GENES FROM GENOMIC SEQUENCES

The use of large databases with various computerized search capabilities has blossomed into a new science referred to as bioinformatics (11). Baxevanis and Ouellette (11) categorized gene-finding strategies into three categories. These include mapping and identifying genes, predicting genes from genomic sequences, and determining gene function. Content-based methods analyze a sequence for particular codons and repeats that are known to occur frequently throughout the genomes of several different organisms, including humans. Site-based methods concentrate on finding specific sequences, patterns, or consensus regions, and the methods often involve searching for start and stop codons and polyA tracts. The comparative method searches for regions of homology between the query sequence and known protein sequences. Searching for an unknown gene in a known human genomic sequence seems simple. However, there are no direct methods for finding genes, because there are no landmarks for the beginnings or endings of them. This may help to understand the high incidence of false positive and false negative results of some search programs. In searching for a gene, one initially identifies open reading frames (ORFs), which are long stretches of several thousand bp without a stop codon, with the hope of finding protein coding sequences. The start site of translation from mRNA is always the codon AUG, which in the genomic sequence would be ATG. Unfortunately, many ATG codons are not start sites for genes and do not initiate ORFs. A gene's 3' end contains both a stop codon of either TAA, TAG, or TGA and the sequence AATAAA, which is the polyadenylation signal. In genomic sequences, these stop codons are often distributed at random and are not necessarily at the end of an ORF or gene.

In searching for genes, GenBank and other databases look for genomic sequences such as ORFs, start and stop codons, and polyadenylation signals. They also look for consensus sequences for transcription factor binding sites, intron splice sites, and genomic sequences rich in CpG nucleotides. Consensus sequences for the binding of transcription factors are sequences, such as the TATA box, that occur in the 5' promoter region of certain genes. The TATA box is located approx 25–30 bp proximal to the transcription initiation site of most genes. A similar consensus sequence, the CAAT box, is located approx 80 bp proximal to many genes, particularly those expressed in cardiac and skeletal muscle. The consensus sequences GT and AG are the junctions at which splicing of mRNA occurs to remove introns. CpG nucleotides are dinucleotides on the same strand joined together by a phosphodiester bond and are distinct from dinucleotides on different strands bound by complementary hydrogen bonds (e.g., CG). Genomic sequences rich in CpG nucleotides are known as CpG islands *(12)*. In the human genome, nonrandomly distributed CpG islands occur primarily near the first exon of genes or proximal to regions containing genes. It is estimated that CpG dinucleotides account for only 1% of the human genome *(12)*. There are approx 50,000 CpG islands in the human genome. Once a region of genomic sequence is a candidate gene, the target sequence can be amplified by PCR and analyzed for

disease-producing mutations. Maroni *(13)* used a prediction program based on CpG islands, promoter regions, and spliced donor sites to identify the first exon of 68,000 genes. The accuracy of this program was determined by comparing the predicted number of genes with the actual number of genes on chromosome 21 and 22, and the incidence of false positives was 17%. This program does appear more promising than previous programs. Having accurate computerized programs to search for genes is of great importance to scientists in academia and of great value to pharmaceutical and biotechnology companies.

MAPPING AND IDENTIFYING GENES RESPONSIBLE FOR CARDIOVASCULAR DISEASE

One of the greatest accomplishments of the 21st century—possibly even the millennium—will likely be the identification of all human genes and their function. This knowledge has obvious implications regarding the diagnosis, prevention, and treatment of cardiac disorders. Many scientists have compared knowing the full complement of human genes to knowing the complete table of periodic elements. There are two major classes of inherited disorders: Single-gene diseases and polygenic diseases. In Single-gene disorders, one gene predominates in causing a phenotype, whereas in polygenic disorders, multiple genes are required to induce the phenotype. An example of a single-gene disorder is familial hypertrophic cardiomyopathy. Hypertension and atherosclerosis are examples of polygenic disorders.

The conventional approach to identify a disease-producing gene is to find a family in which there is a segregating Single-gene disorder. Single-gene disorders are inherited in specific Mendelian patterns, which include autosomal dominant, autosomal recessive, and sex linked. One prefers to find a multigenerational family with at least 10 affected individuals *(14)*. The DNA of each family member is genotyped for chromosomal DNA markers. Several thousand chromosomal markers that are mapped at 1–2-centimorgan (cM) (1 cM = 1 million bp) intervals throughout the human genome are available *(15–17)* from several commercial sources *(11)*. The Genethon markers are the most commonly used. Usually, one genotypes family members by initially using 300–350 markers selected to span the human genome at about 10-cM intervals. This process of genotyping families to find a Single-gene disorder is usually automated. The genotypes are analyzed for genetic linkage in an attempt to map the chromosomal locus of the gene responsible for the disease. Genes, as defined by Mendel, are units of hereditary that are independently transmitted. An individual has two copies of each gene, one from each parent. Only one copy of a gene can be transmitted from a parent to an offspring, and the transmitted copy is selected is purely by chance, so that each copy has a 50% chance of being transmitted. In a process called recombination, which occurs during prophase of meiosis I, the homologous chromosomes pair and exchange portions of their DNA, and this resorts the genes present on each. The basic principle behind genetic linkage analysis is to determine if a gene responsible for the disease in a particular family is genetically linked to one of the chromosomal markers. Genetic linkage refers to two genes or DNA sequences on the same chromosome that are in such close physical proximity that they tend not to separate and are coinherited. Thus, genetic linkage analysis searches for the exception: genes or DNA sequences that are not independently inherited. If one or more chromosomal markers are found in affected individuals at a frequency that is greater than expected by chance, it indicates that the marker and the gene responsible for the disease are on the same chromosome in close physical proximity. The known location of the marker enables one to determine the locus of the gene. A gene may be 10–40 cM from the marker to which it is linked. The next step in mapping the gene's locus is to analyze additional closely spaced markers (1–2 cM apart) and narrow the region by flanking the gene with closely spaced markers. One would aim to narrow the region to 1–2 million bp.

Prior to completion of the HGP, to clone and sequence the gene after knowing its locus often required positional cloning, which is cloning the gene knowing only its position relative to the markers. This can be a very tedious process and take years. Today the use of bioinformatics often makes positional cloning unnecessary. Once the locus of the gene is mapped, GenBank and other databases can be used to identify genomic sequences in that locus with the hope of finding ESTs or known genes already mapped to the region. The ESTs can be sequenced as candidate genes to determine if a mutation is present that segregates with the disease and is present only in affected individuals. GenBank usually has information regarding the organ(s) in which an EST is expressed. If the tissue expression profile is not known, it may be preferable to determine prior to analysis whether that particular sequence is expressed in the human heart. It must be emphasized that not all ESTs have accurately been annotated to the appropriate genomic sequence. Many ESTs underwent only a single sequence pass and thus must be interpreted with caution. It is also important to keep in mind that an EST is a region of approx

100–300 bp that were selected from a clone having probably 1000–1500 bp; thus, databases often have redundant ESTs. The NCBI attempts to integrate the various sources and to cluster ESTs as they are annotated within the genomic sequence and chromosomal loci. In general, a cluster of ESTs in a region is greater confimation of a gene than a single EST. The sequences of multiple cDNAs are available from multiple species and can also be used to identify human homologs. If none of the annotated ESTs are shown to have the responsible mutation, one can determine through computerized gene prediction programs whether the genomic sequence of the locus contains genes not yet identified. (See previous section on bioinformatics.) Despite the recent availability of genomic sequences, ESTs, and cDNAs, positional cloning all too often remains the only viable option. This problem will be minimized as more ESTs and genes are mapped to their chromosomal loci. In cases where sufficiently large families with a disease of interest cannot be found, one may select initially to pursue the candidate gene approach (18,19).

DETERMINING THE FUNCTION OF HUMAN GENES THROUGH DATABASE SEQUENCE ANALYSIS

In our quest to utilize genomic information to improve the well being of humankind, determining the function of genes remains paramount. Understanding the pathogenesis of disease and improving its prevention, diagnosis, and treatment will require knowing and manipulating the function of genes. The conventional methods of determining gene function are as follows: (i) expression of normal or mutant genes in cultured cells to observe the effects on cell function; (ii) analysis of the phenotype following expression of the gene in the intact animal, a process known as transgenesis; (iii) analysis of the phenotype following gene elimination through homologous recombination, known as creating a knockout model; or (iv) identification of genes responsible for Single-gene disorders. At a meeting in Cold Spring Harbor a few years ago, we estimated it may take up to a century by conventional techniques to determine the function of human genes. But development of gene and protein databases has markedly accelerated our ability to determine gene function (20).

In addition to the conventional methods for determining gene function, it is now evident that bioinformatics can be used to help determine gene function. In parallel with sequencing the human genome, there has been a major effort to sequence simpler and smaller genomes of single-celled and multicellular organisms. The complete nucleotide genomic sequence of more than 50 organisms is now available in GenBank and other databases. The first genome to be completely sequenced was that of *Haemophilus influenza* in 1995. It consists of 1.4 million bases and 1740 genes. Since that time, the genomes of multicellular organisms have been sequenced—the first was the nematode *Caenorhabditis elegans (21)*. The functions of many of the genes in these organisms are known, and the functions of the remaining genes can be more easily determined in these organisms than in humans. One approach to determine the function of a human gene is to search for sequence homology between it and genes of known function in simpler organisms. For example, an organism such as *C. elegans* has 19,000 genes and consists of 959 cells. The functions of many of these genes are already known. It is not surprising that 36% of the genes in *C. elegans* are homologous to human genes. Experimental confirmation of a suspected function is far more efficient and much less costly than determining gene function by trial and error. By using specialized computerized programs (e.g., BLAST®) to analyze sequence data from such sources as GenBank, human DNA sequences can be aligned with the genomic sequences of single-celled and multicellular organisms to determine the extent of sequence homology. Through this mechanism, it is possible to travel back in evolutionary time to over a billion years ago, which is close to the time of origin of multicellular organisms. It is of note that the genome of geneticists' favored organism, *Drosophila melanogasterer (22)*, has been sequenced recently, and its genes have been identified. The complete sequence of the mouse genome will soon be available *(23)*. It is roughly the size of the human genome and is estimated to have the same number of genes. Furthermore, most of the genes in the mouse and human have similar function, which means much of the information gleaned from mouse genomic data will apply to humans.

In addition to being determine through sequence homology, gene function will be determined through identifying the nucleotide sequences that encode for protein motifs of known function. For example, it is estimated there are over 3000 kinases, and they should all at least share the motif for transfer of high-energy phosphate. It is estimated there are approx 2000 transcriptional factors *(24)*, and each has at least one common DNA binding motif that can be used as a probe to search databases for other members of this family. There are over 1500 known functional motifs *(24)* that have been identified in proteins, and the genomic sequences encoding these motifs are being identified. Given the combination of genomic sequences, cDNA sequences, and protein sequences, a rich complexity of information relating to gene function is available. While the human may have 40,000 genes, it

is highly likely these genes can be grouped into a few thousand gene families. These families of genes are likely to have common functional motifs that could be used to probe the various nucleotide databases to identify other members of the family. Bioinformatics, initially a science related to the storage and retrieval of sequences, is likely to make its greatest contribution in helping determine gene function.

DETERMINING GENE FUNCTION FROM SINGLE GENE DISORDERS

Genomics will significantly help in determining gene function through the mapping and identification of genes responsible for Single-gene disorders *(25)*. While these disorders are rare, they represent many of the more common and acquired forms of disease. A good example is the cholesterol receptor, which was identified *(26)* as a result of studies in patients with familial hypercholesterolemia. These studies provided tangible quantitative evidence for the role of cholesterol in atherosclerosis. Furthermore, they led to discoveries about the network of cholesterol transport, uptake, deposition, and synthesis. And they ultimately led to use of statins, which inhibit cholesterol synthesis and are a common treatment for patients at risk of complications from coronary heart disease.

Another example of a Single-gene disorder is familial hypertrophic cardiomyopathy (HCM) *(27,28)*. Hypertrophy, a hallmark of this disease, is also a known independent risk factor for sudden death and heart failure in acquired forms of the disease. Genetic animal models have been generated using mutant genes known to cause familial HCM in humans *(28–30)*. Analysis of these models has shown hypertrophy and fibrosis to be secondary phenotypes. The mouse model, characterized primarily by cardiac fibrosis, was reversed by losartan, which blocks angiotensin II *(31)*. The rabbit model *(32)*, which exhibits fibrosis and hypertrophy similar to the human phenotype, regressed with the administration of simvastatin *(33)*. Clinical trials are necessary to assess these therapies in patients with familial HCM. In the rabbit model of human HCM, animals with the mutant gene that had not yet developed hypertrophy had abnormal ventricular wall tissue, as determined by Doppler velocities *(34)*. The tissue Doppler technique has also been shown to be sensitive and specific in detecting human familial HCM *(35)*, and it can detect abnormal tissue prior to the development of hypertrophy. This technique can now be used to screen athletes or select members of families with familial HCM who have not yet developed the disease. Therapy could be initiated in these individuals as part of primary prevention. In the next few years, the genes responsible for most Single-gene disorders will be identified. Many of these diseases will serve as models not only to elucidate pathogeneses but also to determine the function of individual genes and improve diagnosis, prevention, and treatment of acquired diseases.

PREDICTING PROTEIN STRUCTURE FROM COMPUTATIONAL GENOMICS

The overall function of a protein is determined by its structure. The primary structure of a protein is determined by the sequence of its amino acids. Whether obtained directly or derived from the nucleotide sequences, the primary structure is intrinsic to the overall structure of the protein. The secondary and tertiary structures of a protein are best determined experimentally by techniques such as X-ray crystallography or nuclear magnetic resonance. These techniques can only be done by highly skilled individuals, are very tedious, and lag behind the progress of protein sequencing. This has created the opportunity for using computational biology to develop three-dimensional protein models from nucleotide and protein sequence data from a variety of organisms. These models can be evaluated in experimental preparations and are often used to develop specific drugs. Genomic sequences that encode known domains such as signaling and transmembrane sequences are essential to creating protein models and determining protein function. To these ends, genomics currently plays a lesser role than proteomics, but predicting protein shape from nucleotide sequences is still a primary goal.

POLYGENIC DISORDERS—THE PROMISE OF SNPS (SINGLE NUCLEOTIDE POLYMORPHISMS) AND GENE CHIPS

Genetic linkage analysis has been extremely successful in identifying genes with Mendelian inheritance patterns that can cause Single-gene disorders. In these disorders, a Single-gene predominates despite the influence from the environment and modifier genes. This makes possible statistical detection of the genes even in a relatively small sample. In contrast, in disorders such as coronary artery disease, diabetes, and hypertension, no one genetic defect predominates, and the effects of an individual genetic defect are further diluted by major environmental influences. One can predict that there are 20–30 genes influencing coronary artery disease, and each contributes less than 5% susceptibility for the disease. The sample size required to detect the influence of just one of these genes is prohibitive. Evidence that

polygenic diseases have an inherited component is well established. In monozygotic twins, in whom there is 100% sharing of genes, the risk of both twins inheriting a polygenic disease is much greater than the risk in dizygotic twins, who share only 50% of their genes. In endemic populations, there is also evidence for inheritance of polygenic diseases. The barriers to identifying genes involved in polygenic diseases are many and prohibitive. The minimum sample size required (36) to identify such genes is several thousand, and a minimum of 500,000 markers, at intervals of a few hundred thousand bp, are required. Such a search would require very-high-throughput genotyping and would cost millions of dollars. One approach in identifying polygenic diseases is to enrich a population for a particular disease. For example, a search for genes that contribute to coronary artery disease would include only individuals with diabetes, hypercholesterolemia, and hypertension. Unfortunately, approaches of this nature have not been productive. Another approach is to select siblings with or without the disease of interest. This approach is likely to be successful only if the effect of a gene is statistically quite significant.

Hope for unraveling polygenic disorders currently rests on the success of using single nucleotide polymorphisms (SNPs). The variation in the human genome nucleotide sequence is believed to be only 0.1% among individuals, with the corollary that 99.9% of genomic sequences are identical (37). This variation is primarily due to single nucleotide polymorphisms, which occur at intervals of 1000 bp and total about 3 million (38,39). Most of these SNPs are in introns with less than 500,000 present in exons. Those present in exons are assumed to have functional significance such as physical differences (for example, height and weight) or disease susceptibility. If an SNP is shown to contribute to a disease, the SNP will be found in people with the disease more commonly than by chance, and the SNP would be detected by a modified form of genetic linkage analysis. Confirmation of the functional significance of the gene and the SNP would be required through biochemical or experimental methods. In the next 5 years, most of the SNPs should be identified, and their effects—if any—on disease will likely be determined through experimental studies, population studies, or genotype/phenotype correlations. At present, the best approach for studying polygenic diseases is to combine SNP technology with high throughput analysis in populations enriched for a particular phenotype.

A recent technique offers further hope for discovering genes involved in polygenic diseases. This approach uses microarrays (40), which are also referred to as gene chips. In a microarray, single-stranded DNA from genes are stuck to small wafers. These arrays can be probed with genes expressed in diseased tissue, such as an atherosclerotic lesion, to search for the complementary sequences. Upon hybridization, a characteristic fluorescence is emitted, and the pattern of fluorescence indicates which genes are active. For certain diseases, one can also assess the temporal sequence of gene activation. While many of the active genes are secondary to the disease process, the technology does provide appropriate candidates genes *(41)*.

It is highly likely that genes contributing to susceptibility toward common cardiac diseases will be identified in the near future. This affords the opportunity to prescribe more appropriate lifestyles and therapies to prevent the development of cardiac diseases. Knowing susceptibility genes will also contribute to our understanding of physiological and pathological pathways and will provide further targets for specific therapies. Knowing these genes may also provide the necessary infrastructure for treating individuals based on their genetic profiles.

ACKNOWLEDGMENTS

The assistance of Brandon Roberts and Debbie Graustein is greatly appreciated. This work is supported by grants from the National Heart, Lung, and Blood Institute; Specialized Centers of Research (P50–HL54313-08); and the National Institutes of Health Training Center in Molecular Cardiology (T32–HLO7706-09).

REFERENCES

1. Fraser C, Norris S, Weinstock G, et al. Complete Genome Sequence of *Treponema pallidum*, the Syphilis Spirochete. Science 1999;281:375–388.
2. Kuo MH, Allis CD. Roles of histone acetyltransfrases and deacetylases in gene regulation. Bio Essays 1998;20:615–626.
3. Lu J, McKinsey TA, Nicol RL, Olson EN. Signal-dependent activation of the MEF2 transcription factor by dissociation from histone deacetylases. Proc Natl Acad Sci USA 2000;97:4070–4075.
4. Fields C, Adams MD, White O, Venter JC. How many genes in the human genome? Nature Genetics 1994;7:345–346.
5. Bestor TH, Bycko B. Creation of genomic methylation patterns. Nature Genetics 1996;12:363–367.
6. Collins FS. Shattuck lecture—medical and societal consequences of the human genome project. N Engl J Med 1999;341:28–37.
7. Cooper NG. *The Human Genome Project: Deciphering the Blueprint of Heredity.* 1st ed. Mill Valley, CA: University Science Books; 1994.
8. Marshall E. A high-stakes gamble on genome sequencing. Science 1999;284:1906–1909.
9. Normile D, Pennisi E. Team wrapping up sequence of first human chromosome. Science 1999;285:2038.
10. Deloukas P, Schuler GD, Gyapay G, et al. A physical map of 30,000 human genes. Science 1998;282:744–746.
11. Baxevanis AD, Ouellette BFF. *Bioinformatics: A Practical Guide to the Analysis of Genes and Proteins.* 2nd ed. New York: Wiley-Interscience, A John Wiley & Sons, Inc; 2001.
12. Davuluri RV, Grosse I, Zhang MQ. Computational identification of promoters and first exons in the human genome. Nature Genetics 2001;29:412–417.
13. Maroni G. The organization of eukaryotic genes. Evol Biol 1996;29:1-19.
14. Towbin JA, Roberts R. Cardiovascular diseases due to genetic abnormalities. In: Fuster V, Alexander RW, O'Rourke RA, Wellens HJJ, eds. *Hurst's the Heart.* 10th ed. New York: McGraw-Hill Professional; 2001:1735–1826.
15. Murray JC, Buetow KH, Weber JL, et al. A comprehensive human linkage map with centimorgan density. Cooperative Human Linkage Center (CHLC). Science 1994;265: 2049–2054.
16. Sheffield VC, Weber JL, Buetow KH, et al. A collection of tri- and tetranucleotide repeat markers used to generate high quality, high resolution human genome-wide linkage maps. Hum Mol Genet 1995;4:1837–1844.
17. Weber JL, May PE. Abundant class of human DNA polymorphisms which can be typed using the polymerase chain reaction. Am J Hum Genet 1989;44:388–396.
18. Li D, Tapscott T, Gonzalez O, et al. Desmin mutation responsible for idiopathic dilated cardiomyopathy. Circulation 1999;100:461–464.
19. Olson TM, Michels VV, Thibodeau SN, Tai Y-S, Keating MT. Actin mutations in dilated cardiomypathy, a heritable form of heart failure. Science 1998;280:750–752.
20. Jasny BR, Roberts L. Genome: Unlocking the Genome. Science 2001;294:81.
21. Hodgkin J, Horowitz RS, Jasny BR, Kimble J. C. elegans: sequence to biology. Science 1998;282:2011.
22. Garza D, Ajioka JW, Burke DT, Hartl DL. Mapping the Drosophila genome with yeast artificial chromosomes. Science 1989;246:641–646.
23. Thomas JW, Summers TJ, Lee-Lin SQ, et al. Comparative genome mapping in the sequence-based era: early experience with human chromosome 7. Genome Res 2000;10:624–633.
24. Brivanlou AH, Darnell J. Signal transduction and the control of gene expression. Science 2002;295:813–818.
25. Vukmirovic OG, Tilghman SM. Exploring genome space. Nature 2000;405:820–822.
26. Brown MS, Goldstein JL. Expression of the familial hypercholesterolemia gene in heterozygotes: mechanism for a dominant disorder in man. Science 1974;185:61–63.
27. Geisterfer-Lowrance AA, Kass S, Tanigawa G, et al. A molecular basis for familial hypertrophic cardiomyopathy: A beta-cardiac myosin heavy chain gene missense mutation. Cell 1990;62:999–1006.
28. Marian AJ, Roberts R. The molecular genetic basis for hypertrophic cardiomyopathy. J Mol Cell Cardiol 2001;33:655–670.
29. Oberst L, Park J-T, Wu Y, et al. Decreased left ventricular ejection fraction, detected by [178]TA radionuclide angiography in transgenic mice expressing a mutant cardiac troponin T-Gln[92]: Altered function precedes structural abnormalities. Circ Res. In press.
30. Geisterfer-Lowrance AA, Christe M, Conner DA, et al. A mouse model of familial hypertrophic cardiomyopathy. Science 1996;272:731–734.
31. Lim DS, Lutucuta S, Bachireddy P, et al. Angiotensin II blockade reverses myocardial fibrosis in a transgenic mouse model of human hypertrophic cardiomyopathy. Circulation 2001;103:789–791.

32. Marian AJ, Wu Y, Lim D-S, et al. A transgenic rabbit model for human hypertrophic cardomyopathy. J Clin Invest 1999;104:1683–1692.

33. Patel R, Nagueh SF, Tsybouleva N, et al. Simvastatin induces regression of cardiac hypertrophy and fibrosis and improves cardiac function in a transgenic rabbit model of human hypertrophic cardiomyopathy. Circulation 2001;104:317–324.

34. Nagueh SF, Kopelen H, Lim DS, Zoghbi WA, Quinones MA, Roberts R. Tissue Doppler imaging consistently detects myocardial contraction and relaxation abnormalities, irrespective of cardiac hypertrophy, in a transgenic rabbit model of human hypertrophic cardiomyopathy. Circulation 2000;102:1346–1350.

35. Nagueh SF, Bachinski LL, Meyer D, et al. Tissue Doppler imaging consistently detects myocardial abnormalities in patients with hypertrophic cardiomyopathy and provides a novel means for an early diagnosis before and independently of hypertrophy. Circulation 2001;104:128–130.

36. Kruglyak L. Prospects for whole-genome linkage disequilibrium mapping of common disease. Nat Genet 1999;22:139–144.

37. Risch N, Merikangas K. The future of genetic studies of complex human diseases. Science 1996;273:1516–1517.

38. Marth G, Yeh R, Minton M, et al. Single-nucleotide polymorphisms in the public domain: how useful are they? Nature Genetics 2001;27:371–372.

39. Weaver TA. High-throughput SNP discovery and typing for genome-wide genetic analysis. Trends Genet 2000;21:36–42.

40. Friend SH, Stoughton R. The magic of microarrays. Scientific Am 2002;286:44–53.

41. Brazma A, Hingamp P, Quackenbush J, et al. Minimum information about a micoarray experiment (MIAME)-toward standards for microarray data. Nat Genet 2001;29:365–371.

4 Gene Therapy and Cardiovascular Diseases

Yi Chu, PhD, Neal L. Weintraub, MD, and Donald D. Heistad, MD

CONTENTS

INTRODUCTION

Gene therapy is a promising new field in modern medicine and holds great potential for the treatment of cardiovascular diseases. This chapter will discuss the principles and methods of gene-based therapy and the use of gene transfer in research and in treatment of cardiovascular diseases.

PRINCIPLE OF GENE TRANSFER

Gene transfer is a procedure in which genetic material, either DNA or RNA, is introduced directly or via a vector into selected somatic cells. The new genetic material contains one or more expression cassettes, or transgenes, that express a functional protein or RNA as the transgene product. Gene transfer can be accomplished in two ways. Ex vivo gene transfer involves the removal of cells, transduction of the removed cells, and implantation of the modified cells in the target environment, whereas in vivo gene transfer allows for the direct delivery of a transgene to cells. In both methods, the goals are for the transduced cells to express the transgene and for the transgene product to produce an autocrine, paracrine, or endocrine effect (Fig. 1).

Gene transfer is a valuable tool for understanding the mechanisms of cardiovascular diseases and may become an integral part of the treatment regimen for patients with cardiovascular disease *(1)*. Gene transfer of plasmid DNA that expresses vascular endothelial growth factor (VEGF) has been used with favorable outcome to treat peripheral arterial disease and coronary heart disease in patients who were not candidates for conventional regimens *(2,3)*. In addition, gene therapy may be developed for common diseases, including hypertension and dyslipidemias *(4,5)*.

METHODS OF GENE TRANSFER

Vectors

Although used successfully in patients for gene transfer into skeletal and cardiac muscle, naked DNA alone is inefficient for transducing most cells or tissues *(2,3)*. Because naked DNA is the safest reagent for gene transfer, efforts are underway to improve its transduction efficiency. Electroporation, or the application of an electric field, increases efficiency of gene transfer 10- to 100-fold after administration of naked DNA *(6)*. Hydrodynamics-based gene delivery, a recent approach to improving naked DNA transfer, involves the rapid intravenous injection of naked DNA in a volume of solution as large as the entire volume of blood in the animal *(7)*. Similarly, inducing high pressure by other means, including inflation of a blood-pressure cuff *(8)* or clamping of a blood vessel *(9)*, has increased the efficiency of gene transfer of naked DNA. The clinical use of these methods is untested, but the safety of naked DNA makes it the preferred method for gene therapy.

From: *Contemporary Cardiology: Principles of Molecular Cardiology*
Edited by: M. S. Runge and C. Patterson @ Humana Press Inc., Totowa, NJ

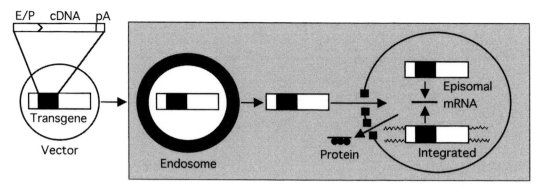

Fig. 1. Gene transfer to (or transduction of) a somatic cell. The vector contains an expression cassette, which contains the DNA segment with the enhancer/promoter (E/P), the gene-encoding sequence (cDNA), and the polyadenylation (pA) sequence. The vector enters the cell through endocytosis. The genome of the vector enters the nucleus and either exists as an episome (e.g., adenovirus) or integrates into the chromosome (e.g., retrovirus). The host transcription factors and RNA polymerase II bind to the E/P region to initiate transcription. Mature mRNA containing pA sequence is transported from the nucleus to cytoplasm to serve as template for synthesis of the transgenic protein. When antisense RNA is the transgene product, transcribed RNA binds to cognate mRNA to inhibit translation.

The use of viral vectors to transduce host cells is an efficient method of gene transfer (Table 1). For viruses to be used as vectors, regions of the viral genome that are critical for viral replication are removed, and one or more expression cassettes for transgenes are inserted. Recombinant virus lacking replication genes is generated and propagated in "packaging cells," which provide the necessary components for viral replication and packaging that the genome of the replication-deficient virus lacks. The ability to achieve a sufficiently high viral titer should be considered when choosing a viral vector.

A retrovirus derived from a murine leukemia virus was the first viral vector used for gene transfer (10). Transduction with a retrovirus occurs via the retroviral receptor PiT-2, which is present on a variety of cells (11). The efficiency of retroviral transduction may be increased by pseudotyping, a technique whereby the viral surface protein that binds to the cell is replaced with another protein, usually vesicular stomatitis virus glycoprotein G (VSV-G). VSV-G binds to a membrane phospholipid, which is present in high concentrations in many cells and in many species (12). After infection, the retrovirus genome is randomly inserted into the host cell chromosome, and the transgene is stably expressed in transduced cells and their progeny—if the promoter or enhancer is not silenced upon insertion. Random insertion into the host chromosome, however, makes insertional mutagenesis possible. An important disadvantage in the use of the retroviral vector in cardiovascular gene transfer is that transduction only occurs in dividing cells, which are few in the adult cardiovascular system. Furthermore, because the retroviral genome is small (approx 10 kilobases [kb]),

the transgene must be small. Used in early experiments in blood vessels (13,14), retroviral vectors are currently being tested in clinical trials of gene therapy for the treatment of cancer, AIDS, multiple sclerosis, and hemophilia (see *The Journal of Gene Medicine* web site: www.wiley.co.uk/genetherapy/clinical/).

Lentiviral vectors, derived from a subgroup of retroviruses including HIV and immunodeficiency viruses in other species, have recently been developed (15,16). The usual specificity of lentiviruses for CD4+ cells is redirected by pseudotyping with VSV-G protein. Major advantages of the lentivirus vector are its ability to transduce both dividing and nondividing cells and the stable expression of transgenes. Concerns about the safety of lentiviruses as vectors and the low viral titers attained with lentiviruses are being addressed (15,16).

Adenovirus vectors are used extensively in gene transfer as research tools and as a means of therapy (17,18). With a large genome of approximately 36 kb, adenoviruses can accommodate a larger transgene than retroviruses (17,18). Furthermore, transduction efficiency is high in both dividing and nondividing cells, and high-titer viral stocks of adenoviral vectors are easily produced. Adenoviruses enter cells via interaction with a cellular receptor, the Coxsackie-adenovirus receptor, combined with help from integrins $\alpha_v\beta_3$ or $\alpha_v\beta_5$ (19,20) and possibly other membrane proteins (21,22). The viral genome remains extrachromosomal in the host cell, which accounts in part for the short duration of expression of the transgene. Although usually a limitation, short duration may be an advantage for treating transient abnormalities associated with some cardiovascular

Table 1
Vectors for Cardiovascular Gene Transfer

Vector	Advantages	Disadvantages
Adenovirus	High transduction efficiency	Highly immunogenic
	Rapid, transient expression	Transient expression
Adeno-associated virus	Safety	Slow expression
	Prolonged expression	
	Low immunogenicity	
Electroporation	Ease and versatility	Unsuitable for internal use
Helper-dependent adenovirus	High transduction efficiency	Difficulty to produce and purify
	Prolonged expression	
	Low immunogenicity	
Lentivirus	Transduce dividing and nondividing cells	Difficulty to produce
	Prolonged expression	Slow expression
Liposome	Ease and versatility	Low transduction efficiency
	Low, short-term toxicity	
Naked DNA	Safety	Immunogenicity due to unmethylated CpG
Retrovirus	Prolonged expression	Transduce only dividing cells
		Slow expression

conditions *(23)*. Immunogenicity is high with adenoviral vectors and may contribute to the short duration of transgene expression. Furthermore, the host immune response elicited by the adenoviral vector may be fatal in some patients. Immunogenicity is reduced, and duration of expression is increased in "helper-dependent" or "gutted" adenoviral vectors in which the entire viral protein-coding sequence is deleted *(24)*. Adenoviral vectors are being used in clinical trials to treat peripheral arterial diseases (www.wiley.co.uk/genetherapy/clinical).

Another promising vector for use in cardiovascular gene transfer is the adeno-associated virus (AAV) vector *(25)*. Major advantages of the AAV vector are safety and long-term expression of the transgene *(25)*. No known human disease has been associated with AAV. AAV-mediated gene transfer has been successful in cardiomyocytes, with sustained expression of a reporter gene without inflammation or necrosis *(26)*. In contrast to adenoviral vectors, transgene expression is usually delayed in onset with AAV vectors. Improvements in genetic technology may help to overcome the disadvantages associated with the use of AAV, which include limited transgene size (<4.5 kb) and difficulty in production of high titers of virus *(27,28)*.

An ideal vector would be safe and efficient and yield high but controllable levels of gene expression. Although a useful vector should have tropism for the targeted tissue or cell, site-selective delivery may be attained by the use of liposome- or viral-mediated gene transfer with attached targeting components *(29,30)*. Furthermore, gene transfer may be regulated by transfering several genes, some with modulatory effects *(31,32)*.

Delivery

LOCAL INJECTION

An effective in vivo approach for gene transfer to blood vessels involves the intraluminal injection of a vector through a catheter *(33,34)*. This method requires that blood flow be stopped, often for many minutes, to allow attachment and uptake of the vector. With intraluminal injection, the transgene is expressed in the endothelium and to a variable extent in the adventitia, presumably through the vasa vasorum that originate in the vascular lumen. One disadvantage of the approach is the potential for reperfusion injury or problems associated with ischemia.

Vectors have been delivered directly into the coronary artery via a specially adapted angioplasty balloon catheter *(35)*. The virus is injected into the arterial wall through many small nipples in the catheter. This approach has been used to alter vasomotor responses and to inhibit vascular remodeling after balloon injury *(36)*.

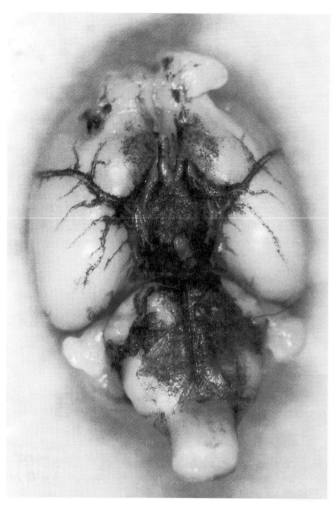

Fig. 2. Expression of β-galactosidase (dark staining) on the ventral surface of the mouse brain 1 day after intracisternal injection of AdCMV-βgal. Transduction occurred in the leptomeninges near the basilar artery, the circle of Willis, the middle cerebral artery, and smaller arteries. Reproduced with permission *(65)*.

To avoid interruption of blood flow, the viral vector may be applied to the adventitia of a vessel. We have observed excellent expression of the transgene in the adventitia after injecting recombinant viruses into the periarterial sheath *(37)*. Others have applied a gel in vivo to the coronary arteries to stimulate angiogenesis *(38)*.

We and others *(39,40)* have injected viral vectors into the pericardium with excellent expression of the transgene in the visceral and parietal pericardium. We unexpectedly observed higher levels of transgene expression in the pericardium over the atria than over the ventricles. Preferential expression over the atria probably results from the presence of more pericardial fluid around the atria than around the potential space over the ventricles. Gene transfer to the pericardium may "bathe" the myocardium in

proteins produced by the transgene. This approach might be useful for gene transfer of VEGF and other proteins that stimulate angiogenesis.

Injecting viral vectors into the cisterna magna produces a wide distribution of transgene expression throughout the subarachnoid space *(41,42)* (Fig. 2). The vector is carried through the cerebrospinal fluid to tissues lining the subarachnoid space, including tissues overlying blood vessels at the base of the brain. After intracisternal injection of virus, the transgene is expressed in the meninges and the adventitia of vessels, but not in brain parenchyma. Transgene expression in the adventitia profoundly alters vasomotor responses *(43,44)*. We have used this approach to prevent cerebral vasospasm after subarachnoid hemorrhage in experimental animals *(45)*.

SYSTEMIC INJECTION

After intravenous injection of adenoviral vectors, the transgene is expressed primarily in the liver in several species *(46–49)*; however, levels of expression in the liver may not be high in humans because of the paucity of Coxsackie-adenovirus receptor in human liver *(50)*. Blood-borne virus probably does not have sufficient time to bind to the endothelium of arterial capillaries or veins, and the virus recirculates until it is trapped in the liver. After expression in the liver, secretable proteins are released into the circulation.

Transgene expression can be targeted to specific tissues after intravenous injection of vectors. For example, liposomes conjugated to a monoclonal antibody that recognizes the extracellular domain of E-selectin bind preferentially to activated endothelium *(29)*. We have demonstrated that adenoviral vectors preferentially bind to endothelial cells that express vascular cell adhesion molecule-1 *(22)*, which may help explain the observation that transgene expression is greater in endothelium overlying atherosclerotic lesions than in normal endothelium *(51,52)*. Strategies to target activated endothelium, especially areas overlying atherosclerotic lesions, may be useful in delivering therapeutic genes to blood vessels.

Angiotensin-converting enzyme (ACE) is expressed at high levels in the endothelium of pulmonary capillaries. Intravenous injection of a bi-specific antibody to ACE has been used for selective delivery of adenoviral vectors to pulmonary endothelium *(53)*.

In the approaches described above, gene transfer is targeted to specific cell surface molecules. An alternative approach is to use a tissue-specific promoter to produce preferential expression in selected tissues. For example, liver-specific promoters may increase expression levels of a transgene in the liver after intravenous injection *(54)*. Several endothelium-specific promoters have been evaluated (55). Intravenous injection of fms-like tyrosine kinase-1 resulted in transgene expression in the endothelium, with very low levels of expression in the liver.

The best overall approach for systemic injection of a viral vector is to use a virus that binds to organ-specific or diseased endothelium without producing significant transduction in the liver. Combining this approach with the use of a tissue-specific promoter should result in the production of high levels of transgene expression in the desired tissues.

INTRAMUSCULAR INJECTION

Intramuscular injection of adenoviral vectors consistently results in long-term expression of the transgene. This finding implies that skeletal muscle is immunoprivileged and that transgene expression may be longer with intramuscular injection of a vector than with intravenous injection. For example, in a study of hypercholesterolemic mice, injection of a solution of hemagglutinating virus of Japan–liposome with a mutated monocyte chemoattractant protein-1(MCP-1) into skeletal muscle resulted in expression of the mutant MCP-1 in the blood for several weeks and the inhibition of atherosclerotic lesions (56). In a similar approach (intramuscular injection), an adenoviral vector that expresses neurotrophic factor-3 produced sustained doses of NT-3 and prevented diabetic neuropathy in rats (57).

GENE TRANSFER IN RESEARCH

Gene Transfer to Cells in Culture

One of the first steps in gene transfer studies is to demonstrate the effects of the transgene on cultured cells. In vitro cell studies are useful for assessing new vectors and for examining the effects of vectors and transgenes on isolated cells. Adenovirus-mediated gene transfer to endothelial cells, smooth muscle cells, and cardiac myocytes in culture results in high levels of transduction when a large amount of virus is used; therefore, the effects of a transgene can easily be demonstrated in this setting. For example, the retinoblastoma gene product significantly inhibits proliferation of vascular smooth muscle cells in culture (58), and gene transfer of copper–zinc or manganese superoxide dismutase to endothelial cells in culture inhibits oxidation of low-density lipoprotein by endothelial cells (59). Gene transfer of catalase significantly inhibits cell proliferation and promotes apoptosis in vascular smooth muscle cells in culture (60). Thus, gene transfer to cells in vitro confirms the functional activity of a vector and allows for the study of biological processes in isolated cells.

Gene Transfer to Blood Vessels

The effects of gene transfer in blood vessels may be examined in vitro and in vivo. For in vitro studies, vascular rings grown in tissue culture medium for one day maintain normal vascular function, including endothelium-mediated vasomotor responses (43). Adenovirus-mediated gene transfer to blood vessels in vitro results in significant transduction in the endothelium and adventitia, but not in the vascular media. However, gene transfer to the media beneath the internal elastic lamina may be achieved by denuding the endothelium (61). Thus, in vitro cell studies may be used to study the effects of a transgene in the different vascular layers. For example, adenovirus-mediated overexpression of endothelial nitric oxide synthase (eNOS) in the adventitia in vitro reduces contractile responses (62) and increases nitric oxide–mediated relaxation (43). The latter finding indicates that the adventitia can be transduced to express nitric oxide–mediated function that had previously been attributed exclusively to the endothelium.

Gene transfer to blood vessels in vivo is usually achieved either by stopping blood flow in the vessel for up to 20 min to allow the vector to enter the cell or by injecting the vector at very high pressure levels (33,63). Because neither approach can be used for delicate vessels such as intracranial arteries, other gene transfer methods have been developed (64). Injection of adenoviral vectors into the cisterna magna allows the virus to diffuse through the cerebrospinal fluid and results in significant transduction in the adventitia and perivascular tissues (41,65). When the transgene product is secreted outside of transduced cells, concentrations sufficient to alter vascular function can be achieved. Another relatively noninvasive method is to inject the virus into the vascular sheath (37). Both of the above approaches, however, limit transduction to the adventitia; thus, the ability of gene transfer to affect vascular function depends on the properties of the transgene product. When the product is diffusible, like nitric oxide, or secreted, like calcitonin gene-related peptide (CGRP) and extracellular superoxide dismutase (ECSOD), vascular function may be altered.

Gene Transfer to the Heart

Gene transfer to isolated cardiomyocytes in vitro has been performed with the use of naked DNA combined with lipofectin, electroporation, and calcium phosphate. Limited success has been achieved with these techniques; the efficiency of gene transfer is about 3–10% for neonatal cardiomyocytes and lower for adult cardiomyocytes (66). Retroviruses are not capable of efficiently transducing terminally differentiated cardiomyocytes (66). Recombinant adenoviruses yield a higher level of transgene expression *(66,67)*. Adenoviruses have several advantages over retroviruses and nonviral approaches. First, adenoviral DNA does not integrate into the host cell DNA, and the large adenoviral genome can accommodate a large transgene. Furthermore, adenoviral vectors are capable of achieving high titers in the host. Recent reports suggest that recombinant AAV, lentiviruses, and Sindbis virus can efficiently transduce cardiomyocytes in vitro *(26,68,69)*.

Several methods of delivery have been used for in vivo myocardial gene transfer; however, the recombinant adenoviral vectors are used most commonly. Although early studies showed that transgene expression could be achieved with direct injection of adenoviruses into the myocardium, expression was limited to the area of administration *(70,71)*.

To produce extensive transgene expression, viral vectors have been delivered to the myocardium via the coronary circulation, without the intramyocardial injury resulting from direct needle injection. However, achieving widespread cardiomyocyte transduction with injection into the coronary vessels is challenging *(63)*, and several novel strategies have been used. For example, cardioplegic arrest increases the efficiency of gene transfer by allowing longer exposure to the viral vectors *(72)*. In addition, increasing vascular permeability by reducing the concentration of calcium in the perfusate or by administering agents such as histamine improves the efficiency of myocardial gene transfer *(73,74)*. Cross-clamping the aorta and pulmonary artery for 10–40 s while injecting the virus into the ventricular apex via a catheter produces homogeneous transduction of cardiomyocytes in the right and left ventricles *(75)*. Although intracoronary delivery of viral vectors results in widespread transduction of cardiomyocytes, the approach is highly invasive.

In a recent study in rabbits, an adenoviral vector was subselectively injected into the left or right coronary artery *(76)*. A high viral titer and a relatively large infusion volume (5×10^{11} viral particles in 2.5 mL) resulted in a high level of transgene expression in the injected ventricle (Fig. 3). Moreover, ventricular function in response to isoproterenol infusion was increased 3–6 d after gene transfer to overexpress the β_2-adrenergic receptor. Another experimental approach for gene transfer to the myocardium is the intrapericardial administration of viral vectors. Initial studies showed that transgene expression was restricted to epicardial cardiomyocytes after intrapericardial injection of recombinant adenovirus *(39,77)*. Later studies in rats and mice showed that co-injection of proteolytic enzymes with adenovirus increased expression of the transgene, presumably by facilitating the diffusion of adenovirus into the myocardial tissue *(78)*. The subxiphoid incision used to deliver

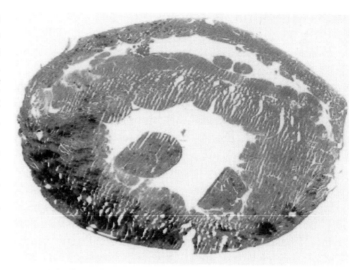

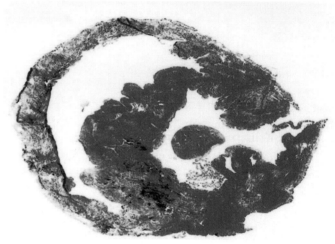

Fig. 3. X-Gal staining to detect expression of β-galactosidase (dark staining) in rabbit myocardium 3 days after adenoviral-mediated gene transfer via selective delivery into the left circumflex (top panel) or right coronary artery (bottom panel). Reproduced with permission *(76)*.

the adenovirus in this study did not affect ventricular function and was well tolerated.

In a novel, noninvasive approach for gene transfer to the heart, adenovirus prepared in albumin-coated microbubbles was injected intravenously, and the albumin microbubbles were destroyed in the heart by ultrasound. This technique resulted in significant transgene expression throughout the myocardium without invasive surgical procedures *(79)*. Some transgene expression occurred in the liver, indicating the difficulty of targeting the vector solely to the heart. A disadvantage with this technique is the possibility of endothelial damage. Nevertheless, the high efficiency of myocardial gene transfer and the noninvasive nature of the approach suggest this technique may be useful in experimental and clinical settings.

GENE THERAPY FOR CARDIOVASCULAR DISEASES

Atherosclerosis

ANGIOGENESIS THERAPY

Gene therapy is a promising approach for treating ischemic heart disease and peripheral vascular disease for several reasons. First, conventional medical therapy and revascularization procedures are not effective for many patients with ischemic heart disease. Second, several methods of delivery for gene therapy are available because of access to the coronary and peripheral vasculature of animals and humans through transvascular (catheter-based), percutaneous, and surgical approaches. Finally, angiogenesis can be induced by transient expression of angiogenic peptides; therefore, long-term expression of the transgene, which is often difficult to achieve, is not required.

Several models and transgenes have been used in experimental studies of angiogenic gene therapy for peripheral vascular disease. Although adenoviral vectors are the most efficient at delivering genes to the vasculature, problems related to immunogenicity limit their use in humans (80); therefore, plasmids have been used in many studies to deliver genes to the peripheral vasculature. However, the efficiency of plasmid-mediated gene transfer is low. Fewer than 1% of target cells express the transgene; nevertheless, physiologically significant levels of the transgene product can be detected in the circulation (81). Moreover, because plasmid DNA remains in an unintegrated, nonreplicative form, the probability of insertional mutagenesis is low, which is an important consideration for clinical use.

Studies conducted in animal models strongly suggest that therapeutic angiogenesis can be achieved with several genes encoding different proteins, including VEGF, fibroblast growth factor, angiopoietin, and hypoxia-inducible factor-1 (HIF-1) (80). In a rabbit model of hind limb ischemia, intraarterial administration of a VEGF plasmid did not produce angiogenesis in remote sites such as the liver, lung, heart, testes, or contralateral limb. This finding suggests that revascularization is restricted primarily to the area of ischemia (82).

To avoid limitations associated with intraarterial transgene delivery, most investigators use intramuscular injections. Expression of angiogenic peptides can be sustained in skeletal muscle cells and in cardiomyocytes after intramuscular plasmid delivery. Presumably, the protein is secreted from transduced muscle cells and diffuses to the local vasculature to promote angiogenesis. For example, intramuscular delivery of VEGF and HIF-1

plasmid constructs in a rabbit model of hind limb ischemia increased the formation of collateral vessels (83). This increase in collateral circulation improved calf blood pressure ratio, angiographic score, resting and maximal regional blood flow, and capillary density. These findings indicate angiogenic therapy has a beneficial effect on limb perfusion.

Angiogenic gene therapy has been used successfully in experimental models of myocardial ischemia. For example, in an ameroid model of porcine myocardial ischemia, intracoronary delivery of an adenovirus containing the cDNA for human fibroblast growth factor-5 increased the number of capillaries in the ischemic region and improved regional cardiac perfusion and function (84). In addition, adenoviral-mediated overexpression of VEGF-121 by direct intramyocardial injection improved regional cardiac perfusion and function in the same model (85). Plasmid transfection of VEGF and hepatocyte growth factor improved myocardial blood flow after intramyocardial delivery in a porcine ameroid model and in a rat model of myocardial infarction (86,87).

Gene therapy to induce angiogenesis may have deleterious effects. For example, sustained overexpression of VEGF by implantation of transduced myoblasts into the mouse heart resulted in formation of intramural vascular tumors resembling hemangiomas (88). Thus, investigators should proceed carefully in initiating gene therapy to promote angiogenesis in humans. Early clinical studies in patients with coronary artery disease and peripheral vascular disease are promising (89,90), but results must be interpreted cautiously in the absence of a control group.

PREVENTION OF POSTANGIOPLASTY RESTENOSIS

Restenosis after percutaneous peripheral arterial and coronary angioplasty is of great interest to basic research and clinical investigators and to cardiologists. The hypothesis that gene therapy might be used to treat postangioplasty restenosis was derived from early studies of cardiovascular gene therapy in which a double balloon catheter was used for gene transfer into the arterial wall (13,91). Arterial injury from the balloon causes excessive proliferation of neointimal smooth muscle cells, which helps in remodeling and contributes to postangioplasty restenosis. Thus, gene therapy for restenosis has been aimed at molecules involved in the signaling pathways that control proliferation and migration of smooth muscle cells. Studies in a rat model of balloon arterial injury have shown that adenovirus-mediated overexpression of the cyclin-dependent kinase inhibitor, p21, inhibits neointimal formation in the carotid artery (92). Similar results were obtained by overexpressing tissue inhibitor of matrix metalloproteinases 1, which inhibits degradation of the extracellular matrix and migration of smooth muscle cells (93).

eNOS helps to maintain vascular homeostasis, in part by reducing the rate of smooth muscle cell proliferation (94). The endothelium is denuded during mechanical injury of the artery, and transduction of cells of the vessel wall with eNOS may help restore nitric oxide production. Overexpression of eNOS by intraarterial delivery of an adenoviral vector or by seeding the arterial wall with syngeneic smooth muscle cells transduced by a retroviral vector inhibits smooth muscle cell proliferation and neointimal formation in the rat carotid artery after balloon injury (95,96). These findings show that vascular gene transfer may be used to study mechanisms that regulate proliferation of vascular cells in pathological states.

The extent of luminal narrowing after balloon injury depends not only on the rate of proliferation of smooth muscle cells but also on the extent of apoptosis of smooth muscle cells. Apoptosis of neointimal smooth muscle cells tends to counterbalance proliferation and to promote remodeling of the arterial wall (97); however, loss of neointimal smooth muscle cells may destabilize the lesion. Downregulation of the anti-apoptotic protein, Bcl-xL, in neointimal smooth muscles cells induces apoptosis and regression of vascular lesions (98). These results suggest that gene therapy to increase apoptosis of neointimal smooth muscle cell may be used to prevent or treat postangioplasty restenosis.

Strategies are being developed to target vectors precisely to the site of vascular injury. In a study of lesion-directed delivery of vectors, Gordon et al. (99) developed a retrovirus vector containing an antisense cyclin G1 construct that was targeted to the exposed collagen found at sites of balloon injury. When injected intraarterially or intravenously, the vector efficiently transduced neointimal cells after balloon injury. Moreover, a low dose of the collagen-targeted construct inhibited neointimal formation better than a untargeted construct. Novel targeting techniques should increase the efficacy, specificity, and safety of gene therapy.

MYOCARDIAL DYSFUNCTION

Gene transfer has been used to study the mechanisms of cardiac function in vivo. The sarcoplasmic reticulum plays a central role in Ca^{2+} movement during contraction and relaxation of cardiomyocytes. Expression of sarcoplasmic reticulum Ca^{2+} ATPase (SERCA2a) and Ca^{2+} uptake into the sarcoplasmic reticulum is reduced in failing hearts (100). The effects of adenoviral-mediated cardiac overexpression of SERCA2a have been examined in transition to heart failure in aortic-banded rats (101).

The virus was delivered into the aortic root via a catheter advanced from the cardiac apex while the aorta and pulmonary artery were cross-clamped for 30 s. Adenoviral gene transfer restored SERCA2a expression and ATPase activity and improved systolic and diastolic function of the left ventricle. Adenoviral-mediated overexpression of a β-adrenergic receptor kinase inhibitor prevented or reversed systolic dysfunction in a rabbit model of myocardial infarction, suggesting that β-adrenergic receptor desensitization and uncoupling contribute to heart failure in this model (102,103).

Reactive oxygen species play an important role in ischemic myocardial dysfunction. In a study in rabbits, adenoviral vectors carrying the ESCOD gene reduced cardiac damage resulting from a 30-min coronary occlusion (104). The adenoviral vector was targeted for hepatocytes, and the protein was released into the circulation from the liver. Intravenous infusion of heparin, which displaces ECSOD from its binding sites on the cell surface, increased the release of the protein, and subsequent infusion of protamine helped to relocate ECSOD to the heart. Transduction is easier with hepatocytes than with cardiomyocytes, and the use of hepatocytes minimizes adenoviral-mediated inflammation in the heart. Moreover, delivery of the transgene product to the myocardium could be more precisely timed by the use of heparin and protamine.

Acute viral myocarditis is a major cause of heart disease and can cause rapidly progressive heart failure. Immune activation, caused in part by release of pro-inflammatory cytokines, contributes to viral myocarditis. In vivo electroporation has been used (105) to transduce skeletal muscle cells in mice with plasmid constructs containing the cDNA for interleukin-1 (IL-1) receptor antagonist and interleukin-10 (IL-10). Treatment with plasmids containing cDNA for IL-1 receptor antagonist and IL-10, both of which are anti-inflammatory proteins, decreased the expression of myocardial cytokines and infiltration by inflammatory cells and improved survival in a mouse model of myocarditis.

Other methods of gene transfer have been used to study disease mechanisms and to treat other forms of heart disease. The effects of overexpression of eNOS during experimental cardiac transplantation were studied by injecting liposome–DNA complexes into the aortic root during cardioplegic arrest (106). Treatment with the eNOS gene reduced endothelial cell activation and leukocyte infiltration and extended graft survival without immunosuppression. Gene therapy administered during cardioplegic arrest may eventually help high-risk patients with heart failure maintain cardiac performance in the early postoperative period after bypass or heart valve surgery, when inotropic therapy is frequently required (107).

Vascular Diseases

HYPERTENSION

Because many antihypertensive drugs are relatively safe and effective, gene therapy for most patients with hypertension may not be used widely for many years. However, conventional drug therapy is frequently ineffective because of noncompliance; therefore, long-acting gene therapy may eventually become part of antihypertensive therapy.

Gene therapy to correct monogenic forms of hypertension will have only limited application, because hypertension is usually polygenic. A more likely goal for gene therapy to treat hypertension will be to reduce vascular resistance and arterial pressure by targeting genes that increase vascular resistance or code for a vasodilator product.

In several experimental models of hypertension, arterial pressure has been modestly reduced by transfer of genes encoding vasodilators including human kallikrein *(108)*. An alternative approach is to interfere with the function of genes whose products increase vascular resistance, such as components of the renin–angiotensin system. For example, systemic or central administration of antisense oligodeoxynucleotides to angiotensinogen or the angiotensin II type 1 (AT1) receptor reduces arterial pressure in hypertensive but not normotensive rats *(109–112)*. Injection of a long segment of cDNA (in antisense orientation) for angiotensinogen, the AT1 receptor, or ACE reduced arterial pressure in spontaneously hypertensive rats for several months *(113,114)*.

Generation of superoxide by angiotensin may contribute to hypertension *(115)*, perhaps in part by inactivation of nitric oxide. We have observed that gene transfer of ECSOD to spontaneously hypertensive rats significantly reduces arterial pressure *(116)*. Gene transfer of ECSOD is an attractive option for treating hypertension for two reasons. First, precise titration, such as that required when using potent vasodilators, may not be required. Second, gene trasfer of ECSOD may protect against vascular injury produced by superoxide and peroxynitrite.

PULMONARY HYPERTENSION

Inhalation of nitric oxide is effective in treating pulmonary hypertension. Studies in rats and mice have shown that inhalation of an adenovirus that expresses eNOS for the production of nitric oxide in the pulmonary circulation attenuates pulmonary hypertension caused by bleomycin *(117)*. Coupling gene transfer of eNOS with administration of a cGMP phosphodiesterase inhibitor is effective against pulmonary hypertension. In addition, inhalation of an adenovirus that expresses CGRP attenuates pulmonary hypertension in mice and inhibits pulmonary vascular remodeling *(118)*. Recent attention has been focused on early treatment of pulmonary hypertension, and the use of gene therapy in early stages of this deadly disease is of particular interest.

STROKE

After the initial injury of stroke, researchers believe that progressive injury occurs primarily in the ischemic "penumbra" at the junction of normal and ischemic tissue. If this hypothesis is correct, administration of appropriate drugs or the use of gene transfer may reduce tissue injury during the days after onset of cerebral ischemia.

An important concern in the use of gene transfer to treat stroke is whether cerebral ischemia might impair synthesis of the transduced protein. However, high levels of expression of the transgene product were observed in studies of the ischemic brain after gene transfer of a recombinant adenovirus carrying a reporter gene *(119)*. This finding indicates cerebral ischemia may not affect gene transfer and expression.

In a pioneering study, an intracerebroventricular injection of an adenovirus that overexpresses the IL-1 receptor antagonist reduces infarct size in rats when given before ischemia *(120)*. In addition, gene transfer of a glial cell line–derived neurotrophic factor *(121)* protected against ischemic infarction. Other candidates for gene therapy for stroke include the anti-inflammatory cytokine IL-10, antioxidants, and agents that inhibit apoptosis.

Subarachnoid hemorrhage accounts for about 10% of strokes and about 25% of deaths from stroke. Cerebral vasospasm, a major problem after subarachnoid hemorrhage, occurs several days after the initial hemorrhage and may often produce stroke. No treatment is currently available to prevent vasospasm after subarachnoid hemorrhage. We have reported that gene transfer of CGRP, which is an extremely potent cerebral vasodilator, prevents vasospasm after subarachnoid hemorrhage in rabbits *(45)*. In addition, gene transfer of eNOS may help prevent cerebral vasospasm.

DYSLIPIDEMIAS

Experimental and clinical studies have established a causal role for hypercholesterolemia in atherosclerotic heart disease. Gene transfer is a valuable tool for studying the pathways of lipoprotein metabolism in vivo, and this technique holds promise as a therapeutic agent in humans *(24)*. Adenoviral-mediated gene transfer to the liver is particularly suitable for determining the effects of overexpression of a transgene product on lipid metabolism. This technique has been used to study several genes believed to increase or decrease atherogenic lipoproteins, such as the genes for scavenger receptor B-1, phospholipid transfer protein, hepatic lipase, 7α-hydroxylase, and apolipoproteins (apo) *(24)*.

Hepatic expression of human apoE carried by an adenoviral vector resulted in rapid regression of atherosclerotic lesions in apoE-deficient mice *(122)*. Macrophages were not transduced in the study, so the investigators concluded that liver-derived apoE entered the circulation, was deposited in atherosclerotic vessels, and reduced atherosclerotic lesions. In another study in apoE-deficient mice, a single injection of a helper-dependent adenoviral vector containing the apoE gene resulted in lifetime correction of hypercholesterolemia *(123)*. The apoE-transduced mice were protected from atherosclerosis for 2.5 yr, which is the natural mouse lifespan.

FUTURE PERSPECTIVE

Since the first studies of gene transfer to blood vessels *(13,14)*, researchers have known that several obstacles must be overcome before gene transfer is widely accepted for use in patients. At least three basic requirements must be met before gene transfer becomes a viable option for the treatement of cardiovascular diseases. The first and most challenging requirement is the development of a safe and effective vector. A safe vector must elicit minimal immune responses and have few side effects. In addition, the vector should be easily produced and efficiently transduced, and the expression of the transgene product should be sufficiently long to enable the protein to produce the desired effect.

A second requirement of effective gene transfer is the delivery of the vector to a target tissue, with preferential expression in the target tissue. Targeting to specific or diseased tissues after intravascular injection of a vector and the use of tissue-specific promoters will allow greater efficacy and the use of lower doses of vectors. For many transgene products, regulation of expression will be necessary to avoid excessive concentrations of the product.

A third requirement is to identify the appropriate genes for gene transfer to achieve the desired effect. Even when an effective gene is identified, an alternative gene may prove to be more advantageous. For example, although gene transfer of CGRP, a potent vasodilator, prevents cerebral vasospasm after subarachnoid hemorrhage *(45)*, a transgene product that inhibits vasoconstriction may be more specific and therefore preferable to a vasodilator.

In summary, this chapter briefly reviews the principle and applications of gene transfer as a research tool and as therapy for cardiovascular diseases. The future of gene transfer and therapy depends on the development of safe and effective vectors, efficient and targeted delivery of vectors and, more fundamentally, a deeper understanding of the mechanisms of diseases and the functions of genes.

REFERENCES

1. Heistad DD. Gene transfer to blood vessels: a research tool and potential therapy. Am J Hypertens 2001;14:28S–32S.
2. Isner JM, Baumgartner I, Rauh G, et al. Treatment of thromboangiitis obliterans (Buerger's disease) by intramuscular gene transfer of vascular endothelial growth factor: preliminary clinical results. J Vasc Surg 1998;28:964–973.
3. Losordo DW, Vale PR, Symes JF, et al. Gene therapy for myocardial angiogenesis: Initial clinical results with direct myocardial injection of phVEGF *(165)* as sole therapy for myocardial ischemia. Circulation 1998;98:2800–2804.
4. Chu Y, Faraci F, Heistad DD. Gene therapy of hypertensive vascular injury. Curr Hypertens Reports 2000;2:92–97.
5. Phillips MI. Gene therapy for hypertension: the preclinical data. Hypertension 2001;38:543–548.
6. Mir L, Bureau M, Gehl J, et al. High-efficiency gene transfer into skeletal muscle mediated by electric pulses. Proc Natl Acad Sci USA 1999;96:4262–4267.
7. Liu D, Knapp JE. Hydrodynamics-based gene delivery. Curr Opin Mol Ther 2001;3:192–197.
8. Zhang G, Budker V, Williams P, Subbotin V, Wolff JA. Efficient expression of naked DNA delivered intraarterially to limb muscles of nonhuman primates. Hum Gene Ther 2001;12:427–438.
9. Liu F, Nishikawa M, Clemens PR, Huang L. Transfer of full-length Dmd to the diaphragm muscle of Dmd (mdx/mdx) mice through systemic administration of plasmid DNA. Mol Ther 2001;4:45–51.
10. Mulligan R. The basic science of gene therapy. Science 1993;260:926–932.
11. Macdonald C, Walker S, Watts M, Ings S, Linch DC, Devereux S. Effect of changes in expression of the amphotropic retroviral receptor PiT-2 on transduction efficiency and viral titer: implications for gene therapy. Hum Gene Ther 2000;11:587–595.
12. Barrette S, Douglas J, Orlic D, et al. Superior transduction of mouse hematopoietic stem cells with 10A1 and VSV-G pseudotyped retrovirus vectors. Mol Ther 2000;1:330–338.
13. Nabel EG, Plautz G, Boyce FM, Stanley JC, Nabel GJ. Recombinant gene expression in vivo within endothelial cells of the arterial wall. Science 1989;244:1342–1344.
14. Wilson JM, Birinyi LK, Salomon RN, Libby P, Callow AD, Mulligan RC. Implantation of vascular grafts lined with genetically engineered endothelial cells. Science 1989;244:1344–1346.
15. Naldini L. Lentiviruses as gene transfer agents for delivery to non-dividing cells. Curr Opin Biotechnol 1998;9:457–463.
16. Kafri T, Van Praag H, Ouyang I, et al. A packaging cell line for lentiviral vectors. J Virol 1999;73:576–584.
17. Gerard RD, Collen D. Adenovirus gene therapy for hypercholesterolemia, thrombosis and restenosis. Cardiovasc Res 1997;35:451–458.
18. Chu Y, Heistad DD. Gene transfer to blood vessels using adenoviral vectors. Methods Enzymol 2002;346:263-276.
19. Roelvink PW, Lizonova A, Lee JG, et al. The coxsackievirus-adenovirus receptor protein can function as a cellular attachment protein for adenovirus serotypes A, C, D, E, and F. J Virol 1998;72:7909–7915.

20. Wickham TJ, Mathias P, Cheresh DA, Nemerow GR. Integrins alpha v beta 3 and alpha v beta 5 promote adenovirus internalization but not virus attachment. Cell 1993;73:309–319.

21. Hong SS, Karayan L, Yournier J, Curiel DT, Boulanger P. Adenovirus type 5 fiber knob binds to MHC class I alpha2 domain at the surface of human epithelial and B lymphoblastoid cells. EMRB J 1997;16:2294–2306.

22. Chu Y, Heistad DD, Cybulsky MI, Davidson BL. Vascular cell adhesion molecule-1 augments adenovirus-mediated gene transfer. Arterioscler Thromb Vasc Biol 2001;21:238–242.

23. Heistad DD, and Faraci FM. Gene Therapy for Cerebral Vascular Disease. Stroke 1996;27:1688–1693.

24. Belalcazar M, Chan L. Somatic gene therapy for dislipidemias. J Lab Clin Med 1999;134:194–214.

25. Flotte TR, Carter BJ. Adeno-associated virus vectors for gene therapy. Gene Ther 1995;2:357–362.

26. Svensson EC, Marshall DJ, Woodard K, et al. Efficient and stable transduction of cardiomyocytes after intramyocardial injection or intracoronary perfusion with recombinant adeno-associated virus vectors. Circulation 1999;99:201–205.

27. Duan D, Yue Y, Engelhardt JF. Expanding AAV packaging capacity with trans-splicing or overlapping vectors: a quantitative comparison. Mol Ther 2001;4:383–391.

28. Cao L, Liu Y, During MJ, Xiao W. High-titer, wild-type free recombinant adeno-associated virus vector production using intron-containing helper plasmids. J Virol 2000;74:11456–11463.

29. Spragg DD, Alford DR, Greferath R, et al. Immunotargeting of liposomes to activated vascular endothelial cells: A strategy for site-selective delivery in the cardiovascular system. Proc Natl Acad Sci USA 1997;94:8795–8800.

30. Kibbe MR, Murdock A, Wickham T, Lizonova A, Kovesdi I, Nie S, Shears L, Billiar TR, Tzeng E. Optimizing cardiovascular gene therapy: increased vascular gene transfer with modified adenoviral vectors. Arch Surg 2000;135:191–197.

31. Lee LY, Zhou X, Polce DR, et al. Exogenous control of cardiac gene therapy: Evidence of regulated myocardial transgene expression after adenovirus and adeno-associated virus transfer of expression cassettes containing corticosteroid response element promoters. J Thorac Cardiovasc Surg 1999;118:26–35.

32. Smith-Arica JR, Williams JC, Stone D, Smith J, Lowenstein PR, Castro MG. Switching on and off transgene expression within lactotrophic cells in the anterior pituitary gland in vivo. Endocrinology 2001;142:2521–2532.

33. Von der Leyen HE, Gibbons GH, Morishita R, et al. Gene therapy inhibiting neointimal vascular lesion: In vivo transfer of endothelial cell nitric oxide synthase gene. Proc Natl Acad Sci 1995;92:1137–1141.

34. Newman KD, Dunn PF, Owens JW, et al. Adenovirus-mediated gene transfer into normal rabbit arteries results in prolonged vascular cell activation, inflammation and neointima hyperplasia. J Clin Invest 1995;96:2955–2965.

35. Morishige K, Shimokawa H, Eto Y, et al. Adenovirus-mediated transfer of dominant-negative Rho-kinase induces a regression of coronary atherosclerosis in pigs in vivo. Arterioscler Thomb Vasc Biol 2001;21:548–554.

36. Morishige K, Shimokawa H, Yamawaki T, et al. Local adenovirus-mediated transfer of C-type natriuretic peptide suppresses vascular remodeling in porcine coronary arteries in vivo. J Am Coll Card 2000;35:1040–1047.

37. Rios CD, Ooboshi H, Piegors DJ, Davidson BL, Heistad DD. Adenovirus-mediated gene transfer to normal and atherosclerotic vessels: A novel approach. Arterioscler Thromb Vasc Biol 1995;15:2241–2245.

38. Lopez JJ, Edelman ER, Stamler A, et al. Angiogenic Potential of Perivascularly Delivered aFGF in a Porcine Model of Chronic Myocardial Ischemia. Am J Physiol 1998;274: H930–H936.

39. Lamping KG, Rios CD, Chun JA, Ooboshi H, Davidson BL, Heistad DD. Intrapericardial Administration of Adenovirus for Gene Transfer. Am J Physiol 1997;41:H310–H317.

40. March KL, Woody M, Mehdi K, Zipes DP, Brantly M, Trapnell BC. Efficient in vivo catheter-based pericardial gene transfer mediated by adenoviral vectors. Clin Cardiol 1999;22:I23–I29.

41. Ooboshi H, Welsh MJ, Rios CD, Davidson BL, Heistad DD. Adenovirus-mediated gene transfer to cerebral blood vessels in vivo. Circ Res 1995;77:7–13.

42. Chen AFY, Jiang S, Crotty TB, et al. Effects of in vivo adventitial expression of recombinant endothelial nitric oxide synthase gene in cerebral arteries. Proc Natl Acad Sci USA 1997;94:12568–12573.

43. Ooboshi H, Chu Y, Rios CD, Faraci FM, Davidson BL, Heistad DD. Altered vascular function following adenovirus-mediated overexpression of endothelial nitric oxide synthase. Am J Physiol 1997;42:H265–H270.

44. Tsuitsui M, Chen AF, O'Brien T, Crotty TB, Katusic Z. Adventitial expression of recombinant eNOS gene restores NO production in arteries without endothelium. Arterioscler Thromb Vasc Biol 1998;18:1231–1241.

45. Toyoda K, Faraci FM, Watanabe J, et al. Gene transfer of CGRP prevents vasoconstriction after subarachnoid hemorrhage. Circ Res 2000;87:818–824.

46. Herz J, Gerard RD. Adenovirus-mediated transfer of low density lipoprotein receptor gene acutely accelerates cholesterol clearance in normal mice. Proc Natl Acad Sci USA 1993;90:2812–2816.

47. Kozarsky KF, McKinley DR, Austin LL, Raper SE, Stratford-Perricaudet LD, Wilson JM. In vivo correction of low density lipoprotein receptor deficiency in the Watanabe heritable hyperlipidemic rabbit with recombinant adenovirus. J Biol Chem 1994;269:13695–13702.

48. Spady DK, Cuthbert JA, Willard MN, Meidell RS. Adenovirus-mediated transfer of a gene encoding cholesterol 7α-hydroxylase into hamsters increases hepatic enzyme activity and reduces plasma total and low density lipoprotein cholesterol. J Clin Invest 1995;96:700–709.

49. Jaffe HA, Danel C, Longenecker G, et al. Adenovirus-mediated in vivo gene transfer and expression in normal rat liver. Nat Genet 1992;1:372–378.

50. Bergelson JM, Cunningham JA, Droguett G, et al. Isolation of a common receptor for coxsackie B virues and adenoviruses 2 and 5. Science 1997;275:1320–1323.

51. Ooboshi H, Rios CD, Chu Y, et al. Augmented Adenovirus-Mediated Gene Transfer to Atherosclerotic Vessels. Arterioscler Thromb Vasc Biol 1997;17:1786–1792.

52. Rekhter MD, Simari RD, Work CW, Nabel GJ, Nabel EG, Gordon D. Gene transfer into normal and atherosclerotic human blood vessels. Circ Res 1998;82:1243–1252.

53. Reynolds PN, Zinn KR, Gavrilyuk VD, et al. A targetable, injectable adenoviral vector for selective gene delivery to pulmonary endothelium in vivo. Molec Ther 2000;2: 562–578.

54. Guo ZS, Wang LH, Eisensmith RC, Woo SL. Evaluation of promoter strength for hepatic gene expression in vivo following adenovirus-mediated gene transfer. Gene Ther 1996;3:802–810.

55. Nicklin SA, Reynolds PN, Brosnan MJ, et al. Analysis of cell-specific promoters for viral gene therapy targeted at the vascular endothelium. Hypertension 2001;38:65–70.

56. Ni W, Egashira K, Kitamoto S, et al. New anti-monocyte chemoattractant protein-1 gene therapy attenuates atherosclerosis in apolipoprotein E-knockout mice. Circulation 2001;103:2096–2101.

57. Pradat PF, Kennel P, Maimi-Sadaoui S, et al. Continuous delivery of neurotrophin 3 by gene therapy has a neuroprotective effect in experimental models of diabetic and acrylamide neuropathies. Hum Gene Ther 2001;12:2237–2249.

58. Chang MW, Barr E, Seltzer J et al. Cytostatic gene therapy for vascular proliferative disorders with a constitutively active form of the retinoblastoma gene product. Science 1995;267:518–522.

59. Fang X, Weintraub NL, Rios CD, et al. Overexpression of human superoxide dismutase inhibits oxidation of low-density lipoprotein by endothelial cells. Circ Res 1998;82:1289–1297.

60. Brown MR, Miller FJ Jr, Li WG, et al. Overexpression of human catalase inhibits proliferation and promotes apoptosis in vascular smooth muscle cells. Circ Res 1999;85:524–533.

61. Rome JJ, Shayani V, Flugelman MY, et al. Anatomic barriers influence the distribution of in vivo gene transfer into the arterial wall: modeling with microscopic tracer particles and verification with recombinant adenoviral vector. Arterioscler Thromb 1994;14:148–161.

62. Chen AFY, O'Brien T, Tsutsui M, et al. Expression and function of recombinant endothelial nitric oxide synthase gene in canine basilar artery. Circ Res 1997;80:327–335.

63. Barr E, Carron J, Kalyuyeh AM, et al. Efficient catheter-mediated gene transfer into the heart using replication-defective adenovirus. Gene Ther 1994;1:51–58.

64. Ooboshi H, Rios CD, Heistad DD. Novel methods for adenovirus-mediated gene transfer to blood vessels in vivo. Mol Cell Biochem 1997;172:37–46.

65. Christenson SD, Lake KD, Ooboshi H, et al. Adenovirus-mediated gene transfer in vivo to cerebral blood vessels and perivascular tissue in mice. Stroke 1998;29:1411–1416.

66. Kirshenbaum LA. Adenovirus mediated-gene transfer into cardiomyocytes. Mol Cell Biochem 1997;172:13–21.

67. Hajar RJ, del Monte F, Matsui T, Rosenzweig A. Prospects for gene therapy for heart failure. Circ Res 2000;86:616–621.

68. Sakoda T, Kasahara N, Hamamori Y, Kedes L. A high-titer lentiviral production system mediates efficient transduction of differentiated cells including beating cardiac myocytes. J Mol Cell Cardiol 1999;31:2037–2047.

69. Datwyler DA, Eppenberger HM, Koller D, Bailey JE, Magyar JP. Efficient gene delivery into adult cardiomyocytes by recombinant Sindbis virus. J Mol Med 1999;77:859–864.

70. Guzman RJ, Lemarchand P, Crystal RG, Epstein SE, Finkel T. Efficient gene transfer into myocardium by direct injection of adenovirus vectors. Circ Res 1993;73:1202–1207.

71. French BA, Wojciech M, Geske RS, Bolli R. Direct in vivo gene transfer into porcine myocardium using replication-deficient adenoviral vectors. Circulation 1994;90:2414–2424.

72. Kypson, AP, Hendrickson, SC, Wilson K, et al. Adenovirus-mediated gene transfer of the β_2-adrenergic receptor to donor hearts enhances cardiac function. Gene Ther 1999;6:1298–1304.

73. Donahue JK, Kikkawa K, Thomas AD, Marban E, Lawrence JH. Acceleration of widespread adenoviral gene transfer to intact rabbit hearts by coronary perfusion with low calcium and serotonin. Gene Ther 1998;5:630–634.

74. Logeart D, Hatem SN, Rucker-Martin C, et al. Highly efficient adenovirus-mediated gene transfer to cardiac myocytes after single-pass coronary delivery. Hum Gene Ther 2000;11:1015–1022.

75. Hajar RJ, Schmidt U, Matsui T, et al. Modulation of ventricular function through gene transfer in vivo. Proc Natl Acad Sci USA 1998;95:5251–5256.

76. Shah AS, Lilly RE, Kypson AP, et al. Intracoronary adenovirus-mediated delivery and overexpression of the beta(2)-adrenergic receptor in the heart: prospects for molecular ventricular assistance. Circulation 2000;101:408–414.

77. Aoki M, Morishita R, Muraishi A, Moriguchi A, Sugimoto T, Maeda K, Dzau VJ, Kaneda Y, Higaki J, Ogihara T. Efficient in vivo gene transfer into the heart in the rat myocardial infarction model using the HVJ (hemagglutinating virus of Japan)-liposome method. J Mol Cell Cardiol 1997;29:949–959.

78. Fromes Y, Salmon A, Wang X, et al. Gene delivery to the myocardium by intrapericardial injection. Gene Ther 1999;6:683–688.

79. Shohet RV, Chen S, Zhou YT, et al. Echocardiographic destruction of albumin microbubbles directs gene delivery to the myocardium. Circulation 2000;101:2554–2556.

80. Baumgartner I, Isner JM. Somatic gene therapy in the cardiovascular system. Annu Rev Physiol 2001;63:427–450.

81. Losordo DW, Pickering JG, Takeshita S, et al. Use of the rabbit ear artery to serially assess foreign protein secretion after site-specific arterial gene transfer in vivo. Evidence that anatomic identification of successful gene transfer may underestimate the potential magnitude of transgene expression. Circulation 1994;89:785–792.

82. Takeshita S, Zheng LP, Brogi E, et al. Therapeutic angiogenesis. A single intraarterial bolus of vascular endothelial growth factor augments revascularization in a rabbit ischemic hind limb model. J Clin Invest 1994;93:662–670.

83. Vincent KA, Shyu K-G, Luo Y, et al. Angiogenesis Is Induced in a Rabbit Model of Hindlimb Ischemia by Naked DNA Encoding an HIF-1/VP16 Hybrid Transcription Factor. Circulation 2000;102:2255–2261.

84. Giordano FJ, Ping P, McKirnan MD, et al. Intracoronary gene transfer of fibroblast growth factor-5 increases blood flow and contractile function in an ischemic region of the heart. Nat Med 1996;2:534–539.

85. Mack CA, Patel SR, Schwarz EA, et al. Biologic bypass with the use of adenovirus-mediated gene transfer of the complementary deoxyribonucleic acid for vascular endothelial growth factor 121 improves myocardial perfusion and function in the ischemic porcine heart. J Thorac Cardiovasc Surg 1998;115:168–176.

86. Tio RA, Tkebuchava T, Scheuermann TH, et al. Intramyocardial gene therapy with naked DNA encoding vascular endothelial growth factor improves collateral flow to ischemic myocardium. Hum Gene Ther 1999;10:2953–2960.

87. Aoki M, Morishita R, Taniyama Y, et al. Angiogenesis induced by hepatocyte growth factor in non-infarcted myocardium and infarcted myocardium: up-regulation of essential transcription factor for angiogenesis, ets. Gene Ther 2000;7:417–427.

88. Lee RJ, Springer ML, Blanco-Bose WE, Shaw R, Ursell PC, Blau HM. VEGF gene delivery to myocardium: deleterious effects of unregulated expression. Circulation 2000;102:898–901.

89. Rosengart TK, Lee LY, Patel SR, et al. Angiogenesis gene therapy: phase I assessment of direct intramyocardial administration of an adenovirus vector expressing VEGF121 cDNA to

individuals with clinically significant severe coronary artery disease. Circulation 1999;100:468–474.

90. Baumgartner I, Pieczek A, Manor O, et al. Constitutive expression of phVEGF165 after intramuscular gene transfer promotes collateral vessel development in patients with critical limb ischemia. Circulation 1998;97:1114–1123.

91. Nabel EG, Plautz G, Nabel GJ. Site-specific gene expression in vivo by direct gene transfer into the arterial wall. Science 1990;249:1285–1288.

92. Chang MW, Barr E, Lu MM, Barton K, Leiden JM. Adenovirus-mediated over-expression of the cyclin/cyclin-dependent kinase inhibitor, p21 inhibits vascular smooth muscle cell proliferation and neointima formation in the rat carotid artery model of balloon angioplasty. J Clin Invest 1995;96:2260–2268.

93. Dollery CM, Humphries SE, McClelland A, Latchman DS, McEwan JR. Expression of tissue inhibitor of matrix metalloproteinases 1 by use of an adenoviral vector inhibits smooth muscle cell migration and reduces neointimal hyperplasia in the rat model of vascular balloon injury. Circulation 1999;99:3199–3205.

94. Garg UC, Hassid A. Nitric oxide-generating vasodilators and 8-bromo-cyclic guanosine monophosphate inhibit mitogenesis and proliferation of cultured rat vascular smooth muscle cells. J Clin Invest 1989;83:1774–1777.

95. Janssens S, Flaherty D, Nong Z, et al. Human endothelial nitric oxide synthase gene transfer inhibits vascular smooth muscle cell proliferation and neointima formation after balloon injury in rats. Circulation 1998;97:1274–1281.

96. Chen L, Daum G, Forough R, Clowes M, Walter U, Clowes AW. Overexpression of human endothelial nitric oxide synthase in rat vascular smooth muscle cells and in balloon-injured carotid artery. Circ Res 1998;82:862–870.

97. Khurana R, Martin JF, Zachary I. Gene therapy for cardiovascular disease: a case for cautious optimism. Hypertension 2001; 38:1210–1216.

98. Pollman MJ, Hall JL, Mann MJ, Zhang L, Gibbons GH. Inhibition of neointimal cell bcl-x expression induces apoptosis and regression of vascular disease. Nat Med 1998;4: 222–227.

99. Gordon EM, Zhu NL, Forney Prescott M, Chen ZH, Anderson WF, Hall FL. Lesion-targeted injectable vectors for vascular restenosis. Hum Gene Ther 2001;12:1277–1287.

100. Hajjar RJ, del Monte F, Matsui T, Rosenzweig A. Prospects of gene therapy for heart failure. Circ Res 2000;86:616–621.

101. Miyamoto MI, del Monte F, Schmidt U, et al. Adenoviral gene transfer of SERCA2a improves left-ventricular function in aortic-banded rats in transition to heart failure. Proc Natl Acad Sci USA 2000;97:793–798.

102. White DC, Hata JA, Shah HS, Glower DD, Lefkowitz RJ, Koch WJ. Preservation of β-adrenergic receptor signaling delays the development of heart failure after myocardial infarction. Proc Natl Acad Sci USA 2000;97:5428–5433.

103. Shah AS, White DC, Emani S, et al. In vivo ventricular gene delivery of a β-adrenergic receptor kinase inhibitor to the failing heart reverses cardiac dysfunction. Circulation 2001;103:1311–1316.

104. Li Q, Bolli R, Qui Li Q, et al. Gene therapy with extracellular superoxide dismutase protects conscious rabbits against myocardial infarction. Circulation 2001;103:1893–1898.

105. Nakano A, Matsumori A, Kawamoto S, et al. Cytokine gene therapy for myocarditis by in vivo electroporation. Hum Gene Ther 2001;12:1287–1297.

106. Iwata A, Sai S, Nitta Y, et al. Liposome-mediated gene transfection of endothelial nitric oxide synthase reduces endothelial activation and leukocyte infiltration in transplanted hearts. Circulation 2001;103:2753–2759.

107. Davidson MJ, Jones JM, Emani SM, et al. Cardiac gene delivery with cardiopulmonary bypass. Circulation 2001;104:131–133.

108. Wang C, Chao L, Chao J. Direct gene delivery of human tissue kallikrein reduces blood pressure in spontaneously hypertensive rats. J Clin Invest 1995;95:1710–1716.

109. Phillips MI, Wielbo D, Gyurko R. Antisense inhibition f hypertension: A new strategy for renin-angiotensin candidate genes. Kidney Int 1994;46:1554–1556.

110. Kotovich MJ, Gelband CH, Reaves P, et al. Reversal of hypertension of angiotensin II type 1 receptor antisense gene therapy in the adult SHR. Am J Physiol 1999;277: H1260–H1264.

111. Raizada MK, Katovich MJ, Wang H, et al. Is antisense gene therapy a step in the right direction in the control of hypertension? Am J Physiol 1999;45:H423–H432.

112. Phillips MI. Is gene therapy for hypertension possible? Hypertension 1999;33:8–13.

113. Phillips MI, Mohuczy-Dominiak D, Coffey M, et al. Prolonged reduction of high blood pressure with an in vivo, nonpathogenic, adeno-associated viral vector delivery at AT1-R mRNA antisense. Hypertension 1997;29:374–380.

114. Wang H, Katovich MJ, Gelband CH, et al. Sustained inhibition of angiotensin I-converting enzyme (ACE) expression and long-term antihypertensive action by virally mediated delivery of ACE antisense cDNA. Circ Res 1999;85:614–622.

115. Landmesser U, Harrison DG. Oxidation stress and vascular damage in hypertension. Coron Artery Dis 2001;12:455–461.

116. Chu Y, Iida S, Lund DD, et al. Gene transfer of extracellular superoxide dismutase reduces arterial pressure in spontaneously hypertensive rats: role of heparin-binding domain. Circ Res 2003;92:461–468.

117. Champion HC, Bivalacqua TJ, D'Souza FM, et al. Gene transfer of endothelial nitric oxide synthase to the lung of the mouse in vivo: Effect on agonist-induced and flow-mediated vascular responses. Circ Res 1999;84:1422–1432.

118. Champion HC, Bivalacqua TJ, Toyoda K, et al. In vivo gene transfer of prepro calcitonin gene-related peptide (CGRP) to the lung attenuates chronic hypoxia-induced pulmonary hypertension in the mouse. Circulation 2000;101:923–930.

119. Ooboshi H, Ibayashi S, Takada J, Yao H, Kitazono T, Fujishima M. Adenovirus-mediated gene transfer to ischemic brain. Ischemic flow threshold for transgene expression. Stroke 2001; 32:1043–1047.

120. Betz AL, Yang GY, Davidson BL. Attenuation of stroke size in rats using an adenoviral vector to induce overexpression of interleukin-1 receptor antagonist in brain. J Cereb Blood Flow Metab 1995;15:547–551.

121. Kitagawa H, Sasaki C, Sakai K, et al. Adenovirus-mediated gene transfer of glial cell line-derived neurotrophic factor prevents ischemic brain injury after transient middle cerebral artery occlusion in rats. J Cereb Blood Flow Metab 1999;19:1336–1344.

122. Tsukamoto K, Tangirala R, Chun SH, Pure E, Rader DJ. Rapid regression of atherosclerosis induced by liver-directed gene transfer of apoE in apoE-deficient mice. Arterioscler Thromb Vasc Biol 1999;19:2162–2170.

123. Kim IH, Jozkowicz A, Piedra PA, Oka K, Chan L. Lifetime correction of genetic deficiency in mice with a single injection of helper-dependent adenoviral vector. Proc Natl Acad Sci USA 2001;98:13282–13287.

5 Stem Cells and Progenitor Cells in Cardiovascular Disease

Jalees Rehman, MD and Keith L. March, MD, PhD

CONTENTS

INTRODUCTION

Few topics in cardiovascular research have generated as much promise and controversy as that of using stem cells or progenitor cells to improve cardiovascular function. The first section of this chapter will discuss general principles of stem and progenitor cell biology and therapy. The second section will illustrate these principles with specific stem and progenitor cell types used or proposed for use in the treatment of cardiovascular disease. Stem cell and progenitor cell therapy function in two ways in the treatment of cardiovascular disease. First, cell therapy is used to improve myocardial function by forming new myocardial tissue or modifying injured tissue in a process known as myocardial regeneration. Second, cell therapy is used to expand the coronary vasculature via vasculogenesis, angiogenesis, or arteriogenesis; the inclusive term angiogenesis will be used for this review.

Until recently, myocardial regeneration and angiogenesis were treated as two distinct therapeutic goals; however, recent studies suggest the two processes may be interrelated. For example, transdifferentiation may occur in relatively immature and mature cells *(1)*, and endothelial cells can transdifferentiate into cardiomyocytes *(2)*. Therefore, cell therapy designed to increase the local number of endothelial cells in blood vessels might also increase the number of cardiomyocytes. An interdependence between cell-induced myocardial regeneration and angiogenesis is suggested by the emerging concept that long-term engraftment and survival of delivered stem cells or progenitor cells depend on adequate vascularization of the transplanted cells.

STEM AND PROGENITOR CELL BIOLOGY AND THERAPY

Definitions

Stem cells are characterized by two key features. First, stem cells have the ability to differentiate into distinct cell lineages, a feature known as pluripotency. Second, stem cells have the ability to be propagated in an undifferentiated form (self-renewal or expandability) *(3)*. Many cells in the embryo meet these criteria; a less common population of stem cells can be found in adults. Although stem cells of embryonic origin can be propagated indefinitely, adult stem cells may have only a limited self-renewal capacity. Progenitor cells are not as clearly defined as stem cells. The term progenitor is used to denote cells that are committed to developing along a single pathway or cell lineage but are not fully differentiated into a mature phenotype.

Autologous (self) or heterologous (donor) cells can be used in stem or progenitor cell therapy. The advantage of autologous cells is the absence of cellular rejection and infections resulting from the transplantation of heterologous

From: *Contemporary Cardiology: Principles of Molecular Cardiology*
Edited by: M. S. Runge and C. Patterson © Humana Press Inc., Totowa, NJ

cells. However, the disadvantage of autologous cells is the possible necessity of ex vivo expansion to achieve adequate cell numbers for clinical use.

Mechanisms of Stem and Progenitor Cell Therapy

The ultimate goal of cardiac cell therapy with stem cells or progenitor cells is to improve myocardial function by either myocardial regeneration or angiogenesis. Stem and progenitor cells may improve cardiovascular function in at least three ways. The most commonly proposed mechanism is that local delivery or transplantation into target tissue may repopulate the diseased heart with healthy cells. In this mode, stem cells or progenitor cells are called "building blocks." Differentiation into the desired cell phenotype can occur either ex vivo (before transplantation into the heart) or in vivo after delivery. In either case, the cells integrate functionally into the surrounding parenchymal tissue under the control of local paracrine or mechanical signals.

The second mechanism by which stem cells and progenitor cells may improve myocardial function is by the endogenous production of growth factors and cytokines (4). These factors increase the local proliferation or survival of cells in the surrounding tissue after delivery. In this mode, stem and progenitor cells function as "factories."

Finally, stem cells or progenitor cells may serve as autologous or heterologous vectors for gene therapy (5). The use of a cell for gene therapy may increase gene targeting because of natural homing or migration mechanisms associated with cell populations.

If the therapeutic goal is to regenerate cardiomyocytes after myocardial infarction, the use of stem or progenitor cells as building blocks would be most appropriate because of the limited proliferative capacity of cardiomyocytes (6). In contrast, the use of stem and progenitor cells as factories or cell vectors for gene therapy may be desirable if the target tissue contains viable cells such as endothelial or smooth muscle cells that can respond appropriately by proliferating. Although each of the three mechanisms may be enhanced by the pluripotentiality and expandability of stem cells, mature differentiated somatic cells can act via these modes. However, few data are available that compare the efficacy of stem and progenitor cell transplantation with that of mature differentiated somatic cells.

Delivery of Stem and Progenitor Cells

Selection of an optimal method of delivery of stem or progenitor cells to a target area such as the heart is important in designing therapies for clinical use. Cells can be delivered into the intravascular or extravascular compartments.

The use of intravascular routes (both intravenous and intracoronary) for local delivery has been limited by poor cardiac extraction. However, this difficulty may be overcome with the delivery of particulate matter such as cells, which may get trapped in capillary beds of the myocardium. For this method of delivery to be effective, the trapped cells would have to emigrate into the myocardial tissue. This method of simple selective coronary delivery may be feasible and requires study.

Direct delivery of either drugs or genes into extravascular compartments is effective and results in minimal washout caused by bloodflow and maximal local delivery. Optimal cell delivery with this method has not yet been defined. Approaches for extravascular delivery include direct intramyocardial injection, retrograde coronary venous delivery under supraphysiologic pressure, and intrapericardial delivery. Intramyocardial injection of cells by either epicardial surgical techniques or endomyocardial catheter-based approaches has been used in many studies. Although delivery is direct and systemic loss is limited, this method appears to limit particulate dispersion because it is based on the creation of focal needle dissections in the myocardium.

Retrograde infusion of cells into the coronary veins, a novel percutaneous method of cardiac cell delivery, appears promising for delivery of gene (7) and protein (8) material. In contrast to intramyocardial needle injection, this method may achieve widespread myocardial distribution of particles and cells (Fig. 1) (9) because of the conduit properties of the branching venous circulation. These preexisting channels conduct injected material to sites at which hydrostatic pressure facilitates access to the extravascular parenchyma, presumably at the level of postcapillary venules. Although intrapericardial delivery is a highly efficient method for placement of genes and drugs around the vessels of the heart (10–12), the survival and effects of cells introduced into the pericardial sac are unknown. The intrapericardial route might be an effective means of delivery when the delivered cells would function as local secretory units.

Limited information is available for directly comparing the efficacy and feasibility of these delivery methods. In addition, long-term survival of cells placed with these delivery methods is unknown.

A distinctive approach to improving the tissue availability of stem or progenitor cells is to increase circulating or local cell numbers by systemic or local treatment with cytokines or chemokines or genes encoding such factors. Increasing the number of appropriate circulating cells may increase local angiogenesis, presumably by providing more cells to respond to endogenous local signals

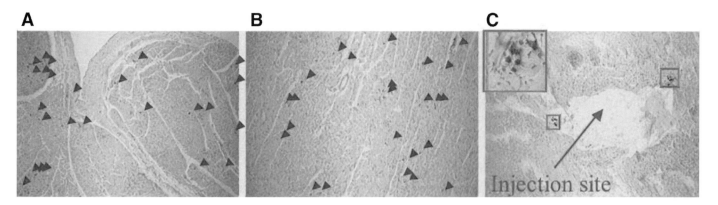

Fig. 1. Retrograde coronary venous delivery of Brd-U-labeled (blue arrows) adipose stromal cells into the porcine heart (endocardial area [**A**]; mid-myocardial area [**B**]) shows widespread distribution of infused cells within the myocardium. Direct myocardial injection creates an artificial channel in the myocardial tissue (**C**). Delivery of similar numbers of cells via retrograde delivery results in local placement of Brd-U-labeled cells around the injection site.

for cell homing to ischemic or injured tissue. Local delivery of chemokinetic signals may increase angiogenesis by recruiting functional cells from the intravascular compartment. Such approaches may partially obviate the need for delivery of exogenous cells. The discovery that extracardiac stem or progenitor cells repopulate the heart in adults *(13,14)* suggests that increasing the circulating stem and progenitor cell number or cardiac homing may be an effective form of endogenous noninvasive cell therapy.

Limitations of Stem and Progenitor Cell Therapy

To date, only preliminary studies have been conducted on the safety and feasibility of using stem and progenitor cell delivery to improve cardiac function in humans *(15,16)*. All published controlled studies showing a beneficial cardiovascular effect of stem and progenitor cell therapy have been conducted in animals. Although clinical trials of cell therapy are being conducted and appear to have promising results, data on long-term safety and efficacy will not be available in the near future. Furthermore, several other important issues need to be addressed before stem and progenitor cell therapy can be used in clinical settings.

In several studies, high numbers of cells have been used to achieve a beneficial effect on cardiac function; 1 to 10×10^6 transplanted cells have been used in mouse or rat models compared with up to 800×10^6 in clinical studies. The number of cells needed for a beneficial effect may affect the clinical feasibility of cell therapy. In addition, the survival time of implanted cells is unknown; therefore, persistence of initial improvements in cardiac function will need to be evaluated carefully.

To avoid rejection of transplanted cells, immunodeficient mice are often used in studies of cell therapy for angiogenesis and arteriogenesis. Baseline angiogenesis is abnormal in immunodeficient mice because of the importance of inflammation in angiogenesis and arteriogenesis; therefore, the benefits of cell therapy may not be replicated in non-immunodeficient recipients with normal angiogenesis.

Recent in vitro studies suggest that embryonic stem cells can fuse with bone marrow cells or cells of the central nervous system to create a hybrid polyploid cell with a mixed phenotype *(17,18)*. This hybrid phenotype is rare (seen in less than 0.1% of cells) and may not apply to all stem cells; however, cell fusion should be excluded when interpreting in vivo studies that demonstrate that transplanted stem cells are able to differentiate into desired mature cell types.

In autologous cell therapy, stem cells or progenitor cells derived from patients with cardiovascular disease may not have the same therapeutic potential as cells from healthy patients. Cell function may be reduced in patients with systemic diseases such as hyperlipidemia or diabetes. In most animal models of stem or progenitor cell transplantation, cells have been obtained from humans or animals without such comorbidities; therefore, the efficacy of autologous cell therapy in certain patient populations is unknown.

STEM AND PROGENITOR CELLS USED TO TREAT CARDIOVASCULAR DISEASE

This section will highlight characteristics of specific types of progenitor and stem cells that have been studied for use in promoting angiogenesis and myocardial regeneration. The classification scheme used here is based on the cell descriptions used by research groups active in this area and is not based on specific biological differences among the cell types. This scheme reflects the diversity of isolation, purification, and differentiation protocols used in cell therapy research. For example, cell therapy with unrefined bone marrow mononuclear cells (BM-MNC) comprises a broad mixture of hemangioblasts, hematopoietic stem cells, endothelial progenitor cells, and mature blood cells. The advantages of using a heterogeneous cell population are twofold. First, the likelihood of delivering multiple types of active angiogenic or myocardiogenic cells to the heart is increased. Second, the time delay required to purify cell populations is avoided. However, the use of a more purified hematopoietic stem cell population may improve efficacy per cell, even though fewer cells will be recovered after purification. Data directly comparing the efficacy and feasibility of the various cell types used in experimental cell therapy are limited.

Blood-Derived Endothelial-Like Cells and Endothelial Progenitor Cells

Blood-derived endothelial-like cells and endothelial progenitor cells (EPCs) have been studied extensively for their angiogenic properties. Blood-derived endothelial-like cells are isolated from peripheral blood by plating and attachment at high density on fibronectin. After culture in an endothelial growth medium that contains growth factors such as vascular endothelial growth factor (VEGF), cells express endothelial surface markers such as vascular/endothelial (VE)-cadherin and platelet/endothelial cell adhesion molecule (PECAM1) (CD31) and exhibit an endothelial phenotype (uptake of low-density lipoprotein [LDL] and binding of Ulex-lectin) (19–21). These cells are frequently called EPCs (19–21); however, most studies in which this type of cell population has been characterized have shown only an endothelial phenotype and not expression of specific progenitor or stem cell markers like AC133 in humans or Sca-1 in mice. The only stem/progenitor cell marker that has been described on peripheral blood–derived cultured cells is CD34, which can also be an endothelial cell marker (22). This method of attachment-based isolation without the use of surface markers for purification results in a cell population of endothelial-like cells, probably comprising a mixture of mature circulating endothelial cells (23), bone marrow–derived EPCs (24–26), and monocytic cells (27–30) that transdifferentiate into endothelial cells. The number of endothelial-like cells that can be obtained with this isolation method is about 1% of the plated mononuclear cells; however, this number can be increased by statin therapy via the nitric oxide/Akt pathway (31–33), by in vivo treat-

ment with recombinant VEGF (34), or by myocardial infarction (35). The clinical use of these observations has not been determined.

Studies in models of hindlimb or myocardial ischemia in immunodeficient rodents have shown that transplantation of about 10^6 peripheral blood-derived endothelial-like cells (20,21) increases angiogenesis. Blood-derived endothelial-like cells home preferentially to ischemic areas and incorporate into foci of neovascularization (20,21). The percentage of delivered cells that home to ischemic areas is unknown. Another potential application for blood-derived endothelial-like cells is the seeding of vessel grafts ex vivo to improve graft patency (36).

Because of their ability to home to ischemic areas, blood-derived endothelial-like cells have been used as vectors to carry the VEGF gene (37). The number of cells required to increase angiogenesis could be reduced 30-fold by using VEGF-transfected cells. Thus, peripheral blood-derived endothelial-like cells exert their angiogenic effect by producing growth factors such as VEGF (factory) and not by supplying additional cell material (building blocks). The length of survival time of these cells after transplantation is unknown. Some studies suggest that the population of blood–derived endothelial-like cells can be expanded before transplantation; however, data supported by direct cell counts have not confirmed this finding.

All published in vivo studies with peripheral blood-derived endothelial-like cells to date have been conducted in animals. Although the use of autologous cells in patients seems promising, 12 L of blood from a patient would be required to isolate enough cells to achieve an angiogenic effect (37). This amount of blood is not readily available in any clinical setting; thus, the use of drugs or genetic agents such as the VEGF gene to improve function in a smaller number of cells may be the only feasible clinical approach.

True EPCs constitute only a small subset of peripheral blood–derived endothelial-like cells. EPCs are characterized by expression of specific stem/progenitor cell markers such as AC133, c-kit, or Sca-1 and coexpression of endothelial markers such as VE-cadherin, PECAM1, or VEGF-receptor 2 (VEGFR-2, kinase insert domain receptor [KDR]). In addition, endothelial phenotype as characterized by LDL uptake is used to identify EPCs. Because mature endothelial cells and hematopoietic cells share several surface markers, the most rigorous definition of human EPCs in regard to surface expression is that of coexpression of AC133 and VE-cadherin (22). EPCs, although rare in peripheral blood (about 0.1% or less of total mononuclear cells), can be isolated in significantly

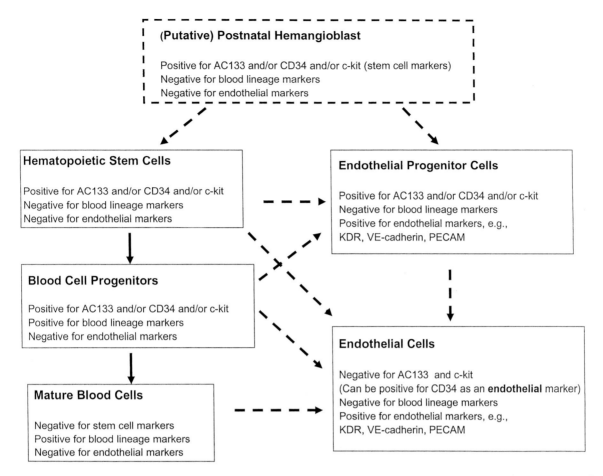

Fig. 2. Schematic representation of the development of endothelial cells and endothelial progenitor cells. Solid arrows indicate classic pathways that have been well established in vitro and in vivo. Dashed arrows represent pathways of cell differentiation that occur ex vivo. The extent to which these pathways contribute to the in vivo formation of endothelial cells is unknown.

higher numbers from umbilical cord blood or bone marrow *(38,39)*. EPCs can be mobilized into peripheral blood by in vivo exposure to granulocyte colony stimulating factor (G-CSF) *(38,40,41)*, or by vascular trauma *(42)* and statin therapy *(32)*. In some studies, CD34 has been used as the stem/progenitor cell marker for EPCs *(26,43)*. Although it has limited specificity, the CD34 marker appears to be a stem/progenitor cell marker and not just an endothelial marker when found in an environment that is rich in stem and progenitor cells like bone marrow, cord blood, or G-CSF–mobilized blood. In these environments, the expression of AC133 and CD34 significantly overlap *(38)*.

Of the EPCs isolated from stem/progenitor cell–rich environments such as bone marrow, it is not clear what percentage is derived from hemangioblasts, which are the putative common precursor of endothelial cells and hematopoietic cells, and what percentage is derived from AC133-positive hematopoietic cells, which have the ability to transdifferentiate into an endothelial phenotype (Fig. 2).

Transdifferentiation occurs in vitro *(39,40,43)* and in vivo *(24)*.

Human EPCs derived from G-CSF–mobilized peripheral blood can proliferate ex vivo. EPCs increased angiogenesis and prevented detrimental myocardial remodeling in a rat infarct model after intravenous injection of 2×10^6 CD34 positive cells into athymic rats *(44)*. Like peripheral blood–derived endothelial-like cells *(21)*, EPCs preferentially home to areas of ischemia *(44)*. Human umbilical cord blood–derived endothelial-like cells, which may have a high percentage of true EPCs, and peripheral blood–derived endothelial-like cells similarly increased angiogenesis in a nude rat model of hindlimb ischemia *(45)*. Although the distinction between EPCs and total peripheral blood–derived endothelial-like cells is of significant scientific interest, no data indicate superiority of EPCs over blood-derived endothelial cells; therefore, until comparative studies are conducted, the decision on which cell type to use for autologous therapy may be guided by factors such as the accessibility of cell type and the sufficiency of cell numbers.

Bone Marrow Mononuclear Cells and Hematopoietic Stem Cells

The mononuclear cell fraction of bone marrow comprises a broad mixture of hematopoietic stem cells, blood progenitor cells, mesenchymal stem cells, endothelial progenitor cells, and other mature differentiated cells. Injection of BM-MNC without purification or differentiation of cells allows for rapid autologous delivery without significant delay between cell extraction and delivery. Furthermore, a mixed cell population may be able to act through multiple synergistic modes and may allow for greater cell plasticity. In addition, the bone marrow may contain beneficial cells not yet identified as significant that may be lost during purification or differentiation steps. These advantages must be weighed against the disadvantages of using unrefined BM-MNC, which include a possible reduction in efficacy because of the proportion of nonactive cells. Several studies have assessed the effects of BM-MNC on cardiovascular function. In a rabbit ischemic hindlimb model, direct injection of about 7×10^6 autologous BM-MNC into the hindlimb resulted in incorporation of fluorescently labeled mononuclear cells into a capillary network and improved hindlimb perfusion as shown by laser Doppler studies, angiography, and histology (46). In pigs, fresh crude autologous bone marrow aspirate was injected intramyocardially without isolation of BM-MNC into sites of chronic ameroid-induced ischemia (47). Cardiac function significantly improved and angiogenesis increased over 3–4 wk. Similar findings were obtained by injection of autologous BM-MNC into pigs with acute myocardial ischemia (48). Furthermore, bone marrow cells in both pig studies secreted angiogenic cytokines in vitro, suggesting that the in vivo benefits may have resulted in part from increased production of growth factors. Labeling studies of BM-MNC cells suggested that the transplanted cells differentiated primarily into endothelial cells and not into cardiomyocytes (48).

The formation of cardiomyocytes by bone marrow cells was assessed in a rat infarction model. Transplantation of freshly isolated bone marrow cells into rat myocardium after infarction increased angiogenesis, but no evidence of cardiomyocyte formation was seen. However, cultured bone marrow–derived mesenchymal stem cells differentiated into cardiomyocytes after exposure to 5-azacytidine (49), which will be discussed in a later section. One approach for potentially increasing the therapeutic efficacy of bone marrow cells while retaining the use of a mixture of

stem and progenitor cells is to isolate cells that are positive for a broad stem/progenitor cell marker while excluding cells that have markers specific for blood cell lineages. This method was used in a study in which labeled enhanced green fluorescent protein (EGFP) bone marrow cells positive for the stem cell marker, c-kit, and negative for specific lineage markers were transplanted into gender-mismatched mice. About 10^4–10^5 c-kit–positive cells were injected into female mice in the area of infarcted myocardium (50). Evaluation of the expression of EGFP and the coexpression of specific differentiation markers showed in vivo differentiation of the cells into cardiomyocytes, endothelial cells, and smooth muscle cells in the area of the myocardial scar after only 9 d. In addition, transplanted cells proliferated in vivo as confirmed by BrdU uptake. Repopulation of the myocardial scar with proliferating cells was accompanied by improved ventricular function.

Another hematopoietic cell type in the bone marrow that has recently been characterized is the side population, as defined by flow cytometry. The side population, which makes up only 0.05% of all bone marrow cells, is described as potent hematopoietic stem cells that are negative for the CD34 marker but positive for c-kit. Bone marrow transplantation of 2000 side population cells into lethally irradiated recipient mice resulted in reconstitution of myocardial tissue and stable engraftment. After transplantation the recipient mice underwent coronary artery ligation. At 2–4 wk after infarction, transplanted side population–derived cells had circulated to the heart and differentiated into either endothelial cells (prevalence, 3%) or cardiomyocytes (prevalence, 0.02%) (51).

A recent case report demonstrated the clinical feasibility of bone marrow mononuclear cell transplantation into the heart. In this report, a patient with coronary artery disease received 1.2×10^7 autologous bone marrow mononuclear cells via an intracoronary catheter. Delivery was well tolerated, and myocardial perfusion and left ventricular function improved at 10 wk after the infusion and stent placement.

Cardiac availability of bone marrow mononuclear cells or hematopoietic stem cells may be increased by injecting cell-mobilizing agents. Subcutaneous injection of rats with the mobilizing agents, stem cell factor and G-CSF, significantly improved survival after myocardial infarction (50). Histologic analysis showed increased repopulation of the infarcted area with proliferating cells in treated animals. In a clinical study, subcutaneous injection of granulocyte macrophage–colony stimulating factor (GM-CSF), which mobilizes BM-MNC and hematopoietic stem cells, improved collateral formation in patients with coronary artery disease when compared with placebo (52); the cellular mechanism of this effect is not known.

Mesenchymal Stem Cells

Mesenchymal stem cells, also referred to as marrow stromal cells, are bone marrow-derived cells that are distinct from bone marrow–derived hematopoietic stem cells. For example, CD34 is expressed on hematopoietic stem cells but not on mesenchymal stem cells. In addition, mesenchymal stem cells belong to the adherent cell fraction of bone marrow cells when cultured on a plastic dish, whereas hematopoietic stem cells do not attach. However, mesenchymal stem cells are true stem cells because they can differentiate into several mature cell phenotypes (adipocytes, chondrocytes, smooth muscle cells, cardiac muscle cells, and others), and they can be propagated in an undifferentiated form (53–55). Murine mesenchymal stem cells can differentiate into cardiomyocytes in vitro (56) and in vivo (57), and they can survive long term in the mouse heart (57).

In a study in rats, autologous bone marrow–derived cells were treated ex vivo with 5-azacytidine, labeled with BrdU, and delivered via direct injection into a cryoinjury scar. The scar area showed evidence of increased capillary density and BrdU-positive cells with a cardiomyocyte phenotype (49). In addition, left ventricular function improved in treated rats.

A new cell type called multipotent adult progenitor cells (MAPCs) has recently been isolated from human bone marrow. MAPCs differ from other mesenchymal stem cells because they can proliferate in low levels of serum in growth medium (58). MAPCs can differentiate into vascular endothelial cells in vitro and into tumor cells in vivo. Because MAPCs can be expanded in vitro for at least 80 population doublings, significant numbers of cells can be generated over time. MAPCs are being evaluated in ischemic models.

Myoblasts

Skeletal myoblasts, also called skeletal muscle satellite cells, are committed but undifferentiated cells in the skeletal muscle tissue that can enter the mitotic cycle and differentiate into myocytes, thus allowing for skeletal muscle regeneration (59). Skeletal myoblasts obtained from a muscle biopsy in humans can proliferate ex vivo in culture (15). Because of their accessibility and expandability, myoblasts may be a clinically feasible option for autologous cell therapy. Skeletal myoblasts can survive for at least 3 mo after transplantation into the heart (60). After injection of myoblasts into a myocardial injury scar in animals, the transplanted cells differentiate into skeletal

myocytes as shown by expression of skeletal myosin heavy chain (61) and myotube formation (62). Although transplanted cells do not usually express cardiac specific markers such as cardiac myosin heavy chain, they can be stimulated to contract ex vivo, which suggests they are functional myocytes (61). Some studies suggest that a subpopulation of engrafted myoblasts have a cardiac phenotype; however, this suggestion has not been confirmed by expression of cardiac specific markers (62,63). In a comparative study, fetal cardiomyocytes (5×10^6 cells), nonautologous skeletal myoblasts (5×10^6 cells), or control medium was injected into a myocardial infarction scar in rats (64). After immunosuppressive treatment, left ventricular function and histology were assessed at 4 wk. Left ventricular ejection fraction improved similarly in both groups treated with cell therapy compared with the control group. The myoblast grafts stained positive for skeletal muscle myosin heavy chain after 1 mo. Cardiac tissue surrounding the graft stained positive for connexin 43, whereas the skeletal myoblast graft did not express this marker. These findings suggest that improvement of cardiac function was related to electromechanical coupling of the graft to the cardiac tissue. Although the mechanism is unknown, myoblast transplantation improves cardiac function by reducing ventricular remodeling and increasing systolic and diastolic function (65–67).

A novel application of myoblast cell therapy is the use of gene-transfected myoblasts. VEGF-transfected myoblasts improve ventricular function and increase capillary density (68). The two therapeutic goals of myocardial regeneration and angiogenesis can be achieved concomitantly by using myoblasts as autologous cell vectors. The clinical feasibility and safety of autologous myoblast therapy has been shown in a case report in which 800×10^6 myoblasts were obtained via muscle biopsy under local anesthesia from a patient with heart failure. Cells were grown in vitro for 2 wk and then implanted into a myocardial infarction scar during a coronary artery bypass graft operation. Follow-up imaging showed new, viable tissue in the scar area after 5 mo. This report, although only in a single patient, indicates the clinical applicability of cardiac myoblast cell therapy, and trials for evaluating this approach are underway.

Adipose Stromal Cells

The discovery of pluripotent cells in the adipose tissue (69) has provided a new source of cells for myocardial regeneration and angiogenesis. The pluripotent cells, which are found in the stromal or non-adipocyte fraction of adipose tissue, can differentiate in vitro into adipocytes, chondrocytes (69), and other cell types. Adipose stromal cells can easily be obtained in large numbers—at least 1–2 million cells/5–10 g of subcutaneous adipose tissue after 5 d of culture *(70)*—and can proliferate extensively in vitro. Liposuction often yields 1000–3000 g of adipose tissue; therefore, 1 to 3×10^9 cells may be readily obtained from subcutaneous adipose tissue. Human safety and feasibility studies for cardiac cell therapy have used fewer than 10^9 cells; therefore, pluripotent adipose stromal cells for autologous cell therapy may be clinically feasible with limited or no in vitro expansion. Adipose stromal cells express smooth muscle alpha-actin after 4–5 d in culture, which suggests that adipose stromal cells either contain significant numbers of smooth muscle cells/myofibroblasts or can differentiate into a smooth muscle cell/myofibroblast phenotype *(70)*. In addition, adipose stromal cells secrete significant amounts of angiogenic growth factors such as VEGF *(70)*. Preliminary data have shown that adipose stromal cells can be transfected successfully with mammalian expression plasmids (J Rehman, MD, and KL March, MD, PhD, unpublished data, 2003). Because of the possible heterogeneity of the adipose stromal fraction, the term stem cells should not be applied until further characterization of the cell fraction. Nevertheless, the adipose stromal fraction contains large numbers of easily expandable, pluripotent cells that secrete angiogenic growth factors. Native or transfected adipose stromal cells could be used for autologous cell therapy to induce angiogenesis and myocardial regeneration. These cells are being studied in ischemic models in animals.

Embryonic Stem Cells

The primary advantage of embryonic stem cells is their virtual immortality and their ability to be propagated in an undifferentiated state without losing the capacity to differentiate into several cell lineages *(71)*. Both animal and human embryonic stem cells have been evaluated in the treatment of cardiovascular disease. Murine embryonic stem cells can differentiate into vascular progenitor cells *(72)* and cardiomyocytes *(73)*, and can survive long-term as differentiated cardiomyocytes in the mouse heart *(73)*. Human embryonic stem cells can differentiate in vitro into cardiomyocytes *(74)* as evidenced by expression of cardiac specific genes and the ability to contract spontaneously. In addition, human embryonic stem cells respond to chronotropic agents such as isoproterenol by increasing contraction frequency. When cultured in an endothelial growth medium, human embryonic stem cells differentiate into an endothelial phenotype and express endothelial markers such as VE-cadherin, PECAM1, or VEGFR-2 and internalize acetylated LDL. Cells isolated for PECAM1 expression form endothelial cord-like structures in vitro and participate in the formation of capillaries when transplanted into immunodeficient mice *(75)*.

Two major concerns are associated with the use of human embryonic stem cells in treating cardiac disease. Ethical issues are the most significant obstacle to using embryonic stem cells in a clinical setting. According to Green *(76)*, these concerns can be summarized in four questions: (1) May we ever intentionally destroy a human embryo? (2) May we benefit from the destruction of human embryos by others? (3) May we create a human embryo for the purpose of destroying it? (4) May we clone human embryos? A universally acceptable answer to these questions has not been proposed. Moreover, society has yet to determine whether human embryonic stem cells should be used in the clinical setting.

The second concern associated with embryonic stem cell use is the possibility of allotransplantation reactions. Because embryonic stem cells are derived from heterologous sources, an immune rejection response may develop in the recipient. Another concern, only theoretical at this point because of lack of supporting data, is that transplantation of immortal cells could result in tumor formation.

CONCLUSIONS

The use of local or systemic cellular approaches for the treatment of cardiovascular disease is an important therapeutic concept that needs further development and investigation. Much remains to be determined about the optimal cell types and methods before cellular approaches become an integral part of clinical medicine. Mature differentiated cells have been used for cell therapy with an efficacy similar to that seen with stem cells and progenitor cells *(77–80)*. Cell-based therapies have significant potential to address the substantial morbidities seen in patients with impaired cardiac function. As with other therapies that require biologic and mechanical considerations, the details such as harvesting, selection, infusion, and potency of cells will determine whether the transition can be made from promise to patient.

REFERENCES

1. Weissman IL, Anderson DJ, Gage F. Stem and progenitor cells: origins, phenotypes, lineage commitments, and transdifferentiations. Annu Rev Cell Dev Biol 2001;17:387–403.
2. Condorelli G, Borello U, De Angelis L, et al. Cardiomyocytes induce endothelial cells to trans-differentiate into cardiac muscle: implications for myocardium regeneration. Proc Natl Acad Sci USA 2001;98:10733–10738.
3. Marshak DR, Gottlieb D, Gardner RL. Introduction: Stem Cell Biology. In: Marshak DR, Gottlieb D, Gardner RL, eds. Stem Cell Biology. Cold Springs, New York: Cold Springs Harbor Laboratory Press; 2001:1–16.

4. Majka M, Janowska-Wieczorek A, Ratajczak J, et al. Numerous growth factors, cytokines, and chemokines are secreted by human CD34(+) cells, myeloblasts, erythroblasts, and megakaryoblasts and regulate normal hematopoiesis in an autocrine/paracrine manner. Blood 2001;97:3075–3085.

5. Nabel EG. Stem cells combined with gene transfer for therapeutic vasculogenesis: magic bullets? Circulation 2002;105:672–674.

6. Soonpaa MH, Field LJ. Survey of studies examining mammalian cardiomyocyte DNA synthesis. Circ Res 1998;83:15–26.

7. Boekstegers P, von Degenfeld G, Giehrl W, et al. Myocardial gene transfer by selective pressure-regulated retroinfusion of coronary veins. Gene Ther 2000;7:232–240.

8. Herity NA, Lo ST, Oei F, et al. Selective regional myocardial infiltration by the percutaneous coronary venous route: A novel technique for local drug delivery. Catheter Cardiovasc Interv 2000;51:358–363.

9. Hou DM, Cates P, Bekkers S, et al. Efficient myocardial delivery of microspheres and endothelial cells via selective retrograde coronary venous delivery [abstract]. J Am Coll Cardiol 2002;39:76A.

10. March KL, Woody M, Mehdi K, Zipes DP, Brantly M, Trapnell BC. Efficient in vivo catheter-based pericardial gene transfer mediated by adenoviral vectors. Clin Cardiol 1999;22:I23–I29.

11. Stoll HP, Carlson K, Keefer LK, Hrabie JA, March KL. Pharmacokinetics and consistency of pericardial delivery directed to coronary arteries: direct comparison with endoluminal delivery. Clin Cardiol 1999;22:I10–I16.

12. Hou D, Rogers PI, Toleikis PM, Hunter W, March KL. Intrapericardial paclitaxel delivery inhibits neointimal proliferation and promotes arterial enlargement after porcine coronary overstretch. Circulation 2000;102:1575–1581.

13. Laflamme MA, Myerson D, Saffitz JE, Murry CE. Evidence for cardiomyocyte repopulation by extracardiac progenitors in transplanted human hearts. Circ Res 2002;90:634–640.

14. Quaini F, Urbanek K, Beltrami AP, et al. Chimerism of the transplanted heart. N Engl J Med 2002;346:5–15.

15. Menasche P, Hagege AA, Scorsin M, et al. Myoblast transplantation for heart failure. Lancet 2001;357:279–280.

16. Strauer BE, Brehm M, Zeus T, et al. Intracoronary, human autologous stem cell transplantation for myocardial regeneration following myocardial infarction. Dtsch Med Wochenschr 2001;126:932–938.

17. Terada N, Hamazaki T, Oka M, et al. Bone marrow cells adopt the phenotype of other cells by spontaneous cell fusion. Nature 2002;416:542–545.

18. Ying QL, Nichols J, Evans EP, Smith AG. Changing potency by spontaneous fusion. Nature 2002;416:545–548.

19. Asahara T, Murohara T, Sullivan A, et al. Isolation of putative progenitor endothelial cells for angiogenesis. Science 1997;275:964–967.

20. Kalka C, Masuda H, Takahashi T, et al. Transplantation of ex vivo expanded endothelial progenitor cells for therapeutic neovascularization. Proc Natl Acad Sci USA 2000;97:3422–3427.

21. Kawamoto A, Gwon HC, Iwaguro H, et al. Therapeutic potential of ex vivo expanded endothelial progenitor cells for myocardial ischemia. Circulation 2001;103:634–637.

22. Rafii S. Circulating endothelial precursors: mystery, reality, and promise. J Clin Invest 2000;105:17–19.

23. Mancuso P, Burlini A, Pruneri G, Goldhirsch A, Martinelli G, Bertolini F. Resting and activated endothelial cells are increased in the peripheral blood of cancer patients. Blood 2001;97:3658–3661.

24. Crosby JR, Kaminski WE, Schatteman G, et al. Endothelial cells of hematopoietic origin make a significant contribution to adult blood vessel formation. Circ Res 2000;87:728–730.

25. Lin Y, Weisdorf DJ, Solovey A, Hebbel RP. Origins of circulating endothelial cells and endothelial outgrowth from blood. J Clin Invest 2000;105:71–77.

26. Shi Q, Rafii S, Wu MH, et al. Evidence for circulating bone marrow-derived endothelial cells. Blood 1998;92:362–367.

27. Fernandez Pujol B, Lucibello FC, Gehling UM, et al. Endothelial-like cells derived from human CD14 positive monocytes. Differentiation 2000;65:287–300.

28. Fernandez Pujol B, Lucibello FC, Zuzarte M, Lutjens P, Muller R, Havemann K. Dendritic cells derived from peripheral monocytes express endothelial markers and in the presence of angiogenic growth factors differentiate into endothelial-like cells. Eur J Cell Biol 2001;80:99–110.

29. Harraz M, Jiao C, Hanlon HD, Hartley RS, Schatteman GC. CD34- blood-derived human endothelial cell progenitors. Stem Cells 2001;19:304–312.

30. Schmeisser A, Garlichs CD, Zhang H, et al. Monocytes coexpress endothelial and macrophagocytic lineage markers and form cord-like structures in Matrigel under angiogenic conditions. Cardiovasc Res 2001;49:671–680.

31. Llevadot J, Murasawa S, Kureishi Y, et al. HMG-CoA reductase inhibitor mobilizes bone marrow—derived endothelial progenitor cells. J Clin Invest 2001;108:399–405.

32. Dimmeler S, Aicher A, Vasa M, et al. HMG-CoA reductase inhibitors (statins) increase endothelial progenitor cells via the PI 3-kinase/Akt pathway. J Clin Invest 2001;108:391–397.

33. Vasa M, Fichtlscherer S, Adler K, et al. Increase in circulating endothelial progenitor cells by statin therapy in patients with stable coronary artery disease. Circulation 2001; 103:2885–2890.

34. Asahara T, Takahashi T, Masuda H, et al. VEGF contributes to postnatal neovascularization by mobilizing bone marrow-derived endothelial progenitor cells. Embo J 1999;18:3964–3972.

35. Shintani S, Murohara T, Ikeda H, et al. Mobilization of endothelial progenitor cells in patients with acute myocardial infarction. Circulation 2001;103:2776–2779.

36. Kaushal S, Amiel GE, Guleserian KJ, et al. Functional small-diameter neovessels created using endothelial progenitor cells expanded ex vivo. Nat Med 2001;7:1035–1040.

37. Iwaguro H, Yamaguchi J, Kalka C, et al. Endothelial progenitor cell vascular endothelial growth factor gene transfer for vascular regeneration. Circulation 2002;105:732–738.

38. Peichev M, Naiyer AJ, Pereira D, et al. Expression of VEGFR-2 and AC133 by circulating human CD34(+) cells identifies a population of functional endothelial precursors. Blood 2000; 95:952–958.

39. Quirici N, Soligo D, Caneva L, Servida F, Bossolasco P, Deliliers GL. Differentiation and expansion of endothelial cells from human bone marrow CD133(+) cells. Br J Haematol 2001;115:186–194.

40. Gehling UM, Ergun S, Schumacher U, et al. In vitro differentiation of endothelial cells from AC133-positive progenitor cells. Blood 2000;95:3106–3112.

41. Takahashi T, Kalka C, Masuda H, et al. Ischemia- and cytokine-induced mobilization of bone marrow-derived endothelial progenitor cells for neovascularization. Nat Med 1999;5:434–438.

42. Gill M, Dias S, Hattori K, et al. Vascular trauma induces rapid but transient mobilization of VEGFR2(+)AC133(+) endothelial precursor cells. Circ Res 2001;88:67–74.

43. Kang HJ, Kim SC, Kim YJ, et al. Short-term phytohaemagglutinin-activated mononuclear cells induce endothelial progenitor cells

from cord blood CD34+ cells. Br J Haematol 2001; 113:962–969.

44. Kocher AA, Schuster MD, Szabolcs MJ, et al. Neovascularization of ischemic myocardium by human bone-marrow-derived angioblasts prevents cardiomyocyte apoptosis, reduces remodeling and improves cardiac function. Nat Med 2001; 7:430–436.

45. Murohara T, Ikeda H, Duan J, et al. Transplanted cord blood-derived endothelial precursor cells augment postnatal neovascularization. J Clin Invest 2000;105:1527–1536.

46. Shintani S, Murohara T, Ikeda H, et al. Augmentation of postnatal neovascularization with autologous bone marrow transplantation. Circulation 2001;103:897–903.

47. Fuchs S, Baffour R, Zhou YF, et al. Transendocardial delivery of autologous bone marrow enhances collateral perfusion and regional function in pigs with chronic experimental myocardial ischemia. J Am Coll Cardiol 2001;37:1726–1732.

48. Kamihata H, Matsubara H, Nishiue T, et al. Implantation of bone marrow mononuclear cells into ischemic myocardium enhances collateral perfusion and regional function via side supply of angioblasts, angiogenic ligands, and cytokines. Circulation 2001;104:1046–1052.

49. Tomita S, Li RK, Weisel RD, et al. Autologous transplantation of bone marrow cells improves damaged heart function. Circulation 1999;100:II247–II256.

50. Orlic D, Kajstura J, Chimenti S, et al. Mobilized bone marrow cells repair the infarcted heart, improving function and survival. Proc Natl Acad Sci USA 2001;98:10344–10349.

51. Jackson KA, Majka SM, Wang H, et al. Regeneration of ischemic cardiac muscle and vascular endothelium by adult stem cells. J Clin Invest 2001;107:1395–1402.

52. Seiler C, Pohl T, Wustmann K, et al. Promotion of collateral growth by granulocyte–macrophage colony-stimulating factor in patients with coronary artery disease: a randomized, double-blind, placebo-controlled study. Circulation 2001;104:2012–2017.

53. Pittenger MF, Marshak DR. Mesenchymal Stem Cells of Human Adult Bone Marrow. In: Marshak DR, Gottlieb D, Gardner RL, eds. Stem Cell Biology. Cold Springs, New York: Cold Springs Harbor Laboratory Press; 2001:349-374.

54. Pittenger MF, Mackay AM, Beck SC, et al. Multilineage potential of adult human mesenchymal stem cells. Science 1999;284:143–147.

55. Minguell JJ, Erices A, Conget P. Mesenchymal stem cells. Exp Biol Med 2001;226:507–520.

56. Fukuda K. Development of regenerative cardiomyocytes from mesenchymal stem cells for cardiovascular tissue engineering. Artif Organs 2001;25:187–193.

57. Toma C, Pittenger MF, Cahill KS, Byrne BJ, Kessler PD. Human mesenchymal stem cells differentiate to a cardiomyocyte phenotype in the adult murine heart. Circulation 2002;105:93–98.

58. Reyes M, Dudek A, Jahagirdar B, Koodie L, Marker PH, Verfaillie CM. Origin of endothelial progenitors in human postnatal bone marrow. J Clin Invest 2002;109:337–346.

59. Campion DR. The muscle satellite cell: a review. Int Rev Cytol 1984;87:225–251.

60. Koh GY, Klug MG, Soonpaa MH, Field LJ. Differentiation and long-term survival of C2C12 myoblast grafts in heart. J Clin Invest 1993;92:1548–1554.

61. Murry CE, Wiseman RW, Schwartz SM, Hauschka SD. Skeletal myoblast transplantation for repair of myocardial necrosis. J Clin Invest 1996;98:2512–2523.

62. Atkins BZ, Lewis CW, Kraus WE, Hutcheson KA, Glower DD, Taylor DA. Intracardiac transplantation of skeletal myoblasts yields two populations of striated cells in situ. Ann Thorac Surg 1999;67:124–129.

63. Chiu RC, Zibaitis A, Kao RL. Cellular cardiomyoplasty: myocardial regeneration with satellite cell implantation. Ann Thorac Surg 1995;60:12–18.

64. Scorsin M, Hagege A, Vilquin JT, et al. Comparison of the effects of fetal cardiomyocyte and skeletal myoblast transplantation on postinfarction left ventricular function. J Thorac Cardiovasc Surg 2000;119:1169–1175.

65. Jain M, DerSimonian H, Brenner DA, et al. Cell therapy attenuates deleterious ventricular remodeling and improves cardiac performance after myocardial infarction. Circulation 2001;103:1920–1927.

66. Suzuki K, Murtuza B, Suzuki N, Smolenski RT, Yacoub MH. Intracoronary infusion of skeletal myoblasts improves cardiac function in doxorubicin-induced heart failure. Circulation 2001;104:I213–I217.

67. Taylor DA, Atkins BZ, Hungspreugs P, et al. Regenerating functional myocardium: improved performance after skeletal myoblast transplantation. Nat Med 1998;4:929–933.

68. Suzuki K, Murtuza B, Smolenski RT, et al. Cell transplantation for the treatment of acute myocardial infarction using vascular endothelial growth factor-expressing skeletal myoblasts. Circulation 2001;104:I207–I212.

69. Zuk PA, Zhu M, Mizuno H, et al. Multilineage cells from human adipose tissue: implications for cell-based therapies. Tissue Eng 2001;7:211–228.

70. Rehman J, Li J, Williams CA, Bekkers S, Considine RV, March KL. Human adipose stromal cells express the angiogenic factor VEGF and its receptor VEGFR-2 [abstract]. Arterioscler Thromb Vasc Biol 2002;22:111.

71. Smith A. Embryonic Stem Cells. In: Marshak DR, Gottlieb D, Gardner RL, eds. Stem Cell Biology. Cold Springs, New York: Cold Springs Harbor Laboratory Press; 2001:205–230.

72. Yamashita J, Itoh H, Hirashima M, et al. Flk1-positive cells derived from embryonic stem cells serve as vascular progenitors. Nature 2000;408:92–96.

73. Klug MG, Soonpaa MH, Koh GY, Field LJ. Genetically selected cardiomyocytes from differentiating embryonic stem cells form stable intracardiac grafts. J Clin Invest 1996;98:216–224.

74. Kehat I, Kenyagin-Karsenti D, Snir M, et al. Human embryonic stem cells can differentiate into myocytes with structural and functional properties of cardiomyocytes. J Clin Invest 2001;108:407–414.

75. Levenberg S, Golub JS, Amit M, Itskovitz-Eldor J, Langer R. Endothelial cells derived from human embryonic stem cells. Proc Natl Acad Sci USA 2002;99:4391–4396.

76. Green RM. Four moral questions for human embryonic stem cell research. Wound Repair Regen 2001;9:425–428.

77. Kim EJ, Li RK, Weisel RD, et al. Angiogenesis by endothelial cell transplantation. J Thorac Cardiovasc Surg 2001;122:963–971.

78. Yau TM, Fung K, Weisel RD, Fujii T, Mickle DA, Li RK. Enhanced myocardial angiogenesis by gene transfer with transplanted cells. Circulation 2001;104:I218–I222.

79. Yoo KJ, Li RK, Weisel RD, et al. Heart cell transplantation improves heart function in dilated cardiomyopathic hamsters. Circulation 2000;102:III204–III209.

80. Yoo KJ, Li RK, Weisel RD, Mickle DA, Li G, Yau TM. Autologous smooth muscle cell transplantation improved heart function in dilated cardiomyopathy. Ann Thorac Surg 2000;70:859–865.

II MYOCARDIAL DISEASE

6 Development of the Vertebrate Heart

Mabelle Ashe and David Bader, PhD

INTRODUCTION

The developmental pattern of heart formation is highly conserved among all vertebrates. Lineage tracing studies of heart precursors in pregastrulating embryos have shown that the earliest identifiable presumptive cardiac cells are located on two patches lateral to the anterior–posterior axis of the epiblast *(1–3)*. In the pregastrulation period, these cells migrate via ingression through to the primitive streak and position themselves within the primitive streak, later undergoing gastrulation to take up position in the antero-lateral mesoderm. These cells eventually become part of the lateral splanchnic mesoderm. The presumptive cardiac cells of the splanchnic mesoderm subsequently form a simple tube consisting of two layers—an inner endocardium and an outer myocardium—separated by a connective tissue–filled space called the cardiac jelly. The cardiac jelly is greatly expanded in the regions of the forming valves.

The primitive heart tube eventually elongates and loops to initiate atrioventricular (AV) patterning that forms the chambers of the heart. Then, cells from the proepicardial organ (PEO), which is a diverticulum from the forming liver, will migrate toward and surround the surface of the developing heart to form the epicardium and cardiovascular structures of the heart.

At the same time, neural crest cells migrate to the heart and contribute connective tissue and smooth muscle cells to form the great vessels and the outflow tract. Thus, cells of differing embryonic origin make up the diverse cardiac progenitors that differentiate to form characteristic heart structures, such as myocytes of the atrial, ventricular, and conduction systems and the cardiovasculature, and local structures, such as valves and septi. The following sections will review the processes that regulate heart formation and the underlying molecular mechanisms that control critical cellular events, such as commitment and differentiation, during cardiac development (Table 1).

HEART MORPHOGENESIS

Early Heart Morphogenesis

The heart is one of the first recognizable organs to develop in the embryo *(4)*. The process of heart formation has been studied extensively in humans, chicks, frogs, fish, *Drosophila*, and mice. Although developmental patterns vary, the origin of cardiac progenitors is highly conserved among vertebrates *(3,5,6)*. Fate map studies have shown that the earliest identifiable heart progenitor cells are located in the distal portion of the epiblast in two small clusters lateral to the anteroposterior axis in the early primitive streak (PS) stage (mouse 7 dpc) of embryogenesis (Fig. 1) *(7)*. At this stage, the presumptive heart field comprises only about 50 epiblast cells with an unspecified cell fate. Studies indicate that these cells remain multipotent until later stages of gastrulation when they commit to a cardiac fate, possibly in response to an inductive signal from surrounding tissues *(8)*.

During mid PS, the primitive streak of the embryo in gastrulation begins to extend anteriorly. At this time,

From: *Contemporary Cardiology: Principles of Molecular Cardiology*
Edited by: M. S. Runge and C. Patterson @ Humana Press Inc., Totowa, NJ

Table 1
Milestones of Early Heart Development in Different Species*

	Mouse	Chick	Human	Frog	Zebrafish
Migration of precardiac cells from epiblast	7 dpc (primitive streak)	HH4 (definitve streak)	15–16 days	Staqe 10	50% epiboly (5.5 hpf)
First evident assembly of myocardial plate	7 dpc (late primitive streak; just presomite)	HH5 Head process (19–22 h)	18 days	Approx stage 13	8–10 somites (approx 13 hpf)
Generation of single heart tube initiated	8 dpc (5–10 somites)	HH9 (7 somites)	22 days (4–10 somites)	Stage 28	20 somites (approx 19 hpf)
Tubular heart starts contraction	8.5 dpc (8–10 somites)	HH10 10 somites	23 days	Approx stage 33	26 somites (22 hpf)
Looping	8.5 dpc	HH11 (11–13 somites)	23 days	Stage 33–36	33 hpf
Cushions form	9.5 dpc	HH17	28 days (30–38 somites)	Approx stage 41	48 hpf

*The mouse data are primarily from Kaufman and Navaratnam (1981) (10), and DeRuiter (1992) (4); the chick data are from Patten (1957) (91), Romanoff (1960) (92), DeHaan (1965) (26), Manasek (1968) (90), Viragh et al. (1989) (93), and Garcia-Martinez (1993) (3); the human data are from Sissman (1970) (95), and Hamilton and Mossman (1972) (94); the frog data are from Sater and Jacobson (1990) (96); and the zebrafish data are from Stanier and Fishman (1992) (97). Adapted from (34).

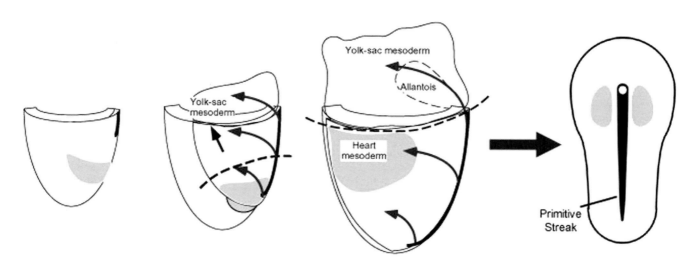

Fig. 1. Lineage tracing of epiblast cells destined for the heart fields. Epiblast cells (shaded) destined for the heart field ingress through the primitive streak at early to mid primitive streak stages. During late primitive streak, the mesodermal layer expands during gastrulation and the heart precursors in the mesoderm are displaced anteriorly and proximally to the cardiogenic region (straight arrow) (1). The precardiac cells continue their anteroproximal migration until they form two heart fields lateral to the primitive streak. The dashed lines represent the approximate border between the embryonic and the extraembryonic mesoderm. Adapted from (7).

the epiblast comprises only one germ layer. By ingression, cells surrounding the primitive streak, including cells of the presumptive heart field, invaginate through the primitive streak to form the nascent endodermal and mesodermal germ layers of the embryo (9). The cardiac precursors migrate laterally from the rostral half of the primitive streak into the presumptive mesoderm (10). The anteroposterior polarity of cardiac precursors has been configured by this stage of development; the anterior cells contribute to the future formation of the bulbus

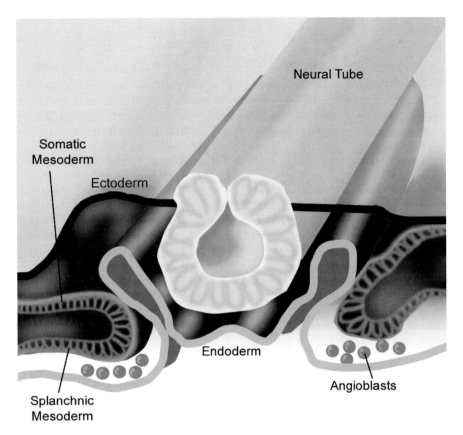

Fig. 2. Anterior cross-section of the precardiac mesoderm at 5–7 somite stage. Before formation of the heart tube, the mesodermal layer splits into somatic and splanchnic mesodermal layers. The splanchnic mesoderm contains the myocardial precursors. The endocardial angioblast precursors are between the splanchnic mesoderm and foregut. Adapted from *(34)*.

cordis, followed by ventricular precursors, which eventually form the ventricles, and the posteriorly positioned cells contribute to the future atrium *(3)*. Immediately after ingression, cardiac precursors localize to the distal portion of the newly formed lateral plate mesoderm (Fig. 2). However, at late PS (mouse 7.5 dpc), cardiac precursors relocate to the anteroproximal region of the mesoderm, which is called the lateral splanchnic mesoderm, and form two distinct clusters of precardial cells, or the heart fields, lateral to the primitive streak *(1)*. At this stage, these migrating cells are already specified and can independently express the cardiac phenotype *(11)*.

Lineage studies have shown that the precardial cells migrating through the primitive streak at mid PS have an anteroposterior alignment that corresponds to their lineage specification at later stages of development *(3)*. However, explants studies have shown that specification of the heart precursors to cardiac cell lineages does not occur until they migrate to the anterior heart field of the embryo. Furthermore, these studies indicate the significance of cell movement and inductive signaling in determining the fate of cardiac precursors *(1,12,13)*. In contrast, Montgomery et al. *(14)* have shown that gastrulation may not be required for specification of cardiac lineage. They collected cardiac progenitors before and after gastrulation and showed that, although both sets of cardiac precursors differentiate when cultured in vitro at high density, only the mesodermal progenitors collected after gastrulation differentiated into cardiomyocytes at low density. This finding suggests that pregastrulating cardiac precursors are not yet specified and still require some degree of inductive signaling, possibly through cell–cell interaction, for differentiation into cardiac lineages. Regardless of the variables that control the fate of cardiac progenitors during development, commitment of precardiac cells requires successful migration into the appropriate position in the embryo to become part of the heart field and inductive signals from the surrounding tissues. Studies indicate that bone morphogenetic protein (BMP-2) and fibroblast growth factor-4 (FGF-4) signaling are critical in the specification of cardiac mesodermal cells *(15)*. Once the cardiac precursors are established in the anterior heart field, this region will become the position of the newly formed heart.

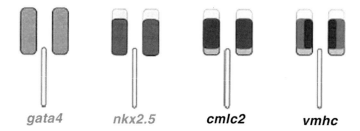

Fig. 3. Differential gene expression patterns reveal subpopulations within the anterior lateral plate mesoderm (ALPM). Schematic comparing overlapping expression patterns at the 15-somite stage, showing dorsal views of the ALPM, with anterior at the top. The notochord is depicted as a white rod. At this stage, *gata4* is expressed in a large part of the ALPM, including the cells that express *nkx2.5* *(98)*, and cmlc2 expression is restricted to the *nkx2.5*-expressing cells located anterior to the tip of the notocord *(99)*. *Vmhc* expression is restricted to a medial subpopulation of the *cmlc2*-expressing cells *(99)*. Adapted from *(89)*.

At this stage, cardiac precursors begin to express the endothelial- and myocardial- specific markers (Fig. 3), specifically flt-1, GATA-4, and Nkx-2.5 *(16,17)*. Nkx-2.5 is a vertebrate homolog of the *Drosophila* transcription factor *tinman* that is required for heart formation. The expression of *Nkx-2.5* is regulated by the transforming growth factor β (TGFβ) member decapentaplegic (dpp), which has a similar expression pattern and activity to BMP-2 derived from endoderm in vertebrates. Therefore, members of both the FGF and TGFβ families are important in early heart morphogenesis, particularly in specification of precardiac mesoderm. However, because these morphogens are required for regulation of other events in early embryogenesis, mutational analysis of their function in cardiogenesis has been limited by early embryonic lethality. Although studies in *Drosophila* have been helpful, the role of FGF and TGFβ members in cardiac lineage specification in vertebrates is unknown *(15)*.

Formation of the Heart Tube

Once the cell lineages have been specified, the precardiac mesodermal cells within the heart fields separate into two distinct populations. The population of cells fated to become endocardium migrates toward the endodermal layer and away from the remaining cellular cluster, which will become myocardial cells *(18)*. The underlying endoderm may send a signal, possibly vascular endothelial growth factor (VEGF), that induces the migration of endocardial-fated precardial cells *(18,19)*. The stage of development in which the fate of these precardial cells is determined is unknown; however, the distinction between endocardial and myogenic lineages probably occurs very early, possibly before gastrulation *(20,21)*.

Once cell fates have been established, the heart fields fuse beneath the foregut to form the cardiac crescent (Fig. 4). The two wings of the cardiac crescent move toward the ventral midline and fuse along the anteroposterior axis to form the heart tube *(22)*. The transcription factor *GATA-4* is critical in the formation of the heart tube. In mice lacking *GATA-4*, the crescent wings do not fuse and develop into two independent lateral heart tubes *(23)*. Interestingly, despite the disruption of proper heart tube formation, the bilateral tubes that *did* form contained differentiated cardiomyocytes, indicating that cardiac determination, or the ability to express a cardiac phenotype, is independent of the cellular environment *(11)*. The stage of heart morphogenesis in which the heart tube forms is brief. Almost as soon as the cardiac crescent comes together to form the bilateral heart tube, the newly formed structure initiates the series of morphological movements that define looping.

The heart tube is attached to the foregut via a broad connection known as the dorsal mesocardium, and to the ventral body wall via the ventral mesocardium *(24)*. At this stage, the tube is almost linear and comprises two layers, the inner endocardium and the outer myocardium, that envelop a central lumen. The cardiac jelly, which is a cushion of extracellular matrix, separates the two layers and is relatively thin in areas other than those that correspond to the forming valves. Lineage tracing studies have shown that although the heart tube is still linear, its tissues make up the primordia of the future trabeculated ventricles and, possibly, part of the future outflow tract *(25)* (Fig. 5).

Shortly after its formation and simultaneously with the descent of the anterior intestinal portal, the heart tube elongates along its anteroposterior axis (Fig. 6A). The elongated heart tube loses its attachment as the ventral mesoderm is absorbed. Only the attachment to the ventral body through the ventral mesocardium disappears. This absorption leaves a deep ventral groove, called the midsagittal furrow, along

St 7   St 10

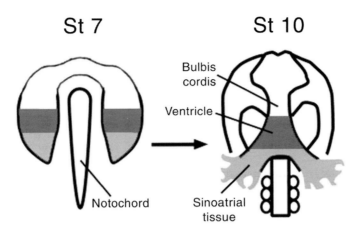

Fig. 4. Formation of the heart tube. Ventral view of cardiac precursors in the embryonic heart fields. Before heart tube formation (murine 7.5 dpc, chick HH7), the two lateral heart fields fuse at the anterior poles to form the cardiac crescent. Fusion continues down the antero-posterior axis to form the definitive heart tube. The relative anterior–to–posterior positions of precardiac cells in the primitive streak are maintained through heart tube formation, as depicted by the shading pattern denoting the eventual contribution of precardiac cells to specific regions of the heart. Adapted from *(34)*.

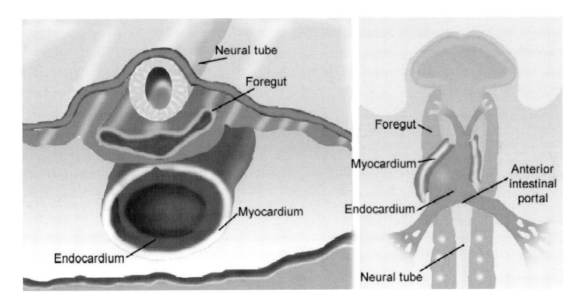

Fig. 5. Cross-section and ventral views of the heart tube Adapted from *(34)*.

the previous point of insertion of the ventral mesoderm into the heart tube. In addition, the formation of two lateral furrows, the interventricular grooves, at this stage divides the elongated heart tube into a cranial and caudal portion, which will give rise to the future right and left ventricles, respectively *(24,25)*. These interventricular grooves will be the initiation sites of the series of movements that make up cardiac looping. Once a closed primitive cardiac structure is established, several modifications must occur before the characteristic four-chambered adult heart is noted. At this stage, the ventricular region and outflow tract are located

anterior to the presumptive atrial region and sinus venosus (SV). This configuration will change with the initiation of cardiac looping.

Cardiac Looping

Once the initial heart tube has formed and polarity has been established, the nascent heart initiates a series of movements, known collectively as cardiac looping, that will reposition the individual heart segments to resemble their final configuration in the adult heart. Cardiac looping (mouse 8.5 dpc, 7 somites) comprises a series of

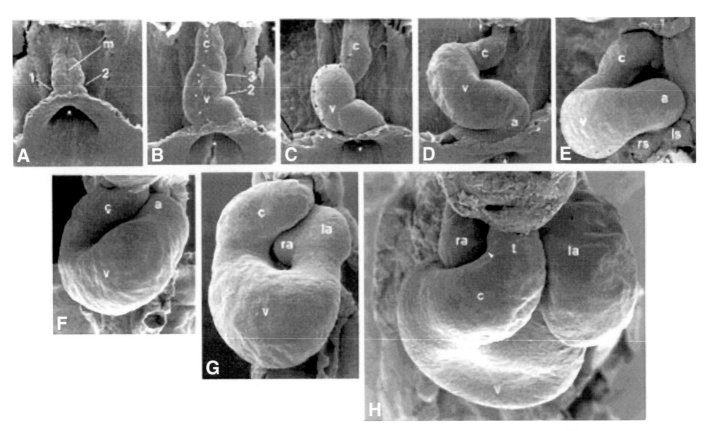

Fig. 6. Positional and morphological changes of the embryonic heart tube during cardiac looping. **(A)** Prelooping stages (murine 8 dpc, chick HH9). Establishment of the heart tube concomitant with descensus of the anterior intestinal portal (asterisks). The ventral midline of the heart tube is marked by the insertion line of the ventral mesocardium (m); the right (1) and left (2) lateral furrows appear. **(B)** Initiation of cardiac looping (murine 8.5 dpc, chick HH10). The right lateral furrow (1, panel A) flattens as the left (2) furrow deepens. The conoventricular sulcus (3) appears. **(C)** The primitive ventricular region (v) bends toward the ventral surface and simultaneously flaps toward the right side. Note that the primitive outflow tract (c) does not bend but remains as a straight tube in its original position. **(D)** As dextral looping ends, the primitive atria (a) appear and the primitive ventricular region is displaced toward the right, causing a kinking of the primitive outflow tract. The period after dextral looping is characterized by two morphological events: **(E)** the shortening of the distance between the primitive outflow tract and the atrial region, and **(F)** the rearrangement of the primitive ventricular bend so it now lies posterior, rather than anterior, to the atrial region. In addition, this timepoint marks the appearance of the sinus venosus and the lateral expansion of the atrial region. Note the general growth of the heart tube. (rs, right horn of the sinus venosus; ls, left horn of the sinus venosus) **(G)** At the end of S-shaped looping (murine 9.5 dpc, chick HH18), the relative positions of, not only the atrial and ventricular regions, but also the left and right atrium and proximal and distal ventricular regions, have changed. **(H)** After completion of looping, the heart undergoes further remodeling, including the appearance of the truncus arteriosus (t) and positional changes in the outflow tract with respect to the atria due to the process of "wedging." ra, right atrium; la, left atrium Adapted from *(78)*.

complicated and highly controlled mechanical maneuvers that correctly position the rudimentary heart segments in relation to one another. Before looping, the heart segments are aligned in reverse order relative to their final positions in the adult heart; the ventricular (arterial) pole segments, such as the sinus venosus and atrial segments, are located anterior to the atrial (venous) pole segments, such as the bulbus cordis and ventricular segments, along the heart tube. However, upon completion of cardiac looping, the linear heart tube undergoes a series of contortions that will correctly align the venous (atrial) pole anterior to the arterial (ventricular) pole (Fig. 7). In addition, remodeling occurs concurrently inside the heart tube. Along with mechanical reshaping, discrete portions of the heart tube undergo diverse morphological changes that define distinct fragments along the tube that are destined to specific structural fates. Morphological transformations and mechanical restructuring during looping create a series of segments separated by constrictions that, from the venous to the arterial

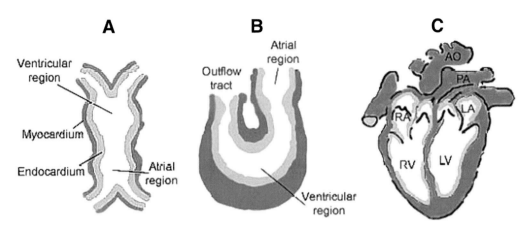

Fig. 7. Key stages in the development of the vertebrate heart. Key stages include the (**A**) heart tube stage, (**B**) cardiac looping , and (**C**) remodeling to produce the adult four-chambered heart. LA, left atrium; LV, left ventricle; RA, right atrium; RV, right ventricle, PA, pulmonary artery; AO, aorta. Adapted from *(34)*.

pole, will eventually develop into the SV, the common atrium, the atrioventricular canal, the primitive ventricular region, and the outflow tract/conus/bulbus arteriosus. Furthermore, the myocardial cells of the primitive heart tube at this stage become electrically coupled and begin to contract in unison *(26)*. Dextral (right-handed) looping comprises movements that are initiated with a series of bends between the segments, beginning with the invagination of the left interventricular groove situated at the border of the primitive right (anterior) and left (posterior) ventricular regions. On the opposite side of the border, the right interventricular groove simultaneously flattens out, producing the initial rightward asymmetrical curvature in the heart tube that places the right ventricular region adjacent, rather than anterior, to the left ventricular region (Fig. 6B).

At this time, segments within the heart tube begin to be defined. For example, the AV junction forms in between the primordial ventricular region and separates the primitive atrial and ventricular segments. In addition, a furrow, known as the primitive conoventricular sulcus, develops between the primitive bulbus (conus) and apical ventricular region, separating the primitive ventricle from the outflow tract. After the conoventricular sulcus develops, the ventricular portion of the heart tube thickens by accelerated myocyte proliferation and elongates faster than the conus portion. These changes cause the primitive ventricular region to bulge out ventrally in a "C" shape *(24)*. Because of this ventricular expansion, the bulging ventricular region flaps toward the right and continues to elongate throughout cardiac looping (Fig. 6C). The conus region remains in a horizontal position until an arterial kink causes the conus to be displaced vertically. Unlike the

ventricular region, the conus region remains a relatively straight, thin-layered tube. At the end of this rightward flapping, dextral looping is complete, and the conus, or primitive outflow tract, has been repositioned in the anterior region of the "C"-shaped heart tube, above the ventricular region *(25)* (Fig. 6D).

After dextral looping, around 9.5 dpc, the embryo undergoes "turning," a process by which the embryo rotates its body around the craniocaudal axis. Turning coincides with a series of movements and morphological changes that define the "S" shape stage of heart looping. These shifts, which reshape the heart tube into a characteristic "S" shape, reposition the specific cardiac segments in their appropriate anatomical and spatial relation with respect to each other. Two pivotal changes occur in the structure of the heart loop during this time to form the characteristic "S" shape. First, the distance between the conus and the caudal primitive atria decreases (Fig. 6E), which initiates the process of "wedging" *(27)*. During wedging, the outflow tract becomes wedged between the two developing ventricular chambers. As the conus and AV regions get closer together, the outflow septum in the conus region converges with the ventricular septum in the AV region and repositions the outflow tract between the ventricular chambers. These regions must converge accurately to ensure proper septation of the outflow tract. Any structural misalignments during wedging can result in ventricular septal defects *(27)*. The second change that occurs during "S" phase is the repositioning of the ventricular region posterior to the primitive atria *(24)* (Fig. 6F). These changes in the spatial orientation of heart tube segments coincide with the disappearance of the dorsal mesocardium and the appearance of remnants of the nascent SV in the posterior portion of the primitive atria.

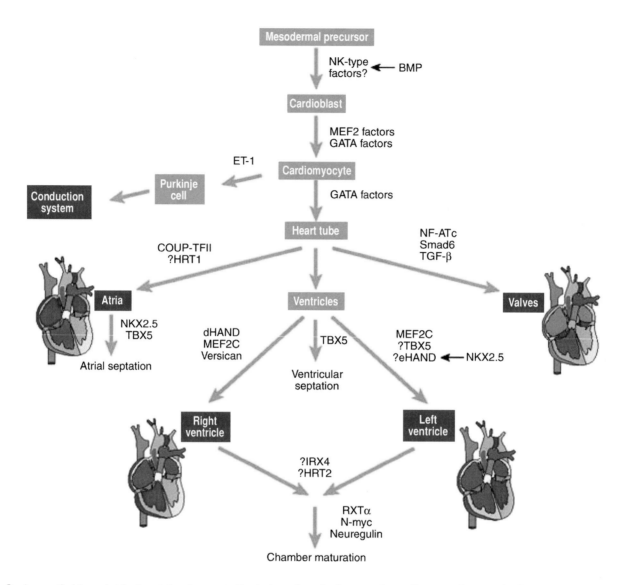

Fig. 8. A genetic blueprint for heart development. Depiction of particular steps in cardiac morphogenesis, focusing on mesodermal contributions. Cardiac regions affected by specific pathways are highlighted in dark boxes. Factors necessary for distinct steps during cardiogenesis in model organisms or humans are indicated beside arrows. Regulatory factors suspected to have region-specific roles are indicated with a "?." Cell types or regions of the heart are indicated in boxes. Adapted from *(54)*.

the atrial region is appropriately positioned above the right and left ventricles, and the primitive outflow tract and SV are located anterior to the nascent cardiac chambers. The shape and structure of the primitive heart tube have been redefined to resemble the relative form and chamber positioning of a mature heart (Fig. 6G).

The biomechanics involved in regulation of looping during cardiogenesis are poorly understood; the results of several studies have been inconclusive. For example, disruption of actin filaments in the chick heart prevented dextral looping, but the reasons for this result are not

known *(28)*. The biomechanical changes during heart formation involve highly regulated shifts in both cellular and extracellular dynamics and behavior and changes that occur in the extracardiac environment. However, much work is necessary to understand the mechanisms that define cardiac looping *(24)*.

Genetic models have been important in identifying potential molecular mechanisms in the process of heart looping (Fig. 8). Recent studies have shown that a group of basic helix-loop-helix (bHLH) and homeobox (Hox) transcription factors may be involved in the regulation of of basic helix-loop-helix (bHLH) and homeobox (Hox) transcription factors may be involved in the regulation of looping of the heart tube. These regulatory elements include *Nkx-2.5* (a vertebrate homolog of the *Drosophila* gene *tinman*), the dHand and eHand genes, and *MEF2C (29)*. Deletion of any of these genes causes defects in cardiac looping *(30)*; however, the mechanisms involved in this process are poorly understood. The involvement of these genes in the regulation of differentiation and laterality indicates the connection of these processes to the complex series of morphogenetic movements in cardiac looping *(29)*. These defects may be secondary to the disruption of a more generalized embryological process such as turning. Genetic ablation of these genes does not exclusively disrupt heart morphogenesis but results in a widespread disruption in body patterning. Furthermore, similar defects in body patterning result from the deletion of various types of genes, which suggests these genes may be involved in regulation of a more universal morphogenic process.

Remodeling the Primitive Heart

Up to this point in the formation of the heart, the epicardium or the coronary vasculature system has not developed. During subsequent stages of looping, at approx 8.5–9 mouse dpc (stage 18 chick), cells from the proepicardial organ migrate as an epithelial sheet toward the heart to the AV sulcus. Then, these cells continue to migrate around the heart tube and envelop the myocardium to form the epicardial layer of the heart *(31)*. Cells from the epicardium undergo epithelial-to-mesenchymal transition (EMT) and penetrate the myocardium to form the structures of the coronary vasculature. These cells that undergo EMT give rise to all the progenitors of the coronary vasculature, including endothelium smooth muscle and fibroblast cells *(32)*.

In addition to the epicardium and the coronary vasculature, the cardiac conduction system has not developed at this stage. Although cardiogenic cells are contractile and electrically coupled very early in development, the cardiac conduction system, which is responsible for regulation of rhythmical cardiac contractions, does not develop until later stages *(26)*. The first sporadic contractions are observed in the future apex of the developing ventricles; however, before looping the cellular basis or origin of the future conduction system is unknown. During "S" looping, differentiated Purkinje fibers of the cardiac conduction system are recruited from working myocytes via signals from the developing coronary system *(33)* and begin to appear in the myocardial layer of the heart tube. The cardiac conduction system will continue to develop and differentiate throughout the later stages of cardiomorphogenesis *(31,34)*.

In addition to the development of nascent cardiac structures such as the epicardium, the coronary vascular system, and the cardiac conduction system, later stages of heart development are defined by further maturation of existing heart segments, including the atria, ventricles, SV, and outflow tracts. Furthermore, new intracardial structures, such as the AV septum, the AV canal, and the truncus arteriosus, form in later stages of development *(4,24)*. Cardiac myocytes continue to proliferate and differentiate until a few days after birth, when they quit dividing. Regulation of cardiomyocyte proliferation during development is poorly understood. Around 4–10 d after birth, murine cardiomyocytes undergo one final round of karyokinesis without cytokinesis, thus forming the binucleated cardiomyocytes characteristic of an adult, terminally differentiated mouse heart *(35)*. At this stage, the heart has all the myocytes it will have for a lifetime. Whether the adult heart contains multipotent or unipotent stem cells is disputed; however, most, if not all, cardiac cells are presumed to have permanently withdrawn from the mitotic phase of the cell cycle and are terminally differentiated after the final karyokinesis *(36)*. After terminal differentiation, cardiac growth occurs primarily through cardiac hypertrophy or cell growth, rather than cell division *(37)*.

The Origin of Heart Progenitors

Although the earliest stages of cardiac development are highly conserved among all vertebrates, the later stages of heart development diverge depending on the particular functions required by the lifestyle of the organisms (Fig. 9). All vertebrate adult hearts have common features that distinguish them from other species: (1) both the heart and its associated vessels are surrounded by a continuous endothelial layer, (2) the heart develops a high-pressure ventricular chamber that generates enough force to infuse blood throughout the entire vertebrate body, (3) atrial/ventricular diversification, and (4) unidirectional blood flow in the heart *(34)*.

These similarities in the adult vertebrate heart result from conservation in morphogenetic patterns and structures between species during early stages of embryogenesis. Early stages of heart development are similar in zebrafish, *Xenopus,* chick, mouse, and human embryos, despite differences in morphology. Whether the early embryo begins as a flattened mass of cells as seen in the chick, or as a spherical blastula as seen in the mouse or *Xenopus,* the origin of cardiac progenitors is conserved for all vertebrates. The population of cells that develops into the vertebrate heart tube has three primary origins: the mesoderm, the PEO, and the neural crest. Cells that

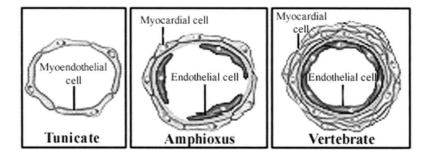

Fig. 9. Schematic of heart structures at later stages of development. By chick stage 15 (approx mouse ED 9.5), the atrial and ventricular regions of the heart tube are morphologically distinct. The ventricular bend thickens due to growth of the myocardial wall and trabeculation. The cardiac jelly separates the myocardium from endocardium and becomes thicker in regions destined to become future cushions and valvular structures, such as the outflow tract and atrioventricular junction. After chick stage 27 (approx mouse ED 12.5), septation of the cardiac chambers occurs, and the trabeculated myocardial layer expands and compacts. The left and right atria and ventricle become distinct with the growth of the atrioventricular cushions and the emergence of the atrial and interventricular septi. A, atrium; AV, atrioventricular canal; LA, left atrium; LV, left ventricle; OFT, outflow tract; RA, right atrium; RV, right ventricle; V, ventricle. Adapted from *(34)*.

eventually form the multichambered heart and most of the great vessels and outflow tract are primarily derived from the lateral mesodermal layer of the embryo. However, the cardiac neural crest is the source for ectomesenchymal precursors that will eventually contribute to outflow tract septation and patterning of the great arteries *(1,27)*. In contrast, the cells that form the coronary vasculature and the epicardium originate from the proepicardial serosa, located just above the liver primordium *(38)*. The specific fate of cardiac progenitors is determined by both their relative position in the developing embryo and the inductive signals from the environment. Inductive signals and movements of the cardiac primordium affect the unique patterning seen during heart development and the diversification and commitment of cardiac tissues.

PATTERNING

The Role of Neural Crest

Ablation studies have been important in studying the contribution of neural crest cells to cardiac morphogenesis. The cardiac neural crest provides precursors for valvuloseptal components of the outflow tract and for the formation of the great arteries (Fig. 10). Specifically, neural crest provides precursors to the three caudal aortic arch pairs, pharyngeal arches 3, 4, and 6, which will eventually form the carotid arteries, the aortic arch, and the ductus arteriosus *(39)*. Ablation of premigratory cardiac neural crest cells in rhombomeres 6–8 in the chick results in severe cardiovascular malformations, including double-outlet right ventricle, inappropriate aortic arch patterning, overriding aorta, decreased myocardial contractility, ventricular septal

defects, tetralogy of Fallot, and persistent truncus arteriosus *(40)*. Partial ablation of cardiac neural crest cells results in similar, but less pronounced, phenotypic defects, with the exception of persistent truncus arteriosus, which occurs after only a threshold number of cells are ablated *(41)*. These findings, in conjunction with lineage tracing analysis of quail–chick chimeras, have shown how the ectomesenchymal cells of the neural crest incorporate into the developing heart, what role they play in outflow tract septation and in patterning of the great arteries, and how these processes relate to the phenotypic malformations seen in neural crest defects. In addition, ablation studies have contributed to an understanding of the pathology of human diseases. For example, patients with DiGeorge syndrome, or the related CATCH-22 syndrome, which is caused by a microsomal deletion in chromosome 22q11, present with similar phenotypic dysmorphogenesis (i.e., tetralogy of Fallot, ventricular septal defects, and truncus arteriosus) as seen in cardiac neural crest–ablated chicks *(42)*. The similar malformations in humans with these congenital defects and in chicks with ablated cardiac neural crest suggest that a defect in cardiac neural crest activity during development underlies the phenotypic malformations. In fact, studies have shown that patients afflicted with DiGeorge syndrome have defects in cardiac neural crest expansion that contribute to manifestations of the disease. In addition, recent studies have associated specific genes with DiGeorge syndrome. For example, deletion of the T-box gene *Tbx1* in mice has resulted in the development of similar defects as those seen with DiGeorge syndrome, including abnormalities in outflow tract development, cleft palate, and glandular hypoplasia *(43)*. Some of the genes within this

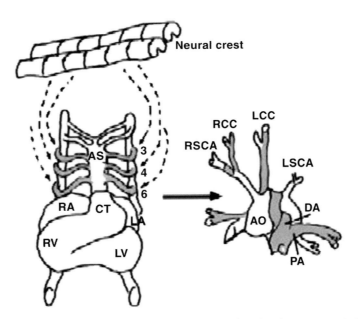

Fig. 10. Evolution of the chordate heart tube, shown in cross section. The presumptive chordate ancestor's heart may have been similar to the tube of modern tunicates, which comprises a single layer of myoendothelial cells with myofibrils in them that functioned at low pressures without any valvular structures. The contractile endostylar artery of ampioxus may be an intermediary form; it generates unidirectional flow and has a discontinuous lining of endothelial cells. In contrast, the vertebrate heart tube generates higher pressures, and has a thicker muscular layer with a continuous endothelial lining. Adapted from *(34)*.

deletion have been identified, and future studies will be aimed at identifying whether these genes are important in cardiac neural crest function during embryonic patterning.

Cardiac neural crest cells play a pivotal role in outflow tract septation during cardiac morphogenesis, and labeling studies have defined the contribution of premigratory neural crest cells to this process. By transplanting quail neural crest cells into the premigratory cardiac neural crest region of chicks, investigators can track the migration of transplanted cells with quail-specific markers to determine the distribution pattern of cardiac neural crest cells in developing cardiac structures. Ectomesenchymal cells first migrate from the cardiac neural crest to pharyngeal arches 3, 4, and 6, and then move toward the developing heart (Fig. 11). Pharyngeal arch 5 disintegrates in the vertebrate embryo and contributes little to this process. Once in the developing heart, neural crest–derived ectomesenchymal cells supply the precursors that form the pulmonary and aortic semilunar valves and infundibuli, and the pulmonary trunk of the outflow tract *(44)*. The ectomesenchymal cells of the outflow tract ridges are finger-like projections that extend from the aortic-pulmonary septum and contribute to the formation of the muscular outflow tract. Evidence indicates these cells induce differentiation of the surrounding cardiac precursors into myocardium *(45)*. Explant studies have

shown that differentiation of the myocardium of outflow tract tissue requires previous exposure to either ectomesenchymal cells from the aortic-pulmonary ridges or conditioned media of ectomesenchymal cells of the aortic-pulmonary ridges. The mechanism by which neural crest precursors signal the surrounding myocardium to differentiate into muscle is unknown.

Although explant and ablation studies have been useful in defining the role of neural crest precursors in heart patterning, genetic models have provided vital clues for the identification of key genes regulating neural crest precursor activity during heart formation. For example, the *Splotch* [2H] (*Sp*[2H]) mouse mutant has been used in studies assessing the role of the Pax3 transcription factor in the specification of cardiac neural crest cells and heart patterning. The *Sp*[2H] mouse mutant, a modification of the *Splotch* mutant, contains an inactivating deletion in the *Pax3* paired homeodomain. The cardiac defects in the *Sp*[2H] mouse mutant, such as truncus arteriosus and ventricular septal defects, are similar to those produced by cardiac neural crest ablation in the chick. Although cardiac neural crest cell migration appears to be unaffected in *Sp*[2H] mutant mice, the number of premigratory cardiac neural crest cells is decreased in the neural folds of these mice at earlier stages of development *(46)*. In addition to the decrease in the number of neural crest precursor cells,

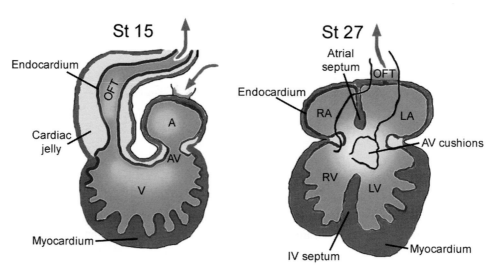

Fig. 11. Schematic of the contribution of neural crest cells to the development of aortic arch structures and pulmonary arteries. Cardiac neural crest cells migrate toward and populate aortic arches 3, 4 and 6, and the aortic sac. These cells will contribute to the formation of aortic arch arteries and the pulmonary arteries (depicted in black). AO, aorta; AS, aortic sac; DA, ductus arteriosus; LA, left atrium; LCC, left common carotid; LSCA, left subclavian artery; LV, left ventricle; PA, pulmonary artery; RA, right atrium; RCC, right common carotid; RSCA, right subclavian artery; RV, right ventricle; RPA, right pulmonary artery; LPA, left pulmonary artery.

the expression of *Wnt-1* is significantly reduced within the neural tube of these embryos. *Wnt-1* is the mammalian homolog of the *Drosophila* gene *wingless* and a member of the larger Wnt family of signaling molecules that are involved in axis induction *(47)*. Expansion of the precursor population of the cardiac neural crest within the neural tube may depend on activation of *Wnt-1* expression. *Pax3* induces transcriptional activation of *Wnt-1* within the neural tube; therefore, the decrease in the population of cardiac neural crest precursors may be caused by disruption of *Pax3*-mediated induction of *Wnt-1* expression in the developing neural tube of these mice *(48)*. Although this finding applies to neural crest, it shows the intimate relationship between diverse cellular components and normal heart development.

The contribution of neural crest to heart patterning is affected by changes in the *Hox* genes, which are important for segmental patterning in *Drosophila* and may be involved in aortic arch patterning during heart development. A craniocaudal gradient of expression of a set of *Hox* genes is seen in ectomesenchymal cells of the pharyngeal arches 3, 4, and 6 during aortic arch patterning *(49)*. If expression of *Hox* genes in chick embryos is disrupted with antisense oligonucleotides in premigratory neural crest cells, and these cells are transplanted into developing pharyngeal arches, patterning of the arches is abnormal and results in malformations of the great arteries *(50)*. In addition, the role of *Hox* genes in pharyngeal arch patterning by neural crest precursors is supported by

studies in mice with null mutations of retinoic acid receptors (RAR), which regulate *Hox* gene expression. Mice with null RAR mutations have abnormal patterning of pharyngeal arch derivatives, similar to the defect seen in mice with neural crest ablation *(51)*.

Mouse models, such as the Sp^{2H} and *Hox* mouse mutants, have contributed significantly to our understanding of the molecular pathways involved in the regulation of the activity of neural crest precursors during the processes of outflow tract septation and aortic arch patterning. Because interfering with the neural crest cell contribution to heart morphogenesis results in similar conotruncal defects, the molecular pathways involved in regulation of neural crest activity may be linked to a common universal developmental pathway. Therefore, these models are tools for the study of the pathological basis of conotruncal heart malformations and will improve our understanding of the genetic and pathological basis of human congenital heart defects, specifically those associated with the more common syndromes such as DiGeorge and CATCH-22.

Chamber Specification

The individual heart chambers become compartmentalized early during cardiac morphogenesis. Although the process by which cardiac cells determine chamber designation is poorly understood, several chamber-specific markers have been identified. Chamber specification begins in the early stages of cardiac development before

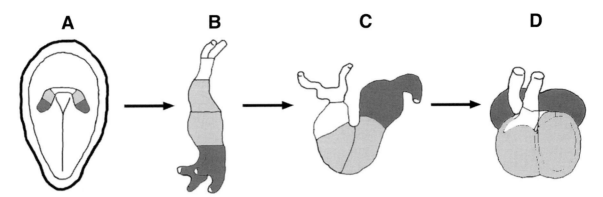

Fig. 12. Summary of major events in cardiac development. (**A**) Specification of the heart fields and formation of the cardiac crescent. (**B**) Heart tube formation. (**C**) Cardiac looping. (**D**) Cardiac remodeling. The conservation of compartmentalization at different stages of development is shown by differential shading of specified regions, including conotruncus (light) ventricular (medium) and atrial (dark) regions. Adapted from *(100)*.

segmentation of the heart tube *(52)*. Although cardiac precursors are destined to a particular segment of the heart tube before gastrulation, the earliest evidence of chamber-specific restriction is seen before heart tube formation. In the chick, differential expression of atrial- and ventricular-specific myosin heavy chain (MHC) genes is observed between anterior and posterior cardiac precursors as early as stage *(8)*. Shortly after the cardiac wings fuse, precardiac cells differentiate along the anteroposterior axis of the heart tube to define the primitive atrial and ventricular regions as seen by the localized expression of contractile proteins in the heart tube. Cells at the posterior pole of the heart tube begin to express atrial MHC, which is an atrial-specific marker, and precardiac cells in the anterior preventricular region of the nascent heart tube almost simultaneously begin to express ventricular myosin light chain (Fig. 3). Expression of these genes is the first evidence of chamber specification within the heart *(8,34)*.

After this initial specification of cardiac precursors, factors with broad expression patterns throughout the heart tube become restricted at later stages of heart looping. In the mouse, contractile proteins MHCα and MHCβ are expressed throughout the heart tube at early stages of heart looping but, at later stages, their expression becomes restricted to the atrium and the ventricle, respectively *(34)*. Other genes become more restricted in their expression pattern and after down-regulation show laterality in their chamber-specific expression. For example, expression of the bHLH genes *dHAND* is restricted primarily to the right ventricle and *eHAND* to the left ventricle. However, expression patterns of contractile protein genes are highly variable among species during chamber specification. Although chamber-specific expression of these contractile protein genes suggests these genes are

involved in chamber differentiation, studies have not shown a definitive role for these factors in regionalization of cardiac precursors. Because many of these genes are homogeneously expressed in precardial cells before regionalization, targeted mutagenesis has not been helpful in defining the function of these genes during chamber specification *(15)*.

The primitive atrial and ventricular regions undergo divergent pathways of differentiation that define their distinctive morphological and physiological characteristics (Fig. 12). As the heart tube develops, the size of the ventricular region drastically expands, and the myocardium undergoes characteristic thickening. In contrast, the atrial region remains relatively small with a thin myocardium. Much more is known about the molecular processes involved in ventricular maturation than those that underlie atrial maturation. As the ventricles mature, the ventricular wall becomes trabeculated, acquires finger-like extensions that project into the lumen, and thickens to form the compact layer.

Mice lacking *RAR* genes have severe morphological defects, specifically those associated with cardiac neural crest patterning. In mice lacking retinoid X receptor *(RXRα)*, the observed cardiac defects include not only neural crest–associated deficiencies, but also underdeveloped ventricles characterized by a thin compact layer, disorganized trabeculation, and incomplete ventricular septation. Cardiac neural crest cells of the aortic sac in the outflow region of the heart signal to the developing myocardium and induce myocardialization; therefore, the lack of ectomesenchymal signaling to the ventricular myocardium may result in the ventricular defects seen in null mice *(53)*. Other signaling pathways involved in ventricular maturation include neuregulin signaling from the endocardium to the neuregulin receptors erbB2 and erbB4, which are expressed specifically in the ventricular myocardium. Genetic ablation of genes for neuregulin receptors in mice produces defects similar to those seen in RXR null mice in ventricular myocyte maturation, including lack of trabeculation and altered contractility (15). In addition, the transcription factor gene *MEF2C* may be involved in ventricular maturation. Ventricular hypoplasia is seen in mice deficient in *MEF2C*. However, the mechanism by which *MEF2C* regulates ventricular development is unknown (54).

Molecular mechanisms of atrial maturation, although not well defined, have been studied in patients with Holt–Oram syndrome, which is characterized by defects in atrial septation and limb formation. The syndrome occurs because of a mutation in the "T-box" gene *TBX5*. *TBX5* is expressed in the developing atrial wall and, subsequently, in the developing atrial septum during cardiogenesis. However, the function of *TBX5* in atrial maturation is unknown (55).

The AV canal, which is the constriction between the ventricular and atrial segments of the heart tube, separates the presumptive atria and ventricles. The left and right atrial and ventricular chambers are formed by changes in the ventricular myocardium caused by inductive signaling from the endocardium and, possibly, the cardiac neural crest (in the ventricle). The AV canal undergoes drastic morphological and physiological changes to form the mature tricuspid and mitral valves and to separate the atria from the ventricles. The formation of the AV septum begins with a thickening of the cardiac jelly surrounding the AV canal. Signals from the myocardium induce EMT transition of the endocardium (56). The mesenchymal cells migrate into the cardiac jelly and proliferate, forming the endocardial cushions and chordae tendineae. The endocardial cushions eventually join to form the prospective valvular structures (Fig. 12). The TGFβ family plays a significant role in this process (57). Studies suggest that TGFβ secreted from the myocardium interacts with TGFβ receptors in the endocardium and signals these cells to undergo EMT transition during AV cushion formation (58). AV septal defects are frequently seen in humans with trisomy 21 (Down's syndrome). However, the correlation between this chromosomal aberration and the defects in endocardial cushion formation is unknown (15).

Defects in ventricular and septal maturation are common in congenital heart malformations. Many mutations cause thinning of the ventricular wall, lack of compaction, and ventricular septal defects, which suggests that these mutations disrupt a common developmental process rather than a specific process of heart development. Whether chamber formation is directed by a systemic or heart-specific

morphological and/or physiological phenomena (or both) is unknown.

Laterality

Differences are clearly seen between the right and left sides of the heart, including the relative thickness of the ventricles and differences in AV valves. Lateral differences are apparent early in cardiac development. Although differences in left and right axes are seen as early as gastrulation, cardiac looping is one of the first physiological events to establish definitive left–right (L–R) asymmetry during organogenesis. To establish proper "situs," or handedness, the heart must be accurately positioned in the left hemithorax and must have characteristic rightward looping. The correct lateral positioning of the heart and other organs in the thoracoabdominal cavities (including lungs, liver, and gut) is known as "situs solitus" (34). Recent studies have shown that several genes are involved in specification of laterality of visceral organs, particularly the heart. Precision L–R patterning of the heart is crucial for proper alignment of the circulatory components of the heart, and any abnormalities in the process can lead to congenital heart defects.

The signaling mechanisms that control laterality begin at gastrulation. At gastrulation, the embryo begins to institute L–R asymmetry around Henson's node by initiating lateral expression of several common morphogens, such as *BMPs*, *Sonic Hedgehog* (Shh), and *Nodal*, in the lateral plate mesoderm, which is the future source of many visceral organs including the heart. During cardiac crescent formation, expression of the left-sided genes, *Nodal* and *Lefty-2*, is repressed in the lateral plate mesoderm (59). An asymmetric expression pattern is established whereby *Shh* and *BMP-4* expression is restricted to the right, and *Nodal* and *Lefty-2* to the left, of the lateral plate mesoderm. The left-sided expression of *Nodal* induces asymmetric expression of the bicoid-related homeodomain protein *Pitx-2* in the developing heart tube and the gut (60,61).

The role of these genes and signaling pathways in regulation of L–R patterning has been studied in mouse models of lateral randomization defects. A mouse strain with inversion of embryonic turning (inv/inv) was produced by a random insertion into chromosome 4 (62). In inv/inv mice, the laterality of the visceral organs is reversed, a condition called complete situs inversus. The left-sided markers, *Lefty-1*, *Lefty-2*, and *Nodal*, are expressed on the right in these mutant mice, which suggests that expression of *Nodal* and *Lefty* control the lateral positioning of the visceral organs. The mutated gene(s) responsible for aberrant expression of *Nodal* and *Lefty* in inv/inv mice is *inversin*; however, the only information about this gene is that it functions upstream of these factors to direct the left-sided expression pattern (63).

Inverse viscerum (iv/iv) mice, produced by a mutation in chromosome 12, have lateral defects characterized by random sidedness. This chromosomal aberration disrupts the *left-right dynein* (*Lrd*) gene responsible for L–R polarity around Henson's node (64). iv/iv and legless mice (produced by a chromosomal deletion) have similarly disrupted *Lrd* genes that result in phenotypes characterized by normal (situs solitus), reversed (situs inversus), or random (situs ambiguous) asymmetry. Disruption of *Lrd* results in ciliary abnormalities that lead to dysregulated expression of lateral genes. Without the proper laterality around Henson's node, the patterning of asymmetric signals becomes randomized. Therefore, various lateral phenotypes are seen when these genes are expressed normally, abnormally (similar to inv/inv mice), or not at all (61).

Patients with Kartegener's syndrome, also called primary ciliary dyskinesia (PCD), have ciliary abnormalities that result in randomized situs, similar to that seen in iv/iv mice. However, ciliary defects in patients with PCD are also seen in the lungs, sinus cavity, and reproductive tract, and can cause respiratory symptoms and male infertility (55). The gene responsible for PCD has not been identified, but a mutated dynein may be involved because of similarities between the phenotype of PCD and iv/iv mice (60). Cardiac situs abnormalities, which are usually not heart-specific, occur secondary to a more general situs defect during development and probably involve molecular processes involved in general body patterning rather than heart morphogenesis.

Cardiac Myogenesis and Differentiation

Three pivotal stages define cardiomyogenesis: (1) the existence of the myocardium as an epithelium, (2) trabeculation of the myocardial lining facing the lumen, and (3) compaction of the basal layers of trabeculated myocardium. Differentiation of myocardium, defined by the expression of cardiac contractile genes, is initiated at the early heart tube stage before contraction. At this stage, the myocardium, seen as a one- to two-cell epithelial layer, surrounds the inner endocardium. The signals involved in specification of myocardium are not well defined. Explant studies suggest that anterior endoderm signaling, required at later stages of differentiation, is not required for early myocardial specification, possibly because of the lack of inductive signals from the neural crest cells that have not yet populated this region (65,66). The differentiation of myocardial cells is propogated in a wave-like manner along the anterioposterior axis of the heart tube. Differentiated myocardial cells express sarcomeric proteins and initiate organization of myofibrils into visible striated myofilaments.

Once cardiac looping is completed, the myocardial layer initiates the series of morphological changes that define trabeculation (Fig. 12). Myocardial trabeculation increases surface area, facilitates contractility, and channels circulation in the ventricular chambers. Trabeculation is initiated along the elongated outer curvature of the ventricular region of the cardiac primordium. Although the inner curvature is smooth, the myocardial layer of the outer curvature develops trabecular ridges that run in a dorsal–ventral pattern. These ridges appear to form as the myocardium "buckles" from compression of the myocardial layer at the deep bend of the outer curvature (67). With continuing stress, the ridges elongate into finger-like projections with ends facing the inner lumen of the ventricular region. To this point, the differentiation of the myocardial layer is relatively uniform throughout the ventricular region; however, as the ventricular septum forms, the left and right ventricles develop their characteristic morphology. The ventricular septum elongates as a thick compact layer of muscle that divides the ventricular region into the left and right ventricles. After ventricular septation, the trabeculae of the left ventricle become thicker and more randomly distributed than those of the right ventricle. Neuregulin and its receptors, erbB2 and erbB4, contribute to the process of trabeculation (68). Disruption of any of the neuregulin genes and their receptors in mice results in lack of trabeculation and contractile defects, which may be a secondary effect of the lack of trabeculation (15).

The trabeculae remodel throughout cardiogenesis in response to differentiative and hemodynamic signals. In remodeling, the trabeculae reorganize so that the apical ends face the ventricular lumen. In addition, the trabecular apices congeal and undergo further reorganization to create the honeycomb-like appearance characteristic of mature trabeculated myocardium. Surrounding presumptive valvular and papillary structures, the trabeculated myocardium becomes compact to form the musculature portion of these structures (69).

The initial compact layer arises from the thin one- to two-cell myocardial sheath as a result of two phenomena: (1) the proliferation of cardiomyocytes and (2) the compaction of the basal portion of the trabeculated layer. Most proliferating myocardial cells are found at the base of the trabecular layer because the myocardial cells at the apical ends of the trabeculae are terminally differentiating and, consequently, withdrawing from the cell cycle. Thus, an apicobasal gradient develops along the trabecular projections; myocardial cells at the apical ends have increased potential to differentiate and decreased potential to proliferate, as compared with those at the basal end. FGF may be involved in stimulation of cell division during this process. Blocking FGF receptor function in vivo decreases myocardial proliferation (70). However, most of the thickness of the compact layer is achieved by subsequent compaction of the basal portion of the trabeculae.

The molecular mechanisms involved in compaction are unknown, but the RXRα gene may contribute to this process. Ventricular maturation is defective in RXRα null mice; specifically, they have a thin compact layer. However, the effect of RXRα on compaction is unknown, and whether this result is a systemic problem or associated with neural crest function is unknown (53). As compaction occurs, cells from the epicardium delaminate and invade the compact layer. These epicardial-derived cells will eventually give rise to the coronary vasculature. Species lacking a compact layer do not form coronary vessels, suggesting an intimate connection between these two processes (69).

Myocardial cells, unlike skeletal muscle cells, do not withdraw from the cell cycle before differentiation. Myocardial cells continue to proliferate while differentiating throughout cardiogenesis. Shortly after birth in mice, between neonatal d 4 and 10, cardiomyocytes terminally differentiate and permanently withdraw from the cell cycle. At this stage, heart growth changes from hyperplastic to hypertrophic, which signals the end of cardiogenesis (35).

Although more is known about the process of skeletal myogenesis than cardiac myogenesis, recent studies have identified several genes involved in the specification and differentiation of cardiac myocytes. One of these genes is DMEF2 (myocyte enhancing binding factor) in Drosophila. The MEF2 genes belong to the MADS box family of transcription factors. Although the mouse has four MEF2, Drosophila has only one, DMEF2. Inactivation of this gene in Drosphila results in lack of muscle differentiation, including differentiation of cardiomyocytes, and causes early death. The effect of MEF2 on myocyte differentiation in higher vertebrates is unknown; however, because the MEF2 genes have a muscle-specific pattern similar to that seen in Drosophila, these genes may have a similar function in muscle differentiation (71).

DIVERSIFICATION

The Cardiac Conduction System

Propagation of electrical impulses from the apex of the right atrium to the base of the left ventricle during cardiac contraction ensures proper hemodynamic expulsion. An intricate conduction network that coordinates the rhythmic contractions of the heart controls the propagation of impulses. The cardiac conduction system (CCS) comprises the central CCS, which includes the sinoatrial (SA) node, the AV node, and the AV bundles, and the peripheral CCS, which includes the Purkinje fibers and the atrial conduction system. Little is known about the origin, specification, and differentiation of the CCS, which has been studied mainly in avian models. The point at which cells initially commit to a CCS fate has not been well established; lineage-tracing studies have shown the origin of cells, and particularly Purkinje fibers, that make up specific components of the CCS. These studies have shown that cardiac conduction cells are probably not derived from neural crest precursors, as previously believed, but that recruited bipotential myocardial precursors are involved in the development of conduction cells (72) (Fig. 13). Several morphological and physiological characteristics distinguish differentiated conduction cells from other myocardial cells. Expression of some muscle-specific genes, such as TnI and desmin, is reduced in myocardial precursors that differentiate into Purkinje fibers (32). Gene expression patterns of conduction cells resemble skeletal and neural tissues more than myocardial tissues. Conduction cells develop distinct ion channels, gap junctions, and neurofilaments necessary for coordinated conduction of electrical impulses through the heart (73). Recent studies have suggested that signaling from the surrounding coronary vasculature induces the differentiation of myocardial precursors into Purkinje fibers. In studies in which coronary vascularization was inhibited, Purkinje fiber formation was significantly reduced, and stimulation of ectopic coronary vascularization increased induction of Purkinje fibers (74). These studies suggest that paracrine signaling from the coronary vasculature may induce differentiation of cardiomyocyte precursors into Purkinje fibers. In vitro studies have shown that endothelin-1 can signal cultured myocardial cells to differentiate into a conductive phenotype. However, an in vivo mechanism of paracrine signaling from the coronary vessels has not been identified (75). Many components of the CCS, specifically the central CCS, are intact before the recruitment of cardiomyocytes for Purkinje fiber formation, although the source of cardiomyocyte recruitment unknown (32).

One of the earliest signs of coordination of electrical impulses is seen after the formation of the tubular heart when blood is propelled through the heart by a series of peristaltic contractions. As the tube becomes segmented, conductivity becomes fast in the atrial and ventricular

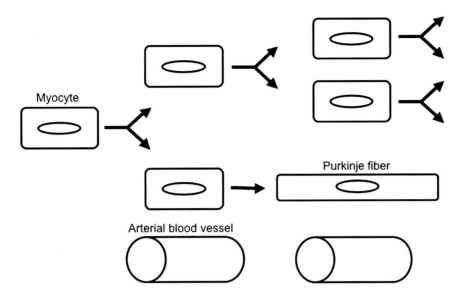

Fig. 13. Contribution of the myocyte lineage to coronary vasculature and cardiac conduction system. Vasculogenic formation of coronary blood vessels occurs mainly in the post-septation phase of heart development. Only subpopulations of the clonally related, beating myocytes differentiate into Purkinje fibers in the perivascular region of developing coronary arteries. Myocardial cells continue dividing, whereas Purkinje cells withdraw from the cell cycle. Adapted from *(32)*.

regions, whereas conductivity is slow in the intermediate primitive inflow tract, the AV canal, and the outflow tract. This alternating arrangement of fast and slow conducting segments prevents backflow through the tubular heart in the absence of valvular structures. However, a more sophisticated system is needed once chamber formation is complete. One of the first components of the CCS to form is the SA node, or the "leading pacemaker." Initially developed from cells derived from the inflow tract and AV canal, the SA node relocates to the left side of the developing heart tube once the SV forms at the late stage of cardiac looping. The AV node and ring located at the atrial septum, along with the associated AV bundles, become morphologically distinguishable in the AV canal segment shortly after the SA node develops. Cardiac impulses responsible for contraction are generated at the SA node and are propagated through the atrial chambers. These impulses converge at the AV node and AV ring and then are passed through the AV bundles to the Purkinje fibers innervating the ventricular chambers. Stimulation of the Purkinje fibers induces the contraction of the ventricular chambers, and blood is ejected through the outflow tracts and into the body *(32,72)*.

Once the primary CCS network has been established, CCS remodeling may occur as a result of signaling from the coronary vasculature to the surrounding myocytes to differentiate in response to hemodynamic changes. In the chick, formation of the complete CCS, including a lead-ing pacemaker, the AV node, and connecting bundles, may occur primarily during myocardial compaction *(72)*. However, recent reports suggest that development of the CCS differs in the mouse heart. Using a combination of lineage trace analysis with a reporter gene and optical mapping, Rentschler et al visualized the process of maturation of the murine CCS in vivo *(76)*. Their findings suggest that the CCS begins to develop much earlier than previously thought, possibly at the early stages of cardiac looping (approx 8.5 dpc), and that components of the murine CCS develop simultaneously rather than sequentially as seen in the chick. In addition, the mouse CCS is almost intact before perfusion of the coronary vessels, suggesting that cardiovascular hemodynamics do not influence remodeling of the CCS in mice as is seen in the chick.

Formation of the Coronary Vasculature

The development of elaborate multilayered cardiac chambers in higher vertebrates has necessitated the formation of an intricate vascular network capable of supplying oxygen and nutrients to all myocardial cells, including those within the thick myocardial walls of the heart *(24)*. Vascularization of the heart is first seen during chamber formation. Coronary vessel development is unique because it is distinct from the development of the great vessels and systemic vascular development. Precursors of the coronary vasculature originate from the proepicardial serosa, which is an extracardiac outgrowth of the liver primordium

(38,77). The proepicardial serosa, which includes the PEO, is the primary contributor of precursor cells for the coronary vascular system. Derived from the liver diverticulum and parts of the liver primordium, the PEO is a continuous convoluted epithelial layer that resembles a cluster of grapes. Cells from the PEO migrate as an epithelial sheet toward the dorsal myocardium and form a connecting bridge, called the sinu-ventricular ligament, between the dorsal wall of the myocardium and the ventral wall of the SV that will serve as a thoroughfare for cells migrating toward the heart *(78).* Once the cells reach the heart and adhere to the AV groove, they migrate cranially over the myocardium and envelop the entire surface of the heart up until the proximal portion of the outflow tract, forming the epicardial layer of the cardiac primordium.

Although little is known about the signaling mechanisms involved in the targeting and adherence of the epicardium to the myocardial layer, recent studies indicate the involvement of cell adhesion molecules, particularly vascular cellular adhesion molecule-1 (VCAM-1) and α4 integrin. VCAM-1 is expressed on the surface of the myocardium, whereas α4 integrin is expressed in the developing epicardium. The formation of the epicardial layer is defective in mice deficient for either VCAM-1 or α4 integrin. Although the development of the epicardium initially seems unaffected by the absence of VCAM-1 or α4 integrin, the epicardial layer disintegrates by 11.5 dpc, suggesting that these cell adhesion molecules may be required for maintenance of the epicardium, rather than for its adhesion to the myocardial wall *(24).* Some epicardial cells undergo EMT, at which time they delaminate from the surface of the epicardium and invade the underlying subepicardial layers. Recent studies have shown that a FOG-2–dependent signaling pathway may be involved in this process. In mice deficient in *FOG-2,* epicardial formation is normal, but the cells do not undergo EMT and do not delaminate *(79).* Epicardial EMT strongly resembles mesenchymalization of cells in the AV cushion during valve formation. EMT of the endothelial cells of the AV cushion occurs almost simultaneously with EMT of epicardial cells. The simultaneous EMT of these cardiac layers in approximately the same cardiac region indicates that these two events are related. In fact, the mechanisms that direct EMT of epicardial cells are similar to those that control EMT of endocardial cells during AV cushion formation *(24).* These processes not only show a spatiotemporal relationship, but also share similar gene expression patterns, including upregulation of genes such as *Bves (80), slug (81),* and *ets-1 (82),* all of which regulate EMT during embryogenesis *(80,81,83) .* Once the cells become mobilized, they migrate through the myocardium and populate the interstitial spaces in the myocardial compact layer. Then, the mesenchymal cells differentiate into fibroblastic cells and the smooth muscle and endothelial components of the coronary vasculature *(38,84).*

The rudimentary coronary vascular network begins as a series of discontinuous channels dispersed throughout the myocardium and subepicardium. To form a mature, continuous vascular network that includes arteries, veins, arterioles, venules, and capillary beds, these sinusoids must undergo extensive fusion and remodeling. Two distinct processes are involved in the formation of this network: (1) vasculogenesis, or *de novo* formation of capillary networks, and (2) angiogenesis, or the formation of blood vessels from outgrowth and sprouting of preexisting blood vessels. The coronary vascular network is expanded by *de novo* recruitment of vascular precursor cells and pericytes to sites of nascent vascular channels, and by proliferation, migration, and differentiation of existing sinusoids *(85).* The rudimentary coronary vascular plexus undergoes extensive remodeling, depending on the demands of the cardiac tissue for oxygen and nutrients *(86).* Although the signaling molecules involved in coronary vascular remodeling are unknown, conservation between peripheral and coronary blood vessel formation is logical, and the same factors that control peripheral angiogenesis and vasculogenesis may also regulate coronary vascularization. The VEGFs are important in regulating blood vessel formation. Embryonic death caused by defects in blood vessel formation is seen in mice deficient in VEGFs or their receptors. The spatiotemporal expression patterns of VEGFs vary with the isoform *(87).* A deficiency in the VEGF splice variants, *VEGF164* and *VEGF188,* impairs angiogenesis during coronary vascularization, resulting in early embryonic lethality due to cardiac ischemia *(88).*

Once the coronary vessels have undergone remodeling, the epicardium detaches from the myocardial layer to form the subepicardial space. The deposition of cellular matrix components drastically expands the thickness and size of the epicardial space. In addition, the capillaries at the proximal end of the aorta fuse to form the coronary arterial orifice, which then connects to the aorta. This connection provides oxygenated blood to the coronary vascular plexus via the peripheral vascular system *(38).*

REFERENCES

1. Parameswaran M. Regionalisation of cell fate and morphogenetic movement of the mesoderm during mouse gastrulation. Dev Gen 1995;17:16–28.
2. Lawson KA. Clonal analysis of epiblast fate during germ layer formation in the mouse embryo. Development (Suppl) 1991;113:891–911.

3. Garcia-Martinez V. Primitive-streak origin of the cardiovascular system in avian embryos. Dev Biol 1993;159:706–719.

4. DeRuiter MC. The development of the myocardium and endocardium in mouse embryos. Fusion of two heart tubes? Anat Embryol 1992;185:461–473.

5. Tam PP. Mapping vertebrate embryos. Curr Biol 1996;6:104–106.

6. Schoenwolf GC. Molecular genetic control of axis patterning during early embryogenesis of vertebrates. Ann NY Acad Sci 2000;919:246–260.

7. Tam PP. The allocation of epiblast cells to the embryonic heart and other mesodermal lineages: the role of ingression and tissue movement during gastrulation. Nat Genet 1997;16:174–178.

8. Yutzey KE. Diversification of cardiomyogenic cell lineages during early heart development. Circ Res 1995;77:216–219.

9. Hogan B. Manipulating the Mouse Embryo: A Laboratory Manual. Plainview, NY: Cold Spring Harbor Laboratory Press, 1994:xvii, 497.

10. Kaufman MH, Navaratnam V. Early differentiation of the heart in mouse embryos. J Anat 1981;133:235–246.

11. Slack JMW. From Egg to Embryo. Cambridge, U.K.: Cambridge University Press, 1991.

12. Nascone N. An inductive role for the endoderm in Xenopus cardiogenesis. Development (Suppl) 1995;121:515–523.

13. Schultheiss TM. Induction of avian cardiac myogenesis by anterior endoderm. Biochem Biophys Res Commun 1995;217:1120–1127.

14. Montgomery MO. Staging of commitment and differentiation of avian cardiac myocytes. Dev Biol 1994;164:63–71.

15. Sucov HM. Molecular insights into cardiac development. Ann Rev Physiol 1998;60:287–308.

16. Heikinheimo M. Localization of transcription factor GATA-4 to regions of the mouse embryo involved in cardiac development. Dev Biol 1994;164:361–373.

17. Lyons GE. Vertebrate heart development. Br J Anaesth 1996;76:680–684.

18. Sugi Y, Markwald RR. Formation and early morphogenesis of endocardial endothelial precursor cells and the role of endoderm. Dev Biol 1996;175:66–83.

19. Dumont DJ, Jussila L, Taipale J, et al. Cardiovascular failure in mouse embryos deficient in VEGF receptor-3. Science 1998;282:946–949.

20. Cohen-Gould L, Mikawa T. The fate diversity of mesodermal cells within the heart field during chicken early embryogenesis. Dev Biol 1996;177:265–273.

21. Fernandez JE, Melguizo C, Prados J, Marchal JA, Alvarez L, Aranega A. Production and characterization of a new monoclonal antibody, GR-ICOR-2, recognizing sarcomeric actin: analysis of the expression in the developing chick heart. Histol Histopathol 1994;9:765–771.

22. Stalsberg H. Regional mitotic activity in the precardiac mesoderm and differentiating heart tube in the chick embryo. Dev Biol 1969;20:18–45.

23. Molkentin JD, Lin Q, Duncan SA, Olson EN. Requirement of the transcription factor GATA4 for heart tube formation and ventral morphogenesis. Genes Devel 1997;11:1061–1072.

24. Manner J. Cardiac looping in the chick embryo: a morphological review with special reference to terminological and biomechanical aspects of the looping process. Anat Rec 2000;259:248–262.

25. de la Cruz MV, Castillo MM, Villavicencio L, Valencia A, Moreno-Rodriguez RA. Primitive interventricular septum, its primordium, and its contribution in the definitive interventricular septum: in vivo labelling study in the chick embryo heart. Anat Rec 1997; 247:512–520.

26. DeHaan RL. Development of pacemaker tissue in the embryonic heart. Ann NY Acad Sci 1965;127:7–18.

27. Kirby ML. Neural crest and cardiovascular patterning. Circ Res 1995; 77:211–215.

28. Itasaki N. Actin bundles on the right side in the caudal part of the heart tube play a role in dextro-looping in the embryonic chick heart. Anat Embryol 1991;183:29–39.

29. Srivastava D. Genetic assembly of the heart: implications for congenital heart disease. Annu Rev Physiol 2001;63:451–469.

30. Baldwin HS. Advances in understanding the molecular regulation of cardiac development. Curr Opin Pediatr 1999;11:413–418.

31. Komiyama M. Origin and development of the epicardium in the mouse embryo. Anat Embryol 1987;176:183–189.

32. Mikawa T. The polyclonal origin of myocyte lineages. Annu Rev Physiol 1996;58:509–521.

33. Cheng G LW, Cole GJ, Mikawa T, Thompson RP, Gourdie RG. Development of the cardiac conduction system involves recruitment within a multipotent cardiomyogenic lineage. Development 1999;126:5041–5049.

34. Fishman MC, Olson EN. Parsing the heart: genetic modules for organ assembly. Cell 1997;91:153–156.

35. Soonpaa MH, Kim KK, Pajak L, Franklin M, Field LJ. Cardiomyocyte DNA synthesis and binucleation during murine development. Am J Physiol 1996; 271:H2183–2189.

36. Anversa P, Leri A, Kajstura J, Nadal-Ginard B. Myocyte growth and cardiac repair. J Mol Cell Cardiol 2002;34:91–105.

37. Li F, Wang X, Capasso JM, Gerdes AM. Rapid transition of cardiac myocytes from hyperplasia to hypertrophy during postnatal development. J Mol Cell Cardiol 1996;28:1737–1746.

38. Mikawa T. Pericardial mesoderm generates a population of coronary smooth muscle cells migrating into the heart along with ingrowth of the epicardial organ. Dev Biol 1996;174:221–232.

39. Manner J, Seidl W, Steding G. The formal pathogenesis of isolated common carotid or innominate arteries: the concept of malseptation of the aortic sac. Anat Embryol 1997;196:435–445.

40. Waldo K. A novel role for cardiac neural crest in heart development. J Clin Invest 1999;103:1499–1507.

41. Nishibatake M. Pathogenesis of persistent truncus arteriosus and dextroposed aorta in the chick embryo after neural crest ablation. Circulation 1987;75:255–264.

42. Payne RM, Johnson MC, Grant JW, Strauss AW. Toward a molecular understanding of congenital heart disease. Circulation 1995;91:494–504.

43. Jerome LA, Papaioannou VE. DiGeorge syndrome phenotype in mice mutant for the T-box gene, Tbx1. Nature Genetics 2001; 27:286–291.

44. van den Hoff MJ, Moorman AF. Cardiac neural crest: the holy grail of cardiac abnormalities? Cardiovasc Res 2000; 47:212–216.

45. van den Hoff MJ. Myocardialization of the cardiac outflow tract. Dev Biol 1999;212:477–490.

46. Epstein DJ. Splotch (Sp2H), a mutation affecting development of the mouse neural tube, shows a deletion within the paired homeodomain of Pax-3. Genomics 1991;10:356–364.

47. Moon RT, Kimelman D. From cortical rotation to organizer gene expression: toward a molecular explanation of axis specification in Xenopus. Bioessays 1998;20:536–545.

48. Conway SJ. Decreased neural crest stem cell expansion is responsible for the conotruncal heart defects within the splotch (Sp(2H))/Pax3 mouse mutant. [see comments.]. Biochimica et Biophysica Acta 2000;1466:315–327.

49. Hunt P. Homeobox genes and models for patterning the hindbrain and branchial arches. Nature 1991;353:861–864.

50. Kirby ML. Abnormal patterning of the aortic arch arteries does not evoke cardiac malformations. Dev Dyn 1997;208:34–47.

51. Mendelsohn C. Function of the retinoic acid receptors (RARs) during development (II). Multiple abnormalities at various stages of organogenesis in RAR double mutants. Development (Suppl) 1994;120:2749–2771.

52. Harvey RP. Seeking a regulatory roadmap for heart morphogenesis. Sem Cell Dev Biol 1999;10:99–107.

53. Gruber PJ. RXR alpha deficiency confers genetic susceptibility for aortic sac, conotruncal, atrioventricular cushion, and ventricular muscle defects in mice. Ann Emerg Med 1996;28:273–277.

54. Srivastava D. A genetic blueprint for cardiac development. Australasian Radiology 2000;44:285–289.

55. Brennan P. Congenital heart malformations: aetiology and associations. Semin Neonatol 2001;6:17–25.

56. Nakajima Y, Yamagishi T, Hokari S, Nakamura H. Mechanisms involved in valvuloseptal endocardial cushion formation in early cardiogenesis: roles of transforming growth factor (TGF)-beta and bone morphogenetic protein (BMP). Anat Rec 2000;258:119–127.

57. Markwald R, Eisenberg C, Eisenberg L, Trusk T, Sugi Y. Epithelial-mesenchymal transformations in early avian heart development. Acta Anatomica 1996;156:173–186.

58. Brown CB. Antibodies to the Type II TGFbeta receptor block cell activation and migration during atrioventricular cushion transformation in the heart. Dev Biol 1996;174:248–257.

59. Yost HJ. Establishment of left-right asymmetry. Int Rev Cytol 2001;203:357–381.

60. Goldstein AM. Patterning the heart's left-right axis: from zebrafish to man. J Pediatr Surg 1998;33:756–758.

61. Kathiriya IS. Left-right asymmetry and cardiac looping: implications for cardiac development and congenital heart disease. Development (Suppl) 2000; 127:2133–2142.

62. Morishima M, Yasui H, Nakazawa M, Ando M, Ishibashi M, Takao A. Situs variation and cardiovascular anomalies in the transgenic mouse insertional mutation, inv. Teratology 1998;57:302–309.

63. McQuinn TC, Miga DE, Mjaatvedt CH, Phelps AL, Wessels A. Cardiopulmonary malformations in the inv/inv mouse. Anat Rec 2001;263:62–71.

64. Supp DM, Brueckner M, Kuehn MR, et al. Targeted deletion of the ATP binding domain of left-right dynein confirms its role in specifying development of left-right asymmetries. Development (Suppl) 1999;126:5495–5504.

65. Gannon M. Initiation of cardiac differentiation occurs in the absence of anterior endoderm. Am J Physiol 1995;269:E231–238.

66. Farrell M. A novel role for cardiac neural crest in heart development. Trends Cardiovasc Med 1999;9:214–220.

67. Taber LA. Mechanical aspects of cardiac development. Prog Biophys Mol Biol 1998;69:237–255.

68. Carraway KL III. Involvement of the neuregulins and their receptors in cardiac and neural development. Bioessays 1996; 18:263-266.

69. Sedmera D. Developmental patterning of the myocardium. Anat Rec 2000;258:319–337.

70. Mima T. Fibroblast growth factor receptor is required for in vivo cardiac myocyte proliferation at early embryonic stages of heart development. Proc Nat Acad Sci USA 1995;92:467–471.

71. Gilman V, Khanzenzon N, Lesche R, et al. Activation of the MEF2 transcription factor in skeletal muscles from myotonic mice. Mol Cell Biol 2002;22:3842–3851.

72. Moorman AF. Development of the conduction system of the heart. PACE Pacing Clin Electrophysiol 1997;20:2087–2092.

73. Gourdie RG. Conducting the embryonic heart: orchestrating development of specialized cardiac tissues. Trends Cardiovasc Med 1999;9:18–26.

74. Hyer J. Induction of Purkinje fiber differentiation by coronary arterialization. Proc Nat Acad Sci USA 1999;96:13214–13218.

75. Gourdie RG. Terminal diversification of the myocyte lineage generates Purkinje fibers of the cardiac conduction system. Development (Suppl) 1995; 121:1423–1431.

76. Rentschler S. Visualization and functional characterization of the developing murine cardiac conduction system. Development (Suppl) 2001;128:1785–1792.

77. Manner J. Does the subepicardial mesenchyme contribute myocardioblasts to the myocardium of the chick embryo heart? A quail-chick chimera study tracing the fate of the epicardial primordium. Anat Rec 1999;255:212–226.

78. Manner J. The origin, formation and developmental significance of the epicardium: a review. Ann Anat 2001;183:261–265.

79. Tevosian SG. FOG-2, a cofactor for GATA transcription factors, is essential for heart morphogenesis and development of coronary vessels from epicardium. Development (Suppl) 2000;127:2031–2040.

80. Wada AM. Bves: prototype of a new class of cell adhesion molecules expressed during coronary artery development. Development (Suppl) 2001; 128:2085–2093.

81. Carmona R, Mercado JM. Immunolocalization of the transcription factor Slug in the developing avian heart Affinity for inorganic carbon of Gracilaria tenuistipitata cultured at low and high irradiance. Anat Embryol 2000;201:103–109.

82. Macias D. Immunoreactivity of the ets-1 transcription factor correlates with areas of epithelial-mesenchymal transition in the developing avian heart. Dev Biol 1998;200:57–68.

83. Fafeur V. The ETS1 transcription factor is expressed during epithelial-mesenchymal transitions in the chick embryo and is activated in scatter factor-stimulated MDCK epithelial cells. Histochem J 1998;30:627–634.

84. Dettman RW. Common epicardial origin of coronary vascular smooth muscle, perivascular fibroblasts, and intermyocardial fibroblasts in the avian heart. Cell Growth Differ 1997;8:655–665.

85. Tomanek RJ. Vascular endothelial growth factor expression coincides with coronary vasculogenesis and angiogenesis. Am J Physiol 1999;276:H350–358.

86. Zelis R, Flaim SF, Liedtke AJ, Nellis SH. Cardiocirculatory dynamics in the normal and failing heart. Ann Rev Physiol 1981;43:455–476.

87. Carmeliet P, Collen D. Molecular basis of angiogenesis. Role of VEGF and VE-cadherin. Fibroblast growth factor-1 stimulates branching and survival of myocardial arteries: a goal for therapeutic angiogenesis? [letter; comment.]. Ann NY Acad Sci 2000;902:249–62; Discussion 262–264.

88. Carmeliet P. Impaired myocardial angiogenesis and ischemic cardiomyopathy in mice lacking the vascular endothelial growth factor isoforms VEGF164 and VEGF188. [see comments.]. J Clin Invest 1999;103:475–482.

89. Yelon D. Cardiac patterning and morphogenesis in zebrafish. Devel Dyn 2001;222:552–563.

90. Manasek FJ. Embryonic development of the heart. I. A light and electron microscopic study of myocardial development in the early chick embryo. J Morphol 1968;125:329–365.

91. Patten BM. Early embryology of the chick. New York: McGraw-Hill;1957.

92. Romanoff AL. The heart. In: The Avian Embryo. New York: Macmillan; 1960:681–780.

93. Viragh S, Szabo E, Challice CE. Formation of the primitive myo- and endocardial tubes in the chick embryo. J. Mol Cell Cardiol 1989;21:123–137.

94. Hamilton WJ, Mossman HW. Hamilton, Boyd and Mossman's Human Embryology. Cambridge:W Heffer & Sons;1972.

95. Sissman MJ. Developmental landmarks in cardiac morphogenesis: comparative chronology. Am J Cardiol 1970;25:141–148.

96. Sater AK, Jacobson AG. The restriction of the heart morphogenetic field in Xenopus laevis. Development 1990;108: 461–470.

97. Stainier DYR, Fishman MC. Patterning the zebrafish heart tube: acquisition of anteroposterior polarity. Dev. Biol 1992;153:91–101.

98. Serbedzija GN, Chen JN, Fishman MC. Regulation in the heart field of zebrafish. Development 1998;125:1095–1101.

99. Yelon D, Stainier DY. Patterning during organogenesis: genetic analysis of cardiac chamber formation Semin Cell Dev Biol. 1999;10:93–98.

100. Olson EN, Srivastava D. Molecular pathways controlling heart development. Science 1996;3;272:671–676.

101. Fishman MC, Olson EN. Parsing the heart: genetic modules for organ assembly. Cell 1997;19:153–516.

7 Inherited Myocardial Diseases

Elizabeth M. McNally, MD, PhD

CONTENTS

OVERVIEW: GENETIC CONSIDERATIONS

Almost half of all patients with congestive heart failure (CHF) present with evidence of reduced cardiac function or cardiomyopathy (1–3). Of patients with cardiomyopathy, nearly half have nonischemic cardiomyopathy (4). Nonischemic cardiomyopathy may arise from hypertension or valvular disease; however, a significant number of cardiomyopathies have a heritable component. In the last decade, considerable progress has been made in understanding the inheritance patterns and the molecular defects associated with the development of cardiomyopathies (5).

Genetic studies have correlated genetic polymorphisms with cardiomyopathic phenotypes and have revealed the broad genetic heterogeneity that underlies heritable cardiomyopathies. Mutations at multiple alleles in a single gene may be associated with a particular cardiomyopathic phenotype, and allelic heterogeneity can be used to indicate clinical outcome. Correlations between genotype and phenotype can be useful in screening and treating family members. Genetic data, combined with clinical and experimental data, have been helpful in assessing the function of mutant gene products; therefore, dissection of the genetics of the cardiomyopathies has provided insight not only

for the clinician but also for the basic scientist in determining the functional defects that result from these mutations.

However, genetic studies in humans have limitations. Genetic studies establish statistically significant associations between a genetic polymorphism and a particular phenotype. Results from genetic studies are strengthened by identifying additional mutations or multiple cases of the same mutation. However, demonstrating a causal nature of a mutation often requires supplemental studies. For example, in vitro studies of the normal and mutated gene product can be used to indicate function of a gene product. Developing an animal model by using gene insertion or gene disruption techniques can help identify the causative nature of gene mutations. But even when in vitro and in vivo studies are used to evaluate the effects of a mutation, the complete cellular function of a gene product may not be identified. Mutations in animal models may not recapitulate the human findings. Thus, the clinician must assess all the data before informing the patient or the patient's family of the prognosis.

Many inherited hypertrophic and dilated cardiomyopathy syndromes have an autosomal dominant pattern of inheritance (6). In examination of multiple generations in a patient's family history, fewer than half of family members

From: *Contemporary Cardiology: Principles of Molecular Cardiology*
Edited by: M. S. Runge and C. Patterson @ Humana Press Inc., Totowa, NJ

are usually affected. Males and females tend to be affected equally, and father-to-son transmission excludes mitochondrial and X-linked inheritance. These findings are influenced, in part, by ascertainment bias because only large multigenerational families are suitable for genetic studies. An important genetic feature of the inherited cardiomyopathies is age-dependent expressivity or penetrance; signs and symptoms of cardiomyopathy are often absent in younger patients, despite the presence of the mutated allele. Variable penetrance and expressivity complicate genetic studies because even subjects with gene mutations may appear entirely normal. The hypertrophic and dilated cardiomyopathies are genetically heterogeneous. Mutations in different genes may produce an identical cardiomyopathy phenotype. In some cases the gene products may interact in a macromolecular complex, but in other cases, the relationship between gene products is less clear.

HYPERTROPHIC CARDIOMYOPATHY

Sarcomeric Gene Mutations

Hypertrophic cardiomyopathy is defined by an increase in the thickness of the left or right ventricular wall or of both walls (7). Hypertrophy may often be asymmetrical and tends to affect, in descending order, the interventricular septum, the posterior or anterior wall, or the apex (Fig. 1). The overall ventricular volume is normal or reduced, and a pressure gradient caused by septal hypertrophy may be established within the ventricle. The clinical correlates of these anatomic findings are primarily arrhythmias and CHF. The range of arrhythmias seen in hypertrophic cardiomyopathy is wide and includes sudden cardiac death, ventricular and atrial tachyarrhythmias, and bradyarrhythmias. The estimated incidence of hypertrophic cardiomyopathy is 1:500 (8), with a significant percentage resulting from inherited disease (9). The prevalence of hypertrophic cardiomyopathy and familial hypertrophic cardiomyopathy (FHC) varies considerably according to geographic location, age of the population, and diagnostic technique. Myofibrillar disarray, which may be seen on histopathologic study, has limited diagnostic use because it affects only a small portion of the myocardium.

FHC is characterized by an autosomal dominant inheritance pattern and age-dependent penetrance and expressivity. Mutations in 10 different genes have been associated with the development of FHC (Table 1). Most genes associated with FHC encode proteins of the sarcomere (10–12). The sarcomere, which is the fundamental unit of contraction of striated muscle (Fig. 2), is composed

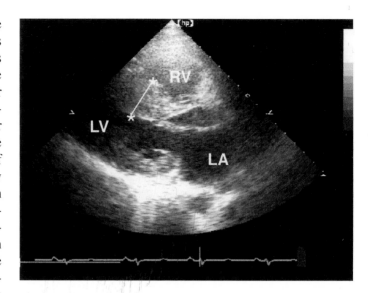

Fig. 1. Long-axis view of a two-dimensional echocardiogram of hypertrophic cardiomyopathy (HCM). Note the marked thickening of the interventricular septum (asterisks and white line), a characteristic finding in HCM. Septal thickening can lead to gradients in the outflow tract. LA, left atrium; LV, left ventricle; RV, right ventricle.

of thick and thin filaments. The thick filaments are composed of myosin and myosin binding protein C (MyBPC), whereas the thin filaments include actin and the two regulatory proteins, troponin and tropomyosin. The near crystalline array found within striated muscle permits thin filaments to slide along thick filaments in response to changes in intracellular calcium. Myosin hydrolyzes ATP to create a force, or powerstroke, that allows thin filaments to slide along thick filaments.

The β-myosin heavy chain (βMyHC) gene, also known as MYH7, was the first gene associated with FHC mutations (13,14). Myosin is a hexamer composed of two heavy chains and four light chains (two regulatory light chains and two essential light chains). Proteolysis was initially used to separate myosin into a globular head region and an elongated rod region. Located within the head domain are sequences specified for interacting with actin, hydrolyzing ATP, and producing force. The rod region directs the assembly of thick filaments and forms the backbone from which myosin heads protrude. βMyHC, which is the primary myosin heavy chain of the human ventricle, accounts for the enzymatic and motor function that underlies muscle contraction in the ventricle. More than 50 different mutations in the βMyHC gene have been associated with FHC (10–12). Based on analyses of a three-dimensional crystal structure of βMyHC's myosin head, many of the mutations associated with FHC are located in regions that dictate ATPase and actin binding activity (15).

Table 1
Genetic Regions and Genes Associated with Familial Hypertrophic Cardiomyopathy

Disease	OMIM no.	Gene product (gene name)	Chromosome location
CMH1	192600	β-Myosin heavy chain* (MYH7)	14q12
CMH2	115195	Cardiac troponin T* (TNNT2)	1q32
CMH3	115196	α-Tropomyosin* (TPM1)	15q22.1
CMH4	115197	Myosin binding protein C* (MYBPC3)	11p11.2
CMH6	600858	γ subunit AMP-activated protein kinase† (PRKAG2)	7q3
CMH7	191044	Troponin I* (TNNI3)	19q13.4
CMH8	160790	Myosin light chain 1* (MYL1)	3p
CMH9	188840	Titin* (TTN)	2q24.3
CMH10	160781	Myosin light chain 2* (MYL2)	12q23–24
	102540	Cardiac actin* (ACTC)	15q14
	160710	α-Myosin heavy chain* (MYH6)	14q12

OMIM, Online Mendelian Inheritance in Man (http://www.ncbi.nlm.nih.gov/Omim/); CMH, hypertrophic cardiomyopathy.
*Sarcomeric gene product.
†Non-sarcomeric gene product.

A common βMyHC mutation, R403Q, is present in multiple families with FHC and is located near the region of myosin that interfaces with actin (14). The R403Q mutation was generated in the mouse by creating an allele in the endogenous αMyHC gene, which is the primary gene expressed in the mouse myocardium (16). The R403Q mutant mice develop hypertrophic cardiomyopathy with sudden death. This model and another mouse model that expresses a mutant αMyHC from a transgene (17) have shown the usefulness of mice in studying mechanisms of cardiomyopathy. Although useful, mouse models have technical limitations because of the small size of the mouse heart and the rapid heart rate (600 beats per minute in the unanesthetized state) (20). A larger animal model of FHC, which allows for hemodynamic and pharmacologic studies, was generated by inserting mutant transgenes into fertilized rabbit oocytes. These transgenes direct expression of mutant βMyHC specifically in the hearts of rabbits (18,19).

Pathogenic features of mutant MyHC molecules have been studied with in vitro motility assays (10,21). By using purified actin and myosin, the velocity of thin filament sliding can be measured, indicating the in vivo properties of muscle contraction (22). Results of such studies indicate that mutations in the βMyHC gene can reduce or increase the velocity of thin filament sliding (23–27). Thus, different mutations in the βMyHC gene may result in different pathogenetic mechanisms. In dominant diseases such as FHC, both the normal and the abnormal alleles are expressed, which means hybrid myosins may be generated with heads that function at different rates. These hybrid myosins may contribute to the development of FHC.

Because of the large size of the βMyHC gene, and the laborious screening process (28,29), mutation screens have concentrated mainly on those exons that encode the head region of βMyHC. Only recently was the entire βMyHC gene more fully examined, and FHC mutations within the βMyHC rod region identified (30). Mutations that map outside of the myosin force-producing region and to the rod region may produce a hypertrophic phenotype through mechanisms different from those in the myosin head. Such mutations may affect thick filament assembly, thereby altering force transmission or other properties of the sarcomere.

Although rare, mutations have been identified in both the regulatory and essential light chain myosin genes in patients with FHC (31–33). Mutations in the gene encoding the essential myosin light chain (MLC) 1/3 are associated with hypertrophy of the midportion of the ventricle, whereas mutations in the gene encoding regulatory MLC2 are associated with concomitant skeletal muscle disease (see below). The function of myosin light chains in striated muscle is not fully understood. In crystallographic studies, the light chains are located near the head–rod junction where they may modulate the powerstroke (34).

MyBPC interacts with myosin along myosin's rod region (35). More than 30 different mutations in the gene encoding MyBPC have been identified in FHC patients (36–38). About 15–30% of FHC patients have mutations within the MyBPC gene. MyBPC has nine immunoglobulin domains and three fibronectin domains. A unique region, found only in cardiac MyBPC, can be phosphorylated (39). At its carboxyl-terminus, MyBPC binds both myosin and titin, and many of the known mutations would likely produce a

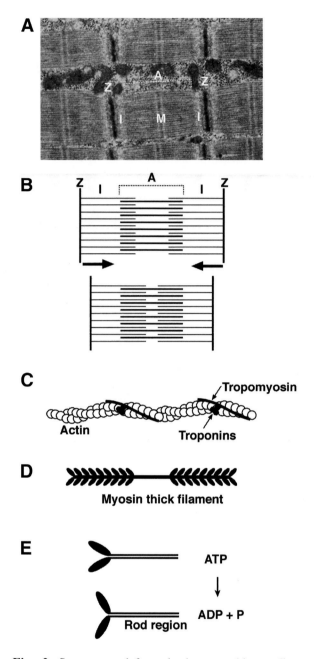

truncated MyBPC. MyBPC may help organize and stabilize sarcomeres *(40)*. Many MyBPC mutations described in humans with FHC produce a milder phenotype that includes both CHF and arrhythmias associated with hypertrophic cardiomyopathy *(41)*. Age of onset is much later and sudden cardiac death is less frequent in patients with MyBPC gene mutations than in patients with βMyHC gene mutations. Gene targeting and transgenesis have been used to develop mouse models of MyBPC mutations in FHC *(42–44)*. Mice with MyBPC mutations have abnormal cardiac function and a milder form of hypertrophic cardiomyopathy than mice with sarcomere-associated cardiomyopathy.

Mutations in the cardiac troponin T (cTnT) and cardiac troponin I genes have been described in FHC patients *(45–47)*. The thin filaments of striated muscle, which are composed of actin, tropomyosin, and troponin subunits, provide a backbone against which myosin heads move. In addition, troponin and tropomyosin regulate calcium at the actomyosin interface. cTnT, a 37-kDa protein, binds along the length of α-tropomyosin and can be phosphorylated. The binding of cTnT to α-tropomyosin is regulated by calcium. cTnT mutations appear to be associated with less hypertrophy than mutations in other hypertrophy-related genes but with an increased risk of sudden cardiac death *(48)*. In mice with mutant cTnT, sudden death occurs with only a modest degree of hypertrophy *(49–51)*, and pathologic studies indicate a dominant negative mode of action. Cardiomyocytes expressing mutant cTnT are hypersensitive to calcium *(52)*, and in vitro studies suggest that mutations in thin filament proteins increase the sliding velocity and may adversely alter crossbridge dynamics *(53)*. The clinician should suspect cTnT mutations in patients with FHC who present with minimal hypertrophy and a prominent family history of sudden cardiac death. Mutations in cardiac troponin C have been reported in patients with FHC, but additional studies are needed to confirm the pathogenic nature of troponin C mutations *(54)*.

Mutations in the α-Tropomyosin gene associate with FHC *(45,47)*. α-Tropomyosin, which is expressed and alternatively spliced in cardiac and skeletal muscle, is an elongated rod-like protein that lies along the major groove

Fig. 2. Sarcomere defects in hypertrophic cardiomyopathy (HCM). (**A**) An electron micrograph of a sarcomere. The thin filaments, which constitute the I band, insert into the Z lines. The A band represents both thin and thick filaments. The H band (not shown) represents the midportion of the sarcomere and is composed only of thick filaments. The M band is in the center of the sarcomere. The resting length of a sarcomere is 2 μm. (**B**) Upon contraction, the sarcomere shortens. The A band remains a constant length, but the I bands and the distance between the Z lines shorten. (**C**) Thin filaments are composed of actin filaments, tropomyosin that binds along the major groove of the actin filaments, and the three troponin subunits. Troponin and tropomyosin allow calcium to regulate the actin–myosin interaction. (**D**) The thick filament, which is composed of myosin and myosin-binding

Fig. 2. *(Continued)* protein C, is a large assembly of myosin molecules in an antiparallel array. The center region of the thick filament is devoid of myosin heads. (**E**) A single myosin molecule (shown) is composed of two heavy chains and four light chains (not shown). Proteolysis splits myosin into the S1 head region and the rod region. The S1 head hydrolyzes ATP and binds actin. The myosin light chains bind at the head–rod junction.

of actin filaments. The clinical course in patients with α-tropomyosin mutations is relatively severe and is similar to that seen in patients with βMyHC mutations (45,47,55). Studies in mice suggest a dominant negative mode of function in which mutant forms of α-tropomyosin interfere with normal function of the thin filament (56).

Non-Sarcomeric Gene Mutations

A variant of FHC has recently been associated with mutations in the γ2 regulatory subunit of AMP-activated protein kinase, PRKAG2 (57,58). PRKAG2 regulates the level of ATP in the cell through kinase activity when AMP/ATP ratios favor AMP. Mutations in the γ2 subunit may limit enzymatic activation and essentially mimic a condition of energy depletion. In FHC patients with PRKAG2 mutations, preexcitation similar to what is found in Wolff–Parkinson–White syndrome may be seen (58). With PRKAG2 mutations, the surface electrocardiogram (ECG) may show a shortened PR interval and/or a widened QRS or may reveal left bundle branch block. Defects in the conduction system may appear before hypertrophy develops. The similar constellation of arrhythmias and CHF symptoms eventually dominate the clinical picture. Identifying additional PRKAG2 mutations and associating a genotype with a phenotype may indicate whether the hypertrophic phenotype can be separated from the preexcitation aspects of the phenotype. Whether PRKAG2 FHC and sarcomeric-associated FHC have the same pathogenetic mechanism is unknown. Because mutations in PRKAG2 appear to alter energy production, force production is indirectly altered. However, myocardium from patients with PRKAG2 mutations has an abnormal accumulation of glycogen, which is similar to that seen with storage diseases (59). In children, glycogen storage diseases such as Pompe's disease (see below) can lead to hypertrophic cardiomyopathy. Genetic heterogeneity underlies the Wolff–Parkinson–White syndrome, and additional genetic mechanisms that contribute to this arrhythmia disorder will be identified, which should clarify the underlying pathology and molecular mechanisms.

Clinical Implications

In evaluating a patient with FHC, the clinician should obtain a careful family history with particular emphasis on relatives with sudden death. Early family history of sudden death in a symptomatic FHC patient may warrant implantation of a cardiac defibrillator, potentially even in asymptomatic patients. For those patients with a family history that suggests a milder course, the decision to implant a cardiac defibrillator may be deferred until symptoms develop. The clinician should consider the clinical and genetic

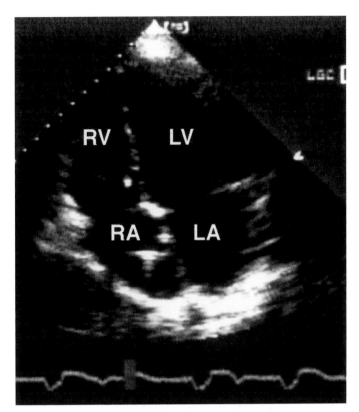

Fig. 3. A four-chamber, two-dimensional echocardiogram of dilated cardiomyopathy showing enlargement of all four chambers and the presence of a pacemaker (white region in the RA). LA, left atrium; LV, left ventricle; RA, right atrium; RV, right ventricle.

information before deciding on device implantation. Automatic defibrillators are an effective means of controlling ventricular arrhythmias that frequently accompany hypertrophic cardiomyopathy (60,61).

DILATED CARDIOMYOPATHY

Dilated cardiomyopathy is classified as four-chamber enlargement with contractile dysfunction (Fig. 3) (7). The definition of dilated cardiomyopathy excludes significant preexisting ischemic, valvular, pericardial, and congenital disease as a cause. Clinical manifestations include systolic and diastolic dysfunction and arrhythmias (both tachyarrhythmias and bradyarrhythmias). The incidence of dilated cardiomyopathy, estimated at 36.5 per 100,000, varies considerably depending on the geographic location of the population (62). The etiology is heterogeneous and includes toxic (e.g., ethanol, adriamycin) and infectious (e.g., Coxsackie virus, Chagas disease) agents. Other associated illnesses or medical conditions such as hypertension and pregnancy may contribute to the development of cardiomyopathy, and the mechanisms may be under

Table 2
Genetic Regions and Genes Associated with Familial Dilated Cardiomyopathy

Disease (ref.)	OMIM no.	Gene product (gene name)	Chromosome location	Clinical features
CMD1A (97–99)	115200	Lamin A/C (LMNA)	1q21	MD, LD
CMD1B (167)	600884		9q13	
CMD1C (141,142)	601493		10q21–23	
CMD1D (95)	601494	Troponin T	1q32	
CMD1E (168)	601154	Sodium channel (SCN5A)	3p25–22	
CMD3F (169)	602067		6q23	MD
CMD1G (91)	604145	Titin	2q24.3–34	
CMD1H (170)	604288		2q22–22	
CMD1I (122)	604765	Desmin (DES)	2q35	
CMD1J (171)	605362		6q23–24	deafness
CMD1K (172)	605182		6q12	
CMD1L (87)	606685	δ-Sarcoglycan (SGCD)	5q33	
CMD1M (90)	607482	MLP (CSRP3)	11p15	
CMD1N (90)	607487	Tcap/telethonin (Tcap)	17q12	
CMD1O (173)	608569	Sulfonylurea receptor 2 (ABCC9)	12p12	
(92)	102540	Cardiac actin (ACTC)	15q14	
(174)	172405	Phospholamban (PLB)	6q22	
(94)	106760	β-Myosin heavy chain	14q12	
(145)	605676	Desmoplakin (DSP)	6q24	WHK
XLCM (69,70	302045	Dystrophin	Xq21	MD
CDM3A(160)	300069	Tafazzin	Xq28	neutropia

OMIM, Online Mendelian Inheritance in Man (http://www.ncbi.nlm.nih.gov/Omim/); CMD, dilated cardiomyopathy; XLCM, X-linked dilated cardiomyopathy; MD, muscular dystrophy; LD, lipodystrophy; WHK wooly hair, keratoderma.

genetic control. In this chapter, cardiac-intrinsic causes of dilated cardiomyopathy will be discussed. Studies of first-degree relatives have shown that 35% of patients with idiopathic dilated cardiomyopathy may actually have an inherited form of cardiomyopathy or familial dilated cardiomyopathy (FDC) (63–65).

Assessing genetic diseases requires ascertainment of large families, which is difficult and can lead to bias. The genetic heterogeneity of dilated cardiomyopathy is illustrated by the identification of at least 19 different genetic regions significantly associated with FDC (6) (Table 2). In some cases, the gene product affected by the mutation has been identified, but in many cases the gene product is unknown. In the next several years, genetic etiologies of FDC will be uncovered, identifying gene products that play a role in myocardial stability.

Cytoskeletal Gene Mutations

The dystrophin gene on the X chromosome is best known for its association with Duchenne/Becker muscular dystrophy, the most common X-linked disorder. Affecting one in 3500 liveborn males, Duchenne/Becker muscular dystrophy, which usually presents in childhood, is characterized by progressive proximal muscle weakness. Although cardiomyopathy frequently accompanies the muscular dystrophies (66,67), mutations in the dystrophin gene have been associated with cardiomyopathy that occurs in the absence of overt muscle degeneration and muscular dystrophy (68–70). In these cases, affected males present with four-chamber enlargement, CHF, and tachy- and bradyarrhythmias in the second or third decade of life. Cardiac transplantation has been used successfully to treat these patients. In these families, carrier females may develop dilated cardiomyopathy in the fifth or sixth decade (71), although earlier onset has been described (72). Cardiomyopathy of early or late-onset in these women may be caused by a skewing of X-inactivation that preferentially maintains the mutant X-chromosome. Alternatively, the chimeric state of dystrophin-normal cardiomyocytes adjacent to dystrophin-abnormal cardiomyocytes may

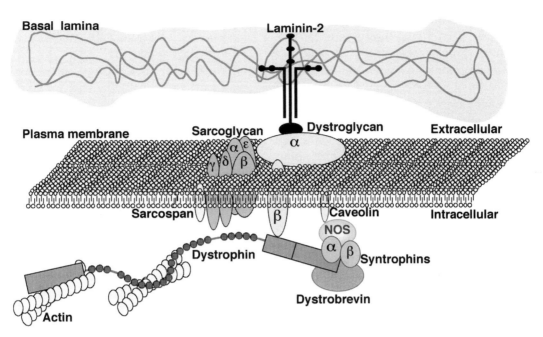

Fig. 4. The dystrophin–glycoprotein complex (DGC) is a mechanosignaling complex that stabilizes the plasma membrane in heart and skeletal muscle. Dystrophin, an elongated cytoskeletal protein that sits beneath the plasma membrane, binds cytoskeletal actin. In addition, dystrophin forms the dystrophin glycoprotein complex by binding a complex of transmembrane and membrane-associated proteins. Dystroglycan is composed of α and β subunits and binds directly to dystrophin in the cytoplasm and laminin 2 in the extracellular matrix, thus forming a link between the cytoskeleton, the membrane, and the extracellular matrix. The sarcoglycan complex is composed of several different subunits (α–ε) and may serve to strengthen the interaction between the dystroglycan subunits. Mutations in the sarcoglycan genes lead to cardiomyopathy and muscular dystrophy. Caveolin, neuronal nitric oxide synthase (NOS), the syntrophins, and dystrobrevin are part of the dystrophin glycoprotein complex.

contribute to the development of cardiomyopathy. Several different mechanisms may explain why cardiac muscle cells are affected more than skeletal muscle cells. Mutations that alter dystrophin's 5′ regulatory regions may eliminate expression in cardiomyocytes but not in skeletal myocytes *(73)*. Alternatively, the role of dystrophin in cardiac and skeletal muscle cells may differ, and regions of dystrophin may be more important in cardiac cell than in skeletal muscle cell function *(70)*.

In skeletal muscle, the dystrophin protein is found at the periphery of the myofiber in a submembranous position *(74)*. Dystrophin binds a complex of transmembrane proteins in skeletal and cardiac muscle and forms the dystrophin–glycoprotein complex (DGC) (Fig. 4) *(75)*. These transmembrane proteins are secondarily destabilized when dystrophin is mutated. The proposed role of the DGC is to provide mechanical stability to the muscle membrane during the repeated forces associated with contraction. This hypothesis is supported by the interaction of dystrophin with cytoskeletal actin in its amino terminus and along its rod region *(76,77)*. At its carboxyl end, dystrophin binds to dystroglycan, which is a widely expressed protein that binds to the extracellular

matrix protein laminin-2 (merosin) *(78)*. Thus, the DGC forms a mechanical link that connects the cytoskeleton to the membrane and the extracellular matrix. Mutations in dystrophin and DGC proteins lead to membrane instability and abnormal membrane permeability *(75)*. Eccentric contraction in dystrophin-deficient skeletal muscle and pressure overload hypertrophy in dystrophin-deficient hearts increase membrane damage, a finding that emphasizes the role of dystrophin as mechanical stabilizer *(79,80)*. In cardiac muscle, dystrophin and the DGC are associated with the plasma membrane and the T tubule system *(81,82)*.

Coxsackie B virus is a significant cause of myocarditis and virally mediated cardiomyopathy *(83)*. Badorff and colleagues showed that the 2A protease produced by the Coxsackie B3 strain can recognize and cleave dystrophin in cardiomyocytes *(84)*. Furthermore, this cleavage can be inhibited by a substrate that resembles dystrophin *(85)*. These findings suggest that membrane instability caused by dystrophin cleavage may mediate cardiomyopathy that accompanies Coxsackie infection; therefore, dystrophin defects may contribute to more than only inherited forms of dilated cardiomyopathy.

δ-Sarcoglycan is a transmembrane component of the DGC. Mutations in δ-sarcoglycan are a rare cause of autosomal recessive limb-girdle muscular dystrophy *(86)*. Two different mutations have been identified in the δ-sarcoglycan gene in a large cohort of patients with dilated cardiomyopathy from three different families *(87)*. These patients have only a single mutated δ-sarcoglycan allele, a pattern consistent with autosomal dominant inheritance. Because these mutations encode missense amino acid substitutions and a microdeletion, they may be dominant interfering or dominant negative. In mice, disrupting the smooth muscle sarcoglycan complex causes vasospasm and results in cardiomyopathy *(88,89)*. Although studies are limited, no evidence of vasospasm has been found in cardiomyopathy patients with mutant δ-sarcoglycan *(87)*. This finding may be explained by different inheritance patterns and by the presence of a normal δ-sarcoglycan allele in these subjects. Additional studies of patients with δ-sarcoglycan gene mutations are needed to establish the role of δ-sarcoglycan in dilated cardiomyopathy.

Titin is a large cytoskeletal protein that interacts with the sarcomere and membrane-associated proteins in muscle and heart. Titin may help maintain the integrity of cardiomyocytes and skeletal myofibers and contributes to the elastic recoil that occurs after muscle contraction. Together with muscle LIM protein (MLP) and telethonin, titin participates in the passive stretch mechanism in cardiomyocytes *(90)*. Titin interacts directly with MyBPC. Because the titin gene is large, screening for mutations is difficult; however, mutations in the titin gene associate with FDC *(91)*.

Cardiac actin is a component of the sarcomere, and mutations in the gene for cardiac actin are a rare cause of inherited dilated cardiomyopathy *(92)*. Olson et al. screened a cohort of patients with dilated cardiomyopathy, finding two different actin gene mutations in small families with DCM *(92)*. In more recent studies, Olson et al. *(93)* identified mutations in the cardiac actin gene in families with hypertrophic and/or dilated cardiomyopathic phenotypes. The mutant amino acids were modeled in the three-dimensional crystal structure of actin, and these changes map to the area of actin that interacts with myosin. Mutations in other areas of the actin molecule may alter force transmission and lead to dilated cardiomyopathy. Hypertrophic cardiomyopathy often progresses to a dilated phenotype. The regulation of the progression from hypertrophic to dilated cardiomyopathy is not well understood, and genetic control may influence this transition. Supporting this hypothesis is the recent association between FDC and mutations in βMyHC, α-tropomyosin, and cTnT *(94,95)*. Studying these mutations may help our understanding of the role of genes in the progression from a hypertrophic to a dilated state and the progression of cardiomyopathy and CHF.

Defects in the nuclear cytoskeleton may contribute to the genesis of cardiomyopathy and arrhythmias (Fig. 5) *(96)*. Mutations in the nuclear intermediate filament protein lamin A/C have been associated with a constellation of symptoms that includes dilated cardiomyopathy, heart block at the level of atrioventricular node (AV), and muscular dystrophy *(97–99)*. Lamin A/C, which is associated with the inner nuclear membrane, provides structure to the nucleus. Lamin A and lamin C are alternative splice forms of the same gene. When the lamin A/C gene is mutated, forces of contraction against a weakened nuclear membrane may produce disease in a manner similar to the mechanism by which cytoskeletal defects lead to instability of the plasma membrane. Alternatively, the nuclear cytoskeleton creates a scaffold for heterochromatin *(100)*; in this model, lamin A/C may regulate gene expression or DNA replication directly or indirectly. Both lamin A and C share the amino terminal globular region with two α-helical rod domains. Mutations that create missense amino acid substitutions along the rod portions of lamin A/C have been associated with cardiomyopathy *(99)*, whereas missense mutations that alter a small region of the second α-helical domain lead to an unusual disorder of adipocyte wasting and lipid abnormalities known as Dunnigan-type familial partial lipodystrophy *(101,102)*. The differential effects of mutations in lamin A/C, with some leading to cardiac and muscle disease and others leading to adipocyte wasting, are not understood. Lamin A/C is found in the nucleus of many differentiated cell types. One mechanism by which mutations may lead to tissue-specific phenotypes is by disrupting tissue specific protein-protein interactions. Because lamin A/C may help regulate gene expression by scaffolding heterochromatin regions, protein–DNA interactions may be disrupted in a tissue-specific manner.

ASSOCIATED SKELETAL MUSCLE DISEASE

Because many of the same genes are expressed in both cardiac and skeletal muscle, mutations that lead to intrinsic cardiac disease may also lead to intrinsic skeletal muscle disease. The most common example of this duality is the combination of cardiac disease and a muscular dystrophy, although muscle weakness may be mild. For patients with cardiomyopathy, measuring serum levels of skeletal muscle enzymes such as creatine kinase (CK) may be helpful in diagnosing muscular dystrophy. Serum levels of CK may be 2–10 times higher than normal in

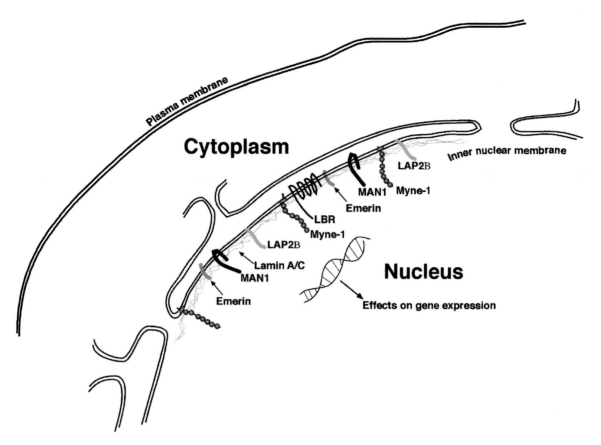

Fig. 5. The nuclear membrane. Several proteins in the inner nuclear membrane are involved in cardiomyopathy, heart block, and muscular dystrophy. Lamin A/C is an intermediate protein that provides structure to the nucleus, and emerin, which is the product of the gene involved in Emery–Dreifuss muscular dystrophy, binds to lamin A/C. Together, these proteins along with other inner nuclear membrane proteins such as MAN1, lamin-associated protein (LAP) 2β, the lamin B receptor (LBR), and myne-1(nesprin-1α), may form a complex that scaffolds heterochromatin and thereby regulates gene expression.

patients with mild forms of muscular dystrophy. CK-MB levels are often increased in muscular dystrophy patients because cardiac specific forms of many enzymes are expressed during the regeneration of skeletal muscle, which is a hallmark of the muscular dystrophies. Serum aldolase is a relatively specific but insensitive skeletal muscle marker that may indicate skeletal muscle-specific damage. Biopsy of skeletal muscle can be helpful because centrally located nuclei, variable fiber size, and increased fibrosis are seen in mild forms of muscular dystrophy. Patients may not report weakness but may be considered relatively unathletic. CHF symptoms may limit exercise tolerance, which would prevent complaints of muscle weakness.

Preferential involvement of the respiratory musculature can be seen in Duchenne and Becker muscular dystrophy and the limb-girdle muscular dystrophies and should be evaluated when considering cardiac transplantation in these patients *(103)*. MRI can be used to assess muscle damage. Severe skeletal muscle disease alone can possibly lead to cardiomyopathy *(104)*; hypoventilation and hypoxemia from respiratory muscle dystrophy may lead to right ventricular involvement as shown by ECG and echocardiograph findings and ultimately to the development of cor pulmonale. Cardiac and skeletal muscle disease may progress at different rates in muscular dystrophies, which may account for the presence of skeletal muscle disease without significant cardiomyopathy and vice versa *(105)*.

Severe skeletal muscle disease that limits physical activity may also limit CHF symptoms. Nonetheless, standard pharmacologic treatment including angiotensin-converting enzyme inhibitors or receptor blockade plus β blockade should be considered along with surveillance for and treatment of arrhythmias *(106)*. Not all muscular dystrophy patients develop cardiomyopathy. For example, mutations in the genes for calpain and dysferlin often cause autosomal recessive muscular dystrophy, but cardiomyopathy usually does not develop in these patients. Of muscular dystrophy patients, those with DGC gene mutations, Emery–Dreifuss muscular dystrophy, or myotonic dystrophy are most likely to show cardiomyopathy.

Mutations in the genes encoding the DGC are common causes of muscular dystrophy, and cardiomyopathy and arrhythmias often develop in patients with DGC mutations *(67,105)*. Frank cardiac dilation often develops later in the disease after significant progression of skeletal muscle dystrophy. This finding suggests that the DGC is more important for normal skeletal muscle function than cardiac muscle function, which is paradoxical given DGC's hypothesized role as a mechanical stabilizer. Cardiac muscle is under considerable, almost constant, force and, unlike skeletal muscle, has limited to no regenerative potential. Thus, the delayed onset of clinical cardiomyopathy after the progression of skeletal muscle dystrophy is surprising. Cardiac muscle has possibly developed additional mechanisms by which to protect against the membrane instability associated with dystrophin and sarcoglycan gene mutations. The dystrophin homolog utrophin may substitute for dystrophin in heart *(107,108)*. Mice with mutations in the genes for both dystrophin and utrophin have a more severe cardiomyopathy (and skeletal muscle dystrophy) than mice with a mutation in either of the genes.

In the lamin A/C-mediated muscular dystrophy/cardiomyopathy syndrome, cardiomyopathy is more prominent, with skeletal muscle dystrophy ranging from mild to asymptomatic *(98,99)*. Disease of the cardiac conduction system, such as AV nodal heart block, can be an early presentation of lamin A/C mutations. Treatment with pacemakers reduced the incidence of sudden death in a large cohort of patients with lamin A/C mutations *(109)*. Because pacemaker implantation did not eliminate sudden death, a significant percentage of sudden deaths may result from ventricular tachyarrhythmias; therefore, implantable cardiac defibrillators should be considered in these patients.

Mutations in the gene for the nuclear protein emerin lead to Emery–Dreifuss muscular dystrophy *(110)*, which is an X-linked recessive disease. Like lamin A/C mutations, emerin mutations are associated with progressive muscular dystrophy, AV nodal heart block, and cardiomyopathy. Lamin A/C and emerin can interact at the nuclear membrane *(111,112)*. The clinical picture associated with mutations in lamin A/C is referred to as autosomal dominant Emery Dreifuss because of the overlap in the phenotypic presentation of lamin A/C and emerin gene mutations.

Myotonic dystrophy arises from a trinucleotide repeat expansion at chromosome 19q1 *(113)*. The normal chromosome may have from 5 to 30 copies of this CTG repeat. An increase to more than 50 copies of the CTG repeat is associated with the development of myotonic dystrophy, which may be accompanied by muscle weakness that is progressive and mild, AV nodal heart block, cardiomyopathy, temporal wasting, cataracts, testicular atrophy, and neuropsychiatric defects. A relatively common genetic disorder, myotonic dystrophy is found in 1:8000 subjects. Myotonic dystrophy is inherited in an autosomal dominant fashion, and subsequent generations tend to have more CTG repeats and earlier onset of disease consistent with genetic anticipation, that is, earlier onset in succeeding generations. The repeat expansion leads to abnormal nuclear retention of mRNAs including the mRNA encoding myotonic dystrophy protein kinase (DMPK). Mice in which the DMPK gene has been deleted have abnormalities of the cardiac conduction system *(114)*. Recent data demonstrate that abnormal nuclear accumulation of the mRNA encoding only the CTG expansion contributes significantly to the pathology in myotonic dystrophy *(115)*.

RESTRICTIVE CARDIOMYOPATHIES

The information on the genetics of restrictive cardiomyopathies is limited, in part, because these disorders are rarer than dilated or hypertrophic cardiomyopathies. Restrictive cardiomyopathies are characterized by decreased myocardial compliance with increased filling pressures *(116,117)*. Hypertrophy affecting both ventricles can be detected by echocardiography or MRI. Symptoms of CHF may accompany increases in intracardiac pressures and in the size of the atria. As with other inherited myopathies, conduction system disease and arrhythmias are an important clinical concern. Infiltrative processes, which occur secondary to metabolic or genetic derangements and include amyloidosis, sarcoidosis, or hemochromatosis, may also arise as an intrinsic defect in the myocyte.

A major pathologic characteristic of intrinsic restrictive cardiomyopathies is an increase in the type III intermediate filament protein desmin *(118)*, which is best seen using electron microscopy. Desmin, which is part of the cytoskeleton and nuclear cytoskeleton, is important for the stability of lateral interactions within sarcomeres *(119)*. An accumulation of desmin disrupts the sarcomere and probably impedes the generation of force and its transmission within the sarcomere. Mutations in the desmin gene, which maps to chromosome 2q35, have been found in families with restrictive cardiomyopathies as well as in individuals *(120–122)*. Mice with a transgene expressing a desmin sequence with a small deletion of seven amino acids serve as a model for desmin myopathy *(123)*. These mice develop a restrictive physiology with impaired relaxation, thus supporting the role of desmin mutations in restrictive cardiomyopathies. Desmin is expressed in skeletal muscle, and desmin mutations have been associated with skeletal muscle myopathies *(120,121)*. In skeletal disease, an abnormal accumulation of intracellular aggregates of desmin can be seen on electron microscopy.

Like other cardiomyopathies, restrictive cardiomyopathies are genetically heterogeneous. Not all desmin-related myopathies, which are defined as those characterized by an increase in desmin, arise from mutations in the gene for desmin. For example, in a large family with an autosomal recessive desmin-related myopathy, the gene for desmin was normal, and the mutation mapped to chromosome 11q21-q23, where the CRYAB gene is located *(124)*. CRYAB encodes α B-crystallin, a small heat shock protein that aids in protein folding and that binds both cytoplasmic actin and desmin. A missense mutation in CRYAB, R120G, was associated with myopathy *(124)*. When the mutant CRYAB gene is introduced into muscle cell lines, desmin and α B-crystallin accumulate within the cells *(125)*. Moreover, mice that overexpress R120G α B-crystallin in cardiac tissue develop restrictive physiology with impaired relaxation and evidence of intracellular accumulation of aggregates composed of desmin and α B-crystallin *(126)*.

The genetic heterogeneity that underlies these disorders extends beyond the desmin and CRYAB genes. In a large four-generation family with mild ventricular hypertrophy, enlarged atria, CHF symptoms, and desmin accumulation *(127)*, many family members developed atrial fibrillation and venous hypertension. Genetic analysis of this large family excluded the involvement of the desmin and α B-crystallin genes. Therefore, there are additional genetic regions associated with restrictive cardiomyopathies. Because of their progressive characteristics, restrictive cardiomyopathies may overlap phenotypically with both hypertrophic and dilated cardiomyopathies.

ARRHYTHMOGENIC RIGHT VENTRICULAR CARDIOMYOPATHY

In the cardiac-intrinsic disorder arrhythmogenic right ventricular cardiomyopathy (ARVC), cardiomyocytes in the right ventricle are replaced by fibrofatty infiltration in a pathologic process similar to that seen in the muscular dystrophies *(128)*. Patients with ARVC, frequently referred to as arrhythmogenic right ventricular dysplasia, present with ventricular tachyarrhythmias, ventricular fibrillation, and sudden death. ARVC is usually seen in the late second or early third decade of life and may be more common than previously thought, given the results

of a study of sudden death in athletes *(129)*. However, this study was conducted in Italy and its results may have been influenced by geographic and genetic variation. Increased awareness of ARVC among physicians may lead to more effective screening for both ARVC and hypertrophic cardiomyopathy. Because ARVC is difficult to detect by standard two-dimensional echocardiography, the best diagnostic technique is MRI, which has increased ability to detect infiltrative process within the myocardium *(130)*.

Mutations in seven chromosomal locations have been associated with the development of ARVC *(131–137)* (Table 3). The mode of inheritance is autosomal dominant in all cases of ARVC. By using positional candidate cloning, it has been shown that families with ARVC type 2 have missense mutations in the cardiac ryanodine receptor (RYR2) *(138)*. The ryanodine receptor, which is a large protein found in the sarcoplasmic reticulum of cardiomyocytes, regulates calcium handling within the cell. Mutations in the RYR2 gene have been associated with catecholaminergic polymorphic ventricular tachycardia, which indicates the allelic nature of ARVC and other inherited arrhythmia syndromes *(139,140)*. The ryanodine receptor is a large protein with diverse functions and regulatory mechanisms, and mutations that alter different aspects of ryanodine function may account for the overlapping phenotypes of primary arrhythmia and infiltrative disease. The identification of additional human mutations and studies in mice will help in mapping the structure and function of the ryanodine receptor.

A single large Swedish family was identified with a syndrome that included a myofibrillar skeletal myopathy, cardiomyopathy, and ARVC, and genetic evidence has suggested linkage to chromosome 10q22.3 *(137)*. Histologic study of skeletal muscle biopsy specimens showed myopathic changes, rimmed vacuoles, and intracellular accumulation of cytoskeletal proteins including desmin. Thus, the ARVCs and desmin-related myopathies may overlap pathologically. The genetic region associated with this disorder overlaps with the locus for dilated cardiomyopathy, CMD1C *(141,142)*, so these two disorders may be allelic.

The ARVC phenotype can include epidermal disease in addition to the usual cardiac findings. A mutation in the gene encoding the cytoskeletal protein plakoglobin has been associated with an autosomal recessive ARVC-type pathology that includes abnormalities of the skin and hair called Naxos disease or woolly hair disease *(143,144)* (Table 3). In these patients, fibrofatty infiltration is seen in the right ventricle, and clinical symptoms include ventricular tachyarrhythmias and congestive

Table 3
Arrhythmogenic Right Ventricular Cardiomyopathies

Disease (ref.)	OMIM no.	Gene product	Chromosome location
Autosomal dominant			
ARVC1 *(131)*	107970		14q23–q24
ARVC2 *(132,138)*	600996	Ryanodine receptor	1q42–q43
ARVC3 *(134)*	602086		14q12–q22
ARVC4 *(133)*	602087		2q32.1–q32.3
ARVC5 *(135)*	604400		3p23
ARVC6 *(136)*	604401		10p14–p12
Myofibrillar myopathy/ARVC *(137)*			10q22.3
Autosomal recessive			
Naxos *(143)* (woolly hair, keratoderma, ARVC)	601214	Plakoglobin	17q21

OMIM, Online Mendelian Inheritance in Man (http://www.ncbi.nlm.nih.gov/Omim/); ARVC, arrhythmogenic right ventricular cardiomyopathies.

cardiomyopathy. Plakoglobin (γ-catenin) is found in the desmosome, which is a specialized structure found in most cells that functions in intracellular connections. In the heart, the desmosome may be particularly important at the intercalated disk where gap junction proteins such as connexins are located. In addition, desmosomal integrity is critical to the epidermis: mutant plakoglobin results in woolly hair and keratoderma. A mutation in the desmosomal protein desmoplakin leads to dilated cardiomyopathy, arrhythmia, woolly hair disease, and keratoderma *(145)*. Although rare, these mutations show the importance of cell-to-cell integrity in maintaining normal function of the heart.

MITOCHONDRIAL GENE MUTATIONS AND CARDIOMYOPATHY

Mitochondrial gene mutations contribute to the development of both hypertrophic and dilated cardiomyopathy *(146)*. Some mitochondrial proteins are encoded by the maternally inherited mitochondrial genome. Additional mitochondrial proteins are encoded by maternally and paternally inherited genes in the nucleus. The mitochondrial genome encodes components of the respiratory chain, which provides cells with energy and is an especially important component of cells that have a high energy demand, such as cardiac and skeletal muscle cells. Because each cell has multiple copies of the mitochondrial genome and each of those copies can independently acquire mutations, the mitochondrial genomes within a single cell

can be different, a condition known as heteroplasmy. This genetic heterogeneity can complicate the assessment of mitochondrial mutations in cardiac and skeletal myopathies. Both inherited and sporadic mutations within the mitochondria can lead to cardiac muscle dysfunction. Classic histologic findings such as red ragged fibers may be present in skeletal muscle but not in cardiac muscle. Because of the genetic heterogeneity in the mitochondrial genome, considerable phenotypic heterogeneity is present.

Mitochondria generate ATP through oxidative phosphorylation and the electron transport chain. The electron transport chain comprises four membrane-associated complexes and a fifth complex that completes the synthesis of ATP from ADP. The mitochondrial genome is 16.5 kb in length and has 37 genes that encode components of the mitochondrial translation system and 13 other proteins. Disorders of the mitochondrial complex II are associated with a broad range of phenotypes, including hypotonia, growth retardation, cardiomyopathy, myopathy, neuropathy, organ failure, and metabolic derangement. Heteroplasmic deletions in the mitochondrial genome can lead to the Kearns–Sayre syndrome, which includes pigmentary retinopathy, external ophthalmoplegia, cardiac conduction system disease, and cardiomyopathy and can have early onset *(147)*. In patients with Kearns–Sayre syndrome, intraventricular conduction system disease and AV nodal heart block can be successfully treated with pacemaker implantation *(148)*.

Familial cardiomyopathy phenotypes have been associated with specific point mutations in the mitochondrial genome, including A3260G, C3303T, and *A4300G (149–151)*. With each of these mutations, the hypertrophic phenotype dominates the clinical picture, although the age of onset and the extent of muscle weakness may vary. The MELAS (mitochondrial encephalopathy, lactic acidosis, and stroke-like episodes) syndrome may be associated with the A3243G polymorphism in the *tRNA^LEUUUR* gene *(152)*. Patients with MELAS present with symptoms similar to those seen in patients with the *PRKAG2* gene mutation; 20% to 30% of MELAS patients develop cardiomyopathy that may appear hypertrophic with a preexcitation component *(57,58)*. This highlights the importance of ATP production and utilization in the development of hypertrophic cardiomyopathy associated with conduction system disease.

STORAGE DISEASES

The storage diseases, which are usually seen in children and infants, are characterized by a thickened ventricle cardiomyopathy and evidence of metabolic abnormalities *(153)*. Most storage diseases are glycogen storage diseases, in which an increased number of glycogen vacuoles can affect liver and brain function. Cardiomyopathy and skeletal myopathy often occur with evidence of increased glycogen content in intracytoplasmic vacuoles. Strict adherence to dietary recommendations to avoid hypoglycemia can reduce the pathologic progression of these disorders. Although usually diagnosed early in life, storage disorders occasionally present later in life. Pompe's disease, an autosomal recessive disorder of the acid maltase gene at chromosome 17q25, is a lysosomal storage disease characterized by an accumulation of glycogen *(154)*, usually accompanied by a hypertrophic cardiomyopathy possibly with Wolff–Parkinson–White findings of preexcitation. An X-linked lysosomal glycogen storage disease, Danon disease is characterized by cardiomyopathy, myopathy, and mental retardation with intracytoplasmic vacuoles without acid maltase deficiency *(155)*. Mutations in the enzyme lysosomal-associated membrane protein (LAMP) 2 have been found in patients with Danon disease. Both sarcolemmic and basement membrane proteins are found within the intracytoplasmic vacuoles, indicating a defect in "metabolism" of the structural protein products within the cell.

SYNDROMES WITH CARDIOMYOPATHIES

Several genetic syndromes are associated with the development of cardiomyopathy. When managing patients with cardiomyopathy, clinicians may treat symptoms ranging from CHF to arrhythmias and may consider patient suitability for cardiac transplantation. Identifying the gene products responsible for cardiomyopathy syndromes will provide relevant information on pathways involved in myocardiocyte viability and function.

Friedreich's ataxia, an autosomal recessive disorder, is characterized by ataxia and abnormal findings in the spinocerebellar tracts, the dorsal columns, the pyramidal tracts, and the cerebellum. Most patients with Friedreich's ataxia will develop cardiac dysfunction; the hypertrophic cardiomyopathy seen in early phases progresses to a dilated phenotype. The frataxin gene on chromosome 9q13, which encodes an 18-kDa protein necessary for iron metabolism, is mutated in patients with Friedreich's ataxia *(156,157)*. In most of these patients, a trinucleotide repeat in the first exon of the frataxin gene is expanded and results in the absence of the frataxin protein, which is associated with abnormal accumulation of iron in the mitochondria. The length of the repeat expansion correlates with left ventricular wall thickness *(158)*. Chelating agents may be effective for treating Friedreich's ataxia. In a mouse model, ablating the frataxin gene in myocardium leads to cardiomyopathy *(159)*.

Barth syndrome, which is associated with mutation in the tafazzin gene (also known as G4.5), is an X-linked disorder characterized by neutropenia, skeletal myopathy, cardiomyopathy, and endocardial fibroelastosis *(160,161)*. The tafazzin gene is thought to encode an acyltransferase enzyme that alters glycophospholipids of the inner mitochondrial membrane. Mutations in tafazzin have been associated with left ventricular noncompaction, a disorder characterized by an abnormally hypertrabeculated and thin-walled myocardium *(162)*. Left ventricular noncompaction is usually seen in children, but these findings suggest a clinical continuum from left ventricular noncompaction to endocardial fibroelastosis and dilated cardiomyopathy.

Noonan syndrome is an autosomal dominant syndrome that includes dysmorphic facial features, short stature, pulmonic stenosis, and hypertrophic cardiomyopathy *(163)*. A relatively common genetic syndrome, Noonan syndrome has an incidence of 1 in 2500 live births, and the genetic defect maps to chromosome 12q24. Mutations in the gene PTPN11, which encodes the non–receptor-type protein tyrosine phosphatase SHP-2 (src homology region 2-domain phosphatase-2), have been associated with Noonan syndrome *(164)*. SHP-2 is recruited in response to receptor–ligand interactions and interacts with several signaling pathways, including the JAK–STAT (janus kinase–signal transducer and activator of transcription), ERK (extracellular-regulated kinase), JNK (c-Jun amino-terminal kinase), and the NF-κB (nuclear factor κB) cascades. Genetically engineered mice that lack SHP-2 die early in development with defective semilunar valves *(165)*. In patients with Noonan syndrome, nine different missense mutations have been described and may result in increased activity of the SHP-2 protein. The three-dimensional crystal structure of SHP-2 has been described *(166)*, and defining the molecular pathways in myocyte development and maturation that are altered by SHP-2 mutations may be facilitated by the genetic heterogeneity of Noonan syndrome.

MOLECULAR DIAGNOSTICS

Molecular diagnostics are just beginning to make an impact on the diagnosis and treatment of the inherited myocardial disorders. Although the molecular mechanisms of FHCs are among the best understood, the genetic and allelic heterogeneity that underlie these disorders hamper mutation detection. New, cost-effective strategies for detecting common and unique mutations will lead to increases in the collection of known mutations and to improved diagnoses. However, molecular diagnostics play an ancillary role in the diagnosis of inherited myocardial disorders, which currently relies on clinical and pathologic findings. Obtaining a thorough family history is an essential part of evaluating patients with cardiomyopathies and affects the management of patients with inherited cardiomyopathy. For example, patients with a family history of sudden death may be more likely to undergo placement of an internal defibrillator.

As the human genome project progresses, the number of genes associated with the development of cardiomyopathies will increase, and our understanding of the genetic mechanisms that lead to cardiac muscle dysfunction should broaden. In addition, the role of genetic modifier loci will be better understood. In many of the inherited cardiomyopathy syndromes, variable penetrance and expressivity suggest that certain changes in DNA carry an increased but not certain risk of developing cardiomyopathy. As the use of diagnostic DNA technology increases, our understanding of how additional genetic loci contribute to an increased risk of cardiomyopathy will improve. Until then, DNA diagnostic technology should be used cautiously, and the implications of DNA mutations should not be overstated. The role of the cardiovascular genetic counselor will expand to accommodate the needs created by the evolving database of genetic and clinical information *(122,142,170,171)*.

REFERENCES

1. Eriksson H. Heart failure: a growing public health problem. J Intern Med 1995;237:135–141.
2. Senni M, Tribouilloy CM, Rodeheffer RJ, et al. Congestive heart failure in the community: trends in incidence and survival in a 10-year period. Arch Intern Med 1999;159:29–34.
3. Senni M, Tribouilloy CM, Rodeheffer RJ, et al. Congestive heart failure in the community: a study of all incident cases in Olmsted County, Minnesota, in 1991. Circulation 1998;98:2282–2289.
4. Felker GM, Thompson RE, Hare JM, et al. Underlying causes and long-term survival in patients with initially unexplained cardiomyopathy. N Engl J Med 2000;342:1077–1084.
5. Seidman JG, Seidman C. The genetic basis for cardiomyopathy: from mutation identification to mechanistic paradigms. Cell 2001;104:557–567.
6. Franz WM, Muller OJ, Katus HA. Cardiomyopathies: from genetics to the prospect of treatment. Lancet 2001;358:1627–1637.
7. Richardson P, McKenna W, Bristow M, et al. Report of the 1995 World Health Organization/International Society and Federation of Cardiology Task Force on the Definition and Classification of cardiomyopathies. Circulation 1996;93:841–842.
8. Maron BJ, Gardin JM, Flack JM, Gidding SS, Kurosaki TT, Bild DE. Prevalence of hypertrophic cardiomyopathy in a general population of young adults. Echocardiographic analysis of 4111 subjects in the CARDIA Study. Coronary Artery Risk Development in (Young) Adults. Circulation 1995;92:785–789.
9. Maron BJ, Olivotto I, Spirito P, et al. Epidemiology of hypertrophic cardiomyopathy-related death: revisited in a large non-referral-based patient population. Circulation 2000;102:858–864.
10. Bonne G, Carrier L, Richard P, Hainque B, Schwartz K. Familial hypertrophic cardiomyopathy: from mutations to functional defects. Circ Res 1998;83:580–593.
11. Marian AJ, Roberts R. The molecular genetic basis for hypertrophic cardiomyopathy. J Mol Cell Cardiol 2001;33: 655–670.
12. Seidman CE, Seidman JG. Molecular genetic studies of familial hypertrophic cardiomyopathy. Basic Res Cardiol 1998;93:13–16.
13. Jarcho JA, McKenna W, Pare JA, et al. Mapping a gene for familial hypertrophic cardiomyopathy to chromosome 14q1. N Engl J Med 1989;321:1372–1378.
14. Geisterfer-Lowrance AA, Kass S, Tanigawa G, et al. A molecular basis for familial hypertrophic cardiomyopathy: a beta cardiac myosin heavy chain gene missense mutation. Cell 1990;62:999–1006.
15. Rayment I, Holden HM, Sellers JR, Fananapazir L, Epstein ND. Structural interpretation of the mutations in the beta-cardiac myosin that have been implicated in familial hypertrophic cardiomyopathy. Proc Natl Acad Sci USA 1995;92: 3864–3868.
16. Geisterfer-Lowrance AA, Christe M, Conner DA, et al. A mouse model of familial hypertrophic cardiomyopathy. Science 1996; 272:731–734.
17. Vikstrom KL, Factor SM, Leinwand LA. Mice expressing mutant myosin heavy chains are a model for familial hypertrophic cardiomyopathy. Mol Med 1996;2:556–567.
18. Marian AJ, Wu Y, Lim DS, et al. A transgenic rabbit model for human hypertrophic cardiomyopathy. J Clin Invest 1999;104: 1683–1692.
19. Patel R, Nagueh SF, Tsybouleva N, et al. Simvastatin induces regression of cardiac hypertrophy and fibrosis and improves cardiac function in a transgenic rabbit model of human hypertrophic cardiomyopathy. Circulation 2001;104:317–324.

20. Dalloz F, Osinska H, Robbins J. Manipulating the contractile apparatus: genetically defined animal models of cardiovascular disease. J Mol Cell Cardiol 2001;33:9–25.

21. Redwood CS, Moolman-Smook JC, Watkins H. Properties of mutant contractile proteins that cause hypertrophic cardiomyopathy. Cardiovasc Res 1999;44:20–36.

22. Kron SJ, Spudich JA. Fluorescent actin filaments move on myosin fixed to a glass surface. Proc Natl Acad Sci USA 1986;83:6272–6276.

23. Cuda G, Fananapazir L, Zhu WS, Sellers JR, Epstein ND. Skeletal muscle expression and abnormal function of beta-myosin in hypertrophic cardiomyopathy. J Clin Invest 1993; 91:2861–2865.

24. Cuda G, Fananapazir L, Epstein ND, Sellers JR. The in vitro motility activity of beta-cardiac myosin depends on the nature of the beta-myosin heavy chain gene mutation in hypertrophic cardiomyopathy. J Muscle Res Cell Motil 1997;18:275–283.

25. Palmiter KA, Tyska MJ, Haeberle JR, Alpert NR, Fananapazir L, Warshaw DM. R403Q and L908V mutant beta-cardiac myosin from patients with familial hypertrophic cardiomyopathy exhibit enhanced mechanical performance at the single molecule level. J Muscle Res Cell Motil 2000;21:609–620.

26. Tyska MJ, Hayes E, Giewat M, Seidman CE, Seidman JG, Warshaw DM. Single-molecule mechanics of R403Q cardiac myosin isolated from the mouse model of familial hypertrophic cardiomyopathy. Circ Res 2000;86:737–744.

27. Sweeney HL, Straceski AJ, Leinwand LA, Tikunov BA, Faust L. Heterologous expression of a cardiomyopathic myosin that is defective in its actin interaction. J Biol Chem 1994;269: 1603–1605.

28. Jaenicke T, Diederich KW, Haas W, et al. The complete sequence of the human beta-myosin heavy chain gene and a comparative analysis of its product. Genomics 1990;8:194–206.

29. Liew CC, Sole MJ, Yamauchi-Takihara K, et al. Complete sequence and organization of the human cardiac beta-myosin heavy chain gene. Nucleic Acids Res 1990;18:3647–3651.

30. Blair E, Redwood C, de Jesus Oliveira M, et al. Mutations of the light meromyosin domain of the beta-myosin heavy chain rod in hypertrophic cardiomyopathy. Circ Res 2002;90:263–269.

31. Poetter K, Jiang H, Hassanzadeh S, et al. Mutations in either the essential or regulatory light chains of myosin are associated with a rare myopathy in human heart and skeletal muscle. Nat Genet 1996;13:63–69.

32. Flavigny J, Richard P, Isnard R, et al. Identification of two novel mutations in the ventricular regulatory myosin light chain gene (MYL2) associated with familial and classical forms of hypertrophic cardiomyopathy. J Mol Med 1998;76: 208–214.

33. Lee W, Hwang TH, Kimura A, et al. Different expressivity of a ventricular essential myosin light chain gene Ala57Gly mutation in familial hypertrophic cardiomyopathy. Am Heart J 2001; 141:184–189.

34. Rayment I, Rypniewski WR, Schmidt-Base K, et al. Three-dimensional structure of myosin subfragment-1: a molecular motor. Science 1993;261:50–58.

35. Freiburg A, Gautel M. A molecular map of the interactions between titin and myosin-binding protein C. Implications for sarcomeric assembly in familial hypertrophic cardiomyopathy. Eur J Biochem 1996;235:317–323.

36. Bonne G, Carrier L, Bercovici J, et al. Cardiac myosin binding protein-C gene splice acceptor site mutation is associated with familial hypertrophic cardiomyopathy. Nat Genet 1995; 11:438–440.

37. Watkins H, Conner D, Thierfelder L, et al. Mutations in the cardiac myosin binding protein-C gene on chromosome 11 cause familial hypertrophic cardiomyopathy. Nat Genet 1995;11:434–437.

38. Rottbauer W, Gautel M, Zehelein J, et al. Novel splice donor site mutation in the cardiac myosin-binding protein-C gene in familial hypertrophic cardiomyopathy. Characterization Of cardiac transcript and protein. J Clin Invest 1997;100:475–482.

39. Gautel M, Zuffardi O, Freiburg A, Labeit S. Phosphorylation switches specific for the cardiac isoform of myosin binding protein-C: a modulator of cardiac contraction? Embo J 1995; 14:1952–1960.

40. Gruen M, Gautel M. Mutations in beta-myosin S2 that cause familial hypertrophic cardiomyopathy (FHC) abolish the interaction with the regulatory domain of myosin-binding protein-C. J Mol Biol 1999;286:933–949.

41. Charron P, Dubourg O, Desnos M, et al. Clinical features and prognostic implications of familial hypertrophic cardiomyopathy related to the cardiac myosin-binding protein C gene. Circulation 1998;97:2230–2236.

42. Yang Q, Sanbe A, Osinska H, Hewett TE, Klevitsky R, Robbins J. A mouse model of myosin binding protein C human familial hypertrophic cardiomyopathy. J Clin Invest 1998;102:1292–1300.

43. Yang Q, Osinska H, Klevitsky R, Robbins J. Phenotypic deficits in mice expressing a myosin binding protein c lacking the titin and myosin binding domains. J Mol Cell Cardiol 2001;33:1649–1658.

44. McConnell BK, Fatkin D, Semsarian C, et al. Comparison of two murine models of familial hypertrophic cardiomyopathy. Circ Res 2001;88:383–389.

45. Thierfelder L, Watkins H, MacRae C, et al. Alpha-tropomyosin and cardiac troponin T mutations cause familial hypertrophic cardiomyopathy: a disease of the sarcomere. Cell 1994;77:701–712.

46. Forissier JF, Carrier L, Farza H, et al. Codon 102 of the cardiac troponin T gene is a putative hot spot for mutations in familial hypertrophic cardiomyopathy. Circulation 1996;94:3069–3073.

47. Watkins H, McKenna WJ, Thierfelder L, et al. Mutations in the genes for cardiac troponin T and alpha-tropomyosin in hypertrophic cardiomyopathy. N Engl J Med 1995;332:1058–1064.

48. Moolman JC, Corfield VA, Posen B, et al. Sudden death due to troponin T mutations. J Am Coll Cardiol 1997;29:549–555.

49. Tardiff JC, Factor SM, Tompkins BD, et al. A truncated cardiac troponin T molecule in transgenic mice suggests multiple cellular mechanisms for familial hypertrophic cardiomyopathy. J Clin Invest 1998;101:2800–2811.

50. Tardiff JC, Hewett TE, Palmer BM, et al. Cardiac troponin T mutations result in allele-specific phenotypes in a mouse model for hypertrophic cardiomyopathy. J Clin Invest 1999;104:469–481.

51. Oberst L, Zhao G, Park JT, et al. Dominant-negative effect of a mutant cardiac troponin T on cardiac structure and function in transgenic mice. J Clin Invest 1998;102:1498–1505.

52. Chandra M, Rundell VL, Tardiff JC, Leinwand LA, De Tombe PP, Solaro RJ. Ca(2+) activation of myofilaments from transgenic mouse hearts expressing R92Q mutant cardiac troponin T. Am J Physiol Heart Circ Physiol 2001;280:H705–H713.

53. Homsher E, Lee DM, Morris C, Pavlov D, Tobacman LS. Regulation of force and unloaded sliding speed in single thin filaments: effects of regulatory proteins and calcium. J Physiol 2000;524:233–243.

54. Hoffmann B, Schmidt-Traub H, Perrot A, Osterziel KJ, Gessner R. First mutation in cardiac troponin C, L29Q, in a patient with hypertrophic cardiomyopathy. Hum Mutat 2001;17:524.

55. Coviello DA, Maron BJ, Spirito P, et al. Clinical features of hypertrophic cardiomyopathy caused by mutation of a "hot

spot" in the alpha-tropomyosin gene. J Am Coll Cardiol 1997; 29:635–640.

56. Prabhakar R, Boivin GP, Grupp IL, et al. A familial hypertrophic cardiomyopathy alpha-tropomyosin mutation causes severe cardiac hypertrophy and death in mice. J Mol Cell Cardiol 2001; 33:1815–1828.

57. Blair E, Redwood C, Ashrafian H, et al. Mutations in the gamma(2) subunit of AMP-activated protein kinase cause familial hypertrophic cardiomyopathy: evidence for the central role of energy compromise in disease pathogenesis. Hum Mol Genet 2001;10:1215–1220.

58. Gollob MH, Green MS, Tang AS, et al. Identification of a gene responsible for familial Wolff-Parkinson-White syndrome. N Engl J Med 2001;344:1823–1831.

59. Arad M, Benson DW, McKenna WJ, et al. Mutations in PRKAG2 cause Wolff Parkinson White and Hypertrophic Cardiomyopathy. Circulation 2001;104:11–21.

60. Hauer RN, Aliot E, Block M, et al. Indications for implantable cardioverter defibrillator (ICD) therapy. Study Group on Guidelines on ICD of the Working Group on Arrythmias and the Working Group on Cardiac Pacing of the European Society of Cardiology. Europace 2001;3:169–176.

61. Maron BJ, Shen WK, Link MS, et al. Efficacy of implantable cardioverter-defibrillators for the prevention of sudden death in patients with hypertrophic cardiomyopathy. N Engl J Med 2000;342:365–373.

62. Codd MB, Sugrue DD, Gersh BJ, Melton LJ III. Epidemiology of idiopathic dilated and hypertrophic cardiomyopathy. A population-based study in Olmsted County, Minnesota, 1975–1984. Circulation 1989;80:564–572.

63. Grunig E, Tasman JA, Kucherer H, Franz W, Kubler W, Katus HA. Frequency and phenotypes of familial dilated cardiomyopathy. J Am Coll Cardiol 1998;31:186–194.

64. Mestroni L, Rocco C, Gregori D, et al. Familial dilated cardiomyopathy: evidence for genetic and phenotypic heterogeneity. Heart Muscle Disease Study Group. J Am Coll Cardiol 1999;34:181–190.

65. Baig MK, Goldman JH, Caforio AL, Coonar AS, Keeling PJ, McKenna WJ. Familial dilated cardiomyopathy: cardiac abnormalities are common in asymptomatic relatives and may represent early disease. J Am Coll Cardiol 1998;31:195–201.

66. Perloff JK, Roberts WC, de Leon AC, Jr., O'Doherty D. The distinctive electrocardiogram of Duchenne's progressive muscular dystrophy. An electrocardiographic-pathologic correlative study. Am J Med 1967;42:179–188.

67. Perloff JK. Cardiac rhythm and conduction in Duchenne's muscular dystrophy: a prospective study of 20 patients. J Am Coll Cardiol 1984;3:1263–1268.

68. Berko BA, Swift M. X-linked dilated cardiomyopathy. N Engl J Med 1987;316:1186–1191.

69. Muntoni F, Cau M, Ganau A, et al. Brief report: deletion of the dystrophin muscle-promoter region associated with X-linked dilated cardiomyopathy. N Engl J Med 1993;329: 921–925.

70. Ortiz-Lopez R, Li H, Su J, Goytia V, Towbin JA. Evidence for a dystrophin missense mutation as a cause of X-linked dilated cardiomyopathy. Circulation 1997;95:2434–2440.

71. Mirabella M, Servidei S, Manfredi G, et al. Cardiomyopathy may be the only clinical manifestation in female carriers of Duchenne muscular dystrophy. Neurology 1993;43:2342–2345.

72. Melacini P, Fanin M, Angelini A, et al. Cardiac transplantation in a Duchenne muscular dystrophy carrier. Neuromuscul Disord 1998;8:585–590.

73. Bastianutto C, Bestard JA, Lahnakoski K, et al. Dystrophin muscle enhancer 1 is implicated in the activation of non-muscle isoforms in the skeletal muscle of patients with X-linked dilated cardiomyopathy. Hum Mol Genet 2001;10:2627–2635.

74. Towbin JA. The role of cytoskeletal proteins in cardiomyopathies. Curr Opin Cell Biol 1998;10:131–139.

75. Hack AA, Groh ME, McNally EM. Sarcoglycans in muscular dystrophy. Microsc Res Tech 2000;48:167–180.

76. Rybakova IN, Patel JR, Ervasti JM. The dystrophin complex forms a mechanically strong link between the sarcolemma and costameric actin. J Cell Biol 2000;150:1209–1214.

77. Ervasti JM, Campbell KP. Dystrophin and the membrane skeleton. Curr Opin Cell Biol 1993;5:82–87.

78. Jung D, Yang B, Meyer J, Chamberlain JS, Campbell KP. Identification and characterization of the dystrophin anchoring site on beta-dystroglycan. J Biol Chem 1995;270:27305–27310.

79. Petrof BJ, Shrager JB, Stedman HH, Kelly AM, Sweeney HL. Dystrophin protects the sarcolemma from stresses developed during muscle contraction. Proc Natl Acad Sci USA 1993; 90:3710–3714.

80. Danialou G, Comtois AS, Dudley R, et al. Dystrophin-deficient cardiomyocytes are abnormally vulnerable to mechanical stress-induced contractile failure and injury. Faseb J 2001;15:1655–1657.

81. Frank JS, Mottino G, Chen F, Peri V, Holland P, Tuana BS. Subcellular distribution of dystrophin in isolated adult and neonatal cardiac myocytes. Am J Physiol 1994;267:C1707–C1716.

82. Kostin S, Scholz D, Shimada T, et al. The internal and external protein scaffold of the T-tubular system in cardiomyocytes. Cell Tissue Res 1998;294:449–460.

83. Kereiakes DJ, Parmley WW. Myocarditis and cardiomyopathy. Am Heart J 1984;108:1318–1326.

84. Badorff C, Lee GH, Lamphear BJ, et al. Enteroviral protease 2A cleaves dystrophin: evidence of cytoskeletal disruption in an acquired cardiomyopathy. Nat Med 1999;5:320–326.

85. Badorff C, Berkely N, Mehrotra S, Talhouk JW, Rhoads RE, Knowlton KU. Enteroviral protease 2A directly cleaves dystrophin and is inhibited by a dystrophin-based substrate analogue. J Biol Chem 2000;275:11191–11197.

86. Nigro V, de Sa Moreira E, Piluso G, et al. Autosomal recessive limb-girdle muscular dystrophy, LGMD2F, is caused by a mutation in the delta-sarcoglycan gene. Nat Genet 1996; 14:195–198.

87. Tsubata S, Bowles KR, Vatta M, et al. Mutations in the human delta-sarcoglycan gene in familial and sporadic dilated cardiomyopathy. J Clin Invest 2000;106:655–662.

88. Coral-Vazquez R, Cohn RD, Moore SA, et al. Disruption of the sarcoglycan-sarcospan complex in vascular smooth muscle: a novel mechanism for cardiomyopathy and muscular dystrophy. Cell 1999;98:465–474.

89. Hack AA, Lam MY, Cordier L, et al. Differential requirement for individual sarcoglycans and dystrophin in the assembly and function of the dystrophin-glycoprotein complex. J Cell Sci 2000;113:2535–2544.

90. Knoll R., Hoshijima M, Hoffman HM, et al. The cardiac mechanical stretch sensor machinery involves a Z disc complex that is defective in a subset of human dilated cardiomyopathy. Cell 2002;111:943–955.

91. Gerull B, Gramlich M, Atherton J, et al. Mutations of TTN, encoding the giant muscle filament titin, cause familial dilated cardiomyopathy. Nat Genet 2002;30:201–204.

92. Olson TM, Michels VV, Thibodeau SN, Tai YS, Keating MT. Actin mutations in dilated cardiomyopathy, a heritable form of heart failure. Science 1998;280:750–752.

93. Olson TM, Doan TP, Kishimoto NY, Whitby FG, Ackerman MJ, Fananapazir L. Inherited and de novo mutations in the cardiac actin gene cause hypertrophic cardiomyopathy. J Mol Cell Cardiol 2000;32:1687–1694.

94. Kamisago M, Sharma SD, DePalma SR, et al. Mutations in sarcomere protein genes as a cause of dilated cardiomyopathy. N Engl J Med 2000;343:1688–1696.

95. Li D, Czernuszewicz GZ, Gonzalez O, et al. Novel cardiac troponin T mutation as a cause of familial dilated cardiomyopathy. Circulation 2001;104:2188–2193.

96. Wilson KL, Zastrow MS, Lee KK. Lamins and disease: insights into nuclear infrastructure. Cell 2001;104:647–650.

97. Bonne G, Di Barletta MR, Varnous S, et al. Mutations in the gene encoding lamin A/C cause autosomal dominant Emery-Dreifuss muscular dystrophy. Nat Genet 1999;21:285–288.

98. Bonne G, Mercuri E, Muchir A, et al. Clinical and molecular genetic spectrum of autosomal dominant Emery-Dreifuss muscular dystrophy due to mutations of the lamin A/C gene. Ann Neurol 2000;48:170–180.

99. Fatkin D, MacRae C, Sasaki T, et al. Missense mutations in the rod domain of the lamin A/C gene as causes of dilated cardiomyopathy and conduction-system disease. N Engl J Med 1999;341:1715–1724.

100. Wilson KL. The nuclear envelope, muscular dystrophy and gene expression. Trends Cell Biol 2000;10:125–129.

101. Cao H, Hegele RA. Nuclear lamin A/C R482Q mutation in canadian kindreds with Dunnigan-type familial partial lipodystrophy. Hum Mol Genet 2000;9:109–112.

102. Shackleton S, Lloyd DJ, Jackson SN, et al. LMNA, encoding lamin A/C, is mutated in partial lipodystrophy. Nat Genet 2000;24:153–156.

103. Sivak ED, Shefner JM, Sexton J. Neuromuscular disease and hypoventilation. Curr Opin Pulm Med 1999;5:355–362.

104. Megeney LA, Kablar B, Perry RL, Ying C, May L, Rudnicki MA. Severe cardiomyopathy in mice lacking dystrophin and MyoD. Proc Natl Acad Sci USA 1999;96:220–225.

105. Politano L, Nigro V, Passamano L, et al. Evaluation of cardiac and respiratory involvement in sarcoglycanopathies. Neuromuscul Disord 2001;11:178–185.

106. Shaddy RE, Tani LY, Gidding SS, et al. Beta-blocker treatment of dilated cardiomyopathy with congestive heart failure in children: a multi-institutional experience. J Heart Lung Transplant 1999;18:269–274.

107. Grady RM, Teng H, Nichol MC, Cunningham JC, Wilkinson RS, Sanes JR. Skeletal and cardiac myopathies in mice lacking utrophin and dystrophin: a model for Duchenne muscular dystrophy. Cell 1997;90:729–738.

108. Deconinck AE, Rafael JA, Skinner JA, et al. Utrophin-dystrophin-deficient mice as a model for Duchenne muscular dystrophy. Cell 1997;90:717–727.

109. Nelson SD, Sparks EA, Graber HL, et al. Clinical characteristics of sudden death victims in heritable (chromosome 1p1-1q1) conduction and myocardial disease. J Am Coll Cardiol 1998;32:1717–1723.

110. Nagano A, Koga R, Ogawa M, et al. Emerin deficiency at the nuclear membrane in patients with Emery-Dreifuss muscular dystrophy. Nat Genet 1996;12:254–259.

111. Clements L, Manilal S, Love DR, Morris GE. Direct interaction between emerin and lamin A. Biochem Biophys Res Commun 2000;267:709–714.

112. Vaughan A, Alvarez-Reyes M, Bridger JM, et al. Both emerin and lamin C depend on lamin A for localization at the nuclear envelope. J Cell Sci 2001;114:2577–2590.

113. Caskey CT, Pizzuti A, Fu YH, Fenwick RG, Jr., Nelson DL. Triplet repeat mutations in human disease. Science 1992;256: 784–789.

114. Berul CI, Maguire CT, Aronovitz MJ, et al. DMPK dosage alterations result in atrioventricular conduction abnormalities in a mouse myotonic dystrophy model. J Clin Invest 1999; 103:R1–R7.

115. Mankodi A, Logigian E, Callahan L, et al. Myotonic dystrophy in transgenic mice expressing an expanded CUG repeat. Science 2000;289:1769–1773.

116. Kushwaha SS, Fallon JT, Fuster V. Restrictive cardiomyopathy. N Engl J Med 1997;336:267–276.

117. Denfield SW, Rosenthal G, Gajarski RJ, et al. Restrictive cardiomyopathies in childhood. Etiologies and natural history. Tex Heart Inst J 1997;24:38–44.

118. Goebel HH. Desmin-related myopathies. Curr Opin Neurol 1997;10:426–429.

119. Banwell BL. Intermediate filament-related myopathies. Pediatr Neurol 2001;24:257–263.

120. Goldfarb LG, Park KY, Cervenakova L, et al. Missense mutations in desmin associated with familial cardiac and skeletal myopathy. Nat Genet 1998;19:402–403.

121. Sjoberg G, Saavedra-Matiz CA, Rosen DR, et al. A missense mutation in the desmin rod domain is associated with autosomal dominant distal myopathy, and exerts a dominant negative effect on filament formation. Hum Mol Genet 1999;8:2191–2198.

122. Li D, Tapscoft T, Gonzalez O, et al. Desmin mutation responsible for idiopathic dilated cardiomyopathy. Circulation 1999; 100:461–464.

123. Wang X, Osinska H, Dorn GW II, et al. Mouse model of desmin-related cardiomyopathy. Circulation 2001;103:2402–2407.

124. Vicart P, Caron A, Guicheney P, et al. A missense mutation in the alphaB-crystallin chaperone gene causes a desmin-related myopathy. Nat Genet 1998;20:92–95.

125. Perng MD, Muchowski PJ, van Den IP, et al. The cardiomyopathy and lens cataract mutation in alphaB-crystallin alters its protein structure, chaperone activity, and interaction with intermediate filaments in vitro. J Biol Chem 1999;274:33235–33243.

126. Wang X, Osinska H, Klevitsky R, et al. Expression of R120G-alphaB-crystallin causes aberrant desmin and alphaB-crystallin aggregation and cardiomyopathy in mice. Circ Res 2001; 89:84–91.

127. Zhang J, Kumar A, Stalker HJ, et al. Clinical and molecular studies of a large family with desmin-associated restrictive cardiomyopathy. Clin Genet 2001;59:248–256.

128. Fontaine G, Fontaliran F, Hebert JL, et al. Arrhythmogenic right ventricular dysplasia. Annu Rev Med 1999;50:17–35.

129. Corrado D, Basso C, Schiavon M, Thiene G. Screening for hypertrophic cardiomyopathy in young athletes. N Engl J Med 1998;339:364–369.

130. van der Wall EE, Kayser HW, Bootsma MM, de Roos A, Schalij MJ. Arrhythmogenic right ventricular dysplasia: MRI findings. Herz 2000;25:356–364.

131. Rampazzo A, Nava A, Danieli GA, et al. The gene for arrhythmogenic right ventricular cardiomyopathy maps to chromosome 14q23-q24. Hum Mol Genet 1994;3:959–962.

132. Rampazzo A, Nava A, Erne P, et al. A new locus for arrhythmogenic right ventricular cardiomyopathy (ARVD2) maps to chromosome 1q42-q43. Hum Mol Genet 1995;4: 2151–2154.

133. Rampazzo A, Nava A, Miorin M, et al. ARVD4, a new locus for arrhythmogenic right ventricular cardiomyopathy, maps to chromosome 2 long arm. Genomics 1997;45:259–263.

134. Severini GM, Krajinovic M, Pinamonti B, et al. A new locus for arrhythmogenic right ventricular dysplasia on the long arm of chromosome 14. Genomics 1996;31:193–200.

135. Ahmad F, Li D, Karibe A, et al. Localization of a gene responsible for arrhythmogenic right ventricular dysplasia to chromosome 3p23. Circulation 1998;98:2791–2795.

136. Li D, Ahmad F, Gardner MJ, et al. The locus of a novel gene responsible for arrhythmogenic right-ventricular dysplasia characterized by early onset and high penetrance maps to chromosome 10p12-p14. Am J Hum Genet 2000;66:148–156.

137. Melberg A, Oldfors A, Blomstrom-Lundqvist C, et al. Autosomal dominant myofibrillar myopathy with arrhythmogenic right ventricular cardiomyopathy linked to chromosome 10q. Ann Neurol 1999;46:684–692.

138. Tiso N, Stephan DA, Nava A, et al. Identification of mutations in the cardiac ryanodine receptor gene in families affected with arrhythmogenic right ventricular cardiomyopathy type 2 (ARVD2). Hum Mol Genet 2001;10:189–194.

139. Laitinen PJ, Brown KM, Piippo K, et al. Mutations of the cardiac ryanodine receptor (RyR2) gene in familial polymorphic ventricular tachycardia. Circulation 2001;103:485–490.

140. Priori SG, Napolitano C, Tiso N, et al. Mutations in the Cardiac Ryanodine Receptor Gene (hRyR2) Underlie Catecholaminergic Polymorphic Ventricular Tachycardia. Circulation 2001;103: 196–200.

141. Bowles KR, Abraham SE, Brugada R, et al. Construction of a high-resolution physical map of the chromosome 10q22-q23 dilated cardiomyopathy locus and analysis of candidate genes. Genomics 2000;67:109–127.

142. Bowles KR, Gajarski R, Porter P, et al. Gene mapping of familial autosomal dominant dilated cardiomyopathy to chromosome 10q21-23. J Clin Invest 1996;98:1355–1360.

143. McKoy G, Protonotarios N, Crosby A, et al. Identification of a deletion in plakoglobin in arrhythmogenic right ventricular cardiomyopathy with palmoplantar keratoderma and woolly hair (Naxos disease). Lancet 2000;355:2119–2124.

144. Protonotarios N, Tsatsopoulou A, Anastasakis A, et al. Genotype-phenotype assessment in autosomal recessive arrhythmogenic right ventricular cardiomyopathy (Naxos disease) caused by a deletion in plakoglobin. J Am Coll Cardiol 2001;38:1477–1484.

145. Norgett EE, Hatsell SJ, Carvajal-Huerta L, et al. Recessive mutation in desmoplakin disrupts desmoplakin-intermediate filament interactions and causes dilated cardiomyopathy, woolly hair and keratoderma. Hum Mol Genet 2000;9:2761–2766.

146. Santorelli FM, Tessa A, D'Amati G, Casali C. The emerging concept of mitochondrial cardiomyopathies. Am Heart J 2001; 141:E1.

147. Lestienne P, Ponsot G. Kearns-Sayre syndrome with muscle mitochondrial DNA deletion. Lancet 1988;1:885.

148. Polak PE, Zijlstra F, Roelandt JR. Indications for pacemaker implantation in the Kearns-Sayre syndrome. Eur Heart J 1989; 10:281–282.

149. Zeviani M, Gellera C, Antozzi C, et al. Maternally inherited myopathy and cardiomyopathy: association with mutation in mitochondrial DNA tRNA(Leu)(UUR). Lancet 1991;338:143–147.

150. Bruno C, Kirby DM, Koga Y, et al. The mitochondrial DNA C3303T mutation can cause cardiomyopathy and/or skeletal myopathy. J Pediatr 1999;135:197–202.

151. Casali C, d'Amati G, Bernucci P, et al. Maternally inherited cardiomyopathy: clinical and molecular characterization of a large kindred harboring the A4300G point mutation in mitochondrial deoxyribonucleic acid. J Am Coll Cardiol 1999;33:1584–1589.

152. Ciafaloni E, Ricci E, Shanske S, et al. MELAS: clinical features, biochemistry, and molecular genetics. Ann Neurol 1992;31: 391–398.

153. Wolfsdorf JI, Holm IA, Weinstein DA. Glycogen storage diseases. Phenotypic, genetic, and biochemical characteristics,

and therapy. Endocrinol Metab Clin North Am 1999;28: 801–823.

154. Kohlschutter A, Hausdorf G. Primary (genetic) cardiomyopathies in infancy. A survey of possible disorders and guidelines for diagnosis. Eur J Pediatr 1986;145:454–459.

155. Nishino I, Fu J, Tanji K, et al. Primary LAMP-2 deficiency causes X-linked vacuolar cardiomyopathy and myopathy (Danon disease). Nature 2000;406:906–910.

156. Koenig M, Mandel JL. Deciphering the cause of Friedreich ataxia. Curr Opin Neurobiol 1997;7:689–694.

157. Durr A, Cossee M, Agid Y, et al. Clinical and genetic abnormalities in patients with Friedreich's ataxia. N Engl J Med 1996;335:1169–1175.

158. Isnard R, Kalotka H, Durr A, et al. Correlation between left ventricular hypertrophy and GAA trinucleotide repeat length in Friedreich's ataxia. Circulation 1997;95:2247–2249.

159. Puccio H, Simon D, Cossee M, et al. Mouse models for Friedreich ataxia exhibit cardiomyopathy, sensory nerve defect and Fe-S enzyme deficiency followed by intramitochondrial iron deposits. Nat Genet 2001;27:181–186.

160. Bione S, D'Adamo P, Maestrini E, Gedeon AK, Bolhuis PA, Toniolo D. A novel X-linked gene, G4.5. is responsible for Barth syndrome. Nat Genet 1996;12:385–389.

161. D'Adamo P, Fassone L, Gedeon A, et al. The X-linked gene G4.5 is responsible for different infantile dilated cardiomyopathies. Am J Hum Genet 1997;61:862–867.

162. Ichida F, Tsubata S, Bowles KR, et al. Novel gene mutations in patients with left ventricular noncompaction or Barth syndrome. Circulation 2001;103:1256–1263.

163. Noonan JA. Hypertelorism with Turner phenotype. A new syndrome with associated congenital heart disease. Am J Dis Child 1968;116:373–380.

164. Tartaglia M, Mehler EL, Goldberg R, et al. Mutations in PTPN11, encoding the protein tyrosine phosphatase SHP-2, cause Noonan syndrome. Nat Genet 2001;12:12.

165. Chen B, Bronson RT, Klaman LD, et al. Mice mutant for Egfr and Shp2 have defective cardiac semilunar valvulogenesis. Nat Genet 2000;24:296–299.

166. Hof P, Pluskey S, Dhe-Paganon S, Eck MJ, Shoelson SE. Crystal structure of the tyrosine phosphatase SHP-2. Cell 1998;92:441–450.

167. Krajinovic M, Pinamonti B, Sinagra G, et al. Linkage of familial dilated cardiomyopathy to chromosome 9. Heart Muscle Disease Study Group. Am J Hum Genet 1995;57: 846–852.

168. McNair WP, Ku L, Taylor MR, et al SCN5A mutation associated with dilated cardiomyopathy conduction disorder, and arrhythmia. Circulation 2004; 110:2163–2167.

169. Messina DN, Speer MC, Pericak-Vance MA, McNally EM. Linkage of familial dilated cardiomyopathy with conduction defect and muscular dystrophy to chromosome 6q23. Am J Hum Genet 1997;61:909–917.

170. Jung M, Poepping I, Perrot A, et al. Investigation of a family with autosomal dominant dilated cardiomyopathy defines a novel locus on chromosome 2q14-q22. Am J Hum Genet 1999;65:1068–1077.

171. Schonberger J, Levy H, Grunig E, et al. Dilated cardiomyopathy and sensorineural hearing loss: a heritable syndrome that maps to 6q23-24. Circulation 2000;101:1812–1818.

172. Sylvius N, Tesson F, Gayet C, et al. A new locus for autosomal dominant dilated cardiomyopathy identified on chromosome 6q12-q16. Am J Hum Genet 2001;68:241–246.

173. Bienengraeber M, Olson T M Selivanov VA et al. ABCC9 mutations identified in human dilated cardiomyopathy disrupt catalytic K(ATP) channel gating. Nat Genet 2004;36:382-387.

174. Schmitt JP, Kamisago M, Asahi M e al. Dilated cardiomyopathy and heart failure caused by a mutation in phospholamban. Science 2003;299:1410–1413.

8

Receptor-Signaling Pathways in Heart Failure

*Shayela Suvarna, PhD, Liza Barki-Harrington, PhD,
Miwako Suzuki, MD, PhD, Philippe Le Corvoisier, MD,
and Howard A. Rockman, MD*

CONTENTS

INTRODUCTION

Heart failure, a progressive disorder characterized by deterioration of cardiac function and premature myocardial cell death, results from several common heart diseases such as coronary atherosclerosis, hypertension, and valvular diseases *(1,2)*. With almost 550,000 new cases diagnosed each year, heart failure affects an estimated 4.7 million Americans, and costs associated with the disease range from $10 billion to $40 billion per year *(3)*. The aggregate 5-year mortality of patients with heart failure is about 50%, while the 1-year mortality of patients with advanced disease may exceed 50% *(3)*. To maintain adequate myocardial contractility in response to injury, the heart uses several mechanisms, including hypertrophy of myocardial cells, changing the energetics of myocardial cell contraction, and upregulating transcription of several genes *(4,5)*.

Often a prelude to heart failure, myocardial hypertrophy is a pathophysiologic response of the heart to an increased work demand. Because myocardial cells are terminally differentiated in adults, cardiac growth during hypertrophy results from an increase in the size of individual myocardial cells and not from a change in cell number *(5)*. Myocyte cell growth is regulated by the activation of multiple plasma membrane receptor–mediated signals that connect the extracellular and intracellular environments. Stimulation of key effector molecules transmits the signal to the cell nucleus via a complex interacting network of protein kinases, phospholipid kinases, and protein phosphatases *(6–9)*. Increased hemodynamic load results in marked changes in cardiac gene expression, including genes for contractile proteins, myofilament organization, ion channels, cell surface receptors, transporters, and genes for enzymes involved in signaling pathways, cardiac energetics, and cell survival *(5,6)*. In addition, embryonic markers, such as atrial natriuretic factor, α-skeletal actin, and β-myosin heavy chain, are often re-expressed *(5,6)*.

Although cardiac hypertrophy is initially compensatory, over time the heart undergoes myocardial decompensation. The mechanisms responsible for the transition from stable compensated hypertrophy to myocardial dysfunction are not well understood. The following hypotheses have been suggested for the progression of myocardial dysfunction: (1) alterations in Ca^{2+} availability *(10)*, (2) abnormalities in the myocyte cytoskeleton such as microtubular polymerization *(11)*, (3) alterations in intracellular signaling pathways *(6–8)*, (4) decreased volume fraction of cardiomyocyte myofibrils *(12)*, and (5) aberrations in G protein–coupled receptor signaling *(13)*.

From: *Contemporary Cardiology: Principles of Molecular Cardiology*
Edited by: M. S. Runge and C. Patterson @ Humana Press Inc., Totowa, NJ

According to classic theories, myocardial hypertrophy is a long-term adaptive response of cardiac muscle to increased mechanical loading that prevents heart failure (5,14,15). The increase in wall thickness is thought to normalize wall stress as described by the law of Laplace. In fact, more than 100 years ago, Osler described cardiac hypertrophy as a compensatory process with an increase in thickness of the muscular walls (16). Although cardiac hypertrophy may normalize wall stress, epidemiologic data have shown an association between ventricular hypertrophy and increased cardiac mortality, casting doubt on the validity of the wall stress hypothesis (17,18). Recent studies in genetically engineered mice with a blunted hypertrophic response to hemodynamic stress have shown that hypertrophy, not increased wall stress, may trigger cardiac decompensation (19,20). These studies also highlight the importance of intracellular signaling pathways in the development of heart failure.

This chapter will explore the cellular mechanisms underlying cardiac hypertrophy and heart failure, with emphasis on the involvement of G protein–coupled receptors (GPCRs) and their signaling pathways in these processes. In addition, several therapeutic approaches based on molecular intervention will be presented.

G PROTEIN–COUPLED RECEPTOR SIGNALING IN HYPERTROPHY AND HEART FAILURE

Most hormones and neurotransmitters involved in cardiac signaling initiate cellular responses by binding to receptors that couple to guanine nucleotide binding proteins (G proteins) (21). GPCRs comprise a family of seven transmembrane–α helical receptors that mediate responses to a vast array of ligands (13,22). The basic unit of GPCR receptor signaling is composed of three parts: a receptor, the heterotrimeric G protein, and an effector molecule such as a G-protein–regulated enzyme or an ion channel (Fig. 1) (13,22).

The heterotrimeric G protein comprises three subunits: α, β, and γ (Fig. 1). The α subunit has a single high-affinity binding site for guanine nucleotides (GDP or GTP) as well as independent GTPase activity that is responsible for termination of signaling. Binding of extracellular ligand to the receptor induces a conformational change that favors productive coupling of the receptor with the G protein, thereby catalyzing the exchange of GDP with GTP on the Gα subunit, and the dissociation of GαGTP from G$\beta\gamma$ subunits. Both GαGTP and G$\beta\gamma$ are signaling molecules that modulate the activity of specific effector molecules. The G$\beta\gamma$ complex interacts with effector molecules

such as the muscarinic K$^+$ channel I$_{k,Ach}$, adenylyl cyclase, phospholipase C β, and the G protein–coupled receptor kinases (GRKs) (23). The G$\beta\gamma$ subunits help regulate mitogen-activated protein kinase (MAPK) pathways involved in cell growth and differentiation (24).

G proteins are divided into the following four major families based on amino acid similarity of the α subunits: Gαs, Gαi, Gαq/11, and Gα12/13. Members of the Gαs subfamily stimulate adenylyl cyclase to generate the second-messenger cAMP, which leads to activation of cAMP-dependent protein kinase (PKA). PKA-dependent phosphorylation of the L-type Ca^{2+} channel increases the release of Ca^{2+} from the sarcoplasmic reticulum, which increases cardiac contractility (25–27). In addition, PKA phosphorylates transcription factors such as c-fos, which results in changes in gene expression (28). G proteins of the Gαi family are usually activated by ligands that reduce downstream signals. Cholinergic stimulation of the heart leads to Gαi coupling, which results in a decrease in cAMP production. G proteins of the Gαq family activate phospholipase Cβ, which generates the second messengers diacylglycerol and inositol 1,4,5-triphosphate (IP3). Diacylglycerol, together with increased levels of calcium, activates the serine/threonine protein kinase C (PKC), which functions in many signaling pathways. When IP3 binds to the IP3 receptor in the sarcoplasmic reticulum, Ca^{2+} is released and Ca^{2+}/calmodulin kinase and calcineurin are activated, thereby increasing transcription of hypertrophic genes (7). Receptors that couple to Gαq include α1-adrenergic, angiotensin II, and endothelin-1 receptors.

Although the stimulation of receptors by ligand binding activates many cellular processes, elaborate mechanisms are in place to turn off the signal, a process known as desensitization. During receptor desensitization, the responsiveness of the receptor wanes despite continuing agonist stimulation. The following three families of regulatory molecules are involved in the desensitization of GPCRs: (1) second messenger–regulated kinases (e.g., PKA and PKC), (2) GRKs (e.g., β-adrenergic receptor kinase (1), and (3) the arrestins. Activation of PKA and PKC by Gαs and Gαq-coupled receptors results in the phosphorylation of serine and threonine residues located primarily on the third intracellular loop of the receptor (22). These events directly alter conformation of the receptor and uncouple the receptor from the G protein. This type of receptor regulation is called heterologous desensitization because any stimulant that increases second messengers can potentially cause the phosphorylation and desensitization of any GPCR containing an appropriate PKA and/or PKC consensus phosphorylation site (22).

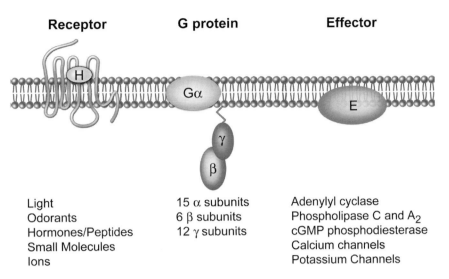

Fig. 1. Summary of G protein–coupled receptor signaling. The basic unit of G protein–coupled receptor signaling comprises: a seven-transmembrane-spanning receptor, a heterotrimeric G protein, and an effector molecule, such as an enzyme or ion channel. Reprinted with permission (13).

Another type of desensitization of the GPCR, called homologous desensitization, involves rapid, agonist-specific desensitization of the receptor. In homologous desensitization, agonist-dependent phosphorylation of the receptor by GRK is followed by recruitment of an arrestin protein, which sterically uncouples the receptor from the G protein. After arrestin binds, many GPCRs undergo agonist-promoted endocytosis via clathrin-coated vesicles or non-coated vesicle pathways (Fig. 2) (22,29). Receptor internalization is important because GPCRs must undergo dephosphorylation and resensitization before being recycled back to the plasma membrane (30,31). Downregulation of receptors after prolonged exposure to agonist begins with internalization of the receptors. The net loss of receptors from the cell surface during downregulation may be due to decreased receptor synthesis, destabilization of receptor mRNA, or increased receptor degradation.

In addition to its classic role in uncoupling the receptor–G protein complex, arrestin may help mediate receptor internalization via clathrin-coated vesicles. The mechanism is not fully understood, but arrestin appears to serve as an adaptor protein that links the receptors to clathrin, the clathrin adaptor AP2, and other elements of the internalization system (32). Arrestins also facilitate the activation and subcellular localization of signaling proteins involved in complex heptahelical receptor-stimulated pathways (32,33).

β-Adrenergic Receptors

By releasing epinephrine and norepinephrine, the autonomic nervous system plays an important role in rapid changes of both chronotropy (heart rate) and inotropy (force of contraction). Norepinephrine and epinephrine, which bind both to α- and β-adrenergic receptors in myocytes, trigger the intracellular signaling pathways that activate contractile forces and the pathways involved in growth of the heart muscle (34).

β-Adrenergic receptors (βARs) belong to the superfamily of GPCRs. Three subtypes of βARs have been identified in the human heart: β1, β2, and β3 (35). The β1AR subtype is predominant and maintains a ratio of 80:20 β1 to β2 (36). Located primarily in the atria, the ventricles, and the conduction system, activation of β1ARs increase heart rate, contractility, and conduction velocity. Although present on cardiac myocytes, β2ARs are located predominantly on smooth muscle cells of vascular walls, on skeletal muscle cells, and on cells of the bronchial, gastrointestinal, and urinary systems where they regulate smooth muscle relaxation and glycogenesis. β3ARs regulate lipolysis and thermogenesis and may have a direct, negative inotropic effect on the heart (37,38).

Increased sympathetic activity following injury to the heart leads to elevated plasma levels of norepinephrine in patients with symptomatic and asymptomatic left ventricular dysfunction. Elevated levels of catecholamines are strongly correlated to increased mortality in patients with chronic heart failure (39). Accumulating evidence suggests that chronic activation, not short-term activation, of the sympathetic system can have long-term adverse affects on the function of the myocardium through downregulation of βARs (40).

Desensitization   Internalization

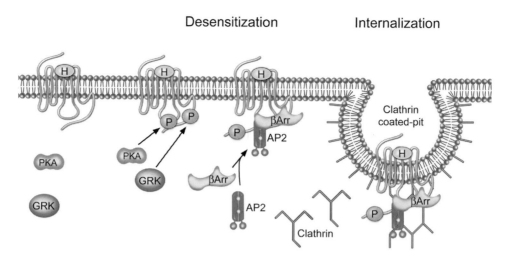

Fig. 2. Molecular mechanisms involved in the G protein–coupled receptor kinase (GRK)- and β-arrestin–dependent desensitization and internalization of G protein–coupled receptors (GPCRs). GPCR activation leads to GRK-dependent phosphorylation of intracellular serine and threonine residues that facilitate the translocation and binding of β-arrestin proteins to the receptor. β-Arrestins, via their association with the β2-adaptin subunit of the AP_2 heterotetrameric adaptor complex, target GPCRs to clathrin-coated pits. In addition to binding β2-adaptins, β-arrestins bind clathrin. The GPCR is subsequently internalized via clathrin-coated vesicles. AP_2, AP_2 heterotetrameric adaptor complex; βArr, β-arrestin; E, effector; G, G protein; H, hormone; P, phosphate group.

Heart failure is characterized by a reduced responsiveness of receptors to agonist stimulation. This reduced responsiveness results from a decrease in the number of receptors caused by downregulation of the receptor and from impaired function of receptors caused by uncoupling of the receptor (41,42), both of which may contribute to abnormal contractile function in heart failure. Selective downregulation of βARs results in a shift in the β1AR:β2AR ratio from 80:20 in the normal heart to 60:40 in the failing heart (43,44). This ratio shift may affect activation of specific intracellular signaling pathways (45).

The development of transgenic technology along with the availability of cardiac-specific promoters has allowed researchers to study the role of the βAR system in the failing heart by overexpressing components of this system in the myocardium. Transgenic mice with overexpression of either β1AR or β2AR in the ventricle have significantly different phenotypes, indicating differences in function of these two receptor subtypes in the myocardium. A 5- to 15-fold overexpression of β1ARs produces dilated cardiomyopathy, with pathologic changes similar to those caused by chronic stimulation of catecholamines (46) (Fig. 3A). In contrast, moderate overexpression of β2ARs in mice does not cause significant cardiomyopathy and may increase contractile function (47,48) (Fig. 3B). However, extremely high levels of β2AR expression cause rapid and progressive cardiomyopathy (47,49). These studies indicate that moderate expression of β2AR may improve heart function, whereas high levels of overexpression will exacerbate the disease.

Gene knockout studies in mice have demonstrated the differences between β1ARs and β2ARs in regulating cardiac function. Knockout of β1ARs causes embryonic death in most homozygous mice (50). Mice that do survive the absence of β1ARs have normal resting heart rate and blood pressure and, despite the presence of β2ARs in the heart, show no contractility response to β-agonist stimulation (50). In contrast, β2AR knockout mice are healthy and viable. The only physiological effects of the absence of β2ARs are altered vascular tone and energy metabolism seen only during the stress of exercise (51). These data suggest that β1ARs are essential to cardiac development in mice and act as a central mediator of inotropy and chronotropy in response to catecholamines (50). In contrast, β2ARs seem to have little effect on resting cardiac function in mice (51). The different mechanisms involved in receptor coupling of β1AR and β2AR to G proteins and the activation of different signaling pathways may explain, in part, the distinct phenotypes in transgenic mice caused by overexpression of the two receptors. Coupling of β2ARs to both Gαs and Gαi proteins activates signaling pathways that promote cell differentiation and survival, whereas coupling of β1ARs to Gαs primarily activates apoptotic pathways (52–54).

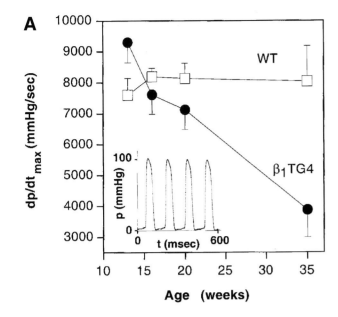

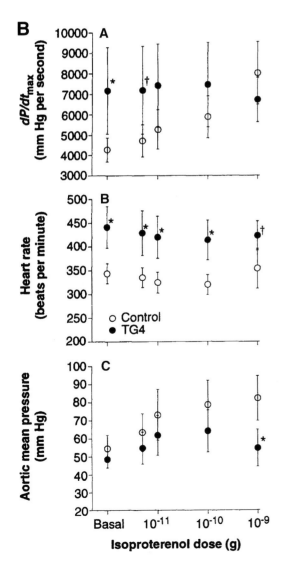

Angiotensin II Receptors

Angiotensin II is a biologically active neuropeptide that stimulates myocardial growth responses, new protein synthesis, and myocardial hypertrophy. The complex signaling initiated by angiotensin II is mediated primarily through the Gq-coupled angiotensin II type 1 receptor (AT1R), and to some extent, the angiotensin II type 2 receptor (AT2R) (32,55). Downstream signals from the angiotensin II–bound receptors activate MAPKs, which help regulate cell growth and differentiation (56–59) (Fig. 4).

Pressure overload on the left ventricle increases the expression of angiotensinogen mRNA, which leads to cardiac hypertrophy (60); however, hypertrophy can be blocked by angiotensin-converting enzyme (ACE) inhibitors and angiotensin receptor blockers (61). These findings suggest that endogenous angiotensin II plays a role in cardiac hypertrophy, possibly through an autocrine mechanism (62,63). In vivo studies have shown that administration of angiotensin II induces collagen deposition in the myocardium and causes myocyte hypertrophy and increased left ventricular mass (64–68). ACE inhibitors and angiotensin II receptor blockers prevent or reverse hypertension-induced increases in left ventricular mass and collagen deposition in murine models of hypertension (65,67,68).

Studies of transgenic mice with a cardiac-specific overexpression of the AT1R or AT2R suggest that AT2R-mediated signaling cascades modulate growth of cardiac myocytes (55,69). However, studies in AT1R knockout mice have shown that activation of the $AT1_AR$, a subtype of AT1R, is not required to trigger load-induced hypertrophy in the adult cardiomyocyte (64,70). This finding indicates a possible role for the $AT1_BR$ subtype in the hypertrophic response. Although the function of AT2Rs in the heart is not well understood, studies suggest that upregulation of cardiac AT2Rs during chronic left ventricular hypertrophy, serve as an antigrowth signal to inhibit the effects of angiotensin II on the immediate growth response in the adult heart (71). Despite the controversy regarding the role of the AT1R subtype(s) as a

Fig. 3. (A) Left ventricular contractility (dP/dt_{max}) in wild-type (WT) mice and mice overexpressing β1adrenergic receptors (β1TG4). Overexpression of β1-adrenergic receptors leads to a marked decrease in contractility. Reprinted with permission (46). **(B)** In vivo assessment of left ventricular function in mice overexpressing β1adrenergic receptors and in wild type mice at baseline and after β adrenergic receptor stimulation. Reprinted with permission (46).

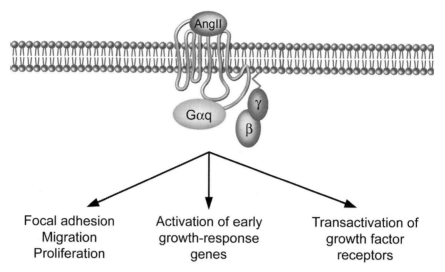

Fig. 4. Model illustrating the different pathways involved in angiotensin II (Ang II)–mediated signal transduction via the angiotensin II type 1 receptor.

signal transducer or modulator of the hypertrophic response, evidence indicates that they are important in the transduction of mechanical load in pressure-overload hypertrophy.

α1-Adrenergic Receptors

In the normal human heart, the ratio of βAR to α1-adrenergic receptors is 10:1. However, even this small number of cardiac α1-adrenergic receptors can produce a positive inotropic response. Norepinephrine and phenylephrine increase coupling of α1-adrenergic receptors to Gαq, which increases calcium levels in the myocyte, thereby producing a positive inotropic response and an increase in growth. Furthermore, overexpression of $\alpha1_A$-adrenergic receptors in the mouse heart increases cardiac contractility without inducing hypertrophy (72). However, transgenic mice with an overexpression of a constitutively active mutant of the $\alpha1_B$-adrenergic receptor have a phenotype consistent with cardiac hypertrophy (73), whereas mice with an overexpression of wild-type $\alpha1_B$-adrenergic receptors have left ventricular dysfunction (74).

Endothelin Receptors

Endothelin is a powerful constrictor of vascular smooth muscle cells and a strong inducer of myocardial hypertrophy (75,76). It also mediates several physiological effects, such as positive inotropy, acceleration of catecholamines, secretion of aldosterone, and inhibition of renin secretion. Of the three isoforms of endothelin, endothelin-1 is expressed in the cardiovascular system and is released by myocytes during mechanical stress–induced hypertrophy (77). In rats,

synthesis of endothelin-1 and its receptor, Gq-coupled ET_A, are upregulated during the development of heart failure (78). Long-term treatment with the endothelin receptor antagonist, BQ-123, significantly improves survival in rats with chronic heart failure (79). BQ-123 inhibits stretch-induced activation of MAPK and protein synthesis suggesting that endothelin-1 is involved in an autocrine/paracrine mechanism of hypertrophy, similar to the effects of angiotensin II in the heart (77).

Gαq-Mediated Signaling

In vitro studies have linked the Gαq signaling pathway with the initiation of cardiac hypertrophy. Several Gq-coupled receptor ligands, such as norepinephrine/phenylephrine (80,81), angiotensin II (63), and endothelin-1 (82), produce hypertrophic responses in cultured neonatal cardiomyocytes. The role of Gαq in hypertrophy has been assessed in studies of transgenic mice with cardiac-specific overexpression of a Gαq inhibitory peptide, which interferes with the receptor-Gq/11 interaction. Overexpression of the Gαq inhibitor peptide in a mouse model of pressure overload (83) blocked signaling through Gq-coupled receptors (84), significantly decreased the development of cardiac hypertrophy (84), blocked the activation of downstream signaling pathways (85), and reduced the development of left ventricular dysfunction (19) (Fig. 5). In contrast, moderate overexpression of wild-type Gαq (86) or a constitutively active mutant of Gαq (87) produced a phenotype of cardiac hypertrophy and modest cardiac dysfunction in transgenic mice, whereas marked overexpression of Gαqs lead to overt

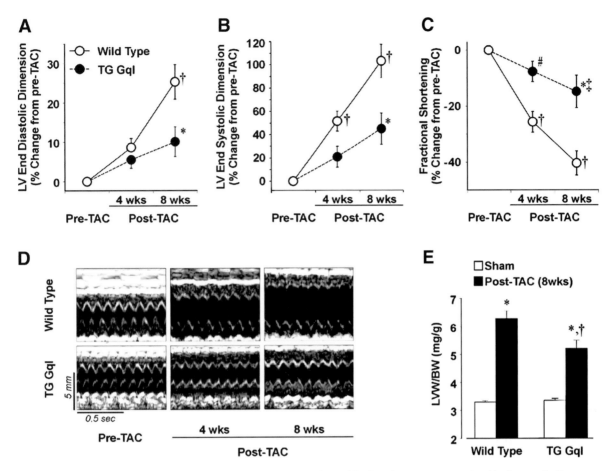

Fig. 5. Serial echocardiography in conscious wild-type and Tg Gq1 mice with chronic pressure overload before and after transverse aortic constriction (TAC). Reprinted with permission *(19)*.

heart failure *(86)*. Moreover, when transgenic mice with overexpression of Gαq were stressed by transverse aortic constriction, eccentric hypertrophy with progressive worsening of ventricular function developed *(88)*. Together, these data indicate that activation of Gq/G11 signaling pathways plays a critical role in the development of cardiac hypertrophy and heart failure.

The Role of G Protein–Coupled Receptor Kinases in Heart Failure

The main mechanism of GPCR desensitization is agonist-dependent phosphorylation of the receptor by GRKs. Phosphorylation is followed by recruitment of arrestin, which sterically interferes with the coupling of the receptor and the G protein. Of the seven members of the GRK family (GRK 1–7), GRK2 (commonly known as βAR kinase 1 [βARK1]) and GRK5 are expressed most frequently in the heart *(89)*. GRK3 and GRK6 have been identified in cardiac tissue, but its mRNA expression levels are significantly lower than those of βARK and GRK5 *(89)* (Fig. 6).

GRK-mediated desensitization of βAR may be an important mechanism for decreasing the catecholamine responsiveness seen in the failing heart. The importance of βARK1 in heart disease is supported by studies showing that increased expression of βARK1 is associated with hypertension *(90)*, ventricular hypertrophy *(91)*, and heart failure *(43)*.

The development of transgenic mice with cardiac-targeted overexpression of full-length βARK1 protein or a peptide inhibitor of βARK1 (βARK1ct), and mice with the βARK1 gene ablated *(92,93)*, provide a powerful tool to study heart failure. The 194-amino-acid βARK1ct peptide encodes the Gβγ-binding domain of βARK1, and the peptide that is formed competes with endogenous βARK1 for Gβγ-mediated membrane translocation and activation *(94)*. In transgenic mice overexpressing βARKct, βARK activity is inhibited. The pathophysiology of heart failure has been studied by mating transgenic mice overexpressing βARKct with mice from various mouse models *(95–97)*, including

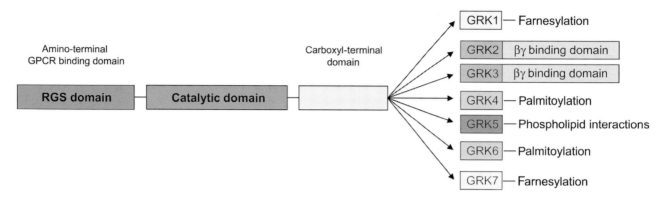

Fig. 6. Schematic representation of the domain architecture for G protein–coupled receptor kinases (GRK) 1–7. The amino-terminal G protein–coupled receptor-binding domain of GRK1–GRK7 contains a conserved regulators of G protein signaling (RGS) domain. The targeting of each GRK to the plasma membrane is mediated by distinct mechanisms that involve the carboxyl-terminal domains. GRK1 and GRK7 are farnesylated at carboxyl terminal CAAX motifs. The carboxyl-terminal domains of GRK2 and GRK3 contain a βγ-subunit binding domain that exhibits sequence homology to a pleckstrin homology domain. The GRK5 carboxyl-terminal domain contains a stretch of 46 basic amino acids that mediate interactions with phospholipids of the plasma membrane. GRK4 and GRK6 are palmitoylated at cysteine residues.

skeletal muscle LIM protein knockout mice *(97,98)*, transgenic mice with cardiac overexpression of calsequestrin *(99)*, and transgenic mice with overexpression of a mutant cardiac α-myosin heavy chain *(100)*. In each case, cardiac overexpression of the βARKct prevented hypertrophy and progressive deterioration in cardiac dysfunction, improved exercise tolerance, corrected the classical biochemical alterations of βAR function *(40)*, and improved survival (Fig. 7A, B). Moreover, effects on survival were synergistic with improved survival achieved by βAR blocker treatment *(99)*, a finding that supports clinical data showing improved survival in patients with chronic heart failure treated with β-blockers *(101–104)*.

Knockout of the βARK1 gene in mice leads to death of all embryos by d 15.5 of gestation *(92)*. Mice heterozygous for the βARK1 gene have no obvious developmental abnormalities, despite a 50% reduction in the level of βARK1 protein and GRK activity *(92)*. Heterozygous animals grow into normal adults but have increased contractile responses to isoproterenol stimulation *(105)*. Studies have shown that the level of βARK1 activity determines the response to catecholamine stimulation and the level of contractile function in the normal heart *(93,105)*. These findings have important implications for treatment of diseases characterized by increased βARK1 activity because even partial inhibition of βARK1 may improve cardiac function in response to catecholamine stimulation *(13)*.

Studies in larger animal models have shown that in vivo delivery of an adenovirus encoding the βARKct

transgene can improve cardiac function. In rabbits with heart failure, delivery of the βARKct transgene prevented the development of biochemical abnormalities in the βAR system, delayed the onset of hemodynamic heart failure, and reversed the development of heart failure after myocardial infarction *(84,106,107)*.

The functional role of GRK5 and GRK3 has also been determined with the use of genetically engineered mice. Overexpression of GRK5 resulted in desensitization of βARs *(108)*, whereas overexpression of GRK3 attenuated thrombin-mediated signaling *(109)*.

Phosphoinositide 3-Kinase Pathways and Heart Failure

Phosphoinositide 3-kinases (PI3Ks), a conserved family of lipid kinases, comprise three classes based on substrate specificity. Class 1 PI3Ks, which includes PI3Kα, β, γ, and δ, regulates many fundamental cellular functions, including proliferation and transformation of cells and antiapoptotic effects *(110)*. The activation of PI3K in response to pressure overload depends on released Gβγ subunits *(111)*. Furthermore, activation of PI3K under conditions of hypertrophy is primarily mediated through stimulation of Gq-coupled receptors because cardiac-specific overexpression of a Gq inhibitor peptide eliminates PI3K activation in transgenic mice *(111)*.

Studies of the role of PI3K in βAR internalization have shown an important link between the activation of PI3K and GPCR function. These studies have shown that βARK1 and PI3K form an interacting complex in the cytosol *(112,113)*. Upon agonist stimulation, βARK1

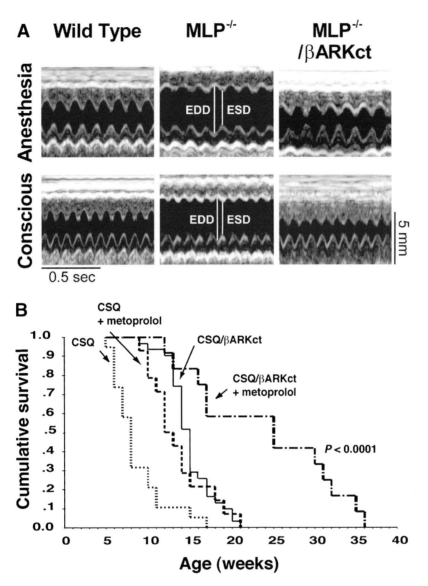

Fig. 7. (A) Echocardiography in conscious and anesthetized wild type mice, muscle LIM protein knockout mice (MLP$^{-/-}$), and MLP$^{-/-}$/β-adrenergic receptor kinase-1 inhibitor (βARKct) mice. Representative M-mode echocardiographic tracings are shown for the same mouse under anesthesia and in the conscious state. The white lines indicate left ventricular end-diastolic dimension (EDD) and end-systolic dimension (ESD). Although the MLP$^{-/-}$ mouse shows an enlarged chamber with reduced cardiac performance under both conscious and anesthetized conditions, chamber diameter and cardiac performance are normal in the MLP$^{-/-}$/βARKct mouse. Reprinted with permission *(96)*. (B) Improved survival of transgenic mice overexpressing calsequestrin (CSQ) through inhibition of βARK by overexpressing the βARKct peptide. Kaplan–Meier analysis of the survival probability between the specified genotypes of mice either untreated or chronically treated with the selective β1adrenergic receptor antagonist metoprolol. The mean survival age of CSQ/βARKct mice is significantly higher than that of CSQ transgenic littermates ($p<0.0001$). Moreover, treating CSQ/βARKct with metoprolol further improves survival, indicating a synergism between the two therapeutic modalities. Reprinted with permission *(99)*.

mediates agonist-dependent translocation of PI3K to the membrane, enabling PI3K to co-localize with the GPCR and regulate receptor internalization. Phospholipids generated by the action of PI3K are required for efficient receptor internalization and for recruitment of adaptor proteins involved in targeting the receptor complex to clathrin-coated pits *(113)* (Fig. 8). In vivo studies of hypertrophied hearts have shown that high levels of βARK1 increase P3K activity *(112)* and receptor desensitization *(91)*. These studies suggest that alterations in

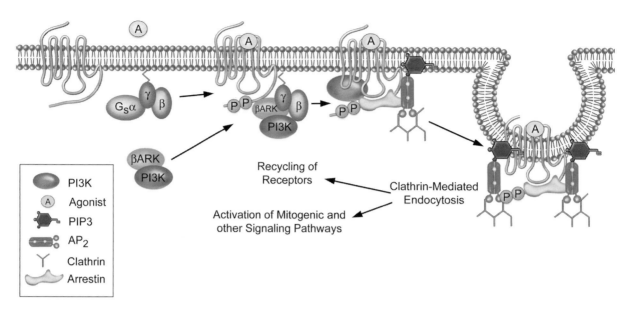

Fig. 8. Schematic representation of putative steps involved in the β-adrenergic receptor kinase (βARK1)–mediated translocation of G protein–coupled receptors (GPCRs) after agonist stimulation. Agonist binding to β adrenergic receptor causes the dissociation of heterotrimeric G proteins into Gα-GTP and G βγ subunits. Gβγ-dependent translocation of βARK1 recruits phosphoinositide 3-kinase (PI3K) to the membrane, which initiates two processes: βARK1-mediated receptor phosphorylation and activation of PI3Kγ. Activation of PI3Kγ increases the local concentration of D-3 phosphoinositides in the region of the activated GPCR. Generation of D-3 phosphoinositides initiates endocytic invagination of the phosphorylated receptor, which is mediated by phosphoinositide binding to β-arrestin and AP2 adaptin protein molecules. Thus, PI3K may promote nucleation of clathrin-coated pits around the newly activated GPCRs, providing additional internalization sites to those already present in the preformed clathrin-coated pits.

PI3K activation and recruitment may contribute to abnormalities in βAR function.

Taken together, the evidence supports the hypothesis that the loss of βAR signaling, the *sine qua non* of the heart failure phenotype, contributes to the pathogenesis of the failing heart. Furthermore, these data suggest that genetic techniques to restore βAR signaling may be a new therapeutic approach for treating heart failure.

GROWTH FACTOR RECEPTORS IN HYPERTROPHY AND HEART FAILURE

In addition to GPCR signaling, several endocrine factors affect the hypertrophic growth response. Two of these endocrine factors, the receptor tyrosine kinases and cytokines, are characterized by their ability to alter cell growth and function.

Receptor Tyrosine Kinases

Growth factors control cell growth, proliferation, and division *(114)*. Receptors for growth factors are comprised of a dimer between two single transmembrane domain units with an extracellular hormone-binding site

and a cytosolic tyrosine kinase domain, which becomes autophosphorylated upon ligand binding *(115)* (Fig. 9).

Several growth factors, such as fibroblast growth factor (FGF) and insulin-like growth factor-1 (IGF), are involved in the pathogenesis of cardiac hypertrophy. FGF mediates a hypertrophic response induced by pressure overload in mice, and targeted disruption of the FGF-2 gene prevents the development of myocardial hypertrophy *(116)*. Similarly, IGF-1 levels are increased in pressure-overloaded cardiomyocytes *(117–119)*. The downstream signaling pathways that transduce the FGF-induced hypertrophic response are partially mediated by activation of MAPK pathways *(120)*.

Members of the transforming growth factor β (TGFβ) family also play an important role in the myocardial response to hypertrophic stimuli *(121)*. Levels of TGFβ1 mRNA increase in response to pressure overload *(122,123)* and may upregulate expression of fetal genes, such as β-myosin heavy chain and α-skeletal actin genes *(124)*. Moreover, the increase in the levels of TGFβ1/2 in response to pressure overload or cytokine-induced heart failure involves the deposition of extracellular matrix (ECM) proteins and increased myofibrillar collagen content *(122,125)*.

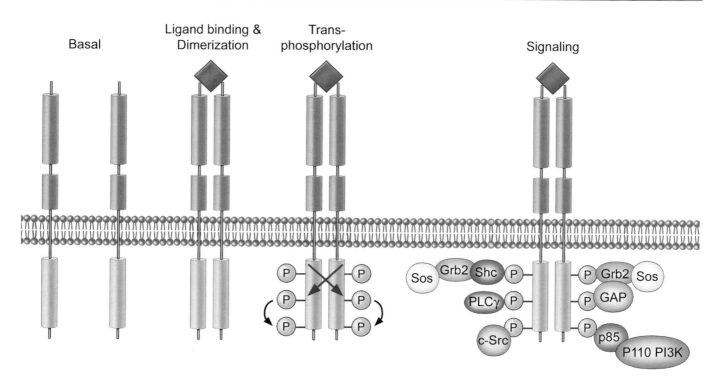

Fig. 9. Receptor tyrosine kinases are single transmembrane domain proteins that undergo dimerization and transphosphorylation upon ligand binding. Autophosphorylation promotes association of the receptor with phosphotyrosine binding or SH2 domain–containing adaptor proteins such as Shc and Grb2, and signaling proteins such as c-Src, PLCγ, RasGTPase, and p85-p110 PI3K, to form a membrane-associated complex.

Cytokines

Although cytokines act primarily on cells that are involved in the immune response, studies show that they affect the structure and function of the myocardium. One of the multiple pathways activated by cytokines that was shown to be linked to the heart is the Janus kinase–signal transducer and activator of transcription (JAK–STAT) signaling pathway, which is activated by the ciliary neurotrophic/leukemia inhibitory factor/interleukin 6 (IL-6)/cardiotrophin-1 through the gp130 transmembrane receptor *(126)*. Activation of the JAK–STAT pathway transmits signals from the membrane to the nucleus *(127)* resulting in changes in gene expression. Other pathways activated by cytokines include c-Src tyrosine family kinases, MAPK, and PI3K *(128)*.

Several lines of evidence indicate the importance of gp130 in the development of cardiac hypertrophy. Cardiac-specific disruption of gp130 induces heart failure in response to mechanical stress by increasing apoptosis *(129)*. In addition, expression of constitutively active gp130

in transgenic mice leads to ventricular hypertrophy *(130)*, whereas hypertrophy is markedly inhibited in mice with a negative expression of gp130 *(131)*. Cardiotrophin-1 of the IL-6 family contributes to cardiomyocyte hypertrophy by inducing cell enlargement, sarcomeric organization, and embryonic gene expression *(132)*. Cardiotrophin-1 also increases myocyte survival in vitro by preventing apoptosis *(133)*.

Another important cytokine, tumor necrosis factor-α (TNFα), may also play a role in myocardial disease. Plasma levels of TNFα and other cytokines were found to be elevated in patients with heart failure, particularly in patients with end-stage heart failure compared to those with the recent onset of symptoms *(134–136)* (Fig. 10). This finding suggests that cytokine secretion occurs relatively late in the pathogenesis of heart failure *(137)*. In experimental systems, biomechanical stress increased endogenous production of TNFα by myocytes *(138)*. Furthermore, cardiac-specific overexpression of TNFα in mice resulted in ventricular dilatation with fibrosis, poor cardiac contractility, reduced response to βAR receptor stimulation, re-expression of fetal genes, and premature death *(139–141)*.

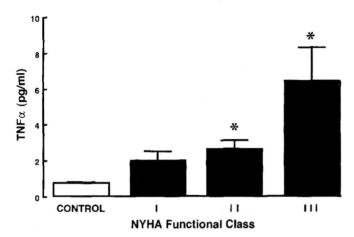

Fig. 10. Levels of tumor necosis factor α (TNFα) in normal subjects and in patients with heart disease. TNFα levels were determined from frozen plasma samples from age-matched subjects without heart disease and from patients with asymptomatic and symptomatic left ventricular dysfunction. TNFα levels were higher in patients with heart failure than age-matched controls and increased proportionally with severity of heart failure. Reprinted with permission *(191)*.

INTRACELLULAR SIGNALING PATHWAYS IN HYPERTROPHY AND HEART FAILURE

Growth signals received by the cell are transmitted to the nucleus through a complex and intricate network of pathways. The following three signaling pathways integrate signals from different receptor molecules (as discussed above) and are involved in myocardial hypertrophy: (1) MAPK, (2) JAK–STAT, and (3) calmodulin/calcineurin.

Mitogen-Activated Protein Kinases

MAPK signaling pathways are involved in a wide range of cellular programs, including cell differentiation, migration, division, and death *(142)*. The ubiquitous superfamily of serine/threonine kinases, which is activated by tyrosine and threonine phosphorylation, helps regulate gene expression and cytoplasmic activities. The MAPK signaling cascade comprises a three-kinase module: an MAPK, an MAPK activator (MAPKK), and an MAPKK activator (MAPKKK) *(57,76,142,143)* (Fig. 11). The signal is transmitted by sequential phosphorylation and activation of the components of the cascade (Fig. 11). Activated MAPKs phosphorylate downstream kinases (e.g., MAPK-activated protein kinase 2 and p90RSK) and intranuclear gene products, such as c-jun and c-myc. Activation of MAPKs leads to cell proliferation and differentiation *(144)*. Three main subfamilies of MAPKs are found in mammalian cells: the extracellular regulated

kinases (ERKs), the stress-activated protein kinases/c-Jun N-terminal kinases (SAPKs/JNKs), and the p38 MAPKs *(57,56,142,143)*. Evidence suggests that all members of the MAPK family contribute to the development of cardiac hypertrophy and possibly to the progression to heart failure *(19,58,85,121,145–147)*.

EXTRACELLULAR-REGULATED KINASES

Of the six subtypes of ERKs (ERK 1 to 6) in the MAPK family, ERK1 (44 kDa) and ERK2 (42 kDa) are the predominant isoforms found in the heart *(148)*. The ERK pathway can be stimulated by mitogens, including hormones, growth factors, and cytokines *(58)*. The major upstream activator of the ERK pathway is the small G protein, Ras. Ras activates c-Raf-1, followed by the sequential phosphorylation of MEK and ERK (Fig. 11). Activated ERKs then phosphorylate and regulate the activity of transcription factors that modulate the expression of target genes *(58,149)*.

Ligand stimulation of Gq-coupled receptors activates ERK pathways in vitro in cultured myocytes *(150)* and in vivo in pressure overload hypertrophy *(85,147)*. Transgenic mice with increased ERK activity caused by constitutive expression of MEK1 develop concentric hypertrophy and die prematurely *(151)*. Furthermore, overexpression of the constitutively active mutant of TGF-β-activated kinase, a member of the MAPK kinase kinase (MAP-KKK) family, leads to cardiac hypertrophy and dysfunction in transgenic mice *(121)*. However, under certain conditions, ERK activation may provide cardioprotection from ischemia/reperfusion and other apoptotic stimuli *(151,152)*.

JNK-SAPKS

The three isoforms of the JNK family, JNK1 (SAPKγ), JNK2 (SAPKα), and JNK3 (SAPKβ), are activated primarily by physiological stresses, such as changes in pH and oxidative or ultraviolet stress *(153)*. The Rho family of small G proteins such as Rac and cdc42 are thought to activate the JNK pathways. JNKs are directly phosphorylated by MEK4 and MEK7, which are, in turn, activated by MEK kinase (MEKK) 1 and 2 *(76,143,153–155)*. By interacting selectively with transcription factors, JNKs can target specific transcription factors *(156)*. In vitro studies have shown that phenylephrine, endothelin-1, and angiotensin II activate JNK in myocytes *(157,158)* (Fig. 11). In cardiomyocytes from neonatal rats, expression of wild type and constitutively active forms of MKK7 activates JNK pathways without activating either ERK or p38 pathways, and this selective activation of JNK results in cellular hypertrophy *(159)*. Moreover, in vivo studies in mice

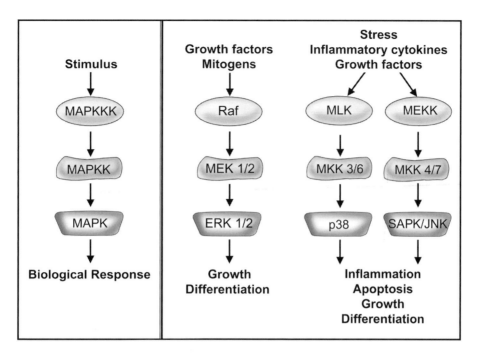

Fig. 11. Mitogen-activated protein kinase (MAPK) signaling pathways. MAPK signaling cascades are organized hierarchically into three-tiered modules. MAPKs are phosphorylated and activated by MAPK-kinases (MAPKKs), which in turn are phosphorylated and activated by MAPKK-kinases (MAPKKKs).

show that JNK activity increases in response to pressure overload *(19,85,147)*. This increase in JNK activity can be inhibited by the overexpression of either a dominant inhibitory mutant of SEK-1 or an inhibitor of Gq. In addition, a lack of circulating norepinephrine and epinephrine can inhibit a pressure overload–induced increase in JNK activity in mice *(85,147,160)*.

p38

Of the four isoforms in the p38 MAPK family (p38α, p38β, p38γ, and p38δ), p38α and p38β are the ones primarily expressed in the heart *(161)*. p38 MAPKs are activated by mechanical, osmotic, and chemical stress as well as radiation and GPCR activation *(162)*. Several GPCR agonists, such as phenylephrine *(163)*, endothelin-1 *(157)*, and angiotensin II *(164)*, can activate p38 both in vitro and in vivo. In cultured rat neonatal cardiomyocytes, p38α and p38β have distinct functions. p38α is involved in programmed cell death, or apoptosis, whereas p38β and the upstream activator of p38, MKK6, induce hypertrophy as measured by an increased cell surface area, enhanced organization of sarcomeric proteins, and induction of atrial natriuretic factor expression *(165,166)*. Pressure overload hypertrophy induced by aortic banding activates both p38 isoforms, with short-term hemodynamic stress resulting primarily from the activation of non-Gq coupled receptor pathways *(85,147,165)*.

The role of MAPK pathways in the progression of heart failure is complex because various pathways are activated at different stages of the disease and because of differences in species. For example, in wild type mice with pressure overload, acute activation of JNK is followed by activation of p38α/p38β and ERK at 7 d *(85)*, and JNK pathways remain activated as cardiac function deteriorates *(19)*. In contrast, JNK activity is significantly increased without changes in ERK or p38 activity in spontaneously hypertensive rats *(167,168)*. In human failing hearts with ischemic disease, JNK and p38 activity are increased, but protein levels in MAPK pathways are not altered *(169)*. In the hearts of patients with compensated hypertrophy, none of the MAPKs are activated, whereas all MAPKs are significantly increased in the hearts of patients with advanced heart failure *(170)*.

Taken together, these studies indicate that MAPK pathways are important in the development of cardiac hypertrophy and the subsequent transition to decompensation. Further study is required to determine which molecule(s) are responsible for detrimental signals and which molecules can be protective.

JAK–STAT Pathways

Originally described as the signal-transducing pathway of interferons, the JAK–STAT signaling pathway participates in the signaling of several immune and non-immune

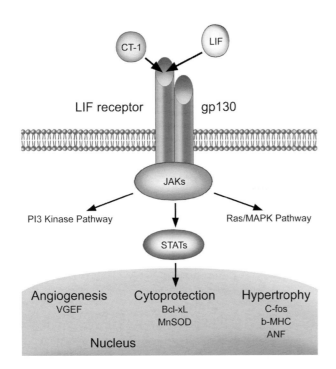

Fig. 12. Schematic model of gp130-dependent signaling in cardiac myocytes and the role of STAT in cardiac remodeling.

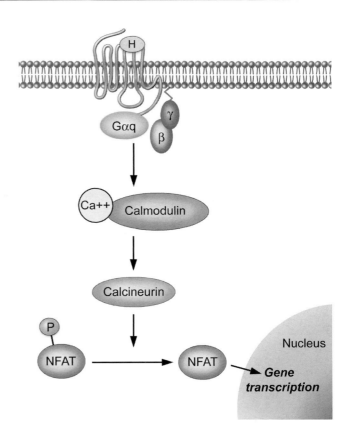

Fig. 13. Calcineurin signaling pathway in cardiomyocytes. Calcineurin is activated by calcium bound to calmodulin, which in turn leads to dephosphorylation of nuclear factor of activated T cells (NFAT) and its subsequent translocation to the nucleus.

mediators *(171–173)*. Cytokines and interferons activate JAK kinases, which then undergo tyrosine phosphorylation. After phosphorylation, JAK kinases activate STAT proteins, which become dimerized *(171–173)*. STAT proteins are subsequently translocated to the nucleus, where they function as transcription factors and modulate expression of target genes *(171–173)* (Fig. 12).

Aggregated cytokines bind to receptors that activate JAK and phosphorylate gp130. JAK-catalyzed tyrosine kinase activates multiple signal-transducing pathways, including STAT, the Ras-MAPK pathway, and PI3K pathways, which then in turn transmit intracellular signals to the nucleus *(128)*. Cytokines activated by gp130 may play an important role in heart failure *(127)*. Transgenic mice with cardiac-specific overexpression of STAT3 have lower levels of doxorubicin-induced apoptosis in the myocardium than wild-type mice, indicating that STAT3 may have a cytoprotective effect *(174)*. Thus, STAT3 not only activates hypertrophic signals but also protects against heart failure by inhibiting myocardial cell death *(174)*.

Ca²⁺-Sensitive Signaling Pathways: Calmodulin and Calcineurin

Calcium regulates the interaction between actin and myosin in crossbridge formation and the contraction of muscle cells. Changes in the intracellular concentration of calcium affect the ability of cardiomyocytes to contract

and influence Ca^{2+}-sensitive signaling pathways for hypertrophy *(9)*. Initiation of mechanical or agonist-induced cardiac hypertrophy activates Ca^{2+} signaling pathways through the binding of Ca^{2+} to intracellular binding proteins, such as calmodulin. The interaction of Ca^{2+} with binding proteins activates Ca^{2+}/calmodulin-dependent protein kinases and protein phosphatase 2B, known as calcineurin. Calcineurin is a serine/threonine phosphatase comprising a catalytic subunit calcineurin A, a calcium-binding protein calcineurin B, and calmodulin *(175)*. Calcineurin regulates transcription by dephosphorylating transcription factors, such as the nuclear factor of activated T cells (NFATs). Once activated, calcineurin binds to NFATs in the cytoplasm, where they are dephosphorylated and translocated to the nucleus. Once in the nucleus, NFATs bind to the DNA and increase the rate of gene transcription *(176)* (Fig. 13). NFATs can directly induce cardiac hypertrophy in mice *(177)*. Cardiac-specific overexpression of calcineurin in mice causes marked hypertrophy with progressive enlargement of the heart and possible sudden death *(178)*. Experimental hypertrophy can be reversed in

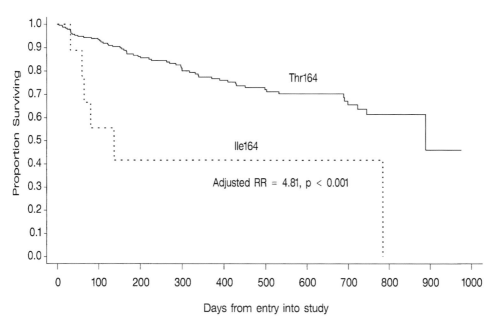

Fig. 14. Kaplan–Meier survival curve for patients with congestive heart failure who have the wild-type β2adrenergic receptor (Thr164) or the Ile 164 polymorphism, which was found only in the heterozygous state. Survival is defined as the proportion of patients who have not died or who have not undergone cardiac transplantation. The risk of death or transplantation was higher for patients with the Ile 164 polymorphism (*n* = 10) than for patients with the Thr 164 receptor (*n* = 247). Reprinted with permission *(188)*.

some models by agents such as cyclosporine A and FK506 that inhibit calcineurin and prevent nuclear translocation of NFATs *(9,179)*. Although evidence indicates that calcineurin is an important regulator of the cardiac hypertrophic response in vivo, the use of calcineurin inhibitory agents in the treatment of hypertrophy requires further study *(7,9)*.

GENETIC POLYMORPHISMS AND HEART FAILURE

Genetics play an important role in disease progression and prognosis in chronic diseases such as hypertension and heart failure. The clinical heterogeneity of complex diseases such as heart failure stems from the effects of environmental and genetic factors on the penetrance (percentage of patients with a specific genotype that expresses the corresponding phenotype) and expressivity (differences in the degree of a phenotype in patients with the same genotype) of genes. Genes that affect phenotypic expression of a disease are called modifier genes because they affect the development of the disease once it has occurred. One of the modifier genes that affect outcome of heart disease is an insertion/deletion polymorphism in the gene for ACE, which significantly affects plasma and myocardial levels of ACE *(180)*. In fact,

studies have shown that ACE polymorphism is associated with an increased risk of myocardial infarction and death, even in otherwise low-risk subjects *(181,182)*. Furthermore, ACE polymorphism affects long-term survival *(183)* and β-blocker therapy *(184)* in patients with congestive heart failure. However, genetic differences may not be a risk factor for the development of atherosclerosis or hypertension *(181)*. Another example of genetic polymorphism affecting outcome is the common variant of the gene for adenosine monophosphate deaminase 1, which is associated with prolonged survival without cardiac transplantation in patients with advanced heart failure *(185)*.

Genetic heterogeneity has been identified in the structure and function of β2 and β1ARs in humans *(186,187)*. Basal and agonist-stimulated adenylyl cyclase activities were reduced in cells with β2ARs containing a Thr to Ile substitution at amino acid 164 in the fourth transmembrane-spanning domain because of defective coupling of the receptor to Gs *(187)*. In heart failure patients with the Ile 164 allele, survival *(188)* and exercise capacity *(189)* are significantly reduced (Fig. 14). Genetic polymorphisms in βARs may account for differences in the pathophysiological characteristics of patients with chronic heart failure and may eventually be used clinically to identify high risk patients *(190)*.

CONCLUSION

Over the past decade, our knowledge of the membrane receptors and intracellular signaling pathways that mediate abnormal responses of the myocyte to disease states has increased significantly. Although scientists have made great progress, our understanding of the complexity of the intricate web of intersecting pathways is incomplete. A better understanding of how key signaling molecules interact in the cell, under both normal physiological conditions and in response to overload stress, is critical in designing novel therapeutic strategies to delay or reverse the pathological development of heart failure.

REFERENCES

1. Katz AM, Lorell BH. Regulation of cardiac contraction and relaxation. Circulation 2000;102:IV69–IV74.
2. Towbin JA, Bowles NE. The failing heart. Nature 2002;415: 227–233.
3. 2001 Heart and Stroke Statistical Update. Dallas: American Heart Association. 2001.
4. Alpert NR, Mulieri LA. Increased myothermal economy of isometric force generation in compensated cardiac hypertrophy induced by pulmonary artery constriction in the rabbit. A characterization of heat liberation in normal and hypertrophied right ventricular papillary muscles. Circ Res 1982;50:491–500.
5. Chien KR. Genomic circuits and the integrative biology of cardiac diseases. Nature 2000;407:227–232.
6. MacLellan WR, Schneider MD. Genetic dissection of cardiac growth control pathways. Annu Rev Physiol 2000;62:289–319.
7. Molkentin JD. Calcineurin and beyond: cardiac hypertrophic signaling. Circ Res 2000;87:731–738.
8. Sadoshima J, Izumo S. The cellular and molecular response of cardiac myocytes to mechanical stress. Annu Rev Physiol 1997;59:551–571.
9. Molkentin JD, Dorn IG II. Cytoplasmic signaling pathways that regulate cardiac hypertrophy. Annu Rev Physiol 2001;63: 391–426.
10. Gwathmey JK, Copelas L, MacKinnon R, et al. Abnormal intracellular calcium handling in myocardium from patients with end-stage heart failure. Circ Res 1987;61:70–76.
11. Tsutsui H, Ishihara K, Cooper GT. Cytoskeletal role in the contractile dysfunction of hypertrophied myocardium. Science 1993;260:682–687.
12. Urabe Y, Mann DL, Kent RL, et al. Cellular and ventricular contractile dysfunction in experimental canine mitral regurgitation. Circ Res 1992;70:131–147.
13. Rockman HA, Koch WJ, Lefkowitz RJ. Seven-transmembrane-spanning receptors and heart function. Nature 2002;415:206–212.
14. Chien KR. Stress pathways and heart failure. Cell 1999;98: 555–558.
15. Grossman W, Jones D, McLaurin LP. Wall stress and patterns of hypertrophy in the human left ventricle. J Clin Invest 1975;56: 56–64.
16. Osler W. The Principles and Practice of Medicine. New York:Appleton;1892.
17. Kannel WB, Castelli WP, McNamara PM, McKee PA, Feinleib M. Role of blood pressure in the development of congestive heart failure. The Framingham Study. N Engl J Med 1972;287: 781–787.
18. Levy D, Garrison RJ, Savage DD, Kannel WB, Castelli WP. Prognostic implications of echocardiographically determined left ventricular mass in the Framingham Heart Study. N Engl J Med 1990;322:1561–1566.
19. Esposito G, Rapacciuolo A, Naga Prasad SV, et al. Genetic alterations that inhibit in vivo pressure-overload hypertrophy prevent cardiac dysfunction despite increased wall stress. Circulation 2002;105:85–92.
20. Hill JA, Karimi M, Kutschke W, et al. Cardiac hypertrophy is not a required compensatory response to short-term pressure overload. Circulation 2000;101:2863–2869.
21. Gudermann T, Nurnberg B, Schultz G. Receptors and G proteins as primary components of transmembrane signal transduction. Part 1. G-protein-coupled receptors: structure and function. J Mol Med 1995;73:51–63.
22. Lefkowitz RJ. G protein-coupled receptors. III. New roles for receptor kinases and beta-arrestins in receptor signaling and desensitization. J Biol Chem 1998;273:18677–18680.
23. Clapham DE, Neer EJ. G protein beta gamma subunits. Annu Rev Pharmacol Toxicol 1997;37:167–203.
24. Gutkind JS. The pathways connecting G protein-coupled receptors to the nucleus through divergent mitogen-activated protein kinase cascades. J Biol Chem 1998;273:1839–1842.
25. Kamp TJ, Hell JW. Regulation of cardiac L-type calcium channels by protein kinase A and protein kinase C. Circ Res 2000; 87:1095–1102.
26. Marx SO, Reiken S, Hisamatsu Y, et al. PKA phosphorylation dissociates FKBP12.6 from the calcium release channel (ryanodine receptor): defective regulation in failing hearts. Cell 2000;101:365–376.
27. Tada M, Toyofuku T. SR Ca(2+)-ATPase/phospholamban in cardiomyocyte function. J Card Fail 1996;2:S77–S85.
28. Osaki J, Haneda T, Sakai H, Kikuchi K. cAMP-mediated c-fos expression in pressure-overloaded acceleration of protein synthesis in adult rat heart. Cardiovasc Res 1997;33:631–640.
29. Ferguson SS. Evolving concepts in G protein-coupled receptor endocytosis: the role in receptor desensitization and signaling. Pharmacol Rev 2001;53:1–24.
30. Sibley DR, Strasser RH, Benovic JL, Daniel K, Lefkowitz RJ. Phosphorylation/dephosphorylation of the beta-adrenergic receptor regulates its functional coupling to adenylate cyclase and subcellular distribution. Proc Natl Acad Sci USA 1986;83:9408–9412.
31. Yu SS, Lefkowitz RJ, Hausdorff WP. Beta-adrenergic receptor sequestration. A potential mechanism of receptor resensitization. J Biol Chem 1993;268:337–341.
32. Luttrell LM, Roudabush FL, Choy EW, et al. Activation and targeting of extracellular signal-regulated kinases by beta-arrestin scaffolds. Proc Natl Acad Sci USA 2001;98:2449–2454.
33. McDonald PH, Chow CW, Miller WE, et al. Beta-arrestin 2: a receptor-regulated MAPK scaffold for the activation of JNK3. Science 2000;290:1574–1577.
34. Koch WJ, Lefkowitz RJ, Rockman HA. Functional consequences of altering myocardial adrenergic receptor signaling. Annu Rev Physiol 2000;62:237–260.
35. Caron MG, Lefkowitz RJ. Catecholamine receptors: structure, function, and regulation. Recent Prog Horm Res 1993;48: 277–290.
36. Brodde OE. Beta-adrenoceptors in cardiac disease. Pharmacol Ther 1993;60:405–430.

37. Gauthier C, Leblais V, Kobzik L, et al. The negative inotropic effect of beta3-adrenoceptor stimulation is mediated by activation of a nitric oxide synthase pathway in human ventricle. J Clin Invest 1998;102:1377–1384.

38. Gauthier C, Tavernier G, Charpentier F, Langin D, Le Marec H. Functional beta3-adrenoceptor in the human heart. J Clin Invest 1996;98:556–562.

39. Cohn JN, Levine TB, Olivari MT, et al. Plasma norepinephrine as a guide to prognosis in patients with chronic congestive heart failure. N Engl J Med 1984;311:819–823.

40. Bristow MR. Why does the myocardium fail? Insights from basic science. Lancet 1998;352:8–14.

41. Bristow MR, Ginsburg R, Minobe W, et al. Decreased catecholamine sensitivity and beta-adrenergic-receptor density in failing human hearts. N Engl J Med 1982;307:205–211.

42. Bristow MR, Hershberger RE, Port JD, Minobe W, Rasmussen R. Beta 1- and beta 2-adrenergic receptor-mediated adenylate cyclase stimulation in nonfailing and failing human ventricular myocardium. Mol Pharmacol 1989;35:295–303.

43. Ungerer M, Bohm M, Elce JS, Erdmann E, Lohse MJ. Altered expression of beta-adrenergic receptor kinase and beta 1-adrenergic receptors in the failing human heart. Circulation 1993;87:454–463.

44. Bristow MR, Minobe WA, Raynolds MV, et al. Reduced beta 1 receptor messenger RNA abundance in the failing human heart. J Clin Invest 1993;92:2737–2745.

45. Lefkowitz RJ, Rockman HA, Koch WJ. Catecholamines, cardiac beta-adrenergic receptors, and heart failure. Circulation 2000;101:1634–1637.

46. Engelhardt S, Hein L, Wiesmann F, Lohse MJ. Progressive hypertrophy and heart failure in beta1-adrenergic receptor transgenic mice. Proc Natl Acad Sci USA 1999;96:7059–7064.

47. Liggett SB, Tepe NM, Lorenz JN, et al. Early and delayed consequences of beta(2)-adrenergic receptor overexpression in mouse hearts: critical role for expression level. Circulation 2000;101:1707–1714.

48. Milano CA, Allen LF, Rockman HA, et al. Enhanced myocardial function in transgenic mice overexpressing the beta 2-adrenergic receptor. Science 1994;264:582–586.

49. Dorn GW II, Tepe NM, Lorenz JN, Koch WJ, Liggett SB. Low- and high-level transgenic expression of beta2-adrenergic receptors differentially affect cardiac hypertrophy and function in Galphaq- overexpressing mice. Proc Natl Acad Sci USA 1999;96:6400–6405.

50. Rohrer DK, Desai KH, Jasper JR, et al. Targeted disruption of the mouse beta1-adrenergic receptor gene: developmental and cardiovascular effects. Proc Natl Acad Sci USA 1996;93:7375–7380.

51. Chruscinski AJ, Rohrer DK, Schauble E, Desai KH, Bernstein D, Kobilka BK. Targeted disruption of the beta2 adrenergic receptor gene. J Biol Chem 1999;274:16694–16700.

52. Xiao RP, Avdonin P, Zhou YY, et al. Coupling of beta2-adrenoceptor to Gi proteins and its physiological relevance in murine cardiac myocytes. Circ Res 1999;84:43–52.

53. Zhu WZ, Zheng M, Koch WJ, Lefkowitz RJ, Kobilka BK, Xiao RP. Dual modulation of cell survival and cell death by beta(2)-adrenergic signaling in adult mouse cardiac myocytes. Proc Natl Acad Sci USA 2001;98:1607–1612.

54. Geng YJ, Ishikawa Y, Vatner DE, et al. Apoptosis of cardiac myocytes in Gsalpha transgenic mice. Circ Res 1999;84:34–42.

55. Wollert KC, Drexler H. The renin-angiotensin system and experimental heart failure. Cardiovasc Res 1999;43:838–849.

56. Touyz RM, Schiffrin EL. Signal transduction mechanisms mediating the physiological and pathophysiological actions of angiotensin II in vascular smooth muscle cells. Pharmacol Rev 2000;52:639–672.

57. Sugden PH, Clerk A. Regulation of the ERK subgroup of MAP kinase cascades through G protein-coupled receptors. Cell Signal 1997;9:337–351.

58. Sugden PH, Clerk A. Cellular mechanisms of cardiac hypertrophy. J Mol Med 1998;76:725–746.

59. Haendeler J, Berk BC. Angiotensin II mediated signal transduction. Important role of tyrosine kinases. Regul Pept 2000;95:1–7.

60. Griendling KK, Murphy TJ, Alexander RW. Molecular biology of the renin-angiotensin system. Circulation 1993;87:1816–1828.

61. Rockman HA, Wachhorst SP, Mao L, Ross J Jr. ANG II receptor blockade prevents ventricular hypertrophy and ANF gene expression with pressure overload in mice. Am J Physiol 1994; 266:H2468–H2475.

62. Esther CR, Marino EM, Howard TE, et al. The critical role of tissue angiotensin-converting enzyme as revealed by gene targeting in mice. J Clin Invest 1997;99:2375–2385.

63. Sadoshima J, Xu Y, Slayter HS, Izumo S. Autocrine release of angiotensin II mediates stretch-induced hypertrophy of cardiac myocytes in vitro. Cell 1993;75:977–984.

64. Harada K, Komuro I, Shiojima I, et al. Pressure overload induces cardiac hypertrophy in angiotensin II type 1A receptor knockout mice. Circulation 1998;97:1952–1959.

65. Kim S, Iwao H. Molecular and cellular mechanisms of angiotensin II-mediated cardiovascular and renal diseases. Pharmacol Rev 2000;52:11–34.

66. Kim S, Ohta K, Hamaguchi A, Yukimura T, Miura K, Iwao H. Angiotensin II induces cardiac phenotypic modulation and remodeling in vivo in rats. Hypertension 1995;25:1252–1259.

67. Lijnen P, Petrov V. Antagonism of the renin-angiotensin system, hypertrophy and gene expression in cardiac myocytes. Methods Find Exp Clin Pharmacol 1999;21:363–374.

68. Lijnen P, Petrov V. Antagonism of the renin-angiotensin-aldosterone system and collagen metabolism in cardiac fibroblasts. Methods Find Exp Clin Pharmacol 1999;21:215–227.

69. Lorell BH. Role of angiotensin AT1, and AT2 receptors in cardiac hypertrophy and disease. Am J Cardiol 1999;83:48H–52H.

70. Kudoh S, Komuro I, Hiroi Y, et al. Mechanical stretch induces hypertrophic responses in cardiac myocytes of angiotensin II type 1a receptor knockout mice. J Biol Chem 1998;273: 24037–24043.

71. Bartunek J, Weinberg EO, Tajima M, Rohrbach S, Lorell BH. Angiotensin II type 2 receptor blockade amplifies the early signals of cardiac growth response to angiotensin II in hypertrophied hearts. Circulation 1999 99:22–25.

72. Lin F, Owens WA, Chen S, et al. Targeted alpha(1A)-adrenergic receptor overexpression induces enhanced cardiac contractility but not hypertrophy. Circ Res 2001;89:343-350.

73. Milano CA, Dolber PC, Rockman HA, et al. Myocardial expression of a constitutively active alpha 1B-adrenergic receptor in transgenic mice induces cardiac hypertrophy. Proc Natl Acad Sci USA 1994;91:10109–10113.

74. Grupp IL, Lorenz JN, Walsh RA, Boivin GP, Rindt H. Overexpression of alpha1B-adrenergic receptor induces left ventricular dysfunction in the absence of hypertrophy. Am J Physiol 1998;275:H1338–H1350.

75. Yanagisawa M, Kurihara H, Kimura S, et al. A novel potent vasoconstrictor peptide produced by vascular endothelial cells. Nature 1988;332:411–415.

76. Clerk A, Pham FH, Fuller SJ, et al. Regulation of mitogen-activated protein kinases in cardiac myocytes through the small G protein Rac1. Mol Cell Biol 2001;21:1173–1184.

77. Yamazaki T, Komuro I, Kudoh S, et al. Endothelin-1 is involved in mechanical stress-induced cardiomyocyte hypertrophy. J Biol Chem 1996;271:3221–3228.

78. Sakai S, Miyauchi T, Sakurai T, et al. Endogenous endothelin-1 participates in the maintenance of cardiac function in rats with congestive heart failure. Marked increase in endothelin-1 production in the failing heart. Circulation 1996;93:1214–1222.

79. Sakai S, Miyauchi T, Kobayashi M, Yamaguchi I, Goto K, Sugishita Y. Inhibition of myocardial endothelin pathway improves long-term survival in heart failure. Nature 1996; 384:353–355.

80. Knowlton KU, Michel MC, Itani M, et al. The alpha 1A-adrenergic receptor subtype mediates biochemical, molecular, and morphologic features of cultured myocardial cell hypertrophy. J Biol Chem 1993;268:15374–15380.

81. Simpson P. Norepinephrine-stimulated hypertrophy of cultured rat myocardial cells is an alpha 1 adrenergic response. J Clin Invest 1983;72:732–738.

82. Shubeita HE, McDonough PM, Harris AN, et al. Endothelin induction of inositol phospholipid hydrolysis, sarcomere assembly, and cardiac gene expression in ventricular myocytes. A paracrine mechanism for myocardial cell hypertrophy. J Biol Chem 1990;265:20555–20562.

83. Rockman HA, Ross RS, Harris AN, et al. Segregation of atrial-specific and inducible expression of an atrial natriuretic factor transgene in an in vivo murine model of cardiac hypertrophy. Proc Natl Acad Sci USA 1991;88:8277–8281.

84. Akhter SA, Luttrell LM, Rockman HA, Iaccarino G, Lefkowitz RJ, Koch WJ. Targeting the receptor-Gq interface to inhibit in vivo pressure overload myocardial hypertrophy. Science 1998; 280:574–577.

85. Esposito G, Prasad SV, Rapacciuolo A, Mao L, Koch WJ, Rockman HA. Cardiac overexpression of a G(q) inhibitor blocks induction of extracellular signal-regulated kinase and c-Jun NH(2)-terminal kinase activity in in vivo pressure overload. Circulation 2001;103:1453–1458.

86. D'Angelo DD, Sakata Y, Lorenz JN, et al. Transgenic Galphaq overexpression induces cardiac contractile failure in mice. Proc Natl Acad Sci USA 1997;94:8121–8126.

87. Mende U, Kagen A, Cohen A, Aramburu J, Schoen FJ, Neer EJ. Transient cardiac expression of constitutively active Galphaq leads to hypertrophy and dilated cardiomyopathy by calcineurin-dependent and independent pathways. Proc Natl Acad Sci USA 1998;95:13893–13898.

88. Sakata Y, Hoit BD, Liggett SB, Walsh RA, Dorn GW, 2nd. Decompensation of pressure-overload hypertrophy in G alpha q-overexpressing mice. Circulation 1998;97:1488–1495.

89. Inglese J, Freedman NJ, Koch WJ, Lefkowitz RJ. Structure and mechanism of the G protein-coupled receptor kinases. J Biol Chem 1993;268:23735–23738.

90. Gros R, Benovic JL, Tan CM, Feldman RD. G-protein-coupled receptor kinase activity is increased in hypertension. J Clin Invest 1997;99:2087–2093.

91. Choi DJ, Koch WJ, Hunter JJ, Rockman HA. Mechanism of beta-adrenergic receptor desensitization in cardiac hypertrophy is increased beta-adrenergic receptor kinase. J Biol Chem 1997;272:17223–17229.

92. Jaber M, Koch WJ, Rockman H, et al. Essential role of beta-adrenergic receptor kinase 1 in cardiac development and function. Proc Natl Acad Sci USA 1996;93:12974–12979.

93. Koch WJ, Rockman HA, Samama P, et al. Cardiac function in mice overexpressing the beta-adrenergic receptor kinase or a beta ARK inhibitor. Science 1995;268:1350–1353.

94. Koch WJ, Hawes BE, Inglese J, Luttrell LM, Lefkowitz RJ. Cellular expression of the carboxyl terminus of a G protein-coupled receptor kinase attenuates G beta gamma-mediated signaling. J Biol Chem 1994;269:6193–6197.

95. Freeman K, Lerman I, Kranias EG, et al. Alterations in cardiac adrenergic signaling and calcium cycling differentially affect the progression of cardiomyopathy. J Clin Invest 2001;107:967–974.

96. Esposito G, Santana LF, Dilly K, et al. Cellular and functional defects in a mouse model of heart failure. Am J Physiol Heart Circ Physiol 2000;279:H3101–H3112.

97. Rockman HA, Chien KR, Choi DJ, et al. Expression of a beta-adrenergic receptor kinase 1 inhibitor prevents the development of myocardial failure in gene-targeted mice. Proc Natl Acad Sci USA 1998;95:7000–7005.

98. Arber S, Hunter JJ, Ross J, Jr., et al. MLP-deficient mice exhibit a disruption of cardiac cytoarchitectural organization, dilated cardiomyopathy, and heart failure. Cell 1997;88:393–403.

99. Harding VB, Jones LR, Lefkowitz RJ, Koch WJ, Rockman HA. Cardiac beta ARK1 inhibition prolongs survival and augments beta blocker therapy in a mouse model of severe heart failure. Proc Natl Acad Sci USA 2001;98:5809–5814.

100. Freeman K, Colon-Rivera C, Olsson MC, et al. Progression from hypertrophic to dilated cardiomyopathy in mice that express a mutant myosin transgene. Am J Physiol Heart Circ Physiol 2001;280:H151–H159.

101. The Cardiac Insufficiency Bisoprolol Study II (CIBIS-II): a randomised trial. Lancet 1999;353:9–13.

102. Effect of metoprolol CR/XL in chronic heart failure: Metoprolol CR/XL Randomised Intervention Trial in Congestive Heart Failure (MERIT-HF). Lancet 1999;353:2001–2007.

103. Packer M, Coats AJ, Fowler MB, et al. Effect of carvedilol on survival in severe chronic heart failure. N Engl J Med 2001;344:1651–1658.

104. Packer M, Bristow MR, Cohn JN, et al. The effect of carvedilol on morbidity and mortality in patients with chronic heart failure. U.S. Carvedilol Heart Failure Study Group. N Engl J Med 1996;334:1349–1355.

105. Rockman HA, Choi DJ, Akhter SA, et al. Control of myocardial contractile function by the level of beta-adrenergic receptor kinase 1 in gene-targeted mice. J Biol Chem 1998;273:18180–18184.

106. White DC, Hata JA, Shah AS, Glower DD, Lefkowitz RJ, Koch WJ. Preservation of myocardial beta-adrenergic receptor signaling delays the development of heart failure after myocardial infarction. Proc Natl Acad Sci USA 2000;97:5428–5433.

107. Shah AS, White DC, Emani S, et al. In vivo ventricular gene delivery of a beta-adrenergic receptor kinase inhibitor to the failing heart reverses cardiac dysfunction. Circulation 2001; 103:1311–1316.

108. Rockman HA, Choi DJ, Rahman NU, Akhter SA, Lefkowitz RJ, Koch WJ. Receptor-specific in vivo desensitization by the G protein-coupled receptor kinase-5 in transgenic mice. Proc Natl Acad Sci USA 1996;93:9954–9959.

109. Iaccarino G, Rockman HA, Shotwell KF, Tomhave ED, Koch WJ. Myocardial overexpression of GRK3 in transgenic mice: evidence for in vivo selectivity of GRKs. Am J Physiol 1998;275:H1298–H1306.

110. Rameh LE, Cantley LC. The role of phosphoinositide 3-kinase lipid products in cell function. J Biol Chem 1999;274:8347–8350.

111. Naga Prasad SV, Esposito G, Mao L, Koch WJ, Rockman HA. Gbetagamma-dependent phosphoinositide 3-Kinase activation in hearts with in vivo pressure overload hypertrophy. J Biol Chem 2000;275:4693–4698.

112. Naga Prasad SV, Barak LS, Rapacciuolo A, Caron MG, Rockman HA. Agonist-dependent recruitment of phosphoinositide 3-Kinase to the membrane by beta -adrenergic receptor kinase 1. A role in receptor sequestration. J Biol Chem 2001;276:18953–18959.

113. Naga Prasad SV, Laporte SA, Chamberlain D, Caron MG, Barak L, Rockman HA. Phosphoinositide 3-kinase regulates beta2-adrenergic receptor endocytosis by AP-2 recruitment to the receptor/beta-arrestin complex. J Cell Biol 2002; 158:563-75.

114. Waltenberger J. Modulation of growth factor action: implications for the treatment of cardiovascular diseases. Circulation 1997;96:4083–4094.

115. Schlessinger J, Ullrich A. Growth factor signaling by receptor tyrosine kinases. Neuron 1992;9:383–391.

116. Schultz JE, Witt SA, Nieman ML, et al. Fibroblast growth factor-2 mediates pressure-induced hypertrophic response. J Clin Invest 1999;104:709–719.

117. Calderone A, Takahashi N, Izzo NJ, Jr., Thaik CM, Colucci WS. Pressure- and volume-induced left ventricular hypertrophies are associated with distinct myocyte phenotypes and differential induction of peptide growth factor mRNAs. Circulation 1995;92:2385–2390.

118. Li RK, Li G, Mickle DA, et al. Overexpression of transforming growth factor-beta1 and insulin-like growth factor-I in patients with idiopathic hypertrophic cardiomyopathy. Circulation 1997;96:874–881.

119. Serneri GG, Modesti PA, Boddi M, et al. Cardiac growth factors in human hypertrophy. Relations with myocardial contractility and wall stress. Circ Res 1999;85:57–67.

120. Bogoyevitch MA, Glennon PE, Andersson MB, et al. Endothelin-1 and fibroblast growth factors stimulate the mitogen-activated protein kinase signaling cascade in cardiac myocytes. The potential role of the cascade in the integration of two signaling pathways leading to myocyte hypertrophy. J Biol Chem 1994;269:1110–1119.

121. Zhang D, Gaussin V, Taffet GE, et al. TAK1 is activated in the myocardium after pressure overload and is sufficient to provoke heart failure in transgenic mice. Nat Med 2000;6:556–563.

122. Villarreal FJ, Dillmann WH. Cardiac hypertrophy-induced changes in mRNA levels for TGF-beta 1, fibronectin, and collagen. Am J Physiol 1992;262:H1861-H1866.

123. Takahashi N, Calderone A, Izzo NJ, Jr., Maki TM, Marsh JD, Colucci WS. Hypertrophic stimuli induce transforming growth factor-beta 1 expression in rat ventricular myocytes. J Clin Invest 1994;94:1470–1476.

124. Parker TG, Packer SE, Schneider MD. Peptide growth factors can provoke "fetal" contractile protein gene expression in rat cardiac myocytes. J Clin Invest 1990;85:507–514.

125. Sivasubramanian N, Coker ML, Kurrelmeyer KM, et al. Left ventricular remodeling in transgenic mice with cardiac restricted overexpression of tumor necrosis factor. Circulation 2001;104:826–831.

126. Kishimoto T, Taga T, Akira S. Cytokine signal transduction. Cell 1994;76:253–262.

127. Yamauchi-Takihara K, Kishimoto T. A novel role for STAT3 in cardiac remodeling. Trends Cardiovasc Med 2000;10:298–303.

128. Hirano T, Nakajima K, Hibi M. Signaling mechanisms through gp130: a model of the cytokine system. Cytokine Growth Factor Rev 1997;8:241–252.

129. Hirota H, Chen J, Betz UA, et al. Loss of a gp130 cardiac muscle cell survival pathway is a critical event in the onset of heart failure during biomechanical stress. Cell 1999;97:189–198.

130. Hirota H, Yoshida K, Kishimoto T, Taga T. Continuous activation of gp130, a signal-transducing receptor component for interleukin 6-related cytokines, causes myocardial hypertrophy in mice. Proc Natl Acad Sci USA 1995;92:4862–4866.

131. Uozumi H, Hiroi Y, Zou Y, et al. gp130 plays a critical role in pressure overload-induced cardiac hypertrophy. J Biol Chem 2001;276:23115–23119.

132. Pennica D, King KL, Shaw KJ, et al. Expression cloning of cardiotrophin 1, a cytokine that induces cardiac myocyte hypertrophy. Proc Natl Acad Sci USA 1995;92:1142–1146.

133. Sheng Z, Knowlton K, Chen J, Hoshijima M, Brown JH, Chien KR. Cardiotrophin 1 (CT-1) inhibition of cardiac myocyte apoptosis via a mitogen-activated protein kinase-dependent pathway. Divergence from downstream CT-1 signals for myocardial cell hypertrophy. J Biol Chem 1997;272:5783–5791.

134. Habib FM, Springall DR, Davies GJ, Oakley CM, Yacoub MH, Polak JM. Tumour necrosis factor and inducible nitric oxide synthase in dilated cardiomyopathy. Lancet 1996;347:1151–1155.

135. Levine B, Kalman J, Mayer L, Fillit HM, Packer M. Elevated circulating levels of tumor necrosis factor in severe chronic heart failure. N Engl J Med 1990;323:236–241.

136. Torre-Amione G, Kapadia S, Benedict C, Oral H, Young JB, Mann DL. Proinflammatory cytokine levels in patients with depressed left ventricular ejection fraction: a report from the Studies of Left Ventricular Dysfunction (SOLVD). J Am Coll Cardiol 1996;27:1201–1206.

137. Kubota T, Miyagishima M, Alvarez RJ, et al. Expression of proinflammatory cytokines in the failing human heart: comparison of recent-onset and end-stage congestive heart failure. J Heart Lung Transplant 2000;19:819–824.

138. Sack MN, Smith RM, Opie LH. Tumor necrosis factor in myocardial hypertrophy and ischaemia—an anti-apoptotic perspective. Cardiovasc Res 2000;45:688–695.

139. Kadokami T, McTiernan CF, Kubota T, Frye CS, Feldman AM. Sex-related survival differences in murine cardiomyopathy are associated with differences in TNF-receptor expression. J Clin Invest 2000;106:589–597.

140. Kubota T, McTiernan CF, Frye CS, et al. Dilated cardiomyopathy in transgenic mice with cardiac-specific overexpression of tumor necrosis factor-alpha. Circ Res 1997;81:627–635.

141. Li X, Moody MR, Engel D, et al. Cardiac-specific overexpression of tumor necrosis factor-alpha causes oxidative stress and contractile dysfunction in mouse diaphragm. Circulation 2000;102:1690–1696.

142. Seger R, Krebs EG. The MAPK signaling cascade. Faseb J 1995;9:726–735.

143. Garrington TP, Johnson GL. Organization and regulation of mitogen-activated protein kinase signaling pathways. Curr Opin Cell Biol 1999;11:211–218.

144. Davis RJ. The mitogen-activated protein kinase signal transduction pathway. J Biol Chem 1993;268:14553–14556.

145. Force T, Pombo CM, Avruch JA, Bonventre JV, Kyriakis JM. Stress-activated protein kinases in cardiovascular disease. Circ Res 1996;78:947–953.

146. Ramirez MT, Sah VP, Zhao XL, Hunter JJ, Chien KR, Brown JH. The MEKK-JNK pathway is stimulated by alpha1-adrenergic receptor and ras activation and is associated with in vitro and in vivo cardiac hypertrophy. J Biol Chem 1997;272:14057–14061.

147. Rapacciuolo A, Esposito G, Caron K, Mao L, Thomas SA, Rockman HA. Important role of endogenous norepinephrine

and epinephrine in the development of in vivo pressure-overload cardiac hypertrophy. J Am Coll Cardiol 2001;38:876–882.

148. Boulton TG, Nye SH, Robbins DJ, et al. ERKs: a family of protein-serine/threonine kinases that are activated and tyrosine phosphorylated in response to insulin and NGF. Cell 1991;65:663–675.

149. Sadoshima J, Izumo S. Mechanical stretch rapidly activates multiple signal transduction pathways in cardiac myocytes: potential involvement of an autocrine/paracrine mechanism. Embo J 1993;12:1681–1692.

150. Bogoyevitch MA, Ketterman AJ, Sugden PH. Cellular stresses differentially activate c-Jun N-terminal protein kinases and extracellular signal-regulated protein kinases in cultured ventricular myocytes. J Biol Chem 1995;270:29710–29717.

151. Bueno OF, De Windt LJ, Tymitz KM, et al. The MEK1-ERK1/2 signaling pathway promotes compensated cardiac hypertrophy in transgenic mice. Embo J 2000;19:6341–6350.

152. Wang LX, Ideishi M, Yahiro E, Urata H, Arakawa K, Saku K. Mechanism of the cardioprotective effect of inhibition of the renin-angiotensin system on ischemia/reperfusion-induced myocardial injury. Hypertens Res 2001;24:179–187.

153. Davis RJ. Signal transduction by the JNK group of MAP kinases. Cell 2000;103:239–252.

154. Coso OA, Chiariello M, Yu JC, et al. The small GTP-binding proteins Rac1 and Cdc42 regulate the activity of the JNK/SAPK signaling pathway. Cell 1995;81:1137–1146.

155. Minden A, Lin A, Claret FX, Abo A, Karin M. Selective activation of the JNK signaling cascade and c-Jun transcriptional activity by the small GTPases Rac and Cdc42Hs. Cell 1995; 81:1147–1157.

156. Gupta S, Barrett T, Whitmarsh AJ, et al. Selective interaction of JNK protein kinase isoforms with transcription factors. Embo J 1996;15:2760–2770.

157. Nemoto S, Sheng Z, Lin A. Opposing effects of Jun kinase and p38 mitogen-activated protein kinases on cardiomyocyte hypertrophy. Mol Cell Biol 1998;18:3518–3526.

158. Kudoh S, Komuro I, Mizuno T, et al. Angiotensin II stimulates c-Jun NH2-terminal kinase in cultured cardiac myocytes of neonatal rats. Circ Res 1997;80:139–146.

159. Wang Y, Su B, Sah VP, Brown JH, Han J, Chien KR. Cardiac hypertrophy induced by mitogen-activated protein kinase kinase 7, a specific activator for c-Jun NH2-terminal kinase in ventricular muscle cells. J Biol Chem 1998;273:5423–5426.

160. Choukroun G, Hajjar R, Fry S, et al. Regulation of cardiac hypertrophy in vivo by the stress-activated protein kinases/c-Jun NH(2)-terminal kinases. J Clin Invest 1999;104:391–398.

161. Jiang Y, Gram H, Zhao M, et al. Characterization of the structure and function of the fourth member of p38 group mitogen-activated protein kinases, p38delta. J Biol Chem 1997;272:30122–30128.

162. Paul A, Wilson S, Belham CM, et al. Stress-activated protein kinases: activation, regulation and function. Cell Signal 1997;9:403–410.

163. Lazou A, Sugden PH, Clerk A. Activation of mitogen-activated protein kinases (p38-MAPKs, SAPKs/JNKs and ERKs) by the G-protein-coupled receptor agonist phenylephrine in the perfused rat heart. Biochem J 1998;332:459–465.

164. Meloche S, Landry J, Huot J, Houle F, Marceau F, Giasson E. p38 MAP kinase pathway regulates angiotensin II-induced contraction of rat vascular smooth muscle. Am J Physiol Heart Circ Physiol 2000;279:H741–H751.

165. Wang Y, Huang S, Sah VP, et al. Cardiac muscle cell hypertrophy and apoptosis induced by distinct members of the p38

166. mitogen-activated protein kinase family. J Biol Chem 1998;273:2161–2168.

166. Zechner D, Thuerauf DJ, Hanford DS, McDonough PM, Glembotski CC. A role for the p38 mitogen-activated protein kinase pathway in myocardial cell growth, sarcomeric organization, and cardiac-specific gene expression. J Cell Biol 1997;139:115–127.

167. Izumi Y, Kim S, Murakami T, Yamanaka S, Iwao H. Cardiac mitogen-activated protein kinase activities are chronically increased in stroke-prone hypertensive rats. Hypertension 1998;31:50–56.

168. Izumi Y, Kim S, Zhan Y, Namba M, Yasumoto H, Iwao H. Important role of angiotensin II-mediated c-Jun NH(2)-terminal kinase activation in cardiac hypertrophy in hypertensive rats. Hypertension 2000;36:511–516.

169. Cook SA, Sugden PH, Clerk A. Activation of c-Jun N-terminal kinases and p38-mitogen-activated protein kinases in human heart failure secondary to ischaemic heart disease. J Mol Cell Cardiol 1999;31:1429–1434.

170. Haq S, Choukroun G, Lim H, et al. Differential activation of signal transduction pathways in human hearts with hypertrophy versus advanced heart failure. Circulation 2001;103:670–677.

171. Imada K, Leonard WJ. The Jak-STAT pathway. Mol Immunol 2000;37:1–11.

172. Leonard WJ. Role of Jak kinases and STATs in cytokine signal transduction. Int J Hematol 2001;73:271–277.

173. Igaz P, Toth S, Falus A. Biological and clinical significance of the JAK-STAT pathway; lessons from knockout mice. Inflamm Res 2001;50:435–441.

174. Kunisada K, Negoro S, Tone E, et al. Signal transducer and activator of transcription 3 in the heart transduces not only a hypertrophic signal but a protective signal against doxorubicin-induced cardiomyopathy. Proc Natl Acad Sci USA 2000;97:315–319.

175. Crabtree GR. Generic signals and specific outcomes: signaling through Ca2+, calcineurin, and NF-AT. Cell 1999;96:611–614.

176. Rao A, Luo C, Hogan PG. Transcription factors of the NFAT family: regulation and function. Annu Rev Immunol 1997;15:707–747.

177. Kolodziejczyk SM, Wang L, Balazsi K, DeRepentigny Y, Kothary R, Megeney LA. MEF2 is upregulated during cardiac hypertrophy and is required for normal post-natal growth of the myocardium. Curr Biol 1999;9:1203–1206.

178. Molkentin JD, Lu JR, Antos CL, et al. A calcineurin-dependent transcriptional pathway for cardiac hypertrophy. Cell 1998;93: 215–228.

179. Klee CB, Ren H, Wang X. Regulation of the calmodulin-stimulated protein phosphatase, calcineurin. J Biol Chem 1998; 273:13367–13370.

180. Rigat B, Hubert C, Alhenc-Gelas F, Cambien F, Corvol P, Soubrier F. An insertion/deletion polymorphism in the angiotensin I-converting enzyme gene accounting for half the variance of serum enzyme levels. J Clin Invest 1990;86:1343–1346.

181. Cambien F, Evans A. Angiotensin I converting enzyme gene polymorphism and coronary heart disease. Eur Heart J 1995;16:13–22.

182. Cambien F, Poirier O, Lecerf L, et al. Deletion polymorphism in the gene for angiotensin-converting enzyme is a potent risk factor for myocardial infarction. Nature 1992;359:641–644.

183. Andersson B, Sylven C. The DD genotype of the angiotensin-converting enzyme gene is associated with increased mortality in idiopathic heart failure. J Am Coll Cardiol 1996;28:162–167.

184. McNamara DM, Holubkov R, Janosko K, et al. Pharmacogenetic interactions between beta-blocker therapy and the angiotensin-

converting enzyme deletion polymorphism in patients with congestive heart failure. Circulation 2001;103:1644–1648.

185. Loh E, Rebbeck TR, Mahoney PD, DeNofrio D, Swain JL, Holmes EW. Common variant in AMPD1 gene predicts improved clinical outcome in patients with heart failure. Circulation 1999;99:1422–1425.

186. Podlowski S, Wenzel K, Luther HP, et al. Beta1-adrenoceptor gene variations: a role in idiopathic dilated cardiomyopathy? J Mol Med 2000;78:87–93.

187. Green SA, Cole G, Jacinto M, Innis M, Liggett SB. A polymorphism of the human beta 2-adrenergic receptor within the fourth transmembrane domain alters ligand binding and functional properties of the receptor. J Biol Chem 1993;268: 23116–23121.

188. Liggett SB, Wagoner LE, Craft LL, et al. The Ile164 beta2-adrenergic receptor polymorphism adversely affects the outcome of congestive heart failure. J Clin Invest 1998;102:1534–1539.

189. Wagoner LE, Craft LL, Singh B, et al. Polymorphisms of the beta(2)-adrenergic receptor determine exercise capacity in patients with heart failure. Circ Res 2000;86:834–840.

190. Collins FS. Shattuck lecture–medical and societal consequences of the Human Genome Project. N Engl J Med 1999;341:28–37.

191. Torre-Amione G, Kapadia S, Benedict C, Oral H, Young JB, Mann DL. Proinflammatory cytokine levels in patients with depressed left ventricular ejection fraction: a report from the Studies of left Ventricular Dysfunction (SOLVD). J Am Coll Cardiol 1996;27:1202–1206.

9

Recent Insights into the Molecular Pathophysiology of Viral Myocarditis

Tony Tran, MD, Roger D. Rossen, MD, and Douglas L. Mann, MD

CONTENTS

OVERVIEW OF VIRAL MYOCARDITIS

Myocarditis, defined as inflammation of the heart muscle, occurs in response to a wide variety of agents *(1)*. Infectious organisms, a major cause of myocarditis, can have direct cardiomyopathic effects or can predispose to infection with cardiotropic viruses. Viruses can infect cardiac muscle cells or other supporting cells within the heart and cause myocarditis. Coxsackievirus B, adenoviruses, and herpesviruses are important causes of viral myocarditis, especially in North America and Europe *(2)*, and human immunodeficiency virus (HIV) has recently been added to the list of infectious agents that cause myocarditis *(3)* (Table 1). The overall prevalence of myocarditis in patients with suspected viral illness ranges from 2.3% to 5% *(4)*; however, the incidence of viral myocarditis is difficult to determine because of the limited methods for identifying viral infection of the heart.

Characterized by different phases with distinct mechanisms and clinical manifestations, myocarditis is a complex and poorly understood disease. Liu and Mason *(5)* recently suggested that myocarditis be viewed as a continuum comprising three separate phases: acute viral infection (phase I), autoimmunity (phase II), and dilated cardiomyopathy (phase III). The pathogenesis, diagnosis, and treatment differ considerably for each phase. In this chapter, we will review the pathophysiological basis and the best therapeutic approach for each phase of myocarditis.

PHASE I: THE VIRAL STAGE

The early phase of viral myocarditis is triggered by the entry and proliferation of the causative virus in the myocardium and ends with activation of the immune system (Fig. 1). Many viruses infect the heart by binding to specific receptors on cardiac myocytes. In animal models, viral particles can be detected in cardiac myocytes several hours after infection *(6)*. Enteroviruses, such as Coxsackievirus types B3 and B4, are frequently detected by serologic or molecular techniques in clinical myocarditis *(7)*. The Coxsackievirus–adenoviral receptor (CAR) is a recently identified common receptor for Coxsackieviruses and adenoviruses. The presence of this receptor on cardiac myocytes helps explain the high percentage of Coxsackieviruses and adenoviruses found in clinical myocarditis *(8)*. Coxsackievirus B binds to the cardiac myocyte and is internalized via CAR (Fig. 2). As a member of the immunoglobulin superfamily, CAR probably functions as an adhesion molecule. CAR acts as a multifunctional receptor for binding and internalizing Coxsackieviruses and other enteroviruses because of its

From: *Contemporary Cardiology: Principles of Molecular Cardiology*
Edited by: M. S. Runge and C. Patterson @ Humana Press Inc., Totowa, NJ

Table 1
Viral Causes of Dilated Cardiomyopathy

Coxsackievirus types A and B

Poliomyelitis virus

Influenza virus types A and B

Human immunodeficiency virus (HIV)

Adenovirus

Echovirus

Cytomegalovirus

Epstein–Barr virus

Rubeola virus

Respiratory syncytial virus

Varicella–zoster virus

Rabies virus

Hepatitis virus

Yellow fever virus

Lymphocytic choriomeningitis virus

Epidemic hemorrhagic fever virus

Dengue virus

ability to interact with certain co-receptors, which can increase the efficiency of binding of virus to target cells (9). The complement deflecting protein, decay accelerating factor (DAF, CD55), functions as a co-receptor for Coxsackievirus B and forms a receptor complex with CAR (Fig. 2). The presence of DAF significantly increases the binding efficiency of Coxsackievirus B onto the DAF–CAR receptor complex and facilitates the internalization of the virus (10). In contrast, adenoviruses use a different set of co-receptors, including integrin $\alpha_{v\beta3}$ and integrin $\alpha_{v\beta5}$ (11).

Cytopathogenic Effects

Viruses can produce direct toxic effects in the heart through a variety of mechanisms. Damage to infected host cells often results from a viral-induced decrease in the production of important host proteins. Transcription and translation of endogenous host proteins are decreased in cardiac myocytes transfected with non-replicating cDNA from Coxsackievirus B3. These infected cells leak lactic dehydrogenase, suggesting that production of low levels of viral proteins has a cytopathic effect (12). The intracellular production of viral proteinases used to cleave viral proteins may hydrolyze key second messenger proteins necessary for production of essential host proteins such as contractile proteins or proteins required for homeostasis (13). Another protein targeted for reduction by viral infection is the class I

major histocompatibility (MHC) protein, which is displayed on the cell surface and marks the infected cell for attack by natural killer (NK) cells. In addition to reducing protein production, viral infection of the heart may lead to spasm of the coronary microvasculature and secretion of cardiotoxic cytokines such as interleukin-1 and tumor necrosis factor (TNF) (14). These mechanisms may act singly or in concert to produce direct toxic effects on the myocardium (6).

Treatment Considerations

In phase I of myocarditis, the presence of viral infection and replication is often difficult to prove in sufficient time to initiate appropriate antiviral therapies. Several factors contribute to the difficulty in obtaining a timely diagnosis of the viral phase of myocarditis. First, time and expense must be considered. Serologic tests for viral infection take a minimum of 4 d, and culture from myocardial biopsy may take 3 wk or more. Moreover, obtaining a positive culture is often difficult, and obtaining serial viral titers is impractical. Furthermore, no rapid, noninvasive screening tool is available for the immediate detection of viral protein or genetic material. A second complicating feature is that the initial phase of the illness is often subclinical until signs and symptoms of congestive heart failure supervene. Thus, treatment of phase I of viral myocarditis primarily involves avoiding the use of potentially harmful immunosuppressive medications, which may increase viral loads and worsen outcome. In the rare instance in which the infecting organism is known or the myocarditis occurs in the context of a known viral epidemic, direct antiviral therapy may help. For example, ribavirin (Virazole, 1-β-D-ribofuranosyl-1,2,4-triazole-3carboxamide), a synthetic nucleoside analog, has broad antiviral activity against RNA and DNA viruses. In mice infected with encephalomyocarditis virus, early administration of ribavirin decreased viral replication in the heart, reduced myocardial damage, and decreased mortality (15). Furthermore, when recombinant human leukocyte IFN was administered before or simultaneously with infection with encephalomyocarditis virus or Coxsackievirus B, virus replication was inhibited, and the inflammatory response and myocardial damage were reduced (16,17). Clinical trials are ongoing in Europe (The European Study of Epidemiology and Treatment of Cardiac Inflammatory Disease) to determine the efficacy of antiviral therapy in patients with cytomegalovirus and enterovirus-induced myocarditis (18). Other potentially effective strategies for treating the early viral stage of myocarditis include the use of immune globulin to

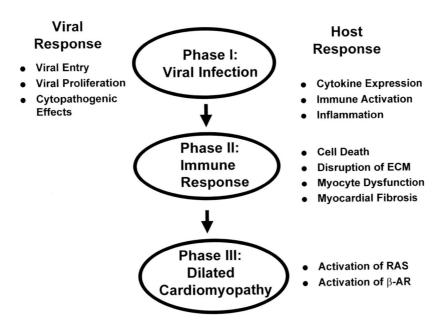

Fig. 1. Viral and host responses during the three phases of myocarditis. β-AR, β-adrenergic system; ECM, extracellular matrix; and RAS, renin angiotensin system. Modified from *(5)*.

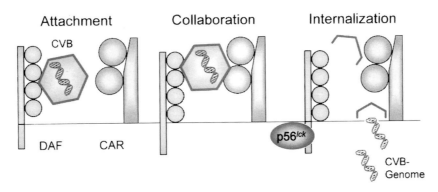

Fig. 2. Cooperation between the coxsackie-adenoviral receptor (CAR) present on cardiac myocytes and the co-receptor, decay accelerating factor (DAF), allows binding of coxsackievirus B (CVB) to the cell surface and subsequent internalization of the virus. Reproduced with permission from the American Heart Association *(5)*.

boost the intrinsic immune response *(19–21)* and the administration of agents that can block entry of the virus through the CAR receptor *(22)*.

PHASE II: IMMUNE-MEDIATED MYOCARDIAL INJURY

The second phase of viral myocarditis begins with the activation of the host immune system, which is intended to decrease viral proliferation and kill virus-infected cells. However, immune activation may have deleterious consequences for the host because of collateral tissue damage that occurs during the process of killing virus-laden cells.

Immune Response

Innate immune responses defend against viral infection even before infected cells can be recognized as antigenically distinct from normal cardiac myocytes. Circulating NK cells promptly kill infected cardiac myocytes after recognizing distinctive viral-induced changes in MHC type I molecules on the surface of myocytes *(23)*. Later, after virus-specific antibodies and T lymphocytes are produced in the infected host, NK cells play a second role in host defense. NK cells kill cardiac myocytes that have been targeted by virus-specific IgG antibodies. Cell death ensues after perforin molecules released by NK cells insert into the cell membrane and form non-selective ion channels that allow water and sodium ions to move freely into the cytoplasm, causing cellular edema and cytolysis *(24,25).* Lodge et al. *(26)* have shown that infection with Coxsackievirus B in mice deficient in NK cell responses increases virus titers and cardiac inflammation. Godeny et al. *(27)* reported that depletion of NK cells significantly increased the severity of infection in mice with myocarditis caused by coxsackievirus B. These findings illustrate the important role of NK cells in defense against viral myocarditis.

The second wave of tissue-infiltrating cells includes antigen specific T lymphocytes, which peak between 4 and 14 d after onset of infection *(28).* CD4+ helper T lymphocytes recognize degraded viral peptide fragments presented by MHC class II molecules, whereas CD8+ cytotoxic T lymphocytes recognize viral antigens bound to MHC class I molecules on target cells. After binding to the antigen–MHC complex, T lymphocytes become activated via stimulation of a biochemical pathway involving phospholipase C and inositol triphosphate, which leads to an increase in intracellular levels of Ca^{2+}. Increased cytoplasmic levels of Ca^{2+}, acting through calcineurin, stimulate nuclear factor of activated T cells (NFAT) to activate transcription of lymphokine genes, resulting in cytokine production. T cells are then able to lyse virus-infected cardiac cells either by membrane insertion of perforin or by apoptosis induced by binding of the Fas–Fas ligand. In addition, granzyme B, a serine protease released from granules of cytotoxic T cells, can mediate apoptosis by penetrating the nucleus of infected cardiomyocytes via perforin-created channels. In murine models of myocarditis, myocardial injury is increased in mice with severe combined immunodeficiency and in mice treated with FK506, an immunosuppressant drug that inhibits the effect of calcineurin on NFAT *(29,30).* Thus, an effective immune response can destroy virus-infected cardiac myocytes and limit the extent and severity of cardiac injury caused by viral infection, but often at the expense of myocardial injury.

Many murine models of myocarditis have shown the significant role of lymphocytes in the immune response. Although cytotoxic lymphocytes assist in clearing virus from the infected heart, the cost is significant. Infiltrating antigen-specific T cells cause significant myocardial damage in the process. Henke et al. *(31)* have reported that Coxsackievirus B3–infected mice deficient in CD4+ lymphocytes have lower mortality and viral titers, but more myocardial inflammation than control mice. However, mice lacking both CD4+ and CD8+ T cells have an even greater decrease in mortality and myocardial inflammatory infiltrates than CD4+ knockout mice and immunocompetent control mice *(31).* These studies support the view that under certain conditions T lymphocytes can increase the severity of myocarditis. In addition, T lymphocytes may destroy normal cardiac cells through an autoimmune reaction; normal host myocardial proteins may share epitopes with viral proteins (molecular mimicry). These host epitopes that resemble viral antigens can be recognized as foreign by activated T cells, resulting in lysis of normal myocardial cells *(32).* The loss of immunological tolerance that results from the presentation of normal host cell cardiac antigens by antigen-presenting cells (APC) that have also processed and express viral antigens is a major problem. These APC express co-stimulatory molecules such as CD86 (B7.2) or CD80 (B7.1) that provide the critical second signal needed to activate potentially autoreactive T lymphocytes. Monocytes migrate alongside T lymphocytes into infected myocardial tissue and accumulate and differentiate into tissue macrophages at sites of inflammation. At these sites, activated tissue macrophages remove tissue debris produced by necrotic and apoptotic cardiac cells. These macrophages are a principal source of proinflammatory cytokines, which are capable of inducing further myocyte dysfunction and tissue damage.

Proinflammatory Cytokines

Increased levels of TNF, interleukin-1 alpha (IL-1α), and interleukin-1 beta (IL-1β) have been observed in patients with myocarditis *(33).* Secreted by inflammatory cells in the heart and by myocytes, cytokines have multiple immunoregulatory roles, including clonal expansion of cytotoxic lymphocytes and regulation of antibody production *(34).* In addition to having a protective role in the immune response, cytokines may have detrimental effects on the heart, such as a direct negative inotropic effect and blunting of the catecholamine response *(35).* Proinflammatory cytokines (e.g., TNF) can increase production of matrix metalloproteinases, which cause matrix degradation and cardiac dilation. Furthermore, profibrotic cytokines contribute to progressive myocardial fibrosis *(36,37).* In addition to their direct effects on the heart, TNF and IL-1β stimulate the expression of the inducible isoform of nitric oxide synthase (iNOS) in infiltrating inflammatory cells and cardiac myocytes. Although nitric oxide has antiviral properties, increased expression of nitric oxide may result in contractile dysfunction, myocyte apoptosis, and myocyte necrosis *(38–40).* Thus, mediators of the immune system can contribute to heart failure after viral myocarditis.

Cross-Reacting Antibodies

Cross-reacting antibodies may contribute to disease progression during transition to the third phase of myocarditis: dilated cardiomyopathy. In patients with histologically proven myocarditis or familial dilated cardiomyopathy, autoreactive antibodies to components of the myocardium are often present. These autoantibodies cross-react with G-protein–linked receptors (such as β_1-adrenoreceptors and muscarinic receptors), mitochondrial antigens, adenosine diphosphate, adenosine triphosphate carrier proteins and cardiac myosin heavy chain (41–44). Some autoantibodies have cardiodepressant (45,46) or cardiostimulatory effects (47).

Duality of the Immune Response

Although activation of the immune system is initially beneficial by limiting the spread of infection, the immune response may act as a double-edged sword; excessive immune responses can lead to disease progression independent of the initial viral infection (Fig. 1). This duality of the effects of the immune system is illustrated in a recent study in mice lacking the proinflammatory cytokine TNF (TNF −/−) (48). In this study, mortality rates were higher in TNF−/− mice infected with encephalomyocarditis virus than in infected wild-type mice (TNF +/+) (48). Furthermore, exogenous administration of TNF prevented the increase in encephalomyocarditis-induced mortality. Thus, the lack of TNF prevented activation of the immune system, which allowed the virus to multiply unchecked, leading ultimately to an increase in mortality. However, increased expression of TNF may be overtly deleterious. Studies have shown that transgenic mice with overexpression of TNF in the cardiac compartment develop florid myocarditis and progressive myocardial fibrosis without challenge with a cardiotropic virus (49,50). Finally, exogenous administration of TNF can aggravate myocarditis, whereas neutralization of TNF by antibodies or soluble receptors can attenuate viral myocarditis (51,52). Taken together, these observations suggest that the same immune responses that are critical in promoting host defenses often lead to unwanted tissue damage in the host organism (53).

Treatment Considerations

Unlike phase I of myocarditis, phase II can be definitively diagnosed by endomyocardial biopsy. The diagnosis is definitive when made a few days to weeks after resolution of a symptomatic viral infection and when many foci of lymphocytic infiltrating cells are seen on histologic sections. The diagnosis is less definitive when the viral prodrome is remote or absent and when only a small number of inflammatory foci are seen on histologic study. Because host autoimmunity may account for significant cardiac injury in phase II of viral myocarditis, the use of immunosuppressants and immunomodulators as potential therapies for infectious myocardial inflammation has been studied.

IMMUNOSUPPRESSIVE THERAPY

Immunosuppressive therapy has not been effective in animal models of viral myocarditis. This lack of efficacy may relate to the duality of the effects of the immune system as described above. For example, corticosteroids increased viral titers in the early phase of viral murine myocarditis, and cyclosporine increased mortality and cardiac insufficiency in mice infected with encephalomyocarditis virus (54,55). However, FTY720, a new immunosuppressant, has shown efficacy in encephalomyocarditis-infected mice. Miyamoto et al. (56) observed that FTY720-treated infected mice survived longer and had fewer cellular infiltrates in the heart than mice treated with cyclosporine or diluent. The mechanism of FTY720 may involve sequestering circulating mature lymphocytes in lymph nodes and Peyer's patches, thereby reducing the number of peripheral lymphocytes available to infiltrate tissues (56). Although anecdotal evidence and small case studies have suggested that patients with viral myocarditis might benefit from early steroidal or immunosuppressive therapy, results of the Myocarditis Treatment Trial indicate that a 24-wk regimen of immunosuppressive therapy (prednisone plus cyclosporine or prednisone plus azathioprine) in patients with biopsy-documented myocarditis did not improve ejection fraction more than did conventional therapy (57). The major limitation of this study was the unexpectedly low rate of positive biopsy specimens (less than 10%), and the extension of enrollment to 2 yr after the initial clinical presentation. Thus, the disease may have already progressed in many patients from immune-mediated cardiac injury to dilated cardiomyopathy, and no form of therapy would have been effective in that setting (57).

IMMUNOMODULATORY THERAPY

Several immunomodulatory therapies have been proposed for treating the autoimmune phase of viral myocarditis. Kishimoto et al. (58) reported that immunoglobulin treatment suppressed Coxsackievirus B3-induced myocarditis in mice and increased survival in C3H/He mice after infection with encephalomyocarditis virus. Immunoglobulin therapy has reduced levels of several inflammatory markers, including TNF, IFN-α, IFN-γ, macrophage inflammatory protein-2, interleukin-6 (IL-6), plasma catecholamines, and soluble intercellular adhesion molecule-1 (59). Exogenous immunoglobulins modulate diverse immune response mechanisms; however, the exact mechanisms by which immunoglobulins affect myocarditis remain to be determined. In a prospective placebo-controlled trial in patients with recent-onset dilated cardiomyopathy or myocarditis, treatment with intravenous immune globulin did not improve left ventricular function when compared with placebo treatment *(60)*. Treatment of mice with intraperitoneal administration of recombinant human interleukin-10 (IL-10) at the same time as infection with encephalomyocarditis virus prolonged survival, decreased myocardial inflammation, and reduced cardiac levels of TNF, IL-2, and iNOS RNA when compared with treatment of control mice with vehicle only *(61)*. IL-10, an immunomodulating cytokine, inhibits T helper type 1 (Th1) cells and macrophages and suppresses the production of proinflammatory cytokines *(62,63)*.

A unique form of immunomodulatory therapy currently under study in clinical trials is immunoadsorption. The technique of immunoadsorption initially gained popularity for treating patients with familial heterozygous hypercholesterolemia *(64)*; however, Wallukat et al. *(65)*, in an uncontrolled pilot study, first reported the use of immunoadsorption in patients with dilated cardiomyopathy who develop autoantibodies against the β_1-adrenoreceptor. In immunoadsorption, autoantibodies are removed by passing a patient's plasma over columns that contain immobilized antibodies against immunoglobulin kappa and lambda light chains and IgG heavy chains. Immunoadsorption depletes several types of circulating immunoglobulins, including autoantibodies, alloantibodies (antibodies directed against antigens from a genetically distinct member of the same species), and circulating immune complexes. Immunoadsorption has been shown to improve ejection fraction and New York Heart Association class in patients with dilated cardiomyopathy *(66,67)*. Felix et al. *(68)* showed that immunoadsorption and administration of intravenous IgG significantly improved left ventricular function and decreased systemic vascular resistance in patients with idiopathic dilated cardiomyopathy, whereas these variables did not change significantly in control patients.

No form of immunosuppressive therapy has proved effective in the clinical setting, although immunomodulatory treatments are promising. Thus, routine immunosuppressive therapy is not recommended for myocarditis patients with a stable clinical course. However, many clinicians recommend aggressive immunosuppressive therapy for patients with fulminant myocarditis or a deteriorating clinical course.

PHASE III: DILATED CARDIOMYOPATHY

The third phase of viral myocarditis begins with the onset of left ventricular dysfunction, which may result from the cytopathogenic effects of the invading virus (phase I) or from the inflammatory effects of immune-mediated mechanisms or autoimmunity (phase II).

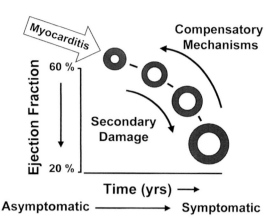

Fig. 3. Pathogenesis of dilated cardiomyopathy. During the initial period of heart failure, several compensatory mechanisms are activated, including the adrenergic nervous system, the renin angiotensin system and the cytokine system. For a short time, these systems can restore cardiovascular function to normal, allowing the patient to remain asymptomatic. However, the sustained activation of these systems can lead to secondary end-organ damage within the ventricle, accompanied by worsening left ventricular remodeling and subsequent cardiac decompensation. During this phase, patients begin to experience symptoms of heart failure. Modified from *(76)*.

Frequently, the third phase of myocarditis results in the onset of overt congestive heart failure.

Viral-induced myocardial damage disrupts the ability of the myocardium to generate force, thereby leading to left ventricular dysfunction and the progression of dilated cardiomyopathy (Fig. 3). For example, the cytopathogenic effects of the invading virus may reduce the number of functioning myocytes or cause myocyte necrosis or apoptosis. In addition, viral infection may lead to alterations in myocardial structure that prevent the generation of force and cause myocardial dilations. Badorff et al. *(68)* have shown that a Coxsackieviral protease can directly modify the sarcoglycan complex in myocytes. As noted above, virus-induced cytokine production may contribute to left ventricular dilation by altering matrix metalloproteinases such as gelatinase, collagenases, and elastases *(69)* and by upregulating profibrotic cytokines, such as transforming growth factor-β. In addition to the above mechanisms, evidence suggests that persistence of viral genomic particles in the myocardium may worsen heart failure and cause early death or the need for transplantation *(70)*. The mechanisms whereby heart failure occurs in this situation are unknown; however, ongoing viral replication may cause cardiac damage through immune-mediated mechanisms, and gene expression of viral particles or proteins may injure cardiocytes, possibly by interfering with contractile function *(71)*. Once left ventricular dysfunction supervenes, heart failure progresses along previously recognized mechanisms that activate compensatory mechanisms that sustain and modulate left ventricular function for months to years. These mechanisms include activation of the sympathetic nervous system and retention of salt and water to preserve cardiac output *(72,73)*, and the production of vasodilatory molecules, such as the prostaglandins *(74)*, proinflammatory cytokines *(75)*, and nitric oxide *(76)*.

Treatment Considerations

The treatment regimen for patients who develop chronic dilated cardiomyopathy as a result of viral myocarditis should not differ from the regimen for patients with idiopathic or ischemic dilated cardiomyopathy. In the absence of chronic viral infection or demonstrable autoimmune activity, patients in phase III, like patients with idiopathic dilated cardiomyopathy and congestive heart failure, should be treated with diuretics, angiotensin-converting enzyme inhibitors, and β-blockers *(76)*. Selected patients should be monitored for recrudescence of viral infection or autoimmunity at specialized centers equipped for such a task.

SUMMARY

Viral myocarditis is a poorly understood disease that progresses insidiously through stages with distinct mechanisms and clinical manifestations. We have reviewed the three distinct phases of viral myocarditis: viral infection (phase I), immune-mediated injury (phase II), and dilated cardiomyopathy (phase III). Both the host response to virus-specific antigens and autoimmune responses may contribute to immune-mediated injury in phase II of viral myocarditis. Although dividing viral myocarditis into three phases may help in understanding the underlying pathophysiological mechanisms, the three stages may not always be distinct and may, in fact, overlap considerably. For example, viral infection may persist into the phase of dilated cardiomyopathy. Important and unique interactions between the host genome and the viral genome affect host phenotype. Current advances in gene and protein-based therapies coupled with increased diagnostic capabilities herald an exciting new era in the understanding and treatment of viral myocarditis.

ACKNOWLEDGMENTS

The authors gratefully acknowledge Mary Soliz for secretarial assistance and Dr. Andrew I. Schafer for his past and present support and guidance. This research was supported by research funds from the N.I.H. (KO8 HL-03560, P50 HL-O6H and RO1 AG-17022, RO1 HL58081-01, RO1 HL61543-01, HL-42250-10/10; RO1 AI46825) MH 63035 and the Department of Veterans Affairs.

REFERENCES

1. Pisani B, Taylor D, Mason JW. Inflammatory myocardial diseases and cardiomyopathies. Am J Med 1997;102:459–469.
2. Savoia MC, Oxman MN. Myocarditis and pericarditis. In: Mandell GL, Bennett JE, Dolin R, eds. Principles and Practice of Infectious Diseases. Philadelphia, PA: Churchill Livingston, 2000:925–941.
3. Rerkpattanapipat P, Wongpraparut N, Jacobs LE. Cardiac manifestations of acquired immunodefiency syndrome. Arch Intern Med 2000;160:602–608.
4. Kishimoto C, Kurnick JT, Fallon JT, Crumpacker CS, Abelmann WH. Characteristics of lymphocytes cultured from murine viral myocarditis specimens. J Am Coll Cardiol 1989;14:799–802.
5. Liu PP, Mason JW. Advances in the understanding of myocarditis. Circulation 2001;104:1076–1082.
6. Woodruff JF. Viral myocarditis. Am J Pathol 1980;101:427–479.
7. Klingel K, Hohenadl C, Canu A, et al. Ongoing enterovirus-induced myocarditis is associated with persistent heart muscle infection: quantitative analysis of virus replication, tissue damage, and inflammation. Proc Natl Acad Sci USA 1992;89:314–318.
8. Bergelson JM, Cunningham JA, Droguett G, et al. Isolation of a common receptor for Coxsackie B viruses and adenoviruses 2 and 5. Science 1997;275:1320–1323.
9. Martino TA, Petric M, Weingartl H, et al. The coxsackie-adenovirus receptor (CAR) is used by reference strains and clinical isolates representing all six serotypes of coxsackievirus group B and by swine vesicular disease virus. Virology 2000;271:99–108.
10. Martino TA, Petric M, Brown M, et al. Cardiovirulent coxsackieviruses and the decay-accelerating factor (CD55) receptor. Virology 1998;244:302–314.
11. Clapham PR, Weiss RA. Immunodeficiency viruses. Spoilt for choice of co-receptors. Nature 1997;388:230–231.
12. Wessely R, Henke A, Zell R, Kandolf R, Knowlton KU. Low-level expression of a mutant coxsackieviral cDNA induces a myocytopathic effect in culture: an approach to the study of enteroviral persistence in cardiac myocytes. Circulation 1998; 98:450–457.
13. Lamphear BJ, Yan R, Yang F, et al. Mapping the cleavage site in protein synthesis initiation factor eIF-4 gamma of the 2A proteases from human coxsackievirus and rhinovirus. J Biol Chem 1993;268:19200–19203.
14. Martino TA, Liu P, Sole MJ. Viral infection and the pathogenesis of dilated cardiomyopathy. Circ Res 1994;74:182–188.
15. Matsumori A, Wang H, Abelmann WH, Crumpacker CS. Treatment of viral myocarditis with ribavirin in an animal preparation. Circulation 1985;71:834–839.
16. Matsumori A, Crumpacker CS, Abelmann WH. Prevention of viral myocarditis with recombinant human leukocyte interferon alpha A/D in a murine model. J Am Coll Cardiol 1987;9: 1320–1325.
17. Lutton CW, Gauntt CJ. Ameliorating effect of IFN-beta and anti-IFN-beta on coxsackievirus B3–induced myocarditis in mice. J Interferon Res 1985;5:137–146.
18. Maisch B, Hufnagel G, Schonian U, Hengstenberg C. The European Study of Epidemiology and Treatment of Cardiac

Inflammatory Disease (ESETCID). Eur Heart J 1995;16 (Suppl O):173–175.

19. McNamara DM, Rosenblum WD, Janosko KM, et al. Intravenous immune globulin in the therapy of myocarditis and acute cardiomyopathy. Circulation 1997;95:2476–2478.

20. Drucker NA, Colan SD, Lewis AB, et al. Gamma-globulin treatment of acute myocarditis in the pediatric population. Circulation 1994;89:252–257.

21. Bozkurt B, Villaneuva FS, Holubkov R, et al. Intravenous immune globulin in the therapy of peripartum cardiomyopathy. J Am Coll Cardiol 1999;34:177–180.

22. See DM, Tilles JG. Treatment of coxsackievirus A9 myocarditis in mice with WIN 54954. Antimicrob Agents Chemother 1992;36:425–428.

23. Rossen RD, Mann DL. Myocardial inflammation. In: Rich RR, Fleisher WT, Shearer WT, Kotzin BL, Schroeder W, eds. Clinical Immunology: Principles and Practice. London: Mosby, 2001:80.1–80.15.

24. Seko Y, Shinkai Y, Kawasaki A, Yagita H, Okumura K, Yazaki Y. Evidence of perforin-mediated cardiac myocyte injury in acute murine myocarditis caused by coxsackie virus B3. J Pathol 1993;170:53–58.

25. Barry WH. Cellular and molecular basis of inflammatory myocardial disease. J Nucl Cardiol 2001;8:499–505.

26. Lodge PA, Herzum M, Olszewski J, Huber SA. Coxsackievirus B-3 myocarditis. Acute and chronic forms of the disease caused by different immunopathogenic mechanisms. Am J Pathol 1987;128:455–463.

27. Godeny EK, Gauntt CJ. Involvement of natural killer cells in coxsackievirus B3–induced murine myocarditis. J Immunol 1986;137:1695–1702.

28. Matsumori A, Kawai C. An animal model of congestive (dilated) cardiomyopathy: dilatation and hypertrophy of the heart in the chronic stage in DBA/2 mice with myocarditis caused by encephalomyocarditis virus. Circulation 1982;66:355–360.

29. McManus BM, Chow LH, Wilson JE, et al. Direct myocardial injury by enterovirus: a central role in the evolution of murine myocarditis. Clin Immunol Immunopathol 1993;68:159–169.

30. Schreiber SL, Crabtree GR. The mechanism of action of cyclosporin A and FK506. Immunol Today 1992;13:136–142.

31. Henke A, Huber S, Stelzner A, Whitton JL. The role of CD8+ T lymphocytes in coxsackievirus B3–induced myocarditis. J Virol 1995;69:6720–6728.

32. Oldstone MB. Molecular mimicry and autoimmune disease. Cell 1987;50:819–820.

33. Matsumori A, Sasayama S. Immunomodulating agents for the management of heart failure with myocarditis and cardiomyopathy—lessons from animal experiments. Eur Heart J 1995; 16(Suppl O):140–143.

34. Smith KA. Interleukin-2: inception, impact, and implications. Science 1988;240:1169–1176.

35. Barry WH. Mechanisms of immune-mediated myocyte injury. Circulation 1994;89:2421–2432.

36. Sivasubramanian N, Coker ML, Kurrelmeyer K, DeMayo F, Spinale FG, Mann DL. Left ventricular remodeling in transgenic mice with cardiac restricted overexpression of tumor necrosis factor. Circulation 2001;104:826–831.

37. Li YY, Feng YQ, Kadokami T, et al. Myocardial extracellular matrix remodeling in transgenic mice overexpressing tumor necrosis factor alpha can be modulated by anti- tumor necrosis factor alpha therapy. Proc Natl Acad Sci USA 2000;97: 12746–12751.

38. Mikami S, Kawashima S, Kanazawa K, et al. Expression of nitric oxide synthase in a murine model of viral myocarditis induced by coxsackievirus B3. Biochem Biophys Res Commun 1996;220:983–989.

39. Hirono S, Islam MO, Nakazawa M, et al. Expression of inducible nitric oxide synthase in rat experimental autoimmune myocarditis with special reference to changes in cardiac hemodynamics. Circ Res 1997;80:11–20.

40. Ishiyama S, Hiroe M, Nishikawa T, et al. Nitric oxide contributes to the progression of myocardial damage in experimental autoimmune myocarditis in rats. Circulation 1997;95:489–496.

41. Limas CJ, Goldenberg IF, Limas C. Autoantibodies against b-adrenoceptors in human idiopathic dilated cardiomyopathy. Circ Res 1989;64:97–103.

42. Klein R, Maisch B, Kochsiek K, Berg PA. Demonstration of organ specific antibodies against heart mitochondria (anti-M7) in sera from patients with some forms of heart diseases. Clin Exp Immunol 1984;58:283–292.

43. Caforio ALP, Grazzini M, Mann JM, et al. Identification of α- and β-cardiac myosin heavy chain isoforms as major autoantigens in dilated cardiomyopathy. Circulation 1992;85:1734–1742.

44. Schultheiss HP, Bolte HD. Immunological analysis of autoantibodies against the adenine nucleotide translocator in dilated cardiomyopathy. J Mol Cell Cardiol 1985;17:603–617.

45. Schulze K, Becker BF, Schauer R, Schultheiss HP. Antibodies to ADP-ATP carrier—an autoantigen in myocarditis and dilated cardiomyopathy—impair cardiac function. Circulation 1990; 81:959–969.

46. Fu ML, Schulze W, Wallukat G, Hjalmarson A, Hoebeke J. A synthetic peptide corresponding to the second extracellular loop of the human M2 acetylcholine receptor induces pharmacological and morphological changes in cardiomyocytes by active immunization after 6 months in rabbits. Clin Immunol Immunopathol 1996;78:203–207.

47. Wallukat G, Wollenberger A, Morwinski R, Pitschner HF. Anti-beta 1-adrenoceptor autoantibodies with chronotropic activity from the serum of patients with dilated cardiomyopathy: mapping of epitopes in the first and second extracellular loops. J Mol Cell Cardiol 1995;27:397–406.

48. Wada H, Saito K, Kanda T, et al. Tumor necrosis factor-α (TNF-α) plays a protective role in acute viral myocarditis in mice: a study using mice lacking TNF-α. Circulation 2000;103:743–749.

49. Kubota T, McTiernan CF, Frye CS, et al. Dilated cardiomyopathy in transgenic mice with cardiac specific overexpression of tumor necrosis factor-alpha. Circ Res 1997;81:627–635.

50. Bryant D, Becker L, Richardson J, et al. Cardiac failure in transgenic mice with myocardial expression of tumor necrosis factor-α (TNF). Circulation 1998;97:1375–1381.

51. Yamada T, Matsumori A, Sasayama S. Therapeutic effect of anti-tumor necrosis factor-alpha antibody on the murine model of viral myocarditis induced by encephalomyocarditis virus. Circulation 1994;89:846–851.

52. Kubota T, Bounoutas GS, Miyagishima M, et al. Soluble tumor necrosis factor receptor abrogates myocardial inflammation but not hypertrophy in cytokine-induced cardiomyopathy. Circulation 2000;101:2518–2525.

53. Mann DL. Tumor necrosis factor and viral myocarditis: the fine line between innate and inappropriate immune responses in the heart. Circulation 2001;103:626–629.

54. Monrad ES, Matsumori A, Murphy JC, Fox JG, Crumpacker CS, Abelmann WH. Therapy with cyclosporine in experimental

murine myocarditis with encephalomyocarditis virus. Circulation 1986;73:1058–1064.

55. Tomioka N, Kishimoto C, Matsumori A, Kawai C. Effects of prednisolone on acute viral myocarditis in mice. J Am Coll Cardiol 1986;7:868–872.

56. Miyamoto T, Matsumori A, Hwang MW, Nishio R, Ito H, Sasayama S, Therapeutic effects of FTY720, a new immuno-suppressive agent, in a murine model of acute viral myocarditis. J Am Coll Cardiol. 2001 May; 37(6):1713–8.

57. Mason JW, O'Connel JB, Herskowitz A, et al. A clinical trial of immunosuppressive therapy for myocarditis. N Engl J Med 1995;333:269–275.

58. Kishimoto C, Takada H, Kawamata H, Umatake M, Ochiai H. Immunoglobulin treatment prevents congestive heart failure in murine encephalomyocarditis viral myocarditis associated with reduction of inflammatory cytokines. J Pharmacol Exp Ther 2001;299:645–651.

59. Kishimoto C, Takada H, Kawamata H, Umatake M, Ochiai H. Immunoglobulin treatment prevents congestive heart failure in murine encephalomyocarditis viral myocarditis associated with reduction of inflammatory cytokines. J Pharmacol Exp Ther 2001;299:645–651.

60. McNamara DM, Holubkov R, Starling RC, et al. Controlled trial of intravenous immune globulin in recent-onset dilated cardiomyopathy. Circulation 2001;103:2254–2259.

61. Nishio R, Matsumori A, Shioi T, Ishida H, Sasayama S. Treatment of experimental viral myocarditis with interleukin-10. Circulation 1999;100:1102–1108.

62. Nakano A, Matsumori A, Kawamoto S, Tahara H, Yamato E, Sasayama S, Miyazaki JI. Cytokine gene therapy for myocarditis by in vivo electroporation. Hum Gene Ther 2001;12:1289–1297.

63. Cunha FQ, Moncada S, Liew FY. Interleukin-10 (IL-10) inhibits the induction of nitric oxide synthase by interferon-gamma in murine macrophages. Biochem Biophys Res Commun 1992;182:1155–1159.

64. Richter WO, Jacob BG, Ritter MM, Suhler K, Vierneisel K, Schwandt P. Three-year treatment of familial heterozygous hypercholesterolemia by extracorporeal low-density lipoprotein immunoadsorption with polyclonal apolipoprotein B antibodies. Metabolism 1993;42:888–894.

65. Wallukat G, Reinke P, Dorffel WV, et al. Removal of autoantibodies in dilated cardiomyopathy by immunoadsorption. Int J Cardiol 1996;54:191–195.

66. Schultheiss HP, Schwimmbeck P, Bolte HD, Klingenberg M. The antigenic characteristics and the significance of the adenine nucleotide translocator as a major autoantigen to antimitochondrial antibodies in dilated cardiomyopathy. Adv Myocardiol 1985;6:311–327.

67. Felix SB, Staudt A, Dorffel WV, et al. Hemodynamic effects of immunoadsorption and subsequent immunoglobulin substitution in dilated cardiomyopathy: three-month results from a randomized study. J Am Coll Cardiol 2000;35:1590–1598.

68. Badorff C, Lee GH, Lamphear BJ, et al. Enteroviral protease 2A cleaves dystrophin: evidence of cytoskeletal disruption in an acquired cardiomyopathy [see comments]. Nat Med 1999;5:320–326.

69. Ono K, Matsumori A, Shioi T, Furukawa Y, Sasayama S. Cytokine gene expression after myocardial infarction in rat hearts: possible implication in left ventricular remodeling. Circulation 1998;98:149–156.

70. Why HJ, Meany BT, Richardson PJ, et al. Clinical and prognostic significance of detection of enteroviral RNA in the myocardium of patients with myocarditis or dilated cardiomyopathy. Circulation 1994;89:2582–2589.

71. Wessely R, Klingel K, Santana LF, et al. Transgenic expression of replication-restricted enteroviral genomes in heart muscle induces defective excitation–contraction coupling and dilated cardiomyopathy. J Clin Invest 1998;102:1444–1453.

72. Eisenhofer G, Friberg P, Rundqvist B, et al. Cardiac sympathetic nerve function in congestive heart failure. Circulation 1996;93:1667–1676.

73. Hasking GJ, Esler MD, Jennings GL, Burton D, Korner PI. Norepinephrine spillover to plasma in patients with congestive heart failure: evidence of increased overall and cardiorenal sympathetic nervous activity. Circulation 1986;73:615–621.

74. Dzau VJ, Packer M, Lilly LS, Swartz SL, Hollenberg NK, Williams GH. Prostaglandins in severe congestive heart failure: relation to activation of the renin–angiotensin system and hyponatremia. N Engl J Med 1984;310:347–352.

75. Torre-Amione G, Kapadia S, Benedict CR, Oral H, Young JB, Mann DL. Proinflammatory cytokine levels in patients with depressed left ventricular ejection fraction: a report from the studies of left ventricular dysfunction (SOLVD). J Am Coll Cardiol 1996;27:1201–1206.

76. Mann DL. Mechanisms and models in heart failure: a combinatorial approach. Circulation 1999;100:999–1088.

10 Genetic Underpinnings of Cardiogenesis and Congenital Heart Disease

Vidu Garg, MD, and Deepak Srivastava, MD

CONTENTS

INTRODUCTION

Congenital heart disease (CHD), the leading noninfectious cause of death in infants, occurs in nearly 1% of live births and causes 10% of spontaneous abortions *(1)*. Diagnosis and treatment of CHD have improved, and surgical palliation for many defects has resulted in an increasing population of adults surviving with complex CHD. Some forms of adult-onset heart disease originate in cardiac developmental defects. The most notable of these defects, aortic valve stenosis, is usually associated with a congenital bicuspid aortic valve and is seen in 1% of the population.

Although the etiology of CHD is poorly understood, the complex process of heart development involves a combination of hemodynamic forces and morphogenetic events that are sensitive to mild perturbations. Infants born with CHD usually have isolated cardiovascular defects that affect only one chamber, septum, or valve of the heart; therefore, the molecular developmental programs for each specific region of the heart may function independently. In recent years, the genes involved in cardiogenesis have been examined in human and animal studies and have provided insight into the genetic pathogenesis of CHD. In this chapter, we review aspects of cardiac morphogenesis that are relevant to CHD, describe animal model systems used to study cardiac development, and provide examples of genes that have regional effects on the cardiovascular system.

MORPHOGENESIS OF THE CARDIOVASCULAR SYSTEM

By the middle of the third week of gestation, a functional cardiovascular system is required to meet the nutritional requirements of the developing human embryo. Soon after gastrulation, cardiac progenitor cells within the anterior lateral plate mesoderm commit to becoming cardiogenic in response to an inducing signal from the adjacent endoderm *(2)*. The specific signaling molecules responsible for this commitment are unknown, but members of the transforming growth factor (TGF)-β and fibroblast growth factor (FGF) family are necessary for this commitment *(3)*. In addition, recent studies have shown that inhibition of a signaling molecule, Wnt, in the anterior lateral mesoderm is necessary for cardiogenesis *(4,5)*. The bilaterally symmetric heart primordia migrate to the midline and fuse to form a single beating heart tube (Fig. 1). The straight heart tube has an outer myocardium and an

From: *Contemporary Cardiology: Principles of Molecular Cardiology*
Edited by: M. S. Runge and C. Patterson © Humana Press Inc., Totowa, NJ

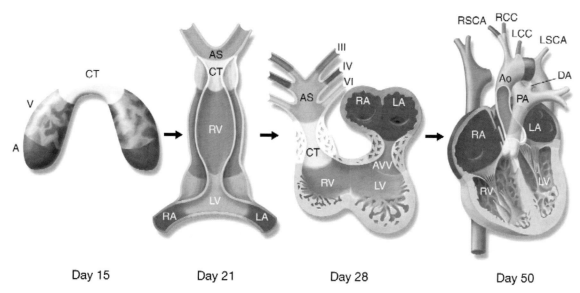

Fig. 1. Schematic of cardiac morphogenesis. Ventral view of cardiac development with morphologically related regions. Cardiogenic precursors form a crescent (left panel, d 15) that will give rise to specific segments of the linear heart tube, which is patterned along the A-P axis to form the various regions and chambers of the looped and mature heart. Each cardiac chamber balloons from the outer curvature of the looped heart tube in a segmental fashion. Neural crest cells populate the bilaterally symmetric aortic arch arteries (III, IV, and VI) and aortic sac (AS) that together contribute to specific segments of the mature aortic arch. Mesenchymal cells form the cardiac valves from the conotruncal (CT) and atrioventricular valve (AVV) segments. Corresponding days of human embryonic development are indicated. A, atrium; Ao, aorta; DA, ductus arteriosus; LA, left atrium; LCC, left common carotid; LSCA, left subclavian artery; LV, left ventricle; PA, pulmonary artery; RA, right atrium; RCC, right common carotid; RSCA, right subclavian artery; V, ventricle. Reproduced with permission *(80)*.

inner endocardium that are separated by an extracellular matrix (ECM) called the cardiac jelly. The linear heart tube is organized along an anterior–posterior (A–P) axis to form the future regions of the four-chambered heart. Rightward looping of the heart tube converts the A–P polarity to a left–right (L–R) polarity. The ventricular chambers mature by ballooning from the outer curvature of the looped heart, whereas the inner curvature undergoes extensive remodeling to align the inflow and outflow portions of the heart with the appropriate ventricular chambers. Further septation and remodeling eventually lead to the four-chambered heart.

A population of migratory neural crest cells known as the cardiac neural crest contributes significantly to the development of the heart. Found in the aortic sac, these neural crest cells are necessary for septation of the truncus arteriosus into the aorta and pulmonary artery and for formation of the semilunar valves and the superior portion of the ventricular septum. In addition, cardiac neural crest cells populate the bilaterally symmetric aortic arch arteries; the cells are necessary for proper remodeling of the aortic arch arteries into a left aortic arch with normal branching of the head and neck vessels. Each aortic arch artery contributes to a specific segment of the mature arch (Fig. 1).

Based on molecular and genetic studies over the last decade, heart development has emerged as a paradigm for organogenesis. Multiple animal models have been used to study molecular mechanisms involved in CHD because pathways of cardiogenesis are highly conserved across species as diverse as flies and humans. The genes for cardiomyocyte formation are similar in humans and in the fruit fly, *Drosophila*, which has a primitive linear heart tube known as a dorsal vessel. *Drosophila* has the advantages of having a rapid breeding time, a simple genome, and DNA that can be chemically mutated in a random fashion. Searching for flies with abnormal hearts and identifying the responsible mutations (reverse genetics) can lead to the identification of genes that are associated with specific developmental defects. However, the form and function of the vertebrate heart differs from that of the fruit fly. Vertebrates share many organotypic features, and genetic pathways for higher-order structures such as chambers are conserved.

Like *Drosophila*, zebrafish can be studied by using chemical mutagenesis, phenotype analysis, and reverse genetics; however, zebrafish have the advantage of being vertebrates with two-chambered hearts. In addition, cardiovascular defects can be visualized in live zebrafish because a functioning circulatory system is not necessary until the late stages of embryonic development.

Chick and mouse model systems have also been used to study four-chambered hearts. Because of easily accessible embryos, chicks are useful for surgical and molecular manipulation; however, the chick system is limited because genomic technology does not exist for true genetic studies. Mice are mammals and have a cardiovascular system nearly identical to that of humans, which allows for elegant in vivo genetic manipulation. Direct gene targeting techniques have been used to develop models for CHD in mice. Each model has unique advantages and has provided important insights into the development of the human heart.

In experimental studies, most cardiac phenotypes result from homozygous mutations of critical cardiac developmental genes and result in death of the embryo. In contrast, infants born with CHD often have heterozygous mutations of one or more critical genes that predispose to the observed phenotype.

DEFECTS OF ATRIAL AND VENTRICULAR DEVELOPMENT

Evidence for chamber-specific molecular developmental programs is seen in the presentation of infants with CHD. For example, in infants with hypoplastic right ventricle, only the right ventricle does not develop properly, whereas the left ventricle and atria have normal structure and function. Several transcription factors are expressed in a chamber-specific pattern. Two members of the basic helix-loop-helix family of transcription factors, dHAND and eHAND (deciduum/extraembryonic membrane, heart, autonomic nervous system, neural crest–derived tissues), are predominantly expressed in the right and left ventricles, respectively (6,7). Deletion of the *dHAND* gene in mice results in hypoplasia of the right ventricle, which indicates that mutation of a single gene can ablate an entire chamber (7). dHAND appears to regulate survival of ventricular cells, although the downstream targets of dHAND that regulate right ventricular survival have not been identified (8).

Another mechanism by which gene transcription is regulated in the developing heart may involve epigenetic factors that alter higher-order chromatin structure through covalent histone modifications. Acetylation, deacetylation, methylation, or phosphorylation of specific residues in histone tails activates or represses transcription of nearby genes. mBop is a muscle-restricted transcriptional repressor that interacts with histone deacetylases and contains a SET domain, which harbors histone methyltransferase activity

in other proteins. dHAND expression in the precardiac mesoderm depends on mBop; mice lacking mBop develop hypoplasia of the right ventricle. This finding suggests a hierarchical relationship during ventricular development.

Myocyte enhancer binding factor-2 (MEF2) is another transcription factor that plays a critical role in ventricular development. Initially studied in *Drosophila*, MEF2 has four orthologues in mammals that are expressed in precursors of the cardiac, skeletal, and smooth muscle lineages in vertebrates (9–11). Targeted deletion of one of the orthologues, MEF2C, in mice results in hypoplasia of the right and left ventricles, but not of the atria (12). The chamber-specific role of MEF2C, despite its homogeneous expression in the heart, suggests that MEF2C is a necessary cofactor for other ventricular-restricted regulatory proteins.

The ECM is also critical in ventricular development. Normal development of the right ventricle depends on two ECM proteins: versican, which is a chondroitin sulfate proteoglycan, and hyaluronan synthase-2 (Has2). Both proteins are expressed in the endocardial cushions and in the ventricular myocardium. Disruption of either the versican or Has2 gene in mice results in hypoplastic right ventricle, whereas the left ventricle is less affected (13,14). The mechanism involved is unknown.

Defects of the atrial or ventricular septum are the most common types of CHD. Genetic linkage analyses of families with autosomal dominant inheritance of CHD have shown that two transcription factors, Nkx2.5 and Tbx5, are important in the genesis of septal defects. In humans, point mutations of Nkx2.5 cause familial atrial septal defects, conduction abnormalities, and sporadic cases of other types of CHD such as tetralogy of Fallot and Ebstein's anomaly (15,16). Nkx2.5 is a homeodomain protein whose orthologue in *Drosophila*, tinman, is necessary for formation of the dorsal vessel in fruit flies (17). In mice, targeted disruption of Nkx2.5 results in the arrest of heart formation after the straight tube stage in homozygous-null embryos (18,19), and careful analysis of heterozygotes has identified abnormalities of the atrial septum and the conduction system (20). Analysis of the mutated gene products in humans has shown important structure–function relationships of the Nkx2.5 protein (21), but the mechanisms that cause CHD are still unknown.

The transcription factor Tbx5 is mutated in patients with the Holt–Oram syndrome, which is characterized by ventricular and atrial septal defects and limb anomalies (22). Tbx5 is expressed in large amounts in the septum and in the future left ventricular segment during mouse embryogenesis (23). Targeted deletion of the gene Tbx5 in mice results in death of homozygous embryos, whereas heterozygous mice have atrial and ventricular septal defects and limb anomalies *(24)*. The mechanism of Tbx5 regulation of ventricular and septal formation is unknown.

DEFECTS IN CONOTRUNCAL AND AORTIC ARCH DEVELOPMENT

Defects of the cardiac outflow tract or the aortic arch account for 20–30% of all cases of CHD *(25)*. Tetralogy of Fallot, persistent truncus arteriosus, and double-outlet right ventricle are examples of defects of the cardiac outflow tract, whereas aortic arch defects include coarctation, interrupted aortic arch, and patent ductus arteriosus *(25)*. The 22q11 deletion syndrome (del22q11), which is the most common gene deletion syndrome and the second most common genetic cause of CHD after trisomy 21, has been important in studying the molecular pathways involved in conotruncal (CT) and aortic arch defects *(26)*. Of patients with del22q11, 75% have defects of the conotruncus and/or the aortic arch, both of which are derived from the cardiac neural crest. Many also have defects of the pharyngeal arch, including cleft palate, dysmorphic facial features, thymic hypoplasia, and hypoparathyroidism *(27–30)*. Furthermore, 85–90% of patients with del22q11 have a monoallelic microdeletion of chromosome 22q11 that spans about 3Mb and contains nearly 30 genes *(31)*. Despite extensive study, the critical genes involved in del22q11 have not been identified; however, mouse models have been generated with deleted syntenic portions of the commonly deleted region on 22q11 *(32–34)*. In studies of these mouse models, the gene for Tbx1, a transcription factor expressed in the pharyngeal arches *(35)*, has been proposed as a likely candidate for the del22q11 syndrome because mice heterozygous for the Tbx1 gene have anomalies of the fourth aortic arch artery, including interrupted aortic arch, type B, and anomalous right subclavian artery *(34,36,37)*. However, most features of del22q11 have not been reproduced in mice. Tbx1 is regulated by the signaling molecule Sonic hedgehog (Shh) in the developing pharyngeal arches *(38)*, and mice with mutations in Shh have aortic arch defects similar to those observed in Tbx1 mutants (Erik N. Meyers, MD, Personal Communication, 2003).

Additional genes in the 22q11 region probably contribute to the del22q11 phenotype in humans, particularly given the absence of Tbx1 point mutations in patients without del22q11. A patient with the del22q11 phenotype has been described with a small deletion in UFD1, a gene involved in an ubiquitin-dependent pathway, and in CDC45, a gene involved in regulation of the cell cycle *(39)*. Homozygous deletion of either gene results in early death

of the embryo; however, the role of either gene in development is unknown *(33,40)*. In addition, homozygous deletion of Crkl, a gene in the 22q11 locus encoding for a signaling adaptor protein, results in a phenotype similar to the Tbx1 homozygous null mouse and produces many features of del22q11 *(41)*. Whether the genes in this locus function independently or in combination is unknown.

Numerous other genes involved in conotruncal and craniofacial development have been identified in targeted disruption studies in mice. Mice lacking endothelin-1 (ET-1) or its receptor, ET_A, have post-migratory neural crest defects similar to those seen in del22q11 *(42,43)*. dHAND and eHAND are down-regulated in neural crest–derived tissues in ET-1- and ET_A-deficient mice, suggesting that the HAND transcription factors function downstream of this signaling cascade *(45)*. A recently identified neural crest–specific enhancer for dHAND is a target for activation by the ET-1 signaling pathway *(45)*. Targeted deletion of dHAND results in programmed cell death of the post-migratory neural crest cells, which suggests that dHAND is necessary for survival of these neural crest–derived cells. Targeted deletion of neuropilin-1, a downstream target of dHAND that is expressed in neural crest–derived tissues, results in a phenotype similar to del22q11 *(8,46)*. Neuropilin-1 is a semaphorin and vascular endothelial growth factor receptor, and mice lacking semaphorin 3C have defects of the cardiac neural crest, suggesting a ligand–receptor interaction *(47)*. Similarly, mutations in the Pax3 gene cause persistent truncus arteriosus in mice, whereas disruption of the gene for the forkhead transcription factor, Mfh1, results in interruption of the aortic arch *(48,49)*. Dissection of these and other molecular pathways may help define the basis for cardiovascular developmental defects.

The zebrafish mutation, gridlock, has no circulation to the posterior trunk and tail because of a blockage in the dorsal aorta where the bilateral aortae fuse *(50)*. This phenotype is similar to aortic coarctation in humans. Positional cloning has shown mutations in a gene encoding a hairy-related transcription factor (HRT) similar to the mammalian HRT2/Hey2 gene *(51,52)*, which is involved in signaling by the Notch pathway. Further study of gridlock in zebrafish has shown that the hairy-related transcription factor is involved in early segregation of endothelial cells into either arterial or venous cell fate *(53)*. Aortic coarctation has a high rate of familial recurrence, and it will be interesting to determine if mutations of gridlock are present in a subset of these affected patients.

Genetic studies in humans have identified the gene responsible for Alagille syndrome, a condition characterized by biliary atresia and conotruncal defects. Mutations have been identified in Jagged-1, a membrane-bound ligand that was originally identified in *Drosophila (54,55)*. In addition, Jagged-1 mutations have been identified in patients with isolated pulmonary stenosis or tetralogy of Fallot *(56)*. Jagged-1 is a ligand for the transmembrane receptor, Notch, which is involved in embryonic patterning and cellular differentiation. Whether HRT proteins mediate Jagged-1 signaling remains to be determined.

The ductus arteriosus is derived from the sixth aortic arch artery, and failure of the ductus arteriosus to close after birth results in patent ductus arteriosus, the third most common form of CHD. Pedigree analysis of individuals with familial patent ductus arteriosus has identified heterozygous mutations of the transcription factor TFAP2B *(57)*, which suggests a role for TFAP2B or its downstream targets in the normal closure of the ductus after birth.

DEFECTS IN VALVE DEVELOPMENT

Congenital abnormalities of the cardiac valves are commonly seen in infants and children. The cardiac valves develop from regional swellings of the ECM known as the cardiac cushions. Reciprocal signaling between the endocardial and myocardial cell layers transforms endocardial cells into mesenchymal cells. The transformed cells then migrate into the cushions and differentiate into the fibrous tissue of the valves. In addition, these cells are responsible for septation of the common atrioventricular (AV) canal into separate right- and left-sided orifices. Trisomy 21, or Down's syndrome, is often associated with incomplete septation of the AV valves. A mouse model of trisomy 21 has been generated *(58)*, but the gene(s) on chromosome 21 that are involved in Down's syndrome have not been identified.

Nuclear factor of activated T cells-c (NFATc), a transcription factor required for the expression of cytokine genes in activated lymphocytes, is controlled by calcineurin, a calcium-regulated phosphatase. In the heart, NFATc expression is restricted to the endocardium. Gene targeting studies in mice have shown that NFATc is necessary for formation of the semilunar valves and, to some extent, the AV valves *(59,60)*.

Although lack of cardiac valve leaflets is a rare cardiac anomaly, thickened valve leaflets resulting in stenotic valves is a common form of CHD. In mouse models, dysplastic semilunar valves have been associated with the absence of PTPN11, which encodes the protein tyrosine phosphatase Shp-2 and is involved in a signaling pathway mediated by the epidermal growth factor receptor *(61)*. The identification of point mutations in PTPN11 in patients with Noonan syndrome, which often includes pulmonic valve stenosis, suggests the importance of PTPN11 in CHD *(62)*.

The Smad proteins are intracellular transcriptional mediators of signaling initiated by TGF-β ligands. Smad-6 is specifically expressed in the AV cushions and outflow tract during cardiogenesis and is a negative regulator of TGF-β signaling. Targeted disruption of Smad-6 in mice results in thickened and gelatinous AV and semilunar valves, similar to those seen in human disease *(63)*. When mutated, other genes in the TGF-β signaling pathway may also result in stenotic and hyperplastic valves. Inhibition of such pathologic processes may be an effective therapy for recurrent valvar stenosis refractory to valvuloplasty.

DEFECTS OF CARDIAC LOOPING AND LEFT–RIGHT ASYMMETRY

Abnormal cardiac looping underlies several types of CHD. Proper folding of the straight heart tube aligns the atrial chambers with the appropriate ventricles and the right ventricle with the pulmonary artery and the left ventricle with the aorta. The atrioventricular septum, which divides the common AV canal into a right and left AV orifice, moves to the right to a position over the ventricular septum. The conotruncus simultaneously septates into the aorta and pulmonary artery and moves to the left to position the conotruncal septum over the ventricular septum (Fig. 2). This movement converts the two-chambered heart into a four-chambered heart.

Arrested or incomplete movement of the AV septum or conotruncus may result in malalignment of the inflow and outflow tracts (Fig. 2). Failure of the AV septum to shift to the right results in both AV orifices emptying into the left ventricle (double-inlet left ventricle), whereas failure of the conotruncus to shift to the left results in both the aorta and pulmonary artery arising from the right ventricle (double-outlet right ventricle). Fog-2, a zinc finger protein, may contribute to this process. Deletion of Fog-2 in mice results in pulmonic stenosis and absence of the coronary vasculature, and embryos with this deletion have a single AV valve that empties into the left ventricle *(64,65)*. The morphologic defects in Fog-2 mutants probably occur because of improper folding of the heart tube, which results in malalignment of the inflow and outflow tracts. Defects in folding may occur because myocardial cells fail to evacuate the inner curvature of the heart and migrate into the cushions, a process called myocardialization.

Abnormalities in the process of cardiac looping are often observed in the setting of randomized L–R patterning of the heart, lungs, and visceral organs. The heart is the

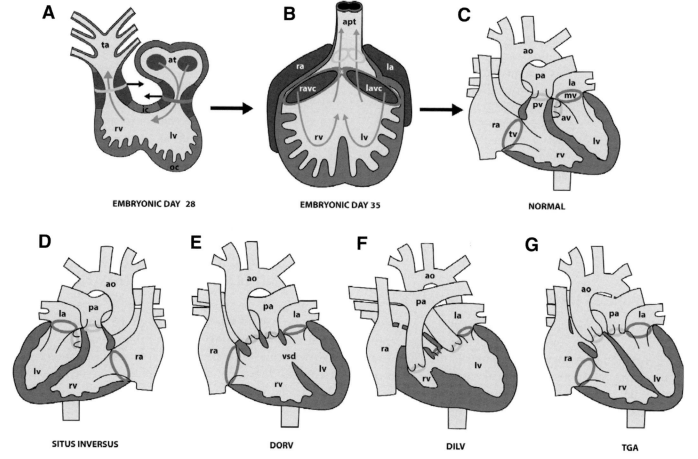

Fig. 2. Normal and abnormal cardiac morphogenesis associated with left–right (L-R) signaling. **(A)** As the linear heart tube loops rightward with inner curvature (ic) remodeling and outer curvature (oc) proliferation, the endocardial cushions of the inflow and outflow tracts become adjacent to one another. Then, the atrioventricular (av) septum shifts to the right, and the aortopulmonary trunk (apt) shifts to the left. **(B)** The inflow tract is divided into the right atrioventricular canal (ravc) and left atrioventricular canal (lavc) by the av septum (*). The outflow tract, known as the truncus arteriosus (ta), becomes the apt upon septation. **(C)** The left atrium (la) and right atrium (ra) are eventually aligned with the left ventricle (lv) and right ventricle (rv), respectively. The lv aligns with the aorta (ao) and the rv with the pulmonary artery (pa) after the great vessels rotate 180°. **(D)** Situs inversus results from a coordinated reversal of the determinants of the left-right axis. **(E)** Double outlet right ventricle (DORV), in which the rv is aligned with both the aorta and pulmonary artery, occurs when the apt fails to shift to the left. **(F)** Similarly, if the av septum fails to shift to the right, both atria communicate with the lv in a condition known as double inlet left ventricle (DILV). **(G)** In transposition of the great arteries (TGA), the apt fails to twist, and the rv communicates with the ao and the lv with the pa. mv, mitral valve; pulmonary valve; tv, tricuspid valve; vsd, ventricular septal defect. Reproduced with permission *(73)*.

first organ to break the bilateral symmetry in the early embryo. A cascade of signaling molecules that regulates L–R asymmetry has been identified and provides a framework in which to consider human L–R defects (Fig. 3). Asymmetric expression of Shh leads to expression of the TGF-β members, nodal and lefty, in the left lateral plate mesoderm *(66)*. The left-sided expression of nodal induces rightward looping of the straight heart tube. In the right-lateral mesoderm, Shh and nodal are inhibited by an activin-receptor mediated pathway. In contrast, the snail-related zinc finger transcription factor is expressed in the right lateral mesoderm and is repressed by Shh on the left *(67)*. The

activin- and nodal-dependent pathways result in expression of the transcription factor, Pitx2, on the left side of visceral organs *(68)*. The asymmetric expression of Pitx2 is sufficient for the establishment of L–R asymmetry in the heart, lungs, and gut.

Recent studies have shown how the initial asymmetry of molecules such as Shh might be established. Henson's node contains ciliary processes that beat in a vortical fashion, creating a leftward movement of morphogens around the node *(69)*. In mice homozygous for the inversus viscerum (iv) mutation, L–R orientation of the heart and viscera is randomized *(70)*. The iv gene encodes for L–R dynein,

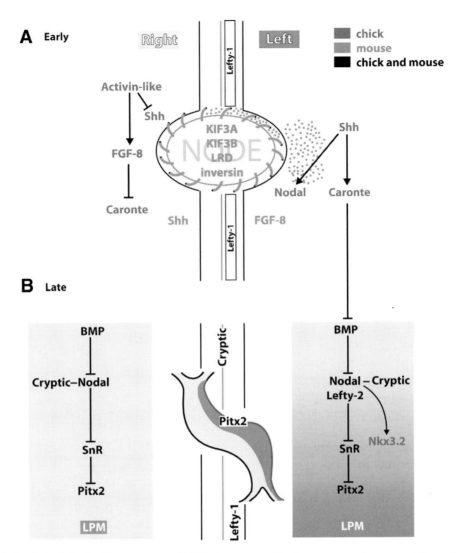

Fig. 3. Cascades regulating left–right (L–R) asymmetry. **(A)** Early asymmetrical gene expression around the node results in activation or repression of Sonic hedgehog (Shh) or fibroblast growth factor (FGF) -8 dependent pathways on the right or left (ventral view). The early roles of Shh and FGF-8 are reversed in mouse and chick. Leftward flow of morphogens (dots) by nodal cilia establishes the asymmetric gradient around the node in mice. Expression of Lefty-1 near the midline may serve as a barrier to maintain left-sided asymmetry of morphogens. At later stages of organogenesis, L-R asymmetric information at the node is transferred to the lateral plate mesoderm (LPM) by Caronte. **(B)** Caronte relieves bone morphogenic protein (BMP) inhibition on the left, initiating a cascade of events that culminates in expression of Pitx2 in the left LPM and in the left side of the heart tube. Consequently, a "leftness" signal appears to be actively propagated to overcome a default "rightness" program. Reproduced with permission *(73)*.

which may act as a force-generating component in cilia located in the node *(71,72)*. In mice with situs inversus totalis (inv) L-R asymmetry is completely reversed, but the function of the inv gene is unknown. These findings suggest a mechanism for situs inversus in Kartagener's syndrome, also known as immotile cilia syndrome.

In patients with heterotaxy syndromes, the cardiac, pulmonary, and gastrointestinal situs is random, whereas a well-coordinated reversal of L-R asymmetry is seen in patients with situs inversus totalis. Disruption of the signaling cascades on the left or right side of the embryo results in randomized cardiac looping and often leads to bilateral right-sidedness (asplenia syndrome) or left-sidedness (polysplenia syndrome). In humans, point mutations of several genes involved in the L-R signaling cascade have been identified: ZIC3, a zinc finger transcription factor; activin receptor IIB; and cryptic, a cofactor of nodal *(73)*.

CARDIOMYOCYTE SPECIFICATION AND DIFFERENTIATION

In contrast to the progress made in identifying genes that control cardiac morphogenesis, relatively little is known about the initial steps in heart formation and how mesodermal cells commit to the cardiac lineage and differentiate to form contractile cardiomyocytes. This phase of cardiac development is difficult to study, in part, because of the functional redundancy among the genes that control these early processes in vertebrates. For example, tinman is required for heart formation in *Drosophila*, but several tinman orthologues in vertebrates are coexpressed in the developing heart *(74)*. The best characterized of these orthologue genes, Nkx2.5, appears to have a role in vertebrate embryos analogous to that of tinman in flies, and gene replacement studies have shown that the mouse Nkx2.5 gene can substitute for some functions of tinman when introduced into Drosophila embryos *(75,76)*. However, the initial steps in cardiac development occur normally in mice lacking Nkx2.5 *(19)*, which suggests that other members of this family of homeobox genes may share common functions with NKX2.5. The finding that abnormalities in cardiac morphogenesis are not seen until later in the development of mice (and humans) with Nkx2.5 mutations suggests that the cardiac-expressed Nk-type homeobox genes function in later developmental stages or, more likely, that subtle cardiac abnormalities become more apparent as the heart begins to function under a hemodynamic load. Further evidence that Nkx2.5 may share common early functions with other members of this multigene family comes from the observation that forced expression of dominant negative versions of Nkx2.5 in frog or fish embryos results in severe early effects on the heart not seen with single gene mutations *(77,78)*.

The recent discovery of a potent muscle-specific coactivator, myocardin, may help in understanding the transcriptional regulation of early cardiogenic commitment *(79)*. Myocardin activates cardiac genes by interacting with the serum response factor, a ubiquitous transcription factor that binds the promoters of numerous cardiac genes. Frog embryos injected with a dominant negative mutant of myocardin fail to form a heart or to activate cardiac gene expression. The role, if any, of myocardin in later stages of heart development is unknown, but the expression of myocardin throughout the heart from embryogenesis to adulthood underscores its potential importance at multiple developmental stages.

The identification of early cardiac control genes such as myocardin may yield insight into the molecular mechanisms of heart formation and may provide opportunities for cardiac regeneration through the ectopic expression of such genes in noncardiac cells. Although approaches are still conceptual, genes that specify cardiac cell identity may soon be used to repair abnormalities resulting from CHD and cardiac disease in adults.

SUMMARY

The early findings described here have identified some of the genes and molecular mechanisms involved in heart development, but the etiology of CHD is complex. CHD is probably caused by a combination of genetic and environmental influences. Several new genes critical for cardiac development have been identified in multiple animal models. Genetic analyses in humans with CHD have identified point mutations in some of these critical genes. Identifying mutated genes in patients with CHD is only the first step because similar genetic abnormalities result in a spectrum of phenotypes in humans. Other genetic and environmental influences probably contribute to differences in phenotype. The challenge in the coming years will be to identify environmental and epigenetic factors that result in CHD in the setting of appropriated genetic susceptibility. Ultimately, some forms of CHD may be prevented by identifying the gene and altering the environment.

REFERENCES

1. Hoffman JI. Incidence of congenital heart disease: II. Prenatal incidence. Pediatr Cardiol 1995;16:155–165.
2. Schultheiss TM, Xydas S, Lassar AB. Induction of avian cardiac myogenesis by anterior endoderm. Development 1995; 121:4203–4214.
3. Schultheiss TM, Burch JB, Lassar AB. A role for bone morphogenetic proteins in the induction of cardiac myogenesis. Genes Dev 1997;11:451–462.
4. Schneider VA, Mercola M. Wnt antagonism initiates cardiogenesis in Xenopus laevis. Genes Dev 2001;15:304–315.
5. Marvin MJ, Di Rocco G, Gardiner A, Bush SM, Lassar AB. Inhibition of Wnt activity induces heart formation from posterior mesoderm. Genes Dev 2001;15:316–327.
6. Srivastava D, Cserjesi P, Olson EN. A subclass of bHLH proteins required for cardiac morphogenesis. Science 1995; 270:1995–1999.
7. Srivastava D, Thomas T, Lin Q, Kirby ML, Brown D, Olson EN. Regulation of cardiac mesodermal and neural crest development by the bHLH transcription factor, dHAND. Nat Genet 1997;16:154–160.
8. Yamagishi H, Olson EN, Srivastava D. The basic helix-loop-helix transcription factor, dHAND, is required for vascular development. J Clin Invest 2000;105:261–270.
9. Nguyen HT, Bodmer R, Abmayr SM, McDermott JC, Spoerel NA. D-mef2: a Drosophila mesoderm-specific MADS box-containing gene with a biphasic expression profile during embryogenesis. Proc Natl Acad Sci USA 1994;91:7520–7524.
10. Lilly B, Zhao B, Ranganayakulu G, Paterson BM, Schulz RA, Olson EN. Requirement of MADS domain transcription factor D-MEF2 for muscle formation in Drosophila. Science 1995;267:688–693.
11. Black BL, Olson EN. Transcriptional control of muscle development bymyocyte enhancer factor-2 (MEF2) proteins. Ann Rev Cell Dev Biol 1998;14:167–196.
12. Lin Q, Schwarz J, Bucana C, Olson EN. Control of mouse cardiac morphogenesis and myogenesis by transcription factor MEF2C. Science 1997;276:1404–1407.

13. Yamamura H, Zhang M, Markwald RR, Mjaatvedt CH. A heart segmental defect in the anterior-posterior axis of a transgenic mutant mouse. Dev Biol 1997;186:58–72.

14. Camenisch TD, Spicer AP, Brehm-Gibson T, et al. Disruption of hyaluronan synthase-2 abrogates normal cardiac morphogenesis and hyaluronan-mediated transformation of epithelium to mesenchyme. J Clin Invest 2000;106:349–360.

15. Schott JJ, Benson DW, Basson CT, et al. Congenital heart disease caused by mutations in the transcription factor NKX2-5. Science 1998;281:108–111.

16. Benson DW, Silberbach GM, Kavanaugh-McHugh A, et al. Mutations in the cardiac transcription factor NKX2.5 affect diverse cardiac developmental pathways. J Clin Invest 1999;104:1567–1573.

17. Bodmer R. The gene tinman is required for specification of the heart and visceral muscles in Drosophila. Development 1993;118:719–729.

18. Tanaka M, Chen Z, Bartunkova S, Yamasaki N, Izumo S. The cardiac homeobox gene Csx/Nkx2.5 lies genetically upstream of multiple genes essential for heart development. Development 1999;126:1269–1280.

19. Lyons I, Parsons LM, Hartley L, et al. Myogenic and morphogenetic defects in the heart tubes of murine embryos lacking the homeo box gene Nkx2-5. Genes Dev 1995;9:1654–1666.

20. Biben C, Weber R, Kesteven S, et al. Cardiac septal and valvular dysmorphogenesis in mice heterozygous for mutations in the homeobox gene Nkx2-5. Circ Res 2000;87:888–895.

21. Kasahara H, Lee B, Schott JJ, et al. Loss of function and inhibitory effects of human CSX/NKX2.5 homeoprotein mutations associated with congenital heart disease. J Clin Invest 2000;106:299–308.

22. Basson CT, Bachinsky DR, Lin RC, et al. Mutations in human Tbx5 cause limb and cardiac malformation in Holt-Oram syndrome. Nat Genet 1997;15:30–35.

23. Bruneau BG, Logan M, Davis N, et al. Chamber-specific cardiac expression of Tbx5 and heart defects in Holt-Oram syndrome. Dev Biol 1999;211:100–108.

24. Bruneau BG, et al. A murine model of Holt-Oram syndrome defines roles of the T-Box transcription factor Tbx5 in cardiogenesis and disease. Cell 2001;106:709–721.

25. Fyler DC. Trends. In: Fyler DC, ed. Nadas' Pediatric Cardiology. Philadelphia:Hanley & Belfus;1992: 273–280.

26. Scambler PJ. The 22q11 deletion syndromes. Hum Mol Genet 2000;9:2421–2426.

27. Ryan AK, Goodship JA, Wilson DI, et al. Spectrum of clinical features associated with interstitial chromosome 22q11 deletions: a European collaborative study. J Med Genet 1997;34:798–804.

28. DiGeorge AM. Discussion on a new concept of the cellular basis of immunology. J Pediatr 1965;67:907.

29. Shprintzen RJ, Goldberg RB, Lewin ML, et al. A new syndrome involving cleft palate, cardiac anomalies, typical facies, and learning disabilities: Velo-cardio-facial syndrome. Cleft Palate J 1978;15:56–62.

30. Kinouchi A, Mori K, Ando M, Takao A. Facial appearance of patients with conotruncal anomalies. Pediatrics (Japan) 1976;17:84.

31. Driscoll DA, Budarf ML, Emanuel BS. A genetic etiology for DiGeorge syndrome: consistent deletions and microdeletions of 22q11. Am J Hum Genet 1992;50:924–933.

32. Puech A, Saint-Jore B, Merscher S, et al. Normal cardiovascular development in mice deficient for 16 genes in 550 kb of the velocardiofacial/DiGeorge syndrome region. Proc Natl Acad Sci USA 2000;97:10090–10095.

33. Lindsay EA, Botta A, Jurecic V, et al. Congenital heart disease in mice deficient for the DiGeorge syndrome region. Nature 1999;401:379–383.

34. Merscher S, Funke B, Epstein JA, et al. Tbx1 is responsible for cardiovascular defects in velo-cardio-facial/DiGeorge syndrome. Cell 2001;104:619–629.

35. Chapman DL, Garvey N, Hancock S, et al. Expression of the T-box family genes, Tbx1-Tbx5, during early mouse development. Dev Dyn 1996;206:379–390.

36. Lindsay EA, Vitelli F, Su H, et al. Tbx1 haploinsufficiency in the DiGeorge syndrome region causes aortic arch defects in mice. Nature 2001;410:97–101.

37. Jerome LA, Papaioannou VE. DiGeorge syndrome phenotype in mice mutant for the T-box gene, Tbx1. Nat Genet 2001;27:286–291.

38. Garg V, Yamagishi C, Hu T, Kathiriya IS, Yamagishi H, Srivastava D. Tbx1, a DiGeorge syndrome candidate gene, is regulated by Sonic Hedgehog during pharyngeal arch development. Dev Biol 2001;235:62–73.

39. Yamagishi H, Garg V, Matsuoka R, Thomas T, Srivastava D. A molecular pathway revealing a genetic basis for human cardiac and craniofacial defects. Science 1999;283:1158–1161.

40. Yoshida K, Kuo F, George EL, Sharpe AH, Dutta A. Requirement of CDC45 for postimplantation mouse development. Mol Cell Biol 2001;21:4598–4603.

41. Guris LD, Fantes J, Tara D, Druker BJ, Imamoto A. Mice lacking the homologue of the human 22q11.2 gene CRKL phenocopy neurocristopathies of DiGeorge syndrome. Nat Genet 2001;27:238-40.

42. Kurihara Y, Kurihara H, Oda H, et al. Aortic arch malformations and ventricular septal defect in mice deficient in endothelin-1. J Clin Invest 1995;96:293–300.

43. Clouthier DE, Hosoda K, Richardson JA, et al. Cranial and cardiac neural crest defects in endothelin-A receptor-deficient mice. Development 1998;125:813–824.

44. Thomas T, Kurihara H, Yamagishi H, et al. A signaling cascade involving endothelin-1, dHAND and msx1 regulates development of neural-crest-derived branchial arch mesenchyme. Development 1998;125:3005–3014.

45. Charité J, McFadden DG, Merlo G, et al. Role of Dlx6 in regulation of an endothelin-1-dependent, dHAND branchial arch enhancer. Genes & Dev 2001 15:3039–3049.

46. Kawasaki T, Kitsukawa T, Bekku Y, et al. A requirement for neuropilin-1 in embryonic vessel formation. Development 1999;126:4895–4902.

47. Feiner L, Webber AL, Brown CB, et al. Targeted disruption of semaphorin 3C leads to persistent truncus arteriosus and aortic arch interruption. Development 2001;128:3061–3070.

48. Epstein DJ, Vogan KJ, Trasler DG, Gros P. A mutation within intron 3 of the Pax-3 gene produces aberrantly spliced mRNA transcripts in the splotch (Sp) mouse mutant. Proc Natl Acad Sci USA 1993;90:532–536.

49. Iida K, Koseki H, Kakinuma H, et al. Essential roles of the winged helix transcription factor MFH-1 in aortic arch patterning and skeletogenesis. Development 1997;124:4627–4638.

50. Zhong TP, Rosenberg M, Mohideen MPK, Weinstein B, Fishman MC. Gridlock, an HLH gene required for assembly of the aorta in zebrafish. Science 2000;287:1820–1824.

51. Nakagawa O, Nakagawa M, Richardson J, Olson EN, Srivastava D. HRT1, HRT2, and HRT3: A new subclass of bHLH transcription

factors marking specific cardiac, somatic, and branchial arch segments. Dev Biol 1999;216:72–84.

52. Nakagawa ON, McFadden DG, Nakagawa M, et al. Members of the HRT family of bHLH proteins act as transcriptional repressors downstream of Notch signaling. Proc Natl Acad Sci USA 2000;97:13655–13660.

53. Zhong TP, Childs S, Leu JP, Fishman MC. Gridlock signalling pathway fashions the first embryonic artery. Nature 2001;414:216–220.

54. Li L, Krantz ID, Deng Y, et al. Alagille syndrome is caused by mutations in human Jagged1, which encodes a ligand for Notch1. Nat Genet 1997;16:243–251.

55. Oda T, Elkahloun AG, Pike BL, et al. Mutations in the human Jagged1 gene are responsible for Alagille syndrome. Nat Genet 1997;16:235–242.

56. Krantz ID, Smith R, Colliton RP, et al. Jagged1 mutations in patients ascertained with isolated congenital heart defects. Am J Med Genet 1999;84:56–60.

57. Satoda M, Zhao F, Diaz GA, et al. Mutations in TFAP2B cause Char syndrome, a familial form of patent ductus arteriosus. Nat Genet 2000;25:42–46.

58. Cox DR, Smith SA, Epstein LB, Epstein CJ. Mouse trisomy 16 as an animal model of human trisomy 21 (Down syndrome): production of viable trisomy 16 diploid mouse chimeras. Dev Biol 1984;101:416–424.

59. Ranger AM, Grusby MJ, Hodge MR, et al. The transcription factor NFATc is essential for cardiac valve formation. Nature 1998;392:186–190.

60. de la Pompa JL, Timmerman LA, Takimoto H, et al. Role of the NFATc transcription factor in morphogenesis of cardiac valves and septum. Nature 1998;392:182–186.

61. Chen B, Bronson RT, Klaman LD, et al. Mice mutant for Egfr and Shp2 have defective cardiac semilunar valvulogenesis. Nat Genet 2000;24:296–299.

62. Tartaglia M, Mehler EL, Goldberg R, et al. Mutations in PTPN11, encoding the protein tyrosine phosphatase SHP-2, cause Noonan syndrome. Nat Genet 2001;29:465–468.

63. Galvin KM, Donovan MJ, Lynch CA, et al. A role for Smad6 in development and homeostasis of the cardiovascular system. Nat Genet 2000;24:171–174.

64. Svensson EC, Huggins GS, Lin H, et al. A syndrome of tricuspid atresia in mice with a targeted mutation of the gene encoding Fog-2. Nat Genet 2000;25:353–356.

65. Tevosian SG, Deconinck AE, Tanaka M, et al. FOG-2, a cofactor for GATA transcription factors, is essential for heart morphogenesis and development of coronary vessels from epicardium. Cell 2000;101:729–739.

66. Levin M, Johnson RL, Stern CD, Kuehn M, Tabin C. A molecular pathway determining left-right asymmetry in chick embryogenesis. Cell 1995;82:803–814.

67. Isaac A, Sargent MG, Cooke J. Control of vertebrate left-right asymmetry by a snail-related zinc finger gene. Science 1997;275:1301–1304.

68. Piedra ME, Icardo JM, Albajar M, Rodriguez-Rey JC, Ros MA. Pitx2 participates in the late phase of the pathway controlling left-right asymmetry. Cell 1998;94:319–324.

69. Nonaka S, Tanaka Y, Okada Y, et al. Randomization of left-right asymmetry due to loss of nodal cilia generating leftward flow of extraembryonic fluid in mice lacking KIF3B motor protein. Cell 1998;95:829–837.

70. Brueckner M, D'Eustachio P, Horwich AL. Linkage mapping of a mouse gene, iv, that controls left-right asymmetry of the heart and viscera. Proc Natl Acad Sci USA 1998;86:5035–5038.

71. Supp DM, Witte DP, Potter SS, Brueckner M. Mutation of an axonemal dynein affects left-right asymmetry in inversus viscerum mice. Nature 1997;389:963–966.

72. Supp DM, Brueckner M, Kuehn MR, et al. Targeted deletion of the ATP binding domain of left-right dynein confirms its role in specifying development of left-right asymmetries. Development 1999;126:5495–5504.

73. Kathiriya IS, Srivastava D. Left-right asymmetry and cardiac looping: implications for cardiac development and congenital heart disease. Am J Med Genet 2001;97:271–279.

74. Harvey RP. NK-2 homeobox genes and heart development. Dev Biol 1996;178:203–216.

75. Ranganayakulu G, Elliott D, Harvey R, Olson E. Divergent roles for NK-2 class homeobox genes in cardiogenesis in flies and mice. Development 1998;125:3037–3048.

76. Park M, Lewis C, Turbay D, et al. Differential rescue of visceral and cardiac defects in Drosophila by vertebrate tinman-related genes. Proc Natl Acad Sci USA 1998;95:9366–9371.

77. Fu Y, Yan W, Mohun TJ, Evans SM. Vertebrate tinman homologues XNkx2-3 and XNkx2-5 are required for heart formation in a functionally redundant manner. Development 1998;125: 4439–4449.

78. Grow MW, Kreig PA. Tinman function is essential for vertebrate heart development: elimination of cardiac differentiation by dominant inhibitory mutants of the tinman-related genes, XNks2-3 and XNkx2-5. Dev Biol 1998;204:87–196.

79. Wang D-Z, Chang PS, Wang Z, Sutherland L, Richardson JA, Small E, Krieg PA, Olson EN. Activation of cardiac gene expression by myocardin, a transcriptional cofactor for serum response factor. Cell 2001;105:851–862.

80. Srivastava D, Olson EN. A genetic blueprint for cardiac development. Nature 2000;407:221–226.

III CORONARY ARTERY DISEASE

11 Coronary Artery Development

Mark W. Majesky, PhD

CONTENTS

INTRODUCTION

Lineage mapping studies have shown an extracardiac origin for the coronary vasculature. Mesothelial cells arising from septum transversum mesenchyme contact the developing myocardium via a transient structure called the proepicardial organ (PEO). Proepicardial cells first extend over the surface of the heart to form the epicardial layer. Then, a subset of epicardial cells transform from epithelial to mesenchymal cells, migrate into the myocardial wall, and serve as progenitor cells for formation of the coronary vessels. Epicardial-derived mesenchymal cells (EPDCs) produce soluble factors that stimulate proliferation of myocardial cells in the compact zone of ventricular myocardium. Genetic studies have begun to identify the molecules that control and coordinate this complex process that ensures adequate perfusion of the myocardium during development of the heart.

CORONARY VESSELS ARISE FROM PROEPICARDIAL CELLS

Embryonic myocardium, initially avascular, receives oxygen and nutrients by diffusion from a common atrioventricular chamber. As the myocardial wall thickens, trabeculations form to maintain nutrient supply to the wall by diffusion. With continued growth of the outer compact layer of myocardium, the trabeculations are eventually replaced by a vascular network that develops within the heart wall to nourish the working myocytes. This vascular network is produced by cells that are recruited from sources outside the heart itself *(1–4)*. A major source of extracardiac vascular progenitor cells is located around the sinus venosus in the region of the developing liver primordium *(5–7)* (Fig. 1). Around E8.5 to 9.0 in the mouse, a population of mesothelial cells originating from septum transversum mesenchyme form villus-like projections that extend toward the exposed atrioventricular sulcus of the myocardial wall *(8,9)*. In the chick, a similar population of cells overlying the sinus venosus region appears around stage 14 *(10)*. Together, these mesothelial cell projections form the PEO, and the entire extracardiac primordium is called the proepicardial serosa *(4)* (Fig. 2). Mesothelial cells reach the heart via these proepicardial villi, either by direct physical contact (avian embryos) or by release of free-floating vesicles or cysts that travel through the cardiac coelom and attach to the outer surface of the myocardium (most mammalian species) *(11)*. After the proepicardial villi contact the

From: *Contemporary Cardiology:Principles of Molecular Cardiology*
Edited by: M. S. Runge and C. Patterson © Humana Press Inc., Totowa, NJ

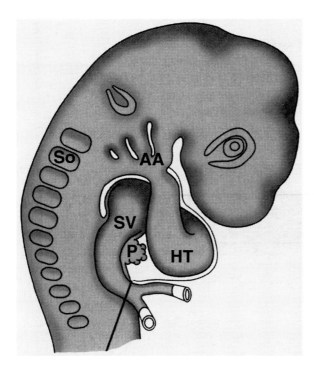

Fig. 1. Origins of the coronary vasculature: Lineage mapping studies show that coronary vessels arise from progenitor cells in the proepicardial organ (P), a transient structure that forms at the junction of the sinus venosus (SV) with the inflow tract of the looped heart tube (HT). AA, aortic arches; So, somites.

myocardium, the outer surface of the heart becomes covered by a single layer of mesothelial cells, which forms the epicardium (Fig. 3). All vertebrates examined so far have an epicardium that arises mainly from extracardiac mesothelial cells that extend from the sinus venosus–liver primordium region. A second source of epicardium-forming mesothelial cells surrounds the distal portion of the outflow tract and arises from pericardial mesothelium at the junction between the outflow tract and the wall of the pericardial cavity (12). This second source of epicardial cells can partially compensate for failure of the PEO-derived epicardial layer to fully form after ablation of the PEO during cardiac development (12). This partial compensation, however, is not sufficient to prevent death in embryos from a loss of signaling from the epicardium to the myocardium.

EPICARDIAL CELLS UNDERGO EPITHELIAL TO MESENCHYMAL TRANSFORMATION

Epicardial cells derived from the PEO initially attach directly to the outer surface of myocardium. A subepicardial space forms between the epicardial covering and the myocardium, and the space widens in the

sulci separating the atrial and ventricular chambers and in the interventricular canal (6). In the sulci and interventricular canal, myocardium-derived signals stimulate an epithelial to mesenchymal transformation (EMT) of the epicardial cells that forms a population of epicardium-derived mesenchymal cells (EPDCs) that enter into and migrate throughout the heart wall (3,13,14). The myocardial-derived factors that direct epicardial EMT have not been identified, but their production in the developing heart appears to be dependent on GATA-4–friend of GATA 2 (FOG2) transcriptional controls (15,16). Studies in chick–quail chimera and lineage tracing methods have shown that EPDCs differentiate into procollagen-producing cardiac fibroblasts, valvular and septal mesenchymal cells, interstitial cells within the aorticopulmonary septum, coronary adventitial fibroblasts, endothelial cells, and coronary smooth muscle cells (CoSMCs) (Fig. 4). In addition, fate mapping studies have shown that EPDCs are abundant in ventricular myocardium and valvuloseptal tissues, but are rare in the walls of the atria and outflow tract (17). A close relationship has been described between coronary vessels and neural crest–derived cells that enter the heart through the sinus venosus region to form cardiac nerves and parasympathetic ganglia (18). Capillary-like vessels form a peritruncal coronary vascular plexus that surrounds the outflow tract. Vessels that arise from this peritruncal ring eventually grow into the aortic wall, make contact with the aortic lumen, and form two opposing right and left main coronary stems (19,20). As directional blood flow through the coronary circuit begins, CoSMCs are recruited to form a media (21) (Fig. 5). Two main coronary stems that usually arise from the sinuses of Valsalva facing the pulmonary artery persist (22).

ORIGINS OF CORONARY ENDOTHELIAL CELLS

The origin of coronary endothelial cells has not been completely defined. In the chick embryo, lineage analysis studies have shown that coronary endothelium originates within the proepicardium, but whether a distinct subpopulation of angioblasts exists in the PEO is not clear (13,17,23). The description of blood island–like structures within the subepicardium of various species (1,7,22,24), including humans (25,26), suggests that coronary vessels arise by a process known as vasculogenesis (Fig. 4). In vasculogenesis, endothelial cells originate from precursor cells called angioblasts rather than from preexisting endothelial cells. Bipotential cells, called hemangioblasts, which can form either endothelial cells or

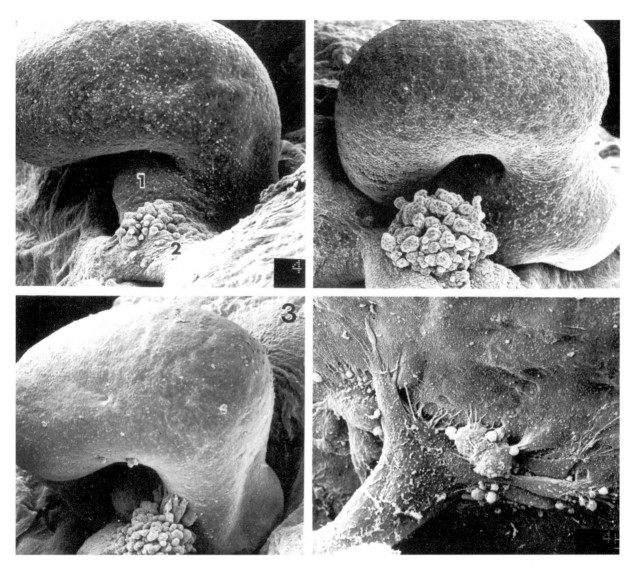

Fig. 2. Formation of the proepicardial organ: Scanning electron micrographs show the origins of proepicardial cells from coelomic mesothelium (upper left) at the junction of the inflow tract of the heart tube *(1)* with the sinus venosus *(2)* in Hamburger-Hamilton (HH) stage 15 chick embryo. Proepicardial cell villi consist of mesothelial cells on the outer surface overlying a proteoglycan-rich extracellular matrix interior (upper right, HH stage 17). Proepicardial cells reach the heart via attachment of proepicardial villus tips to the myocardium (lower left) and extension of pseudopodia over the exposed myocardial surface (lower right, HH stage 18). Reprinted with permission *(10)*.

blood cells, are found in certain areas of the embryo, such as the yolk sac or aorta–gonad–mesonephros region. Hematopoiesis occurs within the subepicardial space and contributes blood cells to the nascent coronary vasculature. Various researchers have suggested that endocardial cells may give rise to endothelial cells in the subepicardial mesenchyme via deep invaginations of the endocardial layer within highly trabeculated myocardium. Although rare, direct physical contact between the endocardium and the subepicardial vascular network can occasionally be detected in the outflow segment of the right ventricle *(22)*. However, dye transfer studies and intraluminal vascular casts suggest that little or no direct communication occurs between the cardiac chambers and subepicardial vessels.

Another source of coronary endothelial cells is the sinus venosus. Continuity between the endothelial lining of the sinus venosus and capillary-like vessels extending through the sinoventricular ligament, which is the remnant of the PEO after it attaches to the myocardium, has been reported *(18,22)*. At the same time, a contribution to coronary endothelium is also made by single cells or small clusters of cells that are not part of a luminized vessel. These cells stain strongly with the QH1 antibody, which is a marker

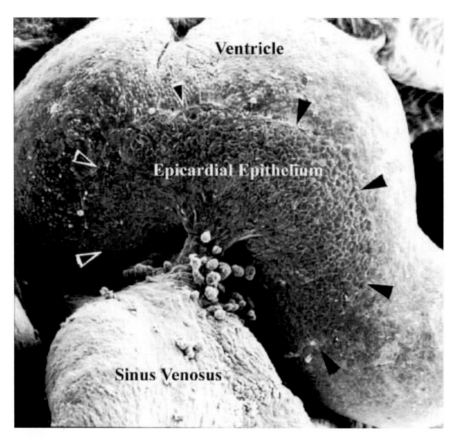

Fig. 3. Formation of the epicardium: Scanning electron micrograph of epicardial cells spreading over the surface of the heart tube in an HH stage 20 chick embryo. Arrows mark the leading edge of the migrating sheet of epicardium. Reprinted with permission *(10)*.

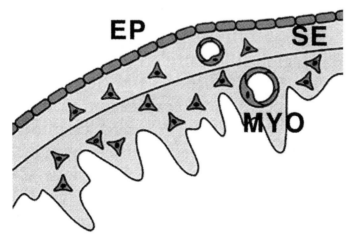

Fig. 4. Epicardial-derived mesenchymal cells (EPDCs): Shortly after the epicardial layer (EP) has formed, myocardial-derived signals stimulate an epithelial to mesenchymal transformation (EMT) that is particularly active in the atrioventricular groove region of the developing heart. The EPDCs thus formed (triangles) actively migrate within the subepicardial layer (SE) and enter the trabeculated myocardium (MYO) where they are recruited to form coronary endothelial cells (vessel profiles), coronary smooth muscle cells, and adventitial fibroblasts.

of angioblasts and endothelial cells in quail embryos. Thus, proepicardial cells may have the properties of a vasculogenic stem cell, which could give rise not only to CoSMCs and adventitial fibroblasts but also to endothelial cells and, possibly, blood cells. This idea is supported by the findings of blood island–like structures in the subepicardial space *(22)* and the observations that coelomic mesothelial cells in the paraaortic region undergo EMT, migrate to the lateroventral regions of the dorsal aorta, and contribute to the hemangioblastic progenitors in this region *(27,28)*. Also derived from the coelomic mesothelium, proepicardial cells may have retained hemangioblastic potential shared by their counterparts in the paraaortic region. However, the clonal analysis studies of Mikawa and Fishman *(23)* do not support this possibility; they found no evidence of a common progenitor for coronary endothelial cells and CoSMCs or for CoSMCs and adventitial fibroblasts. These authors concluded that proepicardial cells are already committed to individual lineages of various vascular cell types when the epicardial layer develops *(23,27)*. Identification of a small number of smooth muscle caldesmon-positive

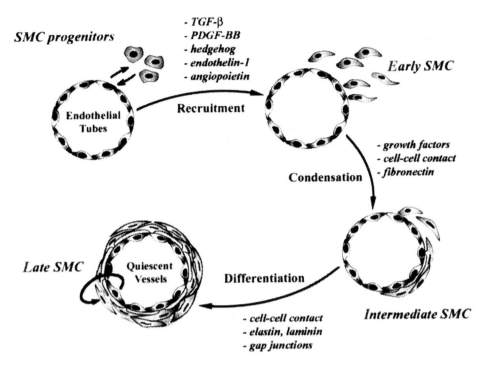

Fig. 5. Formation of the coronary vessel wall: Formation of endothelial tubes from angioblasts followed by recruitment of a pericyte or smooth muscle layer define the major steps in coronary vessel wall formation. Vascular endothelial growth factor (VEGF) and angiopoietin-1 direct the formation of a capillary-like vascular plexus within the subepicardial layer. These nascent coronary vessels penetrate the myocardium and form a peritruncal ring around the aortic root. Establishment of connections with the aortic lumen leads to formation of two primary coronary stems. Initiation of blood flow through the coronary circuit stimulates endothelial cells to recruit smooth muscle cells (SMCs) from nearby epicardial-derived mesenchymal cells (EPDCs). Evidence suggests that secreted factors upregulated by increased coronary blood flow play key roles in SMC recruitment. Such factors include transforming growth factor-β1 (TGF-β1), platelet-derived growth factor-BB (PDGF-BB) and endothelin-1. This interaction is bidirectional since various SMC-derived factors (VEGF, angiopoietin-1, fibroblast growth factors) are known to affect endothelial cell proliferation and differentiation. Distal coronary vessels recruit their SMC layers from upstream arterial sources via the chemotactic actions of PDGF-BB. Maturation of the newly formed vessel wall requires production of an appropriate basement membrane (collagen IV, laminin, nidogen); production of an elastin-rich, fibrillar collagen-type ECM (elastin, fibrillin, collagen I), and signaling events involving biomechanical forces and ECM interactions.

cells within the PEO further supports this proposal *(2)*. Additional studies are required to clarify the origins of coronary endothelial cells and to determine whether and to what extent vasculogenesis in the subepicardial layer contributes to coronary vessel formation.

ORIGINS OF CORONARY SMOOTH MUSCLE CELLS

Most CoSMCs in the heart originate from mesothelial cells of the proepicardial villi. Studies in chick-quail chimeras and dye-labeling studies have shown that the EMT of epicardial cells in the atrioventricular canal and interventricular sulcus results in a population of EPDCs that migrate throughout the heart wall and serve as progenitors for CoSMCs *(3,13)* (Fig. 4). A second source of CoSMCs

was identified by use of a Wnt1-cre recombinase transgenic mouse line *(29)*. The Wnt1 regulatory elements limit expression of the transgene to the dorsal neural tube, including the cardiac neural crest *(30)*. In Wnt1-cre transgenic mice crossed with Rosa26 reporter mice carrying a floxed lacZ allele, the beta-galactosidase reporter gene is expressed only in cells of neural crest origin, and gene expression is sustained throughout the animal's life. These lineage tagging studies have shown that the proximal coronary stems in mice are composed of smooth muscle cells that originate from cardiac neural crest cells, whereas the remainder of the subepicardial and penetrating coronary arteries are made up of epicardium-derived smooth muscle cells. Whether CoSMCs that have embryonic origins in neural crest cells differ in adaptive responses to stimuli or in wound repair from CoSMCs that arise in proepicardial mesothelium may be important to understand the development of atherosclerotic lesions later in life.

In similar studies, aortic smooth muscle cells derived from cardiac neural crest cells clearly differ in response to a common stimulus from aortic smooth muscle cells derived from splanchnic mesoderm. For example, neural crest–derived aortic smooth muscle cells (NC-SMCs) exposed to transforming growth factor-βα1 (TGF-βα1) stimulate protein kinase C (PKC) activity, translocate PKC to the plasma membrane, and increase production of diacylglycerol (31). In contrast, when mesoderm-derived aortic smooth muscle cells (Mes-SMCs) isolated from the same vessels and cultured under identical conditions showed no effect of TGF-β1, neither diacylglycerol production nor PKC activation are affected (31). Similarly, Topouzis and Majesky (32) showed that treatment with TGF-β1 stimulated proliferation of NC-SMCs but not proliferation of Mes-SMCs. Moreover, stimulation of NC-SMCs with TGF-β1 produced 12-fold increases activity of a luciferase reporter construct driven by the human plasminogen activator inhibitor type 1 (PAI-1) promoter, whereas only threefold stimulation was noted for Mes-SMCs. Crosslinking studies with ^{125}I-TGF-β1 showed a positive correlation between SMC stimulation of smooth muscle cell growth, PAI-1 transcriptional activation, and underglycosylation of the type II TGF-β receptor (32). Finally, Gadson et al. (33) reported that expression of the c-myb gene in NC-SMCs but not in Mes-SMCs, and antisense oligonucleotides to c-myb abolished TGF-β1-mediated increases in DNA synthesis and α1-procollagen mRNA levels in NC-SMCs but not in Mes-SMCs. These findings suggest that different smooth muscle cell populations within a common vessel wall respond in lineage-dependent ways to factors involved in vascular development, adaptation, and disease.

GENETIC ANALYSIS OF CORONARY DEVELOPMENT

Methods of modifying the mouse germline by gene targeting have been used to study coronary vessel development and to describe the molecular genetics of the formation and remodeling of the coronary vasculature (Table 1). However, phenotypes obtained from gene disruption studies described below must be interpreted with caution. Formation of the coronary system is tightly coupled to cardiac, vascular, and placental development in the whole embryo. Primary defects in development of one or more of these organ systems can indirectly produce defects in coronary vessel formation. Nevertheless, introducing specific mutations in the mouse germline has provided important insight into coronary development.

α4 Integrin

Integrins are transmembrane proteins that dimerize to form combinations with binding specificity for individual extracellular matrix proteins or cell adhesion molecules. The main ligands for α4β1 integrin are vascular cell adhesion molecule (VCAM)-1 and fibronectin. Mice deficient in expression of α4 integrin have multiple developmental defects that result in embryonic death (34). About 50% of the α4 integrin–deficient mice die before E11.0 because the chorion fails to fuse with the allantois, which is a critical step in formation of the placenta. The remaining 50% die of multiple cardiac defects around E12.5 (34); in these embryos, the proepicardium forms, but vesicle formation and release into the pericardial cavity are decreased (35). However, the few proepicardial vesicles that do reach the surface of the heart do not migrate properly over the myocardium (35). α4 Integrin is normally expressed on proepicardial cells, and its expression is maintained as epicardial cells cover the heart. The myocardium expresses VCAM-1, whereas the subepicardium and PEO express fibronectin; therefore, α4β1 integrin may interact with fibronectin in the PEO and with fibronectin and/or VCAM-1 as epicardial cells attach and migrate over the surface of the heart. The finding that the absence of VCAM-1 in knockout animal models results in a similar defect in epicardium formation lends support for this latter possibility. Fibronectin-null embryos die much earlier in development than either VCAM-1 or α4 integrin–deficient mice, which indicates the importance of fibronectin in cell adhesion and migration during gastrulation. This early embryonic death precludes a detailed analysis of the role of fibronectin in coronary development. Other sites of α4 integrin expression in the heart, such as the endocardial cushions and the outflow tract, are not affected in the α4 integrin–null mouse.

Vascular Cell Adhesion Molecule 1

Two major defects have been seen in VCAM-1–deficient mice. First, the placenta fails to form properly because the allantois does not fuse with the chorion in about VCAM-1–deficient embryos (36). Second, most of the remaining VCAM-1–deficient embryos die around E12.5 because of epicardial defects very similar to those seen in α4 integrin–deficient mice (36). The only known counterrecep-

Table 1
Targeted Mutations Disrupting Coronary Development

Gene (ref)	Phenotype
α4 Integrin (34)	Epicardial & coronary defects
Brain-derived neurotrophic factor (74)	Coronary endothelial defects
Erythropoietin (61)	Myocardial & erythroid defects
Friend of GATA2 (15)	Coronary vessel defects
Notch2 (66)	Vascular & myocardial defects
Platelet-derived growth factor-B (71)	Pericyte recruitment defects
Platelet-derived growth factor B-receptor (72)	Coronary smooth muscle defects
Retinaldehyde dehydrogenase2 (56)	Cardiac & outflow tract defects
Retinoid X receptor α (50)	Epicardial & myocardial defects
VCAM-1 (36,37)	Epicardial & coronary defects
Vascular endothelial growth factor-A (80)	Failure of vascular development
Vascular endothelial growth factor-B (84)	Coronary function defects
Vascular endothelial growth factor-120 (79)	Coronary angiogenesis defects
Wilms' tumor-1 (41)	Epicardial & cardiac defects

VCAM-1, vascular cell adhesion molecule-1.

tor for VCAM-1 is α4 integrin; therefore, the similarity in phenotypes between VCAM-1 knockout mice and α4 integrin knockout mice indicates that VCAM-1 is the major ligand for α4-integrin during epicardial covering of the heart. However, the conclusion that VCAM-1–deficient embryos die around E12.5 because of a lack of epicardial cell adhesion to underlying myocardium is complicated by the possibility that the formation or function of the placenta may not be sufficient to supply nutrients and oxygen to the working embryonic heart (37). Therefore, lack of nutrient supply rather than defective cell adhesion may be the basis for epicardial failure in VCAM-1 null mice.

Wilms' Tumor Protein-1

Wilms' tumor protein-1 (WT1) is a zinc finger–containing DNA binding protein that can act as either an activator or repressor of transcription, depending on the context of its binding site on DNA (38). Deletions and mutations within the WT1 gene have been associated with sporadic cases of Wilms' tumors and with urogenital abnormalities, which suggests that WT1 is involved in the development of the urogenital system (39). WT1 is expressed strongly in the PEO, in epicardial cells, and in EPDCs, but is absent from the myocardium (17). Expression of WT1 is reduced as EPDCs differentiate into coronary endothelial cells and smooth muscle cells and is absent in EPDCs that have migrated into cushion tissue mesenchyme. WT1-deficient mice die at midgestation (40), probably of cardiac failure caused by incomplete formation or mesenchymal transformation of the epicardium. In WT1-deficient mice, coronary vessels do not form, the compact

layer of myocardium fails to expand, and myocardial mass does not increase with the growth of the embryo. Furthermore, the epicardium forms initially but does not undergo mesenchymal transformation to produce precursors of coronary vessels (41). Restoration of WT1 expression by introduction of a yeast artificial chromosome (YAC) containing the WT1 locus into WT1-null mice prevents epicardial defects and restores formation of the coronary arteries (41). However, introduction of the YAC does not restore normal kidney development, a finding that suggests one copy of WT1 is insufficient to support kidney development.

Loss of expression of WT1 within the developing myocardial wall, either by gene deletion or physical ablation of the PEO, leads to the same cardiac phenotype as WT1-deficient mice. The most characteristic feature associated with deletion or ablation of the PEO is a thin ventricular myocardial wall. Much evidence suggests that expansion of the compact layer of ventricular myocardium depends upon cell–cell signaling interactions between cardiac myocytes and EPDCs. Fate mapping studies show that most EPDCs are located within the compact zone of ventricular myocardium; a few are found in the trabeculated myocardium and fewer still in the atrial myocardium (17). Tissue explant studies show that proepicardial cells secrete a mitogen for cardiac myocytes. An absence of EPDCs results in a lack of mitogenic signaling for cardiac myocytes in the compact zone, which in turn results in a thin ventricular wall prone to cardiac failure. Because WT1 expression is decreased when EPDCs differentiate into coronary wall cell types the role of WT1 in cardiac development may be to maintain a sufficient number of mitogenic EPDCs to support myocardial cell proliferation during formation of the ventricles. These studies suggest that WT1 function is required for EPDC formation or survival within the myocardium.

Friend of GATA-2

GATA factors, which are zinc finger–containing transcriptional regulators, play an important role in cell type specification during erythrogenesis, cardiogenesis, and differentiation of visceral endoderm (42). FOG1 was identified as a GATA-1 binding protein in a yeast two-hybrid protein interaction screen (43). Both GATA-1 and FOG1 are essential for erythropoiesis (44). FOG2 was identified by screening of expressed sequence tag databases with the FOG1 sequence (15,43,45,46). The physical interaction of FOG2 with the amino-terminal zinc finger of GATA-4, which occurs both in vitro and in vivo, appears to activate or repress GATA-4–dependent transcription from several different cardiac-restricted promoters in transient transfection assays (43,46). FOG2-deficient mouse embryos die at midgestation with cardiac defects including a thin ventricular myocardium, dilated atria, rounded ventricular apex, common atrioventricular canal, and tetralogy of Fallot (47). In these mice, the coronary vasculature is absent, and expression of endothelial-specific genes, including platelet-endothelial cell adhesion molecule (PECAM) and intercellular adhesion molecule (ICAM)-2, is decreased (15,47). Immunostaining with Flk1/vascular endothelial growth factor (VEGF)-R2 has confirmed an intact endocardium in the absence of coronary endothelium. In FOG2-deficient embryos, the epicardium forms normally, and expression of the epicardial genes WTI1, endoglin, capsulin, and retinaldehyde dehydrogenase (RALDH) is normal. These findings suggest that defects in coronary vessel formation are caused by failure of the epicardial cells either to undergo mesenchymal transformation or to differentiate into coronary endothelium. Other malformations in FOG2-deficient embryos, such as underdeveloped lungs and small livers, may be secondary to cardiac failure.

To determine whether FOG2 functions autonomously in epicardial cells, chimeric mice with a mixture of FOG2 +/+ and FOG2 –/– cells were produced. In these chimeric mice, the absence of FOG2 –/– cells in a given tissue suggests that FOG2 is required for formation of the specific tissue or for survival once the tissue has formed. Specifically, FOG2 –/– cells were found in the epicardium and subepicardial space, indicating that FOG2 function is not required in epicardial cells. To test whether replacing FOG2 in the myocardium could restore the FOG2 null phenotype to normal, α-myosin heavy chain–FOG2 transgenic mice were developed with a FOG2 null background. Expression of FOG2 in the myocardium fully restored coronary vessel formation and heart development (15). The authors concluded that the interaction between FOG2 and GATA is required in the myocardium to generate a signal that directs epicardial cells to undergo EMT and enter the heart to become coronary vessel precursors. Identifying the myocyte-derived signal that controls epicardial cell fate in heart development is an important direction for future work. VEGF is not that signal because its expression levels are unchanged in FOG2 –/– hearts.

To determine which GATA factor binds FOG2 for normal cardiac development, Crispino et al. (16) developed mice with a single amino acid replacement in GATA4 (valine to glycine at position 217) that prevents direct binding of GATA4 to FOG2 but does not alter GATA4 binding to DNA. Homozygous GATA4-V217G mice die around E12.5 and have the phenocopy of FOG2 –/– mice. Pale and edematous, GATA4-V217G mice frequently exhibit pericardial hemorrhage. Whole mount immunostaining for the vascular endothelial markers ICAM-2 and Flk-1 showed a significant loss of coronary vessels in mice with reduced FOG2-GATA4 interactions. As in FOG2-deficient mice, the basic helix-loop-helix transcription factor E-Hand was downregulated in GATA4-V217G mice. However, more defects were found in GATA4-V217G mice than in FOG2 –/– mice, which suggests that GATA4 also interacts with FOG1 or other FOG-like proteins that contribute to the development of the heart (16). Equally likely is the suggestion that FOG2 may interact with other cardiac-restricted transcription factors. The findings of Huggins et al. (48) support this possibility; they used a yeast two-hybrid interaction screen to identify COUP–TF2 (chicken ovalbumin upstream promoter–transcription factor-2) and COUP–TF3 as binding partners for FOG2 (48). The interactions of FOG2 with COUP–TF2 and COUP–TF3 are specific because these interactions are eliminated by cysteine to serine mutations of the fifth and sixth zinc fingers of FOG2 and because FOG2 does not interact with RXRα (retinoid X receptor α), peroxisome proliferating antigen receptor γ, or glucocorticoid receptor (48). FOG2 represses GATA4-dependent transcription and increases the repression of GATA4-dependent transcription by COUP–TF2. These results support the conclusion that FOG2 interacts with multiple cardiac transcription factors to control the complex sequence of events required for vertebrate heart formation.

Retinoic Acid Receptor-α

Retinoic acid (RA) is essential for vertebrate embryonic development (49). RA affects embryonic cell fate and differentiation by binding to and activating a family of DNA binding proteins called retinoic acid receptors (RARs) and retinoid X receptors (RXRs), which are members of the steroid hormone receptor superfamily. RARs act in combination with a variety of co-activators and co-repressors to regulate transcription of retinoid-responsive target genes. In a mouse knockout model for the RXRα gene, cardiac failure is accompanied by significant structural defects of the heart (50). On histologic examination, RXRα-deficient hearts were hypoplastic with a thin ventricular free wall and had defects in the interventricular septum and valvular tissues. In RXRα-deficient embryos, expression of the myosin light chain-2a gene in the ventricles persists abnormally, which suggests a lack of maturation of the ventricular myocardium or mis-specification of the ventricle into an atrial fate (51). To determine if the cardiac defects indicated a requirement for retinoic acid signaling in developing myocytes, the RXRα gene was conditionally deleted in the myocardium by using only myosin light chain–2V promoter sequences to drive Cre recombinase (52). These mice developed normally, suggesting the requirement for RXRα function lies outside the myocardial lineage itself; RXRα activity may possibly be required in the epicardial lineage or for placenta formation, or both. Lineage-specific studies with selective gene deletion in each of these two embryonic tissues will help answer these questions.

Retinaldehyde Dehydrogenase 2

RALDH activity is the rate-limiting step in the in vivo synthesis of RA. Three members of the RALDH gene family have been identified; RALDH2, a nicotinamide adenine dinucleotide (NAD)–dependent dehydrogenase (53), is the first form of the enzyme expressed during embryonic development. Strongly expressed in the epicardium as it covers the heart tube (54,55), RALDH2 continues to be expressed by EPDCs in the subepicardial mesenchyme. The expression of RALDH2 decreases as EPDCs differentiate into coronary endothelial cells, fibroblasts, and smooth muscle cells (17). RALDH2-deficient mice die in utero beginning at E9.5 (56). The embryonic heart tube forms initially, but fails to undergo rightward looping. This failure of cardiac looping is accompanied by abnormal chamber formation, failure of trabeculation of the myocardium, precocious myocyte differentiation, outflow tract septation defects, and lack of development of endocardial cushions (57). These multiple cardiac defects can be restored to normal by incorporating RA in the mother's diet between E6.5 and E10.5. This finding indicates that the developmental defects are caused by lack of catalytic activity of RALDH2 rather than some other property of the protein. Another speculation is that cardiac defects in RALDH2 –/– embryos result from an absence of retinoid-producing EPDCs within the myocardial wall. The lack of improvement of outflow tract defects by exogenous RA is difficult to interpret. A higher concentration or more precise timing of RA delivery may be required to restore cardiac neural crest defects during heart development.

Erythropoietin and the Erythropoietin Receptor

Erythropoietin is an essential growth factor that regulates production of erythrocytes in mammals (58). In addition, erythropoietin is important in megakaryocyte differentiation and endothelial cell proliferation and acts as a neuronal survival factor (59). Erythropoietin-null mice die around E13.5 with multiple developmental defects, including cardiac defects. Failure of erythropoiesis in the fetal liver is caused by alterations in proliferation, survival, and differentiation of erythroid progenitors (60). Erythropoietin –/– mice are hypoxic, but the hypoxia alone cannot explain developmental defects in the myocardium. Both erythropoietin –/– and erythropoietin receptor (EPOR) –/– embryos are characterized by ventricular hypoplasia, particularly within the compact layer, and by defective formation of the interventricular septum (61). However, loss of erythropoietin receptor function in the myocardium alone does not produce cardiac developmental defects, because the hearts of these erythropoietin receptor –/– mice have a normal phenotype. This finding suggests that erythropoietin induces proliferation of cardiac myocytes by an indirect pathway, possibly by activating erythropoietin receptor on the endocardium or epicardium. The compact layer of myocardium is the most severely affected by the absence of erythropoietin signaling; therefore, the epicardium may be the source of a myocyte growth factor activity that is controlled by erythropoietin signaling. A similar role for an epicardial-derived myocardial mitogen was proposed for RA signaling, because cardiac myocyte–specific knockout of RXRα had no effect on cardiac development (52).

Alternatively, the effects of erythropoietin/erythropoietin receptor deficiency may affect either the establishment of the epicardial layer itself, which is frequently detached in mice lacking erythropoietin or erythropoietin receptors, or the development of subepicardial vessels, which are required to nourish the outer compact layer and meet its metabolic requirements for high rates of cell proliferation.

Because erythropoietin is mitogenic for endothelial cells, the lack of erythropoietin signaling may prevent normal coronary vasculogenesis, possibly by interfering with endothelial cell proliferation or survival, tube formation, or recruitment of a supporting pericyte or mural cell layer in the subepicardial space.

Notch2

The Notch family of proteins comprises four members (Notch 1–4). Notch protiens are evolutionarily conserved transmembrane receptors that interact with membrane-bound ligands encoded by the delta, serrate, and jagged genes. When a ligand binds to the extracellular domain of the notch protein, a signal is transmitted intracellularly by a process involving proteolysis of the receptor and nuclear translocation of the intracellular domain of the notch protein (63). Notch1 mutant embryos, which die around E9.5, are characterized by severe growth retardation, disorganized somite formation, and pyknotic neuroepithelium (64). In addition, angiogenic remodeling is defective in mice lacking Notch1 (65). Notch2 –/– mice die around E11.5 with similar growth retardation and widespread apoptosis. A Notch2 hypomorphic allele in mice resulted in death within 24 hours after birth and was associated with multiple defects in development of the kidney, including failure of glomerular capillary networks to form (66). About 40% of Notch2 hypomorphic embryos die around E11.5 with significant cardiac developmental defects, including a thin ventricular wall, reduced trabeculation, and hemorrhage into the pericardial sac. Because Notch2 is not expressed in the myocardium, these cardiac defects may be secondary to effects on neighboring cells. In this respect, the embryonic lethal cardiac phenotype of Notch2 mutants strongly resembles that resulting from ablation of the PEO in the chick embryo (3), deletion of the RXRα gene in mice, or several other targeted mutations that affect development and differentiation of the epicardium and its derivatives (Table 1).

Studies in zebrafish have shown that Notch signaling in the developing vasculature is required for proper arterial–venous differentiation (67). Thus, loss of Notch signaling leads to loss of expression of artery-specific markers and ectopic expression of venous markers within the dorsal aorta. In contrast, increased Notch signaling leads to repression of venous cell fate and corresponding defects in blood vessel formation associated with the loss of arterial–venous identity. Disruption of Notch signaling in zebrafish embryos causes ectopic formation of arteriovenous shunts between the dorsal aorta and cardinal vein and aberrant branching of the intersomitic vessels (67). In studies of bovine microvascular endothelial cells grown on a collagen gel, addition of an antisense jagged oligomer markedly increased invasion and tube formation in the underlying gel in response to fibroblast growth factor (FGF), but not VEGF (68). These findings suggest that jagged-notch signaling can regulate FGF-induced endothelial cell migration, which occurs early during angiogenesis in vivo.

Platelet-Derived Growth Factors and Receptors

Platelet-derived growth factors (PDGFs) belong to the PDGF/VEGF family of growth factors, which comprises at least seven different members (69). These factors bind to and activate type I transmembrane tyrosine kinase receptors. Newly formed capillaries in the peripheral and coronary vasculature require pericyte recruitment to survive and form a stable vascular network (70), and PDGF signaling is important in this recruitment process. Blood vessels acquire a pericyte or smooth muscle coating by two pathways. The first pathway, which is often independent of PDGF, involves de novo recruitment and differentiation of mesenchymal progenitors from surrounding mesenchyme. In the second pathway, upstream preexisting smooth muscle cells migrate and proliferate along a capillary basement membrane. The second pathway requires intact PDGF-B signaling via the PDGF β-receptor (71).

Expression of PDGF-B by endothelial cells is greater in angiogenic sprouts, or immature endothelial cells, than in mature endothelial cells of stable blood vessels. Moreover, PDGF β-receptor–positive cells are usually found clustered around these PDGF-B–expressing vessels. In PDGF-B –/– embryos, vessels in the brain, heart, skeletal muscle, and lung are deficient in recruiting pericytes and, therefore, are prone to degeneration and rupture. In the heart of embryos deficient for PDGF-B–dependent signaling via the PDGF-β receptor (72), intramyocardial-penetrating coronary arteries completely lack smooth muscle cells. Fewer smooth muscle cells are found in major subepicardial coronary vessels in PDGF β-receptor –/– embryos than in the vessels of wild type mice. These results suggest that penetrating coronary arteries recruit smooth muscle cells primarily by migration from preexisting upstream arteries. In addition, rates of vascular smooth muscle cell proliferation are reduced, suggesting that PDGF-B signaling plays two roles in coronary development (stimulation of SMC proliferation and SMC migration). In major subepicardial vessels, some other mechanism appears to be involved in the initial recruitment of smooth muscle cells (possibly via TGF-β), and PDGF-B provides a mitogenic stimulus for expansion of the smooth muscle cell pool. In penetrating coronary branch vessels, PDGF-B signaling acts as a chemotactant to induce downstream migration of preexisting smooth muscle cells and as a mitogen to stimulate proliferation of newly recruited smooth muscle cells.

Brain-Derived Neurotrophic Factor

Brain-derived neurotrophic factor (BDNF) is a member of the nerve growth factor (NGF) family of neurotrophins, which were first described because of their survival activity for sympathetic neurons (73). Although found in the adult heart, BDNF is expressed only in coronary artery and capillary endothelial cells and not in coronary veins (74). The signaling receptor for BDNF, trk-B, is expressed by endothelial cells and smooth muscle cells of the coronary vasculature, suggesting that BDNF may have both autocrine and paracrine functions. BDNF expression begins around E17.5 during cardiac development and peaks at around postnatal day 2. The time frame for trk-B is similar, but expression begins a day later and reaches high levels in the neonatal heart. BDNF-deficient mice die in the early postnatal period, which indicates that BDNF has other essential functions in addition to its neurotrophic effects (75). The early stages of coronary vasculogenesis in BDNF-null mice are normal, but intramyocardial hemorrhage involving the subepicardial coronary arteries begins around E16.5 (74). Ultrastructural analysis has shown degenerative changes in the coronary endothelium of BDNF −/− mice that selectively involved arterial, not venous, endothelial cells. Apoptosis rates were considerably higher in BDNF −/− coronary endothelial cells than in wild type coronary vessels. Thus, BDNF is important for survival of coronary endothelial cells during development and maturation of the coronary vasculature in vivo.

Vascular Endothelial Growth Factor-A

VEGF-A, originally called vascular permeability factor (VPF), was discovered in the early 1980s by Dvorak and colleagues (76) as a factor that made blood vessels leaky. Several groups later showed that VEGF/VPF also stimulated endothelial cell migration and proliferation and was a potent angiogenic factor in vivo (77,78). Four different VEGF family members (VEGF A–D) have been characterized with different binding selectivities for three VEGF receptor tyrosine kinases, VEGF-R1–3. VEGF-A, a heat-stable, 46 kDa dimeric protein with distant homology to PDGF, is produced as four different isoforms generated by alternative splicing. Two isoforms, VEGF-120 and VEGF-165, are secreted forms of VEGF, whereas the other two isoforms, VEGF-189 and VEGF-221, are membrane-bound.

Carmeliet and coworkers (79) used gene targeting methods to produce mice that make VEGF-120 as their sole form of VEGF-A. These mice are phenotypically normal at birth, suggesting that VEGF-120 alone is sufficient to support early vascular development. In contrast, complete VEGF-A–null mice die in utero around E9.5, and embryonic death occurs even if only one copy of the VEGF-A gene is deleted (80). VEGF-120-deficient mice are born alive, but about half die within a few hours after birth because of hemorrhage in various tissues (79). The other half die of cardiac failure before postnatal day 12. Upon dissection, the hearts of VEGF-120 mice are enlarged and structurally dysmorphic, and they beat weakly. Reduced heart rate, decreased left ventricular output, impaired left ventricular contractility, and periods of spontaneous arrhythmia were observed. In addition, right ventricular failure was found, but renal function, liver function, great vessel anatomy, and the levels of circulating blood cells were normal. On histologic analysis of hearts from VEGF-120 mice, the number of capillaries in myocardial tissue was reduced because angiogenesis failed to keep pace with normal myocardial tissue growth in the postnatal period. As a result, progressive ischemia developed, which led eventually to myocardial necrosis and cell death. Capillary density was similarly reduced in kidney and skeletal muscle. These findings could mean either that too little VEGF-120 was made to maintain normal levels of total VEGF-A activity during tissue growth, or that different VEGF isoforms have different biological activities, and VEGF-120 cannot replace VEGF-165 or VEGF-189. In support of the latter possibility, Soker et al. (81) found that VEGF-165, but not VEGF-120, specifically binds to neuropilin-1. Binding of VEGF-165 to neuropilin-1 activates flk1/VEGF-R2 by VEGF-165 and increases the chemotactic and mitogenic effects of VEGF-165 on endothelial cells.

Neuropilin-1 is a membrane-bound protein that was first described in developing neurons, where it functions in a receptor complex for the class 3 semaphorins, which are inhibitory axon guidance signals. Targeted inactivation of the neuropilin-1 gene in mice showed that neuropilin-1 regulates nerve fiber guidance in embryogenesis (82). Neuropilin-1 is also made by endothelial cells in developing blood vessels, including coronary arteries. Constitutive overexpression of neuropilin-1 in transgenic mice resulted in greater than normal density of capillary-sized vessels, dilation of blood vessels, malformed hearts, and death of embryos at midgestation (83). The production of transgenic mice expressing other isoform-specific variants of VEGF-A as their sole source of VEGF-A will clarify whether each isoform of VEGF has a unique function in angiogenesis.

Vascular Endothelial Growth Factor-B

The importance of genes in coronary vessels is not always demonstrated by developmental defects upon introduction of null alleles into the germline. For example, VEGF-B knockout mice are indistinguishable from wild type mice at birth. Although normal at postnatal day 9 (P9), heart weight to body weight ratios were significantly reduced in VEGF-B −/− mice at P25 *(84)*. Capillary density (2300 *c*apillaries/mm²) in the ventricular myocardium was similar in wild type and VEGF-B −/− mice on histologic examination. However, functional differences in cardiac performance were evident when tested in ex vivo preparations of the perfused working heart. Global ischemia-reperfusion studies showed increased diastolic pressure, increased peak contracture, and decreased recovery of contractile function in VEGF-B −/− hearts. In addition, flow-mediated dilation of coronary vessels was reduced in VEGF-B −/− hearts, which predisposes the working myocytes to hypoxia and ischemic injury *(84)*.

DEVELOPMENT OF CORONARY LYMPHATIC VESSELS

Blood and lymphatic vessels develop along parallel, but independent, pathways to form a complete and functional circulatory system *(85)*. Lymphatic vessels collect the extravasated cells and protein-rich interstitial fluid for transport back into the venous cirulation. The lymphatic system comprises an extensive series of capillaries and collecting vessels and ducts. The larger lymphatic vessels are surrounded by a smooth muscle layer that contracts automatically when the vessel becomes stretched with fluid. In addition, the lymphatic vessels function as part of the immune system by transporting white blood cells within the lymphoid organs (thymus, spleen, lymph nodes, tonsils) and the bone marrow. Lymphatic drainage of the coronary arteries is via the adventitial lymphatic network and the subepicardial lymphatic plexus *(86,87)*. Prelymphatic channels are formed by collagen fibrils in the coronary media and function initially to transport interstitial fluid toward the adventitial and periadventitial lymphatic vessels. The smaller arterioles within the myocardium that branch off from penetrating coronary arteries have many more accompanying lymphatic channels than do the main epicardial coronary arteries. Coronary contraction in the radial and longitudinal directions helps propel coronary interstitial fluid toward drainage via adventitial lymphatics.

VEGF is important in lymphatic vessel development. VEGF-C and VEGF-D are ligands for flt4/VEGF-R3, a receptor with intrinsic, ligand-activated tyrosine kinase activity whose expression is limited mainly to lymphatic endothelial cells. Overexpression of VEGF-C in the skin leads to excessive production of lymphatic vessels in the dermis via activation of VEGF-R3 *(88)*. In the chorioallantoic membrane assay, VEGF-C is a highly specific lymphangiogenic factor, but in other studies VEGF-C stimulates angiogenesis via activation of VEGF-R2 *(89)*. In contrast, VEGF-D is highly selective for VEGF-R3 and is a potent lymphangiogenic factor when overexpressed in the skin *(90)*. Mouse embryos deficient in VEGF-R3 die around embryonic day 9.5 with fluid accumulation in the pericardial cavity and cardiac failure secondary to defective large vessel formation *(91)*.

Interstitial myocardial edema, which occurs in several clinical conditions, is usually associated with decreased left ventricular function. In a model of induced myocardial edema in dogs, left ventricular systolic function was not altered although end-diastolic pressure increased significantly from baseline by 3 hours after induction of lymphedema *(92)*. Thus, interstitial myocardial edema may have a direct causal association with diastolic stiffness but has no clear deleterious effect on systolic function in the left ventricle.

CORONARY DEVELOPMENT AND DISEASE

Coronary Anomalies—A Developmental Basis

Coronary anomalies are defined on the basis of what is generally accepted to be normal coronary anatomy. Because of the range of structure of coronary vessels seen in the population, the term "normal" is defined as the interval that falls between two standard deviations from the mean value. According to the classification scheme proposed by Angelini et al. *(93)*, coronary anomalies can be divided into anomalies of origination and course and anomalies of intrinsic coronary anatomy. In anomalies of origination and course, isolated absence of a left main coronary trunk is defined as the condition in which both the left anterior descending and circumflex arteries originate directly from the center section of the left sinus of Valsalva without having a common trunk. According to a study at the Texas Heart Institute *(94)*, the absence of a left main coronary trunk occurs in 0.5–1.0% of the population. Anomalous origin of a coronary ostium outside the normal aortic sinuses includes ectopic origin of a coronary ostium at or near the noncoronary (right posterior) aortic sinus, ectopic origin arising within the ascending aorta, ectopic origin arising from the left ventricle, ectopic origin arising from the right ventricle, and ectopic origin from the pulmonary artery.

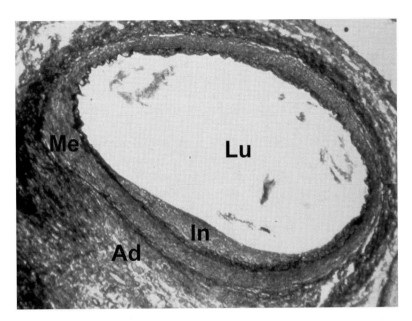

Fig. 6. Intimal thickening in newborn human coronary artery. Smooth muscle cell–containing focal intimal masses are present in human fetal and newborn coronary arteries at sites where atherosclerosis develops later in life. Lu, lumen; In, intima; Me, media; Ad, adventitia.

These anomalous origins occur in 0.1–1.2% of the population *(93)*. Reports of coronary arteries arising from the aortic arch, innominate artery, internal mammary artery, subclavian artery, or descending thoracic aorta are rare *(95,96)*. When a single aortic origin accounts for all coronary blood flow, the condition is usually called single coronary artery *(97)*. With an incidence of about 0.025%, single coronary artery includes a mixture of various coronary origins whose common element is the presence of a single aortic ostium *(98)*.

The category of anomalies of intrinsic coronary anatomy includes coronary arteries that are stenosed or atretic because of a membrane or fibrotic ridge that forms at or near the aortic orifice *(99,100)*. Another intrinsic anomaly, coronary ectasia, can be divided into primary ectasia, in which a localized coronary segment has a disproportionately large diameter, and secondary ectasia, which is defined as a diffuse coronary dilatation in which the entire coronary artery is enlarged secondary to fistulous flow *(101,102)*. Intramural coronary artery is a condition in which the normally subepicardial coronaries and their branches prematurely penetrate the myocardial wall and interventricular septum. Intramural coronary artery occurs in approximately 1% of instances in which it has been examined *(103)*. In rare cases, the right coronary artery, left anterior descending or left circumflex coronary artery takes a subendocardial course after penetrating the myocardium; this condition is an example of a larger category of "coronary malpositions" *(104)*.

Coronary anomalies and their pathophysiological significance have been reviewed extensively elsewhere *(105–107)*.

Coronary Disease—Atherosclerosis

Intimal masses are present in human fetal coronary arteries at sites where atherosclerosis develops later in life (Fig. 6). These intimal masses are initially found in the left anterior descending coronary artery around 6 months gestation and are eccentric in appearance *(108,109)*. By 6 months after birth, the coronary intima has enlarged and become concentric and uniform. Histological evidence of intimal thickening has been reported in 38% of human coronary arteries examined at birth and in 100% of arteries in infants examined at 3 to 6 months of age *(109)*. Intimal/medial ratios increase progressively in the left and right main coronary arteries from 6 months gestation to birth *(110)* and in the left main coronary artery from birth to 2 years of age *(109)*. Intimal tissue comprises mainly smooth muscle cells and associated extracellular matrix proteins; however, macrophages have been seen in the intimal masses by some investigators *(111)* but not others *(109)*. At branch points, coronary vessels develop a complex organization, which includes large pads or intimal cushions composed of a thick intima and many longitudinal muscle bundles (see below). Some coronary vessels have a spiral course at the level of branch origins and form muscle rings around the entrance orifices *(110)*.

Shortly after birth, human coronary arteries develop a second layer of media in which smooth muscle cells are oriented in subintimal longitudinal bundles rather than in the circumferential pattern seen in the outer media *(110,112)*. These longitudinal bundles, which make up the musculoelastic layer *(109)*, are not present in other organs in similar-sized muscular arteries such as the basilar, internal mammary, renal, hepatic, or bronchial arteries. The striking development of this unique longitudinal muscle layer suggests that coronary arteries are subjected to greater mechanical forces in the longitudinal direction than major arteries from other organs. In addition, the formation of this longitudinal muscle layer may allow coronary arteries to contract in the longitudinal direction, which could assist in propelling blood through the coronary circuit. The early appearance of coronary intimal masses and the formation of a pronounced longitudinal smooth muscle layer within the tunica media are unique aspects of coronary development that may predispose these vessels to coronary atherosclerosis and vasospasm later in life.

CONCLUSIONS

Development of the coronary vasculature depends upon progenitor cells that enter the heart from extracardiac sources. Lineage mapping studies have shown that mesothelial cells in the PEO, together with cardiac neural crest–derived mesenchymal cells, give rise to coronary endothelial cells, smooth muscle cells, and adventitial fibroblasts. The process of EMT produces migratory and invasive cells in a highly controlled spatiotemporal pattern and is critical to the generation of both neural crest–derived and proepicardium-derived coronary progenitor cells. These mesenchymal cells enter the myocardial wall and participate in signaling interactions that are necessary for both coronary wall assembly and proliferation of ventricular myocytes within the developing myocardium. The presence of blood island–like structures in the subepicardium suggests that coronary vessels arise by vasculogenesis, first in the subepicardial space and then in the atrioventricular groove region. A coronary plexus subsequently forms around the truncus arteriosus, and coronary vessels from this plexus invade the aortic root to form an arterial connection. This invasion usually produces two persistent coronary stems that form the right and left main coronary arteries. Defects in this invasion process can produce various anomalies of coronary origin, including single coronary artery, ectopic origin from the left ventricle, and ectopic origin from the pulmonary artery. The onset of unidirectional blood flow through the primitive coronary circuit results in recruitment of a supporting smooth

muscle layer to form the tunica media and in extensive remodeling of the coronary network.

Genetic studies of coronary development have identified important roles for specific soluble factors (RA, VEGF-A, BDNF, PDGF-B), adhesion molecules (VCAM-1, α4-integrin), cell surface receptors (Notch2, EPOR, PDGF-B receptor), and transcriptional regulators (WT1, FOG2, GATA4). Future studies in mice and humans will expand this list and define genetic and molecular pathways involved in the complex process of coronary vessel development. In addition, these studies will identify candidate genes for understanding the genetic basis of coronary anomalies. Finally, the striking evidence that intimal masses are present at birth in locations that are predisposed to develop clinically significant coronary atherosclerosis later in life emphasizes the need for a detailed understanding of the cellular and genetic basis of coronary vessel formation during heart development.

ACKNOWLEDGMENTS

I would like to thank Robert J. Tomanek, Takashi Mikawa, Robert J. Schwartz, and Karen K. Hirschi for helpful discussions during preparation of this chapter. This work was supported by grants from the National Institutes of Health and the American Heart Association. The author is an established investigator of the American Heart Association.

REFERENCES

1. Tomanek R. Formation of the coronary vasculature: a brief review. Cardiovasc Res 1996;31:E46–E51.
2. Mikawa T, Gourdie R. Pericardial mesoderm generates a population of coronary smooth muscle cells migrating into the heart along with ingrowth of the epicardial organ. Dev Biol 1996;174:221–232.
3. Gittenberger-de Groot A, Vrancken Peeters M, Mentink M, Gourdie R, Poelmann R. Epicardium-derived cells contribute a novel population to the myocardial wall and the atrioventricular cushions. Circ Res 1998;82:1043–1052.
4. Manner J, Perez-Pomares J, Macias D, Munoz-Chapuli R. The origin, formation and developmental significance of the epicardium: A review. Cells Tissues Organs 2001;169:89–103.
5. Manasek F. Embryonic development of the heart. I. A light and electron microscopic study of myocardial development in the early chick embryo. J Morphol 1968;125:329–365.
6. Viragh S, Challice C. The origin of the epicardium and the embryonic myocardial circulation in the mouse. Anat Rec 1981;201:157–168.
7. Hiruma T, Hirakow R. Epicardial formation in embryonic chick heart. Am J Anat 1989;184:129–138.
8. Viragh S, Challice C. Origin and differentiation of cardiac muscle cells in the mouse. J Ultrastruct Res 1973;42:1–24.
9. Ho E, Shimada Y. Formation of the epicardium studied with the scanning electron microscope. Dev Biol 1978;66:579–585.

10. Manner J. The development of pericardial villi in the chick embryo. Anat Embryol 1992;186:379–385.

11. Komiyama M, Ito K, Shimada Y. Origin and development of the epicardium in the mouse embryo. Anat Embryol 1987;176:183–189.

12. Gittenberger-de Groot A, Vrancken-Peeters M, Bergwerff M, Mentink M, Poelmann R. Epicardial outgrowth inhibition leads to compensatory mesothelial outflow tract collar and abnormal cardiac septation and coronary formation. Circ Res 2000;87:969–971.

13. Dettman R, Denetclaw W, Ordahl C, Bristow J. Common epicardial origin of coronary vascular smooth muscle, perivascular fibroblasts, and intermyocardial fibroblasts in the avian heart. Dev Biol 1998;193:169–181.

14. Perez-Pomares J, Macias D, Garcia-Garrido L, Munoz-Chapuli R. The origin of the subepicardial mesenchyme in the avian embryo: An immunohistochemical and quail-chick chimera study. Dev Biol 1998;200:57–68.

15. Tevosian S, Deconinck A, Tanaka M, et al. FOG-2, a cofactor for GATA transcription factors, is essential for heart morphogenesis and development of coronary vessels from epicardium. Cell 2000;101:729–739.

16. Crispino J, Lodish M, Thurberg B, et al. Proper coronary vascular development and heart morphogenesis depend on interaction of GATA4 with FOG cofactors. Genes Dev 2001;15:839–844.

17. Perez-Pomares J, Phelps A, Sedmerova M, et al. Experimental studies on the spatiotemporal expression of WT1 and RALDH2 in the embryonic avian heart: A model for the regulation of myocardial and valvuloseptal development by epicardially derived cells (EPDCs). Dev Biol 2002;247:307–326.

18. Vrancken Peeters M, Gittenberger-de GA, Mentink M, Hungerford J, Little C, Poelmann R. The development of the coronary vessels and their differentiation into arteries and veins in the embryonic quail heart. Dev Dyn 1997;208:338–348.

19. Bogers A, Gittenberger-de Groot A, Poelmann R, Peault B, Huysmans H. Development of the origin of the coronary arteries, a matter of ingrowth or outgrowth? Anat Embryol 1989;180:437–441.

20. Waldo K, Willner W, Kirby M. Origin of the proximal coronary artery stems and a review of ventricular vascularization in the chick embryo. Am J Anat 1990;188:109–120.

21. Hood L, Rosenquist T. Coronary artery development in the chick: Origin and deployment of smooth muscle cells, and the effects of neural crest ablation. Anat Rec 1992;234:291–300.

22. Poelmann R, Gittenberger-de Groot A, Mentink M, Bokenkamp R, Hogers B. Development of the cardiac coronary vascular endothelium, studied with antiendothelial antibodies, in chicken-quail chimeras. Circ Res 1993;73:559–568.

23. Mikawa T, Fishman D. Retroviral analysis of cardiac morphogenesis: Discontinuous formation of coronary vessels. Proc Natl Acad Sci U S A 1992;89:9504–9508.

24. Viragh S, Gittenberger-de GA, Poelmann R, Kalman F. Early development of quail heart epicardium and associated vascular and glandular structures. Anat Embryol 1993;188:381–393.

25. Hutchins G, Kessler-Hanna A, Moore G. Development of the coronary arteries in the embryonic human heart. Circulation 1988;77:1250–1257.

26. Hirakow R. Epicardial formation in staged human embryos. Kaibogaku Zasshi 1992;67:616–622.

27. Cormier F, Dieterlen-Lievre F. Long-term cultures of chicken bone marrow cells. Exp Cell Res 1990;190:113–117.

28. Munoz-Chapuli R, Perez-Pomares J, Macias D, Garcia-Garrido L, Carmona R, Gonzalez M. Differentiation of hemangioblasts from embryonic mesothelial cells? A model on the origin of the vertebrate cardiovascular system. Differentiation 1999;64:133–141.

29. Jiang X, Rowitch DH, Soriano P, McMahon AP, Sucov HM. Fate of the mammalian cardiac neural crest. Development 2000;127:1607–1616.

30. Echelard Y, Vassileva G, McMahon A. *Cis*-acting regulatory sequences governing *Wnt-1* expression in the developing mouse CNS. Development 1994;120:2213–2224.

31. Wrenn R, Raeuber C, Herman L, Walton W, Rosenquist T. Transforming growth factor-beta: signal transduction via protein kinase C in cultured embryonic vascular smooth muscle cells. In Vitro Cell Dev Biol 1993;29A:73–78.

32. Topouzis S, Majesky M. Smooth muscle lineage diversity in the chick embryo: Two types of aortic SMC differ in growth and receptor-mediated signaling responses to transforming growth factor-beta. Dev Biol 1996;178:430–445.

33. Gadson PJ, Dalton M, Patterson E, et al. Differential response of mesoderm- and neural crest-derived smooth muscle to TGF-beta1: regulation of c-myb and alpha1 (I) procollagen genes. Exp Cell Res 1997;230:169–180.

34. Yang J, Rayburn H, Hynes R. Cell adhesion events mediated by α4 integrins are essential in placental and cardiac development. Development 1995;121:549–560.

35. Sengubusch J, He W, Pinco K, Yang J. Dual functions of α4β1 integrin in epicardial development: initial migration and long-term attachment. J Cell Biol 2002;157:873–882.

36. Kwee L, Baldwin H, Shen H, et al. Defective development of the embryonic and extraembryonic circulatory systems in vascular cell adhesion molecule (VCAM-1) deficient mice. Development 1995;121:489–503.

37. Gurtner G, Davis V, Li H, McCoy M, Sharpe A, Cybulsky M. Targeted disruption of the murine VCAM1 gene: essential role of VCAM-1 in chorioallantoic fusion and placentation. Genes Dev 1995;9:1–14.

38. Armstrong J, Pritchard-Jones K, Bickmore W, Hastie N, Bard J. The expression of the Wilms' tumour gene, WT1, in the developing mammalian embryo. Mech Dev 1993;40:85–97.

39. Hastie N. Life, sex, and WT1 isoforms—three amino acids can make all the difference. Cell 2001;106:391–394.

40. Kriedberg J, Sariola H, Loring J, et al. WT-1 is required for early kidney development. Cell 1993;74:679–691.

41. Moore A, McInnes L, Kreidberg J, Hastie N, Schedl A. YAC complementation shows a requirement for Wt1 in the development of epicardium, adrenal gland, and throughout nephrogenesis. Development 1999;126:1845–1857.

42. Simon M. Gotta have GATA. Nat Genet 1995;11:9–11.

43. Lu J, McKinsey T, Xu H, Wang D, Richardson J, Olson E. FOG-2, a heart- and brain-enriched cofactor for GATA transcription factors. Mol Cell Biol 1999;19:4495–4502.

44. Cantor A, Orkin S. Transcriptional regulation of erythropoiesis: an affair involving multiple partners. Oncogene 2002;21:3368–3376.

45. Tevosian S, Deconinck A, Cantor A, et al. Fog2: A novel GATA-family cofactor related to multitype zinc-finger proteins Friend of GATA and U-shaped. Proc Natl Acad Sci U S A 1999;96:950–955.

46. Svensson E, Tufts R, Polk C, Leiden J. Molecular cloning of FOG-2: A modulator of transcription factor GATA-4 in cardiomyocytes. Proc Natl Acad Sci U S A 1999;96:956–961.

47. Svensson E, Huggins G, Lin H, et al. A syndrome of tricuspid atresia in mice with a targeted mutation of the gene encoding Fog-2. Nature Genet 2000;25:353–356.

48. Huggins G, Bacani C, Boltax J, Aikawa R, Leiden J. Friend of GATA 2 physically interacts with chicken ovalbumin upstream promoter-TF2 (COUP-TF2) and COUP-TF3 and represses COUP-TF2-dependent activation of the atrial natriuretic factor promoter. J Biol Chem 2001;276:28029–28036.

49. Eichele G. A vital role for vitamin A. Nat Genet 1999;21:346–347.

50. Sucov H, Dyson E, Gumeringer C, Price J, Chien K, Evans R. RXR alpha mutant mice establish a genetic basis for vitamin A signaling in heart morphogenesis. Genes Dev 1994;8:1007–1018.

51. Dyson E, Sucov H, Kubalak S, et al. Atrial-like phenotype is associated with embryonic ventricular failure in RXRα–/– mice. Proc Natl Acad Sci U S A 1995;92:7386–7390.

52. Chen J, Kubalak S, Chien K. Ventricular muscle-restricted targeting of the RXRα gene reveals a non-cell-autonomous requirement in cardiac chamber morphogenesis. Development 1998;125:1943–1949.

53. Zhao D, McCaffery P, Ivins K, et al. Molecular identification of a major retinoic-acid-synthesizing enzyme, a retinaldehyde-specific dehydrogenase. Eur J Biochem 1996;240:15–22.

54. Xavier-Neto J, Shapiro M, Houghton L, Rosenthal N. Sequential programs of retinoic acid synthesis in the myocardial and epicardial layers of the developing avian heart. Dev Biol 2000;219:129–141.

55. Niederreither K, Fraulob V, Garnier J, Chambon P, Dolle P. Differential expression of retinoic acid-synthesizing (RALDH) enzymes during fetal development and organ differentiation in the mouse. Mech Dev 2002;110:165–171.

56. Niederreither K, Subbarayan V, Dolle P, Chambon P. Embryonic retinoic acid synthesis is essential for early mouse post-implantation development. Nat Genet 1999;21:444–448.

57. Niederreither K, Vermot J, Messaddeq N, Schuhbaur B, Chambon P, Dolle P. Embryonic retinoic acid synthesis is essential for heart morphogenesis in the mouse. Development 2001;128:1019–1031.

58. Krantz S. Erythropoietin. Blood 1991;77:419–434.

59. Digicaylioglu M, Bichet S, Marti H, et al. Localization of specific erythropoietin binding sites in defined areas of the mouse brain. Proc Natl Acad Sci U S A 1995;92:3717–3720.

60. Lin C, Lim S, D'Agati V, Constantini F. Differential effects of an erythropoietin receptor gene disruption on primitive and definitive erythropoiesis. Genes Dev 1996;10:154–164.

61. Wu H, Lee S, Gao J, Liu X, Iruela-Arispe M. Inactivation of erythropoietin leads to defects in cardiac morphogenesis. Development 1999;126:3597–3605.

62. Asahara T, Chen D, Takahashi T, et al. Tie2 receptor ligands, angiopoietin-1 and angiopoietin-2, modulate VEGF-induced postnatal neovascularization. Circ Res 1998;83:233–240.

63. Artavanis-Tsokonas S, Rand M, Lake R. Notch signaling: cell fate and signal integration in development. Science 1999; 284:770–776.

64. Conlon R, Reaume A, Rossant J. Notch1 is required for the coordinate segmentation of somites. Development 1995;121: 1533–1545.

65. Krebs LT, Xue Y, Norton CR, et al. Notch signaling is essential for vascular morphogenesis in mice. Genes Dev 2000;14:1343–1352.

66. McCright B, Gao X, Shen L, et al. Defects in development of the kidney, heart and eye vasculature in mice homozygous for a hypomorphic Notch2 mutation. Development 2001;128: 491–502.

67. Lawson N, Scheer N, Pham V, et al. Notch signaling is required for arterial-venous differentiation during embryonic vascular development. Development 2001;128:3675–3683.

68. Zimrin AB PM, McMahon GA, Nguyen F, Montesano R, Maciag T. An antisense oligonucleotide to the notch ligand jagged enhances fibroblast growth factor-induced angiogenesis in vitro. J Biol Chem 1996;271:32499–32502.

69. Heldin C, Westermark B. Mechanisms of action and in vivo role of platelet-derived growth factor. Physiol Rev 1999;79: 1283–1316.

70. Benjamin L, Hemo I, Keshet E. A plasticity window for blood vessel remodeling is defined by pericyte coverage of the preformed endothelial network and is regulated by PDGF-B and VEGF. Development 1998;125:1591–1598.

71. Lindahl P, Johansson B, Leveen P, Betsholtz C. Pericyte loss and microaneurysm formation in PDGF-B-deficient mice. Science 1997;277:242–245.

72. Hellstrom M, Kalen M, Lindahl P, Abramsson A, Betsholtz C. Role of PDGF-B and PDGFR-β in recruitment of vascular smooth muscle cells and pericytes during embryonic blood vessel formation in the mouse. Development 1999;126: 3047–3055.

73. Levi-Montalcini R, Booker B. Destruction of the sympathetic ganglia in mammals by an antiserum to the nerve growth factor. Proc Natl Acad Sci U S A 1960;46:384–390.

74. Donovan M, Lin M, Weign P, et al. Brain derived neurotrophic factor is an endothelial cell survival factor required for intramyocardial vessel stabilization. Development 2000;127:4531–4540.

75. Ernfors P, Lee K, Jaenisch R. Mice lacking brain-derived neurotrophic factor develop with sensory deficits. Nature 1994; 368:147–150.

76. Senger D, Galli S, Dvorak A, Perruzzi C, Harvey V, Dvorak H. Tumor cells secrete a vascular permeability factor that promotes accumulation of ascites fluid. Science 1983;219: 983–985.

77. Ferrara N, Henzel W. Pituitary follicular cells secrete a novel heparin-binding growth factor specific for vascular endothelial cells. Biochem Biophys Res Commun 1989;161: 851–855.

78. Connolly D, Heuvelman D, Nelson R, et al. Tumor vascular permeability factor stimulates endothelial cell growth and angiogenesis. J Clin Invest 1989;84:1470–1478.

79. Carmeliet P, Ng Y-S, Nuyens D, et al. Impaired myocardial angiogenesis and ischemic cardiomyopathy in mice lacking the vascular endothelial growth factor isoforms VEGF164 and VEGF188. Nat Med 1999;5:495–502.

80. Carmeliet P, Ferreira V, Breier G, et al. Abnormal blood vessel development and lethality in embryos lacking a single VEGF allele. Nature 1996;380:435–439.

81. Soker S, Takashima S, Miao H, Neufeld G, Klagsbrun M. Neuropilin-1 is expressed by endothelial and tumor cells as an isoform-specific receptor for vascular endothelial growth factor. Cell 1998;92:735–745.

82. Miao H, Soker S, Feiner L, Alonso J, Raper J, Klagsbrun M. Neuropilin-1 mediates collapsin-1/semiohorin III inhibition of endothelial cell motility: functional competition of collapsin-1 and vascular endothelial growth factor-165. J Cell Biol 1999;146:233–242.

83. Kitsukawa T, Shimono A, Kawakami A, Kondoh H, Fujisawa H. Overexpression of a membrane protein, neuropilin, in chimeric mice causes anomalies in the cardiovascular system, nervous system and limbs. Development 1995;121:4309–4318.

84. Bellomo D, Headrick J, Silins G, et al. Mice lacking the vascular endothelial growth factor-B gene (vegfb) have smaller hearts, dysfunctional coronary vasculature and impaired recovery from cardiac ischemia. Circ Res 2000;86:e29–e35.

85. Jussila L, Alitalo K. Vascular growth factors and lymphangiogenesis. Physiol Rev 2002;82:673–700.

86. Eliska O, Eliskova M, Miller A. The morphology of the lymphatics of the coronary arteries in the dog. Lymphology 1999; 32:45–57.

87. Sacchi G, Weber E, Agliano M, Cavina N, Comparini L. Lymphatic vessels of the human heart: precollectors and collecting vessels. A morpho-structural study. J Submicrosc Cytol Pathol 1999;31:515–525.

88. Jeltsch M, Kaipainen A, Joukov V, et al. Hyperplasia of lymphatic vessels in VEGF-C transgenic mice. Science 1997;276: 1423–1425.

89. Cao Y, Linden P, Farnebo J, et al. Vascular endothelial growth factor C induces angiogenesis in vivo. Proc Natl Acad Sci U S A 1998;95:14389–14394.

90. Veikkola T, Jussila L, Makinen T, et al. Signaling via vascular endothelial growth factor receptor-3 is sufficient for lymphangiogenesis in transgenic mice. EMBO J 2001;20: 1223–1231.

91. Dumont D, Jussila L, Taipale J, et al. Cardiovascular failure in mouse embryos deficient in VEGF receptor-3. Science 1998;282:946–949.

92. Miyamoto M, McClure D, Schertel E, et al. Effects of hypoproteinemia-induced myocardial edema on left ventricular function. Am J Physiol 1998;274:H937–H944.

93. Angelini P, Villason S, Chan AJ, Diez J. Normal and anomalous coronary arteries in humans. In: Angelini P, ed. *Coronary Artery Anomalies.* Philadelphia, Pa: Lippincott, Williams & Wilkins; 1999:27–79.

94. Angelini P. Embryology and congenital heart disease. Tex Heart Inst J 1995;22:1–12.

95. Blake H, Manion W, Mattingly T. Coronary artery anomalies. Circulation 1964;30:927–936.

96. Click R, Holmes DJ, Vlietstra R, Kosinski A, Kronmal R. Anomalous coronary arteries: location, degree of atherosclerosis and effect on survival—a report from the Coronary Artery Surgery Study. J Am Coll Cardiol 1990;15:507–508.

97. Hillestad L, Eie H. Single coronary artery. Acta Med Scand 1971;189:409–413.

98. Shirani J, Roberts W. Solitary coronary ostium in the aorta in the absence of other major congenital cardiovascular anomalies. J Am Coll Cardiol 1993;21:137–143.

99. Fortuin N, Roberts W. Congenital atresia of the left main coronary artery. Am J Med 1971;50:385–389.

100. Harada K, Ito T, Suzuki Y. Congenital atresia of left coronary ostium. Eur J Pediatr 1993;152:539–540.

101. Seabra-Gomes R, Somerville J, Ross D, Emanuel R, Parker D, Wong M. Congenital coronary artery aneurysms. Br Heart J 1974;36:329–335.

102. Drexler H, Zeiher A, Wollschlager H, Meinertz T, Just H, Bonzel T. Flow-dependent coronary artery dilatation in humans. Circulation 1989;80:466–474.

103. Reig J, Ruiz de Miguel C, Moragas A. Morphometric analysis of myocardial bridges in children with ventricular hypertrophy. Pediatr Cardiol 1990;11:186–190.

104. Kolodziej A, Lobo F, Walley V. Intra-arterial course of the right coronary artery and its branches. Can J Cardiol 1994;10: 263–267.

105. Angelini P, Velasco J, Flamm S. Coronary anomalies: Incidence, pathophysiology and clinical relevance. Circulation 2002;105:2449–2454.

106. Williams R. The Athlete and Heart Disease: Diagnosis, Evaluation and Management. In: Williams R, ed. Philadelphia: Lippincott, Williams & Wilkins, 1998.

107. Gittenberger de-Groot A, Powlmann R, Bartelings M. Embryology of congenital heart disease. In: Braunwald E, ed. Atlas of Heart Diseases: Congenital Heart Disease. Philadelphia, Pa: Current Medicine;1997:3.1–3.10.

108. Velican D, Velican C. Intimal thickening in developing coronary arteries and its relevance to atherosclerotic involvement. Atherosclerosis 1976;23:345–355.

109. Ikari Y, McManus B, Kenyon J, Schwartz S. Neonatal intima formation in the human coronary artery. Arterioscler Thromb Vasc Biol 1999;19:2036–2040.

110. Velican C, Velican D. Some particular aspects of the microarchitecture of human coronary arteries. Atherosclerosis 1979; 33:191–200.

111. Stary H. Macrophage foam cells in the coronary artery intima of human infants. Ann N Y Acad Sci 1985;454:5–8.

112. Neufeld H, Wagnevoort C, Edwards J. Coronary arteries in fetuses, infants, juveniles and young adults. Lab Invest 1962;11:837–844.

12 Atherosclerosis

George A. Stouffer, MD

CONTENTS

INTRODUCTION AND EPIDEMIOLOGY

Cardiovascular disease, the most common cause of death in the developed world *(1)*, causes more deaths in the United States than the next six leading causes combined. More than 2600 Americans die of cardiovascular disease each day. Furthermore, more than 12 million Americans have coronary artery disease, and more than 4.5 million have suffered a stroke. The American Heart Association (AHA) estimates that 20% of the population has some form of cardiovascular disease *(2)*. These startling statistics are accurate despite a 22% decrease from 1988 to 1998 in death rates from cardiovascular disease.

Clinical Manifestations

Atherosclerosis is a progressive disease of the arterial wall that is characterized by focal thickening and luminal obstruction. Atherosclerotic build-up within the arteries does not cause clinical symptoms (Table 1); rather, symptoms are caused by ischemia to the organ supplied by the atherosclerotic vessel. Thus, coronary artery atherosclerosis (Fig. 1A) presents as angina, myocardial infarction, congestive heart failure, or sudden cardiac death. Carotid atherosclerosis (Fig. 1B) presents as vascular dementia, cerebrovascular accident, or transient ischemic attack.

Atherosclerosis is a systemic disease. About one half of patients with coronary artery disease will have atherosclerotic disease involving the carotid arteries, arteries of the lower extremities, or both. Similarly, one third to two thirds of patients with abdominal aortic aneurysms or lower-extremity arterial disease will also have significant coronary artery disease. The most common cause of death in patients with severe peripheral vascular disease is coronary artery disease *(3)*. Although atherosclerosis generally involves multiple vascular beds, some arteries such as the brachial and internal mammary are spared for reasons that are poorly understood.

Atherosclerotic lesions can be stable or unstable. Lesion stability and the transition from stable to unstable symptoms have been best studied in the coronary system. Stable coronary disease may present as exertional angina in which an atherosclerotic lesion obstructs the arterial lumen and limits blood flow. This situation creates a supply–demand mismatch during periods of increased myocardial metabolism, e.g., during exercise. In contrast, unstable symptoms usually result from a thrombus superimposed on a disrupted atherosclerotic plaque. Thrombus, which can occlude the artery at the site of the lesion or embolize distally to occlude a smaller branch, is initiated by exposure of the blood to components within the plaque that activate the clotting system. Plaque rupture, or disruption of the fibrous cap that isolates the atherosclerotic lesion from the bloodstream, is the most common cause of unstable symptoms.

From: *Contemporary Cardiology: Principles of Molecular Cardiology*
Edited by: M. S. Runge and C. Patterson © Humana Press Inc., Totowa, NJ

Table 1
Clinical Sequelae Associated with Vascular Disease[a]

	Clinical sequelae	
Diseased artery	Obstructive disease	Aneurysmal disease
Carotid/vertebral	Stroke, transient ischemic attack, dementia	Subarachnoid hemorrhage, sudden death
Coronary	Acute coronary syndromes, congestive heart failure, sudden cardiac death, stable angina	
Proximal aorta		Dissection, sudden death, aortic valve insufficiency
Distal aorta	Claudication, hypertension, distal embolization	Rupture, sudden death, distal embolization
Renal arteries	Hypertension, possible chronic renal insufficiency	
Lower extremity arteries	Claudication, distal embolization, limb loss	
Mesenteric	Intestinal angina, poor nutrition, weight loss, ischemic colitis	

[a]Partial list.

Risk Factors

Well-established risk factors for atherosclerosis include cigaret smoking, hypertension, diabetes mellitus, obesity, dyslipidemia, family history of premature vascular disease, and hyperhomocysteinemia. Other factors have been proposed to contribute to atherosclerosis (Table 2). Aging is the most important risk factor from a population perspective; the prevalence of cardiovascular disease increases from 5% in the 20–24-year-old age group to 75% in those older than 75 years (2).

Family history and genetic studies in mice indicate the importance of genetics in the development of atherosclerosis. The presence of premature vascular disease in a first-degree relative is a risk factor for vascular disease, and several gene mutations that lead to premature atherosclerosis have been identified (4). Although common forms of atherosclerosis are multifactorial, several specific gene mutations have been identified that lead to premature atherosclerosis. Mutations in the gene for the low-density lipoprotein (LDL) receptor are associated with familial hypercholesterolemia. Tangier's disease is associated with mutations in the ATP-binding-cassette transporter 1 gene that result in the absence of circulating high-density lipoprotein (HDL). In addition, mutations in the gene for apolipoprotein contribute to atherosclerosis. Despite the identification of single-gene mutations, common forms of atherosclerosis are multifactorial, and identification of genes for the common forms of atherosclerosis and polymorphisms relevant to atherosclerosis is a priority in clinical research.

PATHOLOGY OF ATHEROSCLEROTIC LESIONS

Normal Artery

The normal artery is composed of three layers: the intima, the media, and the adventitia (Table 3, Fig. 2). In larger arteries in humans, the intima comprises a continuous endothelial monolayer on a specialized extracellular matrix called the basement membrane. The internal elastic lamina (IEL), also part of the intima, is an acellular layer rich in connective tissue, especially proteoglycans. In large arteries such as the aorta, a subendothelial layer composed of collagenous bundles, elastic fibrils, smooth muscle cells (SMCs), and some fibroblasts is present. In addition to providing a nonthrombotic surface, the endothelium secretes various agents such as nitric oxide (NO) and endothelin that regulate vascular tone, produce growth factors and cytokines, modify lipoproteins, and regulate attachment of leukocytes and platelets to the blood vessel. Intimal thickening first occurs during fetal development and can be either a pathologic response or a physiologic response to increased blood flow or wall tension.

The media, which extends from the IEL to the external elastic lamina (EEL), is composed primarily of SMCs and extracellular matrix, including type I and type III collagen, fibronectin, proteoglycans, versican, and elastin (in elastic arteries). SMCs are derived locally from individual organ parenchyma during embryogenesis in contrast to the embryonic endothelium that invades the blood vessel.

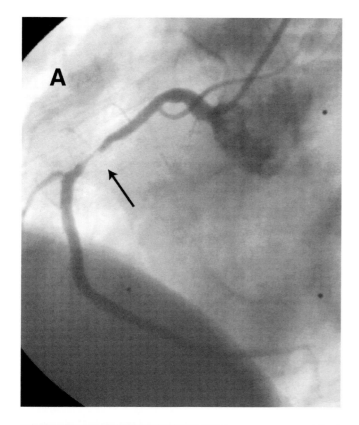

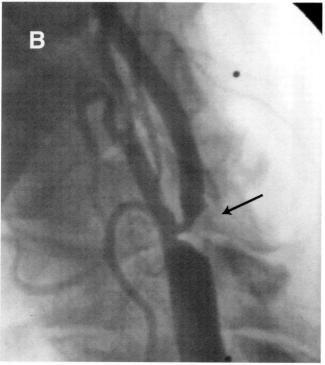

Fig. 1. Angiograms of the right coronary artery (**A**) and left carotid artery (**B**). Arrows indicate area within the artery characterized by the most severe atherosclerotic plaque.

The adventitia is the outermost layer of the vascular wall. The thickness of the adventitia depends on the type and location of the vessel. For example, the cerebral blood vessels almost entirely lack adventitia. The adventitia comprises fibroelastic tissue, composed primarily of fibroblasts. By connecting the blood vessel to its surrounding tissue, the adventitia provides stability and carries nutrients, via the vasa vasorum, to the medial SMCs.

Definition of Atherosclerosis

Atherosclerosis is a chronic disease of the large- and medium-caliber arteries. The hallmarks of atherosclerotic lesions are focal lipid accumulation, cell proliferation, and production of extracellular matrix. The atherosclerotic lesion is initially confined to the intima; however, in advanced atherosclerosis the media and adventitia are also involved. Atheromas usually comprise a necrotic core and a fibrotic cap. The necrotic core is frequently found at the base of the lesion near the IEL. The fibrotic cap is composed of several connective tissue components (especially collagen) and SMCs. The term atherosclerosis is derived from the Greek words for gruel (athero, which corresponds to the necrotic debris at the base of the plaque) and hard (sclerosis, corresponding to the fibrotic cap).

Atherosclerotic lesions tend to evolve at sites characterized by low shear stress and a high flow oscillation (e.g., at bifurcations and along the inner wall of curved segments). The importance of shear stress is evident from studies of endothelial cell morphology. Cells in the regions of arteries where blood flow is uniform and laminar are ellipsoidal in shape and aligned in the direction of flow. Cells where arteries branch or curve and where flow is disturbed have polygonal shapes and no particular orientation, and the endothelial cells in these areas show increased permeability to macromolecules such as LDL *(5)*.

Classification Systems

Several different systems have been used to classify atherosclerotic lesions. The Committee on Vascular Lesions of the Council on Arteriosclerosis of the AHA *(6–8)* has published reports describing a commonly used system in which atherosclerotic lesions are divided into six distinct types. Types I through III are considered preatheromatous lesions, whereas types IV through VI are described as different forms of atheromas (Table 4).

Type I lesions, composed of lipid deposits within the intima, are characterized by the presence of lipid-laden macrophages. These lesions can be detected with microscopy or with biochemical methods. Type II lesions are fatty streaked, small raised yellowish lesions that are visible to the

Table 2
Risk Factors for Coronary Artery Disease

Causal factors for CAD	Factors associated with CAD
Tobacco exposure (both active and passive)	Elevated prothrombotic factors (e.g., fibrinogen, PAI-1, factor VII)
Elevated LDL levels	Markers of infection (e.g., *C. pneumoniae* antibodies)
Decreased HDL levels	
Hypertension	Markers of inflammation (e.g., CRP)
Diabetes mellitus type I	Sedentary lifestyle
Insulin resistance syndromes (diabetes mellitus type II, obesity, physical inactivity)	Elevated lipoprotein [a]
Aging	Post-menopausal state
Elevated homocysteine levels	Psychological factors (e.g., depression)
Premature vascular disease in a first-degree relative	

CAD, coronary artery disease; LDL, low-density lipoprotein; HDL, high-density lipoprotein; PAI-1, plasminogen activator inhibitor-1; CRP, C-reactive protein.

Table 3
Composition of the Vessel Wall in Non-Diseased Large Arteries

Wall layer	Cell type	Extracellular matrix
Intima	Endothelial monolayer	Type IV collagen, laminin, perlecan, syndecan
Media	Smooth muscle cells	Type I collagen, type III collagen, fibronectin, proteoglycans, versican, elastin (in elastic arteries)
Adventitia	Fibroblasts	

naked eye. The hallmark of the fatty streak is the foam cell, which is a macrophage or SMC that is engorged with lipid. Type III lesions are characterized by multiple extracellular lipid pools that do not form a clearly defined acellular lipid core. In arteries with type I through III lesions, the arterial wall is not appreciably thickened and blood flow is not obstructed. The primary mechanism of plaque growth for type I through IV lesions is accumulation of lipid in the vessel wall.

In type IV through VI lesions (Fig. 3), atheromas can be identified, and the histological appearance is characterized by cholesterol clefts, calcification, and an acellular necrotic core. In these lesions, the intimal structure is disrupted by an extensive accumulation of extracellular lipid located in the deep intima (the lipid core). Type V lesions are differentiated from type IV lesions by the presence of a fibrous cap in which the luminal surface of the intima is thickened by deposits of collagen and other fibrous tissue. The mechanism of growth for type V lesions is an increase in SMCs and extracellular matrix. Type VI lesions are characterized by fissuring or disruption of the surface, including ulcers, hematoma, and thrombi. Characteristics of type II (lipid-laden macrophages and SMCs), type IV

(a core of extracellular lipid), and often type V (layers of newly formed fibrous connective tissue) lesions are seen in type VI lesions.

Type IV and V lesions may be silent or overt, depending on the degree of obstruction. In type IV lesions, the degree of luminal obstruction is determined primarily by the amount of lipid. The cap in type IV lesions consists only of preexisting intima, which at highly susceptible arterial sites is relatively thick (adaptive intimal thickening), but less obstructive than fibrous caps seen in type V lesions. In type VI lesions, thrombosis can be superimposed upon the atherosclerotic lesion. The chief growth mechanism for type VI lesions is thrombosis and hematoma.

Most acute clinical manifestations and deaths, and probably most plaque growth, are associated with type VI lesions. Although most clinical symptoms occur with type VI lesions, not all plaque disruption leads to clinical symptoms. Lesion ulceration and thrombosis, as seen in type VI lesions, may occur without clinical symptoms, and a lesion may repeatedly pass through a type VI stage. Traditionally, atherosclerotic vascular disease was thought to result from a gradual accumulation of lipids and cells and progressive

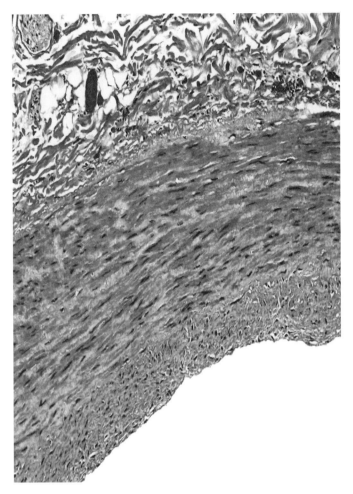

Fig. 2. Photomicrograph of a normal artery. (Image courtesy of Scott Smith, MD, University of North Carolina.)

growth of plaques within the intima of vessels. However, recent thought is that plaque size can change dramatically and that repeated cycles of plaque rupture and healing contribute to plaque growth.

Type I and II lesions can occur in infants, children, and adults. These lesions are distinct from adaptive intimal thickening, which occurs naturally from birth, particularly at bifurcations. Pathological lesions are thicker and may contain lipid deposits. Over time, the lipid accumulation increases and atherosclerotic lesions develop. Fatty streaks can usually be found in the aorta in the first decade of life, in the coronary arteries in the second decade, and in the cerebral arteries in the third or fourth decades. Type IV lesions may frequently be seen from the third decade of life. After the third decade, types V and VI lesions begin to appear and, in some individuals, become the predominant lesion types.

The classification scheme proposed by the Council on Arteriosclerosis of the AHA has been criticized for several reasons. The primary reason involves the nature of the difference between type IV and V lesions. The AHA scheme implies an orderly, linear progression in the development of atherosclerosis and a direct relationship between lesion number and clinical manifestations. Virmani et al. *(9)* proposed a modified AHA classification scheme that further subdivided lesions in categories IV through VI. These "progressive atherosclerotic lesions" were divided into seven categories: intimal xanthoma, intimal thickening, pathological intimal thickening, fibrous cap atheroma, thin fibrous cap atheroma, calcified nodule, and fibrocalcific

Table 4
Classification Scheme for Atherosclerosis (Proposed by the Committee on Vascular Lesions of the Council on Arteriosclerosis, American Heart Association) *(6–8)*

Lesion type	Lesion name	Description of lesion	Subtype
I	Initial lesion	Isolated macrophage foam cells; lesion not visible to the naked eye	
II	Fatty streak	Smooth muscle cells, foam cells, intra- and extracellular lipid	IIa: progression prone IIb: progression resistant
III	Preatheroma	Type II lesions with microscopic evidence of tissue injury and increased extracellular lipid, increased wall thickness	
IV	Atheroma	Significantly thickened intima, cholesterol clefts, calcification, acellular necrotic core	Atheroma with lipid core Atheroma with necrotic core
V	Fibroatheroma	Fibrotic changes, increased smooth muscle cells, formation of fibrous cap	Va: multilayered multiple lipid cores Vb: calcific Vc: fibrotic
VI	Complicated atheroma	Type IV or V lesion, with disruptions to the surface	VIa: disruption of surface fissure ulceration VIb: hematoma VIc: thrombosis

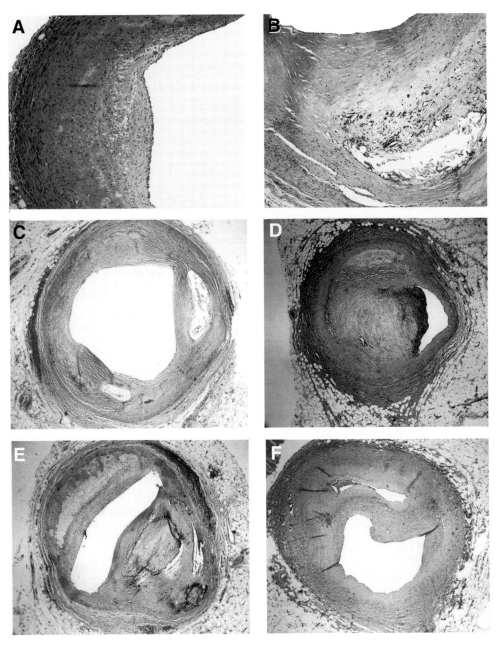

Fig. 3. Photomicrographs showing mild atherosclerosis (**A**) and moderate atherosclerosis (**B** and **C**). Note severe atherosclerosis seen as a superimposed thrombus (**D** and **F**), calcific changes (**E**), and a recanalization channel (**F**).[Images courtesy of Scott Smith, MD.]

plaque. In another modification of the AHA classification scheme proposed by Stary *(10)*, fibroatheroma was designated type V; calcific lesions, type VII; and fibrotic lesions with little or no lipid, type VIII. Lesions listed as types Vb and Vc in the AHA classification are similar to those designated types VII and VIII in Stary's classification *(11)*.

Aneurysms

Aneurysms are defined as a localized dilation of an artery (Fig. 4) and are usually associated with type VI lesions in which the intimal surface is greatly eroded. Aneurysms often contain both acute and chronic thrombi that are layered in long-standing aneurysms. Thrombus may fill the aneurysm, but a lumen that approximates the dimensions of the original vessel is usually preserved.

For aneurysms to occur, matrix degradation or synthesis is altered. The expansion of an abdominal aortic aneurysm is characterized by inflammation, loss of elastin, and increased turnover of collagen in the aortic wall. The inflammatory reaction is characterized by an

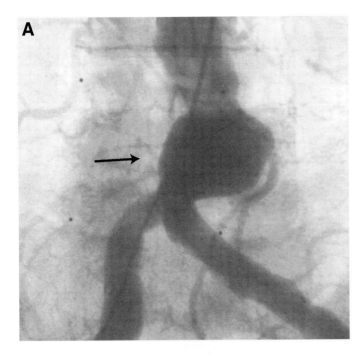

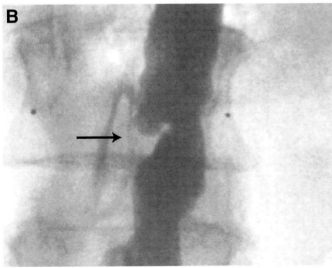

Fig. 4. Aortic angiograms showing aneurysmal (**A**) and obstructive (**B**) disease.

found in aneurysmal wall. Carrell et al. *(15)* used reverse transcriptase polymerase chain reaction (PCR) to show the differential expression of MMPs in vascular diseases. Certain types of MMPs are expressed at higher levels in abdominal aortic aneurysms than in abdominal aortas with obstructive disease. Furthermore, not all types of MMPs were detected in abdominal aortic aneurysms. MMPs are discussed in more detail later in this chapter.

DEVELOPMENT AND PROGRESSION OF ATHEROSCLEROTIC LESIONS

Several theories have been proposed to explain the origin of atherosclerotic disease. An early theory, the thrombogenic or incrustation theory proposed by von Rokitansky in 1852 *(16)*, stated that the organization of fibrin deposits by fibroblasts, with secondary lipid enrichment, led to intimal thickening. Then, in 1856, Virchow described atherosclerosis as "endarteritis deformans." According to Virchow, atheromas resulted from vascular injury that led to inflammation within the intima, and fibrous thickening resulted from proliferating connective tissue cells. Early in the 20th century, the lipidic theory proposed that increased transudation of plasma lipids caused an accumulation of lipids within the arterial wall. Increased plasma levels of lipids, combined with a higher rate of lipid deposition than lipid removal, resulted in an excessive build-up of lipid in the arterial wall. Later theories have indicated the importance of immunologic mechanisms, viruses, aging processes, and clonal proliferation of SMCs. First proposed during the latter part of the 20th century, the response to injury theory, a modification of Virchow's original theory, is currently the dominant theory regarding the pathogenesis of atherosclerosis.

A general paradigm of atherosclerosis formation has been developed. The first observable change in the arterial wall is the accumulation within the intima of lipoprotein particles and their aggregates. Next, cellular adhesion molecules are upregulated, and monocytes adhere to the surface of the endothelium. Vascular cell adhesion molecule-1 (VCAM-1), upregulated early in experimental atherosclerosis, facilitates binding of monocytes and T lymphocytes to endothelial cells *(17)*. Monocytes then transmigrate into the intima, proliferate, and differentiate into macrophages. The macrophages express scavenger receptors, which enable them to ingest lipids to form foam cells. The foam cells die and contribute their lipid-filled contents to the necrotic core of the lesion, which leads to further recruitment of monocytes in a cyclical fashion. SMCs migrate from the medial layer and secrete extracellular matrix, which leads

influx of B and T lymphocytes, plasma cells, and macrophages *(12)*. The activity of collagenase and elastase increases in rapidly enlarging and ruptured aneurysms *(13,14)*. Enzyme activity or experimental enzymatic destruction of the matrix architecture of the aorta results in dilation and rupture. In experimental studies, mechanical injury with destruction of medial lamellar architecture results in aneurysm formation, particularly in the presence of hyperlipidemia. The matrix metalloproteinases (MMPs) are a group of enzymes produced by a wide range of cell types, including fibroblasts, SMCs, and inflammatory cells to the formation of a fibrous cap. The lesion continues to grow by recruiting more mononuclear cells from the blood, which, in turn, causes the proliferation of macrophages and SMCs, the accumulation of intracellular and extracellular lipids, and the production of extracellular matrix *(18)*. This paradigm was derived primarily from experimental studies of abnormal lipid metabolism, including studies of mice deficient in apolipoprotein E or the LDL receptor. Thus, these findings may not be applicable to all clinical cases of atherosclerosis.

Pathogenesis of Atherosclerosis

Several of the current theories regarding the development and progression of atherosclerosis are briefly outlined below. Although the theories are presented separately, extensive overlap exists. The following pathogenic mechanisms may contribute to the development of atherosclerosis but are not discussed here: (1) the autoimmune theory, (2) the clonal-senescence theory (focuses on relationship of age to atherosclerosis), (3) the thrombogenic theory (proposes that plaque is initiated by the organization of small mural thrombi and that thrombus formation is the chief mechanism of atherosclerotic development), and (4) the response to retention theory (proposes that excess accumulation of vascular proteoglycans is detrimental).

Despite our progress in understanding the pathogenesis of atherosclerosis, many of the processes involved remain poorly characterized. Studies of atherosclerosis in humans are limited by the complexity of the cellular and molecular mechanisms that contribute to the process and the long time periods involved (decades in most individuals). Furthermore, significant interindividual variability is seen in pathogenetic mechanisms.

RESPONSE TO INJURY HYPOTHESIS

The response to injury hypothesis was originally proposed by Virchow in 1856, but was extensively updated by Ross *(19)*. The most recent version of this hypothesis emphasizes two major points: (1) atherosclerosis is a chronic inflammatory disease and (2) endothelial dysfunction is important in initiating the process. The endothelium is a single-cell lining that covers the internal surface of blood vessels. Normal endothelium serves many functions, including providing a nonthrombogenic surface, controlling arterial tone, modifying lipoproteins, providing a permeability barrier, and producing cytokines and growth factors. Endothelial cells may become "injured" by various factors (e.g., cigaret smoking, hypertension, diabetes, homocysteine, and infectious agents) that lead to endothelial dysfunction.

When the normal homeostatic properties of the endothelium are altered, multiple changes can occur: (1) upregulation of cellular adhesion molecules that increase adhesion of monocytes or platelets to the endothelium, (2) increased permeability of the endothelium to blood-borne molecules, and (3) endothelial production of procoagulants, vasoactive molecules, cytokines, and growth factors.

Production of nitric oxide (NO), which is an important endothelium-derived relaxing factor, is impaired in damaged endothelial cells. This change in NO production alters the balance between endothelium-derived relaxing and contracting factors that maintain vascular homeostasis. In addition to being a potent vasodilator, NO regulates expression of VCAM *(20)* and maintains the vascular smooth muscle in a nonproliferative state. The synthesis of NO from L-arginine is regulated by the enzyme nitric oxide synthase.

A central tenet of the response to injury hypothesis is that endothelial injury is the proximate cause of atherosclerosis. When the endothelium is damaged, the vasculature becomes more prone to inflammation, thrombosis, and vasoconstriction. If the endothelial injury is not repaired and the stimulus is not removed, the inflammatory response becomes chronic resulting in increasing numbers of macrophages and T lymphocytes. Mononuclear leukocytes multiply within the lesion and release hydrolytic enzymes, cytokines, chemokines, and growth factors that cause further damage and eventual focal necrosis. Chronic persistent endothelial damage and the resulting inflammatory response cause migration and proliferation of SMCs, accumulation of mononuclear cells and lipids, and the formation of fibrous tissue, all of which lead to enlargement of the lesion.

Studies in humans have shown that endothelial dysfunction impairs vasodilatory responses and may become clinically significant before obstructive atheroma develops. Reduced NO production decreases dilation of the coronary arteries and decreases myocardial blood flow in response to hyperemic stimuli. Endothelial dysfunction is measured clinically as a loss of vasodilatory responses to direct intraarterial injection of an NO stimulus such as acetylcholine. Conditions associated with endothelial dysfunction include atherosclerosis, ischemia-reperfusion, transplant atherosclerosis, cardiopulmonary bypass, congestive heart failure, and left ventricular hypertrophy *(21)*. In addition, endothelial function may be affected by risk factors for the development of atherosclerosis, including diabetes mellitus, hypercholesterolemia, hypertension, homocysteinemia, aging, metabolic syndrome, postmenopausal state, smoking, and renal disease.

Treatment with HMG Co-A reductase inhibitors (statins) and angiotensin-converting enzyme (ACE) inhibitors improves endothelial function. Both classes of drugs reduce the progression of atherosclerosis and the occurrence of clinical events in patients with established coronary artery disease (22,23); however, a causal relationship has not been established between improvements in endothelial function and a reduction in cardiovascular events.

OXIDATION HYPOTHESIS

The oxidation hypothesis states that the oxidative modification of LDL or other lipoproteins is central to the atherogenic process (24). Experimental evidence indicates several mechanisms for the atherogenic effects of oxidatively modified LDLs (25). These mechanisms include the recruitment of circulating monocytes and T lymphocytes to the intima, the formation of foam cells from macrophages that bind oxidatively modified LDL via scavenger receptors, the induction of mitogenic responses in SMCs, and the alteration of gene expression in vascular cells (including the upregulation of cellular adhesion molecules). In addition, oxidative processes may have other effects on the growth, proliferation, and death of cells in the arterial wall. The involvement of oxidatively modified LDL in atherogenesis is further supported by the finding that LDL from atherosclerotic plaques formed in vivo is similar to LDL that was oxidatively modified in vitro (26).

An important corollary of this theory is that inhibition of LDL oxidation should reduce the progression of atherosclerosis. Several large-scale prospective observational studies have examined the relationship between the intake of antioxidant vitamins and cardiovascular morbidity and mortality. The effects of all three of the major antioxidant vitamins—vitamin E, vitamin C, and β-carotene—on cardiovascular health have been studied in six large observational trials in which participants were divided into groups according to the estimated intake of the vitamins. A significant cardiovascular benefit was seen with an increase in vitamin E intake in four of the six studies (27).

In contrast to the observational trials, randomized controlled trials have failed to show a cardiovascular benefit from supplementation with vitamin E or β-carotene (28). Of the three trials assessing the effects of β-carotene and/or vitamin E supplementation on the primary prevention of cardiovascular events, no benefit was found for either agent. In secondary prevention trials, vitamin E supplementation reduced nonfatal myocardial infarction in patients with prior myocardial infarction (29) and in patients with angiographically

proven coronary artery disease (30); however, this finding was not confirmed in either the Gruppo Italiano per lo Studio della Sopravvivenza nell'Infarto miocardico (GISSI)-Prevenzione Trial (31) or the Heart Outcomes Prevention Evaluation (HOPE) (22) study. Moreover, none of the studies showed that vitamin E improved cardiovascular or all-cause mortality. The results for β-carotene supplementation were even more concerning. Supplementation with β-carotene failed to show benefit in any of the trials, and in two studies, β-carotene may actually have worsened patient outcome (29,32). No major randomized controlled trials have evaluated the effect of vitamin C supplementation on cardiovascular disease.

The lack of clinical benefit of antioxidant vitamins in the randomized trials does not invalidate the oxidation hypothesis. Numerous potential factors have been suggested to explain the lack of efficacy: (1) vitamin treatment was initiated too late in the disease process to show any preventive benefit, (2) the relative antioxidant deficiency of some patients is greater than that of others, and a clinical measurement of oxidative stress burden may identify patient groups that would benefit from antioxidant supplementation (33), and (3) the type of antioxidant used was inadequate.

INFLAMMATORY HYPOTHESIS

According to classic theory, the role of the macrophage in the arterial wall was to remove fat particles that had infiltrated the intima by phagocytosing lipids. Thus, atherosclerosis was seen primarily as a lipid disorder characterized by the excessive influx of lipids into the arterial wall. However, the role of the macrophage has been expanded in the more recent inflammatory hypothesis in which the function of the macrophage is to mediate an inflammatory response (34). Macrophages are recruited from the bloodstream by an interaction between cellular adhesion molecules on monocytes and endothelial cells. Monocytes transmigrate into the subintimal space and differentiate into macrophages in the presence of macrophage colony stimulating factor (M-CSF), a cytokine that is produced not only by macrophages but also by vascular and stromal cells. Macrophages within atheromas produce free oxygen radicals, proteases, complement factors, growth factors, and cytokines and initiate adaptive immune responses by presenting foreign antigens to T lymphocytes. In addition, macrophages may transform into foam cells by ingesting modified lipoproteins (35).

According to the inflammatory hypothesis, the best way to control atherosclerotic lesions is to regulate the inflammatory response. Factors proposed as triggers for vascular inflammation include oxidized lipoproteins, angiotensin II, diabetes mellitus, and infection (34). Despite being separated into different theories, both lipids and inflammatory mediators contribute to the atherogenic process. For example, the secretion of inflammatory mediators such as MMPs by macrophages is regulated by the lipid content within the cell.

The inflammatory hypothesis has been further supported by the identification of T lymphocytes within atherosclerotic lesions (36). In fact, plaque stability may correlate with the concentration of T lymphocytes. Most T lymphocytes in atherosclerotic lesions are CD4+ cells, and a large proportion of T lymphocytes within randomly sampled plaques present the very late activation antigen VLA-1 and HLA-DR molecules. Studies of surface markers on T lymphocytes in plaque indicate that they are memory cells in a state of chronic activation. Most of the T lymphocytes are T helper cells (Th1), which produce interferon-γ, interleukin-2 (IL-2), tumor necrosis factor-α (TNF-α), tumor necrosis factor-β (TNF-β), and lymphotoxin. In addition, Th1 cells direct cell-mediated immune responses that eliminate intracellular pathogens. Interferon-γ may affect plaque morphology by regulating the synthesis of extracellular matrix and inhibiting the proliferation of SMCs (37). These findings suggest that IFN-γ–producing T lymphocytes may contribute to plaque destabilization by reducing the fibrous cap.

The expression of IL-2 receptors on T lymphocytes may be a marker of plaque activation. In coronary lesions in asymptomatic patients, few T lymphocytes express IL-2 receptors, whereas IL-2 receptor expression is increased in plaque samples from patients with unstable symptoms. In one study of atherectomy specimens obtained from patients with angina pectoris, the number of lesions containing IL-2 receptor-positive T lymphocytes was 50% in patients with stable symptoms and 90% in patients with unstable symptoms. Furthermore, the number of T lymphocytes and the percentage of IL-2 receptor-positive T lymphocytes was higher in patients with acute coronary syndromes than in those with stable symptoms (38).

INFECTIOUS AGENT HYPOTHESIS

The hypothesis that atheromas derive from an infectious agent relates closely to the inflammatory hypothesis. Bacteria and viruses have been proposed as atherogenic agents. In studies of Marek's disease, infection with an avian herpes virus caused atherosclerosis in chickens. In humans, three infectious agents that have been studied as possible causes of atherosclerosis: Chlamydia pneumoniae, cytomegalovirus (CMV), and Helicobacter pylori.

C. pneumoniae is an obligate intracellular organism that has been found in human atherosclerotic lesions by using electron microscopy, immunohistochemistry, and PCR. In addition, the organisms have been cultured from atherosclerotic plaques. However, no association has been found between the type of lesion and the presence of C. pneumoniae. The organism is found in the same frequency in mild and severe lesions. C. pneumoniae may be present in normal vessels but at a lesser frequency than in atheromas. The presence of high antibody titers to C. pneumoniae may have prognostic value (39,40).

Several studies have examined the effects of treatment for C. pneumoniae infection on vascular pathology. The Intracoronary Stenting or Angioplasty for Restenosis-3 (ISAR-3) study found that roxithromycin did not reduce restenosis after coronary stenting in a nonselected group of 1010 patients; however, roxithromycin reduced the rate of restenosis in a subgroup of patients with high C. pneumoniae titers (41). Conflicting results have been reported in other studies in patients with stable coronary artery disease. In a study of 202 patients with non–Q-wave coronary syndromes, roxithromycin reduced major ischemic events (40), whereas azithromycin had no effect in 302 patients with coronary artery disease (42).

Conflicting reports on the efficacy of antibiotic treatment do not necessarily exclude a role for C. pneumoniae in atherosclerosis. C. pneumoniae disseminates systemically within monocytes and can persist intracellularly, which renders antichlamydial treatment ineffective (43). Although studies are ongoing, no direct evidence that C. pneumoniae can cause atherosclerotic lesions in animals or humans has been found.

Two lines of evidence suggest a role for CMV in atherosclerosis. First, CMV has been detected in atherosclerotic plaques by the use of immunohistochemistry, in situ hybridization, and PCR (44). Second, a weak association between atherosclerosis and the presence of anti-CMV antibodies has been found in some but not all seroepidemiologic studies (45). Few data directly implicate CMV in the development of atherosclerosis, and no study has examined the effect of treatment of CMV on progression of atherosclerosis. Although the role of H. pylori in atherosclerosis has been studied, no compelling data indicate a causal relationship (45,46).

MONOCLONAL HYPOTHESIS

The monoclonal theory, originally proposed by Benditt and Benditt (47), states that atherosclerotic lesions result from proliferation of a clonal SMC population. In this theory, SMC proliferation in an atherosclerotic lesion relates more closely to neoplastic growth than to a response to vascular injury. The original support for this theory came from studies of women with a genetic deficiency of glucose-6 phosphate dehydrogenase in which 80% of atherosclerotic plaques were found to be monoclonal *(47,48)*. Another study *(49)* reported that 89.7% of fibrous plaques were monoclonal, whereas only 17.8% of fatty streaks were monoclonal. In a more recent study of PCR amplification of the DNA of an X-inactivated gene from microdissected tissue, the monoclonal origin of the SMCs was confirmed, and monoclonal expansion was also found in nonatherosclerotic intima and media *(50)*.

Vascular Calcification

Vascular calcification, which contributes significantly to cardiovascular morbidity and mortality, can occur in the intima or media. The calcified material consists primarily of calcium apatite. In a clinical setting, calcification is observed in coronary (Fig. 5) and peripheral arteries. In addition to affecting plaque rupture, calcification is a major determinant of complications associated with revascularization procedures. Calcification of the aorta, aortic valve, and mitral annulus can cause severe symptoms or even death in some cases.

Studies of the expression of bone genes in human blood vessels and mouse gene knockout studies have shown that calcification is an active, regulated process and not caused by passive crystallization. Similarities have been found between atherosclerotic lesions and the calcification process in bone. For example, bone regulatory factors and all major components of bone osteoid are found within the arterial wall. In addition, cells that retain osteoblastic lineage are seen within the arterial lining *(51)*. Intimal calcification is an active process in which pericyte-like cells secrete a matrix scaffold that becomes calcified in a similar manner to bone formation. This calcification process, seen as early as the second decade of life in association with fatty streaks, occurs only within atherosclerotic plaques and is associated with lipid deposits, macrophages, and SMCs. Intimal calcium appears as aggregates of calcium crystals, and these deposits can coalesce to produce larger crystals. Furthermore, intimal calcification occasionally has the characteristics of true bone.

Medial calcification occurs independently of intimal calcification and is not associated with atherosclerosis. Appearing as linear deposits usually along the elastic lamellae, medial calcification occurs in the absence of inflammation or lipid deposition. Medial calcification occurs in otherwise healthy elderly patients (Mönckeberg's sclerosis) and in patients with diabetes mellitus and end-stage renal disease.

Vascular calcification may be initiated by several factors, including apoptotic bodies derived from SMCs, lipids, and lipoproteins and the production of bone-associated

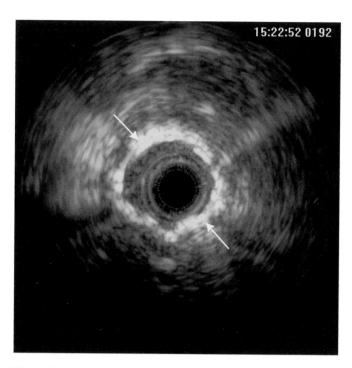

Fig. 5. Intravascular ultrasound image showing severe, concentric calcification.

proteins by SMCs. In addition, increased local concentrations of calcium and phosphate ions in atherosclerotic plaques may contribute to calcification. SMCs can adopt an osteogenic phenotype in culture and express several calcification-regulating proteins, including osteopontin, matrix Gla protein, osteocalcin, osteonectin, collagen, alkaline phosphatase, bone sialoprotein, and bone morphogenic proteins. Several mouse models with medial calcification have been generated, including knock-outs of osteoprotegerin, klotho, carbonic anhydrase II, matrix Gla protein, and Smad 6. In addition, vascular calcification may be induced by feeding vitamin D and calcium or warfarin to normal animals or by fat-feeding mice null for apoE or the LDL-receptor *(52)*.

Arterial Remodeling

The size of the EEL was traditionally thought to be fixed, and plaque growth was thought to lead invariably to luminal narrowing. However, it has now been recognized that the media and EEL of arteries can increase or decrease under physiologic conditions (e.g., closure of the ductus arteriosus and development of collateral vessels) and that the size of the artery changes to protect lumen size during the early phases of atherosclerosis. However, this adaptive mechanism, called remodeling, has limitations. If the atherosclerotic lesion continues to progress, the size of the lumen eventually decreases.

The term arterial remodeling refers to changes in vascular dimensions, such as the cross-sectional area within the EEL. Positive remodeling, also referred to as outward remodeling, is the expansion of the EEL during the development of atherosclerotic plaques. First described in necropsy specimens (53), positive remodeling has been confirmed with intravascular ultrasound (54). In their landmark study of 136 hearts obtained at autopsy, Glagov et al. (53) reported that the lumen area of the left main coronary artery did not decrease in arteries with atherosclerotic lesions involving 0–40% of the cross-sectional area. In contrast, lumen size decreased markedly in vessels with more than 40% of the area involved, and the decrease related closely to the percentage of stenosis. Necropsy (55) and ultrasound (54) studies have extended these findings to other arteries.

The mechanisms of remodeling are being identified. In normal arteries, positive remodeling restores normal shear stress and wall tension in response to changes in flow, wall stretch, and humoral factors (56). Positive remodeling depends on shear-responsive endothelial production of NO and the production of MMPs by inflammatory cells. Remodeling is affected by the location of the vascular bed. For example, positive remodeling is more common in coronary, common carotid, and renal arteries than in arteries of the lower extremities (55). In addition, patient characteristics, such as insulin use, smoking, and cholesterol levels, may affect remodeling. These factors, however, have limited because remodeling response often varies significantly along the same artery (55,57).

In addition to positive remodeling, negative remodeling or inward remodeling can occur in atherosclerotic lesions. Using intravascular ultrasound, Mintz et al. (57) found that negative remodeling was present in 15% of lesions in patients with stable angina. Mintz's group defined negative remodeling as the area of EEL at an atherosclerotic lesion that is less than or equal to 78% of EEL area in the control group. Smits et al. (58), using a less stringent definition of negative remodeling, found negative remodeling in 50% of patients with stable angina.

Negative remodeling has been reported to occur after percutaneous transluminal coronary angioplasty (PTCA). After PTCA, the remodeling response is biphasic. Early after angioplasy, positive remodeling occurs, followed by late shrinkage of the vessel (59). The EEL area rarely decreases below the pre-intervention size; the early positive remodeling reverses to return the vessel to the original size. This late negative remodeling occurs in most patients. In one study (60), 73% of late luminal loss was caused by negative remodeling, whereas only 27% resulted from neointimal proliferation. Balloon angioplasty may induce a focal fibrotic response, which results in inward remodeling. Recently, Dangas et al. (61) found that evidence of positive remodeling before a nonstent interventional procedure predicted higher rates of target lesion revascularization than in arteries with negative or no remodeling.

TRANSITION FROM STABLE TO UNSTABLE CORONARY SYNDROMES

Clinical atherosclerotic disease may manifest as stable or unstable (sudden onset of symptoms) syndromes. The initial presentation of coronary artery disease in the Framingham Study (62) was stable angina in 32% of men and 47% of women, acute coronary syndromes (myocardial infarction and unstable angina) in 36% of men and 25% of women, unrecognized myocardial infarction in 16% of men and 14% of women, and sudden cardiac death in 16% of men and 14% of women. Only 20% of patients who presented with an acute coronary syndrome had antecedent angina. Atherosclerotic disease in the cerebral vessels can manifest as unstable (e.g., transient ischemic attack or cerebrovascular accident) or stable. Similarly, atherosclerosis in the arteries of the lower extremities can be either stable (stable claudication) or unstable (acute thrombosis).

Thrombosis

Intracoronary thrombus plays an important role in the transition from stable to unstable coronary syndromes (63,64). Coronary thrombosis is found in about 70–80% of cases of fatal myocardial infarction (65). Patients with unstable angina have increased levels of D-dimer, plasminogen activator inhibitor-1 (PAI-1), prothrombin fragment 1+2, and fibrinopeptide-A, all of which suggest an ongoing thrombotic process (66). Although thrombus is visible on angiogram in only a few patients with unstable angina, 70% of lesions have the typical characteristics of a thrombus-containing lesion (67). The more sensitive technique of angioscopy has shown that 55–100% (68–70) of lesions in patients with unstable angina have an associated thrombus.

The importance of thrombosis in acute coronary syndromes has been supported by the success of thrombolytic, anticoagulant, and antiplatelet therapy in the treatment of these syndromes. Treatment with aspirin, the most widely used platelet inhibitor, reduces mortality in patients with unstable angina (71–74) and in patients having an acute myocardial infarction (75). In addition, aspirin reduces the transition from stable to unstable vascular disease. The Antiplatelet Trialists Collaboration (76,77), in a meta-analysis of 145 trials involving more than 100,000 patients, found that antiplatelet therapy reduced the occurrence of vascular events by 20–30% in patients with a history of myocardial infarction, transient ischemic attack, stable angina, or peripheral vascular disease. The success of thrombolytic therapy in restoring vessel patency and in reducing mortality in patients with myocardial infarctions associated with ST elevation is well documented (78,79). Antithrombin agents, including unfractionated heparin, low molecular weight heparin, and hirudin derivatives, reduce the incidence of myocardial (re-) infarction and death in patients with acute coronary syndromes. More recently, intravenous glycoprotein IIb/IIIa inhibitors have been shown to protect against myocardial (re-) infarction when used in conjunction with aspirin and heparin in patients with non–Q wave myocardial infarctions and unstable angina (80–82).

Pathogenesis of Acute Coronary Syndromes

Rupture of an atherosclerotic plaque, which initiates thrombus formation, is currently thought to be the proximate cause of most acute coronary syndromes. Plaque rupture occurs primarily at the junction of the atheroma and the normal vessel, a region known as the shoulder of the lesion. In the shoulder area, the fibrous cap is thinnest; activated macrophages and foam cells accumulate; and the level of apoptotic cells is high. Once the plaque ruptures, intravascular hemorrhage and thrombus formation occur. The thrombus, which can extend into the lumen, may be occlusive or nonocclusive, depending on thrombogenic and hemodynamic factors.

Several lines of evidence suggest that plaque rupture precedes most acute coronary syndromes. First, the morphology of the lesion on angiogram and angioscopy is usually irregular and eccentric, a finding that is consistent with plaque disruption (63,67). Second, a high percentage of patients with sudden death have evidence of plaque rupture at autopsy (83). Third, coronary occlusion and myocardial infarction frequently evolve from mild or moderate stenoses (84). A compilation of four angiographic studies found that 65% of myocardial infarctions arose from lesions that were less than 50% stenotic, and 85% of myocardial infarctions arose from lesions less than 70% stenotic based on angiograms done several months before the acute event (85). This finding suggests that less obstructive plaques are more lipid rich and vulnerable to rupture than larger plaques.

Although plaque rupture is thought to cause most acute coronary syndromes, only a minority of cases of plaque rupture results in clinical symptoms. The disruption of plaque is asymptomatic, and the associated rapid plaque growth does not usually cause clinical symptoms. Autopsy data indicate that 9% of healthy, asymptomatic persons have disrupted plaques in the coronary arteries; the percentage increases to 22% in patients with diabetes or hypertension (86). Thrombosed and non-thrombosed disrupted plaques are present in the coronary arteries of many patients who die from ischemic heart disease (87).

One small study suggested that plaque rupture may occur several days before symptoms develop; the study group comprised 20 patients who had undergone coronary angiography within 1 week before having an acute myocardial infarction. When compared with a group of patients who had undergone coronary angiography 6–18 months before having a myocardial infarction, the study group was more likely to have a significant stenosis of greater than 50% and Ambrose's type II eccentric lesions, which indicates plaque rupture and/or thrombi. The control group was more likely to develop a myocardial infarction from a mild stenosis of less than 50%, with rare Ambrose's type II eccentric lesions (88). This last finding confirms those of previous studies (85).

In rare cases, fatal thrombosis in coronary arteries results from a superficial erosion of the intima, without a frank rupture through the fibrous cap of the plaque. In contrast to ruptured plaques, eroded plaques have a base rich in SMCs and proteoglycans. In a study of patients with sudden death caused by thrombosis of the coronary artery, Farb et al. (89) found that the thrombus communicated with a lipid pool in 56% of the cases, but in the remaining cases, the thrombi were attached to a superficial erosion. The attached lesions were more common in women and in smokers.

After plaque disruption or erosion, the following four factors determine the thrombotic response: (1) the character and extent of plaque substrate exposed to the bloodstream, (2) local flow disturbances (e.g., the degree of stenosis and surface irregularities), (3) the depth of arterial injury, and (4) the balance between endogenous pro- and anticoagulant systems (87). For example, the concentration of tissue factors is higher in unstable plaques than in stable plaques and is associated with increased amounts of thrombin generation across the plaque (90). In addition, plaque rupture can cause vasospasm, which leads to stasis and further increases thrombus formation.

Sudden cardiac death from coronary disease may occur in the absence of coronary thrombosis. Burke et al. (91) performed autopsies on the hearts of 113 men with coronary disease who died suddenly, and acute coronary thrombus was found in 59 men. Of the 59 cases of thrombus, 41 resulted from plaque rupture and 18 resulted from superficial erosion. Severe narrowing of the coronary artery by an atherosclerotic plaque without acute thrombosis was found in 54 men. The men without coronary thrombosis were more likely to be older and hypertensive, whereas thrombosis was more common in young smokers with dyslipidemia.

Pathophysiology of Plaque Rupture

Advanced atherosclerotic plaque comprises SMCs, inflammatory cells (macrophages and T lymphocytes), and intracellular and extracellular lipid. The stability of the plaque depends upon a balance between SMCs, the only cells capable of synthesizing the structurally important collagens I and III, and inflammatory cells. Chance of rupture depends on the size of the atheromatous core, the thickness and collagen content of the fibrous cap, and inflammation within the cap. Atherosclerotic plaques with the following characteristics are particularly prone to rupture: (1) large lipid cores, (2) increased numbers of macrophages, (3) increased activity of matrix metalloproteinases, (4) low numbers of SMCs, (5) increased apoptosis of SMCs, and (6) thinner, more friable caps.

Plaque rupture usually occurs at the plaque shoulder because of hemodynamic factors and the spatial distribution of atheroma constituents. Computer models show that the presence of a lipid pool or an intramural hemorrhage within the vessel wall reduces its tensile strength. These shape distortions, together with the degree of stenosis and thickness of the fibrous cap, cause major changes in the distribution of wall stress, which is usually greatest at the junction of the atheroma and the normal vessel wall.

The cellular constituents of atheroma have a typical spatial distribution. T lymphocytes and SMCs are found at the shoulder of the plaque, whereas macrophages are found in the lipid core. Plaques that rupture have increased numbers of activated T lymphocytes and mast cells, but reduced numbers of SMCs at the rupture site. Traditionally, the numbers of SMCs within the atherosclerotic plaque were thought to correlate with the formation of the lesion; however, SMCs are now thought to help maintain the integrity of the plaque. Because they synthesize components of the fibrous cap, SMCs may help stabilize the plaque.

The type and extent of arterial remodeling is associated with clinical presentation and, possibly, with plaque rupture. The EEM and plaque areas are significantly larger in unstable patients than in stable patients. In unstable patients, lesions have larger, softer plaques with larger lipid cores, higher macrophage counts, and more positive remodeling, whereas lesions in patients with stable angina are usually fibrous and calcified, with negative remodeling (54,92).

MMPs, a family of endopeptidases that includes collagenases, gelatinases, and stromelysins, are important in both positive remodeling and plaque rupture. MMPs can be found in soluble and cell membrane–bound forms, both of which have zinc present in the active site, depend on Ca^{2+} for activity, and can react with specific tissue inhibitors of MMPs (TIMPs) to form enzymatically inactive complexes. The soluble form is synthesized as an inactive zymogen that can undergo inactivation, whereas the membrane-bound form (known as membrane-type MMP) is synthesized in an active form and functions in the proteolytic activation of the soluble MMPs (93). The soluble MMPs degrade a broad spectrum of matrix proteins, including collagen, proteoglycans, elastin, gelatin, and fibronectin. In atherosclerotic tissue, the four primary MMPs are interstitial collagenase (MMP-1), gelatinase A (MMP-2), stromelysin (MMP-3), and gelatinase B (MMP-9) (94). In culture, normal SMCs produce MMP-2; however, SMCs in atherosclerotic lesions produce MMP-1, MMP-2, MMP-3, and MMP-9. In addition to SMCs, macrophages can secrete MMPs. The production of MMPs by both macrophages and SMCs is increased by exposure to cytokines such as tumor necrosis factor-α (TNFα) and IL-1. Increased MMP activity, which results in excessive degradation of the fibrous cap, is a major cause of plaque rupture. Thus, a major effort is underway to identify factors that regulate MMP production within atheromas and to develop drugs that inhibit the actions of MMPs.

REFERENCES

1. Yusuf S, Reddy S, Ounpuu S, Anand S. Global Burden of Cardiovascular Diseases: Part I: General Considerations, the Epidemiologic Transition, Risk Factors, and Impact of Urbanization. Circulation 2001;104:2746–2753.
2. American Heart Association. 2002 Heart and Stroke Statistical Update. 2001. Dallas, TX.
3. Hiatt WR. Medical treatment of peripheral arterial disease and claudication. N Engl J Med 2001;344:1608–1621.
4. Breslow JL. Mouse models of atherosclerosis. Science 1996;272:685–688.
5. Gimbrone MA Jr. Vascular endothelium, hemodynamic forces, and atherogenesis. Am J Pathol 1999;155:1–5.
6. Stary HC, Chandler AB, Dinsmore RE, et al. A definition of advanced types of atherosclerotic lesions and a histological classification of atherosclerosis. A report from the Committee on Vascular Lesions of the Council on Arteriosclerosis, American Heart Association. Circulation 1995;92:1355–1374.
7. Stary HC, Chandler AB, Glagov S, et al. A definition of initial, fatty streak, and intermediate lesions of atherosclerosis. A report from the Committee on Vascular Lesions of the Council on Arteriosclerosis, American Heart Association. Circulation 1994;89:2462–2478.
8. Stary HC, Blankenhorn DH, Chandler AB, et al. A definition of the intima of human arteries and of its atherosclerosis-prone regions. A report from the Committee on Vascular Lesions of the Council on Arteriosclerosis, American Heart Association. Circulation 1992;85:391–405.

9. Virmani R, Kolodgie FD, Burke AP, Farb A, Schwartz SM. Lessons from sudden coronary death: a comprehensive morphological classification scheme for atherosclerotic lesions. Arterioscler Thromb Vasc Biol 2000;20:1262–1275.

10. Stary HC. Composition and classification of human atherosclerotic lesions. Virchows Arch A Pathol Anat Histopathol 1992;421:277–290.

11. Stary HC. Natural history and histological classification of atherosclerotic lesions: an update. Arterioscler Thromb Vasc Biol 2000;20:1177–1178.

12. Pasquinelli G, Preda P, Gargiulo M, et al. An immunohistochemical study of inflammatory abdominal aortic aneurysms. J Submicrosc Cytol Pathol 1993;25:103–112.

13. Newman KM, Malon AM, Shin RD, Scholes JV, Ramey WG, Tilson MD. Matrix metalloproteinases in abdominal aortic aneurysm: characterization, purification, and their possible sources. Connect Tissue Res 1994;30:265–276.

14. Newman KM, Ogata Y, Malon AM, et al. Identification of matrix metalloproteinases 3 (stromelysin-1) and 9 (gelatinase B) in abdominal aortic aneurysm. Arterioscler Thromb 1994;14:1315–1320.

15. Carrell TW, Burnand KG, Wells GM, Clements JM, Smith A. Stromelysin-1 (matrix metalloproteinase-3) and tissue inhibitor of metalloproteinase-3 are overexpressed in the wall of abdominal aortic aneurysms. Circulation 2002;105:477–482.

16. Von Rokitansky C. A manual of pathological anatomy. Berlin: Sydenham Society; 1852.

17. Li H, Cybulsky MI, Gimbrone MA Jr, Libby P. Inducible expression of vascular cell adhesion molecule-1 by vascular smooth muscle cells in vitro and within rabbit atheroma. Am J Pathol 1993;143:1551–1559.

18. Lusis AJ. Atherosclerosis. Nature 2000;407:233–241.

19. Ross R. Atherosclerosis—an inflammatory disease. N Engl J Med 1999;340:115–126.

20. De Caterina R, Libby P, Peng HB, et al. Nitric oxide decreases cytokine-induced endothelial activation. Nitric oxide selectively reduces endothelial expression of adhesion molecules and proinflammatory cytokines. J Clin Invest 1995;96:60–68.

21. Verma S, Anderson T. Fundamentals of endothelial function for the clinical cardiologist. Circulation 2002;105:546–549.

22. Yusuf S, Dagenais G, Pogue J, Bosch J, Sleight P. Vitamin E supplementation and cardiovascular events in high-risk patients. The Heart Outcomes Prevention Evaluation Study Investigators. N Engl J Med 2000;342:154–160.

23. Randomised trial of cholesterol lowering in 4444 patients with coronary heart disease: the Scandinavian Simvastatin Survival Study (4S). Lancet 1994;344:1383–1389.

24. Witztum JL, Steinberg D. The oxidative modification hypothesis of atherosclerosis: does it hold for humans? Trends Cardiovasc Med 2001;11:93–102.

25. Parthasarathy S, Santanam N, Ramachandran S, Meilhac O. Oxidants and antioxidants in atherogenesis. An appraisal. J Lipid Res 1999;40:2143–2157.

26. Yla-Herttuala S, Palinski W, Rosenfeld ME, et al. Evidence for the presence of oxidatively modified low density lipoprotein in atherosclerotic lesions of rabbit and man. J Clin Invest 1989; 84:1086–1095.

27. Riley SJ, Stouffer GA. Cardiology Grand Rounds from the University of North Carolina at Chapel Hill. The antioxidant vitamins and coronary heart disease: Part 1. Basic science background and clinical observational studies.. Am J Med Sci 2002; 324:314–320.

28. Riley SJ, Stouffer GA. Cardiology Grand Rounds from the University of North Carolina at Chapel Hill. The antioxidant vitamins and coronary heart disease: Part II. Randomized clinical trials. Am J Med Sci 2003;325:15–19.

29. Rapola JM, Virtamo J, Ripatti S, et al. Randomised trial of alpha-tocopherol and beta-carotene supplements on incidence of major coronary events in men with previous myocardial infarction. Lancet 1997;349:1715–1720.

30. Stephens NG, Parsons A, Schofield PM, et al. Randomised controlled trial of vitamin E in patients with coronary disease: Cambridge Heart Antioxidant Study (CHAOS). Lancet 1996; 347:781–786.

31. Gruppo Italiano per lo Studio della Sopravvivenza nell'Infarto miocardico. Dietary supplementation with n-3 polyunsaturated fatty acids and vitamin E after myocardial infarction: results of the GISSI-Prevenzione trial. Lancet 1999;354:447–455.

32. Omenn GS, Goodman GE, Thornquist MD, et al. Effects of a combination of beta carotene and vitamin A on lung cancer and cardiovascular disease. N Engl J Med 1996;334:1150–1155.

33. Patterson C, Ballinger S, Stouffer GA, Runge MS. Antioxidant vitamins: Sorting out the good and the not so good. J Am Coll Cardiol 1999;34:1216–1218.

34. Libby P, Ridker PM, Maseri A. Inflammation and atherosclerosis. Circulation 2002;105:1135–1143.

35. Kruth HS. Macrophage foam cells and atherosclerosis. Front Biosci 2001;6:D429–D455.

36. Hansson GK, Jonasson L, Seifert PS, Stemme S. Immune mechanisms in atherosclerosis. Arteriosclerosis 1989;9:567–578.

37. Hansson GK, Holm J. Interferon-γ inhibits arterial stenosis after injury. Circulation 1991;84:1266–1272.

38. van der Wal AC, Piek JJ, de Boer OJ, et al. Recent activation of the plaque immune response in coronary lesions underlying acute coronary syndromes. Heart 1998;80:14–18.

39. Gupta S, Leatham EW, Carrington D, Mendall MA, Kaski JC, Camm AJ. Elevated Chlamydia pneumoniae antibodies, cardiovascular events, and azithromycin in male survivors of myocardial infarction. Circulation 1997;96:404–407.

40. Gurfinkel E, Bozovich G, Daroca A, Beck E, Mautner B. Randomised trial of roxithromycin in non-Q-wave coronary syndromes: ROXIS Pilot Study. ROXIS Study Group. Lancet 1997;350:404–407.

41. Neumann F, Kastrati A, Miethke T, et al. Treatment of Chlamydia pneumoniae infection with roxithromycin and effect on neointima proliferation after coronary stent placement (ISAR-3): a randomised, double-blind, placebo-controlled trial. Lancet 2001;357:2085–2089.

42. Muhlestein JB, Anderson JL, Carlquist JF, et al. Randomized secondary prevention trial of azithromycin in patients with coronary artery disease: primary clinical results of the ACADEMIC study. Circulation 2000;102:1755–1760.

43. Gieffers J, Fullgraf H, Jahn J, et al. Chlamydia pneumoniae infection in circulating human monocytes is refractory to antibiotic treatment. Circulation 2001;103:351–356.

44. Epstein SE, Zhou YF, Zhu J. Infection and atherosclerosis: emerging mechanistic paradigms. Circulation 1999;100:e20–e28.

45. de Boer OJ, van der Wal AC, Becker AE. Atherosclerosis, inflammation, and infection. J Pathol 2000;190:237–243.

46. Hansson GK. Immune mechanisms in atherosclerosis. Arterioscler Thromb Vasc Biol 2001;21:1876–1890.

47. Benditt EP, Benditt JM. Evidence for a monoclonal origin of human atherosclerotic plaques. Proc Natl Acad Sci USA 1973; 70:1753–1756.

48. Murry CE, Gipaya CT, Bartosek T, Benditt EP, Schwartz SM. Monoclonality of smooth muscle cells in human atherosclerosis. Am J Pathol 1997;151:697–705.

49. Pearson TA, Wang BA, Solez K, Heptinstall RH. Clonal characteristics of fibrous plaques and fatty streaks from human aortas. Am J Pathol 1975;81:379–387.

50. Schwartz SM, Murry CE. Proliferation and the monoclonal origins of atherosclerotic lesions. Annu Rev Med 1998;49:437–460.

51. Proudfoot D, Shanahan CM. Biology of calcification in vascular cells: intima versus media. Herz 2001;26:245–251.

52. Bostrom K, Demer LL. Regulatory mechanisms in vascular calcification. Crit Rev Eukaryot Gene Expr 2000;10:151–158.

53. Glagov S, Weisenberg E, Zarins CK, Stankunavicius R, Kolettis GJ. Compensatory enlargement of human atherosclerotic coronary arteries. N Engl J Med 1987;316:1371–1375.

54. Nissen SE, Yock P. Intravascular ultrasound: novel pathophysiological insights and current clinical applications. Circulation 2001;103:604–616.

55. Pasterkamp G, Schoneveld AH, van Wolferen W, et al. The impact of atherosclerotic arterial remodeling on percentage of luminal stenosis varies widely within the arterial system. A postmortem study. Arterioscler Thromb Vasc Biol 1997;17:3057–3063.

56. Ward MR, Pasterkamp G, Yeung AC, Borst C. Arterial remodeling. Mechanisms and clinical implications. Circulation 2000;102:1186–1191.

57. Mintz GS, Kent KM, Pichard AD, Satler LF, Popma JJ, Leon MB. Contribution of inadequate arterial remodeling to the development of focal coronary artery stenoses. An intravascular ultrasound study. Circulation 1997;95:1791–1798.

58. Smits PC, Pasterkamp G, de Jaegere PP, de Feyter PJ, Borst C. Angioscopic complex lesions are predominantly compensatory enlarged: an angioscopy and intracoronary ultrasound study. Cardiovasc Res 1999;41:458–464.

59. Kimura T, Kaburagi S, Tamura T, et al. Remodeling of human coronary arteries undergoing coronary angioplasty or atherectomy. Circulation 1997;96:475–483.

60. Mintz GS, Popma JJ, Pichard AD, et al. Arterial remodeling after coronary angioplasty: a serial intravascular ultrasound study. Circulation 1996;94:35–43.

61. Dangas G, Mintz GS, Mehran R, et al. Preintervention arterial remodeling as an independent predictor of target-lesion revascularization after nonstent coronary intervention: an analysis of 777 lesions with intravascular ultrasound imaging. Circulation 1999;99:3149–3154.

62. Murabito JM, Evans JC, Larson MG, Levy D. Prognosis after the onset of coronary heart disease. An investigation of differences in outcome between the sexes according to initial coronary disease presentation. Circulation 1993;88:2548–2555.

63. Mizuno K, Satomura K, Miyamoto A, et al. Angioscopic evaluation of coronary-artery thrombi in acute coronary syndromes. N Engl J Med 1992;326:287–291.

64. Falk E. Unstable angina with fatal outcome: dynamic coronary thrombosis leading to infarction and/or sudden death. Autopsy evidence of recurrent mural thrombosis with peripheral embolization culminating in total vascular occlusion. Circulation 1985;71:699–708.

65. Rauch U, Osende JI, Fuster V, Badimon JJ, Fayad Z, Chesebro JH. Thrombus formation on atherosclerotic plaques: pathogenesis and clinical consequences. Ann Intern Med 2001;134:224–238.

66. Gersh BJ, Braunwald E, Rutherford JD. Chronic coronary artery disease. In: Braunwald E, ed. Heart Disease. 5th ed. Philadelphia: W.B. Saunders; 1997:1289–1365.

67. Ambrose JA, Weinrauch M. Thrombosis in ischemic heart disease. Arch Intern Med 1996;156:1382–1394.

68. Silva JA, Escobar A, Collins TJ, Ramee SR, White CJ. Unstable angina. A comparison of angioscopic findings between diabetic and nondiabetic patients. Circulation 1995;92:1731–1736.

69. de Feyter PJ, Ozaki Y, Baptista J, et al. Ischemia-related lesion characteristics in patients with stable or unstable angina. A study with intracoronary angioscopy and ultrasound. Circulation 1995;92:1408–1413.

70. Tabata H, Mizuno K, Arakawa K, et al. Angioscopic identification of coronary thrombus in patients with postinfarction angina. J Am Coll Cardiol 1995;25:1282–1285.

71. Lewis HD, Davis JW, Archibald DG, et al. Protective effects of aspirin against acute myocardial infarction and death in men with unstable angina. N Engl J Med 1983;309:396–403.

72. Cairns JA, Gent M, Singer J, et al. Aspirin, sulfinpyrazone, or both in unstable angina. N Engl J Med 1985;313:1369–1375.

73. Theroux P, Ouimet H, McCans J, et al. Aspirin, heparin or both to treat unstable angina. N Engl J Med 1988;319:1105–1111.

74. The RISC Group. Risk of myocardial infarction and death during treatment with low dose aspirin and intravenous heparin in men with unstable coronary disease. Lancet 1990;336:827–830.

75. ISIS Collaborative Group. Randomized trial of intravenous streptokinase, oral aspirin, both or neither among 17187 cases of suspected acute myocardial infarction: ISIS-2. Lancet 1988;2:349–360.

76. Antiplatelet Trialists' Collaboration. Collaborative overview of randomised trials of antiplatelet therapy—II: Maintenance of vascular graft or arterial patency by antiplatelet therapy. BMJ 1994;308:159–168.

77. Antiplatelet Trialists' Collaboration. Collaborative overview of randomised trials of antiplatelet therapy—I: Prevention of death, myocardial infarction, and stroke by prolonged antiplatelet therapy in various categories of patients. BMJ 1994;308:81–106.

78. Llevadot J, Giugliano RP, Antman EM. Bolus fibrinolytic therapy in acute myocardial infarction. JAMA 2001;286:442–449.

79. Fibrinolytic Therapy Trialists' (FTT) Collaborative Group. Indications for fibrinolytic therapy in suspected acute myocardial infarction: collaborative overview of early mortality and major morbidity results from all randomised trials of more than 1000 patients. Lancet 1994;343:311–322.

80. The PRISM Study Investigators. A comparison of aspirin plus tirofiban with aspirin plus heparin for unstable angina. N Engl J Med 1998;338:1498–1505.

81. The PRISM-PLUS Study Investigators. Inhibition of the platelet glycoprotein IIb/IIIa receptor with tirofiban in unstable angina and non-Q-wave myocardial infarction. N Engl J Med 1998;338:1488–1497.

82. The PURSUIT Trial Investigators. Inhibition of platelet glycoprotein IIb/IIIa with eptifibatide in patients with acute coronary syndromes. Platelet Glycoprotein IIb/IIIa in Unstable Angina: Receptor Suppression Using Integrilin Therapy. N Engl J Med 1998;339:436–443.

83. Davies MJ, Thomas A. Thrombosis and acute coronary-artery lesions in sudden cardiac ischemic death. N Engl J Med 1984;310:1137–1140.

84. Ambrose JA, Tannenbaum MA, Alexopoulos D, et al. Angiographic progression of coronary artery disease and the development of myocardial infarction. J Am Coll Cardiol 1988;12:56–62.

85. Smith SC Jr. Risk-reduction therapy: the challenge to change. Circulation 1996;93:2205–2211.

86. Davies MJ, Bland JM, Hangartner JR, Angelini A, Thomas AC. Factors influencing the presence or absence of acute coronary artery thrombi in sudden ischaemic death. Eur Heart J 1989; 10:203–208.

87. Falk E, Shah PK, Fuster V. Coronary plaque disruption. Circulation 1995;92:657–671.

88. Ojio S, Takatsu H, Tanaka T, et al. Considerable time from the onset of plaque rupture and/or thrombi until the onset of acute myocardial infarction in humans: coronary angiographic findings within 1 week before the onset of infarction. Circulation 2000;102:2063–2069.

89. Farb A, Burke AP, Tang AL, et al. Coronary plaque erosion without rupture into a lipid core. A frequent cause of coronary thrombosis in sudden coronary death. Circulation 1996;93:1354–1363.

90. Ardissino D, Merlini PA, Bauer KA, et al. Thrombogenic potential of human coronary atherosclerotic plaques. Blood 2001;98:2726–2729.

91. Burke AP, Farb A, Malcom GT, Liang YH, Smialek J, Virmani R. Coronary risk factors and plaque morphology in men with coronary disease who died suddenly. N Engl J Med 1997; 336:1276–1282.

92. Varnava AM, Mills PG, Davies MJ. Relationship between coronary artery remodeling and plaque vulnerability. Circulation 2002;105:939–943.

93. Murphy G, Stanton H, Cowell S, et al. Mechanisms for pro matrix metalloproteinase activation. APMIS 1999;107:38–44.

94. Galis ZS, Sukhova GK, Lark MW, Libby P. Increased expression of matrix metalloproteinases and matrix degrading activity in vulnerable regions of human atherosclerotic plaques. J Clin Invest 1994;94:2493–2503.

13   Antiplatelet Drugs

Karlheinz Peter, MD

CONTENTS

PHYSIOLOGICAL AND PATHOPHYSIOLOGICAL ROLE OF PLATELETS

Although Bizzozero identified platelets as a blood component critical for hemostasis in 1882 *(1)*, the central role of platelets in atherogenesis is just now being recognized *(2)*. During atherogenesis, platelets adhere to exposed matrix proteins on denuded vessel walls. Very early in atherogenesis, platelets also adhere to endothelial cells that express an "atherogenic" profile of cell membrane-bound adhesion molecules. The adhering platelets recruit other platelets and white blood cells and secrete growth signals to nearby vessel wall cells, such as smooth muscle cells and fibroblasts. Aggregating platelets, together with other blood cells, are incorporated into the growing atherosclerotic plaque. Finally, the formation of platelet aggregates causes acute vessel closure and severe clinical sequelae, which is the last step in atherogenesis, or acute plaque rupture. Coronary artery disease and acute coronary syndromes are examples of the many manifestations of atherosclerosis. Because platelets play such a central role in the pathogenesis of atherosclerosis, platelet inhibition is a logical therapeutic strategy for acute and chronic treatment of atherosclerosis and its clinical sequelae. The need for efficient inhibition of platelet function is even more evident in the situation of a vascular injury associated with angioplasty

In this chapter, we will discuss three strategies for inhibiting platelet function: (1) inhibition of cyclooxygenase by aspirin; (2) blockade of the $P2Y_{12}$ adenosine diphosphate (ADP) receptor, and (3) blockade of the glycoprotein (GP) IIb/IIIa receptor.

Platelets in Hemostasis

Platelets are anucleate cytoplasmic fragments of bone marrow megakaryocytes that have minimal capacity to synthesize new proteins. The average life span of a platelet is 7–10 days. The basic characteristics of platelets determine the pharmacodynamics of antiplatelet drugs. Vascular injury that includes defects in the endothelial layer results in platelet adhesion on exposed subendothelial matrix components such as collagen or von Willebrand factor *(3)*. The initial adhesion of platelets results in the formation of a platelet monolayer, which initially seals the injured blood vessel. However, the adhesion process itself activates platelets, resulting in the secretion of factors that recruit more platelets and cause platelet aggregation. These factors secreted by platelets, such as thromboxane A_2 (TXA_2) and serotonin, cause vasoconstriction as a part of hemostasis *(4,5)*. Furthermore, membrane constituents on activated platelets, such as tenase- and prothrombinase-complex, initiate and perpetuate the coagulation cascade, finally resulting in the formation of the fibrin network *(6,7)*. Thus, platelets are key initiators and mediators of all phases of physiological hemostasis, which include the cellular, humoral, and vascular phases. The central role of platelets in hemostasis is supported by the presence of bleeding problems in patients with defects in genes that affect platelet function. Examples of

From: *Contemporary Cardiology: Principles of Molecular Cardiology*
Edited by: M. S. Runge and C. Patterson © Humana Press Inc., Totowa, NJ

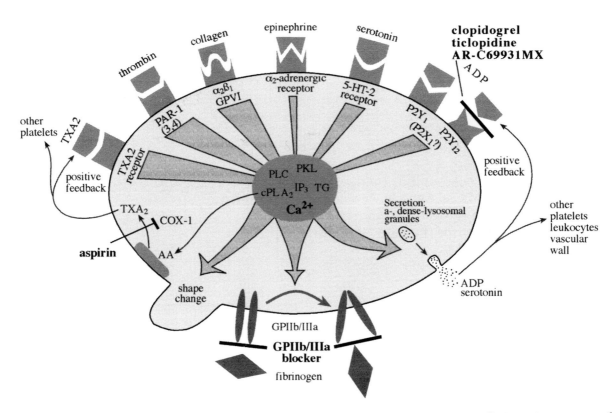

Fig. 1. Major platelet activation pathways and their therapeutic inhibition. AA, arachidonic acid; $\alpha_2\beta_1$ integrin receptor $\alpha_2\beta_1$; ADP, adenosine diphosphate, three types of ADP receptors on platelets: $P2Y_1$, $P2Y_{12}$, $P2X_1$; TG, thromboglobulin; COX-1, cyclooxygenase-1 identical to prostaglandin H synthase with cyclooxygenase and peroxidase activity; $cPLA_2$, cytoplasmic phospholipase A_2; GP, glycoprotein; 5-HT-2 receptor, 5-hydroxytryptamine 2 subtype of serotonin receptor; IP_3, inosityl triphosphate; PAR, protease activated receptor; PLC, phospholipase C; TXA_2, thromboxane A_2.

such defects include the Bernard–Soulier syndrome, which is associated with defects in the von Willebrand receptor (GPIb-IX-V), and Glanzmann thrombasthenia, which is associated with defects in the GP IIb/IIIa receptor. Furthermore, bleeding problems are seen in patients treated with antiplatelet drugs *(8,9)*.

Platelet Activation Pathways

Platelets are activated by agonist binding to surface membrane receptors that are mainly G protein coupled receptors comprising a single polypeptide chain with an extracellular amino-terminus and seven transmembrane domains *(10,11)*. Signaling such as occurs via G proteins results in the activation of the enzymes phospholipase C, protein kinase C, and cytoplasmic phospholipase A_2, and in the formation of second messengers such as diacyl glycerol and inosityl triphosphate (Fig. 1) *(12)*. The intracellular Ca^{2+} concentration, which varies from 0.1 μM in resting platelets to 1 μM in thrombin-activated platelets, is important in platelet signaling *(13)*. Upon platelet activation,

cytosolic Ca^{2+} levels are increased by the release of calcium from the dense tubular system and by the influx of calcium across ligand-gated Ca^{2+} channels such as the $P2X_1$ ADP receptor *(14)*. Complex and mostly unknown signaling mechanisms result in a change in platelet shape and in the secretion and activation of the platelet fibrinogen receptor, GP IIb/IIIa. A direct connection between Ca^{2+} levels and the activation of GP IIb/IIIa via the calcium integrin binding protein has recently been reported *(15)*.

Platelets have unique mechanisms to amplify activating signals. Many of the agents secreted, such as ADP, serotonin, and platelet factor 4, are platelet agonists, which amplify the signal in a positive feedback mechanism (Fig. 1). Another strong amplification system with a positive feedback mode is the TXA_2 signaling pathway. TXA_2 can diffuse across the plasma membrane and can cause not only amplification of the signal, but also recruitment of other platelets into the growing thrombus (Fig. 1). Because of the need to confine this effect locally, the half-life of TXA_2 is brief (about 30 seconds) *(5)*.

ASPIRIN

History of Aspirin

The first medicinal use of acetylsalicylic acid can be traced back to around 500 BCE, when the Chinese used willow bark as a remedy. Around 400 BCE, Hippocrates suggested chewing willow bark to reduce fever and pain, and he recommended tea made from willow bark to ease pain at childbirth. Although willow bark as a remedy was mentioned in Greek and Roman historic writings, this practice seemed to be lost during the Middle Ages. In the 1700s, European settlers encountered Native Americans who used willow bark medicinally. Reverend Edward Stone of Oxford experimented with willow bark as a fever medication, and the Royal Society of London published his results in 1763. In 1828, Leroux isolated the active ingredient of willow bark and named it salicin, after *salix*, the Latin name for the willow tree. Ten years later, a more pure compound was isolated and named salicylic acid.

Extracts of willow bark and chemically synthesized crude preparations of salicylic acids were used for many years as pain relievers; however, major side effects such as stomach problems were associated with these agents. Felix Hoffmann, a chemist at Bayer AG, improved the synthesis process and produced a pure, stable acetylsalicylic acid preparation. In 1899, Bayer AG registered the tradename Aspirin based on the meadowsweet with the Latin name *Spiraea ulmaria (16)*. However, Bayer AG had to relinquish the trademark in 1919 as part of Germany's war reparations at the end of World War I, as per the Treaty of Versailles. More than 50 years later, the Nobel laureate John Vane described the mechanism by which aspirin works: the blocking of the production of hormone-like substances known as prostaglandins *(17)*. Although the effect of aspirin on bleeding time was described in 1956 *(18)*, the antiplatelet effect of aspirin was not widely recognized until the 1980s.

Mechanism of Action

Aspirin inhibits the enzymes cyclooxygenase-1 [COX-1, prostaglandin (PG) H-synthase-1] and cyclooxygenase-2 (COX-2, PG H-synthase-2) in the conversion of arachidonic acid to prostaglandin G_2 (PGG_2) and prostaglandin H_2 (PGH_2) (Fig. 2A) *(19)*. COX-1 is constitutively expressed in most cell types, whereas COX-2 is detectable only after induction in inflammatory cells, endothelial cells, and others. Platelets appear to express only COX-1; however, expression of COX-2 from platelets has been reported in one study *(20)*. Aspirin selectively acetylates the serine residue at position 529 in COX-1, which sterically hinders

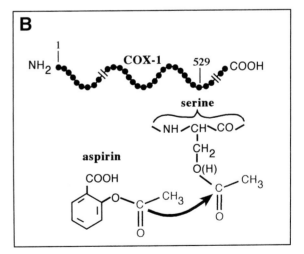

Fig. 2. Aspirin: mechanism of action. **(A)** Cyclooxygenase-1 (COX-1) converts arachidonic acid to prostaglandin G2 (PGG_2), which is converted by the peroxidase activity of COX-1 to prostaglandin H2 (PGH_2). Finally, thromboxane A_2 is synthesized by thromboxane synthase. **(B)** Aspirin inhibits COX-1 by the transfer of its acetyl residue to serine 529 of COX-1, thereby blocking access of arachidonic acid to the catalytic center of COX-1.

arachidonic acid from accessing the catalytic center and results in a permanent loss of cyclooxygenase activity (Fig. 2B). COX-2 is inhibited by the same mechanisms; however, higher doses of aspirin are needed. In human platelets, PGH_2, the product of COX-1, is predominantly metabolized to TXA_2 (Fig. 2A). By its release and binding to the TXA_2-receptor, TXA_2 is part of a positive feedback amplification system (Fig. 1) of platelets that is active with divergent primary platelet agonists (ADP, collagen, thrombin, epinephrine, etc.). Because platelets cannot resynthesize COX-1, the irreversible blockade of COX-1 results in irreversible platelet inhibition. Thus, even though the plasma half-life of aspirin is 15 minutes, platelet inhibition can be seen for about 7–10 days (21).

Clinical Use of Aspirin

The pivotal role of platelets in arterial thrombosis has been established by the beneficial effects of aspirin in patients with myocardial infarction. In the second international study of infarct survival (ISIS-2), administration of aspirin reduced 5-week mortality by 23% in patients with myocardial infarction. The effect of platelet inhibition was equal and additive to the effect of thrombolysis by streptokinase (22). The original benefit of aspirin was still seen at the 10-year follow-up (23). Unstable angina is associated with platelet activation (24), and aspirin reduces the rate of death and myocardial infarction in patients with unstable angina (25–27). In addition, coronary angioplasty is associated with platelet activation, and aspirin significantly reduces the rate of acute vessel closure (28,29). The use of aspirin is essential in these acute clinical situations.

Aspirin has saved the most lives in the secondary prevention of cardiovascular events. In the Antiplatelet Trialists' meta-analysis of approximately 70,000 patients with coronary artery disease, transient ischemic attacks, stroke, or peripheral arterial vascular disease, aspirin reduced the odds ratio for myocardial infarction, stroke, or vascular death by 25% (30). In a recent meta-analysis of 200,000 patients treated with antiplatelet drugs, the benefits of antiplatelet therapy in the secondary prevention of cardiovascular complications were extended to include patients with stable angina pectoris, intermittent claudication, and (if oral anticoagulants are unsuitable) atrial fibrillation (31).

For the primary prevention of cardiovascular events, the increased incidence of hemorrhagic strokes associated with aspirin counteracts the beneficial effect on the rate of myocardial infarction (32–34). In the Physicians Health Study, aspirin increased the rate of stroke by 21% and decreased the rate of myocardial infarction by 44% (32). Nevertheless, no reduction in

mortality from all cardiovascular causes was associated with aspirin (32). When evaluating a patient for aspirin therapy, the physician should carefully weigh the benefits of aspirin in preventing ischemic cardiovascular events against the increased risk of stroke. The higher the risk of cardiovascular disease, the more benefit associated with aspirin. In patients with definite cardiovascular risk factors, especially those with diabetes mellitus, aspirin treatment may be beneficial in the primary prevention of cardiovascular events (35–37).

A consensus has not been reached on the appropriate dose of aspirin. Aspirin-induced gastrointestinal toxicity is dose dependent (38); however, an increase in dose does not increase the antiplatelet effects of aspirin. The Antithrombotic Trialists' Collaborations' meta-analysis has clearly shown that high daily doses (500–1500 mg) of aspirin are not more effective than medium (160–325 mg) or low doses (75–150 mg) (31). Thus, low-dose aspirin produces the full antiplatelet effect with the lowest risk of side effects.

ADP RECEPTOR INHIBITORS

ADP Receptors on Platelets

Although the ability of ADP to induce platelet adhesiveness and platelet aggregation has been known for 40 years (39,40), the cloning of the three ADP receptors on human platelets has just recently been completed. The $P2Y_1$ receptor was the first to be cloned in 1996 (41,42). ADP acts as an agonist for $P2Y_1$, whereas adenosine triphosphate (ATP) acts as an antagonist (Fig. 3) (43). The $P2Y_1$ receptor mediates calcium mobilization and shape change in platelets (44). Although necessary for platelet aggregation in response to ADP, $P2Y_1$ is not sufficient to induce the response (44–46). Biochemical, pharmacological, and genetic data indicated the existence of at least two different ADP receptors on platelets (12,47,48). A second ADP receptor, $P2X_1$, was cloned on human platelets a year later (49). The $P2X_1$ receptor is an ATP-gated ion channel that mediates the rapid entry of calcium into the platelet (within 10 milliseconds) in response to ADP. The role of the $P2X_1$ receptor has not been fully defined; however, $P2X_1$ knock out mice have no abnormalities in hemostasis (14). The third ADP receptor on human platelets, $P2Y_{12}$, was just recently cloned. An expression cloning strategy was used in *Xenopus* oocytes with the goal of detecting Gi-linked receptors (50). The $P2Y_{12}$ receptor seems to be responsible for the positive feedback (see Fig. 1) and thus the amplification of platelet stimuli, especially by weak agonists; therefore, this receptor is central in the final step of aggregation and the stabilization of aggregates (14,51).

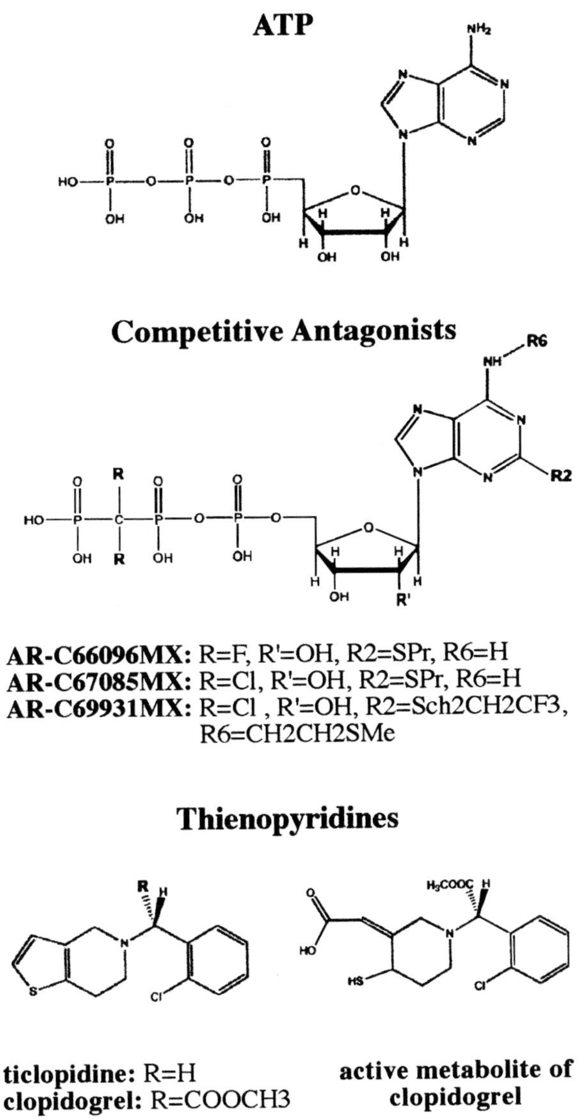

ATP

Competitive Antagonists

AR-C66096MX: R=F, R'=OH, R2=SPr, R6=H
AR-C67085MX: R=Cl, R'=OH, R2=SPr, R6=H
AR-C69931MX: R=Cl , R'=OH, R2=Sch2CH2CF3,
R6=CH2CH2SMe

Thienopyridines

ticlopidine: R=H   **active metabolite of**
clopidogrel: R=COOCH3   **clopidogrel**

Fig. 3. P2Y$_{12}$ ADP receptor inhibition: Thienopyridines and Competitve Antagonists. The new class of competitive antagonists specifically inhibits binding of ADP to P2Y$_{12}$ by its homology to ATP. Thienopyridines are prodrugs that are metabolized in the liver to thiol metabolites, which induce covalent modification of the cysteine residues within P2Y$_{12}$.

Thienopyridines

Although the inhibition of platelet aggregation by the thienopyridine ticlopidine was reported in 1975 (51), significant adverse effects such as skin rash, gastrointestinal symptoms, and bone marrow toxicity with severe and fatal neutropenia prompted the replacement of ticlopidine in clinical use with clopidogrel, another thienopyridine with minimal side effects (52–55). Thienopyridines are prodrugs that have to be metabolized by cytochrome P450 in the liver (Fig. 3). The short-lived active metabolite of clopidogrel was recently identified as being a thiol derivate of the parent agent clopidogrel (Fig. 3) (56). The selectivity of thienopyridines for the P2Y$_{12}$ ADP receptor is caused by a thiol metabolite-induced covalent modification of the cysteine residues, of which four are found in the P2Y$_{12}$ receptor (50,56).

The first significant study for the widespread clinical use of clopidogrel was the Clopidogrel versus Aspirin in Patients at Risk of Ischemic Events (CAPRIE) trial (52), in which clopidogrel was compared with aspirin in the secondary prevention of thromboembolic complications in patients with atherosclerotic disease (prior myocardial infarction, ischemic stroke, or peripheral vascular disease). Clopidogrel was slightly better than aspirin in the CAPRIE trial, and safety and tolerability of clopidogrel and aspirin were similar. In interventional cardiology, the combination of aspirin and clopidogrel after stent placement has become standard treatment because it substantially reduces the risk of a subacute stent thrombosis (55,57–59). Long-term treatment of coronary syndromes with the combination of aspirin and clopidogrel is now becoming part of standard care (60).

Competitive P2Y$_{12}$ Receptor Antagonists

The unique distribution of the P2Y$_{12}$ ADP receptor on platelets, and potentially in the brain, but not in other tissue makes this receptor an excellent pharmacological target with nearly ideal selectivity (50). Clopidogrel blocks all the available P2Y$_{12}$ receptors on platelets and (14) has an excellent safety and tolerability profile (52,54,55). Although a remarkable pharmaceutical agent, clopidogrel has two characteristics that justify the search for other P2Y$_{12}$ ADP receptor inhibitors. First, the full antiplatelet effect of clopidogrel is not seen for at least 2 hours after administration, even with a large loading dose (300 mg) (61). For acute myocardial infarction or urgent coronary interventions, a more rapid antiplatelet effect is needed. Second, the P2Y$_{12}$ receptor is blocked irreversibly, so the antiplatelet effect lasts during the life span of the platelet (62). Because no antagonist is available for clopidogrel, bleeding complications may be a problem.

To overcome these obstacles, a new class of P2Y$_{12}$ ADP receptor inhibitors has been developed (63). Based on the fact that ATP is a competitive antagonist of ADP (Fig. 3), structural homologs have been screened for selectivity against the P2Y$_{12}$ receptor. Several agents have been identified, and some have already been tested in clinical trials (Fig. 3). These agents have the advantage of immediate antiplatelet effects after intravenous application, and because of their short half-life, the antiplatelet effect is rapidly reversed *(63)*. Both intravenous and oral agents are available *(63)*.

GLYCOPROTEIN IIb/IIIa BLOCKERS

Structure of Glycoprotein IIb/IIIa

The term GP IIb/IIIa originates from the description of bands number IIb and IIIa on a gel electrophoresis of platelet proteins *(64)*. GP IIb comprises two chains (heavy chain of 105 kDa and light chain of 25 kDa) that are linked by a disulfide bond (Fig. 4) *(65,66)*. GP IIIa is a single chain protein of 95 kDa (Fig. 4) *(65,66)*. The genes were cloned in the late 1980s, and GP IIb and GP IIIa were located close together on chromosome 17 *(67–70)*. GP IIb/IIIa, the most abundant platelet membrane receptor with 50,000 to 80,000 glycoproteins per platelet, makes up about 2% of the total platelet protein *(71)* and 15% of total surface protein *(72)*. The role of GP IIb/IIIa in fibrinogen binding and platelet aggregation was identified in genetic studies of Glanzmann disease *(73–75)*. Direct binding experiments with fibrinogen *(76,77)*, blocking experiments with monoclonal antibodies *(78)*, and reconstitution of GP IIb/IIIa binding function either after purification of the protein *(79)* or by expression of the transfected cDNA on model cell lines *(80)* provided definite evidence of the binding of fibrinogen and the role of GP IIb/IIIa in platelet aggregation. In addition to fibrinogen, several other ligands (von Willebrand factor, fibronectin, vitronectin, and thrombospondin) have been identified as promoting platelet adhesion *(81)*. The two glycoproteins GP IIb and GP IIIa are identical to the antibody epitopes CD41 and CD61. Finally, GP IIb/IIIa has been identified as a member of the adhesion molecule family called integrins, which have an integrative function between extracellular ligands and the intracellular cytoskeleton (Fig. 4) *(82)*. Integrins have two major functions. First, they mechanically couple the cytoskeleton to the extracellular matrix or to surface receptors of other cells. Second, they transmit signals from the inside of the cell to the outside of the cell and vice versa *(83,84)*. For consistency with the original term GP IIb/IIIa, $\alpha_{IIb}\beta_3$ was chosen as the term within integrin nomenclature *(82–84)*. More than 20 different integrins have been identified, and all have two subunits (α- and β-subunit) that are noncovalently linked to each other. With the exception of α_4, all integrin subunits have a short cytoplasmic tail, one transmembraneous region, and a large extracellular domain. Several integrins have different conformational states *(82–84)*. Upon cell stimulation, integrins can change conformation from a low to a high affinity state for ligand binding (Fig. 1).

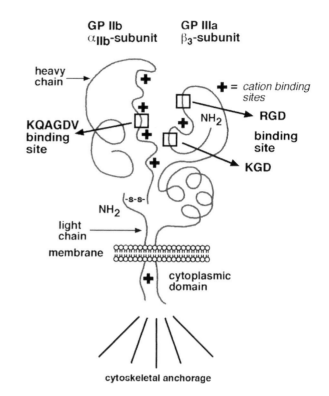

Fig. 4. Structure of GP IIb/IIIa (αIIbβ3, CD41/CD61). Potential binding sites for RGD, KGD, and KQAGVD sequences of fibrinogen are shown. Ca^{2+} binding sites are represented by +.

The Glycoprotein IIb/IIIa Ligand Fibrinogen

Fibrinogen is a 340,000 Da dimeric macromolecule comprising three pairs of disulfide-bonded polypeptide chains, designated Aα-, Bβ-, and γ-chain. Fibrinogen is transformed to fibrin monomers by the cleavage of fibrinopeptides A and B. Because of its symmetrical bivalent structure, fibrinogen serves a bridging function between two GP IIb/IIIa receptors and thereby contributes to platelet aggregation *(85)*. Three sites on fibrinogen are potentially involved in the binding to GP IIb/IIIa (Fig. 4): a sequence of 12 amino acids (HHLGGAKQAGDV) close to the carboxyterminal end of the γ-chain and two RGD sequences within the α-chain *(86)*. The γ-chain sequence seems to be the primary interaction site. Fibrinogen molecules without this sequence do not mediate binding to GP IIb/IIIa and platelet aggregation *(87,88)*. However, recombinant fibrinogen molecules that have RGE sequences instead of the native RGD sequences still support fibrinogen binding and platelet aggregation *(87)*. In addition, blocking experiments with peptide-specific antibodies indicate the primary role of the γ-chain sequence, but not the RGD sequences *(89)*. Nevertheless, peptides based on both sequences block fibrinogen binding to GP IIb/IIIa. Natural GP IIb/IIIa antagonists and pharmaceutically designed drugs are based on the RGD sequence as discussed below.

Glanzmann Thrombasthenia: Glycoprotein IIb/IIIa Blockade

In 1918, Glanzmann first described patients with a hereditary form of hemorrhagic thrombasthenia *(73)*. Abnormalities in GP IIb/IIIa have been identified as the basis of the autosomal recessive disease Glanzmann thrombasthenia *(74)*. Mutations on GP IIb or GP IIIa result either in total loss or significant reduction in platelet surface expression of GP IIb/IIIa or in the expression of nonfunctional GP IIb/IIIa *(9,90,91)*. The clinical features of patients with Glanzmann disease resemble a chronic blockade of GP IIb/IIIa. Most Glanzmann patients have easy bruising, purpura, epistaxis, and gingival bleeding. In women, menorrhagia is a major problem. Gastrointestinal hemorrhage is seen only in a few patients. Intracranial bleeding has been described in case reports of three patients; two patients had bleeding associated with trauma, and circumstances for the third patient were not reported *(9)*. Many patients need blood transfusions at some point. Some patients, especially younger ones, die of hemorrhagic problems, usually associated with trauma *(9)*. No myocardial infarctions or strokes have been reported in these patients *(9)*; however, most of these patients are young. The clinical sequelae of the inability of platelets to aggregate via GP IIb/IIIa are surprisingly mild. Spontaneous bleeding is of minor concern, whereas bleeding associated with trauma (the puncture of arterial vessels for coronary angiography has to be considered as such) is a major problem that can often be managed with blood transfusions. Spontaneous cerebral bleeding in Glanzmann thrombasthenia or in pharmaceutical blockade of GP IIb/IIIa is not a concern. The excellent safety profile is a major reason for the broad use of GP IIb/IIIa blockers.

Development of Glycoprotein IIb/IIIa Blockers

Three types of GP IIb/IIIa blockers have been developed (1) monoclonal antibodies that block ligand binding to GP IIb/IIIa (e.g., abciximab); (2) cyclic peptides based on the R(K)GD sequence (e.g., eptifibatide); and (3) chemical compounds modeled after the RGD structure (e.g., peptidomimetics such as tirofiban and lamifiban). The pharmacology of these three groups of agents differs because of their structural differences. One agent from each group has been approved by the FDA.

ABCIXIMAB (REOPRO®)

Using monoclonal antibody (mAb) techniques that became available in the 1980s, Coller immunized mice

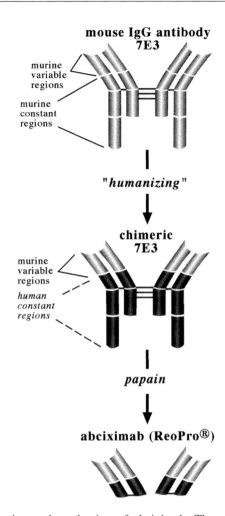

Fig. 5. Design and production of abciximab. The recombinant antibody fragment, abciximab, was made by combining the original mouse anti-GP IIb/IIIa monoclonal IgG antibody sequences of all constant regions with human sequences, followed by digestion with papain.

with human platelets to develop mAbs to test in platelet aggregometry. Coller initially described one of these mAbs, called 7E3, as specific for activated platelets *(92)*. However, 7E3 was eventually shown not to be entirely activation specific; the on- and off-rate of 7E3 binding to platelets was different for nonactivated and activated platelets *(93)*. The antithrombotic effects of mAb 7E3 were identified in a series of animal experiments *(94)*. In initial clinical experiments with 7E3 F(ab)$_2$ fragments, anti-7E3 antibody production in humans was seen *(95,96)*. All mouse antibody sequences of this GP IIb/IIIa blocking antibody, except those of the variable domains of the light and heavy chain, were exchanged with their corresponding human sequences (Fig. 5.) Abciximab, which has been commercially available since December 1994, is a Fab fragment of this 7E3 mAb (Fig. 5) *(97)*.

Because of its small size and minimal number of murine sequences, abciximab was expected to have a low antigenicity *(98)*. Anti-abciximab IgG antibodies are induced with the use of abciximab, but immunological problems such as anaphylactic reactions did not develop in patients who received a second dose *(99)*.

EPTIFIBATIDE (INTEGRILIN®)

Eptifibatide was found by a systematic search of snake venoms with the potential to specifically block the GP IIb/IIIa receptor *(100)*. From the venom of the southeastern pygmy rattlesnake *Sistrurus m. barbouri*, barbourin, a 73-amino-acid polypeptide, was used as a template for the development of a series of peptide compounds tested for the specific inhibition of GP IIb/IIIa *(100,101)*. In contrast to other GP IIb/IIIa blocking agents, which contain RGD sequences, barbourin contained a KGD sequence. The lysine residue seems to provide specificity for GP IIb/IIIa *(100,101)*. RGD sequences present in the fibrinogen α-chain, in fibronectin, and in vitronectin block not only GP IIb/IIIa, but also other integrin receptors such as the fibronectin receptor ($\alpha5\beta1$) and the vitronectin receptor ($\alpha V\beta3$). Therefore, RGD sequences do not specifically block GP IIb/IIIa. However, the KGD sequence may resemble the KQAGDV sequence within the γ-chain of fibrinogen, where the K, G, and D are structurally aligned, and the KGD sequence may thereby specifically block GP IIb/IIIa *(100,101)*. The peptide that was further developed is a cyclic heptapeptide (Fig. 6) *(101)*.

TIROFIBAN (AGGRASTAT®)

In the third strategy to develop GP IIb/IIIa blockers, small molecular weight, non-peptide compounds were identified. The RGD sequence found in the α-chain of fibrinogen, on other integrin ligands, and on most disintegrins (naturally designed to block integrins such as GP IIb/IIIa) was used as a template. The structure of the snake venom echistatin was analyzed, and a tyrosin-like molecule, tirofiban, was developed as an RGD-mimetic (Fig. 6) *(102–104)*.

Specificity of Glycoprotein IIb/IIIa Blockers

GP IIb/IIIa blockers may cross-react with other integrin receptors in addition to GP IIb/IIIa. The two integrin receptors discussed in this context are the vitronectin receptor $\alpha_V\beta_3$ (CD51/CD61) and the leukocyte receptor Mac-1 $\alpha_M\beta_2$ (CD11b/CD18). The vitronectin receptor shares the β_3-subunit with GP IIb/IIIa, and the α_V subunit is highly homologous to the α_{IIb} subunit. Furthermore, like GP IIb/IIIa, $\alpha_V\beta_3$ binds the ligands vitronectin, fibrinogen, von Willebrand factor, fibronectin, and other

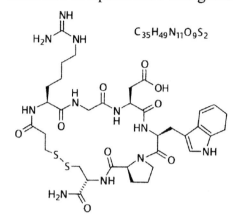

Fig. 6. The structure of tirofiban and eptifibatide. Tirofiban is a chemical RGD analog, and eptifibatide is a KGD peptidomimetic.

RGD-containing ligands. Thus, cross-reactivity of GP IIb/IIIa blockers with $\alpha_V\beta_3$ can be expected.

The clinical role for $\alpha_V\beta_3$ in patients in whom GP IIb/IIIa blockers would be used is unknown. $\alpha_V\beta_3$ is expressed with a high density only on osteoclasts and some tumor cells and with variable density on smooth muscle cells, endothelial cells, polymorphonuclear cells, monocytes, and T-lymphocytes. Small amounts of $\alpha_V\beta_3$ are present on platelets. Platelets can adhere via $\alpha_V\beta_3$ on osteopontin, which is upregulated over atherosclerotic plaques *(105,106)*. Furthermore, the vitronectin receptor is densely expressed on endothelial cells overlying atherosclerotic plaques *(107)*. In experimental models, migration and proliferation of smooth muscle cells and intima hyperplasia after vascular injury were mediated by $\alpha_V\beta_3$ *(108–111)*. Although these data suggest a reduction in restenosis, clinical trials failed to show a reduction in restenosis by the blockade of $\alpha_V\beta_3$ via GP IIb/IIIa blockers *(112)*.

The GP IIb/IIIa blocker abciximab blocks both GP IIb/IIIa and $\alpha_V\beta_3$ with equal affinity *(113)*. For eptifibatide, which was developed to specifically bind GP IIb/IIIa and not other integrins, the data are inconclusive. In initial experiments with purified $\alpha_V\beta_3$, eptifibatide appeared not to bind the vitronectin receptor; however, recent data directly describe functional inhibition of $\alpha_V\beta_3$ by eptifibatide *(114)*.

Although the data are few, tirofiban does not appear to bind and block $\alpha_V\beta_3$ *(115)*.

The integrin Mac-1 is expressed predominately in leukocytes of myeloid and monocytic lineage and in natural killer lymphocytes *(83)*. Mac-1 is a versatile adhesion molecule with ligands of very different biological functions. The interaction of Mac-1 with transmembrane intercellular adhesion molecule-1 (ICAM-1) mediates cell adhesion directly on the endothelium *(83,84)*. By binding the zymogen form of the serine protease factor X, Mac-1 initiates the coagulation serine protease cascade, resulting in thrombin and fibrin formation on cell surfaces *(116)*. In addition, the binding of fibrinogen to Mac-1, which can be part of the coagulation cascade, can mediate cell aggregation and cell adhesion either on immobilized fibrinogen (e.g., demasked on coronary angioplasty) or as a cross-bridge between Mac-1 and ICAM-1 *(117)*. Mac-1 is identical to the complement receptor type 3, which is responsible for the recognition of iC3b-opsonized bacteria and yeast by phagocytes, and thus, the initiation of phagocytosis, degranulation, and respiratory bursts *(118)*. Furthermore, clinically used heparin has recently been identified as a ligand for Mac-1 *(119)*. Therefore, inhibition of Mac-1 may affect coagulation and inflammatory responses both at the atherosclerotic plaques or in reperfusion injury. Data indicate that abciximab binds to Mac-1 and thereby blocks ligand binding *(119–123)*. The cross-reactivity with Mac-1 is unique for abciximab within the group of GP IIb/IIIa inhibitors. However, the clinical advantage of this unique cross-reactivity is unknown.

Pharmacology of Glycoprotein IIb/IIIa Blockers

The antibody fragment abciximab binds to GP IIb/IIIa with high affinity (K_D, 5 nmol/L), the low-molecular-weight GP IIb/IIIa blocker tirofiban has a medium affinity (K_D, 15 nmol/L), and the cyclic peptide eptifibatide has a low binding affinity (K_D, 120 nmol/L) *(124)*. The number of molecules needed to block the receptor should be highest for eptifibatide because the ratio of bound to free molecules is lowest for this agent. The affinity, dissociation rate, body distribution, and elimination route determine the duration of platelet inhibitory effects. The inhibitory effects of abciximab on platelets last for several days *(125,126)*, whereas tirofiban and eptifibatide lose their platelet inhibitory effects within 2–4 hours *(127,128)*. The strategy of antagonism of the GP IIb/IIIa receptor depends on the clinical situation, such as whether acute bleeding may be a problem or whether emergent operation may be necessary. The platelet inhibitory effect of abciximab, which may last for days after cessation of infusion, needs to be antagonized with

platelet transfusions. The antibody fragments will be redistributed within minutes to the transfused platelets, and thus the number of transfused platelets determines the degree of GP IIb/IIIa blockade on the circulating platelets. With the low-molecular-weight GP IIb/IIIa blockers, platelet transfusions are less effective because of the large pool of free GP IIb/IIIa blocker in the plasma, which will immediately block the transfused platelets. The fast clearance will restore platelet function within 2–4 hours after cessation of infusion; therefore, for bridging to a bypass operation, the low molecular weight GP IIb/IIIa blockers are more suitable than the long-acting antibody fragment abciximab.

Dosing of Glycoprotein IIb/IIIa Blockers

The aim of therapy with GP IIb/IIIa blockers is to inhibit platelet aggregation in response to vascular injury, such as angioplasty or the rupture of an unstable atherosclerotic plaque. No laboratory assay is available to indicate the level of platelet inhibition needed for optimal therapeutic success. The standard assay to test for platelet aggregability is light transmission aggregometry with platelet-rich plasma. For this assay, platelets have to be stimulated, but no agreement has been reached on the type or dose of the stimulating agent. Twenty micromoles of ADP is often used; however, thrombin receptor activating peptide (TRAP) or collagen has recently been used *(129)*. Furthermore, test results vary with the anticoagulant *(130)*. The rapid platelet function assay (RPFA), which is a bedside monitoring test that measures the agglutination of fibrinogen-coated beads and TRAP-activated platelets in whole blood, has recently been developed *(131)*. However, no clear correlation has been found in comparative studies of light transmission aggregometry and RPFA *(132)*. The use of flow cytometry to directly determine platelet occupancy by GP IIb/IIIa blockers is least prone to variations caused by differences in stimulating agents and anticoagulants *(126,133)*. However, even though flow cytometry can measure the percentage of occupied GP IIb/IIIa receptors, what percentage needs to be blocked for clinically sufficient platelet inhibition is not known. Although often used, the 80% threshold is not based on strong scientific data. The scope of the dosing problem with GP IIb/IIIa blockers has become evident with the finding that the doses of eptifibatide used in initial trials were probably too low *(130)*. Initial pharmacodynamic studies, done with light transmission aggregometry with sodium citrate anticoagulant, probably overestimated the platelet inhibitory effect of eptifibatide *(130)*. Increasing the dose of eptifibatide may have contributed to favorable outcomes in recent clinical trials *(134)*. In addition, the pharmacological studies used to define dosing of abciximab and tirofiban may be insufficiently large to determine optimal dosing *(132,135)*.

Glycoprotein IIb/IIIa Blocker-Induced Thrombocytopenia

Profound thrombocytopenia has been repeatedly described as an adverse effect in patients treated with GP IIb/IIIa blockers, but its mechanism has not been defined *(136,137)*. The preferred explanation is based on the finding that binding of GP IIb/IIIa blockers to the receptor induces conformational changes in ligand-mimetic properties, thereby exposing ligand-induced binding sites (LIBS) epitopes on GP IIb/IIIa *(138)*. Patients who develop thrombocytopenia during GP IIb/IIIa blocker therapy may have preformed anti-LIBS antibodies that react with the blocker-occupied GP IIb/IIIa and cause a clearance of platelets *(139)*. Furthermore, the complex formed between GP IIb/IIIa blocker and GP IIb/IIIa may be antigenic for preformed antibodies. The incidence of profound thrombocytopenia increases with readministration of abciximab *(99)*, which also indicates the involvement of the immune response. Administration of a second GP IIb/IIIa blocker, eptifibatide, 4 days after abciximab-induced thrombocytopenia did not cause a second thrombocytopenia, which is another finding favoring the existence of antibodies specific for the GP IIb/IIIa blocker *(140)*. Furthermore, binding of anti-LIBS antibodies may cross-link the GP IIb/IIIa receptors that are occupied with GP IIb/IIIa blockers, and the combination may transduce signals to inside the cell, resulting in platelet activation. In one patient with abciximab-induced thrombocytopenia, platelet activation was shown directly *(141)*.

Intrinsic Activating Property of Glycoprotein IIb/IIIa Blockers

Binding of the natural ligand fibrinogen and the ligand mimetic RGD peptide induces conformational changes in GP IIb/IIIa that can be detected by anti-LIBS antibodies *(138,142–145)*. Cyclic peptides derived from the RGD or KGD sequence and chemical compounds that are modeled after the RGD structure bind competitively to the fibrinogen binding pocket within GP IIb/IIIa and are therefore ligand mimetics. In addition, these agents can bind to the nonactivated GP IIb/IIIa on unstimulated platelets and cause a conformational change in GP IIb/IIIa without prior platelet activation *(124,142,143,145)*. All commercially available GP IIb/IIIa blockers unmask the LIBS epitope because of conformational changes *(144,146)*. After dissociation of the GP IIb/IIIa blockers, if the GP IIb/IIIa receptor did not undergo a reverse conformational change,

fibrinogen could bind to the receptor, and platelet aggregation would be induced instead of blocked by GP IIb/IIIa blockers *(143)*. A reverse conformational change might be expected, but the nature of the change has not been defined. Furthermore, GP IIb/IIIa blockers may intrinsically activate platelets via outside-in signaling induced by the binding of GP IIb/IIIa blockers to the GP IIb/IIIa receptor. Outside-in signaling induced by GP IIb/IIIa blockers has been shown by Ca^{2+}-concentration measurements, TXA_2 production, and expression of P-selectin and CD63 *(147–150)*. The intrinsic activating properties of the GP IIb/IIIa blockers seem to be a strategic problem; until now, the ligand mimetic approach has been the only pharmacological strategy for development of GP IIb/IIIa blockers.

Parenteral Use of Glycoprotein IIb/IIIa Blockers

The benefits of GP IIb/IIIa blockade have been assessed in patients undergoing percutaneous coronary interventions (PCI) and in patients with acute coronary syndromes. In the PCI group, GP IIb/IIIa blockade reduced mortality up to 60% in patients undergoing balloon angioplasty and/or stent placement *(151)* and decreased the necessity for repeat revascularization by up to 50% *(151)*. Abciximab data are more robust because abciximab trials included larger numbers of patients. In unstable angina and non-ST segment elevation myocardial infarction, GP IIb/IIIa blockade reduced the risk of death or myocardial infarction by 10–35% *(151)*. The higher the initial risk for the patient, the greater the clinical benefit provided by GP IIb/IIIa blockers. Patients undergoing PCI benefit more than patients treated conservatively, possibly because platelets play a more significant role in patients who sustain vascular wall injury during PCI than in low risk patients with unstable angina. GP IIb/IIIa blockade reduced the risk of death, myocardial infarction, and revascularization within the first 30 days by up to 46% in patients with ST segment elevation myocardial infarction undergoing primary angioplasty *(152)*. In addition, microperfusion as measured by ST segment resolution, peak flow velocity in the coronary arteries, and wall motion improved with abciximab therapy *(153)*. Studies of combined fibrinolysis and GP IIb/IIIa blockade, first done in animals, have recently been completed in a clinical setting. Fibrinolysis and lysed clot material are potent platelet stimuli, so the combination of thrombolysis and potent platelet inhibition seemed ideal. However, two large clinical trials have shown no clinical benefit for the combination of fibrinolysis and GP IIb/IIIa blockade *(154,155)*.

The optimal duration for parenteral GP IIb/IIIa blocker therapy has not been defined and has been decided arbitrarily in most cases. The issue is important because doubling the infusion time for abciximab may worsen outcome *(156)*.

Oral Use of Glycoprotein IIb/IIIa Blockers

The success of parenteral GP IIb/IIIa blockers in the acute inhibition of platelets prompted the development of oral GP IIb/IIIa blockade agents. Aspirin and clopidogrel showed the potential of antiplatelet therapy in primary and secondary prevention of cardiovascular events; therefore, more potent platelet inhibition with the blockade of GP IIb/IIIa would be an important step in cardiovascular medicine. Numerous agents were developed by many pharmaceutical companies. However, results of early large-scale trials with oral GP IIb/IIIa were disappointing, and the initial assessment was that oral GP IIb/IIIa blockers had failed.

For gastrointestinal absorption, oral GP IIb/IIIa blockers are developed as prodrugs that require hepatic conversion to an active moiety. Because of the differences in half life of the agents, the dosing ranged from once a day (roxifiban) to three times a day (xemilofiban). However, significant peaks and troughs in plasma levels were a major problem for oral GP IIb/IIIa blockers *(157,158)*. Large clinical trials with the agents sibrafiban *(159,160)*, xemilofiban *(161)*, and orbofiban *(162)* showed either a trend or a significant difference towards increased mortality with the oral GP IIb/IIIa blockers. The reasons for this failure are not clear. The intrinsic activation property of GP IIb/IIIa blockers has been proposed as a contributing factor. During the peaks and troughs of the plasma levels, low concentrations of GP IIb/IIIa blockers may be prothrombotic. Intrinsic activating properties of these agents were directly shown by an increase in CD63 and P-selectin expression on the platelet surface *(148,149)*. In addition, oral GP IIb/IIIa blockers may have toxic effects, such as direct proapoptotic effects of RGD mimetics *(163–165)*. These toxic effects may not be relevant in short-term treatment with parenteral GP IIb/IIIa blockers, but may become a problem with long-term use of oral GP IIb/IIIa blockers.

CONCLUSIONS

Antiplatelet drugs target different steps in platelet activation pathways. Aspirin and the ADP receptor inhibitors target stimulatory pathways that mediate only weak responses via sole stimulation of their own receptors. However, both pathways are part of a positive feedback mechanism and, thus, are part of the stimulus amplification system in platelets; therefore, independent of the stimulus, both aspirin and ADP receptor inhibitors have significant inhibitory effects on platelet stimulation.

Targeting the GP IIb/IIIa receptor blocks the binding of fibrinogen, the final step common to all platelet activating pathways. Although blocking the GP IIb/IIIa receptor is the most powerful antiplatelet drug strategy available, it may still induce activation pathways in the platelet, as in the secretion of procoagulative agents. In addition to GP IIb/IIIa blockers, aspirin and ADP receptor inhibitors have inhibitory effects on those stimulatory processes. The effects of antiplatelet strategies are additive, and the combination of the three is recommended because of the proven clinical benefits.

Antiplatelet drugs are among the most often used drugs in modern medicine. Aspirin probably saves more lives than any other single drug. Aspirin is recommended for an increasing number of patients because indications for aspirin therapy are extending into other areas, and the number of patients with atherosclerosis and its clinical sequelae is increasing. The newer antiplatelet drugs provide further clinical benefits but are an immense burden on our medical financing systems. Platelet physiology offers many different targets for the inhibition of platelet activation, and several receptors are being studied, such as the thrombin receptor, the von Willebrand receptor, and the TXA_2 receptor, for use in platelet inhibition.

REFERENCES

1. Bizzozero J. Über einen neuen Formbestandteil des Blutes und dessen Rolle bei der Thrombose und Blutgerinnung. Virchows Archiv für Pathologische Anatomie und Physiologie und für Klinische Medizin 1882;90:261–298.
2. Ross R. Atherosclerosis—an inflammatory disease. N Engl J Med. 1999;340:115–126.
3. Ruggeri ZM, Dent JA, Saldivar E. Contributions of distinct adhesive interactions to platelet aggregation in flowing blood. Blood 1999;94:172–178.
4. Bonate PL. Serotonin receptor subtypes: functional, physiological, and clinical correlates. Clin Neuropharmacol 1991; 14:1–16.
5. FitzGerald GA. Mechanisms of platelet activation: thromboxane A_2 as an amplifying signal for other agonists. Am J Cardiol 1991;68:11B–15B.
6. Scandura JM, Ahmad SS, Walsh PN. A binding site expressed on the surface of activated human platelets is shared by factor X and prothrombin. Biochemistry 1996;35:8890–8902.
7. McGee MP, Li LC, Hensler M. Functional assembly of intrinsic coagulation proteases on monocytes and platelets. Comparison between cofactor activities induced by thrombin and factor Xa. J Exp Med 1992;176:27–35.
8. Nurden AT, Didry D, Rosa JP. Molecular defects of platelets in Bernard-Soulier syndrome. Blood Cells 1983;9:333–358.
9. George JN, Caen JP, Nurden AT. Glanzmann's thrombasthenia: the spectrum of clinical disease. Blood 1990; 75:1383–1395.
10. Offermanns S, Toombs CF, Hu YH, Simon MI. Defective platelet activation in G alpha(q)-deficient mice. Nature 1997;389:183–186.

11. Andrews RK, Lopez JA, Berndt MC. Molecular mechanisms of platelet adhesion and activation. Int J Biochem Cell Biol 1997; 29:91–105.

12. Daniel JL, Dangelmaier C, Jin J, Ashby B, Smith JB, Kunapuli SP. Molecular basis for ADP-induced platelet activation. I. Evidence for three distinct ADP receptors on human platelets. J Biol Chem 1998;273:2024–2029.

13. Brass LF. Ca^{2+} homeostasis in unstimulated platelets. J Biol Chem 1984;259:12563–12570.

14. Gachet C. ADP receptors of platelets and their inhibition. Thromb Haemost 2001;86:222–232.

15. Tsuboi S. Calcium integrin-binding protein activates platelet integrin alpha IIbbeta 3. J Biol Chem 2002;277:1919–1923.

16. Dreser H. Herstellung des Aspirins. Archiv fuer die Gesamte Physiologie 1899;76:306–18.

17. Vane JR, Botting RM. Aspirin and other Salicylates. London: Chapman and Hall Medical; 1992.

18. Beaumont JL, Caen J, Bernard J. Influence de l'acide acetyl salicylique dans les maladies hémorrhagiques. Sang 1956; 27:243–248.

19. Patrono C. Aspirin as an antiplatelet drug. N Engl J Med 1994;330:1287–1294.

20. Weber AA, Zimmermann KC, Meyer-Kirchrath J, Schror K. Cyclooxygenase-2 in human platelets as a possible factor in aspirin resistance. Lancet 1999;353:900.

21. Patrono C, Coller B, Dalen JE, et al. Platelet-active drugs: the relationships among dose, effectiveness, and side effect. Chest 2001;119:39S–63S.

22. ISIS-2 (Second International Study of Infarct Survival) Collaborative Group. Randomised trial of intravenous streptokinase, oral aspirin, both, or neither among 17,187 cases of suspected acute myocardial infarction: ISIS-2. Lancet 1988; 2:349–360.

23. Baigent C, Collins R, Appleby P, Parish S, Sleight P, Peto R. ISIS-2: 10 year survival among patients with suspected acute myocardial infarction in randomised comparison of intravenous streptokinase, oral aspirin, both, or neither. The ISIS-2 (Second International Study of Infarct Survival) Collaborative Group. BMJ 1998;316:1337–1343.

24. Fitzgerald DJ, Roy L, Catella F, FitzGerald GA. Platelet activation in unstable coronary disease. N Engl J Med 1986; 315:983–989.

25. Lewis HD Jr, Davis JW, Archibald DG, et al. Protective effects of aspirin against acute myocardial infarction and death in men with unstable angina. Results of a Veterans Administration Cooperative Study. N Engl J Med 1983;309:396–403.

26. Cairns JA, Gent M, Singer J, et al. Aspirin, sulfinpyrazone, or both in unstable angina. Results of a Canadian multicenter trial. N Engl J Med 1985;313:1369–1375.

27. Theroux P, Ouimet H, McCans J, et al. Aspirin, heparin, or both to treat acute unstable angina. N Engl J Med 1988; 319:1105–1111.

28. Barnathan ES, Schwartz JS, Taylor L, et al. Aspirin and dipyridamole in the prevention of acute coronary thrombosis complicating coronary angioplasty. Circulation 1987;76:125–134.

29. Gawaz M, Neumann FJ, Ott I, May A, Schomig A. Platelet activation and coronary stent implantation. Effect of antithrombotic therapy. Circulation 1996;94:279–285.

30. Antiplatelet Trialists' Collaboration. Collaborative overview of randomised trials of antiplatelet therapy—I: Prevention of death, myocardial infarction, and stroke by prolonged antiplatelet therapy in various categories of patients. BMJ 1994;308:81–106.

31. Antithrombotic Trialists' Collaboration. Collaborative meta-analysis of randomised trials of antiplatelet therapy for prevention of death, myocardial infarction, and stroke in high risk patients. BMJ 2002;324:71–86.

32. Peto R, Gray R, Collins R, et al. Randomised trial of prophylactic daily aspirin in British male doctors. Br Med J 1988; 296:313–316.

33. Steering Committee of the Physicians' Health Study Research Group. Final report on the aspirin component of the ongoing Physicians' Health Study. N Engl J Med 1989;321:129–135.

34. ETDRS Investigators. Aspirin effects on mortality and morbidity in patients with diabetes mellitus. Early Treatment Diabetic Retinopathy Study report 14. JAMA 1992;268:1292–1300.

35. Hansson L, Zanchetti A, Carruthers SG, et al. Effects of intensive blood-pressure lowering and low-dose aspirin in patients with hypertension: principal results of the Hypertension Optimal Treatment (HOT) randomised trial. HOT Study Group. Lancet 1998;351:1755–1762.

36. The Medical Research Council's General Practice Research Framework. Thrombosis prevention trial: randomised trial of low-intensity oral anticoagulation with warfarin and low-dose aspirin in the primary prevention of ischaemic heart disease in men at increased risk. Lancet 1998;351:233–241.

37. Avanzini F, Palumbo G, Alli C, et al. Effects of low-dose aspirin on clinic and ambulatory blood pressure in treated hypertensive patients. Collaborative Group of the Primary Prevention Project (PPP)—Hypertension study. Am J Hypertens 2000;13:611–616.

38. Roderick PJ, Wilkes HC, Meade TW. The gastrointestinal toxicity of aspirin: an overview of randomised controlled trials. Br J Clin Pharmacol 1993;35:219–226.

39. Gaarder A, Jonsen L, Laland S, Hellem A, Owren PA. Adenosine diphosphate in red cells as a factor in the adhesiveness of human blood platelets. Nature 1961;192:531–532.

40. Born GV. Aggregation of blood platelets by adenosine diphosphate and its reversal. Nature 1962;194:27–29.

41. Leon C, Vial C, Cazenave JP, Gachet C. Cloning and sequencing of a human cDNA encoding endothelial P2Y1 purinoceptor. Gene 1996;171:295–297.

42. Ayyanathan K, Webbs TE, Sandhu AK, Athwal RS, Barnard EA, Kunapuli SP. Cloning and chromosomal localization of the human P2Y1 purinoceptor. Biochem Biophys Res Commun. 1996;218:783–788.

43. Leon C, Hechler B, Vial C, Leray C, Cazenave JP, Gachet C. The P2Y1 receptor is an ADP receptor antagonized by ATP and expressed in platelets and megakaryoblastic cells. FEBS Lett 1997;403:26–30.

44. Jin J, Daniel JL, Kunapuli SP. Molecular basis for ADP-induced platelet activation. II. The P2Y1 receptor mediates ADP-induced intracellular calcium mobilization and shape change in platelets. J Biol Chem 1998;273:2030–2034.

45. Savi P, Beauverger P, Labouret C, et al. Role of P2Y1 purinoceptor in ADP-induced platelet activation. FEBS Lett 1998;422:291–295.

46. Hechler B, Leon C, Vial C, et al. The P2Y1 receptor is necessary for adenosine 5′-diphosphate-induced platelet aggregation. Blood 1998;92:152–159.

47. Geiger J, Hoenig-Liedl P, Schanzenbacher P, Walter U. Ligand specificity and ticlopidine effects distinguish three human platelet ADP receptors. Eur J Pharmacol 1998;351:235–246.

48. Leon C, Vial C, Gachet C, et al. The P2Y1 receptor is normal in a patient presenting a severe deficiency of ADP-induced platelet aggregation. Thromb Haemost. 1999;81:775–781.

49. Vial C, Hechler B, Leon C, Cazenave JP, Gachet C. Presence of P2X1 purinoceptors in human platelets and megakaryoblastic cell lines. Thromb Haemost 1997;78:1500–1504.

50. Hollopeter G, Jantzen HM, Vincent D, et al. Identification of the platelet ADP receptor targeted by antithrombotic drugs. Nature. 2001;409:202–207.

51. Thebault JJ, Blatrix CE, Blanchard JF, Panak EA. Effects of ticlopidine, a new platelet aggregation inhibitor in man. Clin Pharmacol Ther 1975;18:485–490.

52. CAPRIE Steering Committee. A randomised, blinded, trial of clopidogrel versus aspirin in patients at risk of ischaemic events (CAPRIE). Lancet 1996;348:1329–1339.

53. Bennett CL, Conners JM, Carwile JM, et al. Thrombotic thrombocytopenic purpura associated with clopidogrel. New Engl J Med 2000;342:1773–1777.

54. Bertrand ME, Rupprecht HJ, Urban P, Gershlick AH, for the CLASSICS Investigators. Double-blind study of the safety of clopidogrel with and without a loading dose in combination with aspirin compared with ticlopidine in combination with aspirin after coronary stenting: the clopidogrel aspirin stent international cooperative study (CLASSICS). Circulation 2000;102:624–629.

55. Bhatt DL, Bertrand ME, Berger PB, et al. Meta-analysis of randomized and registry comparisons of ticlopidine with clopidogrel after stenting. J Am Coll Cardiol 2002;39:9–14.

56. Savi P, Pereillo JM, Uzabiaga MF, et al. Identification and biological activity of the active metabolite of clopidogrel. Thromb Haemost 2000;84:891–896.

57. Schomig A, Neumann FJ, Kastrati A, et al. A randomized comparison of antiplatelet and anticoagulant therapy after the placement of coronary-artery stents. N Engl J Med 1996;334:1084–1089.

58. Moussa I, Oetgen M, Roubin G, et al. Effectiveness of clopidogrel and aspirin versus ticlopidine and aspirin in preventing stent thrombosis after coronary stent implantation. Circulation 1999;99:2364–2366.

59. Cosmi B, Rubboli A, Castelvetri C, Milandri M. Ticlopidine versus oral anticoagulation for coronary stenting. Cochrane Database Syst Rev. 2001;4:CD002133.

60. Yusuf S, Zhao F, Mehta SR, Chrolavicius S, Tognoni G, Fox KK, and the Clopidogrel in Unstable Angine to Prevent Recurrent Events Trial Investigators. Effects of clopidogrel in addition to aspirin in patients with acute coronary syndromes without ST-segment elevation. N Engl J Med 2001;345:494–502.

61. Savcic M, Hauert J, Bachmann F, Wyld PJ, Geudelin B, Cariou R. Clopidogrel loading dose regimens: kinetic profile of pharmacodynamic response in healthy subjects. Semin Thromb Hemost 1999;25(Suppl 2):15–19.

62. Weber AA, Braun M, Hohlfeld T, Schwippert B, Tschope D, Schror K. Recovery of platelet function after discontinuation of clopidogrel treatment in healthy volunteers. Br J Clin Pharmacol 2001;52:333–336.

63. Storey F. The P2Y12 receptor as a therapeutic target in cardiovascular disease. Platelets 2001;12:197–209.

64. Phillips DR, Jennings LK, Edwards HH. Identification of membrane proteins mediating the interaction of human platelets. J Cell Biol 1980;86:77–86.

65. Phillips DR, Charo IF, Parise LV, Fitzgerald LA. The platelet membrane glycoprotein IIb-IIIa complex. Blood 1988; 71:831–843.

66. Calvete JJ. Platelet integrin GPIIb/IIIa: structure-function correlations. An update and lessons from other integrins. Proc Soc Exp Biol Med 1999;222:29–38.

67. Bray PF, Rosa JP, Johnston GI, et al. Platelet glycoprotein IIb. Chromosomal localization and tissue expression. J Clin Invest 1987;80:1812–1817.

68. Fitzgerald LA, Steiner B, Rall SC Jr, Lo SS, Phillips DR. Protein sequence of endothelial glycoprotein IIIa derived from a cDNA clone. Identity with platelet glycoprotein IIIa and similarity to "integrin". J Biol Chem 1987;262:3936–3939.

69. Poncz M, Eisman R, Heidenreich R, et al. Structure of the platelet membrane glycoprotein IIb. Homology to the alpha subunits of the vitronectin and fibronectin membrane receptors. J Biol Chem 1987;262:8476–8482.

70. Rosa JP, Bray PF, Gayet O, et al. Cloning of glycoprotein IIIa cDNA from human erythroleukemia cells and localization of the gene to chromosome 17. Blood 1988;72:593–600.

71. Wagner CL, Mascelli MA, Neblock DS, Weisman HF, Coller BS, Jordan RE. Analysis of GPIIb/IIIa receptor number by quantification of 7E3 binding to human platelets. Blood 1996;88:907–914.

72. Jennings LK, Phillips DR. Purification of glycoproteins IIb and III from human platelet plasma membranes and characterization of a calcium-dependent glycoprotein IIb-III complex. J Biol Chem 1982;257:10458–10466.

73. Glanzmann E. Heriditaere haemorrhagische Thrombasthenie: Ein Beitrag zur Pathologie der Blutplaettchen. Jahrbuch fur Kinderheilkunde 1918;88:113–114.

74. Nurden AT, Caen JP. Specific roles for platelet surface glycoproteins in platelet function. Nature 1975;255:720–722.

75. Phillips DR, Agin PP. Platelet membrane defects in Glanzmann's thrombasthenia. Evidence for decreased amounts of two major glycoproteins. J Clin Invest 1977;60:535–545.

76. Mustard JF, Packham MA, Kinlough-Rathbone RL, Perry DW, Regoeczi E. Fibrinogen and ADP-induced platelet aggregation. Blood 1978;52:453–466.

77. Marguerie GA, Plow EF, Edgington TS. Human platelets possess an inducible and saturable receptor specific for fibrinogen. J Biol Chem 1979;254:5357–5363.

78. Bennett JS, Hoxie JA, Leitman SF, Vilaire G, Cines DB. Inhibition of fibrinogen binding to stimulated human platelets by a monoclonal antibody. Proc Natl Acad Sci USA 1983;80:2417–2421.

79. Parise LV, Phillips DR. Reconstitution of the purified platelet fibrinogen receptor. Fibrinogen binding properties of the glycoprotein IIb-IIIa complex. J Biol Chem 1985;260:10698–10707.

80. O'Toole TE, Loftus JC, Du XP, et al. 1990. Affinity modulation of the alpha IIb beta 3 integrin (platelet GP IIb-IIIa) is an intrinsic property of the receptor. Cell Regul 1990;1:883–893.

81. de Groot PG, Sixma JJ. Platelet adhesion. Br J Haematol 1990;75:308–312.

82. Hynes RO. Integrins: a family of cell surface receptors. Cell 1987;48:549–554.

83. Springer TA. Adhesion receptors of the immune system. Nature 1990;346:425–434.

84. Hynes RO. Integrins: versatility, modulation, and signaling in cell adhesion. Cell 1992;69:11–25.

85. Doolittle RF. The structure and evolution of vertebrate fibrinogen. Ann N Y Acad Sci 1983;408:13–27.

86. Andrieux A, Hudry-Clergeon G, Ryckewaert JJ, et al. Amino acid sequences in fibrinogen mediating its interaction with its platelet receptor, GPIIbIIIa. J Biol Chem 1989;264:9258–9265.

87. Farrell DH, Thiagarajan P, Chung DW, Davie EW. Role of fibrinogen alpha and gamma chain sites in platelet aggregation. Proc Natl Acad Sci USA 1992;89:10729–10732.

88. Farrell DH, Thiagarajan P. Binding of recombinant fibrinogen mutants to platelets. J Biol Chem 1994;269:226–231.
89. Liu Q, Matsueda G, Brown E, Frojmovic M. The AGDV residues on the gamma chain carboxyl terminus of platelet-bound fibrinogen are needed for platelet aggregation. Biochim Biophys Acta 1997;1343:316–326.
90. Bray PF. Inherited diseases of platelet glycoproteins: considerations for rapid molecular characterization. Thromb Haemost 1994;72:492–502.
91. French DL, Seligsohn U. Platelet glycoprotein IIb/IIIa receptors and Glanzmann's thrombasthenia. Arterioscler Thromb Vasc Biol 2000;20:607–610.
92. Coller BS. A new murine monoclonal antibody reports an activation-dependent change in the conformation and/or microenvironment of the platelet glycoprotein IIb/IIIa complex. J Clin Invest 1985;76:101–108.
93. Coller BS. Activation affects access to the platelet receptor for adhesive glycoproteins. J Cell Biol 1986;103:451–456.
94. Coller BS, Folts JD, Scudder LE, Smith SR. Antithrombotic effect of a monoclonal antibody to the platelet glycoprotein IIb/IIIa receptor in an experimental animal model. Blood 1986;68:783–786.
95. Gold HK, Gimple LW, Yasuda T, et al. Pharmacodynamic study of F(ab')2 fragments of murine monoclonal antibody 7E3 directed against human platelet glycoprotein IIb/IIIa in patients with unstable angina pectoris. J Clin Invest 1990;86:651–659.
96. Knight DM, Wagner C, Jordan R, et al. The immunogenicity of the 7E3 murine monoclonal Fab antibody fragment variable region is dramatically reduced in humans by substitution of human for murine constant regions. Mol Immunol 1995;32:1271–1281.
97. Coller BS. Platelet GPIIb/IIIa antagonists: the first anti-integrin receptor therapeutics. J Clin Invest 1997;100:S57–S60.
98. Haber E. Antibodies in cardiovascular diagnosis and therapy. Hosp Pract 1986;21:147–157, 161–162, 165–12.
99. Tcheng JE, Kereiakes DJ, Lincoff AM, et al. Abciximab readministration: results of the ReoPro Readministration Registry. Circulation 2001;104:870–875.
100. Scarborough RM, Rose JW, Hsu MA, et al. Barbourin. A GPIIb-IIIa-specific integrin antagonist from the venom of Sistrurus m. barbouri. J Biol Chem 1991;266:9359–9362.
101. Scarborough RM, Naughton MA, Teng W, et al. Design of potent and specific integrin antagonists. Peptide antagonists with high specificity for glycoprotein IIb-IIIa. J Biol Chem 1993;268:1066–1073.
102. Chen Y, Pitzenberger SM, Garsky VM, Lumma PK, Sanyal G, Baum J. Proton NMR assignments and secondary structure of the snake venom protein echistatin. Biochemistry 1991;30:11625–11636.
103. Hartman GD, Egbertson MS, Halczenko W, et al. Non-peptide fibrinogen receptor antagonists. 1. Discovery and design of exosite inhibitors. J Med Chem 1992;35:4640–4642.
104. Egbertson MS, Chang CT, Duggan ME, et al. Non-peptide fibrinogen receptor antagonists. 2. Optimization of a tyrosine template as a mimic for Arg-Gly-Asp. J Med Chem 1994;37:2537–2551.
105. Giachelli CM, Bae N, Almeida M, Denhardt DT, Alpers CE, Schwartz SM. Osteopontin is elevated during neointima formation in rat arteries and is a novel component of human atherosclerotic plaques. J Clin Invest 1993;92:1686–1696.
106. Bennett JS, Chan C, Vilaire G, Mousa SA, DeGrado WF. Agonist-activated alphavbeta3 on platelets and lymphocytes binds to the matrix protein osteopontin. J Biol Chem 1997;272:8137–8140.
107. Hoshiga M, Alpers CE, Smith LL, Giachelli CM, Schwartz SM. Alpha-v beta-3 integrin expression in normal and atherosclerotic artery. Circ Res 1995;77:1129–1135.
108. Srivatsa SS, Fitzpatrick LA, Tsao PW, et al. Selective alpha v beta 3 integrin blockade potently limits neointimal hyperplasia and lumen stenosis following deep coronary arterial stent injury: evidence for the functional importance of integrin alpha v beta 3 and osteopontin expression during neointima formation. Cardiovasc Res 1997;36:408–428.
109. Slepian MJ, Massia SP, Dehdashti B, Fritz A, Whitesell L. Beta3-integrins rather than beta1-integrins dominate integrin-matrix interactions involved in postinjury smooth muscle cell migration. Circulation 1998;97:1818–1827.
110. Stouffer GA, Hu Z, Sajid M, et al. Beta3 integrins are upregulated after vascular injury and modulate thrombospondin- and thrombin-induced proliferation of cultured smooth muscle cells. Circulation 1998;97:907–915.
111. Coleman KR, Braden GA, Willingham MC, Sane DC. Vitaxin, a humanized monoclonal antibody to the vitronectin receptor (alphavbeta3), reduces neointimal hyperplasia and total vessel area after balloon injury in hypercholesterolemic rabbits. Circ Res 1999;84:1268–1276.
112. The ERASER Investigators. Acute platelet inhibition with abciximab does not reduce in-stent restenosis (ERASER study). Circulation 1999;100:799–806.
113. Tam SH, Sassoli PM, Jordan RE, Nakada MT. Abciximab (ReoPro, chimeric 7E3 Fab) demonstrates equivalent affinity and functional blockade of glycoprotein IIb/IIIa and alpha(v)beta3 integrins. Circulation 1998;98:1085–1091.
114. Lele M, Sajid M, Wajih N, Stouffer GA. Eptifibatide and 7E3, but not tirofiban, inhibit alpha(v)beta(3) integrin-mediated binding of smooth muscle cells to thrombospondin and prothrombin. Circulation 2001;104:582–587.
115. Kintscher U, Kappert K, Schmidt G, et al. Effects of abciximab and tirofiban on vitronectin receptors in human endothelial and smooth muscle cells. Eur J Pharmacol 2000;390:75–87.
116. Altieri DC, Morrissey JH, Edgington TS. Adhesive receptor Mac-1 coordinates the activation of factor X on stimulated cells of monocytic and myeloid differentiation: an alternative initiation of the coagulation protease cascade. Proc Natl Acad Sci USA 1988;85:7462–7466.
117. Languino LR, Plescia J, Duperray A, et al. Fibrinogen mediates leukocyte adhesion to vascular endothelium through an ICAM-1-dependent pathway. Cell 1993;73:1423–1434.
118. Todd RF 3rd. The continuing saga of complement receptor type 3 (CR3). J Clin Invest 1996;98:1–2.
119. Peter K, Schwarz M, Conradt C, et al. Heparin inhibits ligand binding to the leukocyte integrin Mac-1 (CD11b/CD18). Circulation 1999;100:1533–1539.
120. Altieri DC, Edgington TS. A monoclonal antibody reacting with distinct adhesion molecules defines a transition in the functional state of the receptor CD11b/CD18 (Mac-1). J Immunol 1988;141:2656–2660.
121. Simon DI, Xu H, Ortlepp S, Rogers C, Rao NK. 7E3 monoclonal antibody directed against the platelet glycoprotein IIb/IIIa cross-reacts with the leukocyte integrin Mac-1 and

blocks adhesion to fibrinogen and ICAM-1. Arterioscler Thromb Vasc Biol 1997;17:528–535.

122. Li N, Hu H, Lindqvist M, Wikstrom-Jonsson E, Goodall AH, Hjemdahl P. Platelet-leukocyte cross talk in whole blood. Arterioscler Thromb Vasc Biol 2000;20:2702–2708.

123. Schwarz M, Kohler B, Nordt T, Ruef J, Bode C, Peter K. Abciximab binds to the leukocyte integrin Mac-1 (CD11b/CD18, αMá2) and thereby results in a functional blockade in vitro and in vivo. Circulation 1999;100:I–33.

124. Scarborough RM, Kleiman NS, Phillips DR. Platelet glycoprotein IIb/IIIa antagonists. What are the relevant issues concerning their pharmacology and clinical use? Circulation 1999;100:437–444.

125. Mascelli MA, Lance ET, Damaraju L, Wagner CL, Weisman HF, Jordan RE. Pharmacodynamic profile of short-term abciximab treatment demonstrates prolonged platelet inhibition with gradual recovery from GP IIb/IIIa receptor blockade. Circulation 1998;97:1680–1688.

126. Peter K, Kohler B, Straub A, et al. Flow cytometric monitoring of glycoprotein IIb/IIIa blockade and platelet function in patients with acute myocardial infarction receiving reteplase, abciximab, and ticlopidine: continuous platelet inhibition by the combination of abciximab and ticlopidine. Circulation 2000;102:1490–1496.

127. Barrett JS, Murphy G, Peerlinck K, et al. Pharmacokinetics and pharmacodynamics of MK-383, a selective non-peptide platelet glycoprotein-IIb/IIIa receptor antagonist, in healthy men. Clin Pharmacol Ther 1994;56:377–388.

128. Harrington RA, Kleiman NS, Kottke-Marchant K, et al. Immediate and reversible platelet inhibition after intravenous administration of a peptide glycoprotein IIb/IIIa inhibitor during percutaneous coronary intervention. Am J Cardiol 1995;76:1222–1227.

129. Gawaz M, Neumann FJ, Schomig A. Evaluation of platelet membrane glycoproteins in coronary artery disease: consequences for diagnosis and therapy. Circulation 1999;99:E1–E11.

130. Phillips DR, Teng W, Arfsten A, et al. Effect of Ca2+ on GP IIb-IIIa interactions with integrilin: enhanced GP IIb-IIIa binding and inhibition of platelet aggregation by reductions in the concentration of ionized calcium in plasma anticoagulated with citrate. Circulation 1997;96:1488–1494.

131. Smith JW, Steinhubl SR, Lincoff AM, et al. Rapid platelet-function assay: an automated and quantitative cartridge-based method. Circulation 1999;99:620–625.

132. Kereiakes DJ, Kleiman NS, Ambrose J, et al. Randomized, double-blind, placebo-controlled dose-ranging study of tirofiban (MK-383) platelet IIb/IIIa blockade in high risk patients undergoing coronary angioplasty. J Am Coll Cardiol 1996;27:536–542.

133. Quinn M, Deering A, Stewart M, Cox D, Foley B, Fitzgerald D. Quantifying GPIIb/IIIa receptor binding using 2 monoclonal antibodies: discriminating abciximab and small molecular weight antagonists. Circulation 1999;99:2231–2238.

134. ESPRIT Investigators. Enhanced Suppression of the Platelet IIb/IIIa Receptor with Integrilin Therapy. Novel dosing regimen of eptifibatide in planned coronary stent implantation (ESPRIT): a randomised, placebo-controlled trial. Lancet 2000;356:2037–2044.

135. Tcheng JE, Ellis SG, George BS, et al. Pharmacodynamics of chimeric glycoprotein IIb/IIIa integrin antiplatelet antibody Fab 7E3 in high-risk coronary angioplasty. Circulation 1994;90:1757–1764.

136. Berkowitz SD, Harrington RA, Rund MM, Tcheng JE. Acute profound thrombocytopenia after C7E3 Fab (abciximab) therapy. Circulation 1997;95:809–813.

137. Giugliano RP. Drug-Induced Thrombocytopenia: Is it a Serious Concern for Glycoprotein IIb/IIIa Receptor Inhibitors? J Thromb Thrombolysis 1998;5:191–202.

138. Frelinger AL 3rd, Lam SC, Plow EF, Smith MA, Loftus JC, Ginsberg MH. Occupancy of an adhesive glycoprotein receptor modulates expression of an antigenic site involved in cell adhesion. J Biol Chem 1988;263:12397–12402.

139. Bednar B, Cook JJ, Holahan MA, et al. Fibrinogen receptor antagonist-induced thrombocytopenia in chimpanzee and rhesus monkey associated with preexisting drug-dependent antibodies to platelet glycoprotein IIb/IIIa. Blood 1999;94:587–599.

140. Rao J, Mascarenhas DA. Successful use of eptifibatide as an adjunct to coronary stenting in a patient with abciximab-associated acute profound thrombocytopenia. J Invasive Cardiol 2001;13:471–473.

141. Peter K, Straub A, Kohler B, Volkmann M, Schwarz M, Kübler W, Bode C. Platelet activation as a potential mechanism of GP IIb/IIIa inhibitor-induced thrombocytopenia. Am J Cardiol 1999;84:519–524.

142. Du XP, Plow EF, Frelinger AL 3rd, O'Toole TE, Loftus JC, Ginsberg MH. Ligands "activate" integrin alpha IIb beta 3 (platelet GPIIb-IIIa). Cell 1991;65:409–416.

143. Peter K, Schwarz M, Ylanne J, et al. Induction of fibrinogen binding and platelet aggregation as a potential intrinsic property of various glycoprotein IIb/IIIa (alphaIIbbeta3) inhibitors. Blood 1998;92:3240–3249.

144. Gawaz M, Ruf A, Neumann FJ, et al. Effect of glycoprotein IIb-IIIa receptor antagonism on platelet membrane glycoproteins after coronary stent placement. Thromb Haemost 1998;80:994–1001.

145. Murphy NP, Pratico D, Fitzgerald DJ. Functional relevance of the expression of ligand-induced binding sites in the response to platelet GP IIb/IIIa antagonists in vivo. J Pharmacol Exp Ther 1998;286:945–951.

146. Leisner TM, Wencel-Drake JD, Wang W, Lam SC. Bidirectional transmembrane modulation of integrin alphaIIbbeta3 conformations. J Biol Chem 1999;274:12945–12949.

147. Honda S, Tomiyama Y, Aoki T, et al. Association between ligand-induced conformational changes of integrin IIbbeta3 and IIbbeta3-mediated intracellular Ca2+ signaling. Blood 1998;92:3675–3683.

148. Holmes MB, Sobel BE, Cannon CP, Schneider DJ. Increased platelet reactivity in patients given orbofiban after an acute coronary syndrome: an OPUS-TIMI 16 substudy. Orbofiban in Patients with Unstable coronary syndromes. Thrombolysis In Myocardial Infarction. Am J Cardiol 2000;85:491–493, A10.

149. Cox D, Smith R, Quinn M, Theroux P, Crean P, Fitzgerald DJ. Evidence of platelet activation during treatment with a GPIIb/IIIa antagonist in patients presenting with acute coronary syndromes. J Am Coll Cardiol 2000;36:1514–1519.

150. Schneider DJ, Taatjes DJ, Sobel BE. Paradoxical inhibition of fibrinogen binding and potentiation of alpha-granule release by specific types of inhibitors of glycoprotein IIb-IIIa. Cardiovasc Res 2000;45:437–446.

151. Topol EJ, Byzova TV, Plow EF. Platelet GPIIb-IIIa blockers. Lancet 1999;353:227–231.

152. Montalescot G, Barragan P, Wittenberg O, et al, for the ADMIRAL Investigators. Abciximab before Direct Angioplasty and Stenting in Myocardial Infarction Regarding Acute and

Long-Term Follow-up. Platelet glycoprotein IIb/IIIa inhibition with coronary stenting for acute myocardial infarction. N Engl J Med 2001;344:1895–1903.

153. Neumann FJ, Blasini R, Schmitt C, et al. Effect of glycoprotein IIb/IIIa receptor blockade on recovery of coronary flow and left ventricular function after the placement of coronary-artery stents in acute myocardial infarction. Circulation 1998;98:2695–2701.

154. Topol EJ, and the GUSTO V Investigators. Reperfusion therapy for acute myocardial infarction with fibrinolytic therapy or combination reduced fibrinolytic therapy and platelet glycoprotein IIb/IIIa inhibition: the GUSTO V randomised trial. Lancet 2001;357:1905–1914.

155. Assessment of the Safety and Efficacy of a New Thrombolytic Regimen (ASSENT)-3 Investigators. Efficacy and safety of tenecteplase in combination with enoxaparin, abciximab, or unfractionated heparin: the ASSENT-3 randomised trial in acute myocardial infarction. Lancet 2001;358:605–613.

156. Simoons ML, and the GUSTO IV-ACS Investigators. Effect of glycoprotein IIb/IIIa receptor blocker abciximab on outcome in patients with acute coronary syndromes without early coronary revascularisation: the GUSTO IV-ACS randomised trial. Lancet 2001;357:1915–1924.

157. Baba K, Aga Y, Nakanishi T, Motoyama T, Ueno H. UR-3216: a manageable oral GPIIb/IIIa antagonist. Cardiovasc Drug Rev 2001;19:25–40.

158. Mousa SA, Bozarth JM, Naik UP, Slee A. Platelet GPIIb/IIIa binding characteristics of small molecule RGD mimetic: distinct binding profile for Roxifiban. Br J Pharmacol 2001;133:331–336.

159. The SYMPHONY Investigators. Sibrafiban versus Aspirin to Yield Maximum Protection from Ischemic Heart Events Post-acute Coronary Syndromes. Comparison of sibrafiban with aspirin for prevention of cardiovascular events after acute coronary syndromes: a randomised trial. Lancet 2000; 355:337–345.

160. Second SYMPHONY Investigators. Randomized trial of aspirin, sibrafiban, or both for secondary prevention after acute coronary syndromes. Circulation 2001;103:1727–1733.

161. O'Neill WW, Serruys P, Knudtson M, et al, for the EXCITE Trial Investigators. Evaluation of Oral Xemilofiban in Controlling Thrombotic Events. Long-term treatment with a platelet glycoprotein-receptor antagonist after percutaneous coronary revascularization. N Engl J Med 2000;342:1316–1324.

162. Cannon CP, McCabe CH, Wilcox RG, et al, for the OPUS-TIMI Investigators. Oral glycoprotein IIb/IIIa inhibition with orbofiban in patients with unstable coronary syndromes (OPUS-TIMI 16) trial. Circulation 2000;102:149–156.

163. Chew DP, Bhatt DL, Sapp S, Topol EJ. Increased Mortality With Oral Platelet Glycoprotein IIb/IIIa Antagonists: A Meta-Analysis of Phase III Multicenter Randomized Trials. Circulation 2001;103:201–206.

164. Buckley CD, Pilling D, Henriquez NV, et al. RGD peptides induce apoptosis by direct caspase-3 activation. Nature 1999;397:534–539.

165. Adderley SR, Fitzgerald DJ. Glycoprotein IIb/IIIa antagonists induce apoptosis in rat cardiomyocytes by caspase-3 activation. J Biol Chem 2000;275:5760–5766.

14 Myocardial Infarction

D. Douglas Miller, MD,CM and Steven C. Herrmann, MD, PhD

CONTENTS

FUNDAMENTAL INJURY–REPAIR PATHWAYS

Myocyte death may be caused by ischemic, metabolic, or toxic injury *(1)*. Necrosis was originally identified as the sole mechanism for ischemic myocardial cell death *(2)*, but we now know that ischemic injury can cause myocardial cell death by necrosis, apoptosis, or both mechanisms. Three major tissue injury–repair pathways have been identified in human biology (Fig. 1). These pathways are recapitulated in the myocardium in response to severe ischemic stress: (1) necrotic cell death with resulting cellular inflammation (infarction) and collagen deposition (fibrosis); (2) changes in chamber shape and geometry to reduce wall stress (remodeling) with wall thinning (aneurysm formation); and (3) hypoxia in the border zone, which promotes macroscopic (collateralization) and microscopic (neovascularization) vessel ingrowth.

These critical cellular and molecular responses to acute ischemic myocardial injury are genetically conserved because of the essential life-sustaining nature of cardiac activity. In mechanical engineering terms, the heart is an auto-cycling, dual-chamber, self-priming impedance pump. Because of this cardiac functional profile, generic tissue injury–repair pathways found in most organ systems are uniquely expressed in the heart after acute injury and during subsequent repair.

ISCHEMIC INJURY

Mechanisms of Myocardial Cell Death

Myocytes usually die of necrosis after acute ischemic injury (Fig. 2). Myocardial energetics are acutely altered during ischemic injury; cardiac high-energy phosphates (phosphocreatine and creatine) *(3)* are depleted, which causes failure of the ionic pump in the plasma membrane. Myocardial levels of ATP are constant or slightly increased during acute ischemia. However, energy is not required for the initial histological sequelae of acute ischemic injury, which include cellular swelling, sarcolemmal disruption, and membrane lysis, with concomitant release of cytoplasmic and nuclear contents. Within 12–24 h after injury, subacute inflammation occurs, and necrotic cells are engulfed by macrophages. Cell degeneration is further characterized by the progressive loss of contractile material and by the replacement of cells with collagen, which results in fibrosis *(4)*. The distribution of ischemia-mediated necrosis and fibrosis in the myocardium is initially patchy and subendocardial.

Apoptosis is an integral part of normal development and tissue homeostasis *(5)*. In healthy human tissue, cell death due to apoptosis is balanced by cell proliferation. The rates of both processes vary by tissue type and age. After ischemic injury, less damaged myocytes may die prematurely by apoptosis *(6)*. The molecular mediators of

From: *Contemporary Cardiology: Principles of Molecular Cardiology*
Edited by: M. S. Runge and C. Patterson © Humana Press Inc., Totowa, NJ

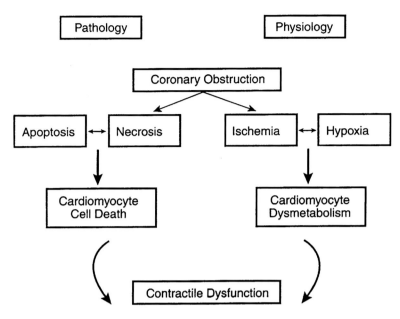

Fig. 1. Myocardial infarction pathophysiology.

apoptosis are under study *(7)*. Although apoptosis can be genetically predetermined or triggered by numerous extracellular mechanisms such as hypoxia, hormones, cytokines, killer T-cell activation, growth factors, and viruses, its final common pathways are energy-requiring and histologically distinct. In addition, apoptosis does not result in local tissue inflammation.

The morphological features of myocyte necrosis and apoptosis overlap *(8)*. Apoptotic cell death is characterized by myocyte shrinkage, chromatin condensation, cytoplasmic blebbing, and cellular fragmentation into small "apoptotic bodies" that undergo phagocytosis by macrophages *(1)*. The fragmented DNA of apoptotic nuclei can be labeled in an assay called terminal transferase–mediated deoxyuridine nucleotide end-labeling (TUNEL) stain *(9)*. Involvement of single cells is not characteristic of apoptosis.

Cardiomyocyte apoptosis is increased in experimental myocardial infarction and occurs paracentric to regions of acute injury *(10)*. In addition, apoptosis contributes to the pathogenesis of left ventricular dysfunction and the associated clinical syndromes of congestive heart failure and cardiac arrhythmias *(1,7)*. Myocardial reperfusion can cause apoptosis as a result of the production of oxygen-free radicals *(7)*. Caspase-3, an essential protease of apoptosis, proteolytically cleaves several programmed death substrates and activates endonucleases, leading to the characteristic fragmentation of internucleosomal DNA, or DNA laddering.

Cellular Events in the Acute Coronary Syndromes

Myocardial infarction was once believed to result from progressive, chronic narrowing of epicardial conduit arteries. Concepts regarding the pathophysiology of acute myocardial infarction have been dramatically revised, and the concept that "vulnerable plaque" causes acute myocardial infarction and necrosis is now widely accepted *(11)*. This understanding has contributed to advances in medical treatment of the major sequelae of transmural infarction, including infarct expansion and ventricular remodeling.

The rupture of plaque in the coronary artery causes partial or complete obstruction of the lumen of the epicardial conduit because platelets and red blood cells aggregate to form a fibrin network (Fig. 3). Sufficient collateral blood flow may be recruited to the area at risk to prevent necrosis. However, without such accessory nutritive blood flow, full thickness, or transmural, necrosis develops in the infarcted area supplied by the occluded vessel. Cellular changes such as decreased glycogen stores, intracellular edema, and distortion of the myocyte sarcoplasmic reticulum and transverse tubular system occur within 20 min of complete occlusion. Mitochondrial swelling and dysfunction occur within the first hour of infarction, when margination of nuclear chromatin is observed.

Within 6 h after myocardial infarction, neutrophils infiltrate the damaged myocardium and release phosphorylase, endopeptidase, and oxidative enzymes to begin the digestion process. By 24 h after infarction, cytoplasmic clumping occurs as the myocyte nucleus becomes

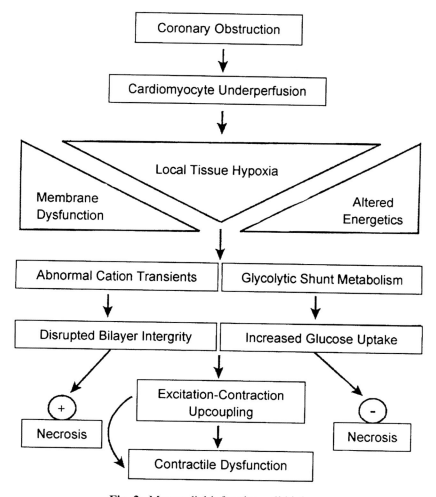

Fig. 2. Myocardial infarction cell biology.

pyknotic or disappears; myofibrils appear stretched under light microscopy. Macrophages infiltrate and remove cellular debris by d 4 after infarction. Granulation tissue appears by d 10 after coronary occlusion, with further collagenization, fibroblast ingrowth, and neovascularization continuing for many weeks. A dense connective tissue scar with interspersed myocytes forms by 6 wk after the initial injury *(12).*

Calcium Handling in Ischemic Left Ventricular Dysfunction

Multiple proteins responsible for contraction compose about 75% of the total volume of the myocardium. Myosin, which consists of two heavy chains and four light chains, forms the thick filaments. The heads of the myosin filaments project from the axis of the α helical tail to form the active crossbridge with the thin filament. Multiple isoforms of myosin and the associated ATPase enzyme are found within the ventricle; the low affinity ATPase, β (V3)

protein, predominates in humans *(13).* Titin (connectin), which is a support protein that extends from the Z-line toward the central M-band, provides elasticity to the sarcomere and tethers the myosin molecules to the Z-line. Titin allows the sarcomere to stretch, thereby contributing to the development of resting sarcomere tension.

The thin filaments comprise F (fibrous) actin molecules arranged in a wrapped, double-stranded helical configuration. Because it can activate myosin ATPase and bind reversibly to myosin, actin plays an important role in cross-bridge formation and muscle contraction. The regulatory troponin complex, with individual subunits known as I (inhibitory), C (calcium), and T (tropomyosin), is found about every 38.5 n*M* along the double helical strand of actin. Tropomyosin, a regulatory protein comprising two α-helices linked together by disulfide bonds, is found in the longitudinal grooves between the actin. Tropomyosin inhibits the head of the myosin molecule from binding to actin and thus forms a cross-bridge for contraction.

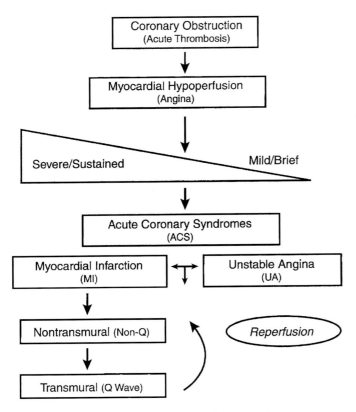

Fig. 3. Myocardial infarction clinical syndromes.

The key ionic mediator of myocyte contraction is calcium. Calcium enters the myocyte through L-type calcium channels and induces release of calcium from the sarco/endoplasmic reticulum calcium-ATPase (SERCA). This "calcium-induced calcium release" causes calcium to interact with troponin C, which reverses the allosteric inhibition of cross-bridge formation by troponin I. The final step of the allosteric interaction involves a shift of tropomyosin into the grooves of the double-stranded actin molecules, thus exposing the actin–myosin binding sites and placing the contractile proteins in their strong binding state. Then, the power-stroke of systole occurs, resulting in myocyte shortening and the development of active force. The subsequent binding and hydrolysis of ATP results in relaxation of the cross-bridges, a decrease in calcium levels, and the inhibition of troponin I.

The calcium flux throughout excitation–contraction coupling is a complex process. Although only small amounts of calcium enter the myocyte through the voltage-sensitive L-type channel during the plateau phase of the action potential, cytosolic calcium increases approximately 10-fold; the balance comes from the calcium-induced release of calcium from the sarcoplasmic reticulum. Small, spontaneous calcium currents, known as "calcium sparks,"

are occasionally released from the sarcoplasmic reticulum, but their function is not clear. Calcium sparks may prompt the graded effect of calcium on myocyte contraction, or they may induce arrhythmias in catecholamine toxicity and during myocardial reperfusion.

Myocardial calcium handling involves an L-type calcium channel, which is associated with a cluster of sarcoplasmic reticulum release channels, called the ryanodine receptor. As the wave of depolarization travels down the T-tubule system, voltage-sensitive L-type channels release calcium into the foot area of the sarcoplasmic reticulum. This small current of calcium induces a conformational change in the calcium-release channels, or the ryanodine receptor, which causes a large flux of calcium into the cytosol and allows the interaction between calcium and troponin C. Calcium is taken back up into the sarcoplasmic reticulum by an active CaATPase (SERCA) protein, which accounts for about 90% of the protein content of the SR.

Myocyte calcium flux is regulated by inositol trisphosphate (IP3) and phospholamban. IP3 activates another calcium-release receptor on the sarcoplasmic reticulum, which increases the concentration of cytosolic calcium. The IP3 receptor shares considerable molecular homology with the ryanodine receptor but has a smaller molecular weight. IP3 receptor activity is increased by α-adrenergic activity, angiotensin II, and probably endothelin. Upregulation of the IP3 calcium system may contribute to the intracellular calcium toxicity seen in heart failure and may promote apoptosis via the Fas pathway (14). Activation and phosphorylation of the β receptor of the SERCA protein phospholamban by c-AMP increases SERCA reuptake of calcium into the sarcoplasmic reticulum. After reuptake, calcium binds within the sarcoplasmic reticulum to calsequestrin and calreticulin, which causes relaxation.

During left ventricular dysfunction, contractile proteins undergo morphologic changes that decrease cardiac contractility. In addition, decreases are seen in the rate of calcium uptake in the SERCA protein (15) and in the level of mRNA for many of the calcium-handling proteins, including the ryanodine receptor (16). The role of calcium fluxes and regulatory proteins in ventricular remodeling has been studied in a mouse model of infarction (17). In this model, the change in calcium concentration induced by L-channel release is decreased, and the force of myocyte contraction and the time to peak contraction are also reduced. In addition, the ability of L-channel calcium influx to induce the release of calcium from the sarcoplasmic reticulum is decreased. These findings suggest that the calcium-induced release of calcium is decreased after myocardial infarction. This reduction in the release of calcium from the sarcoplasmic reticulum is due, at least in part, to the decreased ability of voltage-sensitive channels to induce calcium sparks in the SR. The molecular defect in calcium handling in this mouse infarction model of heart failure is unclear. Multiple mechanisms may be involved. The reorganization and distribution of the L-type calcium channel with the ryanodine receptor would reduce the calcium-induced calcium release. In addition, separation of the T-tubule from the sarcoplasmic reticulum (T-tubule remodeling) and uncoupling of the sarcoplasmic reticulum from the L-type calcium channel would affect calcium handling.

MYOCARDIAL REPERFUSION AFTER ISCHEMIA

Although essential to the preservation of reversibly injured myocardium, early post-infarction reperfusion is associated with additional neutrophil-mediated tissue injury (18). The inflammatory cascade after reperfusion includes endothelial dysfunction, neutrophil sequestration, and complement activation. Both the main complement pathways (classical and alternative) and the lectin-activated pathway are activated during reperfusion. Depleting complement factors with agents such as anti-complement-5 (C-5) monoclonal antibodies and C-1 serine esterase inhibitors protects against reperfusion injury. The lectin pathway is activated by mannose-binding lectin, which interacts with its ligand to activate two mannose-binding lectin-associated serine proteases.

Activation of the cardiac renin–angiotensin system (RAS) correlates with the development of ischemic injury (19). The tissue (autocrine) and systemic (paracrine) effects of RAS have been described. The binding of angiotensin II to AT-1 or AT-2 receptors triggers numerous signal transduction pathways that modulate cardiac function. Activation of RAS localized to cardiac tissue triggers release of second messengers and signaling pathways, including the Janus kinase/signal transducer and activator of transcription (JAK/STAT) pathway. JAK/STAT, a major signal transduction pathway of the cytokine super family, induces apoptosis in ischemic cardiomyocytes by unknown mechanisms. In addition, JAK/STAT activates multiple hypertrophic agonists such as angiotensin II and activates transcription of the angiotensin gene promoter. Ischemia–reperfusion causes activation and translocation of STAT family members (i.e., STAT-5A and STAT-6), which leads to binding to the St domain of the angiotensin promoter gene. This binding increases mRNA levels for angiotensin and activates

JAK2, which causes ischemic–reperfusion cardiac dysfunction by unknown mechanisms.

Any teleological construct for cardiac protection after acute ischemia–reperfusion presupposes that early humans also suffered from acute or chronic arterial vaso-occlusive events, possibly in response to inherited dyslipidemia, chest trauma, or circulating infectious agents. Protein kinase C (PKC), a family of kinases that is conserved in eukaryotic species, transduces a variety of signals critical for cellular function. For example, PKC modulates the actions of nitric oxide (NO) (20). In acute ischemic stress, the production of endothelial nitric oxide synthase (eNOS) causes early cardioprotection via reactive coronary hyperemia. Molecular oxygen increases the levels of reactive oxygen species during the early seconds of reperfusion. Stimulation of protein phosphorylation by reactive oxygen species and other ligands is the probable mechanism for subsequent signal transduction that leads to the expression of stress genes and the production of heat shock proteins (HSP).

Ischemic preconditioning, an adaptive response to a short ischemic period, reduces myocardial injury, ventricular dysfunction, arrhythmias, and cardiomyocyte apoptosis (21). Mediators of preconditioning and ischemia–reperfusion injury include adenosine, acetylcholine, catecholamines, angiotensin II, bradykinin, endothelin, and opiodes. Common delayed responses to several disparate physiologic stressors such as ischemia, reperfusion, hypoxia, or hyperthermia include cellular changes and expression of the genes for HSP, and these responses are mediated by the L-arginine NO pathway. Recovery is improved after ischemia–reperfusion injury in transgenic mice expressing HSP 70 and in rats transfected with HSP 70 (22,23). Reactive oxygen species upregulate the expression of the HSP 72 gene.

Signaling agents for ischemic preconditioning including NO and reactive oxygen species target tyrosine kinase, PKC, and other elements of the kinase cascade. Mitochondrial K-ATP channel openers and the nuclear transcription factor NFκB are probable terminal effectors of ischemic preconditioning (24,25). Experimental data are conflicting on the acute-phase cardioprotective effects of various antioxidant compounds, including manganese superoxide dismutase, catalase, glutathione, and N-2-mercaptoproprionylglycine (MPG) (26). In studies of the effects of oxidative stress, cultured neonatal rat cardiac myocytes were more vulnerable to injury after exposure to catalase and had lower cell-survival rates than cardiac fibroblasts (27). In this setting, p38 mitogen-activated protein kinase (MAPK) and c-jun NH2 terminal linase activation tended to be higher in cardiac myocytes than in fibroblasts. Cellular differences in vulnerability and functional outcome after stress may be due in part to differences in MAPK pathway signaling.

The *Bcl-2* gene, which is an anti-apoptotic gene, and the *Bax* gene, which is a pro-apoptotic gene, are expressed after coronary artery occlusion in rats *(28)*. The differential expression of Bcl-2 and Bax in cardiac myocytes and fibroblasts may account for differences in susceptibility to oxidative stress. Pre-conditioning reduces expression of the *Bax* gene and apoptosis and decreases the accumulation of polymorphonuclear leukocytes in reperfused rat hearts *(29)*.

In animal models of myocardial infarction, administration of nonselective caspase inhibitors reduces infarct size and the rate of apoptotic cell death in the risk area *(30)*. Tetrapeptide Ac-DEVD-CHO, which selectively inhibits caspase 3, improves contractile recovery after ischemia in a rat model of ischemic–reperfused (stunned) myocardium; the mechanisms appear to be independent of suppression of apoptosis *(31)*.

VENTRICULAR GEOMETRY

Scar Formation and Remodeling

In 1935, Tenant and Wiggers *(32)* first described the gross architectural changes in left ventricular geometry after myocardial infarction. These alterations occur in both infarcted and non-infarcted regions (Fig. 4). "Remodeling" of the left ventricle has profound clinical and therapeutic implications. In the initial hours after infarction, the damaged myocardium becomes thinned and the left ventricle dilates. This process, called infarct expansion *(33)*, results from slippage of myocyte bundles. Collagen deposition and fibrosis during scar formation limits infarct expansion by reducing ventricular compliance.

The process of infarct expansion, or ventricular remodeling, is complex and involves multiple cytochemical, hormonal, and autocrine factors. Remodeling is most commonly seen at the ventricular apex, where the radius of curvature is greatest and the ventricular wall is thinnest *(34)*. Thus, occlusion of the left anterior descending coronary artery, especially when accompanied by transmural necrosis, will most likely be associated with unfavorable ventricular remodeling after myocardial infarction. The most adverse result of post-infarction remodeling is aneurysmal formation. One-year mortality after anterior wall infarction is higher in patients with aneurysm formation than in patients with similar ejection fractions without remodeling *(35,36)*.

The dog model is useful in studying regional changes in myocardial function after coronary artery occlusion.

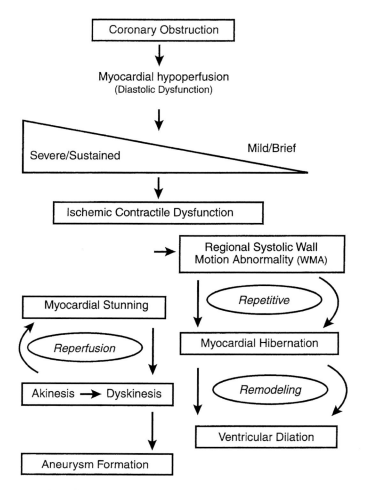

Fig. 4. Myocardial infarction functional syndromes.

Théroux and colleagues *(37)* first showed that infarcted myocardium initially becomes dyskinetic but often improves with time. Areas removed from the injured tissue compensate by becoming hypercontractile, which results in an increase in end-diastolic fiber length. This increased length has been confirmed by both echocardiography *(38)* and contrast ventriculography *(39)*, despite normal filling pressures.

The mechanism of ventricular dilation after infarction is complex (Fig. 5). In a seminal study, Linzbach *(40)* suggested that the total number of muscle fibers in the remodeled section of the heart remains constant, and that ventricular remodeling results primarily from myocyte rearrangement. However, recent studies have introduced the concept of myocyte slippage *(41,42)*. Progressive activation of proteolytic enzymes causes degradation of the collagen extracellular matrix. Matrix metalloproteinases (MMPs) are released from neutrophils within 3 h after myocardial infarction *(43)*. Infarct expansion or remodeling is easily visualized with two-dimensional echocardiography

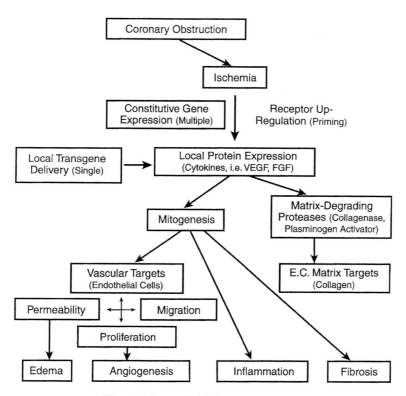

Fig. 5. Myocardial infarction cell biology.

of the infarcted ventricle *(44)*. MMPs require proteolytic cleavage to be activated and to promote a temporal sequence of collagen degradation by MMP1 (collagenase), MMP2, MMP3 (stromelysin), and MMP9 (gelatinase) *(43)*. Degradation of the collagen cross-linking struts results in myocyte slippage, which may be an important mechanism of ventricular remodeling *(45)*.

The activity of MMPs is usually restricted to the area of myocardial damage by tissue inhibitors of MMPs (TIMPs), which form high-affinity, low-molecular-weight complexes with MMPs. TIMPs are induced within 6 h in the infarct zone and return to normal levels at about 14 d post-infarction *(46)*. Recent data suggest that inflammatory proteins, such as C-reactive protein, and blood mononuclear cells may contribute to upregulation of MMPs during myocardial infarction *(47)*. PKC has been implicated as a regulator of MMP gene transcription and receptor upregulation by angiotensin II, endothelin I, catecholamines, and tumor necrosis factor (TNF)-α *(48)*.

Using a transgenic knockout mouse model, Trueblood and coworkers *(49)* studied the role of selective collagen synthesis and osteopontin in geometric ventricular remodeling after infarction. Osteopontin may participate in post-infarction remodeling by promoting local collagen synthesis and accumulation. In Trueblood's study, osteopontin production increased in the infarct zone by d 3 after myocardial infarction in control mice, and a biphasic increase was seen in distant myocardial segments at both d 3 and d 28. Infarct size, heart weight, peak left ventricular pressure, and survival were similar in osteopontin knockout mice and control mice. However, left ventricular dilation was twofold greater in osteopontin knockout mice than in controls. Electron microscopy showed that collagen content was greater in control mice than in knockout mice; type I collagen increased threefold in remote zones and sevenfold in infarcted zones.

Geometric ventricular remodeling has many short- and long-term effects on systolic function. Infarction results in immediate reduction of ventricular systolic function and decreases cardiac output in direct proportion to the amount of injured myocardium. Ventricular dilation, which occurs via the Starling mechanism and in response to increased adrenergic stimulation, increases heart rate and contractility. Ventricular dilation can maintain cardiac output despite infarction involving approximately 20% of the circumferential myocardium *(50)*.

The law of La Place states that increases in ventricular radius increase wall tension. In turn, increased diastolic tension, which represents ventricular afterload, can decrease stroke volume *(51)*. With increasing myocardial oxygen consumption, a mismatch occurs between coronary blood flow and myocardial metabolism that results in further ischemic reduction of systolic function, especially in the endocardium.

Another effect of ventricular remodeling after myocardial infarction is the change in ventricular shape from a prolate ellipse to a more spherical shape. This change in geometry affects the ventricle in two important ways. First, during the systolic phase of normal contraction, ventricle shortening is associated with wall thickening and decreased wall stress. In the elliptical, thinned ventricle, the opposite situation occurs; wall tension increases during systolic contraction, thus limiting stroke volume *(52,53)*. Therefore, geometric remodeling alone can adversely affect cardiac output.

In addition, ventricular dilation affects the papillary muscles and mitral valve apparatus. As the ventricle dilates, the mitral annulus and papillary muscles are stretched to the point where functional mitral regurgitation can occur *(54)*. The adverse effects of mitral regurgitation are twofold. First, forward cardiac output is reduced as blood regurgitates into the left atrium. This situation can cause atrial enlargement and arrhythmias including atrial fibrillation, which can further decrease cardiac output. Furthermore, the regurgitant blood imposes a volume overload on the left ventricle, promoting more dilation and remodeling. The resulting decrease in forward cardiac output with ventricular remodeling and mitral regurgitation exaggerates the hemodynamic defense mechanism, which further distorts the hormonal and cytokine balance in the infarcted ventricle.

Chronic ischemia alters the structure of the myocardium, including a loss of contractile filaments, reduction of sarcoplasmic reticulum, an increase in interstitial fibrillar collagen, the accumulation of glycogen, and increased numbers of small mitochondria. Nevertheless, the ischemic myocardium remains metabolically active *(55)*.

After myocardial infarction, ventricular remodeling occurs in adjacent border zones and in remote myocardial segments where cardiac output is initially preserved and regional wall stress is limited. Ischemic injury alters myocardial function, including increased stiffness, reduced compliance due to fibrosis, left ventricular dilation due to direct myocardial tissue loss (via necrosis and/or apoptosis) and altered hemodynamics (i.e., preload and/or afterload). Additional neurohormonal changes alter wall stress (via Laplace's law) and cause hypertrophy of adjacent normal myocardial segments *(56)*.

Infarcted myocardium may eventually thin due to further fibrosis, and the infarct zone can expand due to myocyte elongation *(57)*. This infarct expansion involves the slippage of myocyte bundles in ischemic and nonischemic regions. Mural realignment of myofibrillar bundles can occur. These maladaptive morphologic and geometric processes begin within days after the acute injury and progress over the ensuing months. Left ventricular dilation and changes in nonellipsoidal shape occur and are associated with cardiac decompensation (i.e., congestive heart failure) and increased mortality (i.e., sudden death) (Fig. 6) *(58)*.

Molecular Remodeling Pathways: Therapeutic Implications

Defining the signaling pathways that control survival and function (i.e., remodeling) of ischemic cardiomyocytes may provide insight into the mechanisms of cardiac injury and help identify potential targets for intervention *(59)*. Many drugs work, at least in part, by modulating apoptosis. Therapeutic strategies are being developed to reduce collateral apoptotic myocardial damage. These "apoptosis blockers" could mitigate post-ischemic myocardial injury and reduce subsequent left ventricular remodeling and ischemic cardiomyopathy (Fig. 7A–C) *(1,60)*.

The serine–threonine kinase known as "Akt" is activated by several cardioprotective ligand–receptor systems, including insulin, insulin-like growth factor-1, and glycoprotein-130 signaling *(59)*. Akt activation reduces TUNEL-positive apoptotic nuclei (DNA fragmentation) in ischemic cardiomyocytes in vivo and in vitro. Apoptosis is blocked in vitro in ischemic rat cardiomyocytes with a constitutively active Akt. Akt activation after gene transfer in a mutant rat model of cardiac ischemia–reperfusion has a powerful cardioprotective effect. This effect involves increased sarcolemmal expression of Glut-4 in vivo and increased glucose uptake in vitro to levels approaching those seen with insulin treatment *(59)*.

In experimental settings, the molecular and metabolic effects of insulin and IGF-1 signaling reduced infarct size and produced functional recovery in post-ischemic wall thickening, contractility ($+dP/dt$), and relaxation ($-dP/dt$). Ischemia-induced cardiac dysfunction and cardiomyocyte apoptosis can be reduced by increased uptake of glucose and more favorable bioenergetics of glycolytic metabolism, both of which were first used with glucose–insulin–potassium infusion to limit infarct size *(61)*. Akt may be an important therapeutic target for intervention in post-infarction injury and ventricular dysfunction.

The mechanism(s) responsible for TNF-induced left ventricular remodeling in the human heart are unknown. MMPs cause collagen degradation *(62)*. Early after ischemic injury,

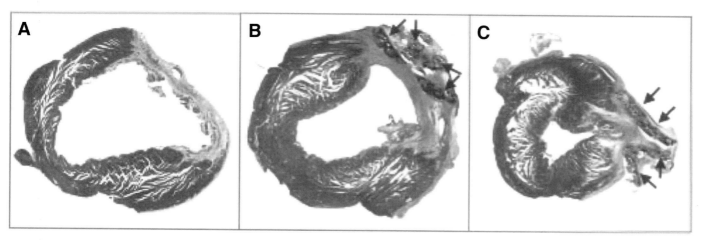

Fig. 6. Masson trichrome–stained transverse sections of a rat left ventricle (LV) 4 wk after surgery to create a left ventricular (LV) aneurysm by left anterior descending artery ligation. Panel **A** is the sham operation with an angiotensin-converting enzyme (ACE) inhibitor showing a dilated LV chamber and large fibrotic scar. Panel **B** illustrates the effect of surgical repair of the LV aneurysm with placebo; the LV chamber size is large, and severe fibrosis has developed beyond the Teflon pledgets (arrows). Panel **C** illustrates the combined effect of LV aneurysm repair plus ACE inhibition, with a small LV chamber and a small area of fibrosis adjacent to the pledgets (arrows). The beneficial effect of remodeling (prevention of LV dilation and maintenance of LV systolic function) was synergistic when suppression of oxidative stress by ACE inhibition (lisinopril 10 mg/kg/d) was combined with surgical repair of the LV aneurysm. Reproduced with permission from *(58)*.

TNF is overexpressed, which, in conjunction with local MMP expression, causes mural thinning *(63)*. The subsequent reduction in local MMP expression is associated with myocardial fibrosis and is inversely related to TIMP-1 levels. TNF-induced fibrosis correlates with increased local levels of transforming growth factor (TGF)-β1 and TGF-β2.

Drugs such as β blockers and angiotensin-converting enzyme (ACE) inhibitors and implanted devices such as the left ventricular assist device (LVAD) favorably influence the remodeling process and improve survival by reducing myocytolysis and the size of the failing heart and by restoring a more normal prolate ellipsoidal shape *(62)*. The LVAD improves function in the chronically failing heart in part by decreasing the activation of collagenolytic enzymes such as MMP and by increasing the local concentration of TIMP *(64)*. In addition, the LVAD may alter expression of genes that affect contractility of the failing heart, such as upregulating gene expression for proteins that regulate sarcoplasmic reticular handling of calcium *(65)*. Whether these events operate in the acute period of remodeling after infarction is unknown.

Experimental data support other gene-modulated therapeutic interventions (Fig. 8) *(66)*. Monoclonal antibodies have been developed against rat mannose-binding lectins. These antibodies block lectin-induced complement activation *(11)* and protect rat hearts from ischemia–reperfusion injury by reducing infarct size, creatine kinase loss, and neutrophil infiltration and by reducing the expression of pro-inflammatory genes such as intercellular adhesion molecule-1, interleukin (IL)-6, and vascular cell adhesion molecule (VCAM)-1.

The JAK/STAT pathway of JAK-2 activation is associated with cardiac dysfunction in ischemic hearts. This pathway is inhibited by cardiac AT-1 receptor antagonism with losartan *(19)*. Activation of the RAS facilitates apoptosis in cardiomyocytes *(67)*. The cardioprotective effect of losartan in humans may involve inhibition of apoptosis.

The decrease in the flux of the creatine kinase reaction in the failing myocardium is associated with reduced levels of the high-energy compounds, phosphocreatine and free creatine. The relation between these changes in myocardial energetics and the pathogenesis of postischemic contractile dysfunction is unknown. Treatment with the creatine analog, β-guanidinoproprionate, reduces cardiac levels of phosphocreatine by 87% and increases experimental mortality after infarction in rats *(3)*. This disruption of myocardial ATP homeostatsis was not associated with incremental impairment of mechanical dysfunction in rat hearts.

NO affects many processes involved in ventricular remodeling *(68)*. NO can increase angiogenesis, decrease cardiac fibrosis, and reduce angiotensin II–mediated cardiomyocyte hypertrophy. NO synthases (NOS), found in

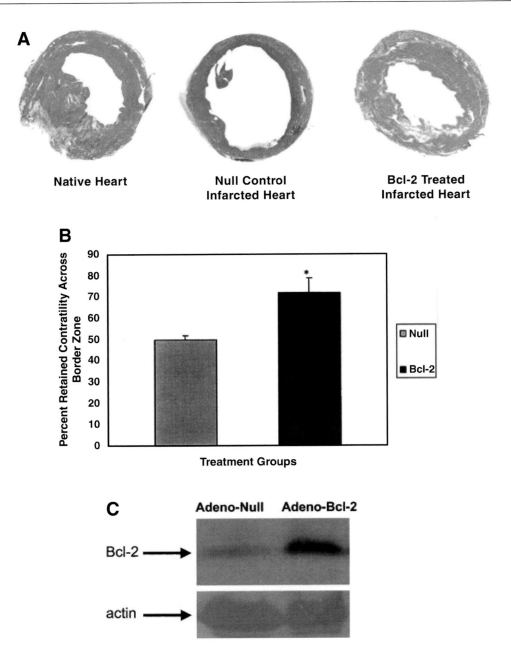

Fig. 7. (A) Three representative sections of a rabbit model of regional ischemia followed by reperfusion (i.e., experimental infarction) at the midchamber level 6 wk following ischemic stress. The "native" heart is uninfarcted and untreated. The "null control–infarcted" heart was untreated with in vivo viral gene transfer of the anti-apoptotic factor (BCL-2). The "BCL-2-treated infarct" heart demonstrated the effect of blocking apoptosis, which results in preservation of ventricular geometry and function (i.e. anti-remodeling effect) as compared to the null control–infarcted heart. **(B)** Sonomicrometry data from BCL-2 untreated (null) and treated animals at 6 wk following experimental infarction demonstrates superior preservation of fractional shortening in the BCL-2 treated group. Results reported are expressed as a percentage of baseline fractional shortening in the reperfused infarct border zone, as compared to the remote viable myocardium (*=$p<0.03$). **(C)** Western blot analysis demonstrating mouse anti-human monoclonal BLC-2 that was utilized to probe tissue samples obtained 6 wk following experimental infarction and reperfusion. Lane 1 is an adeno-null sample, demonstrating no reactivity with BCL-2 or actin (control). Lane 2 is the adeno-null-BCL-2 treated specimen demonstrating increased expression of BCL-2 as compared to controls. Reproduced with permission from *(60)*.

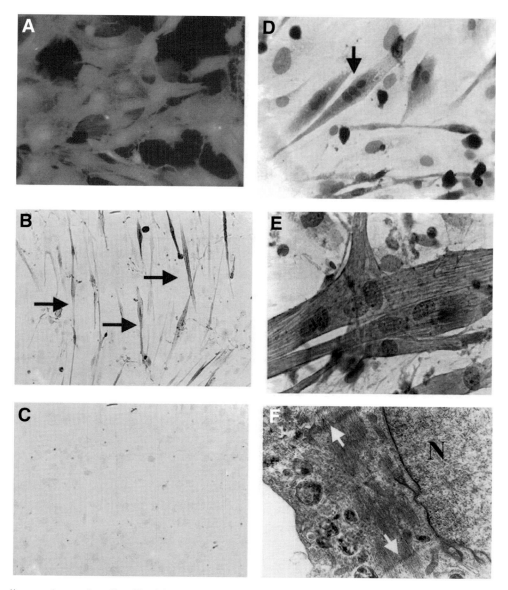

Fig. 8. Cellular cardiomyoplasty of cardiac fibroblasts utilizing adenoviral delivery of myoD results in myogenic differentiation of cultured fibroblasts ex vivo. Primary fibroblasts were isolated from 7-d infarcted rat hearts or rat pericardium and transfected with recombinant adenoviral myoD (a muscle-specific transcription factor master gene that prompts myogenesis in cells, including fibroblasts). Twenty-four hours after transfection, the majority of cultured fibroblasts exhibited expression of a reporter gene (GFP, panel **A**). With serum deprivation, myoD-treated cells differentiate and fuse into multinucleated myotubules (panel **B** arrows) that stain positively for the presence of fast-MHC (myosin heavy chain). These changes were not present in control fibroblasts (panel **C**). Immunostaining for myogenic proteins identified positive cells for fast-MHC (panel **D**, arrows show multinucleated myotubes). Alpha-sarcomeric actin analysis revealed organized sarcomeres with typical cross striation and Z-bands (arrows, N=nucleus, panel **F**). The capacity of myoD to activate myogenesis in fibroblasts (ex vivo) is demonstrated as a possible autologous myogenic cell source for transplantation. Reproduced with permission from *(66)*.

three isoforms, are enzymes that increase local levels of NO. Inhibition of NOS affects myocardial structure and cardiac function. Specifically, inhibition of NOS-3 after myocardial infarction in mice increases left ventricular volume, left ventricular mass, and mortality in an afterload-independent manner. In addition, inhibition of NOS decreases contractility, diastolic function, and capillary density. These findings in mice may have clinical significance. Therapy with NO-donor compounds such as nitrates reduces systemic vascular resistance (preload and afterload), left ventricular remodeling, and cardiac mortality after myocardial infarction *(69)*.

Myocardial Angiogenesis

Restoring myocardial perfusion by promoting local growth of blood vessels has been studied in animal models (70,71) and in patients with chronic myocardial ischemia (72). Few studies have focused on strategies for new vessel growth for acutely infarcted myocardium. Two mechanisms of action have been proposed for the improvement of myocardial perfusion after the administration of angiogenic agents. First, angiogenic agents may cause capillary budding, which promotes formation of a new capillary network; this pathway is called angiogenesis. The second pathway, called arteriogenesis, involves the recruitment, remodeling, and growth of existing muscular arterioles (i.e., epicardial collaterals or R-2 vessels) (73).

Several growth-promoting factors, including recombinant vascular endothelial growth factor (rVEGF) (70) and recombinant fibroblast growth factor-2 (rFGF-2), have been used as angiogenic agents (72,73). In addition, several molecular techniques involving plasmids and adenoviral vectors have been used to transfer the genetic material required to promote local growth factor secretion. These gene-transfer techniques introduce the complementary DNA for growth factors to the affected tissues. Genetically modified proteins can be delivered by intraarterial, intravenous, or direct intramyocardial injection at the time of bypass or via thoracotomy (74). Genetically engineered bioartificial myocytes have been used recently for local delivery of rVEGF (37). Once delivered, the genetic material encoding growth factors must be able to escape immunological detection and be incorporated into local cells such as cardiomyocytes or striated muscle cells.

Multiple benefits can be achieved with local angiogenesis. Cardiac function improves with a decrease in symptoms of ischemia, and normal electromechanical activity of the heart is restored (71,72). In addition, VEGF may provide angiogenesis-independent benefits because of the downstream production of NO, a benefit not seen with FGF-induced angiogenesis (75).

Tissue "priming" may be important to the local efficacy of angiogenic cytokines. VEGF and its two major tyrosine kinase receptors, VEGFR-1 and VEGFR-2, are expressed at high levels in malignant tumors and in angiogenic tissues; however, levels of VEGF and its receptors are very low in normal tissue. Ischemic tissue, which has increased expression of FGF and VEGF receptors, is considered biologically "primed." Unless they are primed, normal tissues may require extended exposure to high levels of growth factors to promote angiogenesis. Normal vessel growth requires the expression and activity of multiple gene products, a condition not produced by therapeutic overexpression of a single gene.

Potential toxicity associated with angiogenesis therapy includes tumor growth, angioma formation, and proliferative retinopathy. The optimal dose range for angiogenic agents is being assessed in phase I and II studies (76). Potential systemic side effects include increased vascular permeability and atherosclerotic plaque mass. Hazards associated with adenoviral vectors include local immune and inflammatory responses. In addition, direct myocardial delivery techniques can cause local inflammation or fibrosis. Moreover, newly formed vessels created by angiogenesis may be functionally abnormal.

Human bone marrow–derived angioblasts have been used experimentally to induce neovascularization in ischemic myocardium (77). Bone marrow from adult humans contains endothelial cell precursors with the phenotypic and functional characteristics of embryonic hemangioblasts. Infarction-bed vasculogenesis and the proliferation of preexisting vasculature (angiogenesis) associated with bone marrow treatment prevent cardiomyocyte apoptosis, reduce remodeling, and improve cardiac function.

Another creative approach to the treatment of postinfarction myocardial dysfunction is the grafting of skeletal myoblasts (78), also known as cell therapy. In a rat infarction model, injecting 1 million myoblasts directly into the infarction zone increased exercise capacity, improved contractile function, and attenuated ventricular dilation. This improvement is associated with survival of the myoblast graft, which during periods of stress results in myotubule differentiation, the formation of new contractile muscle fibers, and the expression of β-MHC molecules (Figs. 9–11) (79–81).

CLINICAL THERAPY FOR LEFT VENTRICULAR REMODELING

Left Ventricular Assist Devices

Left ventricular geometry plays an important role in the reduced systolic function associated with myocardial infarction and end-stage heart failure. LVADs are mechanical pumps implanted into the apex of the left ventricle and the ascending aorta. The LVAD mechanically decompresses the left ventricle while electrical activity continues. The LVAD has been successfully used as a bridge to transplantation in heart failure patients or as primary surgical treatment for heart failure when medical therapy fails.

Studies of endomyocardial biopsies before and after LVAD placement have suggested that left ventricular myocyte function returns toward normal levels after prolonged mechanical rest and decompression. After LVAD placement, changes in left ventricular geometry include

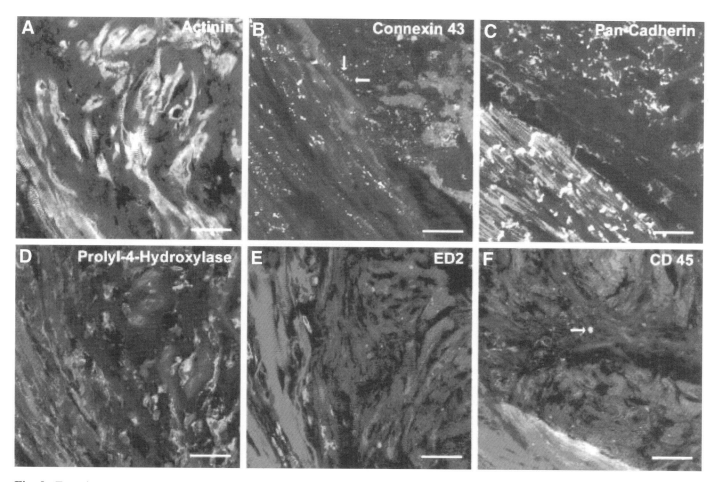

Fig. 9. Experiments demonstrating successful cardiac tissue grafting using engineered heart tissue (EHT) that was reconstituted by mixing cardiac myocytes from neonatal rats with liquid collagen type I. Experiments fitted the EHTs around the circumference of hearts from syngeneic rats, after which implantation was evaluated using echocardiography and special staining techniques. Photomicrographs of sections from the boundary of the host rat myocardium (left) with the grafted EHT myocardium (right) are stained for alpha-sarcomeric actinin **(a)**, connexin 43 **(b)**, cadherins **(c)**, the fibroblast marker prolyl-4-hydroxylase **(d)**, the macrophage marker ED2 **(e)**, and the pan-leukocyte marker CD 45 **(f)**. Actin is labeled with a red stain in all sections **(a–f)**. The arrows in **(b)** indicate possible electrical coupling between EHT-grafted and host cardiac myocytes. The arrow in **(f)** demonstrates a leukocyte within grafted EHT. EHTs may be employed for tissue grafting to repair diseased myocardium. Reproduced with permission from *(79)*.

enlargement of the chamber, reduction in left ventricular mass, and regression of left ventricular hypertrophy *(82,83)*. In addition, both systolic *(84)* and diastolic function *(85)* return toward normal levels after LVAD implantation. Improvements in systolic and diastolic function may be secondary to improvements in the humoral environment responsible for remodeling and to a reduction in wall tension *(86)*. Despite these impressive changes in geometry and cardiac function, long-term ventricular recovery with LVAD explantation is the exception—not the rule *(87,88)*.

Many changes are noted at the cellular level in the myocytes of the remodeled ventricle. Rivello et al. *(89)* have shown that myocytes undergo a process of reverse remodeling after prolonged LVAD implantation, including a reduction in nuclear size and cellular DNA content. This finding suggests that remodeling is a dynamic process and that nuclear changes and abnormal protein expression may be reversible in some cases *(90)*.

Left ventricular dysfunction, increased peak cytosolic calcium transients, and accelerated calcium current decay have been reported in myocytes after LVAD implantation, suggesting improved calcium fluxes during the cardiac action potential and augmented actin–myosin cross-bridge formation. Enhanced production of cyclic-AMP following β-receptor activation with isoproterenol has been described, suggesting improved catecholamine second-messenger signal transduction *(14,84)*.

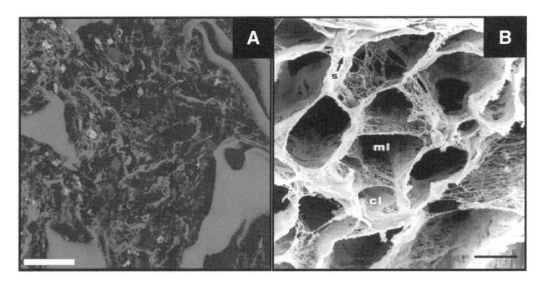

Fig. 10. Demonstration of the effect of mechanical stretch on the formation of bioengineered autologous cardiac muscle grafts, using cultured heart cells from children undergoing tetralogy of Fallot repair. Cells were seeded on a gelatin-matrix scaffold (Gelfoam) and subjected to cyclical mechanical stress (80 cycles/min × 14 d). The confocal scanning micrograph reveals the distribution and organization of fibrillar collagen matrix within the stretched heart cell–seeded Gelfoam (panel **A**). A scanning electron micrograph of the normal endomysial collagen matrix in the human myocardium is illustrated in panel **B**, for comparison. Collagen staining is present (picrosirius staining), and heart cells are shown by autofluorescence. Cyclical stretch enhanced the formation of a three-dimensional tissue engineered cardiac graft by improving proliferation and distribution of human heart cells and by stimulating organized matrix formation. Reproduced with permission from *(80)*.

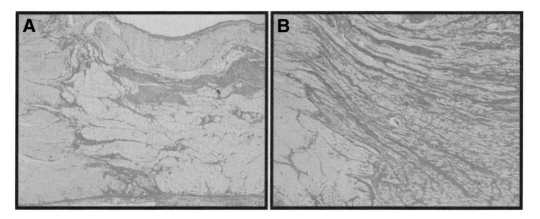

Fig. 11. An experimental model using picrosirius stain of infarction in a control animal (panel **A**) compared with a 4-mo-old scar in a sheep that was engrafted with in-scar injections of autologous skeletal myoblasts. The untreated scar is characterized by white fat deposits (white) and fibrous tissue deposits (dark). The treated scar has a high density of grafted cells, which have replaced the fatty and fibrous tissues. In both panels, normal myocardium is illustrated in the left border of the figure panel. Reproduced with permission from *(81)*.

Calcium metabolism is important in the failing heart after LVAD implantation. Using Northern blot analysis, Heerdt et al. *(65)* reported upregulation in genes for three important calcium-handling proteins: Ca ATP-ase subtype 2a (SERCA-2a), the ryanodine receptor, and the sarcolemma Na-Ca exchanger. However, Western blot analysis showed increased expression of only the SERCA-2a protein. These findings suggest functional improvement of calcium handling by the sarcoplasmic reticulum, and the force–frequency relationship of individual sarcomeres was more favorable after LVAD support.

The dynamic nature of the extracellular matrix has been discussed. After LVAD implantation, MMPs decrease and

TIMPs increase (42). Furthermore, in paired analysis, cross-linking of cellular collagen improved, suggesting stabilization of the extracellular matrix and prevention of myocyte slippage, reducing LV diameter (62).

Other Surgical Interventions

Direct surgical approaches to mitigate left ventricular remodeling have been tried after anterior wall myocardial infarction and in patients with dilated cardiomyopathy (91). Surgical approaches attempt to alter the LaPlace relationship by modifying the radius of curvature and ventricular diameter, thereby returning the remodeled ventricle to a more efficient prolate ellipse. The Batista procedure, or partial ventriculectomy (92), was initially tried with great enthusiasm. Although myocyte wall stress initially improved after surgery, hemodynamics or long-term clinical outcome did not (93). The failure of the Batista procedure to improve clinical status after myocardial infarction or in patients with dilated cardiomyopathy may result from postoperative worsening of the diastolic properties of the ventricle (94).

The surgical anterior ventricular endocardial restoration (SAVER) procedure involves excluding non-contracting, dilated segments of the anterior wall, with or without coronary artery bypass surgery and mitral valve repair or replacement (95). Postoperative ejection fraction increased from 29% to 39%, and left ventricular end-systolic volume decreased from 109 mL/m² to 60 mL/m². After anterior wall myocardial infarction, survival at 18 mo was greater than 85%, and hospital admissions for congestive heart failure were reduced.

Animal studies have suggested surgical therapeutic possibilities other than ventricular resection. McCarthy and colleagues (96) recently published their experience with the Myosplint device (Myocor Inc, Maple Grove, MN). This device is an implantable, polyethylene transventricular splint with two epicardial pads that are adjusted to draw the walls of the left ventricle into close approximation, thereby reducing left ventricular radius and wall tension. Using a tachycardia-mediated cardiomyopathy model, McCarthy's group assessed three-dimensional echocardiographic variables before and after implantation. Ejection fraction increased from 19% to 39% 1 mo after the procedure, whereas both end-diastolic and end-systolic volumes decreased significantly. Cardiac output as assessed by echocardiography increased, but the severity of mitral regurgitation did not change. A similar device has been reported recently to improve hemodynamics in the remodeled ventricle and to increase patient quality of life (97).

Restoration of Flow by Percutaneous Coronary Intervention

Acute myocardial infarction, especially anterior wall transmural injury, is a potent initiating event for myocardial remodeling. Ventricular remodeling is inversely related to prognosis, especially when ejection fraction is reduced after myocardial infarction (98). Landmark trials in thrombolysis for acute infarction suggest that patient survival and residual myocardial function depend on the time elapsed from the onset of symptoms to the restoration of coronary blood flow (99,100). The data for direct primary angioplasty are less clear, although restoration of flow as late as 21 d after the index event can be beneficial (101). The widely held clinical tenets "time is muscle" and "injured muscle remodels unfavorably" are probably correct, regardless of the method used to restore flow to the infarcted myocardium.

Sheiban et al. (102) evaluated left ventricular wall scores and echocardiographic indices of left ventricular volume and remodeling after successful primary angioplasty for acute infarction. Patients were grouped according to time of reperfusion of the infarct-related artery and were followed for 6 mo. In patients in whom TIMI III flow was restored within 4 h, both end-systolic and end-diastolic volumes were reduced at 90 d, whereas patients who underwent revascularization after 6 hours showed no improvement in remodeling indices. Long-term wall motion score was improved in all groups, regardless of the time to flow restoration.

These data (103) support the open artery hypothesis, which suggests that ventricular remodeling may be improved by restoration of coronary blood flow to the infarcted and periinfarct regions (104). Restoring blood flow may improve outcome by preventing dilation of adjacent segments and by returning wall stress to normal levels in the adjacent ventricle via formation of a firmer scar. Improvements in left ventricular geometry should lead to improvements in ejection fraction, thus attenuating many of the hemodynamic and cytokine defense mechanisms. Supporting data from Hara et al. (104) showed that both thallium-201 myocardial scintigraphy injury scores and brain natriuretic peptide levels decrease after elective angioplasty of the infarct-related vessel.

A major limitation of both thrombolytic and angioplasty trials is the failure to address the impact of the microcirculation. Coronary oxygen exchange occurs at the capillary level, not in the epicardial vessels visualized by angiography. Thus, it is not clear whether simple restoration of coronary blood flow in the conduit pipes, with or without improvement in tissue microcirculation flow, has the same remodeling benefits. This discordance between restoration of epicardial flow and lack of microcirculatory integrity has been called the "no-reflow phenomenon" *(105)*. The improvement in clinical outcome with the adjunctive use of glycoprotein IIb/IIIa antagonists during angioplasty may be due in part to the beneficial effect of the antagonists in reducing platelet plugging in the microcirculation.

Using both Doppler echocardiography and video-intensity angiography, Destro et al. *(106)* studied the integrity of the microcirculation after angioplasty and attenuation of ventricular remodeling. When successful angioplasty was associated with increased video intensity (reflecting intact microcirculation) in the area at risk, remodeling and ejection fraction were improved. This benefit occurred in patients in whom angioplasty was deferred, providing support for the open artery hypothesis.

Pharmacologic Therapy for Remodeling

NITRATES

The effects of long-term nitrate therapy after myocardial infarction have been studied in both the Gruppo Italiano per lo Studio della Sopravvienza nell'infarto Miocardico (GISSI-3) *(107)* and the Fourth International Study of Infarct Survival (ISIS-4) trials *(108)*. Neither of these large clinical trials showed an improvement in mortality rates associated with nitrate therapy after myocardial infarction; however, intravenous nitrate therapy has been shown to limit infarct size and expansion for up to 1 yr after the index cardiac event *(109)*. In dogs, prolonged nitrate therapy for 6 wk after myocardial infarction improved ejection fraction and reduced left ventricular volume, cavity expansion, and aneurysm formation *(110)*. Continuous nitrate therapy reduced scar size, collagen content, and ventricular volume and mass more than late perfusion alone *(111)*.

Mahmarian and colleagues *(112)* reported that intermittent nitrate therapy with a transdermal preparation increased ejection fraction and reduced both end-diastolic and end-systolic volume after infarction. These benefits were seen primarily in patients with an ejection fraction of less than 40% and were achieved with a nitrate dose of 0.4 mg/h. End-diastolic and end-systolic volume increased after withdrawal of nitrate therapy.

The mechanism by which nitrate therapy improves ventricular remodeling is not known. In dogs, both left ventricular preload, as estimated by left atrial pressure, and afterload are reduced *(102)*. Thus, stretch-mediated increases in angiotensin II may be reduced, with a subsequent improvement in remodeling and decrease in apoptosis. With reduced afterload, maintenance of stroke volume may decrease the release of catecholamines,

thereby reducing the toxic effects on the myocardium. Another suggested mechanism is that improved coronary blood flow to peri-infarct areas of the myocardium prevents hypertrophy at distant sites via sustained integrity of the extracellular collagen matrix *(103)*.

ANGIOTENSIN CONVERTING ENZYME INHIBITORS AND ANGIOTENSIN RECEPTOR ANTAGONISTS

ACE inhibitors have been studied and used extensively in the prevention of post-infarction ventricular remodeling. In both the Survival and Ventricular Enlargement (SAVE) *(113)* and the Acute Infarction Ramipril Efficacy (AIRE) trials *(114)*, long-term administration of ACE inhibitors improved morbidity and mortality. In patients with an ejection fraction of less than 45% after Q-wave infarction, ACE inhibitors increased stroke volume index and ejection fraction and decreased end-systolic volume *(115)*. End-diastolic volume was lower after anterior wall infarction in patients without clinical heart failure after treatment with captopril at 1 yr of follow-up *(116)*. Although starting ACE inhibitors 1 wk after infarction improves hemodynamics, the improvement is greater if ACE inhibitors are started within 24–48 h after the index event *(117)*. Animal studies, including a rat knockout model for the angiotensin I receptor, have indicated the importance of angiotensin in remodeling and the need for addressing this pathway in the medical treatment of myocardial infarction *(118,119)*.

Early studies in rats showed that ACE inhibitors improve ventricular remodeling after infarction *(120)*. The beneficial effect of ACE inhibitors was initially thought to be independent of the lowering of arterial pressure because hydralazine showed no remodeling benefit at similar reductions in arterial pressure *(121)*. However, ACE inhibitors have a mixed effect on the circulation, and the venodilating properties can cause a decrease in preload and ventricular stretch, which suggests a possible mechanism for improvement in ventricular remodeling after myocardial infarction.

Angiotensin II is a mitogenic hormone that may contribute, possibly in combination with TGF β-1, to the development of fibrosis after infarction *(122)*. In addition, angiotensin II is a potent vasoconstrictor that increases ventricular afterload, thus reducing stroke volume. Kim and colleagues *(123)* described the biochemical changes in the rat model with infusion of angiotensin II. Left ventricular mRNA for β-myosin was increased, suggesting a reversion to a fetal phenotype. After 3 d of infusion, TGF β-1, types I and III collagen, and ventricular mass increased. Blocking the receptor for angiotensin II improved these changes in the myocardium, independent of the effect of receptor blockade on blood. Hanatani et al. *(124)* obtained similar results in the rat infarct model; blocking the angiotensin receptor decreased the expression of β-myosin chain and the level of atrial natriuretic peptide (ANP). Hanatani et al. *(124)* reported no changes in the expression of collagen types I or II. Other studies in the rat infarct model have shown that ACE inhibitors reduce the expression of diacylglycerol kinase phenotypes, which decrease the signaling from diacylglycerol and PKC *(125)*. Taken together, these studies suggest that high levels of circulating angiotensin II can promote cellular and genetic changes in the myocardium after infarction, and that modifications of the cellular matrix may be responsible in part for the role of angiotensin II in ventricular remodeling.

Histopathologic studies have been conducted on the use of ACE inhibitors and angiotensin receptor blockers after myocardial infarction. In a randomized study, Yu and colleagues *(126)* treated rats with fosinopril, valsartan, or combination therapy after myocardial infarction. Both valsartan and combination therapy reduced the level of mRNA for total collagen, type I collagen, and TGF-β. In addition, both valsartan and combination therapy decreased the numbers of myofibroblasts and macrophages in the infarct zone as shown by histomorphometry. ACE inhibition alone was less effective than combination therapy or angiotensin receptor blockade in improving ventricular remodeling after infarction. This observation has not been confirmed in other studies *(127)*.

The difference in the effects of ACE inhibitors and angiotensin receptor blockade in ventricular remodeling suggests a role for bradykinin in this process because receptor antagonists do not increase bradykinin levels. Hu et al. *(128)* treated post-infarction rats with quinapril or losartan with and without the bradykinin receptor antagonist Hoe-14⁰. Both quinapril and losartan reduced left ventricular end-diastolic pressure and left ventricular wall stress in animals with substantial myocardial damage, but neither had an effect on the ventricular pressure–volume relationship. Only quinapril reduced left ventricular weight, and Hoe-14⁰ prevented this effect. These data suggest that post-infarction treatment of ventricular remodeling with ACE inhibitors involves a mechanism that is angiotensin II receptor independent and bradykinin dependent.

Although the role of ACE inhibitors in improving systolic function after infarction has been extensively studied, the effects of these inhibitors on ventricular diastolic properties are less well known. Using the rat infarction model with Doppler echocardiographic indices of diastolic function, Yoshiyama et al. *(129)* showed that the ratio of passive mitral valve filling (E wave) to active atrial mitral valve filling (A wave) increases with infarction, as does the deceleration time of the mitral E wave. These findings suggest that increased left atrial pressure opposes the normal ventricular suction effect of blood across the mitral valve into the normal left ventricle. Treatment of rats with either candesartan or cilazapril improves diastolic variables at 1 and 4 wk follow-up, suggesting a role for ACE inhibitors in the treatment of diastolic dysfunction after myocardial infarction.

β BLOCKERS

The concept of β blocker therapy for heart failure was initially proposed in the early 1970s *(130)*, but was largely ignored because of the advent of inotropic medications for heart failure. However, several landmark clinical trials *(131)* have shown that β blockers such as carvedilol reduce mortality in chronic heart failure patients and improve ejection fraction in long-term follow-up. Although the use of β blockers seems counterintuitive because the failing ventricle is inotropically impaired, new data on the molecular mechanisms of ventricular remodeling may explain the benefits of β blockers for left ventricular dysfunction after myocardial infarction.

With the onset of left ventricular dysfunction after myocardial infarction, plasma catecholamine levels increase progressively via reflexes from the hemodynamic defense mechanism. Biopsy samples obtained from heart failure patients have shown a decrease in the density of β receptors, a reduction in the c-AMP response to isoproterenol, and a decrease in the force induced by exogenous catecholamines *(132)*. Changes in sympathetic activation in the heart primarily reflect local norepinephrine levels in the area of the receptors and the synthesis of the β-1-receptor subpopulation. Regional differences of myocardial β receptor downregulation have been described in rats with post-infarction heart failure *(133)*. The second messenger adenylate cyclase enzyme *(134)* may be uncoupled via phosphorylation of both β1 and β2 receptors by β-adrenergic receptor kinase (BARK), which is upregulated in remodeled ventricles. The reported increase in levels of the inhibitory G protein *(135)* suggests a possible mechanism for β-receptor downregulation and uncoupling.

Catecholamines are cardiotoxic and may contribute to the molecular changes associated with remodeling. In rats, infusion of norepinephrine induces ventricular hypertrophy, a time-dependent increase in the expression of mRNA for IL-6 and IL-1-β, an overexpression of collagen type I and type III *(136)*, and an increase in ANP. Mixed α- and β-receptor blockade with carvedilol prevented the synthesis of both IL-6 and IL-1-β or decreased (attenuated) the synthesis of collagen and ANP. These findings suggest a potential role for receptor-blocking agents in the early stages of remodeling. Grimm et al. *(137)* reported similar findings with carvedilol in an aortic stenosis model of vascular remodeling.

Apoptosis mediated via β1 receptors in the failing ventricle after infarction is an important mechanism for remodeling *(138)*. Mice with genetic overexpression of the β1 receptor exhibit marked apoptosis and ventricular dilation *(139)*. Infusion of isoproterenol for as little as 12 h increased terminal deoxynucleotidyltransferase (TUNEL)–positive myocytes, suggesting an increase in apoptosis. The effect of catecholamine-induced apoptosis appears to be related to β1 receptor activation because norepinephrine-mediated apoptosis is decreased by β1 receptor antagonists and increased by β2 receptor antagonists *(140)*.

The use of β-receptor blockade for reducing ventricular remodeling has not been studied as closely as the use of ACE inhibitors. Yang et al. *(141)* studied the role of carvedilol in post-infarction remodeling in rats. There were three treatment groups: high, intermediate, and low doses of carvedilol. In rats with infarction of 45% of the total myocardium, carvedilol administered for 4 wk after the index event reduced left ventricular weight and volume and end-diastolic pressure in a dose-dependent manner. The decreases in LV weight and volume and end-diastolic pressure were all dose-dependent. Contractility, as estimated by the first derivative of pressure over time *(dP/dt)*, improved in all three treatment groups but was not related to dose. Finally, post-infarction ventricular sphericity (sphericity being abnormal) was affected only in rats who received high doses of carvedilol. Improved sphericity resulted in a less spherical (or more ellipsoidal) ventricular shape.

Ricci et al. *(142)* recently compared ACE inhibition with captopril to β1 receptor blockade with metoprolol alone and in combination with ACE inhibition in the treatment of left ventricular remodeling after infarction. Two hundred fifty consecutive patients experiencing their first myocardial infarction were randomized to receive therapy within 24 h of the index event, and were followed by serial echocardiography at 2 wk, 3 mo, and 6 mo. At 6 mo, left ventricular end-diastolic area index was increased in patients receiving combination therapy, whereas wall motion index was reduced in patients receiving ACE inhibitors alone. The authors concluded that captopril therapy alone improved ventricular remodeling better than combination therapy with β1 receptor blockade after uncomplicated first myocardial infarction.

ALDOSTERONE ANTAGONISTS

Aldosterone, which is a mineralocorticoid steroid hormone linked to the RAS, is released from the zona glomerulosa of the adrenal gland when angiotensin levels increase. Aldosterone binds to steroid receptors in the renal collecting tubule and increases the reabsorption of sodium and water while promoting potassium excretion. Endothelin increases the release of aldosterone, and ANP inhibits aldosterone secretion.

Aldosterone levels are increased in patients with heart failure, presumably as part of the hemodynamic defense mechanism to maintain cardiac output by increasing ventricular filling and stroke volume. In a recent study by Hayashi and colleagues *(143)*, the concentration of aldosterone in the coronary sinus was increased in the acute phase of myocardial infarction, suggesting local production of aldosterone in the myocardium. The level of aldosterone correlates positively with left ventricular end-diastolic index at 1 mo after infarction. In addition, aldosterone levels correlate with levels of plasma procollagen type III aminoterminal peptide, which is a marker for tissue fibrosis.

The role of myocardial aldosterone production in ventricular remodeling is unclear. Levels of both aldosterone synthase mRNA and myocardial angiotensin II increase within 1 month of myocardial infarction *(144)*. Increased aldosterone production and collagen deposition can be reduced by treatment with spironolactone and angiotensin receptor antagonists, and ejection fraction can be increased after infarction with the use of ACE inhibitors and spironolactone *(145)*.

Delyani et al. *(146)* studied the use of aldosterone receptor antagonists to prevent remodeling by comparing ventricular dimensions at 3, 7, and 28 d post-infarction. No difference was observed in collagen deposition or in the derived thinning ratio (measure of remodeling) between controls and antagonist-treated animals at 7 or 28 d. However, the amount of reactive fibrosis was decreased in the viable myocardium in animals treated with aldosterone receptor antagonists, suggesting that aldosterone may play a role in maladaptive remodeling after myocardial infarction. Polymorphisms in the aldosterone synthase gene do not appear to correlate with the propensity for impaired left ventricular function or unfavorable remodeling after myocardial infarction *(147)*.

CONCLUSION

Translational (genomic) and transcriptional (protein synthesis) events, although clinically silent, have a combined effect on patient symptoms, ventricular function, and patient outcome. These endpoints, and the events that precede them, relate closely to the underlying foundation—the cardiovascular health status of the entire organism and the presence of antecedent target organ structural damage at the onset of repair. Otherwise stated, previously normal hearts will respond differently to the many perturbations after coronary artery occlusion than will previously damaged hearts. The processes that occur after acute coronary occlusion and myocardial infarction may evolve slowly over months or years. And all the while, the heart continues its inotropic and chronotropic functions at an average frequency of 72 cycles per minute, often in the face of concomitant drug effects and confounding multiorgan dysfunction.

REFERENCES

1. Dilsizian V. Perspectives on the study of human myocardium: Viability. In Dilsizian V, ed. Myocardial Viability: A Clinical and Scientific Treatise. Armonk, NY: Futura Publishing: 2000:3–22.
2. Reimer KA, Ideker RE. Myocardial ischemia and infarction: anatomic and biochemical substrates for ischemic cell death and ventricular arrhythmias. Hum Pathol 1987;18:462–475.
3. Horn M, Remkes H, Stromer H, Dienesch C, Neubauer S. Chronic phosphocreatine depletion by creatine analogue beta-guanidinoproprionate is associated with increased mortality and loss of ATP in rats after myocardial infarction. Circulation 2001;104:1844–1849.
4. Maes A, Flameng W, Nuyts J, et al. Histological alterations in chronically hypoperfused myocardium: correlation with PET findings. Circulation 1994;90:735–745.
5. Kerr JF, Wyllie AH, Currie AR. Apoptosis: A basic biological phenomenon with wide-ranging implications in tissue kinetics. Br J Cancer 1972;26:239–257.
6. Majno G, Joris I. Apoptosis, oncosis, and necrosis. An overview of cell death. Am J Pathol 1995;146:3–15.
7. Barnes DG, MacKenzie A. Recent recognition and molecular delineation of apoptosis: Beginnings a therapeutic revolution? Ann R Coll Physicians Surg 1999;32:376–382
8. Ohno M, Takemura G, Ohno A, et al. "Apoptotic" myocytes in infarct area in rabbit hearts may be oncotic myocytes with DNA fragmentation: analysis by immunogold electron microscopy combined with in situ nick end-labeling. Circulation 1998;98:1422–1430.
9. Gavrieli Y, Sherman Y, Ben-Sasson SA. Identification of programmed cell death in situ via specific labeling of nuclear DNA fragmentation. J Cell Biol 1992;119:493–501.
10. Vaux DL, Wacker G. Hypothesis: Apoptosis caused by cytotoxins represents a defensive response that evolved to combat intracellular pathogens. Clin Exp Pharmacol Physiol 1995;22:861–863.
11. Libby P. Current concepts of the pathogenesis of the acute coronary syndromes. Circulation 2001;104:365–372.
12. Ramzi S, Cotran RS, Kumar V, Robbins SL. Pathologic Basis of Disease, 4th ed. Philadelphia: Saunders, 1989.
13. Katz AM. Physiology of the Heart, 3rd ed. Philadelphia:Lippincott Williams & Wilkins, 2001.
14. Woodcock EA, Matkovich SJ, Binah O. Ins(1,4,5)P3 and cardiac dysfunction. Cardiovasc Res 1998;40:251–256.
15. Schwinger RH, Munch G, Bolck B, Karczewski P, Krause EG, Erdmann E. Reduced Ca(2+)-sensitivity of SERCA 2a in failing human myocardium due to reduced serin-16 phospholamban phosphorylation. J Mol Cell Cardiol 1999;31:479–491.
16. Arai M, Alpert NR, MacLennan DH, Barton P, Peiasamy M. Alterations in sarcoplasmic reticulum gene expression in human heart failure. A possible mechanism for alterations in systolic and diastolic properties of the failing myocardium. Circ Res 1993;72:463–469.
17. Gomez AM, Guatimosium S, Dilly KW, Vassort G, Lederer WJ. Heart failure after myocardial infarction: altered excitation-contraction coupling. Circulation 2001;104:688–693.
18. Jordan JE, Montalto MC, Stahl GL. Inhibition of mannose-binding lectin reduces postischemic myocardial reperfusion injury. Circulation 2001;104:1413–1418.
19. Mascareno E, El-Shafei M, Maulik N, et al. JAK/STAT signaling is associated with cardiac dysfunction during ischemia and reperfusion. Circulation 2001;104:325–329.
20. Miller MJ. Preconditioning for cardioprotection against ischemia reperfusion injury: the roles of nitric oxide, reactive oxygen species, heat shock proteins, reactive hyperemia and antioxidants. Can J Cardiol 2001;17:1075–1082.
21. Maulik N, Sasaki H, Galang N. Differential regulation of apoptosis by ischemia-reperfusion and ischemia adaptation. Ann NY Acad Sci 1999;874:401–411 (Abstract).
22. Plumier JC, Ross BM, Currie RW. Transgenic mice expressing the human heat shock protein 70 have improved post-ischemic myocardial recovery. J Clin Invest 1995;95:1854–1860.
23. Suzuki K, Sawa Y, Kaneda Y. In vivo gene transfection with heat shock protein 70 enhances myocardial tolerance to ischemia-reperfusion injury in rats. J Clin Invest 1997;99:1645–1650.
24. Cohen MV, Baines CP, Downey JM. Ischemic preconditioning: from adenosine receptor of KATP channel. Ann Rev Physiol 2000;62:79–109.
25. Das D, Engleman R, Maulik N. Oxygen free radical signaling in ischemic preconditioning. Ann NY Acad Sci 1999;874:49–64.
26. Sun JZ, Tang XL, Park SW. Evidence for essential role of reactive oxygen species in the genesis of late preconditioning against myocardial stunning in conscious pigs. J Clin Invest 1996;97:562–576.
27. Zhang X, Azhar G, Nagano K, Wei JY. Differential vulnerability to oxidative stress in rat cardiac myocytes versus fibroblasts. J Am Coll Cardiol 2001;38:2055–2062.
28. Liu L, Azhar G, Gao W, Zhang X, Wei JY. Bcl-2 and Bax expression in adult rat hearts after coronary occlusion: age-associated differences. Am J Physiol 1998;275:R315–R322.
29. Nakamura M, Wang NP, Zhao ZQ, Wilcox JN, Thourani V, Guyton RA. Pre-conditioning decreases Bax expression, PMN accumulation and apoptosis in reperfused rat heart. Cardiovasc Res 2000;45:661–670.
30. Holly TA, Drincic A, Byun Y, et al. Caspase inhibition reduces myocyte cell death induced by myocardial ischemia and reperfusion in vivo. J Mol Cell Cardiol 1999;31:1709–1715.
31. Ruetten H, Badorff C, Ihling C, Zeiher AM, Dimmeler S. Inhibition of caspase-3 improves contractile recovery of stunning myocardium, independent of apoptosis-inhibitory effects. J Am Coll Cardiol 2001;38:2063–2070.
32. Tennant R, Wiggers CJ. The effect of coronary occlusion on myocardial contraction. Am J Physiol 1935;112:351–361.
33. Hutchins GM, Bulkley BH. Infarct expansion versus extension: two different complications of acute myocardial infarction. Am J Cardiol 1978;41:1127–1132.

34. Pfeffer MA, Braunwald E. Ventricular remodeling after myocardial infarction. Experimental observations and clinical implications. Circulation 1990;81:1161–1172.

35. Meizlish JL, Berger HJ, Plankey MA, Errico D, Levy W, Zaret BL. Functional left ventricular aneurysm formation after acute anterior transmural myocardial infarction. Incidence, natural history, and prognostic implications. N Engl J Med 1984;311: 1001–1006.

36. Weisman HF, Healy B. Myocardial infarct expansion, infarct extension, and reinfarction: pathophysiologic concepts. Prog Cardiovasc Dis 1987;30:73–110.

37. Théroux P, Ross J Jr, Franklin D, Covell JW, Bloor Cm, Sasayama S. Regional myocardial function and dimensions early and late after myocardial infarction in the unanesthetized dog. Circ Res 1977;40:158–165.

38. Erlebacher JA, Weiss JL, Eaton LW, Kallman C, Weisfeldt ML, Bulkle BH. Late effects of acute infarct dilation on heart size: a two-dimensional echocardiographic study. Am J Cardiol 1982; 49:1120–1126.

39. McKay RG, Pfeffer MA, Pasternak RC, et al. Left ventricular remodeling after myocardial infarction: a corollary to infarct expansion. Circulation 1986;74:693–702.

40. Linzbach AJ. Heart failure from the point of view of quantitative anatomy. Am J Cardiol 1960;69:370–382.

41. Tyagi SC, Campbell SE, Reddy HK, Tjahja E, Voelker DJ. Matrix metalloproteinase activity expression in infarcted, non-infarcted and dilated cardiomyopathic human hearts. Mol Cell Biochem 1996;155:13–21.

42. Li YY, Feng Y, McTiernan CF, et al. Downregulation of matrix metalloproteinases and reduction in collagen damage in the failing human heart after support with left ventricular assist devices. Circulation 2001;104:1147–1152.

43. Mann DL, Spinale FG. Activation of matrix metalloproteinases in the failing human heart: breaking the tie that binds. Circulation 1998;98:1699–1702.

44. Sutton MG, Sharpe N. Left ventricular remodeling after myocardial infarction pathophysiology and therapy. Circulation 2000;101:2981–2988.

45. Woodiwiss AJ, Tsotetsi OJ, Sprott S, et al. Reduction in myocardial collagen cross-linking parallels left ventricular dilation in rat models of systolic chamber dysfunction. Circulation 2001;103:155–160.

46. Cleutjens JP, Kandala JC, Guarda E, Guntaka RV, Weber KT. Regulation of collagen degradation in the rat myocardium after infarction. J Mol Cell Cardiol 1995;27:1281–1292.

47. Hojo Y, Ikeda U, Ueno S, Arakawa H, Shimada K. Expression of matrix metalloproteinases in patients with acute myocardial infarction. Jpn Circ J 2001;65:71–75.

48. Nagase H. Activation mechanisms of matrix metalloproteinases. Biol Chem 1997;378:151–160.

49. Trueblood NA, Xie Z, Communal C, et al. Exaggerated left ventricular dilation and reduced collagen deposition after myocardial infarction in mice lacking osteopontin. Circ Res 2001;88:1080–1087.

50. Klein MD, Herman MV, Gorlin R. A hemodynamic study of left ventricular aneurysm. Circulation 1967;35:614–630.

51. Mann DL. Mechanisms and models in heart failure, a combinatorial approach. Circulation 1999;100:999–1008.

52. Weber KT, Janicki JS. The heart as a muscle–pump system and the concept of heart failure. Am Heart J 1979;98:371–384.

53. Capasso JM, Li P, Zhang X, Anversa P. Heterogeneity of ventricular remodeling after acute myocardial infarction in rats. Am J Physiol 1992;262:H486-H495.

54. Kono T, Sabbah HN, Rosman H, Alam M, Jafri S, Goldstein S. Left ventricular shape is the primary determinant of functional mitral regurgitation in heart failure. J Am Coll Cardiol 1992;20: 1594–1598.

55. Depre C, Vanoverschelde JJ, Melin JA, et al. Structural and metabolic correlates of the reversibility of chronic left ventricular ischemic dysfunction in humans. Am J Physiol 1995;268: H1265–H1275.

56. Francis GS, McDonald KM, Cohn JN. Neurohormonal activation in preclinical heart failure. remodeling and the potential for intervention. Circulation 1993;87:IV90–IV96.

57. Weisman HF, Bush DE, Mannisis JA, Weisfeldt ML, Healy B. Cellular mechanisms of myocardial infarct expansion. Circulation 1988;78:186–201.

58. Nomoto T, Nishina T, Miwa S, et al. Angiotensin-converting enzyme inhibitor helps prevent late remodeling after left ventricular aneurysm repair in rats. Circulation 2002;106(suppl I): I-115–I-119).

59. Matsui T, Tao T, del Monte F, et al. Akt activation preserves cardiac function and prevents injury after transient cardiac ischemia in vivo. Circulation 2001;104:330–335.

60. Chatterjee S, Steward AS, Bish LT, et al. Viral transfer of the antiapoptotic factor Bcl-2 protects against chronic postischemic heart failure. Circulation 2002(suppl I):I-212–I-217.

61. Malhotra R, Brosius FC III. Glucose uptake and glycolysis reduce hypoxia-induced apoptosis in cultured neonatal rat cardiac myocytes. J Biol Chem 1999;274:12567–12575.

62. Mann DL, Taegtmeyer H. Dynamic regulation of the extracellular matrix after mechanical unloading of the failing human heart: Recovering the missing link in left ventricular remodeling. Circulation 2001;104:1089–1091.

63. Sivasubramanian N, Coker ML, Kurrelmeyer KM, et al. Left ventricular remodeling in transgenic mice with cardiac restricted overexpression of tumor necrosis factor. Circulation 2001;104:826–831.

64. Li YY, Feng Y, McTeirnan C, et al. Downregulation of matrix metalloproteinases and reduction in collagen damage in the failing human heart after support with left ventricular assist device. Circulation 2001;104:1147–1152.

65. Heerdt PM, Holmes JW, Cai B. Chronic unloading by left ventricular assist device reverses contractile dysfunction and alters gene expression in end-stage heart failure. Circulation 2000; 102:2713–2719.

66. Etzion S, Barbash IM, Geinberg MS, et al. Cellular cardiomyopathy of cardiac fibroblasts by adenoviral delivery of MyoD ex vivo: an unlimited source of cells for myocardial repair. Circulation 2002:106(suppl I):I-125–I-130.

67. Ravassa S, Fortuno MA, Gonzales A, et al. Mechanisms of induced susceptibility to angiotensin II-induced apoptosis in ventricular cardiomyocytes of spontaneously hypertensive rats. Hypertension 2000;36:1065–1071.

68. Scherrer-Crosbie M, Ullrich R, Bloch KD, et al. Endothelial nitric oxide limits left ventricular remodeling after myocardial infarction in mice. Circulation 2001;104:1286–1291.

69. Gruppo Italiano per lo Studio della Sopravvivenza nell'infarto Miocardio (GISSI-3): effects of lisinopril and transdermal glyceryl trinitrate singly and together on 6-week mortality and ventricular function after acute myocardial infarction. Lancet 1994; 343:1115–1122.

70. Lu Y, Shansky J, Del Tatto M, Ferland P, Wang X, Vendenburgh H. Recombinant vascular endothelial growth factor secreted from tissue-engineered bioartificial muscles promotes localized angiogenesis. Circulation 2001;104:594–599.

71. Mack CA, Patel SR, Schwartz EA, et al. Biological bypass with the use of adenovirus-mediated gene transfer of the complementary deoxyribonucleic acid for vascular endothelial growth factor 121 improves myocardial perfusion and function in the ischemic porcine heart. J Thorac Cardiovasc Surg 1998;115:168–176.

72. Udelson JE, Dilsizian V, Laham RJ, et al. Therapeutic angiogenesis with recombinant fibroblast growth factor-2 improves stress and rest myocardial perfusion abnormalities in patients with severe symptomatic chronic coronary artery disease. Circulation 2000;102:1605–1610.

73. Schaper W. Collateral vessel growth in the human heart. Role of fibroblast growth factor-2. Circulation 1996;94:600–601.

74. Patterson C, Runge MS. Therapeutic myocardial angiogenesis via vascular endothelial growth factor gene therapy: moving on down the road. Circulation 2000;102:940–942.

75. Ziche M, Morbidelli L, Choudhuri R. Nitric oxide synthase lies downstream from vascular endothelial growth factor–induced but not basic fibroblast growth factor–induced angiogenesis. J Clin Invest 1997;99:2625–2634.

76. Epstein SE. Kornowski R, Fuchs S, Dvorak HF. Angiogenesis therapy: amidst the hype, the neglected potential for serious side effects. Circulation 2001;104:115–119.

77. Kocher A, Schuster M, Szabolcs M, et al. Neovascularization of ischemic myocardium by human bone-marrow-derived angioblasts prevents cardiomyocyte apoptosis, reduces remodeling and improves cardiac function. Nat Med 2001;7:430–436.

78. Jain M, DerSimonian H, Brenner D, et al. Cell therapy attenuates deleterious ventricular remodeling and improves cardiac performance after myocardial infarction. Circulation 2001;103:1920–1927.

79. Zimmermann W-H, Didie M, Wasmeier GH, et al. Cardiac grafting of engineered heart tissue in synergistic rats. Circulation 2002;106(suppl I):I-151–I-157.

80. Akhyari P, Dedak PWM, Weisel RD, et al. Mechanical stretch regimen enhances the formation of bioengineered autologous cardiac muscle grafts. Circulation 2002;106(suppl I):I-137–I-142.

81. Ghostine S, Carrion C, Guarita Souza LC, et al. Long-term efficacy of myoblast transplantation on regional structure and function after myocardial infarction. Criculation 2002;106(suppl I):I-131–I-136.

82. Levin HR, Oz MC, Chen JM, Packer M, Rose EA, Burkhoff D. Reversal of chronic ventricular dilation in patients with end-stage cardiomyopathy by prolonged mechanical unloading. Circulation 1995;91:2717–2720.

83. McCarthy PM, Nakatani S, Vargo R, et al. Structural and left ventricular histologic changes after implantable LVAD insertion. Ann Thorac Surg 1995;59:609–613.

84. Dipla K, Mattiello JA, Jeevanandam V, Houser SR, Margulies KB. Myocyte recovery after mechanical circulatory support in humans with end-stage heart failure. Circulation 1998;97:2316–2222.

85. Barbone A, Oz MC, Burkhoff D, Holmes JW. Normalized diastolic properties after left ventricular assist result from reverse remodeling of chamber geometry. Circulation 2001;104:I229–I232.

86. Young JB. Healing the heart with ventricular assist device therapy: mechanisms of cardiac recovery. Ann Thorac Surg 2001;71:S210–S219.

87. Helman DN, Maybaum SW, Morales DL, et al. Recurrent remodeling after ventricular assistance: is long-term myocardial recovery attainable? Ann Thorac Surg 2000;70:1255–1258.

88. Mann DL, Willerson JT. Left ventricular assist devices and the failing heart: a bridge to recovery, a permanent assist device, or a bridge too far? Circulation 1998;98:2367–2369.

89. Rivello HG, Meckert PC, Vigliano C, Favaloro R, Laguens RP. Cardiac myocyte nuclear size and ploidy status decrease after mechanical support. Cardiovasc Pathol 2001;10:53–57.

90. Baba HA, Grabellus F, August C, et al. Reversal of metallothionein expression is different throughout the human myocardium after prolonged left ventricular mechanical support. J Heart Lung Transplant 2000;19:668–674.

91. Burkhoff D. New heart failure therapy: the shape of things to come? J Thorac Cardiovasc Surg 2001;122:421–423.

92. Batista RJ, Verde J, Nery P, et al. Partial left ventriculectomy to treat end-stage heart disease. Ann Thorac Surg 1997;64:634–638.

93. Franco-Cereceda A, McCarthy PM, Blackstone EH, et al. Partial left ventriculectomy for dilated cardiomyopathy: is this an alternative to transplantation? J Thorac Cardiovasc Surg 2001;121:879–893.

94. Ratcliffe MB, Hong J, Salahieh A, Ruch S, Wallace AW. The effect of ventricular volume reduction surgery in the dilated, poorly contractile left ventricle: a simple finite element analysis. J Thorac Cardiovasc Surg 1998;116:566–577.

95. Athanasuleas CL, Stanley AW Jr, Buckberg GD, Dor V, DiDonato M, Blackstone EH. Surgical anterior ventricular endocardial restoration (SAVER) in the dilated remodeled ventricle after anterior myocardial infarction. RESTORE group. Reconstructive Endoventricular Surgery, returning Torsion Original Radius Elliptical Shape to the LV. J Am Coll Cardiol 2001;37:1199–1209.

96. McCarthy PM, Takagaki M, Ochiai Y, et al. Device-based change in left ventricular shape: a new concept for the treatment of dilated cardiomyopathy. J Thorac Cardiovasc Surg 2001;122:482–490.

97. Konertz WF, Shapland JE, Hotz H, et al. Passive containment and reverse remodeling by a novel textile cardiac support device. Circulation 2001;104:I270–I275.

98. White HD, Norris RM, Brown MA, Brandt PW, Whitlock RM, Wild CJ. Left ventricular end-systolic volume as the major determinant of survival after recovery from myocardial infarction. Circulation 1987;76:44–51.

99. Lee KL, Woodlief LH, Topol EJ, et al for the GUSTO-I Investigators. Predictors of 30-day mortality in the era of reperfusion for acute myocardial infarction. Results from an international trial of 41,021 patients. Circulation 1995;91:1659–1668.

100. Newby LK, Rutsch WR, Califf RM, et al for the GUSTO-I Investigators. Time from symptom onset to treatment and outcomes after thrombolytic therapy. J Am Coll Cardiol 1996;27:1646–1655.

101. Horie H, Takahashi M, Minai K, et al. Long-term beneficial effect of late reperfusion for acute anterior myocardial infarction with percutaneous transluminal coronary angioplasty. Circulation 1998;98:2377–2382.

102. Sheiban I, Fragasso G, Lu C, Tonni S, Trevi GP, Chierchia SL. Influence of treatment delay on long-term left ventricular function in patients with acute myocardial infarction successfully treated with primary angioplasty. Am Heart J 2001;141:603–609.

103. Kim CB, Braunwald E. Potential benefits of late reperfusion of infarcted myocardium. The open artery hypothesis. Circulation 1993;88:2426–2436.

104. Hara Y, Hamada M, Shigematsu Y, et al. Effect of patency from coronary angioplasty during acute myocardial infarction on left ventricular remodeling and levels of natriuretic peptides later. Am J Cardiol 2001;88:683–685.

105. Kloner RA, Ganote CE, Jennings RB. The "no-reflow" phenomenon after temporary coronary occlusion in the dog. J Clin Invest 1974;54:1496–1508.

106. Destro G, Marino P, Barbieri E, et al. Postinfarctional remodeling: increased dye intensity in the myocardial risk area after angioplasty of infarct-related coronary artery is associated with reduction of ventricular volumes. J Am Coll Cardiology 2001;37:1239–1245.

107. GISSI-3. Effects of lisinopril and transdermal glyceryl trinitrate singly and together on 6 week mortality and ventricular function after acute myocardial infarction: Gruppo Italiano per lo Studio della Sopravvienza nell'infarto Miocardico. Lancet 1994;343:1115–1122.

108. ISIS-4 (Fourth International Study of Infarct Survival) Collaborative Group. ISIS-4: a randomized factorial trial assessing early oral captopril, oral mononitrate and intravenous magnesium sulphate in 58,050 patients with suspected acute myocardial infarction. Lancet 1995;345:669–682.

109. Jugdutt BI, Warnica JW. Intravenous nitroglycerin therapy to limit myocardial infarct size, expansion, and complications. Effect of timing, dosage, and infarct location. Circulation 1988;78:906–919.

110. Jugdutt BI, Khan MI. Effect of prolonged nitrate therapy on left ventricular remodeling after canine acute myocardial infarction. Circulation 1994;89:2297–2307.

111. Jugdutt BI, Khan MI, Jugdutt SJ, Blinston GE. Impact of left ventricular unloading after late reperfusion of canine anterior myocardial infarction on remodeling and function using isosorbide-5-mononitrate. Circulation 1995;92:926–934.

112. Mahmarian JJ, Moye LA, Chinoy DA, et al. Transdermal nitroglycerin patch therapy improves left ventricular function and prevents remodeling after acute myocardial infarction: results of a multicenter prospective randomized, double-blind, placebo-controlled trial. Circulation 1998;97:2017–2024.

113. Pfeffer MA, Braunwald E, Moye LA, et al. on behalf of the SAVE Investigators. Effects of captopril on mortality and morbidity in patients with left ventricular dysfunction after myocardial infarction: results of the Survival and Ventricular Enlargement Trial. N Engl J Med 1992;327:669–677.

114. The Acute Infarction Ramipril Efficacy (AIRE) Study Investigators. Effect of ramipril on mortality and morbidity of survivors of acute myocardial infarction with clinical evidence of heart failure. Lancet 1993;342:821–828.

115. Sharpe N, Murphy J, Smith H, Hannan S. Treatment of patients with symptomless left ventricular dysfunction after myocardial infarction. Lancet 1988;1:255–259.

116. Pfeffer MA, Lamas GA, Vaughan DE, Parisi AF, Braunwald E. Effect of captopril on progressive ventricular dilation after anterior myocardial infarction. N Engl J Med 1988;319:80–86.

117. Sharpe N, Smith H, Murphy J, Greaves S, Hart H, Gamble G. Early prevention of left ventricular dysfunction after myocardial infarction with angiotensin-converting-enzyme inhibition. Lancet 1991;337:872–876.

118. Harada K, Sugaya T, Murakami K, Yazaki Y, Komuro I. Angiotensin II type 1A receptor knockout mice display less left ventricular remodeling and improved survival after myocardial infarction. Circulation 1999;100:2093–2099.

119. Youn TJ, Kim HS, Oh BH. Ventricular remodeling and transforming growth factor-beta 1 mRNA expression after nontransmural myocardial infarction in rats: effects of angiotensin-converting enzyme inhabition and angiotensin II type 1 receptor blockade. Basic Res Cardiol 1999; 94:246–253.

120. Pfeffer JM, Pfeffer MA, Braunwald E. Influence of chronic captopril therapy on the infarcted left ventricle of the rat. Circ Res 1985;57:84–95.

121. Raya TE, Gay RG, Aguirre M, Goldman S. Importance of venodilatation in prevention of left ventricular dilatation after chronic large myocardial infarction in rats: a comparison of captopril and hydralazine. Circ Res 1989;64:330–337.

122. Sun Y, Zhang JQ, Zhang J, Ramires FJ. Angiotensin II, transforming growth factor-beta 1 and repair in the infarcted heart. J Mol Cell Cardiol 1998;30:1559–1569.

123. Kim S, Ohta K, Hamaguchi A, Yukimura T, Miura K, Iwao H. Angiotensin II induces cardiac phenotypic modulation and remodeling in vivo in rats. Hypertension 1995;25: 1252–1259.

124. Hanatani A, Yoshiyama M, Kim S, et al. Inhibition by angiotensin II type 1 receptor antagonist of cardiac phenotypic modulation after infarction. J Mol Cell Cardiol 1995;27:1905–1914.

125. Takeda M, Kagaya Y, Takahashi J, et al. Gene expression and in situ localization of diacylglycerol kinase isozymes in normal and infarcted rat hearts: effects of captopril treatment. Circ Res 2001;89:265–272.

126. Yu CM, Tipoe GL, Wing-Hon Lai K, Lau CP. Effects of combination of angiotensin-converting enzyme inhibitor and angiotensin receptor antagonist on inflammatory cellular infiltration and myocardial interstitial fibrosis after acute myocardial infarction. J Am Coll Cardiol 2001;38:1207–1215.

127. Mankad S, d'Amato TA, Reichek N, et al. Combined angiotensin II receptor antagonism and angiotensin-converting enzyme inhibition further attenuates postinfarction left ventricular remodeling. Circulation 2001;103:2845–2850.

128. Hu K, Gaudron P, Anders HJ, et al. Chronic effects of early started angiotensin-converting enzyme inhibition and angiotensin AT1-receptor subtype blockade in rats with myocardial infarction: role of bradykinin. Cardiovasc Res 1998;39:401–412.

129. Yoshiyama M, Takeuchi K, Omura T, et al. Effects of candesartan and cilazapril on rats with myocardial infarction assessed by echocardiography. Hypertension 1999;33:961–968.

130. Waagstein F, Hjalmarson A, Varnauskas E, Wallentin I. Effect of chronic beta-adrenergic receptor blockade in congestive cardiomyopathy. Br Heart J 1975;37:1022–1036.

131. Packer M, Bristow MR, Cohn JN, et al. The effect of carvedilol on morbidity and mortality in patients with chronic heart failure. US Carvedilol Heart Failure Study Group. N Engl J Med 1996;334:1349–1355.

132. Bristow MR. Changes in myocardial and vascular receptors in heart failure. J Am Coll Cardiol 1993;22:61A–71A.

133. Igawa A, Nozawa T, Yoshida N, Jujii N, Tazawa S, Asanoi H. Heterogeneous cardiac sympathetic innervation in heart failure after myocardial infarction of rats. Am J Physiol Heart Circ Physiol 2000;278:H1134–H1141.

134. Bristow MR, Hershberger RE, Port JD, Minobe W, Rasmussen R. Beta 1- and beta 2-adrenergic receptor-mediated adenylate cyclase stimulation in nonfailing and failing human ventricular myocardium. Mol Pharmacol 1989;35:295–303.

135. Kouchi I, Zolk O, Jockenhovel F, et al. Increase in G(i alpha) protein accompanies progression of post-infarction remodeling in hypertensive cardiomyopathy. Hypertension 2000;36:42–47.

136. Barth W, Deten A, Bauer M, Reinohs M, Leicht M, Zimmer HG. Differential remodeling of the left and right heart after norepinephrine treatment in rats: studies on cytokines and collagen. J Mol Cell Cardiol 2000;32:273–284.

137. Grimm D, Huber M, Jabusch HC, et al. Extracellular matrix proteins in cardiac fibroblasts derived from rat hearts with

chronic pressure overload: effects of beta-receptor blockade. J Mol Cell Cardiol 2001;33:487–501.

138. Communal C, Singh K, Sawyer DB, Colucci WS. Opposing effects of beta (1)- and beta(2)-adrenergic receptors on cardiac myocyte apoptois: role of pertussis toxin-sensitive G protein. Circulation 1999;100:2210–2212.

139. Milano CA, Dolber PC, Rockman HA, et al. Myocardial expression of a constitutively active alpha 1β-adrenergic receptor in transgenic mice induces cardiac hypertrophy. Proc Natl Acad Sci USA 1994;91:10109–10113.

140. Colucci WS, Sawyer DB, Singh K, Communal C. Adrenergic overload and apoptosis in heart failure: implication therapy. J Card Fail 2000;6:1–7.

141. Yang Y, Tang Y, Zhang P. Comparative effects of carvediol in large, middle, and small dose in preventing left ventricular remodeling after acute myocardial infarction in rats. Chung-Hua I Hsueh Tsa Chih (Chinese Medical Journal) 2001;81:927–930.

142. Ricci R, Coletta C, Ceci V, et al. Effect of early treatment with captopril and metoprolol singly and together on postinfarction left ventricular remodeling. Am Heart J 2001;142:E5.

143. Hayashi M, Tsutamoto T, Wada A, et al. Relationship between transcardiac extraction of aldosterone and left ventricular remodeling in patients with first acute myocardial infarction: extracting aldosterone through the heart promotes ventricular remodeling after acute myocardial infarction. J Am Coll Cardiol 2001;38:1375–1382.

144. Delcayre C, Silvestre JS, Garnier A, et al. Cardiac aldosterone production and ventricular remodeling. Kidney Int 2000;57: 1346–1351.

145. Rodriguez JA, Godoy I, Castro P, et al. Effects of ramipril and spironolactone on ventricular remodeling after acute myocardial infarction: randomized and double-blind study. Rev Med Chil 1997;125:643–652.

146. Delyani JA, Robinson EL, Rudolph AE. Effect of a selective aldosterone receptor antagonist in myocardial infarction. Am J Physiol Heart Circ Physiol 2001;281:H647–H654.

147. Hengstenberg C, Holmer SR, Mayer B, et al. Evaluation of the aldosternone synthase (CYP11B2) gene polymorphism in patients with myocardial infarction. Hypertension 2000;35: 704-709.

15 Transplant Arteriopathy
Pathology, Pathogenesis, and Prospects for Treatment

Joannis Vamvakopoulos, MS, PhD, Einari Aavik, MS, Daniel du Toit, Pekka Häyry, MD, PhD, and Minnie Sarwal, MD, PhD

CONTENTS

INTRODUCTION

The concept of surgically replacing diseased tissue with healthy tissue to treat end-stage organ failure forms the foundation of clinical transplantation. The science and technique of transplantation trace their origins to the beginning of last century. First tried in the 1950s, solid organ transplantation did not become a credible therapeutic option until the advent of chemical immunosuppression, especially cyclosporine use, in the early 1980s. The recent use of powerful immunosuppressive agents, such as the calcineurin inhibitors cyclosporine A (CsA) and tacrolimus (FK506), in combination with azathioprine or mycophenolate mofetil and steroids has helped to overcome the problem of acute allograft rejection. One-year graft survival rates are currently approximately 90% for most types of transplanted organs. Despite improvements in short-term outcome, the half-life of organ allografts has only marginally increased over the past 20 yr. Long-term organ survival is questionable in patients who have had at least one episode of acute rejection *(1)*. Chronic allograft rejection and drug-related toxicity are the main obstacles to indefinite graft survival.

INCIDENCE OF TRANSPLANT ARTERIOPATHY

The main cause of graft loss after the first year, not including patients who died with a functioning graft, is chronic rejection (CR) (Fig. 1). Cardiovascular complications are the main cause of death in patients with functioning kidney grafts *(2)*. Transplant arteriopathy is an early, almost universal manifestation of CR in solid organ transplants. The annual post-transplant incidence of graft loss due to CR is reported at approximately 3% for liver *(3–6)*, 4% for heart *(7)*, 6–10% for renal *(8)*, and 8% for lung *(9)* allografts. However, graft arterial lesions are seen on coronary angiography in about 9% of heart transplant patients at 1 yr, and about 75% of functioning grafts have lesions at 10 yr *(7)*. Furthermore, intravascular ultrasound (IVUS), considered the "gold standard" for diagnosis of transplant arteriopathy (Fig. 2), has shown intimal thickening in 43% of heart grafts as early as 3 mo after transplantation; the proportion of affected grafts increases to approximately 60% at 1 yr and remains as high thereafter *(11)*. In renal grafts, needle aspiration biopsy studies show chronic graft nephropathy in about 60% of grafts

From: *Contemporary Cardiology: Principles of Molecular Cardiology*
Edited by: M. S. Runge and C. Patterson © Humana Press Inc., Totowa, NJ

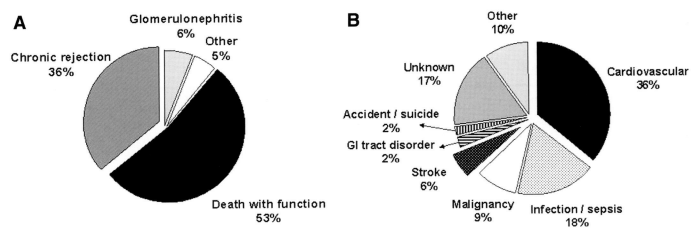

Fig. 1. **(A)** Causes of renal graft loss. Compiled from data provided by Professor LC Paul, European Standard of Care EDTA/ERA and ESOF *(2001)*. **(B)** Causes of death with functioning renal graft. Reproduced with permission *(2)*.

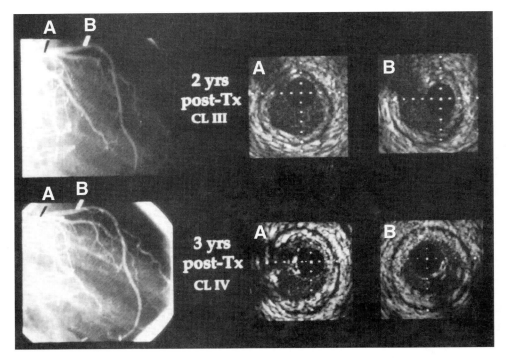

Fig. 2. Detection of transplant arteriopathy using coronary angiography (left) and intravascular ultrasound imaging (IVUS; right). Upper panels show findings in the proximal **(A)** and middle **(B)** portions of the left anterior descending (LAD) coronary artery of the graft at 2 years after transplantation; lower panels show corresponding findings at 3 years after transplantation. Intimal thickness was graded as follows: class (CL) I, none; CL II, minimal; CL III, mild; CL IV, moderate; CL V, severe. Reproduced with permission *(10)*.

surviving more than 3 yr *(12)*. These findings suggest a high incidence of transplant arteriopathy, which is often missed on clinical diagnosis.

Major Risk Factors

Although the etiology and pathogenesis of transplant arteriopathy are not completely understood, several demographic, clinical, and genetic factors are known to influence the risk and timing of graft loss caused by CR.

Acute rejection is the best clinical predictor of CR in both living and cadaveric renal allografts *(13–18)*. The exact mechanism of this predisposition is unknown; however, certain features of acute rejection substantiate its relationship with CR. For example, early rejection episodes (occurring within the first year after transplantation) are deleterious to graft function (12–14), and late acute rejection can be as harmful as early rejection (17,18). Vascular rejection is a strong predictor of graft failure, whereas interstitial rejection is not (13). Vascular rejection involves vascular trauma and probably directly contributes to transplant arteriopathy. In contrast, steroid-responsive acute rejection, which is often promptly treated, does not increase the risk of CR (14,15), although this finding has been challenged (17). Distinct immunological mechanisms may determine the timing and reversibility of acute rejection. For example, early acute rejection, particularly the steroid-resistant type, appears to be associated with increased monocytic inflammation and suppressed production of the interleukin-1 (IL-1) receptor antagonist (19).

Suboptimally treated early acute rejection directly led to CR in a rat model of lung transplantation (20), whereas late acute rejection is a risk factor for CR in human lung allografts (21). Opelz et al. found no detrimental effect of early acute rejection on long-term cardiac graft survival (15). Although this finding may reflect organ-specific susceptibility to immunological trauma and the ensuing loss of function, these authors considered death with a functioning graft as a graft failure. This practice, although widely used, is statistically dubious (22). In smaller studies, angiographic criteria have shown a positive association between early acute rejection and coronary transplant arteriopathy (23).

The effect of donor–recipient human leukocyte antigen (HLA) mismatching on CR has been the focus of considerable debate. Although transplant arteriopathy is certainly promoted by an active alloimmune response, the extent to which immunological events contribute to late graft attrition in the presence of immunosuppression is unknown. In large studies in which serological and DNA typing methods were used, a grade-dependent effect of mismatching at the HLA-A, -B, and -DR loci was seen on long-term cadaveric renal graft survival (24). Similar data have been reported for lung transplants (21). However, the effect of HLA mismatching on survival of cardiac grafts is much less profound than that seen in renal or lung grafts, particularly among black recipients (25). Overall, the strong association of HLA-DR mismatching with acute vascular rejection (13) may account for its predisposing effect on transplant arteriopathy.

Recent studies of syngeneic heart transplantation in lean Zucker rats (26) and allogeneic grafting in rat models of diabetes (27–29) have highlighted a contribution of metabolic factors in the pathogenesis of transplant arteriopathy. While the exact metabolic triggers remain ill-defined, this work has shown that insulin resistance and hyperglycemia are associated with the occurrence of transplant arteriopathy in cardiac grafts independently of the alloimmune response (26,28). Interestingly, metabolic imbalance seems to be particularly detrimental for large vessels (28,29) for reasons that remain to be elucidated.

Active viral infection, in particular infection with cytomegalovirus (CMV), is a potential target for preventive therapy against CR. Both epidemiologic and experimental studies indicate CMV is a risk factor for acute and chronic rejection. Epidemiological evidence links CMV infection to CR for heart (30), renal (31), and liver (32) transplantations. In a rat model of kidney transplantation, CMV infection potentiated graft inflammation and markedly accelerated the development of CR (33,34). CMV-related CR in this model was characterized by prominent monocytic infiltration, transplant arteriopathy, and extensive fibrosis. Similarly, CMV infection accelerated the development of CR in rat models of lung (35) and liver (36) transplantation. Thus, there is a substantial body of evidence implicating CMV as a risk factor for CR; however, the potential importance of other human pathogens less studied in this context should not be underestimated (37).

Several studies have examined the molecular basis of the relationship between CMV infection and CR. Bone marrow–derived cells of the myeloid lineage are reservoirs of latent CMV infection, and putative mechanisms of virus reactivation have been reviewed recently (38). CMV reactivation in response to sepsis, rejection, or administration of antilymphocyte globulin is of particular relevance to transplantation. In these instances, tumor necrosis factor α (TNF-α) appears to play a central role in viral reactivation by inducing nuclear factor κB (NF-κB), a transcription factor that promotes the expression of the immediate early (IE) genes of the CMV genome (39). The presence of CMV DNA, detectable by polymerase chain reaction (PCR), in the serum of cardiac or renal graft recipients coincides with the induction of an antiendothelial antibody response (40). In rat transplantation models, CMV infection was associated with increased expression of adhesion molecules and their ligands (41) and with up-regulation of major histocompatibility complex (MHC) class II antigens, platelet-derived growth factor (PDGF), and PDGF receptor α (PDGFRα) expression (36). Furthermore, in vitro expression of the CMV US28 receptor in primary arterial smooth muscle cells (SMCs) promoted the migration of SMCs in response to chemokines such as RANTES (regulated on activation, normal T cell expressed and secreted) and monocyte chemotactic protein-1 (MCP-1) (42).

Other important clinical and demographic factors that affect the development of CR include donor brain death (43); recipient race and hyperlipidemia for heart transplant patients *(25,44)*; and recipient race, hyperlipidemia, donor age, delayed graft function, and cold ischemic time for cadaveric renal transplant patients *(13,16,45)*. The detrimental effect of prolonged cold ischemic time on graft survival probably relates to the severity of reperfusion injury *(46,47)*.

Transplant arteriopathy often develops insidiously, but CR directly perturbs graft function. In heart graft recipients, functional impairment manifests as reduced exercise tolerance *(7,11)* and worsening performance in clinical function tests, such as dobutamine stress echocardiography *(48)*. These findings probably relate to impaired coronary endothelial function *(11,49)*. Obliterative bronchiolitis, the major manifestation of CR in lung grafts, usually results in shortness of breath and declining forced expiratory volume, despite rejection treatment *(9)*. Chronic graft nephropathy is diagnosed by an intractable decrease in creatinine clearance, a decrease in the glomerular filtration rate (GFR), and the onset of overt proteinuria.

THE PATHOLOGY OF TRANSPLANT ARTERIOPATHY

Histopathology

The histopathology associated with CR is diverse. Transplant arteriopathy, the earliest and most specific manifestation of CR in almost all types of transplanted organs, is histologically characterized by neointimal hyperplasia, which is a diffuse, concentric, fibrous expansion of the intimal lining of graft arteries *(50–53)* (Fig. 3, inset). Growth of this lesion, often accompanied by fragmentation of the internal elastic lamina, results in progressive vascular occlusion, seen as a reduction in the cross-sectional area of the lumen in histological sections or on angiography/IVUS. Neointimal hyperplasia, together with constrictive vascular remodeling, eventually causes complete arterial occlusion (vascular obliteration). Although the neointimal lesion and the fibrous cap of atherosclerotic plaques share few common histologic features, transplant arteriopathy is often referred to as "accelerated arteriosclerosis."

In heart grafts, and presumably in other organ grafts, transplant arteriopathy is often compounded by constrictive (inward) vascular remodeling *(54)*. Transplant arteriopathy in heart grafts is a biphasic process. In the early phase of lesion development, neointimal hyperplasia is the main determinant of coronary stenosis, which is partially counteracted by compensatory vascular enlargement *(54–56)*. Late vascular obliteration is characterized by pronounced vasoconstriction, without further neointimal growth *(54–58)*. Preexisting, donor-transmitted atherosclerotic lesions do not contribute appreciably to this process *(56)*.

The organ-specific histopathology of CR probably results from the ischemia associated with transplant vasculopathy *(53)*. In heart grafts, common histological findings associated with CR include myocardial necrosis and interstitial fibrosis *(59)*. Increased submucosal vascularity *(60)*, interstitial fibrosis, and peribronchial mononuclear cell inflammation (obliterative bronchiolitis) are diagnostic of CR in lung grafts *(51)*. Bile duct obliteration (the "vanishing bile duct" syndrome) is a typical feature of CR in liver grafts *(6)*. Interstitial fibrosis, tubular atrophy, glomerulopathy, peritubular capillary changes, and mesangial fibrosis *(61)* are considered hallmarks of CR in the Banff working classification of kidney transplant pathology *(62)*. However, it is now recognized that not all of these histological findings are specific to CR; some can develop as a response to drug toxicity, hypertension, or infection. Instead, this set of histological findings is said to be collectively indicative of chronic graft nephropathy (CGN) *(52)*.

Cellular Pathology

The histological lesions and functional impairment associated with CR have been reproduced in animal models. The use of knockout and transgenic strains of mice in models of transplant arteriopathy *(63–65)* has facilitated research in the cellular and molecular aspects of CR.

In animal models, although not necessarily in humans, transplant arteriopathy is largely an immune-mediated process *(66,67)* that affects allogeneic grafts only in the presence of peripheral lymphoid tissue *(68)*. Neointimal hyperplasia develops in grafts transplanted across both major and minor histocompatibility barriers *(66)* and affects only the donor vasculature. The relative contribution of cellular versus humoral immunity to the pathology of transplant arteriopathy has been studied extensively. CD4+ T cell–mediated immunity and intact B cell and macrophage function are essential for the development of neointimal hyperplasia in aortic allografts *(67)*. In contrast, CD8+ T cells *(67,69)* and natural killer cells *(67)* appear dispensable. In some studies, heart transplant arteriopathy develops unperturbed in the absence of B cell function *(70)*. In other studies, neointimal lesions have been produced in allogeneic hearts grafted into severe combined immunodeficiency disease (SCID) recipients by administering antiserum directed against the donor alloantigens *(71)*. Antibody-mediated immunity against non-MHC donor antigens has been linked to the pathology of chronic graft nephropathy *(72)*. In this context, the presence of *in situ* complement fixation within the graft may be a reliable indicator of immunologically mediated CR *(73)*. These observations suggest that either component of the adaptive

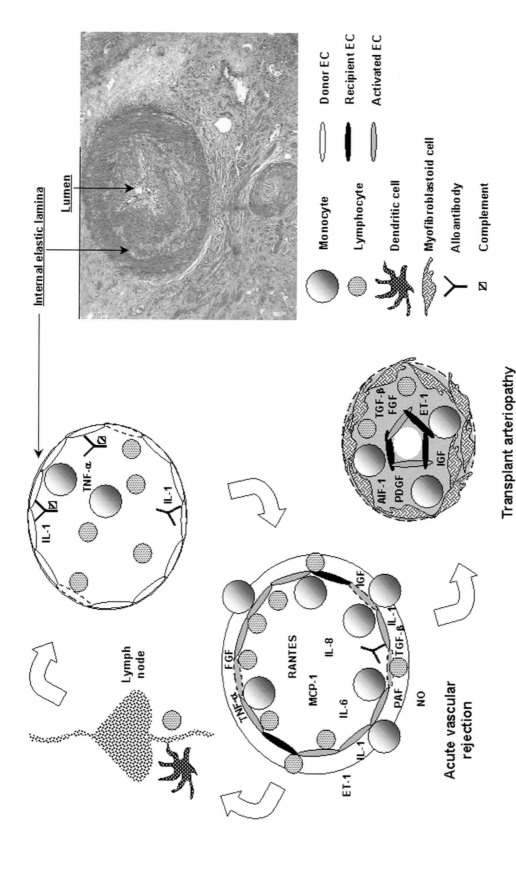

Transplant arteriopathy

Acute vascular rejection

Internal elastic lamina

Lumen

Lymph node

| Donor EC |
| Recipient EC |
| Activated EC |

Monocyte

Lymphocyte

Dendritic cell

Myofibroblastoid cell

Alloantibody

Complement

Fig. 3. Overview of the pathogenesis of transplant arteriopathy. Inset shows two affected intrarenal arteries stained with hematoxylin (100×). AIF-1, allograft inflammatory factor 1; EC, endothelial cell; ET, endothelin; FGF, fibroblast growth factor; IGF, insulin-like growth factor; IL, interleukin; MCP-1, monocyte chemotactic protein-1; NO, nitric oxide; PAF, platelet activating factor; PDGF, platelet-derived growth factor; RANTES, regulated on activation, normal T cell expressed and secreted; TGF-β, transforming growth factor β; TNF-α, tumor necrosis factor α.

247

immune system (cellular or humoral) can independently trigger neointima formation; however, because of the in vivo interaction of cellular and humoral immunity, both branches of the immune response probably cooperate in causing injury to the graft. Neointima formation progresses via a common pathway that appears to require the presence of intact macrophage function.

The typical lesion of transplant arteriopathy comprises cellular elements interspersed between vast deposits of extracellular matrix (ECM) (Fig. 3, inset). The cellular composition of the neointima and the kinetics of cell recruitment into the neointimal lesion have been extensively studied in patients and in animal models (Fig. 3). Donor-derived cells in the neointimal lesion include a few, probably media-derived, vascular SMCs and a variable proportion of endothelial cells. However, most cells of the neointimal population come from the circulating blood of the recipient and include CD4+ lymphocytes, macrophages, and myofibroblast-like cells.

The donor vascular endothelium is the main target of the alloimmune response against vascularized organ grafts (74–76). Endothelial dysfunction, caused by immune trauma or metabolic stress, precipitates the pathological cascade of events that results in neointimal hyperplasia. In studies of sex-mismatched donor–recipient transplant pairs in which both morphological and molecular markers were used, vascular endothelial cells were mostly of donor origin in renal (77), cardiac (78,79), and lung (80) allografts. Significant endothelial cell chimerism has been observed in renal graft peritubular capillaries, particularly after episodes of acute vascular rejection (81). These findings strongly suggest that endothelial trauma initiates neointimal hyperplasia and triggers vascular repair by recipient-derived endothelial cell precursors.

Until recently, the spindle-shaped, proliferating cells that sustain neointimal growth were thought to be donor-derived vascular SMCs (79). In this hypothesis, vascular SMCs normally present in the arterial media were somehow stimulated to detach from, and migrate through, the elastic lamina into the intima (82), where they underwent retro-differentiation into proliferating, ECM-producing cells (83,84). Focal medial necrosis, a frequent histological feature of transplant arteriopathy, was thought to result from irreversible vascular SMC migration out of the media (83). Some investigators argued that only a small proportion of "relatively immature" medial or adventitial vascular SMCs could migrate and undergo proliferation (85). Recent studies, however, have clearly shown that the proliferating myofibroblastoid cells present in neointimal lesions originate primarily from the bone marrow of the graft recipient (86–90). These cells may develop from circulating vascular

SMC progenitors (89) (Fig. 4). Experimental evidence, however, indicates that loss of the donor-derived medial vascular SMCs results in a progressive, irreversible decline of vascular function (91–93), suggesting that such recipient-derived progenitors may never mature into functional vascular SMCs.

Recipient-derived CD4+ and CD8+ lymphocytes infiltrate grafts very early after implantation and reperfusion (80,94). Experiments involving retransplantation of murine hearts into syngeneic hosts after short periods of grafting into allogeneic recipients have shown that the alloreactive T cell load, after just 3 d of primary grafting, could trigger transplant arteriopathy after retransplantation (94). Depletion of both CD4+ and CD8+ cells in the primary (allogeneic) recipient completely prevented subsequent neointimal hyperplasia, indicating that a graft-versus-host disease-like mechanism might initiate transplant arteriopathy in this model. CD4+ T cells persist in occlusive neointimal lesions, and evidence suggests that these long-term alloreactive clones may express a very limited T cell receptor repertoire, making them amenable to specific immunotherapy (95,96).

The kinetics of recipient-derived monocyte migration from the peripheral circulation into the graft are similar to those of lymphocytes (80,97). Retransplantation experiments suggest an initially high monocyte turnover rate, which is followed by an accumulation of recruited monocytes within the graft (98). Monocyte recruitment into the graft is essential for the development of both transplant arteriopathy (67,98,99) and chronic graft nephropathy (100). Furthermore, conditions that promote monocyte activation and extravasation, such as systemic administration of lipopolysaccharide (LPS) (101), IL-1β, or TNF-α (97), markedly accelerate neointimal growth. Like lymphocytes, neointimal monocytes accumulate primarily in the subendothelial space (79), and the extent of monocyte accumulation strongly predicts the development of a neointimal lesion (98,102).

The precise role of monocytes in neointimal hyperplasia is ill-defined. In vitro evidence suggests that macrophages can induce apoptosis in vascular SMCs via Fas–FasL interactions (103). This finding indicates that they may contribute to the pathogenesis of medial necrosis, although other plausible mechanisms have been proposed (104). Some authors have suggested that monocytes may promote the colonization of allograft vessels with the putative vascular SMC precursors that initiate neointimal growth (105). Furthermore, recruited macrophages are the main source of many growth factors expressed in neointimal lesions (106–109). There is also increasing evidence that a subset of human and mouse peripheral blood monocytes may be

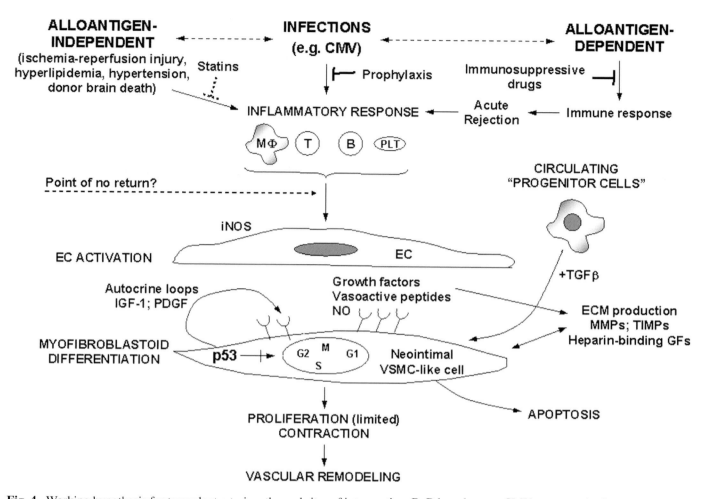

Fig. 4. Working hypothesis for transplant arteriopathy and sites of intervention. B, B lymphocyte; CMV, cytomegalovirus; EC, endothelial cell; ECM, extracellular matrix; GFs, growth factors; IGF-1, insulin-like growth factor-1; iNOS, inducible nitric oxide synthase; MMP, matrix metalloproteinase; Mφ, macrophage; NO, nitric oxide; PDGF, platelet-derived growth factor; PLT, platelet; T, T lymphocyte; TGF-β, transforming growth factor β; TIMP, tissue inhibitor of metalloproteases; VSMC, vascular smooth muscle cell.

able to differentiate into myofibroblast-like cells *(110)*. These observations confirm that monocytes/macrophages are central to the development of transplant arteriopathy and other manifestations of CR and suggest a pleiotropic role for these cells in the relevant pathologies.

Myofibroblasts contribute to the pathology of chronic graft nephropathy *(111,112)* and may be identical to the recipient-derived mesenchymal cells seen in interstitial and neointimal lesions during CR of renal allografts *(113)*. The precise function of myofibroblasts in CR is unknown, but they are probably involved in fibrotic remodeling *(111)*. With the elimination of donor-derived vascular SMCs as the proliferating cell that drives neointimal growth, the myofibroblast may be a suitable candidate.

Moderate numbers of recipient-derived mast cells are known to infiltrate organ allografts *(79)*, but the mast cell

has only recently been identified as contributing to the pathology of transplant arteriopathy. Although intragraft mast cell number correlates with the grade of transplant arteriopathy in rat cardiac grafts *(114)* and with interstitial fibrosis in human renal grafts *(115)*, the exact role of the mast cell in these settings is unknown.

Molecular Pathology

GENOMIC STUDIES

The main goal of genomics is the systematic and comprehensive characterization of gene transcription, which is made possible by recent advances in whole genome sequencing, bioinformatics, and high-throughput transcription profiling technologies. The science of genomics is based on the assumption that net differences in the transcriptomes (the sum of mRNA species and their level of expression) of diseased versus healthy tissue would identify molecular components of disease pathology *(116)*. After being identified, these molecular components could then be targeted for therapy (see Rational Drug Design below). In addition, the identification of all differentially expressed genes for a given disease would allow for the construction of a disease-specific microarray, which, in principle, could be a powerful diagnostic tool.

This large-scale approach to transcript profiling has only just begun in the science of transplantation *(117)*. Saiura and colleagues *(118)* recently published their study of differential gene expression during acute rejection of fully mismatched murine heart allografts, and similar work is being done in humans and nonhuman primates. Insights gained from rodent studies will initially be limited and difficult to interpret because the sequencing of rodent genomes lags behind that of the human genome. In human studies, the limiting factor will be data processing because annotation of the human genome is still in progress.

Challenges are associated with the application of genomics to transplant arteriopathy that are not seen with acute rejection or vascular restenosis (which is also characterized by a fibroproliferative pathology). Gene expression in solid tissue varies considerably over time, and transplant arteriopathy, in both humans and animals, develops gradually through a complex cascade of events and interactions. Furthermore, several risk factors affect the rate of progression of transplant arteriopathy. These limitations may explain in part the lack of data on the genomics of transplant arteriopathy. Nevertheless, studies of differential display PCR have identified a small set of transcripts differentially expressed in fully developed aortic allograft lesions *(119)*.

The application of genomics to transplant arteriopathy will require time-course studies in transcript profiling, guided by firmly established markers of lesion development. Our group is studying correlations between the chronic allograft damage index *(120,121)*, which is a quantitative histological predictor of chronic graft nephropathy, and gene expression during the development of acute rejection and transplant arteriopathy. In a pilot study, we used lympocyte-specific cDNAs spotted on a customized microarray to assess the genomic profile of biopsy specimens from renal allografts. Our results showed distinct gene expression profiles for acute rejection, chronic allograft nephropathy, and healthy renal tissue *(122)*. In addition, we identified novel molecular subtypes of acute rejection, which may be clinically and pathologically homogeneous. This genomic subclassification of acute rejection correlated well with

outcomes such as graft survival, graft function, and the effect of treatment, which implies that individual molecular profiles of acute rejection are biologically relevant and warrant further study. Our findings showed nonspecific genomic signatures of tissue injury and repair in biopsy specimens of chronic allograft nephropathy but did not provide clues to the etiology of this injury (immune versus nonimmune).

To circumvent some of the difficulties associated with genomic studies of transplant arteriopathy, we have focused on the genomics of neointimal hyperplasia and have ignored upstream (alloimmune response) and downstream (chronic interstitial rejection) pathology. We have used three models of vascular remodeling in these studies: (a) endothelial denudation injury *(123)*, (b) arterial allograft *(124)*, and (c) arterial response to lipid-rich diet *(125)*. Because we cannot get cross-sectional vascular biopsy specimens noninvasively from human vessels, we have conducted our studies in nonhuman primates. Ethical considerations have led us to use rodent models in initial interventional studies. We have recently completed our first genomics study in a carotid artery endothelial injury model in baboons *(126)*. In this chapter, we will summarize unpublished results of a pilot study of 9500-clone cDNA microarrays.

The sequence of histological events after denudation injury in the baboon carotid artery has been described elsewhere *(126)*. Briefly, catheter-induced endothelial injury triggers immediate vasoconstriction, followed by vasodilatation, cell migration, and limited proliferation, which result in progressive intimal thickening. Intimal fibrotic changes and ECM deposition are observed as early as 14 d after injury, and the injury response is essentially complete by 3–4 wk.

In our pilot study, we measured vascular gene expression on d 2 and 14 after injury and compared these results with gene expression in healthy, nondenuded baboon carotid arteries. The gene transcripts known to be up-regulated after arterial injury included some involved in cellular apoptosis (interleukin-1β converting enzyme [ICE], DAP kinase-related apoptosis-inducing protein kinases [DRAK]), intracellular signaling (phospholipase C [PLC], protein phosphatase 2A [PP2A], Ras), vasoconstriction (endothelin), migration (basic fibroblast growth factor receptor [bFGFR]), and the removal of damaged tissue (matrix metalloproteinase [MMP] 4) (Table 1). Down-regulation of the tissue inhibitor of metalloproteinases after arterial denudation injury may contribute positively to clearance of damaged tissue (Table 2). Genes involved in cell growth and proliferation (E2F transcription factor 1, CDC-like kinase [CDK] 7, cyclin H, PDGF-B) and the

Table 1
Increase in Gene Transcription 2 and 14 Days After Arterial Denudation

Up-regulated genes	Increase (fold)
Day 2	
Cytochrome p450 cypllB3	27.1
Prostaglandin-endoperoxide synthase 1	21.2
Cytochrome P450-HFLa (IIIA7)	19.3
Insulin-like growth factor binding protein 5	17.4
Transforming growth factor β1	15.3
Cytokine receptor family II	14.5
Phospholipase C	13.8
Interleukin-1β converting enzyme	13.7
β Fibroblast growth factor receptor	12.5
Integrin α2	12.1
Protein phosphatase 2A	11.9
Orphan nuclear hormone receptor	11.8
Cyclin H	11.8
Thyroid hormone receptor α	11.0
Vasoactive intestinal peptide receptor 1	10.9
Endothelin 1	10.9
Cell division cycle (CDC) 21	10.8
Myb	10.6
Ras	9.8
Myocyte-specific enhancer factor 2	9.7
Matrix metalloproteinase 4	9.6
Smooth muscle cell myosin heavy chain	9.1
Disabled homolog 2 (DAB2)	8.9
Early growth response-1	8.7
Day 14	
α1 Type 3 collagen	21.1
α1 Type 2 collagen	17.3
α1 Type 5 collagen	12.9
Dermatopontin	9.6
Caveolin	8.4
α1 Type 6 collagen	6.6
Fibronectin	6.2
Signal sequence receptor α	5.1
Tyr-phosphatase PTPCAAX1	4.7
Platelet-derived growth factor α	4.6
Thrombospondin	4.4
Integrin β1	4.4
Fibronectin	4.4
Insulin growth factor 2	3.9
Annexin I (lipocortin 1)	3.8
Annexin V (endonexin)	3.8

Table 1 *Continued*

Up-regulated genes	Increase (fold)
Actin γ	3.7
Fos	3.6
LIV-1	3.6
Gadd45	2.9
Fibroblast growth factor homologous factor 1	2.8
GATA binding protein 6	2.7
Early growth response-2	2.6
Receptor tyrosine kinase related (RYK)	2.5

establishment of intercellular contacts (thrombospondin, integrins) and genes prominently expressed in intact vascular wall (actin, vimentin) were markedly down-regulated. In contrast, genes involved in cell growth and migration (Egr, IGF, Fos) and ECM deposition and cell attachment (collagen, fibronectin, thrombospondin, dermatopontin, integrins) were up-regulated 2 wk after injury. Gene expression of SMC-associated markers (smooth muscle actin, Sm22α, calponin) and some growth regulators/inhibitors (DR1-associated protein 1 [DRAP1], cell division cycle [CDC] 27) was decreased at 2 wk. The overall gene expression patterns correlated closely with vascular wall histology.

CANDIDATE-MOLECULE STUDIES

Most data on the molecular pathology of transplant arteriopathy are derived from studies of candidate molecules, i.e., those thought to be involved in the pathogenesis of this condition. The goal of these studies has been to identify essential molecular components of transplant arteriopathy by targeted transcript profiling using reverse transcriptase polymerase chain reaction (RT-PCR) followed by specific inhibition of candidate molecules (e.g., by use of receptor antagonists, blocking antibodies, antisense oligonucleotides, or knockout mouse strains). A molecular disease component is defined as essential, or rate-limiting, when its exclusion significantly ameliorates the pathology associated with the disease. In contrast, a vasculoprotective molecule is defined as one whose exclusion exacerbates the disease pathology.

Cells in growing neointimal lesions have an activated, secretory phenotype. Adhesion molecules expressed on these cells and ECM components, such as vasoactive molecules, cytokines, and secreted growth factors, play a role in transplant arteriopathy.

The vascular endothelium of cadaveric grafts, which has an activated phenotype at the time of graft procurement, is characterized by expression of HLA class II

Table 2
Decrease in Gene Transcription 2 and 14 d After Arterial Denudation

Down-regulated genes	Decrease (fold)
Day 2	
Vimentin	0.18
Integrin β3	0.18
Cytochrome P450 IVB1	0.22
Sterol-O-acyltransferase	0.23
Ems 1	0.25
Actin γ	0.27
Afadin	0.31
Stromelysin	0.33
Tissue inhibitor of metalloproteinases-1	0.36
E2F transcription factor 1	0.36
Cyclin-dependent kinase 7	0.40
Thrombospondin 1	0.41
Cyp19 (aromatase)	0.42
Cyclin H	0.43
Epidermal growth factor receptor	0.44
Retinol dehydrogenase	0.45
Smad4/dpc4	0.46
Parotid secretory protein	0.47
Trefoil factor 1	0.49
Phospholipase C, β2	0.50
Retinoic acid receptor α	0.50
Day 14	
Sm22a	0.28
Insulin-like growth factor binding protein 6	0.28
DR1-associated protein 1	0.32
Cell division cycle (CDC) 27	0.34
Insulin-like growth factor binding protein 2	0.34
Aryl hydrocarbon receptor interacting protein	0.35
Cystatin C	0.35
Calponin	0.37
Tetranectin	0.39
11-β dehydrogenase 2	0.40
Integrin β3	0.40
Cyclophilin C	0.40
Erb-b2	0.43
Janus kinase 1	0.44
Vascular endothelial growth factor-B	0.45
Angio-associated, migratory cell protein	0.47
Mitogen-activated protein kinase kinase kinase 5	0.48
Inhibin β-A	0.49
CDC-like kinase 2	0.50
Interleukin-10 receptor	0.50
Smooth muscle cell actin	0.51

molecules and adhesion molecules such as intercellular adhesion molecule (ICAM)-1, vascular cell adhesion molecule (VCAM)-1, and E-selectin *(75)*. This endothelial activation may be triggered by donor brain death, which is associated with systemic cytokine release and an increased risk of early acute rejection *(127)*. Free radical–mediated injury that occurs during graft preservation and reperfusion *(128,129)* and is maintained by the alloimmune response may further increase endothelial activation *(130)*. In a time-course study of adhesion molecule expression during the development of CGN in rats, Kauppinen et al. showed that ICAM-1, VCAM-1, and their respective ligands, leukocyte function-associated antigen-1 (LFA-1) and very late antigen (VLA)-4, are quickly up-regulated early after transplantation and that their expression decreases gradually as tissue injury progresses *(131)*. However, recent studies in knockout mice indicate that ICAM-1 expression is not essential for the development of transplant arteriopathy *(132)*. Similarly, P-selectin expression appears dispensable *(132)*; however, P-selectin seems to be essential for neointimal hyperplasia induced by endothelial denudation *(133)*. These findings illustrate subtle, but potentially crucial, differences between these pathological conditions, which otherwise appear remarkably similar under the microscope. In addition, interactions between the cell and the ECM may contribute to neointimal hyperplasia because blocking the binding of VLA-4 to fibronectin decreases vascular inflammation and prevents transplant arteriopathy *(134)*.

In addition to having a role in regulating leukocyte recruitment, the graft vascular endothelium is both a source and a target of several cytokines that presumably function to sustain endothelial cell activation. Evidence indicates that, despite ongoing immunosuppressive treatment, both peripheral blood and graft-infiltrating leukocytes of allograft recipients actively produce several cytokines *(135)*. Studies in knockout mice indicate that TNFα and IL-1 are involved in neointimal pathology *(136)*. Inhibition of TNFα alone does not prevent transplant arteriopathy *(137)*; however, this finding is not surprising because of the overlapping roles of IL-1 and TNFα in triggering endothelial activation. TNFα and IL-6 may contribute to the pathology of CGN *(138)*. The effect of γ-interferon (γ-IFN) on the development of transplant arteriopathy may be significant. Exogenous administration of γ-IFN to mice with SCID who received xenogeneic vascular grafts resulted in transplant arteriopathy, probably by directly promoting neointimal cell recruitment and proliferation *(139)*.

Activated vascular endothelial cells and macrophages are probably major sources of chemokines and bioactive lipids, which attract and retain recipient mononuclear leukocytes in the growing neointima. Expression of chemokines such as MCP-1, RANTES, and their receptors is crucial for development of the neointimal lesion *(140–143)*. In addition, MCP-1 has recently been implicated in the pathogenesis of obliterative bronchiolitis *(144)*. Generation of the pro-inflammatory lipid platelet-activating factor (PAF), and possibly other related compounds, appears essential for the development of transplant arteriopathy *(145)*.

Several growth factors participate in the pathogenesis of both transplant arteriopathy and chronic interstitial rejection. In neointimal lesions, growth factor expression likely promotes ECM synthesis and the proliferation and differentiation of the myofibroblastoid cells that stimulate lesion growth. Growth factor expression in the graft parenchyma is almost invariably associated with fibrotic remodeling. Macrophages may be the main source of many growth factors found in vascular neointimal lesions. Transforming growth factor (TGF)-β is the most extensively studied growth factor in CR. Distinct patterns of expression of TGF-β in the vascular tissue have been reported in CR of aortic *(146)*, cardiac *(147)*, lung *(148)*, renal *(149,150)*, liver *(151)*, and composite tissue *(152)* allografts. TGF-β is unique among growth factors in having immunomodulatory properties *(153)*; furthermore, both TGF-β1 and its receptor on lymphocytes are upregulated by cyclosporine *(154)*. TGF-β regulates vascular SMC differentiation in vivo *(155)* and promotes the in vitro proliferation of SMCs via an autocrine PDGF-AA loop *(156)*. PDGF is expressed in organ allografts *(157)*. Expression of both TGF-β *(158)* and PDGF *(159–161)* appears essential for neointimal hyperplasia. Other growth factors often found in interstitial and neointimal lesions include allograft inflammatory factor-1 *(162–164)*, thrombospondin-1 *(165)*, and fibroblast growth factor *(166–168)*.

Vasoactive molecules greatly contribute to the pathology of transplant arteriopathy. The activity of potent vasoconstrictors, such as endothelin, is increased in affected graft arteries *(169)*. Recent studies have shown that inhibition of endothelin activity prevents CR in animal models of cardiac *(170)* and renal *(171)* transplantation. In contrast, Shears et al. *(172)* have reported that inhibition of nitric oxide (NO) production aggravates neointimal hyperplasia in aortic allografts, whereas in vivo transfection with inducible NO synthase (iNOS) suppresses it. Other investigators have reported similar results with endothelial NO synthase and have attributed the beneficial effect to inhibition of endothelial activation and leukocyte recruitment *(173)*. Using knockout mice, Koglin et al. *(174)* confirmed the importance of iNOS in preventing neointimal hyperplasia. The local delivery of L-arginine, the amino acid precursor of NO, can also suppress intimal expansion *(175,176)*. Taken together, these findings indicate that endothelin promotes neointimal formation, whereas NO protects against it. In addition, impairment of endothelial L-arginine transport, rather than NOS deficiency, may promote transplant arteriopathy.

Until recently, NO was thought to be the only endogenous gas involved in vascular function. However, the characterization of heme oxygenase *(177)*, together with pioneering work that ascribed biological effects to carbon monoxide (CO) *(178)*, has led to exciting new areas of research in vascular biology. Heme oxygenase-1 (HO-1), an inducible oxidase expressed in vascular tissue, recycles free heme into biliverdin with concurrent generation of CO. Biliverdin is further degraded into bilirubin by the enzyme biliverdin reductase *(179)*. Thus, heme oxygenase mediates vasorelaxation through the production of CO and has potent antioxidant properties because of its heme-scavenging activity and its promotion of bilirubin formation. Hancock et al. *(180)* were the first to link vascular expression of HO-1 with protection of murine cardiac grafts from transplant arteriopathy. In addition, they showed that in vitro induction of HO-1 in endothelial cells prevented the activation of endothelial cells by alloantibody. Paracrine exposure of ischemic endothelial cells to CO down-regulates the release of endothelin-1 and PDGF from these cells *(181)*. Important new evidence suggests that the vasculoprotective properties of HO-1 may have wider therapeutic implications. Adenovirus-mediated HO-1 gene transfer has been reported to inhibit the spontaneous formation of atherosclerotic lesions in both LDL-receptor *(182)* and apoE *(183)* knockout mice. Furthermore, in vivo overexpression of HO-1 reduces neointimal hyperplasia after endothelial denudation injury in rats *(184,185)*. Hence, therapeutic modulation of HO-1 activity or CO bioavailability *(186,187)* may help prevent transplant arteriopathy.

GENETIC POLYMORPHISMS AND SUSCEPTIBILITY TO TRANSPLANT ARTERIOPATHY

Human genetic polymorphism is defined as the existence of multiple variants (polymorphic alleles) of a given genomic DNA sequence in a human population. Many polymorphisms are found throughout the human genome. The frequency of the most common class of polymorphisms, single nucleotide polymorphisms (SNPs), is about 1:1000 base pairs (bp). Because of their high prevalence and fairly uniform distribution,

SNPs are ideal markers for high-resolution mapping of the human genome (188). Furthermore, SNPs can be used in disease association studies because they often occur within genes and gene-associated regions.

Since genetic polymorphisms are essentially mutations, genetic variation may affect disease susceptibility. Certain genetic diseases such as protein deficiencies and some forms of cancer often result from mutations that have deleterious effects on gene or protein structure. Because of the severe morbidity and mortality associated with many genetic diseases, their associated mutations are extremely rare in the general population. In contrast, genetic polymorphisms are found frequently in human populations, which implies that polymorphisms have a more subtle effect on gene or protein function.

The location of a genetic polymorphism can affect disease susceptibility and gene function in different ways (Fig. 5). Polymorphisms that modify binding sites required for transcription factor docking, usually found in gene promoter regions, may affect gene transcription. Polymorphisms located at the 3′ untranslated region may modify polyadenylation signal sequences and other elements, thereby affecting the transport, half-life, or rate of translation of the mRNA (189). Non-synonymous polymorphisms in the first transcribed exon, which often encodes a leader peptide involved in protein compartmentalization and export (190), may affect protein trafficking. Finally, the presence of polymorphisms in exons or intron–exon boundaries (splice junctions) could directly affect both mRNA processing (191) and protein structure. Emerging evidence suggests that allelic variation in gene expression associated with, although not necessarily attributable to, transcribed SNPs is in fact common in the human genome (192).

With the advent of new technologies for high-throughput genotyping, research into the biological implications and clinical relevance of genetic polymorphism is entering a new era. The role of genetic variation in susceptibility to multifactorial human diseases such as cardiovascular disease and cancer is being assessed. The involvement of genetic polymorphisms in human disease, however, should not overshadow the importance of environmental and lifestyle-related risk factors.

The study of genetic polymorphisms is new in the field of transplantation. The best studied putative genetic marker of transplant arteriopathy and CR is a G to C transversion at position +915 of the human TGF-β1 coding sequence. This SNP results in a non-synonymous codon change, Arg25Pro, in the TGF-β1 leader sequence (193,194). Awad et al. (194) showed that in vitro stimulated lymphocytes from carriers of the infrequent C allele released approximately 30% less TGF-β1 than cells from G allele homozygotes. The same group reported an association of G allele homozygosity with both pre- and post-transplant fibrotic lung pathology, as assessed by transbronchial biopsy (194–196). Furthermore, this group recently reported an association of the +915GG genotype with early development of coronary transplant arteriopathy, based on angiographic data (147,197).

We have been unable to reproduce these findings in a smaller but more comprehensive study of thoracic transplant recipient polymorphisms in relation to graft outcome (198). Of the 179 thoracic transplant recipients with well-defined graft outcomes in our study, 96 had lost their grafts due to transplant arteriopathy and related complications within 11 yr after transplantation. Only 83 of the 179 patients retained functioning grafts for longer than 11 yr. We evaluated 11 polymorphisms in eight genes encoding various cytokines, growth factors, and growth factor receptors; our analysis of these data also accounted for several clinical risk factors. Univariate analysis showed that only polymorphisms of the gene encoding the IL-1 receptor antagonist (IL-1Ra), an endogenous inhibitor of IL-1 signaling, were associated with cardiac graft outcome, particularly in those patients with multiple episodes of acute rejection. We confirmed this finding in a logistic regression model. Furthermore, in vitro studies showed that the same polymorphisms of the IL-1Ra gene independently regulate both IL-1Ra and IL-1β release from primary human monocytes in response to LPS (199).

An insertion/deletion polymorphism (200) of the gene encoding the angiotensin-converting enzyme (ACE) may be associated with cardiac graft attrition. Using both angiographic and IVUS data, Pethig et al. (201) found a dose-dependent association of the recipient D allele with the incidence of coronary transplant arteriopathy at 6 yr posttransplant; however, they could not show a significant effect of this polymorphism on either mean neointimal area or ACE plasma levels in the same group of heart transplant recipients. Furthermore, an association between ACE genotype and transplant arteriopathy has not been shown in other studies of heart transplant recipients (202).

The relation between genetic polymorphism and disease susceptibility is complex. In transplantation, additional complexity arises from the interplay between genetically disparate entities (i.e., the graft and the recipient immune system). Ideally, in studying genetic risk factors that affect graft outcome, both donor and recipient genotypes should be analyzed.

The contribution of donor genotype to chronic allograft failure in humans has been examined in only a few

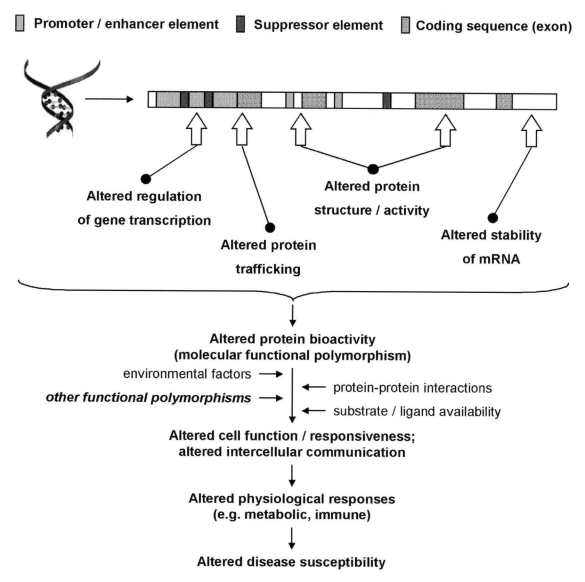

Fig. 5. A paradigm for the relationship between genetic polymorphism and disease susceptibility. The typical structure of a mammalian gene is shown. Block arrows indicate sites within this structure where the occurrence of genetic polymorphisms may result in functional polymorphism (i.e., interindividual differences in the amount of protein produced or in the structure or activity of the protein). In this paradigm, the coordinated effects of other functional polymorphisms and relevant physiological and environmental factors determine the severity of the disease phenotype.

studies, all of these focusing on polymorphisms of genes normally expressed in donor endothelial and vascular smooth muscle tissue. Benza et al. *(203)* examined 48 heart transplant recipients for donor polymorphisms in the genes encoding tissue plasminogen activator (TPA) and plasminogen activator inhibitor 1 (PAI-1), both of which are involved in the regulation of fibrinolysis. Univariate statistical analysis showed a significant association between the PAI-1 polymorphism, an insertion/deletion SNP in the gene promoter, and the incidence

of transplant arteriopathy at 2 yr posttransplant; however, grafts with the PAI-1 2/2 genotype had been exposed to significantly longer ischemic times, which is a potentially confounding factor.

Cunningham et al. *(202)* first studied the ACE insertion/deletion polymorphism in heart graft donor–recipient pairs. Although unable to find an association between recipient ACE genotype and angiographic evidence of transplant arteriopathy at 2 yr posttransplant, they reported an independent association with donor ACE genotype. In another study of heart graft donor–recipient pairs, Borozdenkova et al. *(204)* examined nine polymorphisms in genes encoding cell adhesion molecules (E- and L-selectin, ICAM-1, and platelet endothelial cell adhesion molecule [PECAM]-1). Using univariate statistics, these authors found an association between an exonic ICAM-1 gene polymorphism (469E/K) and angiographic evidence of transplant arteriopathy at 2 yr posttransplant. In this study, the donor 469E allele was associated with protection from transplant arteriopathy, whereas in a previous study of renal transplants the same allele was associated with a faster progression to CGN (205). These observations illustrate the complexity of the genetics of transplant arteriopathy and the need for large studies to confirm putative associations.

MANAGEMENT OF TRANSPLANT ARTERIOPATHY

Immunosuppressive Treatment

Despite their remarkable efficacy in preventing acute rejection, the calcineurin inhibitors cyclosporine and tacrolimus are ineffective in controlling CR. In fact, some studies suggest that cyclosporine may contribute to the pathology of CGN *(8)*, which is not surprising given that long-term use of calcineurin inhibitors is associated with nephrotoxicity *(206)*.

In contrast, a multicenter study *(207)* suggested that a steroid-free CsA/azathioprine regimen was associated with the best long-term graft outcome. However, in this study, the time points after transplantation were relatively early (up to 5 yr), and the authors did not distinguish between causes of graft failure or between actual graft loss and death with a functioning graft. Furthermore, patients on steroid-free immunosuppression in that study had probably been selected on the basis of stable posttransplant course and received a higher mean dose of cyclosporine. High-dose cyclosporine effectively suppresses transplant arteriopathy *(208)*; therefore, the early survival advantage attributed to steroid withdrawal may have been caused by more aggressive cyclosporine dosing.

We recently reported a similar early beneficial effect of complete steroid withdrawal on the incidence of chronic allograft nephropathy in pediatric kidney transplant patients *(209)*. The benefit was partially achieved by higher tacrolimus dosing. Although biopsy-proven tacrolimus toxicity occurred in 40% of steroid-free patients at 1 yr (M Sarwal, MD, PhD, unpublished data, 2003), protocol biopsy specimens showed an absence of CGN in these patients. However, in a recent report of kidney transplant recipients, some clinical benefit was achieved by tapering the steroid dose, but none was observed with complete steroid withdrawal *(210)*. These discrepancies suggest that longer follow-up of steroid-free patients is necessary before drawing firm conclusions on the efficacy of such interventions.

Patient noncompliance with the immunosuppressive regimen precipitates acute rejection of organ allografts and is an obvious behavioral risk factor for CR. Some have postulated that pharmacokinetic risk factors and drug resistance may increase the risk of CR. Kahan et al. *(211)* first proposed that interindividual variability in oral absorption of cyclosporine was a risk factor for CR. Interindividual differences in responsiveness to cyclosporine treatment might pose further risk, even among transplant patients with similar trough levels of the drug *(212)*. Batiuk et al. first showed that calcineurin inhibition by cyclosporine is rapidly reversible in vivo *(213)*, suggesting that an active cellular efflux mechanism might exclude the drug. Lymphocytes express the multidrug resistance protein P-glycoprotein *(214,215)*, and cyclosporine *(216)* and rapamycin *(217)* are substrates for this efflux transporter protein. Although initial reports supported a role for drug resistance in acute and chronic rejection *(218–220)*, these findings have recently been challenged *(221)*, and the issue of immunosuppressive drug resistance after transplantation remains controversial.

Calcineurin inhibitors are unique among immunosuppressive agents in being markedly profibrotic. Both cyclosporine *(154,222–225)* and tacrolimus *(226)* promote TGF-β expression, and cyclosporine regulates expression of the TGF-β receptor in human T lymphocytes *(154)*. Furthermore, cyclosporine directly impairs vascular endothelial function, an effect that is partially reversible by oral administration of L-arginine *(227)*. These biochemical consequences of calcineurin inhibition may contribute to the pathology of CR by promoting both transplant arteriopathy and interstitial fibrosis.

Managing the Risk Factors

Acute vascular rejection is a major clinical risk factor for transplant arteriopathy and CR *(13)*. In recent years, the introduction of rapid, high-resolution, molecular HLA typing methods and flow cytometric cross-matching has facilitated prospective evaluation of organ donors and recipients and has provided a scientific basis for deciding organ allocation. Together with improved diagnostics, such as graft protocol biopsy procedures and the standardization of histological grading systems, these developments should help improve graft outcomes.

New adjunct immunosuppressive agents, such as mycophenolate mofetil *(228,229)*, leflunomide *(230,231)*, and FTY720 *(232)*, should further improve the prevention and treatment of acute allograft rejection. Mycophenolate mofetil, an inhibitor of inosine monophosphate dehydrogenase, suppresses de novo purine biosynthesis, which exclusively fuels lymphocyte proliferation. The use of mycophenolate mofetil substantially reduces the dose of calcineurin inhibitors and is associated with a lower incidence of nephrotoxicity *(233)*; consequently, mycophenolate mofetil is replacing azathioprine in clinical use. Leflunomide, which blocks uridine biosynthesis by inhibiting dihydroorotate dehydrogenase, reduces and in combination with cyclosporine even reverses established transplant arteriopathy in rats *(231)*. Leflunomide inhibits vascular SMC proliferation in vitro, but the inhibition is reversed by uridine supplementation *(230)*. We have observed that FK778, a structural analogue of leflunomide, suppresses neointimal hyperplasia after endothelial denudation injury in rats, even after concurrent uridine administration *(234)*. Another immunosuppressive agent, 15-deoxyspergualin, partially inhibits transplant arteriopathy *(235)*.

In addition to suppressing the immune response, newer agents mitigate transplant arteriopathy by interfering with infiltration and proliferation of the neointimal precursor cells. Rapamycin (sirolimus), a drug recently licensed as an alternative to the calcineurin inhibitors for renal transplantation, is as effective as cyclosporine in preventing acute rejection *(236, 237)*. In animal models, rapamycin reduced neointimal hyperplasia after both alloimmune and endothelial denudation injury *(238,239)*; it also suppressed the development of native atherosclerosis *(240)*. The recent human trials of rapamycin-impregnated stents have been extremely successful on both short- *(241,242)* and long-term *(243,244)* follow-up after stent implantation. Unfortunately, oral rapamycin appears ineffective in controlling vascular restenosis following angioplasty *(245)*. Crucially, however, emerging evidence suggests that oral rapamycin, used as adjunct immunosuppression, does mitigate transplant arteriopathy *(246)*. These beneficial effects of rapamycin are thought to result from inhibition of growth factor–induced proliferation *(247,248)* although other mechanisms have been postulated, including upregulation of vascular NO production *(249)* and interference with certain myeloid differentiation pathways *(250)*. Interestingly, tacrolimus antagonizes the growth-inhibitory activity of rapamycin *(247)*.

Pravastatin, an inhibitor of 3-hydroxy-3-methylglutaryl coenzyme A (HMG-CoA) reductase and a popular antihyperlipidemic agent, was originally shown to reduce both the incidence and progression of transplant arteriopathy in human cardiac *(251)* and renal *(252)* allografts.

In rats, this effect was also associated with a reduction in monocyte infiltration and ECM deposition *(253)*. Statins are now known to exert broad anti-inflammatory and immunomodulatory actions *(254)*, which may account for their vasculoprotective properties. Furthermore, we have recently demonstrated that HMG-CoA reductase inhibition arrests the terminal differentiation of human monocytes into macrophages *(255)*, an essential cellular component of transplant arteriopathy. FTY720, a new immunosuppressant being tested in clinical trials, also reduced transplant arteriopathy in rodents, possibly by interfering with G protein–coupled receptor function *(256,257)*. Finally, multiglycosidorum tripterygii, an experimental compound, may prevent transplant arteriopathy, possibly by suppressing PDGF expression *(258)*. Along with rapamycin, these agents may prove beneficial in the prevention and treatment of transplant arteriopathy. The beneficial effect must be achieved at clinically relevant concentrations, and the pharmacokinetic and safety profiles must be compatible with clinical transplantation.

Effective control of CMV infection minimizes the risk of transplant arteriopathy. With the advent of PCR, latent CMV infection can be readily diagnosed, and relapses can be identified. Nucleoside analogs, such as ganciclovir, are effective against CMV, either as prophylactic therapy or for the acute treatment of active infection. The necessity of intravenous administration of ganciclovir has been overcome with the development of valganciclovir, a novel prodrug formulation of ganciclovir *(259)*. However, the benefit of adding more drugs to an extensive immunosuppressive regimen will have to be weighed against the negative impact of such interventions on patient compliance, quality of life, and the emergence of drug-resistant viral strains.

Rational Drug Design for Controlling Neointimal Hyperplasia

Several studies have shown that the natural history of CR has a "point of no return" (Fig. 4), after which elimination of alloimmune vascular injury no longer stops graft attrition *(260,261)*. In animal models, transplant arteriopathy appears to be self-sustaining early after transplantation *(262,263)* and thereafter gives rise to the same fibrotic sequelae in the absence of alloreactivity and immunosuppression. The point of no return also seems to be a feature of CR in humans (M Sarwal, MD, PhD, unpublished data, 2003). Thus, understanding the early events in transplant arteriopathy is critical because therapeutic intervention may be most effective in early stages. However, solely targeting T cell function would probably not increase graft function further because data from genomic studies suggest that many different metabolic and immunological pathways are involved in long-term pathology. Accordingly, newer agents, such as rapamycin, that mitigate the recruitment and proliferation of the myofibroblastoid neointimal cells and their precursors are more effective than traditional immunosuppression in preventing transplant arteriopathy in rodents (238) and nonhuman primates (264,265).

The process of rational drug design involves using molecular data to identify putative rate-limiting molecular events and using high-throughput technologies to screen, manufacture, and test compounds interfering with these events. Genomics and, in the near future, proteomics offer reliable and comprehensive strategies for obtaining and interpreting molecular data. These strategies should accelerate and optimize the drug discovery process.

PHARMACOGENOMICS: IDENTIFYING RATE-LIMITING GENES

The science of pharmacogenomics involves applying gene transcription data to drug discovery and is an essential component of rational drug design. Transcriptional regulation of a small group of genes may be central to the development of transplant arteriopathy. Rate-limiting genes are not always distinctly regulated; they can be identified in vitro and in vivo by exogenous modulation of their expression at the level of translation (e.g., by means of antisense oligonucleotides) or by manipulating the biological activity of the encoded protein (e.g., through the use of specific receptor agonists/antagonists). Rate-limiting genes that modify the outcome of fibroproliferative vascular disease have been identified with blocking antibodies (266–269), antisense oligonucleotides (270), receptor antagonists (271), and specific receptor tyrosine kinase inhibitors (272,273).

PROMISING DRUG CANDIDATES

We have used rodent models of endothelial denudation to develop compounds to treat fibroproliferative vascular disease. Endothelial denudation results in the formation of neointimal lesions resembling those observed in transplant arteriopathy. The pathologic process of neointimal hyperplasia is remarkably similar in transplant arteriopathy and endothelial denudation, except for the effector mechanism of endothelial trauma (mechanical in denudation versus alloimmune in arteriopathy) and its immediate consequences.

The genes encoding the insulin-like growth factor (IGF)-1 and its receptor have been proposed as rate-limiting for the proliferative component of transplant arteriopathy (274). Suppressing the expression of these genes may help prevent or treat transplant arteriopathy. We have tested this hypothesis by using a synthetic D-amino acid peptide (JB3) that structurally resembles the D-domain of IGF-1 to block the interaction of IGF with its receptor (271). Semiquantitative RT-PCR analysis has shown significant increases in mRNA for IGF-1, PDGF-B, TGF-β1, and epidermal growth factor (EGF) 10 d after carotid artery denudation in rats. These increases in mRNA occurred concomitantly with the induction of intimal cell proliferation and the onset of intimal thickening. Administration of 10–30 µg/kg/d of the D-analog of IGF-1, which is resistant to proteolytic degradation in vivo, reduced intimal cell proliferation by 60–70%. In addition, this peptide suppressed both [^{3}H]thymidine and [^{3}H]glycine incorporation in cultured vascular SMCs by 60–80%, whereas a "scrambled" control peptide had no effect. Thus, blocking the IGF-1/IGF-1R interaction with stable D-peptide analogs of IGF-1 may prevent restenosis after cardiac revascularization procedures and may possibly prevent transplant arteriopathy. In related experiments, the JB3 peptide was equally effective in modulating PDGF-induced vascular SMC growth in vitro, suggesting cross-regulation of the PDGF and IGF-1 receptors on these cells (P Häyry, MD, unpublished observations, 2001). Other reports indicate similar cross-communication between different growth factor receptors (156,275).

Some of the vasoprotective effects attributable to hormones (see below) may involve the regulation of growth factors and their receptors. Estradiol inhibits neointimal hyperplasia in rabbit cardiac allografts. Some authors have associated this beneficial effect with a marked reduction in IGF-1 synthesis in the vascular wall and an inhibition of IGF-1–induced proliferation of aortic SMCs in vitro (276, H Savolainen, MD, unpublished data, 2002). The vasculoprotective effects of somatostatin may be mediated in a manner similar to estradiol. In an early study of rat aortic allografts we showed that angiopeptin (lanreotide) treatment of the recipient rat (80 µg/kg/d by continuous infusion) suppressed the recruitment and proliferation of myofibroblastoid cells in the aortic intima. Although this treatment did not affect IL-1 expression or the release of bioactive lipids, it significantly reduced EGF, IGF-1, and PDGF synthesis (277). In fact, angiopeptin at doses as low as 10 µg/kg (twice daily) inhibited the induction of IGF-1 synthesis on d 1, 2, and 4 after denudation injury in rabbits (278). In humans, the expression of IGF-1 is high in diseased but not in healthy vasculature, and both sandostatin (octreotide) and angiopeptin inhibit the in vitro proliferation of human coronary artery vascular SMCs triggered by IGF-1 or bFGF (279). Finally, treatment with sandostatin reduces mRNA expression of IGF-1 in healthy rat arteries by 70% and prevents the induction of IGF-1 (but not PDGF-A) gene expression after denudation injury (280). Because no change in plasma growth hormone, IGF-1, or glucagon was seen, the effect of sandostatin was likely specific for IGF-1 and mediated locally.

The receptor tyrosine kinase inhibitors may be good candidates for treating transplant arteriopathy. Our group recently evaluated two compounds, CGP-53716 and CGP-57148B, which are highly selective for the PDGFRα,β-associated v-Abl tyrosine kinase. These compounds inhibited not only the formation of acute vascular lesions after denudation injury (272) but also the development of chronic lesions such as those seen in transplant arteriopathy in various transplant models (281). CGP-57148B, recently renamed STI571 (imatinib mesylate), received expedited Food and Drug Administration clearance in the United States for the treatment of certain leukemias and gastrointestinal tumors and is currently marketed as Gleevec® (Novartis). We tested the prescription formulation of this compound and found that Gleevec® was as effective in preventing the development of chronic lesions in rat renal allografts (282) as it was in preventing transplant arteriopathy in rat cardiac allografts (281). While Gleevec® is far less effective than rapamycin in inhibiting neointimal hyperplasia, it is very well tolerated and lacks any immunosuppressive activity. Preliminary data from our laboratory also indicate that Gleevec® may synergize with rapamycin to suppress neointimal hyperplasia (J Vamvakopoulos, MSc, PhD, unpublished data, 2003).

An appealing approach to preventing transplant arteriopathy is to use the vasculoprotective effects of certain human hormones such as estrogens and somatostatin. The vasculoprotective potential of estrogens was originally documented in population studies of hormone replacement therapy (283,284); however, the feminizing side effects of natural estrogens limit their use in clinical transplantation. The prototypical estrogen receptor (ER) α is expressed extensively in the female reproductive organs and elsewhere, but the recently described ERβ (285), which has been the focus of much interest, appears to be the predominant estrogen receptor in baboon (286), rat, and human (287) vascular tissue. Moreover, ERβ is acutely up-regulated after endothelial denudation injury in the rat (288), and its levels (both mRNA and protein) return to normal after the injury response is complete. In a rat model of carotid artery denudation, we studied the vasculoprotective potential of estrogens by evaluating 17β-estradiol, a natural ER ligand, and genistein, a phytoestrogen that preferentially binds to ERβ. Both estrogens reduced intimal thickening in a dose-dependent

manner with equal efficacy (288). However, estradiol, but not genistein, induced uterine hyperplasia. These findings indicate that the vasculoprotective effect of estrogens can be dissociated from their uterotrophic action by targeting ERβ, a fact that has important therapeutic implications.

Somatostatin is a small neuropeptide that signals through five distinct cellular receptors. These receptors have been categorized into two families, somatostatin receptor (SSTR) 1, 4 and SSTR 2, 3, and 5, on the basis of structural similarity and binding affinities for synthetic ligands (289). In a seminal study Rohrer et al. (290) showed that all five SSTRs demonstrate signaling activity (as judged by cyclic AMP accumulation) but that all known actions of somatostatin, such as inhibition of growth hormone, insulin, and glucagon release, were ascribed exclusively to SSTRs 2 and 5. The biological function of the other three receptors is, therefore, unknown. The initial interest in the therapeutic potential of somatostatin was triggered by early animal studies that showed the vasculoprotective properties of the somatostatin analogues octreotide and lanreotide (277–280). However, these compounds did not prevent vascular restenosis in clinical trials (291–293). The lack of clinical efficacy of these analogues may relate to their preferential binding to SSTR subtypes 2 and 5, possibly the wrong targets for such therapy.

This conclusion is supported by our recent finding that SSTRs 1 and 4 are the predominant somatostatin receptors in the vascular wall early after denudation injury in rats, whereas the other SSTRs are expressed at low levels (294). Expression of SSTRs 1 and 4 was three- to four-times higher than that of SSTR 2, whereas expression of SSTR 5 was not induced by vascular injury. We generated and tested three SSTR agonists: CH275 (DesAA1,2,5[D-W8,IAmp9]Somatostatine-14), specific for SSTRs 1 and 4; octreotide, selective for subtypes 2 and 5; and somatostatin-14, which binds with equal affinity to all five SSTRs. Daily injections (50–500 μg/kg/d) of CH275 inhibited the development of neointimal hyperplasia in a dose-dependent manner 14 d after rat carotid denudation injury. In addition, CH275 was more effective in suppressing neointimal growth than either somatostatin-14 or octreotide (295). These findings indicate that somatostatin analogues targeting SSTRs 1 and 4 may be promising candidates for the prevention of transplant arteriopathy.

The Drug Discovery Process

The concept and technologies of rational drug design have recently been reviewed (296). Knowing the molecular conformation of drugs used to target a given protein facilitates the rapid identification of lead compounds.

Molecular structure can be obtained by methods such as protein crystallography and homology modeling, which uses computer simulations of related protein crystal structures as a template for building a model of the protein of interest. Both methods are tedious and have many limitations. For example, not all proteins can form crystals suitable for conformational studies, and assumptions and approximations are used in homology modeling. Furthermore, the structural consequences of physiological protein–protein interactions are not accounted for in either method. Despite the advent of proteomics, less tedious, high-throughput technologies for solving molecular structures have not been developed.

The goal of rational drug design is to generate ligands highly specific for the target protein. The first step in the process is to build a virtual molecular framework (known as a pharmacophore) based on the molecular coordinates of a ligand or set of ligands known to bind to the target protein. The pharmacophore can be further refined; for example, information about protein residues critical for the physiological interactions between ligands and the target protein can be incorporated. Pharmacophores are used to identify new compounds that present a specific arrangement of features responsible for a certain type of activity, and databases of known compound structures are virtually screened to identify pharmacophore matches. Lead compounds can then be rapidly generated by using combinatorial chemistry, an emerging technology that enables high-throughput synthesis of candidate ligands (Fig. 6); subsequently, these are evaluated in vitro and in vivo. Rational discovery of the SSTR 1, 4-specific agonist CH275 (Fig. 7) illustrates the molecular basis of this screening process. The strong affinity of CH275 for human SSTR 1 is due to the hydrophobic interaction of CH275 with a leucine residue in the binding pocket of the receptor; this hydrophobic interaction does not occur with human SSTR 2, causing a substantially reduced binding affinity. Binding affinities to the target protein in each round of compound selection are expected to increase logarithmically; compounds with binding affinities approaching the nanomolar range usually make good drug candidates. After a drug candidate is identified, drug development follows the traditional pathway (preclinical pharmacology and toxicology and galenic formulation) and culminates in clinical trials.

Pharmacogenetics and Individualized Treatment

Although drug discovery has rapidly evolved into a science, finding the right drug for the right patient still embodies the "art of medicine." Extensive interindividual

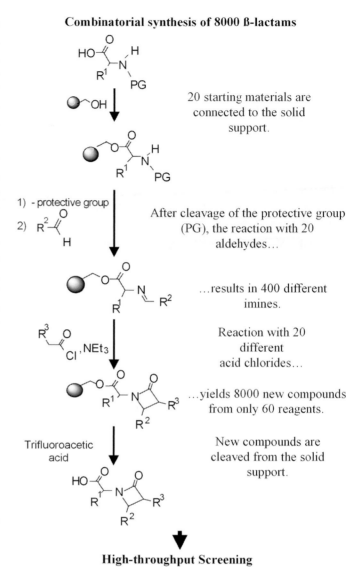

Combinatorial synthesis of 8000 ß-lactams

20 starting materials are connected to the solid support.

After cleavage of the protective group (PG), the reaction with 20 aldehydes...

...results in 400 different imines.

Reaction with 20 different acid chlorides...

...yields 8000 new compounds from only 60 reagents.

New compounds are cleaved from the solid support.

High-throughput Screening

Fig. 6. High-throughput synthesis of bioactive compounds using combinatorial chemistry.

variation in response to pharmacological therapy was first documented almost 50 years ago, and this variation was soon linked with human genetics (297). Because an ideal response to therapy involves not just relief from the symptoms of disease but also from the adverse effects associated with drug treatment, the linking of drug response to genetic polymorphisms has important implications for drug design, testing, and prescribing.

Unlike the emerging field of pharmacogenomics, which uses gene expression data to develop more effective therapies, the science of pharmacogenetics draws from the various SNP mapping projects with the ultimate

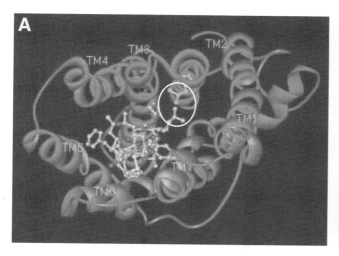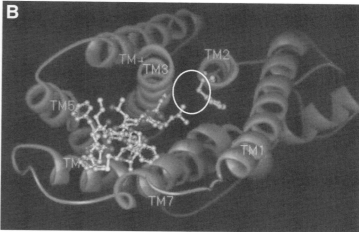

Fig. 7. Structural basis of the specificity of CH275 for the human somatostatin receptor (hSSTR) 1. Homology models of hSSTR 1 (left) and hSSTR 2 (right) are seen in ribbon configuration. CH275 and side chains of hSSTR residues important for the receptor–ligand interactions are displayed as ball-and-stick models. Both receptors contain aspartic acid in the transmembrane (TM)3 domain, and hSSTR 1 has leucine in TM2, whereas hSSTR 2 has phenylalanine at the corresponding position. CH275 was fitted manually into the binding pocket of each receptor to highlight differences in the interactions between receptor and ligand. Note that CH275 interacts with the leucine residue of hSSTR 1 (white circle) but not with the corresponding phenylalanine residue of hSSTR 2. Certain extracellular portions of the receptor have been omitted for clarity. Image courtesy of Dr. A-M Hoffrén (Juvantia Pharma, Biocity Turku, Finland).

aim of understanding the genetic basis of drug responsiveness. Despite confusion about the use of these terms, several authors have recently published reviews on pharmacogenetics *(298–301)*.

SUMMARY

The use of powerful immunosuppressive drugs in clinical transplantation has reduced the incidence of allograft loss by acute rejection. However, transplant arteriopathy and CR are major obstacles to the long-term survival of transplanted organs. Neointimal lesions associated with transplant arteriopathy resemble atherosclerotic plaques; however, atherosclerotic lesions are more localized and nonconcentric and differ in consistency. Transplant arteriopathy affects only the allogenic vasculature, a feature that highlights the importance of alloimmunity in the observed pathology. However, the events triggering vascular injury in this setting are obscure and may involve poorly defined, nonimmune factors such as infection, ischemia, dyslipidemia, hypertension, acute rejection, and drug toxicity. Regardless of the mechanism that precipitates transplant arteriopathy, the end result is cumulative ischemic injury to the graft with progressive loss of function. Recent breakthroughs in understanding the pathology of this condition have led to exciting new avenues of research.

ACKNOWLEDGMENTS

The authors thank Dr A-M Hoffrén (Juvantia Pharma, BioCity Turku) for providing Figure 7.

REFERENCES

1. Hariharan S, Johnson CP, Bresnahan BA, Taranto SE, McIntosh MJ, Stablein D. Improved graft survival after renal transplantation in the United States, 1988 to 1996. N Engl J Med 2000; 342:605–612.
2. Ojo AO, Hanson HA, Wolfe RA, Leichtman AB, Agodoa LY, Port FK. Long-term survival in renal transplant recipients with graft function. Kidney Int 2000;57:307–313.
3. Cho JH, Bhatnagar B, Andreani P, et al. Chronic rejection in pediatric liver transplantation. Transplant Proc 1997;29:452–453.
4. Sellers M, Singer A, Maller E, Olthoff K, Jocobowski D, Shaked A. Incidence of late acute rejection and progression to chronic rejection in pediatric liver recipients. Transplant Proc 1997;29:428–429.
5. Sudan DL, Shaw BW Jr, Langnas AN. Cause of late mortality in pediatric liver transplant recipients. Transplant Proc 1997;29:430–431.
6. Inomata Y, Tanaka K. Pathogenesis and treatment of bile duct loss after liver transplantation. J Hepatobil Pancreat Surg 2001;8:316–322.
7. Grocott-Mason RM, Bustami M, Banner N, et al. Influence of allograft coronary artery disease on survival and cardiac function in the decade following orthotopic cardiac transplantation. Transplant Proc 1997;29:576–577.
8. Hiesse C, Rieu P, Larue JR, et al. Late graft failure and death in renal transplant recipients: analysis in a single-center population of 1500 patients. Transplant Proc 1997;29:240–242.

9. Sundaresan S, Trulock EP, Mohanakumar T, Cooper JD, Patterson GA. Prevalence and outcome of bronchiolitis obliterans syndromes after lung transplantation. Washington University Lung Transplant Group. Ann Thorac Surg 1995;60:1341–1346.

10. Pinto FJ, Chenzbraun A, Botas J, et al. Feasibility of serial intracoronary ultrasound imaging for assessment of progression of intimal proliferation in cardiac transplant recipients. Circulation 1994;90:2348–2355.

11. Julius BK, Attenhofer Jost CH, Sutsch G, et al. Incidence, progression and functional significance of cardiac allograft vasculopathy after heart transplantation. Transplantation 2000; 69:847–853.

12. Kim SI, Kim MS, Kim YS, Jeong HJ, Park K. Biopsy-proven chronic rejection in living donor kidney transplantation—risk factors and graft survival. Transplant Proc 1997;29:100.

13. van Saase JLCM, van der Woude FJ, Thorogood J, et al. The relation between acute vascular and interstitial renal allograft rejection and subsequent chronic rejection. Transplantation 1995;59:1280–1285.

14. Kokado Y, Takahara S, Hatori M, et al. Acute rejection episodes predict long-term renal transplantation survival. Transplant Proc 1997;29:1537–1540.

15. Opelz G, for the Collaborative Transplant Study. Critical evaluation of the association of acute with chronic graft rejection in kidney and heart transplant recipients. Transplant Proc 1997; 29:73–76.

16. Matas AJ, Gillingham KJ, Humar A, Dunn DL, Sutherland DER, Najarian JS. Immunologic and nonimmunologic factors: different risks for cadaver and living donor transplantation. Transplantation 2000;69:54–58.

17. Basadonna GP, Matas AJ, Gillingham KJ, et al. Early versus late acute renal allograft rejection: impact on chronic rejection. Transplantation 1993;55:993–995.

18. Matas AJ, Gillingham KJ, Payne WD, Najarian JS. The impact of an acute rejection episode on long-term renal allograft survival (t1/2). Transplantation 1994;57:857–859.

19. Oliveira JG, Xavier P, Neto S, Mendes AA, Guerra LE. Monocytes-macrophages and cytokines/chemokines in fine-needle aspiration biopsy cultures: enhanced interleukin-1 receptor antagonist synthesis in rejection-free kidney transplant patients. Transplantation 1997;63:1751–1756.

20. Hirt SW, You XM, Moller F, et al. Development of obliterative bronchiolitis after allogeneic rat lung transplantation: implication of acute rejection and the time point of treatment. J Heart Lung Transplant 1999;18:542–548.

21. Kroshus TJ, Kshettry VR, Savik K, John R, Hertz MI, Bolman RM III. Risk factors for the development of bronchiolitis obliterans syndromes after lung transplantation. J Thorac Cardiovasc Surg 1997;114:195–202.

22. West MS, Sutherland DE, Matas AJ. Considering death with function as a graft loss in kidney transplant recipients. Transplant Proc 1997;29:239.

23. Hornick P, Smith J, Pomerance A, et al. Influence of acute rejection episodes, HLA matching, and donor/recipient phenotype on the development of "early" transplant-associated coronary artery disease. Circulation 1997;96:II-148–II-153.

24. Opelz G, Mytilineos J, Scherer S, Schwartz V, for the Collaborative Transplant Study. Clinical implications of DNA typing in organ transplantation. Transplant Proc 1997;29: 1524–1527.

25. Park MH, Tolman DE, Kimball PM. The impact of race and HLA matching on long-term survival following cardiac transplantation. Transplant Proc 1997;29:1460–1463.

26. Cantin B, Wen P, Zhu D, et al. Transplant coronary artery disease: a novel model independent of cellular alloimmune response. Circulation 2001;104:2615–2619.

27. Hoang K, Chen YD, Reaven G, et al. Diabetes and dyslipidemia: a new model for transplant coronary artery disease. Circulation 1998;97:2160–2168.

28. Cantin B, Zhu D, Wen P, et al. Reversal of diabetes-induced rat graft transplant coronary artery disease by metformin. J Heart Lung Transplant 2002;21:637–643.

29. Cantin B, Zhu D, Wen P, et al. Preferential involvement of larger vessels in a rat model of diabetes-induced graft vasculopathy. J Heart Lung Transplant 2002;21:1040–1043.

30. Grattan MT, Moreno-Cabral CE, Starnes VA, Oyer PE, Stinson EB, Shumway NE. Cytomegalovirus infection is associated with cardiac allograft rejection and atherosclerosis. JAMA 1989;261:3561–3566.

31. Peterson PK, Balfour HH, Marker SC, Fryd DS, Howard RJ, Simmons RL. Cytomegalovirus disease in renal allograft recipients: a prospective study of the clinical features, risk factors and impact on renal transplantation. Medicine 1980;59: 283–300.

32. O'Grady JG, Alexander GJ, Sutherland S, et al. Cytomegalovirus infection and donor/recipient HLA antigens: interdependent cofactors in pathogenesis of vanishing bile-duct syndrome after liver transplantation. Lancet 1988;2:302–305.

33. Yilmaz S, Koskinen PK, Kallio E, Bruggeman CA, Häyry PJ, Lemström K. Cytomegalovirus infection-enhanced chronic kidney allograft rejection is linked with intercellular adhesion molecule-1 expression. Kidney Int 1996;50:526–537.

34. Lautenschlager I, Soots A, Krogerus L, et al. Effect of cytomegalovirus on an experimental model of chronic renal allograft rejection under triple-drug treatment in the rat. Transplantation 1997;64:391–398.

35. Koskinen P, Kallio E, Tikkanen J, Bruggenman C, Häyry P, Lemström K. Cytomegalovirus infection accelerates experimental obliterative bronchiolitis via platelet-derived growth factor upregulation. Transplant Proc 1997;29:798.

36. Martelius T, Krogerus L, Hockerstedt K, Mäkisalo H, Bruggeman C, Lautenschlager I. CMV causes bile duct destruction and arterial lesion in rat liver allografts. Transplant Proc 1997;29:796–797.

37. Vamvakopoulos J, Häyry P. Cytomegalovirus and transplant arteriopathy: evidence for a link is mounting, but the jury is still out. Transplantation 2003;75:742–743.

38. Prosch S, Docke WD, Reinke P, Volk HD, Kruger DH. Human cytomegalovirus reactivation in bone-marrow-derived granulocyte/monocyte progenitor cells and mature monocytes. Intervirology 1999;42:308–313.

39. Staak K, Prosch S, Stein J, et al. Pentoxifylline promotes replication of human cytomegalovirus in vivo and in vitro. Blood 1997;89:3682–3690.

40. Toyoda M, Galfayan K, Galera OA, Petrosian A, Czer LSC, Jordan SC. Cytomegalovirus infection induces anti-endothelial cell antibodies in cardiac and renal allograft recipients. Transpl Immunol 1997;5:104–111.

41. Kloover JS, Soots AP, Krogerus LA, et al. Rat cytomegalovirus infection in kidney allograft recipients is associated with increased expression of intracellular adhesion molecule-1,

vascular adhesion molecule-1 and their ligands leukocyte function antigen-1 and very late antigen-4 in the graft. Transplantation 2000;69:2641–2647.

42. Streblow DN, Soderberg-Naucler C, Vieira J, et al. The human cytomegalovirus chemokine receptor US28 mediates vascular smooth muscle cell migration. Cell 1999;99:511–520.

43. Gasser M, Waag AM, Laskowski IA, Tilney NL. The influence of donor brain death on short and long-term outcome of solid organ allografts. Ann Transplant 2000;4:61–67.

44. Eich D, Thompson JA, Ko DJ, et al. Hypercholesterolemia in long-term survivors of heart transplantation: an early marker of accelerated coronary artery disease. J Heart Lung Transplant 1991;10:45–49.

45. Isoniemi H, Nurminen M, Tikkanen MJ, et al. Risk factors predicting chronic rejection of renal allografts. Transplantation 1994;57:68–72.

46. Schneeberger H, Schleibner S, Illner WD, Messmer K, Land W. The impact of free radical-mediated reperfusion injury on acute and chronic rejection events following cadaveric renal transplantation. Clin Transpl 1993;7:219–232.

47. Schneeberger H, Aydemir S, Illner WD, Land W. Nonspecific primary ischemia/reperfusion injury in combination with secondary specific acute rejection-mediated injury of human kidney allografts contributes mainly to development of chronic transplant failure. Transplant Proc 1997;29:948–949.

48. Spes CH, Klauss V, Rieber J, et al. Functional and morphological findings in heart transplant recipients with a normal coronary angiogram: an analysis by dobutamine stress echocardiography, intracoronary Doppler and intravascular ultrasound. J Heart Lung Transplant 1999;18:391–398.

49. Kofoed KF, Czemin J, Johnson J, et al. Effects of cardiac allograft vasculopathy on myocardial blood flow, vasodilatory capacity, and coronary vasomotion. Circulation 1997; 95:600–606.

50. Johnson DE, Gao SZ, Schroeder JS, DeCampli WM, Billingham ME. The spectrum of coronary artery pathologic findings in human cardiac allografts. J Heart Transplant 1989; 8:349–359.

51. Yousem SA, Berry GJ, Brunt EM, et al. A working formulation for the standardization of nomenclature in the diagnosis of heart and lung rejection: Lung Rejection Study Group. J Heart Lung Transplant 1990;9:593–601.

52. Solez K. International standardization of criteria for histologic diagnosis of chronic rejection in renal allografts. ClinTransplant 1994;8:345–350.

53. Radio S, Wood S, Wilson J, Lin H, Winters G, McManus B. Allograft vascular disease: comparison of heart and other grafted organs. Transplant Proc 1996;28:496–499.

54. Lim TT, Liang DH, Botas J, Schroeder JS, Oesterle SN, Yeung AC. Role of compensatory enlargement and shrinkage in transplant coronary artery disease. Serial intravascular ultrasound study. Circulation 1997;95:855–859.

55. Pethig K, Heublein B, Wahlers T, Haverich A. Mechanism of luminal narrowing in cardiac allograft vasculopathy: inadequate vascular remodeling rather than intimal hyperplasia is the major predictor of coronary artery stenosis. Am Heart J 1998; 135:628–633.

56. Wong C, Ganz P, Miller L, et al. Role of vascular remodeling in the pathogenesis of early transplant coronary artery disease: a multicenter prospective intravascular ultrasound study. J Heart Lung Transplant 2001;20:385–392.

57. Kobashigawa J, Wener L, Johnson J, et al. Longitudinal study of vascular remodeling in coronary arteries after heart transplantation. J Heart Lung Transplant 2000;19:546–550.

58. Tsutsui H, Ziada KM, Schoenhagen P, et al. Lumen loss in transplant coronary artery disease is a biphasic process involving early intimal thickening and late constrictive remodeling: results from a 5-year serial intravascular ultrasound study. Circulation 2001;104:653–657.

59. Bieber CP, Stinson EB, Shumway NE, Payne R, Kosek J. Cardiac transplantation in man. VII. Cardiac allograft pathology. Circulation 1970;41:753–772.

60. Zheng L, Ordisa BE, Ward C, et al. Airway vascular changes in lung allograft recipients. J Heart Lung Transplant 1999;18:231–238.

61. Isoniemi HM, Krogerus L, von Willebrand E, et al. Histopathological findings in well-functioning, long-term renal allografts. Kidney Int 1992;41:151–160.

62. Solez K, Axelsen RA, Benediktsson H, et al. International standardization of criteria for the histologic diagnosis of renal allograft rejection: the Banff working classification of kidney transplant pathology. Kidney Int 1993;44:411–422.

63. Shi C, Russell ME, Bianchi C, Newell JB, Haber E. Murine model of accelerated transplant arteriosclerosis. Circ Res 1994; 75:199–207.

64. Koulack J, McAlister VC, Giacomantonio CA, Bitter-Suermann H, MacDonald AS, Lee TD. Development of a mouse aortic transplant model of chronic rejection. Microsurgery 1995;16:110–113.

65. Ensminger SM, Billing JS, Morris PJ, Wood KJ. Development of a combined cardiac and aortic transplant model to investigate the development of transplant arteriosclerosis in the mouse. J Heart Lung Transplant 2000;19:1039–1046.

66. Russell PS, Chase CM, Winn HJ, Colvin RB. Coronary atherosclerosis in transplanted mouse hearts. I. Time course and immunogenetic and immunopathological considerations. Am J Pathol 1994;144:260–274.

67. Shi C, Lee WS, He Q, et al. Immunologic basis of transplant-associated arteriosclerosis. Proc Natl Acad Sci USA 1996; 93:4051–4056.

68. Lakkis FG, Arakelov A, Kinieczny BT, Inoue Y. Immunologic "ignorance" of vascularized organ transplants in the absence of secondary lymphoid tissue. Nat Med 2000;6:686–688.

69. Forbes RD, Zheng SX, Gomersall M, al-Saffar M, Guttman RD. Evidence that recipient CD8+ T cell depletion does not alter development of chronic vascular rejection in a rat heart allograft model. Transplantation 1994;57:1238–1246.

70. Chow LH, Huh S, Jiang J, Zhong R, Pickering G. Intimal thickening develops without humoral immunity in a mouse aortic allograft model of chronic vascular rejection. Circulation 1996; 94:3079–3082.

71. Russell PS, Chase CM, Winn HJ, Colvin RB. Coronary atherosclerosis in transplanted mouse hearts. II. Importance of humoral immunity. J Immunol 1994;152:5135–5141.

72. de Heer E, Davidoff A, van der Wal A, van Geest M, Paul LC. Chronic renal allograft rejection in the rat. Transplantation-induced antibodies against basement membrane antigens. Lab Invest 1994;70:494–502.

73. Mauiyyedi S, Pelle PD, Saidman S, et al. Chronic humoral rejection: identification of antibody-mediated chronic renal allograft rejection by C4d deposits in peritubular capillaries. J Am Soc Nephrol 2001;12:574–582.

74. Salomon RN, Hughes CC, Schoen FJ, Payne DD, Pober JS, Libby P. Human coronary transplantation-associated arteriosclerosis: evidence for a chronic immune reaction to activated graft endothelial cells. Am J Pathol 1991;138:791–798.

75. Taylor PM, Rose ML, Yacoub MH. Coronary artery immunogenicity: a comparison between explanted recipient or donor hearts and transplanted hearts. Transpl Immunol 1993;1:294–301.

76. Hosenpud JD, Everett JP, Morris TE, Mauck KA, Shipley GD, Wagner CR. Cardiac allograft vasculopathy. Association with cell-mediated but not humoral alloimmunity to donor-specific vascular endothelium. Circulation 1995;92:205–211.

77. Sinclair RA. Origin of endothelium in human renal allografts. Br Med J 1972;4:15–16.

78. Sinclair RA. The sex chromatin marker in the endothelium of paraffin-embedded renal and cardiac tissue. J Anat 1972; 112:215–221.

79. Hruban RH, Long PP, Perlman EJ, et al. Fluorescence in situ hybridization for the Y-chromosome can be used to detect cells of recipient origin in allografted hearts following cardiac transplantation. Am J Pathol 1993;142:975–980.

80. Bittman I, Dose T, Baretton GB, et al. Cellular chimerism of the lung after transplantation: an interphase cytogenetic study. Am J Clin Pathol 2001;115:525–533.

81. Lagaaij EL, Cramer-Knijnenburg GF, van Kemenade FL, van Es LA, Bruijn JA, van Krieken JH. Endothelial cell chimerism after renal transplantation and vascular rejection. Lancet 2001; 357:33–37.

82. Hinek A, Boyle J, Tabinovitch M. Vascular smooth muscle cell detachment from elastin and migration through elastic laminae is promoted by chondroitin sulfate-induced "shedding" of the 67-kDa cell surface elastin binding protein. Exp Cell Res 1992; 203:344–353.

83. Geraghty JG, Stoltenberg RL, Sollinger HW, Hullett DA. Vascular smooth muscle cells and neointimal hyperplasia in chronic transplant rejection. Transplantation 1996;62:502–509.

84. Schwartz SM. Smooth muscle migration in vascular development and pathogenesis. Transpl Immunol 1997;5:255–260.

85. Holifield B, Helgason T, Jemelka S, et al. Differentiated vascular myocytes: are they involved in neointimal formation? J Clin Invest 1996;97:814–825.

86. Plissonnier D, Nochy D, Poncet P, et al. Sequential immunological targeting of chronic experimental arterial allograft. Transplantation 1995;60:414–424.

87. Hillebrands J, van den Hurk BM, Klatter FA, Popa ER, Nieuwenhuis P, Rozing J. Recipient origin of neointimal vascular smooth muscle cells in cardiac allografts with transplant arteriosclerosis. J Heart Lung Transplant 2000;19:1183–1192.

88. Hillebrands JL, Klatter FA, van den Hurk BM, Popa ER, Niewenhuis P, Rozing J. Origin of neointimal endothelium and alpha-actin-positive smooth muscle cells in transplant arteriosclerosis. J Clin Invest 2001;107:1411–1422.

89. Saiura A, Sata M, Hirata Y, Nagai R, Makuuchi M. Circulating smooth muscle progenitor cells contribute to atherosclerosis. Nat Med 2001;7:382–383.

90. Shimizu K, Sugiyama S, Aikawa M, et al. Host bone-marrow cells are a source of donor intimal smooth muscle-like cells in murine aortic transplant arteriopathy. Nat Med 2001; 7:738–741.

91. Bigaud M, Schraa EO, Andriambeloson E, et al. Complete loss of functional smooth muscle cells precedes vascular remodeling in rat aorta allografts. Transplantation 1999;68:1701–1707.

92. Skarsgard PL, Wang X, McDonald P, et al. Profound inhibition or myogenic tone in rat cardiac allografts is due to eNOS- and iNOS-based nitric oxide and an intrinsic defect in vascular smooth muscle contraction. Circulation 2000; 101:1303–1310.

93. Andriambeloson E, Pally C, Hengerer B, et al. Transplantation-induced endothelial dysfunction as studied in rat aorta allografts. Transplantation 2001;72:1881–1889.

94. Izutani H, Miyagawa S, Mikata S, Shirakura R, Matsuda H. Essential initial immunostimulation in graft coronary arteriosclerosis induction detected by retransplantation technique in rats: the participation of T cell subsets. Transpl Immunol 1997; 5:11–15.

95. Afshari JT, Hutchinson IV, Kay RA. Long-term alloreactive T cell lines and clones express a limited T cell receptor repertoire. Transpl Immunol 1997;5:122–128.

96. Gange K, Brouard S, Giral M, et al. Highly altered V beta repertoire of T cells infiltrating long-term rejected kidney allografts. J Immunol 2000;164:1553–1563.

97. Kim CJ, Khoo JC, Gillotte-Taylor K, et al. Polymerase chain reaction-based method for quantifying recruitment of monocytes to mouse atherosclerotic lesions in vivo: enhancement by tumor necrosis factor-alpha and interleukin-1beta. Arterioscler Thromb Vasc Biol 2000;20:1976–1982.

98. Kitagawa-Sakakida S, Tori M, Li Z, et al. Active cell migration in retransplanted rat cardiac allografts during the course of chronic rejection. J Heart Lung Transplant 2000;19:584–590.

99. Izutani H, Miyagawa S, Shirakura R, et al. Recipient macrophage depletion reduces the severity of graft coronary arteriosclerosis in the rat retransplantation model. Transplant Proc 1997;29:861–862.

100. Azuma H, Nadeau KC, Ishibashi M, Tilney NL. Prevention of functional, structural and molecular changes of chronic rejection of rat renal allografts by a specific macrophage inhibitor. Transplantation 1995;60:1577–1582.

101. Nagano H, Nadeau KC, Kusaka M, Heeman UW, Tilney NL. Infection-associated macrophage activation accelerates chronic renal allograft rejection in rats. Transplantation 1997; 64:1602–1605.

102. Moreno PR, Bernardi VH, Lopez-Cuellar J, et al. Macrophage infiltration predicts restenosis after coronary intervention in patients with unstable angina. Circulation 1996; 94: 3098–3102.

103. Boyle JJ, Bowyer DE, Weissberg PL, Bennett MR. Human blood-derived macrophages induce apoptosis in human plaque-derived vascular smooth muscle cells by Fas-ligand/Fas interactions. Arterioscler Thromb Vasc Biol 2001; 21:1402–1407.

104. Plissonnier D, Henaff M, Poncet P, et al. Involvement of antibody-dependent apoptosis in graft rejection. Transplantation 2000;69:2601–2608.

105. Kling D, Fingerle J, Harlan JM, Lobb RR, Lang F. Mononuclear leukocytes invade rabbit arterial intima during thickening formation via CD18- and VLA-4-dependent mechanisms and stimulate smooth muscle migration. Circ Res 1995; 77:1121–1128.

106. Alpers CE, Davis CL, Barr D, Marsh CL, Hudkins KL. Identification of platelet-derived growth factors of A and B chains in human renal vascular rejection. Am J Pathol 1996; 148:439–451.

107. Shaddy RE, Hammond EH, Yowell RL. Immunohistochemical analysis of platelet-derived growth factor and basic fibroblast growth factor in cardiac biopsy and autopsy specimens of heart transplant patients. Am J Cardiol 1996;77:1210–1215.

108. Waltenberger J, Akyurek ML, Aurivillius M, et al. Ischemia-induced transplant arteriosclerosis in the rat. Induction of peptide growth factor expression. Arterioscler Thromb Vasc Biol 1996;16:1516–1523.

109. Pilmore HL, Eris JM, Paonter DM, Bishop GA, McCaughan GW. Vascular endothelial growth factor expression in human chronic renal allograft rejection. Transplantation 1999;67:929–933.

110. Abe R, Donnelly SC, Peng T, Bucala R, Metz CN. Peripheral blood fibrocytes: differentiation pathway and migration to wound sites. J Immunol 2001;166:7556–7562.

111. Pedagogos E, Hewitson TD, Walker RG, Nicholls KM, Becker GJ. Myofibroblast involvement in chronic transplant rejection. Transplantation 1997;64:1192–1197.

112. Pilmore HL, Painter DM, Bishop GA, McCaughan GW, Eris JM. Early up-regulation of macrophages and myofibroblasts: a new marker for development of chronic renal allograft rejection. Transplantation 2000;69:2658–2662.

113. Grimm PC, Nickerson P, Jeffery J, et al. Neointimal and tubulointerstitial infiltration by recipient mesenchymal cells in chronic renal-allograft rejection. N Engl J Med 2001; 345:93–97.

114. Koskinen PK, Kovanen PT, Lindstedt KA, Lemström KB. Mast cells in acute and chronic rejection of rat cardiac allografts—a major source of basic fibroblast growth factor. Transplantation 2001;71:1741–1747.

115. Pardo J, Diaz L, Errasti P, et al. Mast cells in chronic rejection of human renal allograft. Virchows Arch 2000;437:167–172.

116. Rubin EM, Tall A. Perspectives for vascular genomics. Nature 2000;407:265–269.

117. Sarwal M, Chang S, Barry C, et al. Genomic analysis of renal allograft dysfunction using cDNA microarrays. Transplant Proc 2001;33:297–298.

118. Saiura A, Mataki C, Maurakami T, et al. A comparison of gene expression in murine cardiac allografts and isografts by means of DNA microarray analysis. Transplantation 2001; 72:320–329.

119. Chen J, Myllärniemi M, Akyurek LM, Häyry P, Marsden PA, Paul LC. Identification of differentially expressed genes in rat aortic allograft vasculopathy. Am J Pathol 1996; 149:597–611.

120. Isoniemi H, Taskinen E, Häyry P. Histological chronic allograft damage index accurately predicts chronic renal allograft rejection. Transplantation 1994;58:1195–1198.

121. Yilmaz S, Nutley M, Taskinen E, Paavonen T, Häyry P. Post-transplantation histology as surrogate marker for long-term kidney allograft outcome. Ann Transplant 2000;5:37–43.

122. Sarwal M, Chua MS, Kambham N, et al. Molecular heterogeneity in acute renal allograft rejection identified by DNA microarray profiling. N Engl J Med 2003;349:125–138.

123. Clowes AW, Collazzo RE, Karnovsky MJ. A morphologic and permeability study of luminal smooth muscle cells after arterial injury in the rat. Lab Invest 1978;39:141–150.

124. Mennander A, Tiisala S, Halttunen J, Yilmaz S, Paavonen T, Häyry P. Chronic rejection in rat aortic allografts. An experimental model for transplant arteriosclerosis. Arterioscler Thromb 1991;11:671–680.

125. Fincham JE, Benade AJ, Kruger M, et al. Atherosclerosis: aortic lipid changes induced by diets suggest diffuse disease with focal severity in primates that model human atheromas. Nutrition 1998;14:17–22.

126. Du Toit D, Aavik E, Taskinen E, et al. Structure of carotid artery in baboon and rat and differences in their response to endothelial denudation angioplasty. Ann Med 2001;33:63–78.

127. Wilhem MJ, Pratschke J, Beato F, et al. Activation of the heart by donor brain death accelerates acute rejection after transplantation. Circulation 2000;102:2426–2433.

128. Azuma H, Nadeau K, Takada M, Tilney NL. Initial ischemia/reperfusion injury influences late functional and structural changes in the kidney. Transplant Proc 1997; 29:1528–1529.

129. Cargnoni A, Ceconi C, Bernocchi P, et al. Changes in oxidative stress and cellular redox potential during myocardial storage for transplantation: experimental studies. J Heart Lung Transplant 1999;18:478–487.

130. Akyurek ML, Funa K, Wanders A, Larsson E, Fellström BC. Expression of CD11b and ICAM-1 in an in vivo model of transplant arteriosclerosis. Transpl Immunol 1995;3:107–113.

131. Kauppinen H, Soots A, Krogerus L, et al. Sequential analysis of adhesion molecules and their ligands in rat renal allografts during the development of chronic rejection. Transpl Int 2000; 13:247–254.

132. Raisky O, Morrison KJM, Obadia JF, McGregor J, Yacoub MH, Rose ML. Acute rejection and cardiac graft vasculopathy in the absence of donor-derived ICAM-1 or P-selectin. J Heart Lung Transplant 2001;20:340–349.

133. Hayashi S, Watanabe N, Nakazawa K, et al. Roles of P-selectin in inflammation, neointimal formation, and vascular remodeling in balloon-injured rat carotid arteries. Circulation 2000; 102:1710–1717.

134. Korom S, Hancock WW, Coito A, Kupiec-Weglinski JW. Blockage of very late antigen-4 integrin binding to fibronectin in allograft recipients. II. Treatment with connecting segment-1 peptides prevents chronic rejection by attenuating arteriosclerotic development and suppressing intragraft T cell and macrophage activation. Transplantation 1998;65:854–859.

135. Wu CJ, Kurbegov D, Lattin B, et al. Cytokine gene expression in human cardiac allograft recipients. Transpl Immunol 1994; 2:199–207.

136. Rectenwald JE, Moldawer LL, Huber TS, Seeger JM, Ozaki CK. Direct evidence for cytokine involvement in neointimal hyperplasia. Circulation 2000;102:1697–1702.

137. Pulkkinen VP, Sihvola RK, Koskinen PK, Lemström KB. Inhibition of tumor necrosis factor-alpha does not prevent cardiac allograft arteriosclerosis in the rat. Transplant Proc 2001;33:347.

138. Heidenreich S, Lang D, Tepel M, Rahn KH. Monocyte activation for enhanced tumour necrosis factor-alpha and interleukin 6 production during chronic renal allograft rejection. Transpl Immunol 1994;2:35–40.

139. Tellides G, Tereb DA, Kirkiles-Smith NC, et al. Interferon-gamma elicits arteriosclerosis in the absence of leukocytes. Nature 2000;403:207–211.

140. Nadeau KC, Azuma H, Tilney NL. Sequential cytokine dynamics in chronic rejection of rat renal allografts: roles for cytokines RANTES and MCP-1. Proc Natl Acad Sci USA 1995; 92:8729–8733.

141. Furukawa Y, Matsumori A, Ohashi N, et al. Anti-monocyte chemoattractant protein-1/monocyte chemotactic and activating factor antibody inhibits neointimal hyperplasia in injured rat carotid arteries. Circ Res 1999;84:306–314.

142. Gao W, Topham PS, King JA, et al. Targeting of the chemokine receptor CCR1 suppresses development of acute and chronic cardiac allograft rejection. J Clin Invest 2000; 105:35–44.

143. Yun JJ, Fischbein MP, Laks H, et al. Early and late chemokine production correlated with cellular recruitment in cardiac allograft vasculopathy. Transplantation 2000;69:2515–2524.

144. Belperio JA, Keane MP, Burdick MP, et al. Critical role for the chemokine MCP-1/CCR2 in the pathogenesis of bronchiolitis obliterans syndrome. J Clin Invest 2001;108:547–556.

145. Crawford SE, Huang L, Hsueh W, et al. Captopril and platelet-activating factor (PAF) antagonist prevent cardiac allograft vasculopathy in rats: role of endogenous PAF and PAF-like compounds. J Heart Lung Transplant 1999;18:470–477.

146. Little DM, Haynes LD, Alam T, Geraghty JG, Sollinger HW, Hullett DA. Does transforming growth factor beta 1 play a role in the pathogenesis of chronic allograft rejection? Transpl Int 1999;12:393–401.

147. Aziz T, Hasleton P, Hann AW, Yonan N, Deiraniya A, Hutchinson IV. Transforming growth factor beta in relation to cardiac allograft vasculopathy after heart transplantation. J Thorac Cardiovasc Surg 2000;119:700–708.

148. El-Gamel A, Awad M, Sim E, et al. Transforming growth factor-beta1 and lung allograft fibrosis. Eur J Cardiothorac Surg 1998;13:424–430.

149. Horvath LZ, Friess H, Schilling M, et al. Altered expression of transforming growth factor-betas in chronic renal rejection. Kidney Int 1996;50:489–498.

150. Brenchley PE, Short CD, Roberts IS. Is persistent TGFbeta1 expression the mechanism responsible for chronic renal allograft loss? Nephrol Dial Transplant 1998;13:548–551.

151. Demirci G, Nashan B, Pichlmayr R. Fibrosis in chronic rejection of human liver allografts: expression patterns of transforming growth factor—TGFbeta1 and TGFbeta3. Transplantation 1996;62:1776–1783.

152. Walgenbach KJ, Llull R, Murase N, Starzl TE, Hirner A. Immunocytes of composite tissue allografts express elevated levels of TGF beta mRNA and protein during chronic rejection. Transplant Proc 1997;29:1542.

153. Nakamura K, Kitani A, Strober W. Cell contact-dependent immunosuppression by CD4+CD25+ regulatory T cells is mediated by cell surface-bound transforming growth factor beta. J Exp Med 2001;194:629–644.

154. Ahuja SS, Shrivastava S, Danielpour D, Balow JE, Boumpas DT. Regulation of transforming growth factor-beta 1 and its receptor by cyclosporine in human T lymphocytes. Transplantation 1995;60:718–723.

155. Grainger DJ, Metcalfe JC, Grace AA, Mosedale DE. Transforming growth factor-beta dynamically regulates vascular smooth muscle differentiation in vivo. J Cell Sci 1998; 111:2977–2988.

156. Battegay EJ, Raines EW, Seifert RA, Bowen-Pope DF, Ross R. TGF-beta induces bimodal proliferation of connective tissue cells via complex control of an autocrine PDGF loop. Cell 1990;63:515–524.

157. Lemström K, Sihvola R, Koskinen P. Expression of platelet-derived growth factor in the development of cardiac allograft vasculopathy in the rat. Transplant Proc 1997; 29: 1045–1046.

158. Yamamoto K, Morishita R, Tomita N, et al. Ribozyme oligonucleotide against transforming growth factor-beta inhibited neointimal formation after vascular injury in a rat model. Circulation 2000;102:1308–1314.

159. Myllärniemi M, Calderon Ramirez L, Lemström K, Buchdunger E, Häyry P. Inhibition of platelet-derived growth factor receptor tyrosine kinase inhibits vascular smooth

160. muscle cell migration and proliferation. FASEB J 1997; 11:1119–1126.

160. Leppanen O, Janjic N, Carlsson MA, et al. Intimal hyperplasia recurs after removal of PDGF-AB and -BB inhibition in the rat carotid artery injury model. Arterioscler Thromb Vasc Biol 2000;20:E89–E95.

161. Noiseux N, Boucher CH, Cartier R, Sirois MG. Bolus endovascular PDGFR-beta antisense treatment suppressed intimal hyperplasia in a rat carotid injury model. Circulation 2000;102:1330–1336.

162. Utans U, Arceci RJ, Yamashita Y, Russell ME. Cloning and characterization of allograft inflammatory factor-1: a novel macrophage factor identified in rat cardiac allografts with chronic rejection. J Clin Invest 1995; 95:2954–2962.

163. Autieri MV, Carbone C, Mu A. Expression of allograft inflammatory factor-1 is a marker of activated human vascular smooth muscle cells and arterial injury. Arterioscler Thromb Vasc Biol 2000;20:1737–1744.

164. Autieri MV, Carbone CM. Overexpression of allograft inflammatory factor-1 promotes proliferation of vascular smooth muscle cells by cell cycle deregulation. Arterioscler Thromb Vasc Biol 2001;21:1421–1426.

165. Zhao XM, Hu Y, Miller GG, Mitchell RN, Libby P. Association of thrombospondin-1 and cardiac allograft vasculopathy in human cardiac allografts. Circulation 2001;103:525–531.

166. Noronha IL, Weis H, Hartley B, Wallach D, Cameron JS, Waldehrr R. Expression of cytokines, growth factors and their receptors in renal allograft biopsies. Transplant Proc 1993;25:917–918.

167. Zhao XM, Citrin BS, Miller GG, et al. Association of acidic fibroblast growth factor and untreated low grade rejection with cardiac allograft vasculopathy. Transplantation 1995;59: 1005–1010.

168. Kouwenhoven EA, Stein-Oakley AN, Maguire JA, Jablonski P, de Bruin RWF, Thomson NM. Increased expression of basic fibroblast growth factor during chronic rejection in intestinal transplant is associated with macrophage infiltrates. Transpl Int 1999;12:42–49.

169. Tanabe S, Uabe M, Han YS, et al. Up-regulation of endothelin-converting enzyme during the development of transplant renal arteriosclerosis in human renal allografts. Transplant Proc 1997;29:1517–1519.

170. Simonson MS, Herman WH, Robinson A, Schulak J, Hricik DE. Inhibition of endothelin-converting enzyme attenuates transplant vasculopathy and rejection in rat cardiac allografts. Transplantation 1999;67:1542–1547.

171. Braun C, Conzelmann T, Vetter S, et al. Prevention of chronic renal allograft rejection in rats with an oral endothelin A receptor antagonist. Transplantation 1999;68:739–746.

172. Shears LL II, Kawaharada N, Tzeng E, et al. Inducible nitric oxide synthase suppresses the development of allograft arteriosclerosis. J Clin Invest 1997;100:2035–2042.

173. Iwata A, Sai S, Nitta Y, et al. Liposome-mediated gene transfection of endothelial nitric oxide synthase reduces endothelial activation and leukocyte infiltration in transplanted hearts. Circulation 2001;103:2753–2759.

174. Koglin J, Glysing-Jenson T, Mudgett JS, Russell ME. Exacerbated transplant arteriosclerosis in inducible nitric oxide-deficient mice. Circulation 1998;97:2059–2065.

175. Niebauer J, Schwarzacher SP, Hayase M, et al. L-arginine delivery after balloon angioplasty reduces monocyte binding and induces apoptosis. Circulation 1999;100:1830–1835.

176. Uemura S, Fathman CG, Torhbard JB, Cooke JP. Rapid and efficient vascular transport of arginine polymers inhibits myointimal hyperplasia. Circulation 2000;102:2629–2635.

177. Maines MD, Trakshel GM, Kutty RK. Characterization of two constitutive forms of rat liver microsomal heme oxygenase. Only one molecular species of the enzyme is inducible. J Biol Chem 1986;261:411–419.

178. Sammut IA, Foresti R, Clark JE, et al. Carbon monoxide is a major contributor to the regulation of vascular tone in aortas expressing high levels of haeme oxygenase-1. Br J Pharmacol 1998;125:1437–1444.

179. Foresti R, Motterlini R. The heme oxygenase pathway and its interaction with nitric oxide in the control of cellular homeostasis. Free Rad Res 1999;31:459–475.

180. Hancock WW, Buelow R, Sayegh MH, Turka LA. Antibody-induced transplant arteriosclerosis is prevented by graft expression of anti-oxidant and anti-apoptotic genes. Nat Med 1998;4:1392–1396.

181. Morita T, Kourembanas S. Endothelial cell expression of vasoconstrictors and growth factors is regulated by smooth muscle cell-derived carbon monoxide. J Clin Invest 1995; 96:2676–2682.

182. Ishikawa K, Sugawara D, Wang X, et al. Heme oxygenase-1 inhibits atherosclerotic lesion formation in LDL-receptor knockout mice. Circ Res 2001;88:506–512.

183. Juan SH, Lee TS, Tseng KW, et al. Adenovirus-mediated heme oxygenase-1 gene transfer inhibits the development of atherosclerosis in apolipoprotein E-deficient mice. Circulation 2001;104:1519–1525.

184. Tulis DA, Durante W, Peyton KJ, Evans AJ, Schafer AI. Heme oxygenase-1 attenuates vascular remodeling following balloon injury in rat carotid arteries. Atherosclerosis 2001;155:113–122.

185. Tulis DA, Durante W, Liu X, Evans AJ, Peyton KJ, Schafer SI. Adenovirus-mediated heme oxygenase-1 gene delivery inhibits injury-induced vascular neointimal formation. Circulation 2001;104:2710–2715.

186. Motterlini R, Clark JE, Foresti R, Sarathchandra P, Mann BE, Green CJ. Carbon monoxide-releasing molecules: characterization of biochemical and vascular activities. Circ Res 2002;90:E17–E24.

187. Motterlini R, Mann BE, Johnson TR, Clark JE, Foresti R, Green CJ. Bioactivity and pharmacological actions of carbon monoxide-releasing molecules. Curr Pharm Des 2003; 9:2525–2539.

188. The International SNP Map Working Group. A map of human genome sequence variation containing 1.24 million single nucleotide polymorphisms. Nature 2001;409:928–933.

189. Conne B, Stutz A, Vassalli JD. The 3' untranslated region of messenger RNA: a molecular 'hotspot' for pathology? Nat Med 2000;6:637–641.

190. Randall LL, Hardy SJS. Unity in function in the absence of consensus in sequence: role of leader peptides in export. Science 1989;243:1156–1159.

191. Proudfoot N. Connecting transcription to messenger RNA processing. Trends Biochem Sci 2000;25:290–293.

192. Lo HS, Wang Z, Hu Y, et al. Allelic variation in gene expression is common in the human genome. Genome Res 2003;13:1855–1862.

193. Derynck R, Rhee L, Chen EY, van Tilburg A. Intron-exon structure of the human transforming growth factor-beta precursor gene. Nucleic Acids Res 1987;15:3188–3189.

194. Awad MR, El-Gamel A, Hasleton P, Turner DM, Sinnott PJ, Hutchinson IV. Transforming growth factor-beta1 gene: association with transforming growth factor-beta1 production,

195. El-Gamel A, Awad M, Sim E, et al. Transforming growth factor-beta1 and lung allograft fibrosis. Eur J Cardiothorac Surg 1998;13:424–430.

196. El-Gamel A, Awad MR, Hasleton PS, et al. Transforming growth factor-beta (TGF-beta1) genotype and lung allograft fibrosis. J Heart Lung Transplant 1999;18:517–523.

197. Densem CG, Hutchinson IV, Cooper A, Yonan N, Brooks NH. Polymorphism of the transforming growth factor-beta 1 gene correlates with the development of coronary vasculopathy following cardiac transplantation. J Heart Lung Transplant 2000;19:551–556.

198. Vamvakopoulos JE, Taylor CJ, Green C, et al. Interleukin 1 and chronic rejection: possible genetic links in human heart allografts. Am J Transplant 2002;2:76–83.

199. Vamvakopoulos J, Green C, Metcalfe S. Genetic control of IL-1beta bioactivity through differential regulation of the IL-1 receptor antagonist. Eur J Immunol 2002;32:2988–2996.

200. Rigat B, Hubert C, Alhenc-Gelas F, Cambien F, Corvol P, Soubrier F. An insertion/deletion polymorphism in the angiotensin I-converting enzyme gene accounting for half of the variance of serum enzyme levels. J Clin Invest 1990;86:1343–1346.

201. Pethig K, Heublein B, Hoffman A, Borlak J, Wahlers T, Haverich A. ACE gene polymorphism is associated with the development of allograft vascular disease in heart transplant recipients. J Heart Lung Transplant 2000;19:1175–1182.

202. Cunningham DA, Crisp SJ, Barbir M, Lazem F, Dunn MJ, Yacoub MH. Donor ACE gene polymorphism: a genetic risk factor for accelerated coronary sclerosis following cardiac transplantation. Eur Heart J 1998;19:319–325.

203. Benza RL, Grenett HE, Bourge RC, et al. Gene polymorphisms for plasminogen activator inhibitor-1/tissue plasminogen activator and development of allograft coronary artery disease. Circulation 1998;98:2248–2254.

204. Borozdenkova S, Smith J, Marshall S, Yacoub M, Rose M. Identification of ICAM-1 polymorphism that is associated with protection from transplant associated vasculopathy after cardiac transplantation. Hum Immunol 2001;62:247–255.

205. McLaren AJ, Marshall SE, Haldar NA, et al. Adhesion molecule polymorphisms in chronic renal graft rejection. Kidney Int 1999;55:1977–1982.

206. Henry ML. Cyclosporine and tacrolimus (FK506): a comparison of efficacy and safety profiles. Clin Transplant 1999; 13:209–220.

207. Opelz G, for the Collaborative Transplant Study. Influence of treatment with cyclosporine, azathioprine and steroids on chronic allograft failure. Kidney Int 1995;48:S89–S92.

208. Koskinen PK, Lemström KB, Häyry PJ. How cyclosporine modifies histological and molecular events in the vascular wall during chronic rejection of rat cardiac allografts. Am J Pathol 1995;146:972–980.

209. Sarwal MM, Yorgin PD, Alexander S, et al. Promising early outcomes with a novel, complete steroid avoidance immunosuppression protocol in pediatric renal transplantation. Transplantation 2001;72:13–21.

210. Sivaraman P, Nussbaumer G, Landsberg D. Lack of long-term benefits of steroid withdrawal in renal transplant recipients. Am J Kid Dis 2001;37:1162–1169.

211. Kahan DB, Welsh M, Schoenberg L, et al. Variable oral absorption of cyclosporine: a biopharmaceutical risk factor for chronic renal allograft rejection. Transplantation 1996; 62:599–606.

212. Clark B, Stoves J, Cole JY, Wortley A, Gooi HC, Newstead CG. Demonstration of the inter-individual variation in cyclosporine A (CsA) responsiveness using an in vitro assay system. Eur J Immunogenet 2000;27:278.

213. Batiuk TD, Pazderka F, Enns J, DeCastro L, Halloran F. Cyclosporine inhibition of calcineurin activity in human leukocytes in vivo is rapidly reversible. J Clin Invest 1995;96:1254–1260.

214. Coon JS, Wang Y, Bines SD, Markham PN, Chong ASF, Gebel HM. Multidrug resistance activity in human lymphocytes. Human Immunol 1991;32:134–140.

215. Chaudhary PM, Mechetner EB, Roninson IB. Expression and activity of the multidrug resistance P-glycoprotein in human peripheral blood lymphocytes. Blood 1992;80:2735–2739.

216. Cumber PM, Jacobs A, Hoy T, Whittaker JA, Tsuruo T, Padua RA. Increased drug accumulation ex vivo with cyclosporin in chronic lymphatic leukemia and its relationship to epitope masking of P-glycoprotein. Leukemia 1991;5:1050–1053.

217. Yacyshyn BR, Bowen-Yacyshyn MB, Pilarski LM. Inhibition by rapamycin of P-glycoprotein 170-mediated export from normal lymphocytes. Scand J Immunol 1996;43:449–455.

218. Kemnitz J, Uysal A, Haverich A, et al. Multidrug resistance in heart transplant patients: a preliminary communication on a possible mechanism of therapy-resistant rejection. J Heart Lung Transplant 1991;10:201–210.

219. Yousem SA, Sartori D, Sonmez-Alpan E. Multidrug resistance in lung allograft recipients: a preliminary communication on a possible mechanism of therapy resistant rejection. J Heart Lung Transplant 1993;12:20–26.

220. Garcia del Moral R, O'Valle F, Andujar M, et al. Relationship between P-glycoprotein expression and cyclosporin A in kidney. An immunohistological and cell culture study. Am J Pathol 1995;146:398–408.

221. Melk A, Daniel V, Weimer R, et al. P-glycoprotein expression is not a useful predictor of acute or chronic kidney graft rejection. Transpl Int 1999;12:10–17.

222. Li B, Sehajpal PK, Khanna A, et al. Differential regulation of transforming growth factor beta and interleukin 2 genes in human T cells: demonstration by usage of novel competitor DNA constructs in the quantitative polymerase chain reaction. J Exp Med 1991;174:1259–1262.

223. Prashar Y, Khanna A, Sehajpal P, Sharma VK, Suthanthiran M. Stimulation of transforming growth factor-beta 1 transcription by cyclosporine. FEBS Lett 1995;358:109–112.

224. Shin GT, Khanna A, Sharma VK, et al. In vivo hyperexpression of transforming growth factor-beta 1 in humans: stimulation by cyclosporine. Transplant Proc 1997;29:284.

225. El-Gamel A, Awad M, Yonan N, et al. Does cyclosporine promote the secretion of transforming growth factor-beta 1 following pulmonary transplantation? Trans Proc 1998;30:1525–1527.

226. Kumano K, He N, Ma P, Endo T, Schiller B. Role of transforming growth factor and monocyte chemoattractant protein in FK506-induced nephropathy in the rat. Transplant Proc 1997;29:1250–1252.

227. Prieto M, Escallada R, Cobo M, et al. Oral arginine restores endothelium-dependent vasodilation in cyclosporine-treated rats. Transplant Proc 1997;29:1244–1245.

228. Danovitch G, Deierhoi M, Ferguson R, Linna J, Monroe S, Tomlanovich S, for The Mycophenolate Mofetil Renal Refractory Rejection Study Group. Mycophenolate mofetil for the treatment of refractory, acute, cellular renal transplant rejection. Transplantation 1996;61:722–729.

229. Tomlanovich S, et al., for the US Renal Transplant Mycophenolate Mofetil Study Group. Mycophenolate mofetil in cadaveric renal transplantation. Am J Kidney Dis 1999; 34:296–303.

230. Nair RV, Cao W, Morris RE. Inhibition of smooth muscle cell proliferation in vitro by leflunomide, a new immunosuppressant, is antagonized by uridine. Immunol Lett 1995;48:77–80.

231. Xiao F, Chong A, Shen J, et al. Pharmacologically induced regression of chronic transplant rejection. Transplantation 1995;60:1065–1072.

232. Brinkman V, Pinschewer D, Chiba K, Feng L. FTY720: a novel transplantation drug that modulates lymphocyte traffic rather than activation. Trends Pharmacol Sci 2000;21:49–52.

233. Weir MR, Anderson L, Fink JC, et al. A novel approach to the treatment of chronic allograft nephropathy. Transplantation 1997;64:1706–1710.

234. Savikko J, Von Willebrand E, Häyry P. Leflunomide analogue FK778 is vasculoprotective independent of its immunosuppressive effect: potential applications for restenosis and chronic rejection. Transplantation 2003;76:455–458.

235. Raisanen-Sokolowski A, Aho P, Tufveson G, Häyry P. Effect of 15-deoxyspergualin on allograft arteriosclerosis and growth factor synthesis in the rat. Transpl Int 1994;7: S376–S377.

236. Groth CG, Backman L, Morales JM, et al., for the Sirolimus European Renal Transplant Study Group. Sirolimus (rapamycin)-based therapy in human renal transplantation: similar efficacy and different toxicity compared with cyclosporine. Transplantation 1999;67:1036–1042.

237. Kreis H, Cisterne JM, Land W, et al., for the Sirolimus European Renal Transplant Study Group. Sirolimus in association with mycophenolate mofetil introduction for the prevention of acute graft rejection in renal allograft recipients. Transplantation 2000;69:1252–1260.

238. Gregory CR, Huie P, Billingham ME, Morris RE. Rapamycin inhibits arterial intimal thickening caused by both alloimmune and mechanical injury. Its effect on cellular, growth factor, and cytokine response in injured vessels. Transplantation 1993;55:1409–1418.

239. Suzuki T, Kopia G, Hayashi S, et al. Stent-based delivery of sirolimus reduces neointimal formation in a porcine coronary model. Circulation 2001;104:1188–1193.

240. Elloso MM, Azrolan N, Sehgal SN, et al. Protective effect of the immunosuppressant sirolimus against aortic atherosclerosis in apoE-deficient mice. Am J Transplant 2003;3:562–569.

241. Sousa JE, Costs MA, Abizaid AC, et al. Sustained suppression of neointimal proliferation by sirolimus-eluting stents: one-year angiographic and intravascular ultrasonic follow-up. Circulation 2001;104:2007–2011.

242. Rensing BJ, Vos J, Smits PC, et al. Coronary restenosis elimination with a sirolimus eluting stent: first European human experience with 6-month angiographic and intravascular ultrasonic follow-up. Eur Heart J 2001;22:2125–2130.

243. Degertekin M, Serruys PW, Foley DP, et al. Persistent inhibition of neointimal hyperplasia after sirolimus-eluting stent implantation: long-term (up to 2 years) clinical, angiographic, and intravascular ultrasound follow-up. Circulation 2002;106:1610–1613.

244. Sousa JE, Costa MA, Sousa AG, et al. Two-year angiographic and intravascular ultrasound follow-up after implantation of sirolimus-eluting stents in human coronary arteries. Circulation 2003;107:381–383.

245. Brara PS, Moussavian M, Grise MA, et al. Pilot trial of oral rapamycin for recalcitrant restenosis. Circulation 2003;107: 1722–1724.
246. Mancini D, Pinney S, Burkhoff D, et al. Use of rapamycin slows progression of cardiac transplantation vasculopathy. Circulation 2003;108:48–53.
247. Cao W, Mohacsi P, Shorthouse R, Pratt R, Morris RE. Effects of rapamycin on the growth factor-stimulated vascular smooth muscle cell DNA synthesis: inhibition of basic fibroblast growth factor and platelet-derived growth factor action and antagonism of rapamycin by FK506. Transplantation 1995;59:390–395.
248. Nair RV, Huang X, Shorthouse R, et al. Antiproliferative effect of rapamycin on growth factor-stimulated human adult lung fibroblasts in vitro may explain its superior efficacy for prevention and treatment of allograft obliterative airway disease in vivo. Transplant Proc 1997;29:614–615.
249. Pham SM, Shears LL, Kawaharada N, Li S, Venkataramanan R, Sehgal S. High local production of nitric oxide as a possible mechanism by which rapamycin prevents transplant arteriosclerosis. Transplant Proc 1998;30:953–954.
250. Woltman AM, de Fijter JW, Kamerling SWA, et al. Rapamycin induces apoptosis in monocyte- and CD34-derived dendritic cells but not in monocytes and macrophages. Blood 2001;98:174–180.
251. Kobashigawa JA, Katznelson S, Laks H, et al. Effect of pravastatin on outcomes after cardiac transplantation. N Engl J Med 1995;333:621–627.
252. Katznelson S, Kobashingawa JA. Dual roles of HMG-CoA reductase inhibitors in solid organ transplantation: lipid lowering and immunosuppression. Kidney Int Suppl 1995; 52:S112–S115.
253. Maggard MA, Ke B, Wang T, et al. Effects of pravastatin on chronic rejection of rat cardiac allografts. Transplantation 1998;65:149–155.
254. Shovman O, Levy Y, Gilburd B, Shoenfeld Y. Antiinflammatory and immunomodulatory properties of statins. Immunol Res 2002;25:271–285.
255. Vamvakopoulos JE, Green C. HMG-CoA reductase inhibition aborts functional differentiation and triggers apoptosis in cultured primary human monocytes: a potential mechanism of statin-mediated vasculoprotection. BMC Cardiovasc Disord 2003;3:6.
256. Hwang MW, Matsumori A, Furukawa Y, et al. FTY720, a new immunosuppressant, promotes long term graft survival and inhibits the progression of graft coronary artery disease in a murine model of cardiac transplantation. Circulation 1999; 100:1322–1329.
257. Nickolova Z, Hof A, Rudin M, Baumlin Y, Kraus G, Hof RP. Prevention of graft vessel disease by combined FTY720/cyclosporine. A treatment in a rat carotid artery transplantation model. Transplantation 2000;69:2525–2530.
258. Hachida M, Zhang X, Lu H, Hoshi H, Koyanagi H. Multiglycosidorum tripterygii, a new immunosuppressant, supresses coronary arteriosclerosis after heart transplantation. J Heart Lung Transplant 1999;18:248–254.
259. Curran M, Noble S. Valganciclovir. Drugs 2001;61:1145–1150.
260. Tullius SG, Hancock WW, Heemann U, Azuma H, Tilney NL. Reversibility of chronic renal allograft rejection. Critical effect of time after transplantation suggests both host immune dependent and independent phases of progressive injury. Transplantation 1994;58:93–99.
261. Brazelton TR, Adams BA, Cheung AC, Morris RE. Progression of obliterative airway disease occurs despite the removal of immune reactivity by retransplantation. Transplant Proc 1997; 29:2613.
262. Izutani H, Miyagawa S, Shirakura R, et al. Evidence that graft coronary arteriosclerosis begins in the early phase after transplantation and progresses without chronic immunoreaction. Histopathological analysis using a retransplantation model. Transplantation 1995;60:1073–1079.
263. Mennander A, Häyry P. Reversibility of allograft arteriosclerosis after retransplantation to donor strain. Transplantation 1996;62:526–529.
264. Ikonen TS, Gummert JF, Hayase M, et al. Sirolimus (rapamycin) halts and reverses progression of allograft vascular disease in non-human primates. Transplantation 2000;70:969–975.
265. Ikonen TS, Gummert JF, Hayase M, et al. Efficacies of sirolimus (rapamycin) and cyclosporine in allograft vascular disease in non-human primates: trough levels of sirolimus correlate with inhibition of progression of arterial intimal thickening. Transpl Int 2000;13:S314–S320.
266. Ferns GA, Raines EW, Sprugle KH, Motani AS, Reidy MA, Ross R. Inhibition of neointimal smooth muscle accumulation after angioplasty by an antibody to PDGF. Science 1991; 253:1129–1132.
267. Jawien A, Bowen-Pope DF, Linder V, Schwartz SM, Clowes AW. Platelet-derived growth factor promotes smooth muscle migration and intimal thickening in a rat model of balloon angioplasty. J Clin Invest 1992;89:507–511.
268. Rutherford C, Martin W, Salame M, Carrier M, Anggard E, Ferns G. Substantial inhibition of neointimal response to balloon injury in the rat carotid artery using a combination of antibodies to platelet-derived growth factor-BB and basic fibroblast growth factor. Atherosclerosis 1997;130:45–51.
269. Hart CE, Kraiss LW, Vergel S, et al. PDGFbeta receptor blockade inhibits intimal hyperplasia in the baboon. Circulation 1999;99:564–569.
270. Sirois MG, Simons M, Edelman ER. Antisense oligonucleotide inhibition of PDGFR-beta receptor subunit expression directs suppression of intimal thickening. Circulation 1997;95:669–676.
271. Häyry P, Myllärniemi M, Aavik E, et al. Stabile D-peptide analog of insulin-like growth factor-1 inhibits smooth muscle cell proliferation after carotid ballooning injury in the rat. FASEB J 1995;9:1336–1344.
272. Myllärniemi M, Calderon L, Lemström K, Buchdunger E, Häyry P. Inhibition of platelet-derived growth factor receptor tyrosine kinase inhibits vascular smooth muscle cell migration and proliferation. FASEB J 1997;11:1119–1126.
273. Banai S, Wolf Y, Golomb G, et al. PDGF-receptor tyrosine kinase blocker AG1295 selectively attenuates vascular smooth muscle cell growth in vitro and reduces neointimal formation after balloon angioplasty in swine. Circulation 1998;97:1960–1969.
274. Saito S, Foegh ML, Lou H, Aras R, Ramwell PW. Oestrogen and transplant vascular disease. Clin Exp Pharmacol Physiol 1999;26:137–143.
275. Smith LE, Shen W, Perruzzi C, et al. Regulation of vascular endothelial growth factor-dependent retinal neovascularization by insulin-like growth factor-1 receptor. Nat Med 1999;5: 1390–1395.
276. Lou H, Zhao Y, Delafontaine P, et al. Estrogen effects on insulin-like growth factor-I (IGF-I)-induced cell proliferation and IGF-I expression in native and allograft vessels. Circulation 1997;96:927–933.

277. Häyry P, Raisanen A, Ustinov J, Mennander A, Paavonen T. Somatostatin analog lanreotide inhibits myocyte replication and several growth factors in allograft arteriosclerosis. FASEB J 1993;7:1055–1060.

278. Howell M, Orskov H, Frystyk J, Flyvberg A, Gronbaek H, Foegh M. Lanreotide, a somatostatin analogue, reduces insulin-like growth factor I accumulation in proliferating aortic tissue in rabbits in vivo. A preliminary study. Eur J Endocrinol 1994; 130:422–425.

279. Grant MB, Wargovich TJ, Ellis EA, Caballero S, Mansour M, Pepine CJ. Localization of insulin-like growth factor I and inhibition of coronary smooth muscle growth by somatostatin analogues in human coronary smooth muscle cells. A potential treatment for restenosis? Circulation 1994;89:1511–1517.

280. Yumi K, Fagin JA, Yamashita M, et al. Direct effects of somatostatin analog octreotide on insulin-like growth factor I in the arterial wall. Lab Invest 1997;76:329–338.

281. Sihvola R, Koskinen P, Myllärniemi M, et al. Prevention of cardiac allograft arteriosclerosis by protein tyrosine kinase inhibitor selective for platelet-derived growth factor receptor. Circulation 1999;99:2295–2301.

282. Savikko J, Taskinen E, von Willebrand E. Chronic allograft nephropathy is prevented by inhibition of platelet-derived growth factor receptor: tyrosine kinase inhibitors as a potential therapy. Transplantation 2003;75:1147–1153.

283. Stampfer MJ, Colditz GA, Willett WC, et al. Postmenopausal estrogen therapy and cardiovascular disease. Ten-year follow-up from the nurses' health study. N Engl J Med 1991;325:756–762.

284. Grady D, Rubin SM, Petitti DB, et al. Hormone therapy to prevent disease and prolong life in postmenopausal women. Ann Intern Med 1992;117:1016–1037.

285. Kuiper GG, Enmark E, Pelto-Huikko M, Nilsson S, Gustafsson JA. Cloning of a novel receptor expressed in rat prostate and ovary. Proc Natl Acad Sci USA 1996;93:5925–5930.

286. Aavik E, du Toit D, Myburgh E, Frösen J, Häyry P. Estrogen receptor beta dominates in baboon carotid after endothelial denudation injury. Mol Cell Endocrinol 2001;182:91–98.

287. Savolainen H, Frösen J, Petrov L, Aavik E, Häyry P. Expression of estrogen receptor sub-types alpha and beta in acute and chronic cardiac allograft vasculopathy. J Heart Lung Transplant 2001;20:1252–1264.

288. Mäkelä S, Savolainen H, Aavik E, et al. Differentiation between vasculoprotective and uterotrophic effects of ligands with different binding affinities to estrogen receptors alpha and beta. Proc Natl Acad Sci USA 1999;96:7077–7082.

289. Patel YC, Greenwood M, Panetta R, et al. Molecular biology of somatostatin receptor subtypes. Metabolism 1996;45:31–38.

290. Rohrer SP, Birzin ET, Mosley RT, et al. Rapid identification of subtype-selective agonists of the somatostatin receptor through combinatorial chemistry. Science 1998;282:737–740.

291. Emanuelsson H, Beatt KJ, Bagger JP, et al. Long-term effects of angiographic restenosis. European Angiopeptin Study Group. Circulation 1995;91:1689–1696.

292. Eriksen UH, Amtorp O, Bagger JP, et al. Randomized double-blind Scandinavian trial of angiopeptin versus placebo for the prevention of clinical events and restenosis after coronary angioplasty. Am Heart J 1995;130:1–8.

293. von Essen R, Ostermaier R, Grube E, et al. Effects of octreotide treatment on restenosis after coronary angioplasty: results of the VERAS study. Circulation 1997;96:1482–1487.

294. Khare S, Kumar U, Sasi R, et al. Differential regulation of somatostatin receptors types 1-5 in rat aorta after angioplasty. FASEB J 1999;13:387–394.

295. Aavik E, Luoto NM, Petrov L, Aavik S, Patel YC, Häyry P. Elimination of vascular fibrointimal hyperplasia by somatostatin receptor 1,4-selective agonist. FASEB J 2002; 16:724–726.

296. Häyry P, du Toit D, Sarwal M, Aavik E, Hoffrén A, Vamvakopoulos J. Rational drug design: making drugs that make a difference. Transplant Proc 2002;34:2000–2002.

297. Kalow W. Pharmacogenetics, pharmacogenomics and pharmacobiology. Clin Pharmacol Ther 2001;70:1–4.

298. Adam GI, Reneland R, Andersson M, Risinger C, Nilsson M, Lewander T. Pharmacogenomics to predict drug response. Pharmacogenomics 2000;1:5–14.

299. McLeod HL, Evans WE. Pharmacogenomics: unlocking the human genome for better drug therapy. Annu Rev Pharmacol Toxicol 2001;41:101–121.

300. Wieczorek SJ, Tsongalis GJ. Pharmacogenomics: will it change the field of medicine? Clin Chim Acta 2001;308:1–8.

301. Schmitz G, Aslanidis C, Lacker KJ. Pharmacogenomics: implications for laboratory medicine. Clin Chem Acta 2001;308:43–45.

16 Thrombolysis

Scientific Basis for Current Therapy

Guy L. Reed III, MD

CONTENTS

INTRODUCTION

Thrombotic occlusion of a coronary artery is the most common cause of myocardial infarction *(1–3)*. In addition, thrombotic vascular occlusion is an important cause of strokes, peripheral arterial occlusion (gangrene), venous thrombosis, and pulmonary embolism. For the last century, these occlusive diseases have been the major causes of death in the United States and are emerging as chief causes of mortality worldwide. The discovery that plasminogen activators enzymatically dissolve thrombi (fibrinolysis) and save patients with myocardial infarction has revolutionized the treatment of cardiovascular disease *(4,5)*. In addition, this discovery has helped to translate results of basic research into clinically useful therapeutic agents that have improved the prevention and treatment of thrombotic vascular diseases.

Thrombus formation is triggered by vascular injury. Damage to endothelial cells and the rupture of arteriosclerotic plaques are the most common causes of coronary artery thrombosis associated with myocardial infarction *(6)*. Thrombi comprise platelet aggregates surrounded by a fibrin meshwork (Fig. 1). Thrombin, the central enzyme in thrombosis, is produced by the coagulation cascade and activates platelets to cause platelet secretion and aggregation, which amplifies the thrombotic process. Fibrinogen, a soluble protein, is converted to the polymer fibrin by thrombin. Furthermore, thrombin activates factor XIII, which covalently cross-links fibrin chains to other fibrin chains, fibrin to α2-antiplasmin (α2AP), and fibrin to thrombin-activatable fibrinolysis inhibitor (TAFI) (Fig. 2). These molecular cross-links increase the mechanical stability of the thrombus and its resistance to fibrinolysis.

By cutting the polymer fibrin into soluble fragments in the process of fibrinolysis, the enzyme plasmin dissolves thrombi in the process of thrombolysis (Fig. 1). Plasmin is generated from the proenzyme (zymogen) plasminogen by plasminogen activators (Fig. 2) such as tissue-type plasminogen activator (t-PA), urinary-type plasminogen activator (u-PA), *Desmodus rotundus* plasminogen activator (DSPA), streptokinase (SK), and staphylokinase (SAK) (Table 1). Physiologic or endogenous fibrinolysis is thought to occur when endogenous plasminogen activators (primarily t-PA) convert fibrin-bound plasminogen to plasmin. Plasmin degrades the various forms of fibrin at different rates; non-cross-linked

From: *Contemporary Cardiology: Principles of Molecular Cardiology*
Edited by: M. S. Runge and C. Patterson © Humana Press Inc., Totowa, NJ

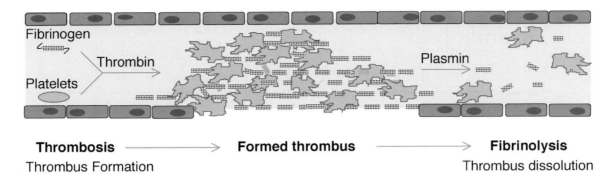

Fig. 1. Overview of thrombosis and fibrinolysis. A thrombus is formed when thrombin (produced by coagulation enzymes) activates platelets to secrete prothrombotic molecules and to aggregate with each other. In addition, thrombin cleaves fibrinogen to fibrin to form the protein matrix of the thrombus. Plasmin, which is generated by plasminogen activators, cleaves fibrin into soluble fragments and dissolves the thrombus in a process known as fibrinolysis.

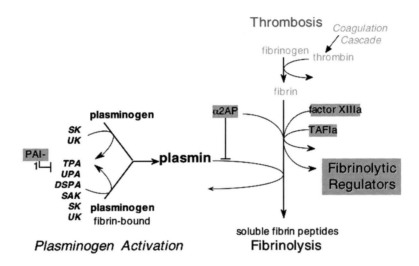

Fig. 2. Molecular regulation of fibrinolysis. Plasmin is generated from plasminogen by the fibrin-dependent plasminogen activators, tissue plasminogen activator (t-PA), urinary-type plasminogen activator (u-PA), *Desmodus rotundus* plasminogen activator (DSPA), and staphylokinase (SAK), and by the fibrin-independent plasminogen activators, streptokinase (SK) and urokinase (UK). Several molecules (fibrinolytic regulators) control the generation or fibrinolytic efficacy of plasmin. Plasminogen activator inhibitor 1 (PAI-1) blocks the activity of t-PA and u-PA. α2-antiplasmin (α2AP) is an extremely fast inhibitor of plasmin that can block fibrinolysis. Activated thrombin activated fibrinolysis inhibitor (TAFIa) cleaves the carboxy terminal lysines of fibrin which prevents the acceleration of fibrinolysis that occurs after early digestion of fibrin by plasmin. Activated factor XIII (factor XIIIa) reduces the fibrinolytic effects of plasmin by cross-linking fibrin chains together and by cross-linking α2AP and TAFI to fibrin.

fibrin lyses quickly while fully cross-linked fibrin resists lysis. Plasminogen accumulates on fibrin at sites of fibrinolysis. The rate of fibrinolysis is related to both the plasminogen bound to fibrin and the plasminogen available in the fluid surrounding the clot *(7–15)*.

Pharmacologic fibrinolysis or thrombolysis occurs when plasmin is generated by an administered plasminogen activator. Important biochemical differences are seen between the plasminogen activators, particularly in how efficiently they activate non-fibrin-bound

and fibrin-bound plasminogen. t-PA, u-PA, DSPA, and SAK activate primarily fibrin-bound plasminogen when used in humans, whereas SK and urokinase (two-chain u-PA) efficiently activate both non-fibrin-bound and fibrin-bound plasminogen (Fig. 2). For both physiologic and pharmacologic plasminogen activation, at least four factors affect the concentration of plasmin available for fibrinolysis: the concentration of plasminogen (particularly the fibrin-bound species), the concentration of plasminogen activator, the concentration

Table 1
Plasminogen Activators Currently Available or In Clinical Trials

Plasminogen activator	Type	Source	Fibrin-dependent?	Trade name
Tissue plasminogen activator	Serine protease	Tissue, R	++	Activase
Reteplase	Serine protease derivative of t-PA	R	+ (89)	Retavase
Lanoteplase	Serine protease derivative of t-PA	R	+	
Tenecteplase	Serine protease mutant of t-PA	R	+++ (94)	TNKase
Single chain urinary-type plasminogen activator (SCUPA)	Serine protease-zymogen	Cells, R	++	Saruplase
Urokinase (UK)	Serine pProtease-cleavage product of SCUPA	Cells, urine, R	No	
	High-molecular weight UK (54 kDa)			
	Low-molecular weight UK (33 kDa)	Abbokinase		
Desmodus rotundus plasminogen activator	Serine protease zymogen	Vampire bats, R	++++	
Staphylokinase	Cofactor	*Staphyococcus sp.*, R	++	*SAK-Star*
Streptokinase	Cofactor activator engineered mutants used in clinical trials (136)	*Streptococcus sp.*, R.	No	Streptase, Kabikinase
Anisoylated plasmin(ogen) streptokinase activator complex	Complex of SK and Lys-plasmin with anisoylated active site (248)	SK and human plasma plasminogen	No	Eminase

t-PA, tissue-type plasminogen activator; R, recombinant.

of plasminogen activator inhibitor-1 (PAI-1), and the amount of α2AP.

Another important biochemical process that determines the efficacy of thrombolysis is the rate of thrombus generation or thrombosis. Preventing the generation of thrombin from prothrombin by inactivating factor Xa, prothrombinase complex, factor VIIa, or other factors can reduce thrombosis. In addition, thrombin may be directly inhibited by hirudin or active site agents, or by heparin, which potentiates its primary physiologic inhibitor antithrombin III.

Fibrinolytic regulation (Fig. 2) is the process that controls the net amount of thrombus lysed by plasmin. Fibrinolytic regulators are molecular factors in the thrombus or in the thrombus milieu that block or impede the net dissolution of thrombi (Table 2). The cellular composition of the thrombus (platelet-rich vs fibrin-rich), the thrombus mass, thrombus age, blood flow, and other factors affect lysis by pharmacologic plasminogen activators (16–18). The amount of functional plasminogen activator available is partially regulated by PAI-1, a potent serine protease inhibitor of t-PA and u-PA (Fig. 2) (19). Studies suggest that PAI-1 is important for regulating the physiologic

lysis of venous and arterial thrombi by endogenous plasminogen activators (19–21). However, PAI-1 probably does not account for the thrombus resistance seen during pharmacologic lysis with SK, which is not inhibited by PAI-1, or with conventional doses of t-PA, where t-PA levels may exceed PAI-1 levels by 100-fold. The rapid inhibitor of plasmin, α2AP, is an important regulator of endogenous fibrinolysis and pharmacologic lysis by plasminogen activators. A serine protease inhibitor, α2AP, instantaneously inactivates non-fibrin-bound plasmin and fibrin-bound plasmin at a slower rate of about 50-fold (22–24). The potent inhibitory effects of α2AP alter the amount of plasmin available for lysis. In addition, activated factor XIII (factor XIIIa) increases the resistance of thrombi to dissolution by plasmin by cross-linking fibrin chains together and linking α2AP and thrombin-activatable fibrinolysis inhibitor (TAFIa) to fibrin (see below). Finally, because it cleaves carboxy-terminal lysine residues from fibrin, TAFIa reduces the fibrinolytic effects of endogenous and pharmacological plasminogen activators (25).

The fibrinolytic system has been studied in mice with targeted gene deletions (Table 3) (26–31). Although mice

Table 2
Critical Pro-fibrinolytic and Anti-fibrinolytic Molecules In Humans

	Function	Source	Size (kDa)	Plasma concentration
Pro-fibrinolytic molecules				
Plasminogen	Fibrinolysis	Liver	90	2 μ*M*
Tissue plasminogen activator	Plasminogen activator	Endothelium, other cells	70	70 p*M*
Urinary-type plasminogen activator (single chain)	Plasminogen activator	Cells, R	50	50 p*M*
Anti-fibrinolytic molecules				
Alpha2-antiplasmin	Plasmin inhibitor	Liver	70	1 μ*M*
Alpha2-macroglobulin	Protease inhibitor	Liver	700	3 μ*M*
Plasminogen activator inhibitor 1	Inhibitor of t-PA and two chain u-PA	Endothelium, Adipocytes, Platelets	50	500 p*M*
Activated factor XIII	Transglutaminase, cross-links molecules to fibrin	A-subunit, bone marrow	310	30 n*M*
Thrombin-activated fibrinolysis inhibitor	Protease cleaves fibrin	Liver	60	75 n*M*

R, recombinant; t-PA, tissue plasminogen activator; u-PA, urinary-type plasminogen activator.

Table 3
Insights from Fibrinolytic Gene Modification In Mice

Gene deletion	Phenotype
Plasminogen	Fibrin accumulation, wasting, ligneous conjunctivitis, abnormal wound healing, increased stroke size *(26–28)*
Tissue plasminogen activator	Impaired fibrinolysis under stress, protection against stroke *(28,29)*
Urinary-type plasminogen activator (single-chain)	Impaired fibrinolysis under stress, slight fibrin deposition *(29)*
Alpha2-antiplasmin	Enhanced endogenous fibrinolysis *(30)*, protection against stroke *(28)*
Alpha2-macroglobulin	No fibrinolytic phenotype described *(31)*
Plasminogen activator inhibitor 1	Mild increase in fibrinolysis under stress *(249)*, increased stroke size *(28)*
Activated factor XIII	Not published
Thrombin-activated fibrinolysis inhibitor	Not published

can survive without plasminogen, they eventually develop fibrin deposits, ligneous conjunctivitis, and abnormal wound healing. Mice can tolerate deletion of the t-PA or u-PA gene, but fibrinolysis is impaired under stress. Endogenous fibrinolysis is increased in mice lacking α2AP, a finding also present in human studies. Loss of the PAI-1 gene slightly increases fibrinolysis under stress.

One study has shown the unexpected effects of the fibrinolytic system on the size of ischemic strokes in mice *(28)*. Mice lacking plasminogen and PAI-1 have larger strokes than those lacking t-PA and α2AP. These results, which need to be confirmed in other models, suggest that

plasmin activity protects against ischemic stroke, and that t-PA activity may be deleterious.

CLINICAL THROMBOLYTIC THERAPY

The optimal use of thrombolytic therapy has been assessed in many clinical trials *(32–34)*. After the seminal GISSI trial showed that plasminogen activator (SK) therapy saved lives in patients with myocardial infarction *(5)*, several trials were designed to establish whether a fibrin-dependent agent such as t-PA (administered by several different regimens) was superior to SK.

Plasminogen Structure

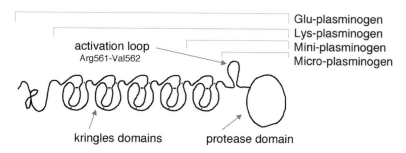

Fig. 3. Plasminogen structure. Plasminogen comprises an amino-terminal peptide, five kringle domains and a protease domain. Various proteolytic fragments of plasminogen are shown that lack one or more of these domains.

Fibrin-dependent plasminogen activators require fibrin for efficient plasminogen activation, and their activity is restricted mainly to the thrombus. Less consumption of clotting factors by plasmin occurs in the circulation. In the Global Utilization of Streptokinase and Tissue plasminogen activator for Occluded coronary arteries (GUSTO) study, mortality was reduced 7.2% by t-PA and 6.3% by SK (35). The superiority of t-PA therapy based on these results has been debated (36,37), but this study helped make t-PA the most extensively used plasminogen activator in the United States. However, SK is the most widely used agent worldwide.

Fibrin-dependent agents have been hypothesized to have fewer bleeding complications because they cause less plasmin-mediated degradation of clotting factors (38). However, the GUSTO trial (35) and several other trials have found that t-PA causes a higher rate of intracranial hemorrhage than SK (0.72% vs 0.49%). The incidence of moderate to severe bleeding was slightly less in patients treated with t-PA (5.4%) than in patients treated with SK (5.8%) (35). A similar level of risk of cerebral hemorrhage has been noted with recombinant plasminogen activator (r-PA) and SK (39). Current data support the hypothesis of Sherry and Marder (40) that patients bleed from sites of vascular injury unmasked by plasminogen activators (e.g., sites of instrumentation) (17,18) and that low fibrinogen levels do not correlate with bleeding (40).

Intense efforts have been focused on improving the therapeutic properties of plasminogen activators, particularly t-PA. Recent trials have compared the efficacy of recombinantly modified t-PAs with SK and t-PA. In a trial comparing tenecteplase to t-PA, no significant differences were seen in mortality or in rates of cerebral hemorrhage between the two agents (41). A large clinical trial established that lanoteplase was equivalent to accelerated alteplase in reducing mortality but that hemorrhagic

stroke rates were significantly higher than alteplase (0.64% alteplase and 1.12% lanoteplase) (42). Reteplase was similar but not superior to SK in reducing mortality. A nonsignificant trend toward greater cerebral hemorrhage was seen with reteplase (43). In the GUSTO III trial, no significant difference in mortality or the incidence of stroke was seen with reteplase and alteplase (44).

MOLECULAR COMPONENTS OF THE FIBRINOLYTIC SYSTEM

Plasminogen and Plasmin

The generation of plasmin from plasminogen is usually tightly controlled. Plasminogen, a 791-amino-acid protein that circulates in the blood at a concentration of about 2 μM, contains an NH_2-terminal peptide region (9 kDa), five homologous kringle structures (9 kDa each), and a protease domain (25 kDa) (Fig. 3) (45). Cleavage of the Arg561-Val562 bond by a plasminogen activator converts plasminogen from a zymogen to the enzyme plasmin (46). Several proteolytic fragments of P(g)-plasmin are generated by this reaction (Fig. 3). Glu-P(g) is the physiologic form of plasminogen found in vivo and contains all plasminogen structures. Glu-P(g) can be proteolytically converted to Lys-P(g) by removal of the NH_2-terminal peptide. Cleavage of plasminogen by the enzyme elastase yields kringles 1–3, kringle 4, and mini-P(g), which contains kringle 5 and the protease domain. Micro (μ)-P(g) consists of the protease domain alone and can be generated by protease cleavage or through recombinant techniques (47–49). Cleavage of Glu-P(g) at other sites by different proteases (e.g., the metalloproteinases) generates fragments that have anti-angiogenic effects (50,51). Glu-P(g) is a highly glycosylated protein, and no crystal or other three-dimensional structure of the full molecule is available. However, structural information on isolated

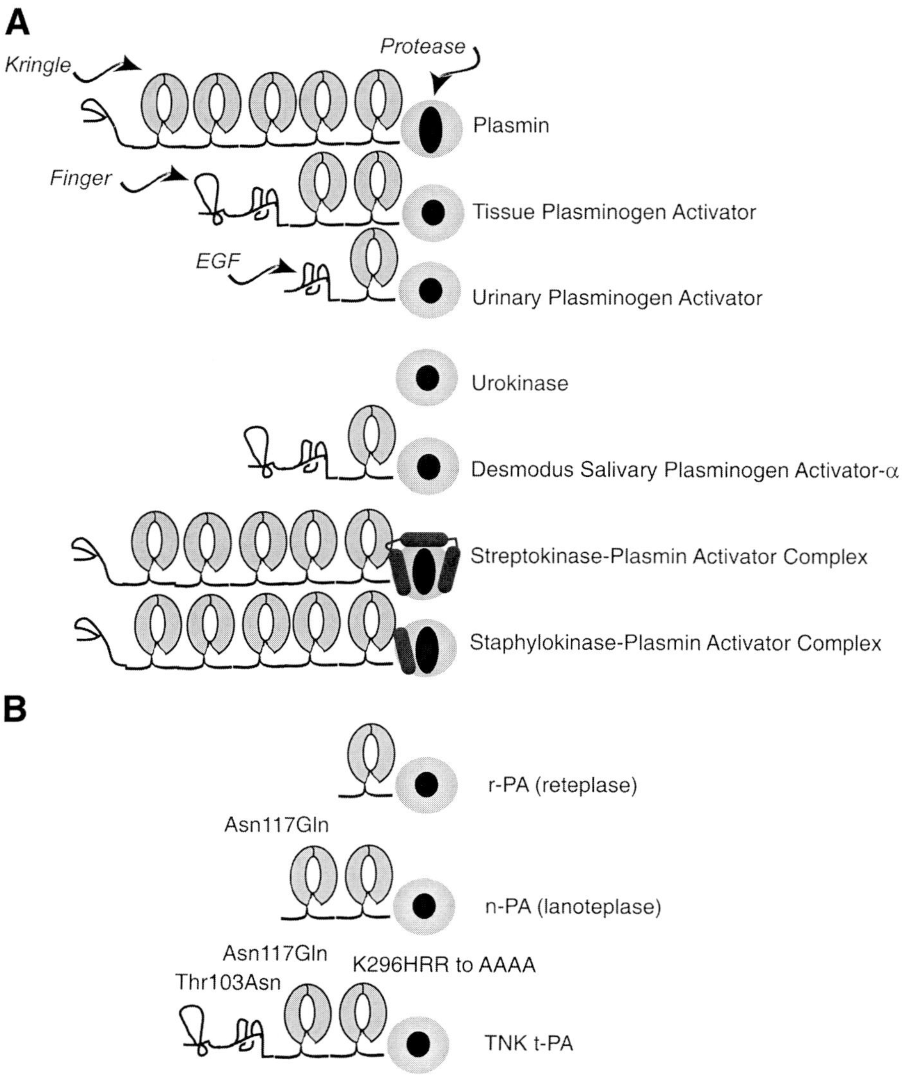

Fig. 4. Structures of plasminogen activators. **(A)** Schematic of the conserved structures of the native plasminogen activators and their recombinant derivatives. Staphylokinase and streptokinase are cofactors that form activator complexes with human plasmin(ogen). **(B).** Structure of newer recombinant tissue plasminogen activator mutants approved or in clinical trials.

domains of plasminogen provides important clues into the structural elements that mediate protein–protein interactions.

The binding of plasminogen to surfaces such as fibrin or cells is important in regulating the function of this enzyme system. Plasminogen binds to cells with low affinity and high capacity via its lysine binding sites, which are associated with its kringle domains and recognize intrapeptide and carboxy-terminal lysines of cell surface proteins (52). The structure, function, and ligand preferences of each of the isolated kringle domains have already been reviewed elsewhere (53–56). The fine structures of the lysine binding sites vary from one kringle to another, and this variation is responsible for the different

ligand affinities of these domains (55,57). The kringles play key roles in the interaction of plasminogen with plasminogen activators (58) and with the primary plasmin inhibitor α2AP.

Plasminogen Acivators

TISSUE PLASMINOGEN ACTIVATOR AND RECOMBINANT DERIVATIVES

t-PA, a serine protease important in endogenous fibrinolysis in mammals (59), is structurally similar to plasminogen, urinary plasminogen activator, and other mammalian plasminogen activators (Fig. 4). t-PA consists of a finger domain (which binds to fibrin), an EGF domain (which may facilitate clearance), two kringle domains (kringle 2 binds fibrin), and a protease domain (which has close homology to thrombin) *(60)*. t-PA is secreted as a single-chain zymogen but is rapidly converted to a two-chain molecule through the cleavage of Arg275-Ile276 by plasmin. Although many cells produce t-PA, endothelial cells may be the most important site of synthesis *(61)*. Most t-PA in the plasma (about 5 ng/mL) circulates in a complex with PAI-1, which is present in excess *(62–64)*.

In contrast to many other zymogens of the fibrinolytic system, single-chain t-PA has a relatively high level of catalytic activity (low zymogenicity) because of a stable salt bridge formed between Lys 156 and Asp 194 *(65)*. T-PA binds directly to fibrin *(66,67)*, and the efficiency of fibrin activation by t-PA increases about 2 logs in the presence of fibrin *(67–69)*. Plasminogen activation by t-PA is significantly increased by fibrinogen and by the DDE fragment of fibrin generated during plasmin-induced fibrinolysis *(70)*. Because of this activation, the fibrin specificity of t-PA is limited, and systemic degradation of fibrinogen increases with increasing doses *(71)*. The sites in fibrin that augment plasminogen activation by t-PA are Aα 148–160, fragment γ chain 311–379 *(72)*, and the α C domains *(73,74)*. Structure–function studies have pinpointed the site of t-PA interaction with PAI-1 to a basic cluster of residues 298–302 that interacts with an acidic cluster of residues in PAI-1 (350–355) *(75–78)*. These studies were used in the design of the new TNK-t-PA mutant, which contains four Ala substitutions of residues 296–299 that render it markedly less susceptible to inhibition by PAI-1.

The clearance of t-PA is mediated largely by receptors on hepatic endothelial cells and Kupffer cells. The mannose receptor and the LRP/α2-macroglobulin receptor are the main pathways for clearance *(79–81)*. The LRP/α2-macroglobulin receptor preferentially binds and clears t-PA/PAI-1 complexes *(82,83)*. In addition, other receptors such as the VLDL receptor (p130) and glycoprotein 330 (LRP-2, megalin P) clear t-PA and t-PA-PAI-1 complexes *(82–86)*. The molecular mechanisms of t-PA clearance have been used to create recombinant molecules (Fig. 2B) with pharmacodynamic properties that simplify dosing and increase thrombolysis *(87)*. In reteplase (r-PA), the finger, EGF, and kringle 1 domains were deleted *(88)*. This deletion increased the plasma half-life of r-PA to four times that of t-PA, but it significantly reduced fibrin binding *(89)*. A large multicenter trial showed that r-PA was equivalent to t-PA (alteplase) *(44)*. In a recent trial, r-PA with adjuvant use of an $\alpha_{IIb}\beta_3$ inhibitor was no better than t-PA alone *(90)*. The main advantage of reteplase over t-PA is the simplified dosing.

In n-PA (lanoteplase), the finger and EGF domains were deleted, and the asparagine 117 glycosylation site was mutated to glutamine *(91)*. Like t-PA, n-PA is produced in eukaryotic cells and is glycosylated. In addition, n-PA has less fibrin binding affinity than t-PA (half-life <5 min) and a markedly longer half-life (37 min), which permits single bolus dosing. In clinical trials, n-PA was equivalent to t-PA (alteplase) but was associated with an increased risk of hemorrhagic stroke *(42)*.

TNK-t-PA (tenecteplase) contains a series of mutations designed to increase the circulating half-life of the molecule, to alter fibrin binding properties, and to induce resistance to PAI-1 *(92,93)*. Threonine 103 in kringle 1 was mutated to asparagine to introduce a new glycosylation site. This mutation increased plasma half-life to 20 min but decreased fibrin binding. This effect was partially overcome by mutating asparagine 117 to glutamine. Although TNK-t-PA binds with slightly lower affinity to fibrin, it is more fibrin-specific than t-PA in clinical trails *(94)*. In a comparative trial of tenecteplase and alteplase, mortality rates or rates of cerebral hemorrhage were the same; therefore, the advantage of tenecteplase over t-PA is limited to simplified dosing *(41)*.

URINARY-TYPE PLASMINOGEN ACTIVATOR AND UROKINASE

U-PA is a serine protease with a mass of 54 kDa. Although produced by several different cell types, u-PA is more abundant in the urine (40–80 ng/mL) than in the plasma (2–4 ng/mL) *(95–97)*. Unlike t-PA, u-PA does not circulate in the blood in a complex with PAI-1. Like t-PA, u-PA has a short half-life (7 min) that may be mediated through hepatic clearance *(98)*. U-PA contains three domains: EGF, kringle (no fibrin affinity), and the protease domain (Fig. 4). Single-chain u-PA is a zymogen with some intrinsic catalytic activity, although the amount of activity has been debated *(99–101)*. Single-chain u-PA is converted to the two-chain u-PA or high-molecular-weight urokinase (HMW-UK) by cleavage at Lys158-Ile159. Although several enzymes cleave at this site, plasmin, factor XIIa, and kallikrein are the most important for fibrinolysis *(102,103)*.

Thrombin and plasmin can cleave two-chain u-PA at Lys135-Lys136 to make low-molecular-weight urokinase (LMW-UK) (Fig. 4). U-PA can be inactivated by being cleaved at the Arg156-Phe bond *(103)*. LMW-UK or urokinase has been used for many years for the treatment of pulmonary embolism, catheter thrombosis, and other thrombotic diseases. UK is a non-fibrin-dependent plasminogen activator that efficiently activates plasminogen in the blood and at the thrombus surface and is well suited for site-directed catheter administration, particularly in patients with peripheral arterial occlusive disease *(104)*.

Single-chain u-PA and plasminogen activate each other in a reciprocal fashion. U-PA converts plasminogen to plasmin which in turn converts single-chain u-PA into two-chain u-PA *(105)*. Single-chain u-PA has some fibrin dependence, even though it does not bind directly to fibrin, rather, it selectively degrades fibrin and spares plasma fibrinogen levels. This fibrin selectivity of single-chain u-PA arises from its high affinity with Glu-P(g) and preferential activation of Glu-P(g) bound to the C-terminal lysines in partially degraded fibrin *(106,107)*. The lag phase usually seen in fibrinolysis by single-chain u-PA may result from the initial degradation of fibrin (initiated by t-PA) that must occur for single-chain u-PA to become functional *(108)*. Subsequent generation of plasmin leads to cleavage of single-chain u-PA to HMW-UK in a process of reciprocal activation. The activity of single-chain u-PA increases nearly 2 logs when it is bound to its receptor on monocytes *(109,110)*.

Despite its fibrin dependence, single-chain u-PA, when used as a thrombolytic agent in humans, is converted to UK and causes widespread activation of the fibrinolytic system with reductions in plasma fibrinogen and $\alpha 2AP$ levels. In the PRIMI trial, thrombolytic reperfusion was greater at 60 min with single-chain u-PA (saruplase) than with SK, but no significant differences were seen at 90 min after initiation of therapy *(111)*. In the PRIMI and COMPASS trials, saruplase was associated with increased intracranial hemorrhage *(111,112)*.

U-PA and u-PA-PAI-1 are cleared through similar mechanisms as t-PA *(113)*, and recombinant modification of u-PA has been used to alter its clearance *(85)*.

DESMODUS SALIVARY PLASMINOGEN ACTIVATOR

A group of plasminogen activators with about 70% homology with t-PA has been cloned from vampire bats (*Desmodus rotundus*) *(114–116)*. Three types of DSPAs have been identified: DSPA gamma, which contains a kringle and a protease domain; DSPA beta, which contains EGF, kringle, and protease domains; and DSPA-α, which contains a finger, EGF, kringle, and protease domains. Only DSPA-α binds to fibrin, which increases the catalytic efficiency of DSPA-α by about 100,000-fold *(117)* or nearly a 1000-fold more than t-PA. The interactions of DSPA with fibrin are more selective than those of t-PA and fibrin because DSPA-α is not significantly stimulated by DDE or DD fragments *(117,118)*. Like t-PA, DSPA-α is an active zymogen but does not require cleavage for full activity *(117)*. Because its circulating half-life is about 10 times longer than t-PA, DSPA can be given as a bolus *(119)*. Although investigators had hoped that DSPA would cause less risk of systemic bleeding because of its fibrin specificity, studies have not confirmed this expectation *(119)*.

STREPTOKINASE

Unlike the direct plasminogen activators t-PA and u-PA, streptokinase (SK) and SAK have no intrinsic enzymatic activity. By forming complexes with plasmin, both SAK and SK serve as cofactors that redirect the substrate specificity of plasmin from the cleavage of fibrin to the cleavage of substrate plasminogen molecules, which increases the total plasmin activity for clot lysis (Fig. 4). This cofactor-induced alteration of the substrate specificity of an enzyme is seen in the interactions of other cofactor proteases that are important in thrombosis such as thrombomodulin–thrombin, tissue factor–factor VIIa, and staphylocoagulase–thrombin *(120)*. SK contains three domains (α, β, and γ) that bind with high affinity to plasminogen (Fig. 4) *(121,122)*. In this stable complex, SK profoundly alters the normal substrate interactions of plasmin by preventing plasmin from cleaving its normal substrates (fibrin, casein, etc.) and protecting it from inhibition by $\alpha 2AP$.

The SK–plasmin(ogen) complex is the most efficient activator of plasminogen described *(123)*. SK is the only plasminogen activator that can convert the plasminogen zymogen to an active enzyme without cleaving the arginine 561-valine 562 bond *(120,122,124–126)*. Because SK–plasminogen or SK–plasmin can activate plasminogen in the presence or absence of fibrin *(49)*, SK is not fibrin-dependent and activates plasminogen in the blood and on the fibrin surface, which may reduce its efficacy as a thrombolytic agent *(49)*. SK is antigenic in humans. Although serious allergic reactions are uncommon, treatment with SK induces the formation of neutralizing antibodies, which makes repeated therapy potentially risky and ineffective *(127–129)*.

STAPHYLOKINASE

Staphylokinase (SAK) is a 136-amino-acid, 15.5-kDa protein secreted by strains of *Staphylococcus aureus* *(130–135)*. The mechanism of plasminogen activation by SAK has been reviewed elsewhere *(136)*. Alone or in a complex with plasminogen, SAK has no enzymatic activity; however, the SAK–plasmin complex activates plasminogen substrates in the blood and on the fibrin surface. In this complex, SAK must be cleaved at Lys10-Lys11 to form a functional plasminogen activator complex *(137)*. SAK preferentially binds to plasmin and fibrin-bound plasminogen, rather than to plasminogen in the blood *(138)*. Although fibrin slightly increases plasminogen activation by the SAK–plasmin complex, the chief mechanism of fibrin-dependent plasminogen activation arises through the susceptibility of the SAK–plasmin complex to inhibition by α2AP. In the presence of fibrin, inhibition of plasmin or the SAK–plasmin complex by α2AP is 50–100 times slower because the lysine binding sites are engaged *(139,140)*. In randomized pilot studies, SAK lysed coronary thrombi in humans with heart attacks but, like SK, induced neutralizing antibodies *(141)*. SAK has a short initial half-life of 6.3 min and a rapid clearance *(142)*, which requires continuous IV infusion or double bolus therapy. Because SAK is highly antigenic in humans, repeated therapy is not advisable because of immune reactions and antibody-mediated neutralization. To reduce antigenicity and clearance rates, SAK has been mutated to permit selective chemical modification with polyethylene glycol *(136)*.

FIBRINOLYTIC REGULATORS

In addition to the plasminogen activators, fibrinolysis is regulated by the serine protease inhibitors α2AP and PAI-1, and fibrin-modifying enzymes, factor XIIIa and TAFI (Fig. 2).

Alpha2-antiplasmin

Alpha2-antiplasmin (α2AP), the dominant, fast-acting inhibitor of plasmin *(22–24)* is critical in regulating physiologic fibrinolysis. Deficiency or inhibition of α2AP causes blood clots to dissolve in vitro *(143,144)*. This spontaneous lysis is due to the unopposed effects of the plasmin generated on the fibrin surface by the endogenous t-PA incorporated into the clot during thrombus formation *(145)*. In addition, deficiency or inhibition of α2AP markedly increases fibrinolysis in vitro and in vivo *(144,146–149)*. Evidence indicates that α2AP, in the blood and cross-linked to the fibrin surface, tightly regulates fibrinolysis and may contribute to the failure of plasminogen activators to completely dissolve thrombi *(146–148)*.

Mature human α2AP is secreted as a 464-amino-acid glycoprotein with a single disulfide bond between Cys43 and Cys116, which is necessary for function *(150)*. The irreversible inactivation of plasmin by α2AP is one of the fastest bimolecular interactions known. The fast initial association between plasmin and α2AP occurs between kringle domains and the carboxy-terminus of α2AP *(151–155)*. The binding of plasmin to fibrin decreases its susceptibility to inhibition by α2AP by 50- to 100-fold. Similarly, removal of the kringle domains of plasmin decreases the reaction rate by about 87-fold *(156,157)*. The kringle domain that mediates the fast initial association

of α2AP with plasmin is debated. Early studies indicated that kringle 1 was responsible, whereas more recent kinetic analyses have suggested that kringle 4 is also required *(155,158–161)*.

The structure of α2AP can be modeled on the recently reported structure of α1-antitrypsin complex *(162)*. In this structure, the active site serine of trypsin reacts with the active center Met 358 of antitrypsin. Then, the cleaved active center loop of antitrypsin (P15-P1) becomes incorporated into the β sheet A of the serpin, causing a large 71 Å "pole to pole" shift in trypsin. The reaction with antitrypsin disrupts the conformation of trypsin and kills the enzyme. A similar mechanism may be responsible for the inhibition of plasmin by α2AP and for the inhibition of plasminogen activators by PAI-1.

Plasminogen Activator Inhibitor-1

PAI-1 is a 52-kDa glycoprotein that circulates in the blood at highly variable concentrations of up to 100 ng/mL *(19,163–165)*. PAI-1 is the major inhibitor of t-PA and two-chain u-PA and contributes to many other processes such as cell adhesion (via its binding to vitronectin) *(166,167)*. After production in megakaryocytes, PAI-1 is usually secreted from human platelets into the bloodstream and is found in an active, latent, and substrate conformation *(168,169)*. The active form of PAI-1 is stabilized by vitronectin and is a fast, stoichiometric inhibitor of t-PA and two-chain u-PA that reacts upon the cleavage of its Arg346-Met347 bond *(19)*. The latent form, which is inactive as an inhibitor, is enriched in platelet releasate *(98)*. The substrate form is cleaved by plasminogen activators. The intermolecular contact sites with t-PA have been localized to an acidic group of residues at 350–355 (Glu-Glu-Ile-Met-Asp) *(78)*. In addition, PAI-1 contains a heparin-binding site in the region 348–370 *(170,171)*. PAI-1 interacts with vitronectin via residues 55, 109, 110, 116, 123 *(172)*.

Lack of PAI-1 increases fibrinolysis in humans and in mice with a deleted PAI-1 gene *(173)*. This finding and the association between high levels of PAI-1 and thrombotic vascular events has led to an effort to identify PAI-1 inhibitors. Recent in vivo studies have suggested that PAI-1 inhibitors may potentiate fibrinolysis *(21,174,175)*.

Plasminogen activator inhibitor-2 (PAI-2) efficiently inhibits two-chain u-PA and slowly inhibits two-chain t-PA. However, almost no PAI-2 is found in normal plasma, which suggests that PAI-2 does not play a key role in the regulation of intravascular fibrinolysis *(176)*.

Thrombin-Activated Fibrinolysis Inhibitor

TAFI is a 423-amino-acid zymogen that migrates as a 60-kDA protein on polyacrylamide gels *(25,177–182)*.

Secreted by the liver, TAF1 circulates in the blood at a concentration of 75 nM *(183)*, although TAFI concentrations differ significantly among individuals *(184)*. Like α2AP, TAFI is cross-linked to the fibrin surface by factor XIIIa *(185)*. TAFI is activated by cleavage at Arg 92 by thrombin, plasmin, trypsin, and kallikrein *(180, 186,187)*. Thrombomodulin, which accelerates the efficiency of thrombin cleavage by about 1000-fold, is the primary physiological activator, although plasmin in the presence of polysaccharides (e.g., unfractionated heparin) is only 10-fold less efficient at activating TAFI *(187)*. This finding suggests that agents such as heparin could have antifibrinolytic effects in the presence of plasminogen activators. TAFIa cleaves the C-terminal lysine residues in fibrin, which significantly reduces the binding of new plasminogen molecules and thereby blocks the marked increase in fibrinolysis that occurs after initial fibrin degradation *(48–53,188–191)*. At saturating levels in vitro, TAFIa prolongs the lysis time by threefold *(25)*, indicating a significant inhibition of fibrinolysis *(187,192)*. TAFIa inhibits fibrinolysis induced by t-PA when Glu-P(g) but not Lys-P(g) is present *(182)*. Recent in vivo studies suggest that inhibition of TAFI can significantly increase lysis in vivo *(193,194)*. Thus, inhibitors of TAFIa may be useful adjuvants to fibrinolytic therapy.

Factor XIIIa

Factor XIII normally circulates in the blood as a zymogen composed of a heterotetramer containing two catalytic a-subunits and two b-subunits *(195)*. Thrombin cleaves an activation peptide from the NH_2-terminus of the a-chain to produce cleaved factor XIII (factor XIII′), which, in the presence of Ca^{2+}, changes conformation to expose a thiol active site and create the active enzyme factor XIIIa *(196)*. Factor XIIIa catalyzes the formation of intermolecular γ-glutamyl-ε-lysyl bonds between adjacent fibrin γ chains and between fibrin α chains *(196)*. These molecular cross-links significantly increase the mechanical strength of the clot and its fibrinolytic resistance to plasmin *(196,197)*. In addition, factor XIIIa cross-links other molecules such as α2AP and TAFI to different sites on the fibrin molecule. Studies of patients with factor XIII deficiency have helped define the hemostatic function of factor XIII. Hemostasis is almost normal in patients with ≥1% factor XIIIa activity, whereas those with <1% activity have delayed bleeding *(198)*. After trauma or injury, patients with factor XIII deficiency form clots normally, but the clot begins to break down and ooze. In these patients, the incidence of hematomas, joint hemorrhage, and

other bleeding episodes, including intracerebral hemorrhage, is increased. Although most of these bleeding episodes follow trauma, a small proportion may be atraumatic or unexplained bleeding. Women with <1% factor XIII activity spontaneously abort after conception, indicating the necessity of factor XIII for a successful pregnancy *(198)*.

Inhibition of factor XIII during clot formation in vitro increases the rate of clot dissolution by plasminogen activators *(199–202)*. Studies of clots made from the blood of patients with partial (>1%) factor XIII deficiency, who are not at risk of delayed bleeding, show that their blood clots lyse faster in vitro *(199)*. Mice have recently been generated in which the catalytic a-subunit has been deleted, but the phenotype has not been fully reported. Moreover, in vivo studies with a potent factor XIIIa inhibitor show that prevention of factor XIIIa–mediated cross-linking causes spontaneous lysis of pulmonary thromboemboli and markedly increases thrombolysis by administered t-PA *(147)*. A common polymorphism in the factor XIIIa subunit (Val34Leu) has been recently associated with a decreased risk of myocardial infarction *(203)*, but the mechanism is not clear.

Alpha2-Macroglobulin

A large 720-kDa protein that inhibits many proteases *(204,205)*, α2-macroglobulin is a homotetramer that circulates in the blood at a concentration of 3 μM. Although a kinetically slower inhibitor of plasmin than α2AP, α2-macroglobulin becomes the primary inhibitor of plasmin during thrombolysis once α2AP is depleted. A "bait region" for different proteases is located in the middle of each subunit of α2-macroglobulin. Once plasmin or another protease cleaves this region, a conformational change occurs in α2-macroglobulin that activates a thioester site, which leads to the formation of a covalent link between glutamate 952 and plasmin (or protease) and traps the protease domain within the cavity of the molecule *(206)*. α2-macroglobulin inhibits t-PA and the SK–plasmin complex *(207)*.

Other Inhibitors

CI inhibitor is a serpin with a molecular mass of 105 kDa that circulates in the blood at concentration of 1.7 μM *(208,209)*. CI inhibitor potently inhibits plasmin, plasma kallikrein, the first component of complement, factors XIa and XIIa, and t-PA *(207)*. Another inhibitor, histidine-rich glycoprotein, with a molecular mass of 75 kDa and a plasma concentration of 1.5 μM *(210)*, binds to the lysine binding region of the first kringle of plasminogen and circulates in the blood in a complex with plasminogen *(211)*;

however, it does not compete efficiently with fibrin or α2AP for binding plasminogen *(212)*.

CONJUNCTIVE ANTITHROMBOTIC THERAPY

The success of thrombolysis is affected by the rate of formation of new thrombus. The original site of vascular injury, the developing thrombotic occlusion, and plasminogen activators can activate the coagulation system and induce thrombus formation. Conjunctive therapy has been proposed to reduce the contribution of platelets and fibrin to continuous thrombus formation during thrombolysis. The conventional adjuvant therapy to plasminogen activators has been heparin and aspirin. Aspirin irreversibly inhibits cyclooxygenase and thereby reduces platelet activation and aggregation by reducing thromboxane formation. The ISIS-2 study showed that aspirin saves lives in patients with acute myocardial infarction and reduces mortality by nearly as much as SK alone *(213)*.

Other inhibitors of platelet function have been developed such as ADP receptor antagonists (clopidogrel) and inhibitors of the platelet aggregation receptor, integrin $\alpha_{IIb}\beta_{III}$. $\alpha_{IIb}\beta_{III}$ inhibitors (e.g., abciximab, integrelin, tirofiban) are being evaluated to determine whether they are more efficacious than aspirin in treating myocardial infarction. Although early results from small studies were promising, a large randomized trial (GUSTO V) showed that a potent $\alpha_{IIb}\beta_{III}$ inhibitor (abciximab), when used in combination with reteplase, did not reduce mortality more than standard therapy with t-PA alone *(214)*. The effects of clopidogrel were additive with those of aspirin in treating patients with non-ST segment elevation myocardial infarctions, but no data support the use of clopidogrel with plasminogen activators *(215)*.

Unfractionated heparin has been used in many clinical trials as an adjunct to plasminogen activators *(216,217)*. Heparin binds to the serine protease inhibitor antithrombin making it a more efficient inhibitor of thrombin. Meta-analyses indicate that heparin is beneficial in patients treated with plasminogen activators who do not receive aspirin *(36)*. In addition, heparin may increase vessel patency in patients treated with aspirin and SK or tissue plasminogen activator *(218,219)*. However, whether the combination of heparin and aspirin adds survival benefits over those seen with aspirin alone in patients with myocardial infarction is unknown *(36)*. Low-molecular-weight heparins may be as effective as unfractionated heparin as adjunctive therapy to plasminogen activators *(220,221)*, but no data show their superiority. In one study hirudin, a direct inhibitor of thrombin, reduced the risk of non-fatal myocardial infarction, but no mortality benefit was seen *(222)*.

NOVEL FIBRINOLYTIC AGENTS AND APPROACHES

Several limitations are associated with current thrombolytic agents. They may induce concurrent thrombosis by activating the coagulation system, and they require an average of 45 min to open arteries. In addition, thromobolytic agents fail to restore normal blood flow in about half of patients (within 90 min), and they are associated with reocclusion in 5–10% of patients within 1 wk after therapy. Intracranial hemorrhage occurs in about 0.3–0.7% of patients treated with thrombolytic agents *(223)*. Because overcoming these limitations would more than double survival rates in patients with myocardial infarction, scientists are searching for novel approaches to fibrinolysis (Table 4).

Fibrin and Platelet Targeting

In fibrin- or platelet-targeting, plasminogen activators are targeted to the thrombus *(224–227)* to increase plasmin generation at the fibrin surface and to increase the efficiency of fibrinolysis. In one successful strategy, the binding domain of a monoclonal anti-fibrin antibody was linked to the catalytic domain of a plasminogen activator such as low-molecular-weight urokinase *(224–228)*. This strategy was further refined by developing a hybrid plasminogen activator capable of activation only by thrombin, thereby further restricting its activity to the thrombus surface *(229)*. Another approach has been to link a plasminogen activator to an anti-platelet antibody with the goal of targeting fibrinolysis to the thrombus *(230,231)*.

Catalytic Targeting

SK forms the most catalytically active plasminogen activator complex, but its therapeutic properties may be limited by its explosive activation and consumption of plasminogen at sites distant from the thrombus. In catalytic targeting, recombinant modification of SK converts it to a fibrin-dependent plasminogen activator that acts only on fibrin-bound plasminogen. This fibrin-dependent SK has greater fibrinolytic potency than the parent protein *(232)*.

Improved Pharmacodynamics

Another approach has been to been to modify plasminogen activators to reduce their in vivo clearance. This method has been applied to t-PA where mutation or deletion of sites that mediate hepatic clearance has resulted in modified recombinant t-PA molecules (lanoteplase, reteplase, and tenecteplase) with prolonged half-lives in humans. The dosing regimens of these agents is simpler

Table 4
Novel Thrombolytic Agents or Approaches

Agent or approach	Rationale	Examples
Platelet or fibrin-targeted plasminogen activators	Increase the binding and concentration of plasminogen activators at the thrombus surface	Single chain u-PA fragment linked to an anti-fibrin or anti-platelet antibody fragment
Catalytic targeting	Restrict plasminogen activation to fibrin-bound plasminogen, prevent plasminogen depletion	Fibrin-dependent SK molecules
Improve pharmacodyamics of plasminogen activators	Simplify dosing Faster therapeutic effects	t-PA derivatives (lanoteplase, reteplase, tenecteplase, see text) Polyethylene glycol modified SAK
PAI-1 inhibitors	Prevent t-PA or two chain u-PA inhibition	Direct PAI-1 inhibitors, tenecteplase-PAI-1-resistant t-PA mutant
Alpha 2-antiplasmin inhibitors	Synergism with plasminogen activators—prevent rapid plasmin and plasminogen activator inhibition	Monoclonal antibodies
Decrease antigenicity of foreign plasminogen activators	Prevent allergic reactions	Modifications of the antigenicity of SAK and SK
TAFIa inhibitors	Increase fibrinolysis by preventing fibrin cleavage by TAFIa	Potato carboxypeptidase inhibitor
Factor XIIIa inhibitors	Increase fibrinolysis by blocking fibrin-fibrin, fibrin-alpha 2-antiplasmin, and fibrin-TAFI cross-linking	Monoclonal antibodies, chemical inhibitors, tridegin
Plasminogen activator chimeras	Combine plasminogen activator and antithromboticfunction in one molecule	Single-chain u-PA and t-PA chimera, Single-chain u-PA fragment fused with hirudin
Thrombolysis and coronary intervention	Increase the rate and extent of reperfusion of thrombotically occluded arteries	Reduced dose plasminogen activator followed by coronary angioplasty or stent
Thrombolysis and ultrasound	Increase plasminogen activator penetration of thrombus, mechanical fragmentation	Conjunctive use of noninvasive low energy ultrasound or ultrasound catheters

PAI-1, plasminogen activator inhibitor-1; SK, streptokinase; TAFI, thrombin activated fibrinolysis inhibitor; t-PA, tissue plasminogen activator; u-PA, urinary-type plasminogen activator.

than t-PA, but clinical data have not shown that the recombinant molecules are superior to t-PA or SK.

Inhibition of Fibrinolytic Regulators

Several molecules regulate fibrinolysis in vivo (Fig. 2). PAI-1 has been a target for drug development because it inactivates t-PA. Several studies have shown that antibodies or other molecular inhibitors of PAI-1 amplify fibrinolysis in vivo (21,175). Mutations in tenecteplase reduce its inhibition by PAI-1 more than 80-fold when compared with t-PA (92). Another major regulator of fibrinolysis in vivo is α2AP. Monoclonal antibodies that prevent α2AP from inhibiting plasmin, combined with t-PA, synergistically amplify fibrinolysis in vitro (144). By

prolonging the half-life of physiologically generated plasmin, α2AP inhibitors cause spontaneous in vivo lysis of experimental thrombi and thromboemboli (146). Inhibitors of α2AP strongly increase fibrinolysis by t-PA in vivo (146,147).

Experimental studies have shown that monoclonal antibody inhibitors of the factor XIII system potently accelerate fibrinolysis in vitro and in vivo (148,201). Because of the rapid cross-linking by factor XIIIa and the short half-life of this enzyme in thrombi, inhibitors of factor XIIIa may be viewed as anti-thrombotic agents (233). The same is true for TAFIa. TAFIa inhibitors can make new thrombi more susceptible to fibrinolysis but will not affect existing fibrin on which TAFI has already acted *(194)*. Limited in vivo experiments suggest that TAFIa inhibitors may increase lysis by plasminogen activators *(92)*.

Modified Plasminogen Activators

Several investigators have tried to create hybrid molecules that combine the functional properties of two plasminogen activators *(234,235)* or the activity of a plasminogen activator with that of an antithrombotic agent. A single-chain u-PA fragment has been fused with hirudin and has been shown to have both fibrinolytic and anticoagulant properties in vitro *(236,237)*. In other studies SAK has been fused with antithrombotic molecules *(238)*.

Plasminogen activators such as DSPA, SAK, and SK are non-human proteins that are antigenic and induce immune reactions. In large clinical trials with SK, non-fatal anaphylaxis occurred in about 0.1% of patients, and episodes of emesis and hypotension were more common. Treatment with SK and SAK induces high levels of antibody production, and repeated therapy with these agents is not advised. To reduce the antigenicity of these agents, the antigenic epitopes have been mapped and mutated *(127,128,232)*.

Maximizing Thrombolytic Therapy

Thrombolytic therapy is clearly most effective at saving lives when used soon after symptoms. In the GUSTO trial, mortality was almost twice as high in patients receiving plasminogen activators 4–6 h after symptoms than in those treated within 2 h after treatment *(35)*. Decreasing the interval from hospital arrival to treatment (door-to-needle time) is important, and efforts have been made to use these agents in ambulances before hospital arrival *(239)*. Plasminogen activators are underutilized in patients with myocardial infarction; current studies suggest that less than half of eligible patients receive them *(240,241)*. Continuing physician education on the proper use of thrombolytic therapy has increased the rates of treatment.

To increase the rate and extent of reperfusion in patients with coronary thrombosis, some experts have advocated the combined use of thrombolytic therapy and percutaneous coronary interventions, such as angioplasty and stenting *(242,243)*, to decrease the time required to restore reperfusion. In addition, some experts have advocated fibrinolytic therapy with adjuvant use of $\alpha_{IIb}\beta_{III}$ inhibitors based on the premise that the fastest and most complete reperfusion should maximize survival *(244)*. Angiographic success is an imperfect correlate of tissue reperfusion *(244,245)*.

Noninvasive low frequency ultrasound accelerates fibrinolysis by increasing the penetration and binding of plasminogen activator *(246,247)*. In addition, microbubbles delivered by catheters may induce mechanical fragmentation of the thrombus *(246)*, which can speed reperfusion.

REFERENCES

1. Chandler AB, Chapman I, Erhardt LR, et al. Coronary thrombosis in myocardial infarction. Report of a workshop on the role of coronary thrombosis in the pathogenesis of acute myocardial infarction. Am J Cardiol 1974;34:823–833.
2. Davies MJ, Woolf N, Robertson WB. Pathology of acute myocardial infarction with particular reference to occlusive coronary thrombi. Br Heart J 1976;38:659–664.
3. DeWood MA, Spores J, Notske R,et al. Prevalence of total coronary occlusion during the early hours of transmural myocardial infarction. N Engl J Med 1980;303:897–902.
4. Rentrop P, Blanke H, Karsch KR, Kaiser H, Kostering H, Leitz K. Selective intracoronary thrombolysis in acute myocardial infarction and unstable angina pectoris. Circulation 1981;63:307–317.
5. (GISSI) GIplSdSnIM. Effectiveness of intravenous thrombolytic treatment in acute myocardial infarction. Lancet 1986;1:397–402.
6. Arbustini E, Dal Bello B, Morbini P, et al. Plaque erosion is a major substrate for coronary thrombosis in acute myocardial infarction. Heart 1999;82:269–272.
7. Alkjaersig N, Fletcher AP, Sherry S. The mechanism of clot dissolution by plasmin. J Clin Invest 1959;38:1086–1095.
8. Sabovic M, Lijnen HR, Keber D, Collen D. Correlation between progressive adsorption of plasminogen to blood clots and their sensitivity to lysis. Thromb Haemost 1990;64:450–454.
9. Rijken DC, Sakharov DV. Basic principles in thrombolysis: regulatory role of plasminogen. Thromb Res 2001;103 Suppl 1:S41–S49.
10. Onundarson PT, Francis CW, Marder VJ. Depletion of plasminogen in vitro or during thrombolytic therapy limits fibrinolytic potential. J Lab Clin Med 1992;120:120–128.
11. Torr SR, Nachowiak DA, Fujii S, Sobel BE. "Plasminogen steal" and clot lysis. J Am Coll Cardiol 1992;19:1085–1090.
12. Stroughton J, Ouriel K, Shortell CK, Cho JS, Marder VJ. Plasminogen acceleration of urokinase thrombolysis. J Vasc Surg 1994;19:298–303; discussion 303–305.
13. Nishino N, Kakkar VV, Scully MF. Influence of intrinsic and extrinsic plasminogen upon the lysis of thrombi in vitro. Thromb Haemost 1991;66:672–677.
14. Tilsner V, Witte G. Effectiveness of intraarterial plasminogen application in combination with percutaneous transluminal angioplasty (PTA) or catheter assisted lysis (CL) in patients with chronic peripheral occlusive disease of the lower limbs (POL). Haemostasis 1988;18 Suppl 1:139–156.
15. Kakkar VV, Sagar S, Lewis M. Treatment of deep-vein thrombosis with intermittent streptokinase and plasminogen infusion. Lancet 1975;2:674–676.
16. Prewitt RM, Downes AM, Gu SA, Chan SM, Ducas J. Effects of hydralazine and increased cardiac output on recombinant tissue plasminogen activator-induced thrombolysis in canine pulmonary embolism. Chest 1991;99:708–714.
17. Marder VJ, Sherry S. Thrombolytic therapy: current status (1). N Engl J Med 1988;318:1512–1520.
18. Marder VJ, Sherry S. Thrombolytic therapy: current status (2). N Engl J Med 1988;318:1585–1595.

19. Loskutoff DJ, Sawdey M, Mimuro J. Type 1 plasminogen activator inhibitor. Prog Hemost Thromb 1989;9:87–115.
20. Robbie LA, Booth NA, Croll AM, Bennett B. The roles of alpha 2-antiplasmin and plasminogen activator inhibitor 1 (PAI-1) in the inhibition of clot lysis. Thromb Haemost 1993;70:301–306.
21. Reilly CF, Fujita T, Hutzelmann JE, Mayer EJ, Shebuski RJ. Plasminogen activator inhibitor-1 suppresses endogenous fibrinolysis in a canine model of pulmonary embolism. Circulation 1991;84:287–292.
22. Collen D. Identification and some properties of a new fast-reacting plasmin inhibitor in human plasma. Eur J Biochem 1976;69:209–216.
23. Moroi M, Aoki N. Isolation and characterization of alpha2-plasmin inhibitor from human plasma. A novel proteinase inhibitor which inhibits activator-induced clot lysis. J Biol Chem 1976;251:5956–5965.
24. Mullertz S, Clemmensen I. The primary inhibitor of plasmin in human plasma. Biochem J 1976;159:545–553.
25. Bajzar L. Thrombin activatable fibrinolysis inhibitor and an antifibrinolytic pathway. Arterioscler Thromb Vasc Biol 2000;20:2511–2518.
26. Ploplis VA, Carmeliet P, Vazirzadeh S, et al. Effects of disruption of the plasminogen gene on thrombosis, growth, and health in mice. Circulation 1995;92:2585–2593.
27. Bugge TH, Flick MJ, Daugherty CC, Degen JL. Plasminogen deficiency causes severe thrombosis but is compatible with development and reproduction. Genes Dev 1995;9:794–807.
28. Nagai N, De Mol M, Lijnen HR, Carmeliet P, Collen D. Role of plasminogen system components in focal cerebral ischemic infarction: a gene targeting and gene transfer study in mice. Circulation 1999;99:2440–2444.
29. Carmeliet P, Schoonjans L, Kieckens L, et al. Physiological consequences of loss of plasminogen activator gene function in mice. Nature 1994;368:419–424.
30. Lijnen HR, Okada K, Matsuo O, Collen D, Dewerchin M. Alpha2-antiplasmin gene deficiency in mice is associated with enhanced fibrinolytic potential without overt bleeding. Blood 1999;93:2274–2281.
31. Umans L, Serneels L, Overbergh L, Lorent K, Van Leuven F, Van den Berghe H. Targeted inactivation of the mouse alpha 2-macroglobulin gene. J Biol Chem 1995;270:19778–19785.
32. Ross AM. New plasminogen activators: a clinical review. Clin Cardiol 1999;22:165–171.
33. Boersma E, Steyerberg EW, Van der Vlugt MJ, Simoons ML. Reperfusion therapy for acute myocardial infarction. Which strategy for which patient? Drugs 1998;56:31–48.
34. Zeymer U, Neuhaus KL. Clinical trials in acute myocardial infarction. Curr Opin Cardiol 1999;14:392–402.
35. GUSTO I. An international randomized trial comparing four thrombolytic strategies for acute myocardial infarction. N Engl J Med 1993;329:673–682.
36. Collins R, Peto R, Baigent C, Sleight P. Aspirin, heparin, and fibrinolytic therapy in suspected acute myocardial infarction. N Engl J Med 1997;336:847–860.
37. Collen D. The plasminogen (fibrinolytic) system. Thromb Haemost 1999;82:259–270.
38. Collen D. Regulation of fibrinolysis: plasminogen activator as a fibrinolytic agent. In: Nnssel HL, ed. Pathobiology of the endothelial cell. New York: Academic Press, 1982:183–189.
39. Inglis AS, Edman P. Mechanism of cyanogen bromide reaction with methionine in peptides and proteins. I. Formation of imidate and methyl thiocyanate. Anal Biochem 1970;37:73–80.
40. Rao AK, Pratt C, Berke A, et al. Thrombolysis in Myocardial Infarction (TIMI) Trial—phase I: hemorrhagic manifestations and changes in plasma fibrinogen and the fibrinolytic system in patients treated with recombinant tissue plasminogen activator and streptokinase. J Am Coll Cardiol 1988;11:1–11.
41. Single-bolus tenecteplase compared with front-loaded alteplase in acute myocardial infarction: the ASSENT-2 double-blind randomised trial. Assessment of the Safety and Efficacy of a New Thrombolytic Investigators. Lancet 1999;354:716–722.
42. Intravenous NPA for the treatment of infarcting myocardium early; In TIME-II, a double-blind comparison of single-bolus lanoteplase vs accelerated alteplase for the treatment of patients with acute myocardial infarction. Eur Heart J 2000;21:2005–2013.
43. Randomised, double-blind comparison of reteplase double-bolus administration with streptokinase in acute myocardial infarction (INJECT): trial to investigate equivalence. International Joint Efficacy Comparison of Thrombolytics. Lancet 1995;346:329–336.
44. Investigators TGUoStOOCAGI. A comparison of reteplase with alteplase for acute myocardial infarction. The Global Use of Strategies to Open Occluded Coronary Arteries (GUSTO III) Investigators. N Engl J Med 1997;337:1118–1123.
45. Ponting CP, Marshall JM, Cederholm-Williams SA. Plasminogen: a structural review. Blood Coagul Fibrinolysis 1992;3:605–614.
46. Robbins KC, Summaria L, Hsieh B, Shah RJ. The peptide chains of human plasmin. Mechanism of activation of human plasminogen to plasmin. J Biol Chem 1967;242:2333–2342.
47. Wang S, Reed GL, Hedstrom L. Deletion of Ile1 changes the mechanism of streptokinase: evidence for the molecular sexuality hypothesis. Biochemistry 1999;38:5232–5240.
48. Wu HL, Chang BI, Wu DH, et al. Interaction of plasminogen and fibrin in plasminogen activation. J Biol Chem 1990;265:19658–19664.
49. Reed GL, Houng AK, Liu L, Parhami-Seren B, Matsueda LH, Wang S, Hedstrom L. A catalytic switch and the conversion of streptokinase to a fibrin-targeted plasminogen activator. Proc Natl Acad Sci USA 1999;96:8879–8883.
50. Pepper MS. Role of the matrix metalloproteinase and plasminogen activator-plasmin systems in angiogenesis. Arterioscler Thromb Vasc Biol 2001;21:1104–1117.
51. Sang QX. Complex role of matrix metalloproteinases in angiogenesis. Cell Res 1998;8:171–177.
52. Plow EF, Herren T, Redlitz A, Miles LA, Hoover-Plow JL. The cell biology of the plasminogen system. Faseb J 1995;9:939–945.
53. Castellino FJ, McCance SG. The kringle domains of human plasminogen. Ciba Found Symp 1997;212:46–60.
54. Chang Y, Mochalkin I, McCance SG, Cheng B, Tulinsky A, Castellino FJ. Structure and ligand binding determinants of the recombinant kringle 5 domain of human plasminogen. Biochemistry 1998;37:3258–3271.
55. Marti DN, Hu CK, An SSA, von Haller P, Schaller J, Llinas M. Ligand preferences of kringle 2 and homologous domains of human plasminogen: canvassing weak, intermediate, and high-affinity binding sites by 1H-NMR. Biochemistry 1997;36:11591–11604.
56. Rejante MR, Byeon IJ, Llinas M. Ligand specificity of human plasminogen kringle 4. Biochemistry 1991;30:11081–11092.
57. Wu TP, Padmanabhan KP, Tulinsky A. The structure of recombinant plasminogen kringle 1 and the fibrin binding site. Blood Coagul Fibrinolysis 1994;5:157–166.

58. Lin LF, Houng A, Reed GL. Epsilon amino caproic acid inhibits streptokinase-plasminogen activator complex formation and substrate binding through kringle-dependent mechanisms. Biochemistry 2000;39:4740–4745.

59. Collen D, Lijnen HR, Todd PA, Goa KL. Tissue-type plasminogen activator. A review of its pharmacology and therapeutic use as a thrombolytic agent. Drugs 1989;38:346–388.

60. van Zonneveld AJ, Veerman H, MacDonald ME, van Mourik JA, Pannekoek H. Structure and function of human tissue-type plasminogen activator (t- PA). J Cell Biochem 1986;32:169–178.

61. Levin EG, Loskutoff DJ. Cultured bovine endothelial cells produce both urokinase and tissue-type plasminogen activators. J Cell Biol 1982;94:631–636.

62. Rijken DC, Juhan-Vague I, de Cock F, Collen D. Measurement of human tissue-type plasminogen activator by a two-site immunoradiometric assay. J Lab Clin Med 1983;101:274–284.

63. Stalder M, Hauert J, Kruithof EK, Bachmann F. Release of vascular plasminogen activator (v-PA) after venous stasis: electrophoretic-zymographic analysis of free and complexed v-PA. Br J Haematol 1985;61:169–176.

64. Booth NA, Walker E, Maughan R, Bennett B. Plasminogen activator in normal subjects after exercise and venous occlusion: t-PA circulates as complexes with C1-inhibitor and PAI-1. Blood 1987;69:1600–1604.

65. Tachias K, Madison EL. Converting tissue type plasminogen activator into a zymogen. Important role of Lys156. J Biol Chem 1997;272:28–31.

66. Thorsen S, Glas-Greenwalt P, Astrup T. Differences in the binding to fibrin of urokinase and tissue plasminogen activator. Thromb Diath Haemorrh 1972;28:65–74.

67. Fears R. Binding of plasminogen activators to fibrin: characterization and pharmacological consequences. Biochem J 1989;261:313–324.

68. Hoylaerts M, Rijken DC, Lijnen HR, Collen D. Kinetics of the activation of plasminogen by human tissue plasminogen activator. Role of fibrin. J Biol Chem 1982;257:2912–2919.

69. Horrevoets AJ, Pannekoek H, Nesheim ME. A steady-state template model that describes the kinetics of fibrin- stimulated [Glu1]- and [Lys78]plasminogen activation by native tissue-type plasminogen activator and variants that lack either the finger or kringle-2 domain. J Biol Chem 1997;272:2183–2191.

70. Weitz JI, Leslie B, Ginsberg J. Soluble fibrin degradation products potentiate tissue plasminogen activator-induced fibrinogen proteolysis. J Clin Invest 1991;87:1082–1090.

71. Collen D, Topol EJ, Tiefenbrunn AJ, Gold HK, Weisfeldt ML, Sobel BE, Leinbach RC, Brinker JA, Ludbrook PA, Yasuda I, et al. Coronary thrombolysis with recombinant human tissue-type plasminogen activator: a prospective, randomized, placebo-controlled trial. Circulation 1984;70:1012–1017.

72. Yonekawa O, Voskuilen M, Nieuwenhuizen W. Localization in the fibrinogen gamma-chain of a new site that is involved in the acceleration of the tissue-type plasminogen activator-catalysed activation of plasminogen. Biochem J 1992;283:187–191.

73. Voskuilen M, Vermond A, Veeneman GH, et al. Fibrinogen lysine residue A alpha 157 plays a crucial role in the fibrin-induced acceleration of plasminogen activation, catalyzed by tissue-type plasminogen activator. J Biol Chem 1987;262:5944–6.

74. Tsurupa G, Medved L. Identification and characterization of novel tPA- and plasminogen- binding sites within fibrin(ogen) alpha C-domains. Biochemistry 2001;40:801–808.

75. Madison EL, Goldsmith EJ, Gerard RD, Gething MJ, Sambrook JF. Serpin-resistant mutants of human tissue-type plasminogen activator. Nature 1989;339:721–724.

76. Madison EL, Goldsmith EJ, Gerard RD, Gething MJ, Sambrook JF, Bassel-Duby RS. Amino acid residues that affect interaction of tissue-type plasminogen activator with plasminogen activator inhibitor 1. Proc Natl Acad Sci USA 1990;87:3530–3533.

77. Tachias K, Madison EL. Variants of tissue-type plasminogen activator that display extraordinary resistance to inhibition by the serpin plasminogen activator inhibitor type 1. J Biol Chem 1997;272:14580–14585.

78. Bennett WF, Paoni NF, Keyt BA, et al. High resolution analysis of functional determinants on human tissue- type plasminogen activator. J Biol Chem 1991;266:5191–5201.

79. Otter M, Barrett-Bergshoeff MM, Rijken DC. Binding of tissue-type plasminogen activator by the mannose receptor. J Biol Chem 1991;266:13931–13935.

80. Andreasen PA, Sottrup-Jensen L, et al. Receptor-mediated endocytosis of plasminogen activators and activator/inhibitor complexes. FEBS Lett 1994;338:239–245.

81. Orth K, Madison EL, Gething MJ, Sambrook JF, Herz J. Complexes of tissue-type plasminogen activator and its serpin inhibitor plasminogen-activator inhibitor type 1 are internalized by means of the low density lipoprotein receptor-related protein/alpha 2-macroglobulin receptor. Proc Natl Acad Sci USA 1992;89:7422–7426.

82. Willnow TE, Goldstein JL, Orth K, Brown MS, Herz J. Low density lipoprotein receptor-related protein and gp330 bind similar ligands, including plasminogen activator-inhibitor complexes and lactoferrin, an inhibitor of chylomicron remnant clearance. J Biol Chem 1992;267:26172–26180.

83. Biessen EA, van Teijlingen M, Vietsch H, et al. Antagonists of the mannose receptor and the LDL receptor-related protein dramatically delay the clearance of tissue plasminogen activator. Circulation 1997;95:46–52.

84. Moestrup SK. The alpha 2-macroglobulin receptor and epithelial glycoprotein-0: two giant receptors mediating endocytosis of multiple ligands. Biochim Biophys Acta 1994;1197:197–213.

85. Kasza A, Petersen HH, Heegaard CW, et al. Specificity of serine proteinase/serpin complex binding to very-low- density lipoprotein receptor and alpha 2-macroglobulin receptor/low- density-lipoprotein-receptor-related protein. Eur J Biochem 1997;248:270–281.

86. Kounnas MZ, Stefansson S, Loukinova E, Argraves KM, Strickland DK, Argraves WS. An overview of the structure and function of glycoprotein 330, a receptor related to the alpha 2-macroglobulin receptor. Ann N Y Acad Sci 1994;737:114–123.

87. Smalling RW. Pharmacological and clinical impact of the unique molecular structure of a new plasminogen activator. Eur Heart J 1997;18 Suppl F:F11–F16.

88. Kohnert U, Rudolph R, Verheijen JH,et al. Biochemical properties of the kringle 2 and protease domains are maintained in the refolded t-PA deletion variant BM 06.022. Protein Eng. 1992;5:93–100.

89. Smalling RW, Bode C, Kalbfleisch J, et al. More rapid, complete, and stable coronary thrombolysis with bolus administration of reteplase compared with alteplase infusion in acute myocardial infarction. RAPID Investigators. Circulation 1995;91:2725–2732.

90. Trial of abciximab with and without low-dose reteplase for acute myocardial infarction. Strategies for Patency Enhancement

in the Emergency Department (SPEED) Group. Circulation 2000;101:2788–2794.

91. Larsen GR, Timony GA, Horgan PG, et al. Protein engineering of novel plasminogen activators with increased thrombolytic potency in rabbits relative to activase. J Biol Chem 1991;266:8156–8161.

92. Keyt BA, Paoni NF, Refino CJ, et al. A faster-acting and more potent form of tissue plasminogen activator. Proc Natl Acad Sci USA 1994;91:3670–3674.

93. Refino CJ, Paoni NF, Keyt BA, et al. A variant of t-PA (T103N, KHRR 296-299 AAAA) that, by bolus, has increased potency and decreased systemic activation of plasminogen. Thromb Haemost 1993;70:313–319.

94. Cannon CP, Gibson CM, McCabe CH, et al. TNK-tissue plasminogen activator compared with front-loaded alteplase in acute myocardial infarction: results of the TIMI 10B trial. Thrombolysis in Myocardial Infarction (TIMI) 10B Investigators. Circulation 1998;98:2805–2814.

95. Husain SS, Gurewich V, Lipinski B. Purification and partial characterization of a single-chain high-molecular-weight form of urokinase from human urine. Arch Biochem Biophys 1983; 220:31–38.

96. Stump DC, Lijnen HR, Collen D. Purification and characterization of single-chain urokinase-type plasminogen activator from human cell cultures. J Biol Chem 1986;261:1274–1278.

97. Darras V, Thienpont M, Stump DC, Collen D. Measurement of urokinase-type plasminogen activator (u-PA) with an enzyme-linked immunosorbent assay (ELISA) based on three murine monoclonal antibodies. Thromb Haemost 1986;56: 411–414.

98. Bachmann F. The plasminogen-plasmin enzyme system. In: Colman RW, Hirsh J, Marder VJ, Clowes AW, George JN, eds. Hemostasis and Thrombosis: Basic Principles and Clinical Practice. Philadelphia: Lippincott Co., 2001:275–320.

99. Pannell R, Gurewich V. Activation of plasminogen by single-chain urokinase or by two-chain urokinase—a demonstration that single-chain urokinase has a low catalytic activity (pro-urokinase). Blood 1987;69:22–26.

100. Petersen LC, Lund LR, Nielsen LS, Dano K, Skriver L. One-chain urokinase-type plasminogen activator from human sarcoma cells is a proenzyme with little or no intrinsic activity. J Biol Chem 1988;263:11189–11195.

101. Lijnen HR, Van Hoef B, De Cock F, Collen D. The mechanism of plasminogen activation and fibrin dissolution by single chain urokinase-type plasminogen activator in a plasma milieu in vitro. Blood 1989;73:1864–1872.

102. Lijnen HR, Stump DC, Collen DC. Single-chain urokinase-type plasminogen activator: mechanism of action and thrombolytic properties. Semin Thromb Hemost 1987;13:152–159.

103. Ichinose A, Fujikawa K, Suyama T. The activation of pro-urokinase by plasma kallikrein and its inactivation by thrombin. J Biol Chem 1986;261:3486–3489.

104. Weber JJ, Chong K. Regional thrombolytic infusion for peripheral arterial occlusion: is urokinase really the drug of choice? Am J Health Syst Pharm 1998;55:2414–2416.

105. Petersen LC. Kinetics of reciprocal pro-urokinase/plasminogen activation—stimulation by a template formed by the urokinase receptor bound to poly(D-lysine). Eur J Biochem 1997;245: 316–323.

106. Longstaff C, Clough AM, Gaffney PJ. Kinetics of plasmin activation of single chain urinary-type plasminogen activator (scu-PA) and demonstration of a high affinity interaction between scu-PA and plasminogen. J Biol Chem 1992;267: 173–179.

107. Lenich C, Pannell R, Gurewich V. The effect of the carboxy-terminal lysine of urokinase on the catalysis of plasminogen activation. Thromb Res 1991;64:69–80.

108. Collen D, Stassen JM, De Cock F. Synergistic effect on thrombolysis of sequential infusion of tissue- type plasminogen activator (t-PA) single-chain urokinase-type plasminogen activator (scu-PA) and urokinase in the rabbit jugular vein thrombosis model. Thromb Haemost 1987;58:943–946.

109. Ellis V, Scully MF, Kakkar VV. Plasminogen activation initiated by single-chain urokinase-type plasminogen activator. Potentiation by U937 monocytes. J Biol Chem 1989;264: 2185–2188.

110. Manchanda N, Schwartz BS. Single chain urokinase. Augmentation of enzymatic activity upon binding to monocytes. J Biol Chem 1991;266:14580–14584.

111. Group. PTS. Randomised double-blind trial of recombinant pro-urokinase against streptokinase in acute myocardial infarction. Lancet 1989;1:863–868.

112. Tebbe U, Michels R, Adgey J, et al. Randomized, double-blind study comparing saruplase with streptokinase therapy in acute myocardial infarction: the COMPASS Equivalence Trial. Comparison Trial of Saruplase and Streptokinase (COMASS) Investigators [see comments]. J Am Coll Cardiol 1998;31: 487–493.

113. van der Kaaden ME, Rijken DC, Kruijt JK, van Berkel TJ, Kuiper J. The role of the low-density lipoprotein receptor-related protein (LRP) in the plasma clearance and liver uptake of recombinant single-chain urokinase-type plasminogen activator in rats. Thromb Haemost 1997;77:710–717.

114. Hawkey C. Plasminogen activator in saliva of the vampire bat Desmodus rotundus. Nature 1966;211:434–435.

115. Gardell SJ, Duong LT, Diehl RE, et al. Isolation, characterization, and cDNA cloning of a vampire bat salivary plasminogen activator. J Biol Chem 1989;264:17947–17952.

116. Kratzschmar J, Haendler B, Langer G, et al. The plasminogen activator family from the salivary gland of the vampire bat Desmodus rotundus: cloning and expression. Gene 1991;105: 229–237.

117. Bringmann P, Gruber D, Liese A, et al. Structural features mediating fibrin selectivity of vampire bat plasminogen activators. J Biol Chem 1995;270:25596–25603.

118. Stewart RJ, Fredenburgh JC, Weitz JI. Characterization of the interactions of plasminogen and tissue and vampire bat plasminogen activators with fibrinogen, fibrin, and the complex of D-dimer noncovalently linked to fragment E. J Biol Chem 1998;273:18292–18299.

119. Schleuning W-D, Donner P. Desmodu rotundus (common vampire bat) salivary plasminogen activator. In: Bachmann F, ed. Fibrinolytics and antifibrinolytics, handbook of experimental pharmacology. Heidelberg: Springer, 2000:447–468.

120. Esmon CT, Mather T. Switching serine protease specificity. Nat Struct Biol 1998;5:933-937.

121. Reed GL, Lin LF, Parhami-Seren B, Kussie P. Identification of a plasminogen binding region in streptokinase that is necessary for the creation of a functional streptokinase-plasminogen activator complex. Biochemistry 1995;34:10266–10271.

122. Wang X, Lin X, Loy JA, Tang J, Zhang XC. Crystal structure of the catalytic domain of human plasmin complexed with streptokinase. Science 1998;281:1662–1665.

123. Lee PP, Wohl RC, Boreisha IG, Robbins KC. Kinetic analysis of covalent hybrid plasminogen activators: effect of CNBr-degraded

fibrinogen on kinetic parameters of Glu1-plasminogen activation. Biochemistry 1988;27:7506–7513.

124. McClintock DK, Bell PH. The mechanism of activation of human plasminogen by streptokinase. Biochem Biophys Res Commun 1971;43:694–702.

125. Reddy KN, Markus G. Mechanism of activation of human plasminogen by streptokinase. Presence of active center in streptokinase-plasminogen complex. J Biol Chem 1972;247:1683–1691.

126. Parry MA, Zhang XC, Bode I. Molecular mechanisms of plasminogen activation: bacterial cofactors provide clues. Trends Biochem Sci 2000;25:53–59.

127. Reed GL, Kussie P, Parhami-Seren B. A functional analysis of the antigenicity of streptokinase using monoclonal antibody mapping and recombinant streptokinase fragments. J Immunol 1993;150:4407–4415.

128. Parhami-Seren B, Keel T, Reed GL. Sequences of antigenic epitopes of streptokinase identified via random peptide libraries displayed on phage. J Mol Biol 1997;271:333–341.

129. Fears R, Ferres H, Glasgow E, et al. Monitoring of streptokinase resistance titre in acute myocardial infarction patients up to 30 months after giving streptokinase or anistreplase and related studies to measure specific antistreptokinase IgG. Br Heart J 1992;68:167–170.

130. Much H. Ueber eine Vorstufe des Fibrinfermentes in Kulturen von Staphylokockkus aurens. Biocehm Ztschr 1908;14:143.

131. Tillet WS, Garner RL. The fibrinolytic activity of hemolytic streptococci. J. Exp. Med. 1933;58:485–502.

132. Gerheim EB. Staphylococcal coagulation and fibrinolysis. Nature 1948;162.

133. Lack CH. Staphylokinase: an activator of plasma protease. Nature 1948;161:559–560.

134. Sako T, Sawaki S, Sakurai T, Ito S, Yoshizawa Y, Kondo I. Cloning and expression of the staphylokinase gene of Staphylococcus aureus in Escherichia coli. Mol Gen Genet 1983;190:271–277.

135. Sako T. Overproduction of staphylokinase in Escherichia coli and its characterization. Eur J Biochem 1985;149:557–563.

136. Collen D. Staphylokinase: a potent, uniquely fibrin-selective thrombolytic agent. Nat Med 1998;4:279–284.

137. Schlott B, Guhrs KH, Hartmann M, Rocker A, Collen D. Staphylokinase requires NH2-terminal proteolysis for plasminogen activation. J Biol Chem 1997;272:6067–6072.

138. Sakharov DV, Lijnen HR, Rijken DC. Interactions between staphylokinase, plasmin(ogen), and fibrin. Staphylokinase discriminates between free plasminogen and plasminogen bound to partially degraded fibrin. J Biol Chem 1996;271:27912–27918.

139. Sakai M, Watanuki M, Matsuo O. Mechanism of fibrin-specific fibrinolysis by staphylokinase: participation of alpha 2-plasmin inhibitor. Biochem Biophys Res Commun 1989;162:830–837.

140. Lijnen HR, Van Hoef B, De Cock F, et al. On the mechanism of fibrin-specific plasminogen activation by staphylokinase. J Biol Chem 1991;266:11826–11832.

141. Vanderschueren S, Barrios L, Kerdsinchai P, et al. A randomized trial of recombinant staphylokinase versus alteplase for coronary artery patency in acute myocardial infarction. The STAR Trial Group. Circulation 1995;92:2044–2049.

142. Collen D, Van de Werf F. Coronary thrombolysis with recombinant staphylokinase in patients with evolving myocardial infarction. Circulation 1993;87:1850–1853.

143. Reed GL III, Matsueda GR, Haber E. Acceleration of plasma clot lysis by an antibody to alpha 2-antiplasmin. Trans Assoc Am Physicians 1988;101:250–256.

144. Reed GLIII, Matsueda GR, Haber E. Synergistic fibrinolysis: combined effects of plasminogen activators and an antibody that inhibits alpha 2-antiplasmin. Proc Natl Acad Sci USA 1990;87:1114–1118.

145. Sakata Y, Eguchi Y, Mimuro J, Matsuda M, Sumi Y. Clot lysis induced by a monoclonal antibody against alpha 2-plasmin inhibitor. Blood 1989;74:2692–2697.

146. Reed GL III, Matsueda GR, Haber E. Inhibition of clot-bound alpha 2-antiplasmin enhances in vivo thrombolysis. Circulation 1990;82:164–168.

147. Butte AN, Houng AK, Jang IK, Reed GL III. Alpha 2-antiplasmin causes thrombi to resist fibrinolysis induced by tissue plasminogen activator in experimental pulmonary embolism. Circulation 1997;95:1886–1891.

148. Reed GL III, Houng AK. The contribution of activated factor XIII to fibrinolytic resistance in experimental pulmonary embolism [see comments]. Circulation 1999;99:299–304.

149. Lijnen HR, Okada K, Matsuo O, Collen D, Dewerchin M. Alpha 2-antiplasmin gene deficiency in mice is associated with enhanced fibrinolytic potential without overt bleeding. Blood 1999;93:2274–2281.

150. Christensen S, Valnickova Z, Thogersen IB, Olsen EHN, Enghild JJ. Assignment of a single disulphide bridge in human alpha 2-antiplasmin: implications for the structural and functional properties. Biochem J 1997;323:847–852.

151. Christensen U, Clemmensen I. Kinetic properties of the primary inhibitor of plasmin from human plasma. Biochem J 1977;163:389–391.

152. Christensen U, Bangert K, Thorsen S. Reaction of human alpha 2-antiplasmin and plasmin stopped-flow fluorescence kinetics. FEBS Lett 1996;387:58–62.

153. Wiman B, Collen D. On the kinetics of the reaction between human antiplasmin and plasmin. Eur J Biochem 1978;84:573–578.

154. Longstaff C, Gaffney PJ. Serpin-serine protease binding kinetics: alpha 2-antiplasmin as a model inhibitor. Biochemistry 1991;30:979–986.

155. Wiman B, Lijnen HR, Collen D. On the specific interaction between the lysine-binding sites in plasmin and complementary sites in alpha 2-antiplasmin and in fibrinogen. Biochim Biophys Acta 1979;579:142–154.

156. Wiman B, Boman L, Collen D. On the kinetics of the reaction between human antiplasmin and a low-molecular-weight form of plasmin. Eur J Biochem 1978;87:143–146.

157. Turner RB, Liu L, Sazonova IY, Reed GL. Structural Elements that Govern the Substrate Specificity of the Clot Dissolving Enzyme Plasmin. submitted.

158. Nilsson T, Sjoholm I, Wiman B. Circular dichroism studies on alpha 2-antiplasmin and its interactions with plasmin and plasminogen. Biochim Biophys Acta 1982;705:264–270.

159. Christensen S, Sottrup-Jensen L, Christensen U. Stopped-flow fluorescence kinetics of bovine alpha 2-antiplasmin inhibition of bovine midiplasmin. Biochem J 1995;305:97–102.

160. Cederholm-Williams SA, De Cock F, Lijnen HR, Collen D. Kinetics of the reactions between streptokinase, plasmin and alpha 2-antiplasmin. Eur J Biochem 1979;100:125–132.

161. Wiman B, Collen D. On the mechanism of the reaction between human alpha 2-antiplasmin and plasmin. J Biol Chem 1979;254:9291–9297.

162. Huntington JA, Read RJ, Carrell RW. Structure of a serpin-protease complex shows inhibition by deformation [In Process Citation]. Nature 2000;407:923–926.

163. Deng G, Curriden SA, Hu G, Czekay RP, Loskutoff DJ. Plasminogen activator inhibitor-1 regulates cell adhesion by binding to the somatomedin B domain of vitronectin. J Cell Physiol 2001;189:23-33.

164. Vaughan DE. Plasminogen activator inhibitor-1: a common denominator in cardiovascular disease. J Investig Med 1998;46: 370–376.

165. Wiman B. Plasminogen activator inhibitor 1 in thrombotic disease. Curr Opin Hematol 1996;3:372–378.

166. Waltz DA, Natkin LR, Fujita RM, Wei Y, Chapman HA. Plasmin and plasminogen activator inhibitor type 1 promote cellular motility by regulating the interaction between the urokinase receptor and vitronectin. J Clin Invest 1997;100:58–67.

167. Chapman HA. Plasminogen activators, integrins, and the coordinated regulation of cell adhesion and migration. Curr Opin Cell Biol 1997;9:714–724.

168. Levin EG, Santell L. Conversion of the active to latent plasminogen activator inhibitor from human endothelial cells. Blood 1987;70:1090–1098.

169. Nar H, Bauer M, Stassen JM, Lang D, Gils A, Declerck PJ. Plasminogen activator inhibitor 1. Structure of the native serpin, comparison to its other conformers and implications for serpin inactivation. J Mol Biol 2000;297:683–695.

170. Kost C, Stuber W, Ehrlich HJ, Pannekoek H, Preissner KT. Mapping of binding sites for heparin, plasminogen activator inhibitor- 1, and plasminogen to vitronectin's heparin-binding region reveals a novel vitronectin-dependent feedback mechanism for the control of plasmin formation. J Biol Chem 1992;267:12098–12105.

171. Ehrlich HJ, Gebbink RK, Keijer J, Pannekoek H. Elucidation of structural requirements on plasminogen activator inhibitor 1 for binding to heparin. J Biol Chem 1992;267:11606–11611.

172. Lawrence DA, Berkenpas MB, Palaniappan S, Ginsburg D. Localization of vitronectin binding domain in plasminogen activator inhibitor-1. J Biol Chem 1994;269:15223–15228.

173. Dieval J, Nguyen G, Gross S, Delobel J, Kruithof EK. A lifelong bleeding disorder associated with a deficiency of plasminogen activator inhibitor type 1. Blood 1991;77:528–532.

174. Friederich PW, Levi M, Biemond BJ, et al. Novel low-molecular-weight inhibitor of PAI-1 (XR5118) promotes endogenous fibrinolysis and reduces postthrombolysis thrombus growth in rabbits. Circulation 1997;96:916–921.

175. Charlton PA, Faint RW, Bent F, et al. Evaluation of a low molecular weight modulator of human plasminogen activator inhibitor-1 activity. Thromb Haemost 1996;75:808–815.

176. Kruithof EK, Gudinchet A, Bachmann F. Plasminogen activator inhibitor 1 and plasminogen activator inhibitor 2 in various disease states. Thromb Haemost 1988;59:7–12.

177. Hendriks D, Wang W, Scharpe S, Lommaert MP, van Sande M. Purification and characterization of a new arginine carboxypeptidase in human serum. Biochim Biophys Acta 1990;1034:86–92.

178. Levin Y, Skidgel RA, Erdos EG. Isolation and characterization of the subunits of human plasma carboxypeptidase N (kininase i). Proc Natl Acad Sci USA 1982;79:4618–4622.

179. Hendriks D, Scharpe S, van Sande M, Lommaert MP. Characterisation of a carboxypeptidase in human serum distinct from carboxypeptidase N. J Clin Chem Clin Biochem 1989;27: 277–285.

180. Eaton DL, Malloy BE, Tsai SP, Henzel W, Drayna D. Isolation, molecular cloning, and partial characterization of a novel carboxypeptidase B from human plasma. J Biol Chem 1991;266: 21833–21838.

181. Campbell W, Yonezu K, Shinohara T, Okada H. An arginine carboxypeptidase generated during coagulation is diminished or absent in patients with rheumatoid arthritis. J Lab Clin Med 1990;115:610–612.

182. Bajzar L, Manuel R, Nesheim ME. Purification and characterization of TAFI, a thrombin-activable fibrinolysis inhibitor. J Biol Chem 1995;270:14477–14484.

183. Bajzar L, Nesheim ME, Tracy PB. The profibrinolytic effect of activated protein C in clots formed from plasma is TAFI-dependent. Blood 1996;88:2093–2100.

184. Mosnier LO, von dem Borne PA, Meijers JC, Bouma BN. Plasma TAFI levels influence the clot lysis time in healthy individuals in the presence of an intact intrinsic pathway of coagulation. Thromb Haemost 1998;80:829–835.

185. Valnickova Z, Enghild JJ. Human procarboxypeptidase U, or thrombin-activable fibrinolysis inhibitor, is a substrate for transglutaminases. Evidence for transglutaminase-catalyzed cross-linking to fibrin. J Biol Chem 1998;273:27220–27224.

186. Mao SS, Cooper CM, Wood T, Shafer JA, Gardell SJ. Characterization of plasmin-mediated activation of plasma procarboxypeptidase B. Modulation by glycosaminoglycans. J Biol Chem 1999;274:35046–35052.

187. Bajzar L, Morser J, Nesheim M. TAFI, or plasma procarboxypeptidase B, couples the coagulation and fibrinolytic cascades through the thrombin-thrombomodulin complex. J Biol Chem 1996;271:16603–16608.

188. Suenson E, Lutzen O, Thorsen S. Initial plasmin-degradation of fibrin as the basis of a positive feed- back mechanism in fibrinolysis. Eur J Biochem 1984;140:513–522.

189. Norrman B, Wallen P, Ranby M. Fibrinolysis mediated by tissue plasminogen activator. Disclosure of a kinetic transition. Eur J Biochem 1985;149:193–200.

190. Fleury V, Angles-Cano E. Characterization of the binding of plasminogen to fibrin surfaces: the role of carboxy-terminal lysines. Biochemistry 1991;30:7630–7638.

191. Pannell R, Black J, Gurewich V. Complementary modes of action of tissue-type plasminogen activator and pro-urokinase by which their synergistic effect on clot lysis may be explained. J Clin Invest 1988;81:853–859.

192. Boffa MB, Wang W, Bajzar L, Nesheim ME. Plasma and recombinant thrombin-activable fibrinolysis inhibitor (TAFI) and activated TAFI compared with respect to glycosylation, thrombin/thrombomodulin-dependent activation, thermal stability, and enzymatic properties. J Biol Chem 1998;273: 2127–2135.

193. Klement P, Liao P, Bajzar L. A novel approach to arterial thrombolysis. Blood 1999;94:2735–2743.

194. Nagashima M, Werner M, Wang M, Zhao L, Light DR, Pagila R, Morser J, Verhallen P. An inhibitor of activated thrombin-activatable fibrinolysis inhibitor potentiates tissue-type plasminogen activator-induced thrombolysis in a rabbit jugular vein thrombolysis model. Thromb Res 2000;98:333–342.

195. Schwartz ML, Pizzo SV, Hill RL, McKee PA. The subunit structures of human plasma and platelet factor XIII (fibrin-stabilizing factor). J Biol Chem 1971;246:5851–5854.

196. Lorand L. Activation of blood coagulation factor XIII. Ann N Y Acad Sci 1986;485:144–158.

197. Gaffney PJ, Whitaker AN. Fibrin crosslinks and lysis rates. Thromb Res 1979;14:85–94.

198. Loewy AG, McDonagh J, Mikkola H, Teller DC, Yee VC. Structure and function of factor XIII. In: Colman RW, Hirsh J, Marder VJ, Clowes AW, George JN, eds. Hemostasis and

Thrombosis: Basic Principles and Clinical Practice. Philadelphia: Lippincott Co., 2001:233–248.

199. Jansen JW, Haverkate F, Koopman J, Nieuwenhuis HK, Kluft C, Boschman TA. Influence of factor XIIIa activity on human whole blood clot lysis in vitro. Thromb Haemost 1987;57:171–175.

200. Lukacova D, Matsueda GR, Haber E, Reed GL III. Inhibition of Factor XIII activation by an anti-peptide monoclonal antibody. Biochemistry 1991;30:10164–10170.

201. Reed GL III, Lukacova D. Generation and mechanism of action of a potent inhibitor of factor XIII function. Thromb Haemost 1995;74:680–685.

202. Seale L, Finney S, Sawyer RT, Wallis RB. Tridegin, a novel peptidic inhibitor of factor XIIIa from the leech, Haementeria ghilianii, enhances fibrinolysis in vitro. Thromb Haemost 1997;77:959–963.

203. Kohler HP, Ariens RA, Mansfield MW, Whitaker P, Grant PJ. Factor XIII activity and antigen levels in patients with coronary artery disease. Thromb Haemost 2001;85:569–570.

204. Williams SE, Kounnas MZ, Argraves KM, Argraves WS, Strickland DK. The alpha 2-macroglobulin receptor/low density lipoprotein receptor- related protein and the receptor-associated protein. An overview. Ann N Y Acad Sci 1994;737:1–13.

205. Roberts RC. Protease inhibitors of human plasma. Alpha-2-macroglobulin. J Med 1985;16:129–224.

206. Kolodziej SJ, Klueppelberg HU, Nolasco N, Ehses W, Strickland DK, Stoops JK. Three-dimensional structure of the human plasmin alpha 2-macroglobulin complex. J Struct Biol 1998;123:124–133.

207. Bennett B, Croll A, Ferguson K, Booth NA. Complexing of tissue plasminogen activator with PAI-1, alpha 2- macroglobulin, and C1-inhibitor: studies in patients with defibrination and a fibrinolytic state after electroshock or complicated labor. Blood 1990;75:671–676.

208. Davis AE, 3rd. Structure and function of C1 inhibitor. Behring Inst Mitt 1989;:142–150.

209. Al-Abdullah IH, Greally J. C1-inhibitor—biochemical properties and clinical applications. Crit Rev Immunol 1985;5:317–330.

210. Leung L. Histidine-rich glycoprotein: an abundant plasma protein in search of a function. J Lab Clin Med 1993;121:630–631.

211. Saez CT, Jansen GJ, Smith A, Morgan WT. Interaction of histidine-proline-rich glycoprotein with plasminogen: effect of ligands, pH, ionic strength, and chemical modification. Biochemistry 1995;34:2496–2503.

212. Ichinose A, Mimuro J, Koide T, Aoki N. Histidine-rich glycoprotein and alpha 2-plasmin inhibitor in inhibition of plasminogen binding to fibrin. Thromb Res 1984;33:401–407.

213. Group. I-SISoISC. Randomised trial of intravenous streptokinase, oral aspirin, both, or neither among 17,187 cases of suspected acute myocardial infarction: ISIS-2. Lancet 1988;2:349–360.

214. Verheugt FW. GUSTO V: the bottom line of fibrinolytic reperfusion therapy. Lancet 2001;357:1898–1899.

215. Yusuf S, Zhao F, Mehta SR, Chrolavicius S, Tognoni G, Fox KK. Effects of clopidogrel in addition to aspirin in patients with acute coronary syndromes without ST-segment elevation. N Engl J Med 2001;345:494–502.

216. Mahaffey KW, Granger CB, Collins R, et al. Overview of randomized trials of intravenous heparin in patients with acute myocardial infarction treated with thrombolytic therapy. Am J Cardiol 1996;77:551–556.

217. Collins R, MacMahon S, Flather M, et al. Clinical effects of anticoagulant therapy in suspected acute myocardial infarction:

218. de Bono DP, Simoons ML, Tijssen J, et al. Effect of early intravenous heparin on coronary patency, infarct size, and bleeding complications after alteplase thrombolysis: results of a randomised double blind European Cooperative Study Group trial. Br Heart J 1992;67:122–128.

219. Investigators GA. The effects of tissue plasminogen activator, streptokinase, or both on coronary-artery patency, ventricular function, and survival after acute myocardial infarction. N Engl J Med 1993;329:1615–1622.

220. Wallentin L, Dellborg DM, Lindahl B, Nilsson T, Pehrsson K, Swahn E. The low-molecular-weight heparin dalteparin as adjuvant therapy in acute myocardial infarction: the ASSENT PLUS study. Clin Cardiol 2001;24:I12–I14.

221. Ross AM, Molhoek P, Lundergan C, et al. Randomized comparison of enoxaparin, a low-molecular-weight heparin, with unfractionated heparin adjunctive to recombinant tissue plasminogen activator thrombolysis and aspirin: second trial of Heparin and Aspirin Reperfusion Therapy (HART II). Circulation 2001;104:648–652.

222. A comparison of recombinant hirudin with heparin for the treatment of acute coronary syndromes. The Global Use of Strategies to Open Occluded Coronary Arteries (GUSTO) IIb investigators. N Engl J Med 1996;335:775–782.

223. Verstraete M. Third-generation thrombolytic drugs. Am J Med 2000;109:52–58.

224. Haber E, Bode C, Matsueda GR, Reed GL III, Runge MS. Antibody targeting as a thrombolytic strategy. Ann N Y Acad Sci 1992;667:365–381.

225. Haber E, Quertermous T, Matsueda GR, Runge MS. Innovative approaches to plasminogen activator therapy. Science 1989;243:51–56.

226. Dewerchin M, Lijnen HR, Van Hoef B, De Cock F, Collen D. Biochemical properties of conjugates of urokinase-type plasminogen activator with a monoclonal antibody specific for cross-linked fibrin. Eur J Biochem 1989;185:141–149.

227. Runge MS, Harker LA, Bode C, et al. Enhanced thrombolytic and antithrombotic potency of a fibrin-targeted plasminogen activator in baboons. Circulation 1996;94:1412–1422.

228. Holvoet P, Laroche Y, Lijnen HR, et al. Characterization of a chimeric plasminogen activator consisting of a single-chain Fv fragment derived from a fibrin fragment D-dimer- specific antibody and a truncated single-chain urokinase. J Biol Chem 1991;266:19717–19724.

229. Yang WP, Goldstein J, Procyk R, Matsueda GR, Shaw SY. Design and evaluation of a thrombin-activable plasminogen activator. Biochemistry 1994;33:606–612.

230. Bode C, Meinhardt G, Runge MS, et al. Platelet-targeted fibrinolysis enhances clot lysis and inhibits platelet aggregation. Circulation 1991;84:805–813.

231. Dewerchin M, Lijnen HR, Stassen JM, et al. Effect of chemical conjugation of recombinant single-chain urokinase- type plasminogen activator with monoclonal antiplatelet antibodies on platelet aggregation and on plasma clot lysis in vitro and in vivo. Blood 1991;78:1005–1018.

232. Reed GL III, Houng AK, Liu L, et al. A catalytic switch and the conversion of streptokinase to a fibrin-targeted plasminogen activator. Proc. Natl. Acad. Sci. (USA) 1999;96: 8879–8883.

233. Robinson BR, Houng AK, Reed GL III. Catalytic life of activated factor XIII in thrombi. Implications for fibrinolytic resistance and thrombus aging. Circulation 2000;102:1151–1157.

234. Kalyan NK, Lee SG, Cheng SM, Hartzell R, Urbano C, Hung PP. Construction and expression of a hybrid plasminogen activator gene with sequences from non-protease region of tissue-type plasminogen activator (t-PA) and protease region of urokinase (u-PA). Gene 1988;68:205–212.

235. Agnelli G, Pascucci C, Nenci GG, Mele A, Burgi R, Heim J. Thrombolytic and haemorrhagic effects of bolus doses of tissue-type plasminogen activator and a hybrid plasminogen activator with prolonged plasma half-life (K2tu-PA: CGP 42935). Thromb Haemost 1993;70:294–300.

236. Lijnen HR, Wnendt S, Schneider J,et al. Functional properties of a recombinant chimeric protein with combined thrombin inhibitory and plasminogen-activating potential. Eur J Biochem 1995;234:350–357.

237. Wnendt S, Janocha E, Steffens GJ, Strassburger W. A strong thrombin-inhibitory prourokinase derivative with sequence elements from hirudin and the human thrombin receptor. Protein Eng 1997;10:169–173.

238. Szarka SJ, Sihota EG, Habibi HR, Wong S. Staphylokinase as a plasminogen activator component in recombinant fusion proteins. Appl Environ Microbiol 1999;65:506–513.

239. Wallentin L. Reducing time to treatment in acute myocardial infarction. Eur J Emerg Med 2000;7:217–227.

240. French JK, Williams BF, Hart HH, et al. Prospective evaluation of eligibility for thrombolytic therapy in acute myocardial infarction. Bmj 1996;312:1637–1641.

241. Boucher JM, Racine N, Thanh TH, et al. Age-related differences in in-hospital mortality and the use of thrombolytic therapy for acute myocardial infarction. Cmaj 2001;164:1285–1290.

242. Ross AM, Coyne KS, Reiner JS, et al. A randomized trial comparing primary angioplasty with a strategy of short-acting thrombolysis and immediate planned rescue angioplasty in acute myocardial infarction: the PACT trial. PACT investigators. Plasminogen-activator Angioplasty Compatibility Trial. J Am Coll Cardiol 1999;34:1954–1962.

243. Brouwer MA, Martin JS, Maynard C, et al. Influence of early prehospital thrombolysis on mortality and event-free survival (the Myocardial Infarction Triage and Intervention [MITI] Randomized Trial). MITI Project Investigators. Am J Cardiol 1996;78:497–502.

244. Herrmann HC. Triple therapy for acute myocardial infarction: combining fibrinolysis, platelet IIb/IIIa inhibition, and percutaneous coronary intervention. Am J Cardiol 2000;85:10C–16C.

245. Matetzky S, Novikov M, Gruberg L, et al. The significance of persistent ST elevation versus early resolution of ST segment elevation after primary PTCA. J Am Coll Cardiol 1999;34:1932–1938.

246. Francis CW. Ultrasound-enhanced thrombolysis. Echocardiography 2001;18:239–246.

247. Siegel RJ, Atar S, Fishbein MC, et al. Noninvasive transcutaneous low frequency ultrasound enhances thrombolysis in peripheral and coronary arteries. Echocardiography 2001;18:247–257.

248. Fears R. Development of anisoylated plasminogen-streptokinase activator complex from the acyl enzyme concept. [Review] [46 refs]. Semin Thromb Hemost 1989;15: 129–139.

249. Carmeliet P, Stassen JM, Schoonjans L, et al. Plasminogen activator inhibitor-1 gene-deficient mice. II. Effects on hemostasis, thrombosis, and thrombolysis. J Clin Invest 1993;92: 2756–2760.

17 Coronary Restenosis

Julius Aitsebaomo, MD, *Martin Moser,* MD, *Susan Smyth,* MD, PhD, *and Cam Patterson,* MD

CONTENTS

INTRODUCTION

Restenosis, usually seen after percutaneous transluminal coronary angioplasty (PTCA), stent placement (in-stent restenosis), or other percutaneous coronary interventions, is a perturbation of the wound healing process that narrows the vessel lumen by more than 50% *(1)*. The benefits of PTCA in patients with coronary artery disease are well established *(2)*, and more than 800,000 procedures are performed yearly in the United States *(3)*. Since the introduction of PTCA, significant advances have been made in interventional cardiology, especially with the use of stenting procedures; however, restenosis is still a major clinical problem that causes significant morbidity and mortality. Up to 20% of all patients undergoing percutaneous interventions require repeated interventional procedures for restenosis (Fig. 1).

Atherosclerosis is the deposition of lipids in the intima of large and medium-sized arteries. When coupled with the destructive properties of hypertension, smoking, and toxic substances in the environment, atherosclerosis causes an inflammatory response within the endothelium *(4)*. The histopathology of restenosis differs from that of primary atherosclerotic lesions, which consist of dense intimal fibrosis with necrotic debris, calcium deposits, foam cells, and cholesterol crystals. In contrast, restenotic lesions contain an underlying chronic atherosclerotic lesion that has undergone mechanical compression with superimposed loose fibroproliferative tissue that is mainly due to smooth muscle–induced intimal hyperplasia *(5)*. This fibroproliferative process occurs both in native vessels and in vein grafts after PTCA, suggesting that the cellular response to vascular injury occurs regardless of the vessel type involved.

Risk factors for restenosis include diabetes mellitus *(1,6)*, high platelet aggregability *(1,7)*, homocysteinemia *(8,9)*, previous cytomegalovirus (CMV) infection *(10–13)*, lesion length before PTCA or stent placement *(14)*, prior restenosis *(15)*, low levels of high-density lipoproteins *(16)*, the presence of multivessel disease *(17)*, and genetic factors *(18–22)*. The diversity of risk factors for restenosis suggests that the pathological fibroproliferative response is exacerbated by multiple forms of cellular injury through a final common pathway.

PATHOPHYSIOLOGY

Most of our understanding of the pathophysiology of restenosis comes from animal models. The endothelial cellular injury caused by transient balloon angioplasty, as well as the foreign materials deployed by stents and the permanent strain the stents apply to the vessel, eventually

From: *Contemporary Cardiology: Principles of Molecular Cardiology*
Edited by: M. S. Runge and C. Patterson © Humana Press Inc., Totowa, NJ

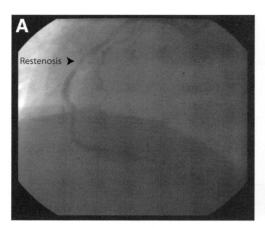 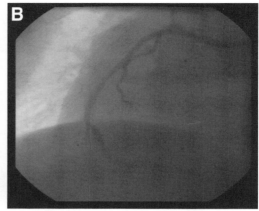

Fig. 1. Angiographic views of a 57-yr-old man who presented 4 mo prior with an acute coronary syndrome due to occlusion of the right coronary artery (RCA) requiring placement of a stent. The patient presented 4 mo after stent placement with similar symptoms caused by in-stent restenosis as shown above: **(A)** pre- and **(B)** postdilatation.

result in endothelial denudation. The presence of a foreign object in the vascular lumen after stent implantation has been shown to produce a chronic inflammatory reaction in experimental systems with stents constructed from various polymer materials (23). Intimal injury, endothelial denudation, and exposure of the thrombogenic subendothelium (24) result in an abrupt onset of rapid, but self-limiting, platelet activation, inflammatory cell infiltration, smooth muscle cell (SMC) proliferation, production of reactive oxygen species and thrombin, and vascular remodeling. Each of these processes may contribute to the formation of restenotic lesions.

The Endothelium

The vascular endothelial cell is an active integrated cell that can detect both humoral and hemodynamic changes within its milieu. Through inter- and intracellular mechanisms, the endothelium can relay signals within the cell and to adjacent cells to synthesize and release substances that affect dynamic changes in the vessel wall. The patency of the lumen after angioplasty is, therefore, determined by the extent of endothelial layer regenerated after balloon or stent injury, the ability of the regenerated endothelium to detect and transduce hemodynamic stimuli that will activate or inhibit growth and migration, and the relative balance between cell growth and cell death. In addition, lumen patency is affected by the plasticity of the remodeled vessel as a result of changes in the extracellular matrix and by the amount of blood flow after the procedure.

Platelets

Immediately after balloon-induced vascular injury or stent implantation, circulating platelets adhere to the endothelium, become activated, and aggregate to one another (25,26) (Fig. 2). The glycoprotein (GP) Ib-IX complex, the collagen receptors GP VI and integrin $\alpha 2\beta 1$, and the platelet fibrinogen receptor GP IIb/IIIa mediate the initial interaction of platelets with various components of the exposed subendothelium. Platelet adhesion, coupled with the local release of mediators at areas of vascular damage, result in platelet activation and GP IIb/IIIa–dependent platelet aggregate formation. After a brief period, the damaged surface becomes quiescent and stops attracting platelets. Platelet deposition along angioplasty-damaged vessels is undetectable by 7 d (27). The presence of an angiographically identifiable thrombus at the time of PTCA is associated with a high rate of restenosis (28). Abnormally high platelet aggregation increases the rate of restenosis twofold (1). In animal models, severe and prolonged thrombocytopenia inhibits neointimal formation after balloon injury (29). However, $\beta 3$-integrin deficient mice, which lack GP IIb/IIIa and $\alpha V\beta 3$ integrin, develop normal levels of intimal hyperplasia after wire-induced endothelial denudation of the femoral artery, despite reduced platelet deposition 1 h after injury (30). Taken together, these results suggest that platelets may contribute to lesion formation in a manner independent of direct platelet–vessel wall interactions.

Activated platelets contribute to the progression of intimal hyperplasia by releasing factors that affect SMCs such as platelet-derived growth factor (PDGF), which promotes growth and migration of SMCs. In addition, activated platelets release transforming growth factor-β_1, serotonin, adenosine diphosphate, and thromboxane A_2, all of which may contribute to intimal hyperplasia (31,32) and to increased extracellular matrix generation (31). Activated

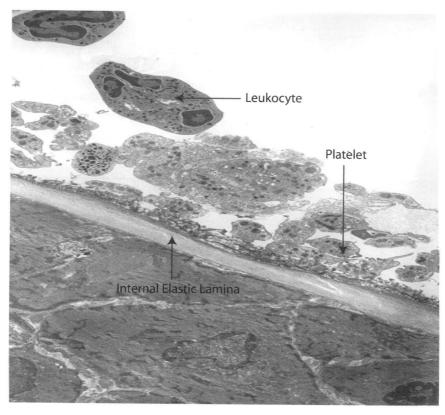

Fig. 2. Electron micrograph of a blood vessel in a mouse 1 h after wire-induced intimal injury; platelet aggregation and leukocyte infiltration, early events in restenosis, are seen.

platelets facilitate the generation of thrombin, a powerful mitogen for SMCs *(33)*. Furthermore, platelets affect the response to injury by recruiting leukocytes to areas of vascular damage and by altering matrix composition through the release of matrix proteins such as thrombospondin, osteopontin, and enzymes that degrade extracellular matrix including matrix metalloproteinases.

Smooth Muscle Cells

The process of vascular lesion formation and vascular remodeling requires both activation of cell growth and apoptotic cell death. Apoptotic cell death, one of the first cellular events induced by balloon angioplasty, occurs in up to 70% of medial SMCs within 30 min of injury *(34,35)*. Unlike medial SMCs, neointimal cells are relatively resistant to apoptotic death induced by angioplasty. This resistance to balloon injury–induced death is associated with a downregulation of the antiapoptotic mediator bcl-x$_L$ in the luminal layers of the media *(34)*. In medial SMCs, apoptosis is followed by a coordinated cellular response that includes PDGF-induced migration of a subpopulation of medial SMCs into the intima, proliferation of intimal and medial SMCs (about 80% of these

migrating cells are in the G1 and S phases of the cell cycle *[36]*), elaboration of extracellular matrix molecules (i.e., chondroitin sulfate and hyaluronan), and vascular remodeling. These events culminate in neointimal hyperplasia (Fig. 3), a defining feature of restenotic lesions. Because SMCs are the major cellular component of restenotic lesions, the mechanisms that elicit their proliferation are important in the pathophysiology of this process.

Leukocytes

Circulating monocytes are among the earliest cells recruited into experimentally induced vascular lesions in animals *(37)* (Fig. 2). Leukocytes are recruited as a precursor to intimal thickening in these models *(38,39)*, and blocking the adhesion molecules that are important for leukocyte recruitment attenuates intimal growth *(40,41)*. The β2 integrin Mac-1, the primary fibrinogen receptor on leukocytes *(42)*, is upregulated after angioplasty *(43,44)*. The blockade or absence of Mac-1 reduces intimal thickening after angioplasty or stent implantation *(41,45)*. Leukocytes that adhere to the vessel walls are seen in the coronary arteries after angioplasty or stent placement in patients *(46)*, and inflammatory cells are

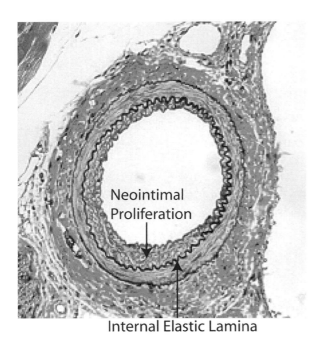

Fig. 3. Photomicrograph of a mouse vessel 4 wk after wire-induced intimal injury showing neointimal hyperplasia, a defining feature of restenosis.

more numerous in restenotic lesions than in de novo lesions *(47)*. Clinical trials indicate that leukocyte activation with platelet adherence can occur despite antiplatelet therapy and that the magnitude of leukocyte activation predicts late clinical events *(43)* and late restenosis *(48)* after angioplasty. These studies suggest that monocytes serve as markers, initiators, and promoters of the restenotic process, perhaps by contributing growth factors that stimulate SMC proliferation.

Growth Factors

Several growth factors are rapidly released from platelets and dying cells after catheter injury. The binding of these growth factors to their respective receptors can lead to transient activation of signal transduction and to activation of early response genes like *c-fos, c-jun,* and *c-myc.* The activation of early response genes triggers a cascade of events that causes the cell to enter the cell cycle. Several cytokines and growth factors derived from platelets, endothelial cells, mononuclear cells, and SMCs play a central role in restenosis. Platelets, for example, are rich in growth factors like PDGF, insulin-like growth factor, transforming growth factor-β_1, and epidermal growth factor *(49)*, each of which is important in the early cellular proliferative events.

Balloon injury–associated trauma to the tunica media causes endothelial denudation of the involved vessel, a process that increases expression of PDGF and its receptor in the vessel wall *(50)*. PDGF has chemotactic *(51)*, migratory *(52)*, and proliferative *(53)* effects on SMCs in the development of the neointima. Uchida et al. *(53)* have shown a sevenfold increase in PDGF-B chain mRNA expression that peaks 7 d after injury in rabbit femoral arteries and persists for at least 21 d. The direct infusion of PDGF-BB into rat carotid arteries induces neointimal formation mainly by stimulating SMC migration *(54)*, and treating rats with neutralizing antibodies to the BB-isoform of PDGF after balloon injury of the carotid artery reduces intimal thickening by 40%. PDGF may act by autophosphorylation of the PDGF receptor, which activates tyrosine kinase and leads to phosphorylation of signaling proteins *(53,55)* that eventually results in new DNA synthesis.

The complex interplay between cytokines and growth factors is oversimplified and underestimated in many animal models, which typically involve a single injury in an artery without preexisting lesions. Moreover, the animals often lack confounding variables, such as hypercholesterolemia, diabetes, or hypertension, that plague most patients the animal models are designed to study. Applying findings from animal models to humans has been unsuccessful, perhaps because of the complexity seen in vivo.

Reactive Oxygen Species

Almost all cells in the vascular wall produce and are regulated by reactive oxygen species (ROS), including superoxide, hydrogen peroxide (H_2O_2), and nitric oxide *(56,57)*. The NAD(P)H oxidase, a membrane-associated enzyme that catalyzes the reduction of oxygen to superoxide, is a major source of ROS production in the vasculature. SMCs and myofibroblasts are major cell sources of ROS in the vessel wall *(25,58,59)*. Factors such as PDGF, angiotensin II, phenylephrine, and thrombin generate intracellular ROS that, in turn, elicit SMC proliferation, survival, hypertrophy, and apoptosis *(60–63)*. These factors generate ROS regardless of whether they signal via tyrosine kinase receptors (e.g., PDGF) *(62)* or via G protein–coupled receptors (e.g., phenylephrine *[64]* and thrombin *[65]*). Growth factors are important in restenosis. PDGF stimulates the production of H_2O_2 in vascular SMCs and leads to SMC growth; suppression of the PDGF-stimulated increase in H_2O_2 blunts this proliferative response *(62)*. Thrombin similarly stimulates H_2O_2 and superoxide production in vascular SMCs, and catalase- or superoxide dismutase–mediated suppression of ROS inhibits thrombin-induced mitogenesis *(65)*. Furthermore, stimulation of SMCs with phenylephrine leads to induction of H_2O_2; suppression of H_2O_2 production inhibits phenylephrine-induced proliferation *(64)*. The proinflammatory mediator angiotensin II, which has a pathophysiologic role in hypertension, atherosclerosis, and restenosis *(66)*, causes vascular SMC hypertrophy via the production of H_2O_2 and superoxide and the activation of p38 mitogen-activated protein kinases *(63,67)*.

In addition to acting as a growth-promoting signaling molecule, ROS can induce programmed cell death under appropriate circumstances. For example, overexpression of the tumor suppressor gene p53 in vascular SMCs leads to an increase in ROS, growth inhibition, and apoptosis *(60)*. Inactivation of p53 by CMV-mediated production of IE84 (one of the viral immediate early genes) is strongly associated with pathologic SMC proliferation in human restenotic lesions *(68)*. These studies suggest that ROS and H_2O_2 mediate not only vascular SMC proliferation, survival, and hypertrophy but also apoptosis of vascular SMCs. This paradox can be partially explained by the differential effects of ROS on cell growth *(69,70)*; the net effect of ROS signaling (cellular proliferation or apoptosis) may be determined by a critical threshold that results from the complex kinetics of the redox milieu.

Lipids

Results from studies in hyperlipidemic mice indicate that hyperlipidemia is associated with more than a twofold increase in neointimal formation *(71)*. The significance of this finding is underscored by the fact that most patients undergoing PTCA are hyperlipidemic *(72)*. However, the association of hyperlipidemia with increased risk of restenosis is not as straightforward as its association with primary coronary atherosclerosis. Low serum levels of high-density lipoproteins (<40 mg/dL) and high cholesterol:high-density lipoprotein ratios correlate with high restenosis rates in small studies *(16,73)*, but in a large prospective trial no association was seen between quantitatively measured restenosis and serum lipid levels. Thus, the association between hyperlipidemia and restenosis may be weak or may be seen only in a subgroup of patients.

Lipid effects on the vascular wall may be due, in part, to interactions with the fibrinolytic system. Studies have shown that inhibition of plasminogen increases the risk of restenosis *(74)*. Lipoprotein(a) [Lp(a)] is a low-density lipoprotein-like particle that contains, in addition to apolipoprotein B, the disulfide-linked apolipoprotein(a) *(75,76)*. Lp(a) has a high degree of homology with plasminogen *(77,78)*, competitively inhibits binding of plasminogen to plasminogen receptors on endothelial cells *(79)*, and inhibits plasminogen activation *(80)* and thrombolysis *(81)*. In addition, Lp(a) interferes with several steps in the fibrinolytic pathway by competing with plasminogen and tissue plasminogen activator for fibrinogen and fibrin binding *(78)*, thus suggesting that patients with high Lp(a) levels may have a greater tendency for thrombosis and coronary restenosis. However, studies have not conclusively shown a link between Lp(a) levels and restenosis. Some studies have not shown a relationship between Lp(a) levels and restenosis *(73)*, whereas others have shown that Lp(a) is significantly higher in patients with restenosis *(82)*. Although the association of serum lipid levels with risk of atherosclerosis is well established, the role of serum lipids in restenosis is not clear.

Thrombin

Thrombin has multiple effects in addition to its role in coagulation and platelet function. Receptors for thrombin are present on vascular SMCs and endothelial cells *(83)*, and thrombin stimulation of the endothelium has prothrombotic *(84)* and proinflammatory *(85)* effects. SMCs undergoing apoptosis, one of the initial events that occur after vascular injury *(34)*, potently activate thrombin. Thrombin activation that occurs after denudation injury persists for up to 10 d *(86)*, and the expression of protease-activated receptor-1, a major thrombin receptor *(87)*, is increased rapidly after injury to the rat carotid artery. Expression of the thrombin receptor remains high during neointimal formation *(88)*. Furthermore, thrombin leads to SMC proliferation *(33)* and migration *(89)*, and stimulates SMCs to synthesize collagen *(90)*, which may contribute to extracellular matrix deposition. Thrombin is both mitogenic and chemotactic for inflammatory cells *(91,92)*. Plasminogen activator inhibitor-1 (PAI-1) can interact with activated thrombin to inhibit thrombin-mediated activity *(93)*, and PAI-1-deficient mice have greater neointimal formation after vascular injury than wild-type mice *(94)*; both of these findings indicate that PAI-1 is critical in lesion formation after vascular injury, probably due in part to its interactions with thrombin. Prolonged administration of hirudin, a potent thrombin inhibitor, in rats *(95)* and short-term administration of hirudin in rabbits *(86)* decreases the vasculoproliferative response. In addition, the vasculoproliferative response is reduced in protease-activated receptor-1 (PAR1)-deficient *(96)* or-inhibited *(97)* mice. These findings of reduced vasculoproliferation associated with thrombin inhibition indicate the central role of thrombin in vascular lesion formation.

VASCULAR REMODELING

Vascular remodeling involves structural alteration of the vessel wall by changes in cell growth, cell death, cell migration, and modulation of the production and degradation of extracellular matrix. Vascular remodeling is an active, adaptive process that occurs in response to the complex interaction between locally generated growth factors, vasoactive substances, and hemodynamic stimuli. Because the vascular endothelium is constantly exposed to humoral factors, inflammatory mediators, and physical forces, the endothelium is strategically located not only to serve as a sensory cell that assesses hemodynamic and humoral signals, but also to act as an effector cell that transduces the signals within the cell and to adjacent cells. These signals cause the synthesis and release or activation of mediators that influence cell growth, cell death, cell migration, or the composition of the extracellular matrix. These events affect the plasticity of the injured vessel and allow the vessel to respond appropriately to stimuli.

The outcome of the remodeling process could be an expansion of the external elastic membrane (commonly referred to as positive remodeling) if the remodeling ratio (the ratio of the lesion to the proximal reference external elastic membrane) is greater than 1.05. In contrast, if the remodeling ratio is less than 0.95, negative remodeling, or constrictive remodeling, occurs (98). Positive remodeling, a form of compensatory enlargement, was first observed in post-mortem studies of human coronary arteries (99). Negative remodeling may be involved in development of luminal stenosis after PTCA (100,101). In rabbits and pigs, arterial remodeling contributes to restenosis after vascular intervention (102,103). Kimura et al. reported a time-dependent, bidirectional remodeling response after percutaneous coronary intervention, with early adaptive enlargement followed by later shrinkage of the vessel (100); these observations were confirmed by Mintz et al. (101). The ability of the injured vessel to regenerate an endothelial layer after intervention may be critical in determining the immediate and late remodeling process and the clinical course of the patient.

IN-STENT RESTENOSIS

Coronary artery stenting is the only procedure that has decreased the incidence of late restenosis when compared with PTCA alone in large studies with sufficient follow-up intervals (104,105). Although the use of stenting has increased dramatically (106), in-stent restenosis is a major medical problem in 10–50% of patients undergoing the procedure in the United States (107,108).

In-stent restenosis is different from restenosis after PTCA (109,110). PTCA-induced restenosis is characterized by elastic recoil of the vessel, constrictive vascular

remodeling, SMC migration and proliferation, excessive extracellular matrix production, and thrombus formation at the site of injury. In contrast, neointimal formation, comprising proliferating SMCs and extracellular matrix formation (111,112), is the major pathological feature of in-stent restenosis (101) because stenting eliminates the vascular elastic recoil and constrictive remodeling seen after PTCA. Increased stent size relative to the proximal reference artery lumen correlates with increased neointimal area (113); therefore, accurate measurement of the reference lumen (perhaps with intravascular ultrasound) may prevent the use of an oversized stent, which would induce restenosis.

The degree of arterial injury induced by stent placement correlates significantly with the extent of inflammation, neointimal thickness, neointimal area, and percent area stenosis (114). Furthermore, a linear relationship exists between the number of monocytes per unit area in the injured segment and the extent of intimal growth (114), suggesting that the inflammatory reaction contributes to neointimal formation during in-stent restenosis.

The role of thrombus in the formation of in-stent restenosis has been debated. Some investigators argue that mural thrombus is the primordial infrastructure that is subsequently reconstituted by activated SMCs (115,116); others have observed that, although thrombus is frequently seen in humans, the extent of thrombosis is limited to less than 5% of the area of the arterial surface (111). Subacute thrombosis after stent placement normally occurs when stent or PTCA damage extends beyond the intima to the media (117). Although the role of thrombus in in-stent restenosis has not been defined, neointimal formation after stent placement may be initiated by the formation of local thrombus adjacent to the stent struts, followed by gradual invasion with macrophages and concomitant deposition of extracellular matrix components.

THERAPEUTIC APPROACHES

As described above, restenosis involves a combination of events: (a) a response to injury with proliferation of SMCs and extracellular matrix formation; (b) platelet deposition and thrombus formation with incorporation of the thrombus overlying the disrupted plaque; and (c) early elastic recoil of the vessel wall followed by significant late constrictive vessel wall remodeling. Because restenosis is irreversible, any therapeutic approach should be prophylactic and should be initiated before or at the time of vessel injury or at least early afterwards (Fig. 4). By the time restenosis is symptomatic, mechanical manipulations such

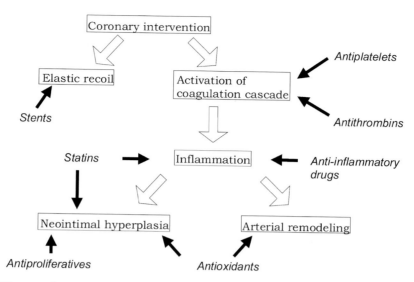

Fig. 4. Therapeutic approaches to inhibit restenosis after coronary artery interventions.

as repeated percutaneous coronary intervention or coronary bypass grafting are usually the only options.

Stent Implantation

The first and most effective antirestenotic tool available, a stent, is a mechanical device consisting of a metallic slotted tube that is implanted by balloon expansion at the site of balloon dilatation. By preventing mechanical recoil, stents reduce the rate of vessel renarrowing at 6 mo *(104)* and the rate of target vessel revascularization at 5-yr follow-up *(118)*. Clinical benefit is greatest when stents are used in vessels such as the left anterior descending artery that tend to have a higher restenosis rate after PTCA *(119)*. With the use of stents, mechanical recoil is limited after balloon dilatation, and the amount of neointimal proliferation, the pathophysiological principle underlying restenosis, does not change. Although stent implantation in percutaneous coronary interventions has decreased restenosis rates, the problem has not been completely resolved. Additional therapies, usually used concurrently with stent placement, are warranted; however, no method to reduce restenosis rates after stent implantation has been widely accepted.

Antiplatelet Strategies

The GP IIb/IIIa receptor is the final common pathway for platelet aggregation. All agonists that induce platelet activation and aggregation activate the GP IIb/IIIa receptor. Upon activation, the conformation of the GP IIb/IIIa complex changes so that soluble fibrinogen can bind to the receptor. One fibrinogen molecule can bind to two platelets, which leads to platelet aggregation.

During platelet activation and aggregation, potent mitogens, such as PDGF and serotonin, are released. These mitogens attract and stimulate SMCs, which is important in the pathogenesis of restenosis *(53)*. Blocking platelet aggregation reduces the release of growth factors *(120)* and, consequently, reduces the proliferative stimulus on cells in the vessel wall that contributes to restenosis.

Three antagonists of the GP IIb/IIIa complex— abciximab, eptifibatide, and tirofiban—are used as therapy for acute coronary syndromes and as prophylaxis of acute ischemic events during PTCA and stent implantation (Table 1). Abciximab is a chimeric antibody fragment that blocks GP IIb/IIIa, whereas eptifibatide and tirofiban are synthetic low-molecular-weight GP IIb/IIIa blockers. In an early trial for high-risk PTCA, abciximab reduced the revascularization rate by 26% when compared with placebo *(121)*. In addition, abciximab was effective in the subgroup of diabetics who underwent elective stent implantation *(122)*. Although the use of GP IIb/IIIa inhibitors as part of an antirestenotic strategy appeared to have potential, other large trials of abciximab as adjunctive therapy for PTCA did not confirm the initial promising results. For example, the Intracoronary Stenting and Antithrombotic Regimen-2 trial examined the effects of abciximab on the incidence of restenosis in patients who underwent stent implantation for acute myocardial infarction. Peri-interventional adjunctive treatment with abciximab did not change the rates of angiographically assessed restenosis after 6 mo *(123)*.

Antiplatelet drugs that do not affect the final common pathway of platelet aggregation, but intervene at earlier steps in platelet activation, have been studied as restenosis

Table 1
Glycoprotein IIb/IIIa Antagonists Approved for Clinical Use

Substance	Abciximab	Epifibatide	Tirofiban
Brand name	Reopro™	Integrilin™	Aggrastat™
Structure	Antibody Fab fragment	Cyclic heptapeptide	Nonpeptide
Molecular weight (kD)	47.6	0.832	0.495
Plasma half-life	10–30 min	Approx 1 h	Approx 2 h
GP IIb/IIIa inhibition	irreversible	reversible	reversible
Approved indications	PCI Refractory unstable angina when PCI is Planned within 24h	Acute coronary syndromes PCI	Acute coronary syndromes

inhibitors; however, none has reduced the rate of restenosis. This group includes the combination of aspirin, dipyridamole (124), ticlopidine (125), clopidogrel (126), and cilostazol, an orally administered phosphodiesterase inhibitor that inhibits platelet activation by increasing cyclic adenosine monophosphate (cAMP) (127). Although abciximab is the most promising antiplatelet agent for inhibiting restenosis, it is not clear if abciximab and the other GP IIb/IIIa inhibitors can reduce clinically relevant restenosis in all patients or only in certain subgroups. In vitro data suggest that abciximab inhibits SMC proliferation and migration, an effect pathophysiologically distinct from platelet aggregation in the development of restenosis. Blocking of the vitronectin receptor, αvβ3 intergin, by abciximab may contriute to the inhibition of SMCs(128).

Antithrombin Therapy

In addition to its role in the coagulation cascade, thrombin has significant non-thrombotic effects on endothelial cells and SMCs, including endothelial cell activation, SMC proliferation and migration, and increased production of extracellular matrix components. All of these effects are factors in restenosis (129). The role of thrombin in lesion formation has been studied in several animal models (89,90). Inhibition of thrombin activation by heparin reduces SMC proliferation and lesion formation in injured arteries (130). Potential mechanisms for this effect, independent of anticoagulant activity (131), include inhibition of nuclear transcription factors downstream of thrombin activation (132), modulation of growth factor activity or receptor binding (133), regulation of extracellular matrix production (134), direct inhibition of SMC proliferation and migration (135), and an anti-inflammatory effect (38). Administration of hirudin, a potent direct thrombin inhibitor, in the periprocedural period reduces neointimal formation

after injury in minipig and rabbit models (136,137). This effect may be caused by prolonged inhibition of thrombin activity within arteries in these animal models by hirudin after short-term administration (86). In contrast, studies in rats have shown that prolonged (but not short-term) administration of hirudin inhibits the vasculoproliferative response (95,138,139). Implantation of heparin-coated stents (38), which provides prolonged local antithrombin activity, or administration of hirudin via adenoviral gene therapy (96), which results in production of hirudin for days, blocks lesion formation in the rat carotid injury model. These experimental studies indicate the importance of thrombin generation in lesion formation, but also emphasize the significance of the time course of thrombin inhibition and the possibility of species-specific responses to thrombin inhibition in the vasculoproliferative process.

Despite their promising results in animal models, thrombin inhibitors have not reduced the incidence of restenosis in human studies. Both unfractionated and—on the basis of longer half-life and greater bioavailability—low-molecular-weight heparin have been studied in patients undergoing balloon angioplasty, and neither has shown an antirestenotic effect (140–144). Similar results have been seen with the potent antithrombin agent hirudin and the bivalent compound hirulog as adjunctive therapy in patients undergoing balloon dilatation (145,146). Furthermore, heparin-coated stents have not protected against the development of restenosis (147). Pharmacologic thrombin inhibitors have not been effective in patients at risk for restenosis; however, the success of these agents in animal models and their failure in human studies suggest that the problem may be dosage or delivery issues rather than application of the thrombin hypothesis.

A second approach to inhibiting thrombin activity—targeting the thrombin receptor PAR1 with inhibitory antibodies—has been considered. This approach has been effective in inhibiting thrombus formation in African green monkeys *(148)* and in blocking neointimal formation after balloon injury in rats *(149)*. Because rodent platelets (in contrast with those in primates) do not express PAR1 and are activated by thrombin in a PAR1-independent manner, these experiments suggest that the effects of thrombin on vascular lesion formation are attributable in part to direct effects of thrombin on vascular cells. The role of thrombin signaling via the PAR1 receptor has been studied more in genetically modified mice that lack the PAR1 receptor. Results from these studies not only confirm previous findings but also suggest a more complex role for this pathway *(150)*. Neointimal and medial areas are decreased in PAR1-deficient mice after denuding injury; however, luminal diameters are also decreased, suggesting that changes in extracellular matrix components in the PAR1-deficient mice may cause adverse remodeling. These studies, combined with the species-specific effects of thrombin inhibitors, show the complexity of this system as it applies to human studies.

Antioxidants

At the site of vascular injury such as seen after balloon dilatation, ROS are produced by cells with tissue damage *(151–153)*. Animal studies have shown a beneficial effect of antioxidants on both cell proliferation and arterial remodeling after balloon angioplasty *(154–157)*. A few small clinical studies have suggested that drugs with antioxidant properties may be beneficial in humans *(154–160)*. A randomized trial in 317 patients who underwent PTCA was stopped early because of a significant antirestenotic effect of probucol, a potent antioxidant with mild lipid-lowering activity *(161)*. These results have been confirmed in other studies *(162–164)*.

The efficacy of probucol, a lipid-lowering agent that was withdrawn from the market because of its modest activity and adverse side effect profile, suggested the possibility that antioxidant strategies may be useful in patients at risk for restenosis. However, other antioxidant regimens have not supported this possibility. In the study of 317 patients mentioned above, a multivitamin regimen of beta-carotene, vitamin C, and vitamin E, which should provide antioxidant activity, had no effect on restenosis *(161)*. Furthermore, carvedilol, a combined α- and β-adrenergic blocker that has stronger antioxidant effects than probucol, had no effect on restenosis after atherectomy *(165)*. Thus, although preclinical data suggest an antirestenotic effect of antioxidant regimens, they have not been effective in human studies. The reasons for this failure are not clear, but additional studies are warranted because of the small

number of studies conducted so far and because of the complexity of oxidative metabolism.

Lipid Modification

Lipid modification may have a role in arresting restenosis because of the association of hyperlipidemia with cardiovascular disease. Although high cholesterol levels are clearly associated with the progression of atherosclerosis, the association between serum lipid levels and the incidence of restenosis has not been confirmed *(166–168)*. These negative findings suggest that lipid-lowering agents would not be beneficial in patients undergoing percutaneous coronary interventions. Nevertheless, several studies have shown that therapy with lipid-lowering drugs reduces the incidence of restenosis *(169,170)*. The effect becomes more significant with a longer period of observation *(171)*; however, reduced restenosis rates have not been reported in all trials *(172,173)*. This issue has not been resolved, but the strategy is promising. The dissociation between lipid levels and restenosis rates suggests that some of the effects of statins on lesion formation may be due to factors other than a reduction in lipid levels.

Cell Cycle Control

Because SMC proliferation is a major determinant of restenosis and many of the upstream mediators of restenosis are potent stimuli for SMC proliferation, antiproliferative therapies have been used to prevent restenosis (Fig. 5). However, inhibiting SMC mitosis by blocking upstream mediators of proliferation has not been successful. In a large clinical trial, trapidil, a PDGF receptor and thromboxane A_2 antagonist, failed to inhibit restenosis *(174)*. Similarly, tranilast, which blocks inflammatory mediators and inhibits the proliferation of SMCs *(175)*, did not prevent restenosis in the large Prevention of REStenosis with Tranilast and its Outcomes (PRESTO) trial *(176)*. One explanation for these results is that inhibition of a single mitogenic pathway may have little consequence given the redundancy of signals that trigger proliferation. Thus, downstream "final common pathway" factors in cell cycle control may be more appropriate antiproliferative targets. The therapeutic options for direct inhibition of the cell cycle increase as more molecules that control the cell cycle are characterized.

Among the low-molecular-weight cell cycle inhibitors, the most promising are rapamycin (Sirolimus) and paclitaxel (Taxol), both of which arrest the cell cycle in G1 and inhibit neointimal proliferation in animals *(177,178)*. In addition, these agents reduce neointimal proliferation in animals when delivered locally via a

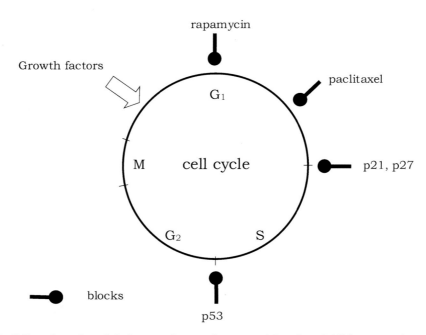

Fig. 5. Cell cycle and modulating agonists used as potential tools to inhibit restenosis.

polymer-coated stent (179,180). Because of their efficacy in animal studies and their clinical safety profiles for use as immunosuppressive agents and cancer chemotherapeutics, rapamycin and paclitaxel are first in line as cell cycle-targeting antirestenotic drugs.

Rapamycin's actions are mediated by binding to its intracellular receptor, the FK506-binding protein FKBP12, which is a member of the immunophilin family of proteins (181). Rapamycin-FKBP12 inhibits a kinase called TOR (target of rapamycin), which is a component in a pathway that regulates cell cycle progression (182). Rapamycin inhibits the proliferation of SMCs by blocking cell cycle progression at the G1/S transition (177). In humans, the implantation of rapamycin-coated stents was recently shown to be safe and effective in inhibiting neointimal formation (183). At 4 mo follow-up, no patient approached greater than 50% vessel narrowing by intravascular ultrasound or quantitative coronary angiography. Although the number of patients studied was small, no edge restenosis or stent thrombosis was observed. At 1 yr follow-up, ultrasound-measured intimal hyperplasia was still low in patients treated with rapamycin-coated stents (184). These data suggest that rapamycin may protect against intimal hyperplasia after stent implantation and thus may reduce the incidence of restenosis. Similar studies are in progress to test the other pharmacologic cell cycle inhibitor, paclitaxel.

Because of the number of molecular targets available for targeting the cell cycle in antirestenosis therapy, gene therapy is a second clinical approach for inhibiting SMC proliferation. Although results from antirestenotic gene therapy trials in humans have not been published, results from animal models are promising. In animal studies, SMC proliferation and neointimal formation have been inhibitied by downregulation of cyclins, which are required for progression of the cell cycle. Cyclins are downregulated by the use of antisense technologies, which rely on the ability of antisense DNA and RNA molecules to bind to a mRNA molecule in a sequence specific fashion to increase the degradation of the RNA (185). Other methods, such as the use of ribozymes, which are catalytic RNA molecules that degrade specific RNAs, are promising. Adenoviral delivery of ribozymes targeting c-myb inhibits neointimal formation in a rat model of balloon dilatation (186).

A second antirestenotic gene therapy that affects the cell cycle makes use of the overexpression of cell-cycle inhibitory molecules. The cyclin-dependent kinase inhibitors p21 and p27 and the antiproliferative transcription factor p53 inhibit neointimal proliferation when delivered by gene therapy in animal models (187–189). In addition, a chimeric p16/p27 molecule has potent antiproliferative activity (190). GAX, a SMC-specific transcription factor, is a promising target for gene overexpression for inhibiting proliferation in vascular disease (191).

Although experimental data support the use of gene therapy as a cell cycle inhibitor, the application of gene therapy to clinical medicine will depend not only on the ability of cell cycle arrest to block restenosis in clinical settings, but also on the demonstration of acceptable safety profiles.

The most promising cell cycle therapy uses the classic pharmacologic approach. Rapamycin-coated stents have been used successfully to prevent restenosis for up to 1 yr in human studies (184). With further work, rapamycin-coated stents can be made broadly available to reduce the incidence of restenosis. In addition, these studies provide evidence of the efficacy of cell cycle inhibitors in human vasculoproliferative disorders and may open the door for other compounds that use gene therapeutic delivery systems based on cell cycle inhibition.

Radiation

Vascular radiotherapy or brachytherapy, which indicates the short distance from the intraluminal radiation source to the vessel wall as the target, is a promising new method for treating restenosis. The radiation can be delivered close to the target—the site of balloon injury—by line sources, liquid sources, gas sources, membrane sources, and radioactive stents. Radiation inhibits SMC proliferation by destroying the integrity of the genomic DNA (192). Both β- and γ-energy emitting isotopes are being used as sources for intravascular radiotherapy.

Electrons, which are the radioactive product emitted by β-sources, have limited penetration; therefore, the greatest therapeutic benefit is achieved within 2–3 mm of the source. Centering the source in the middle of the vessel, which is necessary for equal distribution of radiation throughout the entire target area, is challenging. When the distribution of radiation is not equal, SMCs can be stimulated rather than inhibited. A β-emitting stent and a ^{188}Re liquid-filled balloon technique avoid centering problems but are associated with other risks, such as balloon rupture, which can release radioactive material into the circulation.

Photons, which are emitted by γ-sources, penetrate easily and deeply into tissue, well beyond the vessel wall and its adventitia. Deep penetration is not associated with the problems of equal dose delivery; however, greater side effects due to exposure of non-target tissues are a possibility. In addition, γ-radiation penetrates the standard shield in most cardiac catheterization laboratories. Additional precautions are necessary to reduce exposure to medical personnel.

Results of studies of radiation therapy in animal models of vascular injury are promising (193–195). In most early trials, outcome within 1 mo after radiation treatment was assessed. These studies showed that radiation therapy prevented vascular lesion formation without evidence of necrosis, significant fibrosis, or aneurysm formation. Although these early studies provided the basis for studies in humans, a recent study in which restenosis was measured after radiation therapy in pigs showed increased, rather than decreased, neointimal formation in irradiated arteries when compared with non-irradiated control arteries 6 mo after treatment (196). The disparity between the results in the pig study and those of earlier studies suggests that late effects associated with radiation therapy may adversely affect the vascular response to injury.

Early clinical trials and registries fueled enthusiasm for vascular radiation therapy (197,198). A large trial recently showed that γ-radiation delivered via an intracoronary ribbon inhibited restenosis (108). Although restenosis rates were lower in patients treated with radiation in this study, the incidence of late myocardial infarction was increased in treated patients. This finding illustrates one major drawback associated with radiation therapy—late thrombosis. Thrombosis has been seen in other studies and may relate to implantation of a fresh stent at the time of brachytherapy and early withdrawal of antiplatelet therapy (199). Although not well defined, the mechanisms of late thrombosis may involve delayed reendothelialization, resulting in a sustained local prothrombotic state. Prolonged antiplatelet therapy reduces late thrombosis associated with radiation therapy (200). A second drawback of radiation therapy is edge failure. After brachytherapy, renarrowing of the artery is increased at the edges of the treated area, especially when radioactive stents are used (201). Lower doses of radiation at the edges of the targeted area might stimulate neointimal proliferation (202). This effect might be increased if the area of lower radiation dose has been injured before by PTCA. Edge failure may be avoided with asymmetrical dosing of radioactivity.

Vascular radiotherapy is an effective treatment for in-stent restenosis, especially for patients who have had more than one episode of in-stent restenosis. Thus, patients with multiple restenoses, diabetics, or nondiabetics with a long restenosis area are primary candidates for radiation therapy. In addition, vascular radiotherapy may be indicated for in-stent restenosis within a saphenous vein bypass graft. These conditions are associated with an increased risk of repeat angioplasty. Although promising, radiation therapy is largely experimental, and the long-term consequences of radiation therapy for treatment of vascular disease in humans are unknown. In addition, strategies to prevent delayed reendothelialization and edge failure need to be developed (108).

Endothelial Regeneration

In most hypotheses of restenosis, initial endothelial damage is a trigger for further reactions of the vessel wall at the site of balloon injury. One goal of antirestenotic therapy is to correct endothelial denudation and dysfunction resulting from PTCA or stent implantation as soon as possible *(203)*. Although not well tested in humans, pharmacologic approaches such as the administration of L-arginine and tetrahydrobiopterin, both of which increase nitric oxide release, should be considered.

A second approach that has been considered in animal studies to increase endothelial cell regrowth is the delivery of vascular endothelial growth factor to reduce vessel wall damage after balloon injury *(204)* or stent implantation *(205)*. Another method to accelerate endothelial regeneration is to deliver stem cells that can differentiate into endothelial cells at the site of injury. Although only theoretical, this approach may be used simultaneously with other antirestenotic techniques, either to overcome their side effects (as is the case with radiation therapy) or to provide synergy (as with an antiproliferative strategy).

APPROACHES TO LOCAL DELIVERY

The effective delivery of pharmacologic or gene therapy agents to the site of disease is a challenge in treating vascular disease. Because the site of disease is so close to the bloodstream, the delivered agents rapidly wash out, and the concentration of systemically delivered agents within the arterial wall is never greater than the concentration within the blood compartment. The limitations of systemic delivery are evident in trials of antithrombotic agents. Although these drugs are effective in animal models, effective doses cannot be attained by systemic delivery in humans without adverse side effects. Similarly, cell cycle–targeting drugs such as Taxol and rapamycin have systemic toxicities that may limit their effectiveness unless their delivery can be concentrated specifically at the site of vascular injury.

Two major approaches are under study for targeting drug delivery to the site of vascular lesions. In one method, perfusion catheters are used to administer a pharmacologic agent directly at the site of injury after percutaneous coronary intervention. The drug can be directly applied to the arterial wall with the catheter in several ways, usually through sidehole ports. Potential complications for drug delivery via a perfusion catheter are rapid drug washout and a low delivery ratio. In addition, the duration of the drug effect is limited because the drug is delivered at a single time point. Furthermore, catheter delivery can potentially cause further injury to the vessel wall. This technique can be adapted for pharmacologic and gene therapy approaches, but clinical uses for these catheters have not been established.

Stent-based drug delivery is a second method to target drugs directly to the vessel wall. Stent-based delivery may be advantageous for several reasons. Because stents will be used in the patient regardless, vessel trauma is not increased with an eluting stent. High concentrations can be delivered directly at the site of injury and may be sustained for long periods. However, standard stainless-steel stents have poor absorbency and a low surface area. Coating stents with an eluting vehicle may address these issues, but many of these vehicles elicit an inflammatory response *(206)*. Advances in stent-coating materials have minimized the inflammatory side effects and have improved the eluting properties of the delivery vehicle so that drug-eluting stents are now a practical option in circumstances where delivery and toxicity issues require them *(207)*. Drug-eluting stents can be used for delivery of pharmacologic agents and for gene therapy vectors *(208)*.

Eluting stents have been effective drug delivery devices in large animal studies. Taxol and rapamycin have been delivered efficiently by eluting stents in animal models and have reduced neointimal formation *(179,180)*. In a small uncontrolled registry study in humans, implantation of rapamycin-eluting stents reduced restenosis even at 1 yr follow-up *(184)*. Larger studies with longer follow-up are necessary to verify the use of eluting stents as a tool for targeted drug delivery to inhibit restenosis.

SUMMARY

Although percutaneous coronary interventions have significantly improved the quality of care for patients with coronary artery disease, restenosis is a major limitation. The pathophysiology of restenosis is complex and depends on events in many cellular compartments; thus, the identification of good therapeutic targets is not straightforward. Among potential approaches, stent implantation is an effective strategy to reduce restenosis rates. In addition, data support the use of statins (perhaps even in patients with normal cholesterol levels), radiation therapy, and cell cycle inhibitors such as rapamycin; however, the risk:benefit ratio of these agents and the long-term consequences of their use need to be established.

REFERENCES

1. Bach R, Jung F, Kohsiek I, et al. Factors affecting the restenosis rate after percutaneous transluminal coronary angioplasty. Thromb Res 1994;74(Suppl 1):S55–S67.
2. Gruntzig A. Transluminal dilatation of coronary-artery stenosis. Lancet 1978;1:263.
3. Topol EJ. Coronary-artery stents—gauging, gorging, and gouging. N Engl J Med 1998;339:1702–1704.

4. Ross R. Rous-Whipple Award Lecture. Atherosclerosis: a defense mechanism gone awry. Am J Pathol 1993;143:987–1002.

5. Garratt KN, Edwards WD, Kaufmann UP, Vlietstra RE, Holmes DR Jr. Differential histopathology of primary atherosclerotic and restenotic lesions in coronary arteries and saphenous vein bypass grafts: analysis of tissue obtained from 73 patients by directional atherectomy. J Am Coll Cardiol 1991;17:442–448.

6. Van Belle E, Bauters C, Hubert E, et al. Restenosis rates in diabetic patients: a comparison of coronary stenting and balloon angioplasty in native coronary vessels. Circulation 1997;96:1454–1460.

7. Goel PK, Shahi M, Agarwal AK, Srivastava S, Seth PK. Platelet aggregability and occurrence of restenosis following coronary angioplasty. Int J Cardiol 1997;60:227–231.

8. Morita H, Kurihara H, Kuwaki T, et al. Homocysteine as a risk factor for restenosis after coronary angioplasty. Thromb Haemost 2000;84:27–31.

9. Morita H, Kurihara H, Yoshida S, et al. Diet-induced hyperhomocysteinemia exacerbates neointima formation in rat carotid arteries after balloon injury. Circulation 2001;103:133–139.

10. Blum A, Giladi M, Weinberg M, et al. High anti-cytomegalovirus (CMV) IgG antibody titer is associated with coronary artery disease and may predict post-coronary balloon angioplasty restenosis. Am J Cardiol 1998;81:866–868.

11. Manegold C, Alwazzeh M, Jablonowski H, et al. Prior cytomegalovirus infection and the risk of restenosis after percutaneous transluminal coronary balloon angioplasty. Circulation 1999;99:1290–1294.

12. Speir E, Yu ZX, Takeda K, Ferrans VJ, Cannon RO 3rd. Antioxidant effect of estrogen on cytomegalovirus-induced gene expression in coronary artery smooth muscle cells. Circulation 2000;102:2990–2996.

13. Zhou YF, Leon MB, Waclawiw MA, et al. Association between prior cytomegalovirus infection and the risk of restenosis after coronary atherectomy. N Engl J Med 1996;335:624–630.

14. Kastrati A, Elezi S, Dirschinger J, Hadamitzky M, Neumann FJ, Schomig A. Influence of lesion length on restenosis after coronary stent placement. Am J Cardiol 1999;83:1617–1622.

15. Bresee SJ, Jacobs AK, Garber GR, et al. Prior restenosis predicts restenosis after coronary angioplasty of a new significant narrowing. Am J Cardiol 1991;68:1158–1162.

16. Reis GJ, Kuntz RE, Silverman DI, Pasternak RC. Effects of serum lipid levels on restenosis after coronary angioplasty. Am J Cardiol 1991;68:1431–1435.

17. Gurlek A, Dagalp Z, Oral D, et al. Restenosis after transluminal coronary angioplasty: a risk factor analysis. J Cardiovasc Risk 1995;2:51–55.

18. Amant C, Bauters C, Bodart JC, et al. D allele of the angiotensin I-converting enzyme is a major risk factor for restenosis after coronary stenting. Circulation 1997;96:56–60.

19. Beohar N, Damaraju S, Prather A, et al. Angiotensin-I converting enzyme genotype DD is a risk factor for coronary artery disease. J Investig Med 1995;43:275–280.

20. Ohishi M, Fujii K, Minamino T, et al. A potent genetic risk factor for restenosis. Nat Genet 1993;5:324–325.

21. Ribichini F, Steffenino G, Dellavalle A, et al. Plasma activity and insertion/deletion polymorphism of angiotensin I-converting enzyme: a major risk factor and a marker of risk for coronary stent restenosis. Circulation 1998;97:147–154.

22. Zee RY, Fernandez-Ortiz A, Macaya C, Pintor E, Lindpaintner K, Fernandez-Cruz A. Ace D/I polymorphism and incidence of post-PTCA restenosis: a prospective, angiography-based evaluation. Hypertension 2001;37:851–855.

23. Murphy JG, Schwartz RS, Edwards WD, Camrud AR, Vlietstra RE, Holmes DR Jr. Percutaneous polymeric stents in porcine coronary arteries. Initial experience with polyethylene terephthalate stents. Circulation 1992;86:1596–1604.

24. Block PC. Restenosis after percutaneous transluminal coronary angioplasty—anatomic and pathophysiological mechanisms. Strategies for prevention. Circulation 1990;81:IV2–IV4.

25. Groves PH, Banning AP, Penny WJ, Lewis MJ, Cheadle HA, Newby AC. Kinetics of smooth muscle cell proliferation and intimal thickening in a pig carotid model of balloon injury. Atherosclerosis 1995;117:83–96.

26. LeBreton H, Topol E, Plow EF. Evidence for a pivotal role of platelets in vascular reocclusion and restenosis. Cardiovasc Res 1996;31:235–236.

27. Clowes AW, Reidy MA, Clowes MM. Kinetics of cellular proliferation after arterial injury. I. Smooth muscle growth in the absence of endothelium. Lab Invest 1983;49:327–333.

28. Violaris AG, Melkert R, Herrman JP, Serruys PW. Role of angiographically identifiable thrombus on long-term luminal renarrowing after coronary angioplasty: a quantitative angiographic analysis. Circulation 1996;93:889–897.

29. Friedman RJ, Stemerman MB, Wenz B, et al. The effect of thrombocytopenia on experimental arteriosclerotic lesion formation in rabbits. Smooth muscle cell proliferation and re-endothelialization. J Clin Invest 1977;60:1191–1201.

30. Smyth SS, Reis ED, Zhang W, Fallon JT, Gordon RE, Coller BS. Beta(3)-integrin-deficient mice but not P-selectin-deficient mice develop intimal hyperplasia after vascular injury: correlation with leukocyte recruitment to adherent platelets 1 hour after injury. Circulation 2001;103:2501–2507.

31. Nabel EG, Shum L, Pompili VJ, et al. Direct transfer of transforming growth factor beta 1 gene into arteries stimulates fibrocellular hyperplasia. Proc Natl Acad Sci USA 1993;90: 10759–10763.

32. Pakala R, Willerson JT, Benedict CR. Effect of serotonin, thromboxane A2, and specific receptor antagonists on vascular smooth muscle cell proliferation. Circulation 1997;96: 2280–2286.

33. McNamara CA, Sarembock IJ, Gimple LW, Fenton JW 2nd, Coughlin SR, Owens GK. Thrombin stimulates proliferation of cultured rat aortic smooth muscle cells by a proteolytically activated receptor. J Clin Invest 1993;91:94–98.

34. Perlman H, Maillard L, Krasinski K, Walsh K. Evidence for the rapid onset of apoptosis in medial smooth muscle cells after balloon injury. Circulation 1997;95:981–987.

35. Pollman MJ, Hall JL, Gibbons GH. Determinants of vascular smooth muscle cell apoptosis after balloon angioplasty injury. Influence of redox state and cell phenotype. Circ Res 1999;84:113–121.

36. Yoshida Y, Mitsumata M, Ling G, Jiang J, Shu Q. Migration of medial smooth muscle cells to the intima after balloon injury. Ann N Y Acad Sci 1997;811:459–470.

37. Leibovich SJ, Ross R. The role of the macrophage in wound repair. A study with hydrocortisone and antimacrophage serum. Am J Pathol 1975;78:71–100.

38. Rogers C, Welt FG, Karnovsky MJ, Edelman ER. Monocyte recruitment and neointimal hyperplasia in rabbits. Coupled inhibitory effects of heparin. Arterioscler Thromb Vasc Biol 1996;16:1312–1318.

39. Tanaka H, Sukhova GK, Swanson SJ, et al. Sustained activation of vascular cells and leukocytes in the rabbit aorta after balloon injury. Circulation 1993;88:1788–1803.

40. Barron MK, Lake RS, Buda AJ, Tenaglia AN. Intimal hyperplasia after balloon injury is attenuated by blocking selectins. Circulation 1997;96:3587–3592.

41. Rogers C, Edelman ER, Simon DI. A mAb to the beta2-leukocyteintegrin Mac-1 (CD11b/CD18) reduces intimal thickening after angioplasty or stent implantation in rabbits. Proc Natl Acad Sci USA 1998;95:10134–10139.

42. Wright SD, Weitz JI, Huang AJ, Levin SM, Silverstein SC, Loike JD. Complement receptor type three (CD11b/CD18) of human polymorphonuclear leukocytes recognizes fibrinogen. Proc Natl Acad Sci USA 1988;85:7734–7738.

43. Mickelson JK, Lakkis NM, Villarreal-Levy G, Hughes BJ, Smith CW. Leukocyte activation with platelet adhesion after coronary angioplasty: a mechanism for recurrent disease? J Am Coll Cardiol 1996;28:345–353.

44. Neumann FJ, Ott I, Gawaz M, Puchner G, Schomig A. Neutrophil and platelet activation at balloon-injured coronary artery plaque in patients undergoing angioplasty. J Am Coll Cardiol 1996;27:819–824.

45. Simon DI, Dhen Z, Seifert P, Edelman ER, Ballantyne CM, Rogers C. Decreased neointimal formation in Mac-1(−/−) mice reveals a role for inflammation in vascular repair after angioplasty. J Clin Invest 2000;105:293–300.

46. van Beusekom HM, van der Giessen WJ, van Suylen R, Bos E, Bosman FT, Serruys PW. Histology after stenting of human saphenous vein bypass grafts: observations from surgically excised grafts 3 to 320 days after stent implantation. J Am Coll Cardiol 1993;21:45–54.

47. Moreno PR, Bernardi VH, Lopez-Cuellar J, et al. Macrophage infiltration predicts restenosis after coronary intervention in patients with unstable angina. Circulation 1996;94:3098–3102.

48. Pietersma A, Kofflard M, de Wit LE, et al. Late lumen loss after coronary angioplasty is associated with the activation status of circulating phagocytes before treatment. Circulation 1995;91:1320–1325.

49. Assoian RK, Grotendorst GR, Miller DM, Sporn MB. Celular transformation by co-ordinated action of three peptide growth factors from human platelets. Nature 1984;309:804–806.

50. Lindner V, Giachelli CM, Schwartz SM, Reidy MA. A subpopulation of smooth muscle cells in injured rat arteries expresses platelet-derived growth factor–B chain mRNA. Circ Res 1995;76:951–957.

51. Ferns GA, Raines EW, Sprugel KH, Motani AS, Reidy MA, Ross R. Inhibition of neointimal smooth muscle accumulation after angioplasty by an antibody to PDGF. Science 1991;253:1129–1132.

52. Bornfeldt KE, Raines EW, Nakano T, Graves LM, Krebs EG, Ross R. Insulin-like growth factor-1 and platelet derived growth factor-BB induce direct migration of human arterial smooth muscle cells via signaling pathways that are distinct from those of proliferation. J Clin Invest 1994;93:1266–1274.

53. Uchida K, Sasahara M, Morigami N, Hazama F, Kinoshita M. Expression of platelet-derived growth factor B-chain in neointimal smooth muscle cells of balloon injured rabbit femoral arteries. Atherosclerosis 1996;124:9–23.

54. Jawien A, Bowen-Pope DF, Lindner V, Schwartz SM, Clowes AW. Platelet-derived growth factor promotes smooth muscle migration and intimal thickening in a rat model of balloon angioplasty. J Clin Invest 1992;89:507–511.

55. Grant MB, Wargovich TJ, Ellis EA, Caballero S, Mansour M, Pepine CJ. Localization of insulin-like growth factor I and inhibition of coronary smooth muscle cell growth by somatostatin analogues in human coronary smooth muscle cells. A potential treatment for restenosis? Circulation 1994;89:1511–1517.

56. Griendling KK, Ushio-Fukai M. NADH/NADPH oxidase and vascular function. Trends Cardiovasc Med 1997;7:301–307.

57. Suzuki YJ, Ford GD. Redox regulation of signal transduction in cardiac and smooth muscle. J Mol Cell Cardiol 1999;31:345–353.

58. Pagano PJ, Clark JK, Cifuentes-Pagano ME, Clark SM, Callis GM, Quinn MT. Localization of a constitutively active, phagocyte-like NADPH oxidase in rabbit aortic adventitia: enhancement by angiotensin II. Proc Natl Acad Sci USA 1997;94:14483–14488.

59. Rajagopalan S, Kurz S, Munzel T, et al. Angiotensin II-mediated hypertension in the rat increases vascular superoxide production via membrane NADH/NADPH oxidase activation. Contribution to alterations of vasomotor tone. J Clin Invest 1996;97:1916–1923.

60. Johnson TM, Yu ZX, Ferrans VJ, Lowenstein RA, Finkel T. Reactive oxygen species are downstream mediators of p53-dependent apoptosis. Proc Natl Acad Sci USA 1996;93:11848–11852.

61. Rao GN, Berk BC. Active oxygen species stimulate vascular smooth muscle cell growth and proto-oncogene expression. Circ Res 1992;70:593–599.

62. Sundaresan M, Yu ZX, Ferrans VJ, Irani K, Finkel T. Requirement for generation of H2O2 for platelet-derived growth factor signal transduction. Science 1995;270:296–299.

63. Zafari AM, Ushio-Fukai M, Akers M, et al. Role of NADH/NADPH oxidase–derived H2O2 in angiotensin II–induced vascular hypertrophy. Hypertension 1998;32:488–495.

64. Nishio E, Watanabe Y. The involvement of reactive oxygen species and arachidonic acid in alpha 1-adrenoceptor-induced smooth muscle cell proliferation and migration. Br J Pharmacol 1997;121:665–670.

65. Patterson C, Ruef J, Madamanchi NR, et al. Stimulation of a vascular smooth muscle cell NAD(P)H oxidase by thrombin. Evidence that p47(phox) may participate in forming this oxidase in vitro and in vivo. J Biol Chem 1999;274:19814–19822.

66. Alexander RW. Theodore Cooper Memorial Lecture. Hypertension and the pathogenesis of atherosclerosis. Oxidative stress and the mediation of arterial inflammatory response: a new perspective. Hypertension 1995; 25:155–161.

67. Ushio-Fukai M, Alexander RW, Akers M, Griendling KK. p38 Mitogen-activated protein kinase is a critical component of the redox-sensitive signaling pathways activated by angiotensin II. Role in vascular smooth muscle cell hypertrophy. J Biol Chem 1998;273:15022–15029.

68. Speir E, Modali R, Huang ES, et al. Potential role of human cytomegalovirus and p53 interaction in coronary restenosis. Science 1994;265:391–394.

69. Baas AS, Berk BC. Differential activation of mitogen-activated protein kinases by H2O2 and O2- in vascular smooth muscle cells. Circ Res 1995;77:29–36.

70. Li PF, Dietz R, von Harsdorf R. Differential effect of hydrogen peroxide and superoxide anion on apoptosis and proliferation of vascular smooth muscle cells. Circulation 1997;96:3602–3609.

71. Reis ED, Roque M, Dansky H, et al. Sulindac inhibits neointimal formation after arterial injury in wild-type and apolipoprotein E-deficient mice. Proc Natl Acad Sci USA 2000;97:12764–12769.

72. Popma JJ, Califf RM, Topol EJ. Clinical trials of restenosis after coronary angioplasty. Circulation 1991;84:1426–1436.

73. Cooke T, Sheahan R, Foley D, et al. Lipoprotein(a) in restenosis after percutaneous transluminal coronary angioplasty and coronary artery disease. Circulation 1994;89:1593–1598.

74. Nordt TK, Peter K, Ruef J, Kubler W, Bode C. Plasminogen activator inhibitor type-1 (PAI-1) and its role in cardiovascular disease. Thromb Haemost 1999;82(Suppl 1):14–18.

75. Fless GM, Rolih CA, Scanu AM. Heterogeneity of human plasma lipoprotein (a). Isolation and characterization of the lipoprotein subspecies and their apoproteins. J Biol Chem 1984;259:11470–11478.

76. Gaubatz JW, Heideman C, Gotto AM Jr, Morrisett JD, Dahlen GH. Human plasma lipoprotein [a]. Structural properties. J Biol Chem 1983;258:4582–4589.

77. Eaton DL, Fless GM, Kohr WJ, et al. Partial amino acid sequence of apolipoprotein(a) shows that it is homologous to plasminogen. Proc Natl Acad Sci USA 1987;84:3224–3228.

78. Loscalzo J, Weinfeld M, Fless GM, Scanu AM. Lipoprotein(a), fibrin binding, and plasminogen activation. Arteriosclerosis 1990;10:240–245.

79. Hajjar KA, Gavish D, Breslow JL, Nachman RL. Lipoprotein(a) modulation of endothelial cell surface fibrinolysis and its potential role in atherosclerosis. Nature 1989; 339:303–305.

80. Edelberg JM, Pizzo SV. Lipoprotein(a) inhibits plasminogen activation in a template-dependent manner. Blood Coagul Fibrinolysis 1991;2:759–764.

81. Miles LA, Fless GM, Levin EG, Scanu AM, Plow EF. A potential basis for the thrombotic risks associated with lipoprotein(a). Nature 1989;339:301–303.

82. Horie H, Takahashi M, Izumi M, et al. Association of an acute reduction in lipoprotein(a) with coronary artery restenosis after percutaneous transluminal coronary angioplasty. Circulation 1997;96:166–173.

83. Soifer SJ, Peters KG, O'Keefe J, Coughlin SR. Disparate temporal expression of the prothrombin and thrombin receptor genes during mouse development. Am J Pathol 1994;144:60–69.

84. Hattori R, Hamilton KK, Fugate RD, McEver RP, Sims PJ. Stimulated secretion of endothelial von Willebrand factor is accompanied by rapid redistribution to the cell surface of the intracellular granule membrane protein GMP-140. J Biol Chem 1989;264:7768–7771.

85. Lum H, Malik AB. Regulation of vascular endothelial barrier function. Am J Physiol 1994;267:L223–L241.

86. Barry WL, Gimple LW, Humphries JE, et al. Arterial thrombin activity after angioplasty in an atherosclerotic rabbit model: time course and effect of hirudin. Circulation 1996;94:88–93.

87. Vu TK, Hung DT, Wheaton VI, Coughlin SR. Molecular cloning of a functional thrombin receptor reveals a novel proteolytic mechanism of receptor activation. Cell 1991;64:1057–1068.

88. Wilcox JN, Rodriguez J, Subramanian R, et al. Characterization of thrombin receptor expression during vascular lesion formation. Circ Res 1994;75:1029–1038.

89. Noda-Heiny H, Sobel BE. Vascular smooth muscle cell migration mediated by thrombin and urokinase receptor. Am J Physiol 1995;268:C1195–C1201.

90. Dabbagh K, Laurent GJ, McAnulty RJ, Chambers RC. Thrombin stimulates smooth muscle cell procollagen synthesis and mRNA levels via a PAR-1 mediated mechanism. Thromb Haemost 1998;79:405–409.

91. Bar-Shavit R, Kahn A, Wilner GD, Fenton JW 2nd. Monocyte chemotaxis: stimulation by specific exosite region in thrombin. Science 1983;220:728–731.

92. Bar-Shavit R, Kahn AJ, Mann KG, Wilner GD. Identification of a thrombin sequence with growth factor activity on macrophages. Proc Natl Acad Sci USA 1986;83:976–980.

93. van Meijer M, Smilde A, Tans G, Nesheim ME, Pannekoek H, Horrevoets AJ. The suicide substrate reaction between plasminogen activator inhibitor 1 and thrombin is regulated by the cofactors vitronectin and heparin. Blood 1997; 90:1874–1882.

94. Carmeliet P, Moons L, Lijnen R, et al. Inhibitory role of plasminogen activator inhibitor-1 in arterial wound healing and neointima formation: a gene targeting and gene transfer study in mice. Circulation 1997;96:3180–3191.

95. Gerdes C, Faber-Steinfeld V, Yalkinoglu O, Wohlfeil S. Comparison of the effects of the thrombin inhibitor r-hirudin in four animal models of neointima formation after arterial injury. Arterioscler Thromb Vasc Biol 1996;16:1306–1311.

96. Rade JJ, Schulick AH, Virmani R, Dichek DA. Local adenoviral-mediated expression of recombinant hirudin reduces neointima formation after arterial injury. Nat Med 1996;2:293–298.

97. Andrade-Gordon P, Derian CK, Maryanoff BE, et al. Administration of a potent antagonist of protease-activated receptor-1 (PAR-1) attenuates vascular restenosis following balloon angioplasty in rats. J Pharmacol Exp Ther 2001;298:34–42.

98. Pasterkamp G, Borst C, Gussenhoven EJ, et al. Remodeling of De Novo atherosclerotic lesions in femoral arteries: impact on mechanism of balloon angioplasty. J Am Coll Cardiol 1995; 26:422–428.

99. Glagov S, Weisenberg E, Zarins CK, Stankunavicius R, Kolettis GJ. Compensatory enlargement of human atherosclerotic coronary arteries. N Engl J Med 1987; 316: 1371–1375.

100. Kimura T, Kaburagi S, Tamura T, et al. Remodeling of human coronary arteries undergoing coronary angioplasty or atherectomy. Circulation 1997;96:475–483.

101. Mintz GS, Popma JJ, Pichard AD, et al. Arterial remodeling after coronary angioplasty: a serial intravascular ultrasound study. Circulation 1996;94:35–43.

102. de Smet BJ, van der Zande J, van der Helm YJ, Kuntz RE, Borst C, Post MJ. The atherosclerotic Yucatan animal model to study the arterial response after balloon angioplasty: the natural history of remodeling. Cardiovasc Res 1998;39:224–232.

103. Lafont A, Guzman LA, Whitlow PL, Goormastic M, Cornhill JF, Chisolm GM. Restenosis after experimental angioplasty. Intimal, medial, and adventitial changes associated with constrictive remodeling. Circ Res 1995;76:996–1002.

104. Fischman DL, Leon MB, Baim DS, et al. A randomized comparison of coronary-stent placement and balloon angioplasty in the treatment of coronary artery disease. Stent Restenosis Study Investigators. N Engl J Med 1994;331:496–501.

105. Serruys PW, de Jaegere P, Kiemeneij F, et al. A comparison of balloon-expandable-stent implantation with balloon angioplasty in patients with coronary artery disease. Benestent Study Group. N Engl J Med 1994;331:489–495.

106. Faxon D, Wiliams D, Yeh W, Mehra A, Holubkov R, Detre K. Improved inhospital outcome with expanded use of coronary stents: results from the NHLBI dynamic registry. J Am Coll Cardiol 1999;33(Suppl A):91A.

107. Al Suwaidi J, Berger PB, Holmes DR Jr. Coronary artery stents. JAMA 2000;284:1828–1836.

108. Leon MB, Teirstein PS, Moses JW, et al. Localized intracoronary gamma-radiation therapy to inhibit the recurrence of restenosis after stenting. N Engl J Med 2001;344:250–256.

109. Mach F. Toward new therapeutic strategies against neointimal formation in restenosis. Arterioscler Thromb Vasc Biol 2000;20:1699–1700.

110. Moreno PR, Palacios IF, Leon MN, Rhodes J, Fuster V, Fallon JT. Histopathologic comparison of human coronary in-stent and post-balloon angioplasty restenotic tissue. Am J Cardiol 1999;84:462–466, A9.

111. Kearney M, Pieczek A, Haley L, et al. Histopathology of in-stent restenosis in patients with peripheral artery disease. Circulation 1997;95:1998–2002.

112. Virmani R, Farb A. Pathology of in-stent restenosis. Curr Opin Lipidol 1999;10:499–506.

113. Farb A, Sangiorgi G, Carter AJ, et al. Pathology of acute and chronic coronary stenting in humans. Circulation 1999;99:44–52.

114. Kornowski R, Hong MK, Tio FO, Bramwell O, Wu H, Leon MB. In-stent restenosis: contributions of inflammatory responses and arterial injury to neointimal hyperplasia. J Am Coll Cardiol 1998;31:224–230.

115. Grewe PH, Deneke T, Machraoui A, Barmeyer J, Muller KM. Acute and chronic tissue response to coronary stent implantation: pathologic findings in human specimen. J Am Coll Cardiol 2000;35:157–163.

116. Schwartz RS, Topol EJ, Serruys PW, Sangiorgi G, Holmes DR Jr. Artery size, neointima, and remodeling: time for some standards. J Am Coll Cardiol 1998;32:2087–2094.

117. Komatsu R, Ueda M, Naruko T, Kojima A, Becker AE. Neointimal tissue response at sites of coronary stenting in humans: macroscopic, histological, and immunohistochemical analyses. Circulation 1998;98:224–233.

118. Kiemeneij F, Serruys PW, Macaya C, et al. Continued benefit of coronary stenting versus balloon angioplasty: five-year clinical follow-up of Benestent-I trial. J Am Coll Cardiol 2001;37: 1598–1603.

119. Koning R, Eltchaninoff H, Commeau P, et al, for the BESMART (BeStent in Small Arteries) Trial Investigators. Stent placement compared with balloon angioplasty for small coronary arteries: in-hospital and 6-month clinical and angiographic results. Circulation 2001;104:1604–1608.

120. Reverter JC, Beguin S, Kessels H, Kumar R, Hemker HC, Coller BS. Inhibition of platelet-mediated, tissue factor-induced thrombin generation by the mouse/human chimeric 7E3 antibody. Potential implications for the effect of c7E3 Fab treatment on acute thrombosis and "clinical restenosis". J Clin Invest 1996;98:863–874.

121. Topol EJ, Califf RM, Weisman HF, et al. Randomised trial of coronary intervention with antibody against platelet IIb/IIIa integrin for reduction of clinical restenosis: results at six months. The EPIC Investigators. Lancet 1994;343:881–886.

122. The EPISTENT Investigators. Evaluation of Platelet IIb/IIIa Inhibitor for Stenting. Randomised placebo-controlled and balloon-angioplasty-controlled trial to assess safety of coronary stenting with use of platelet glycoprotein-IIb/IIIa blockade. Lancet 1998;352:87–92.

123. Neumann FJ, Kastrati A, Schmitt C, et al. Effect of glycoprotein IIb/IIIa receptor blockade with abciximab on clinical and angiographic restenosis rate after the placement of coronary stents following acute myocardial infarction. J Am Coll Cardiol 2000;35:915–921.

124. Schwartz L, Bourassa MG, Lesperance J, et al. Aspirin and dipyridamole in the prevention of restenosis after percutaneous transluminal coronary angioplasty. N Engl J Med 1988;318:1714–1719.

125. Kastrati A, Schuhlen H, Hausleiter J, et al. Restenosis after coronary stent placement and randomization to a 4-week combined antiplatelet or anticoagulant therapy: six-month angiographic follow-up of the Intracoronary Stenting and Antithrombotic Regimen (ISAR) Trial. Circulation 1997;96:462–467.

126. Calver AL, Blows LJ, Harmer S, et al. Clopidogrel for prevention of major cardiac events after coronary stent implantation: 30-day and 6-month results in patients with smaller stents. Am Heart J 2000;140:483–491.

127. El-Beyrouty C, Spinler S. Cilostazol for prevention of thrombosis and restenosis after intracoronary stenting. Ann Pharmacother 2001;35:1108–1113.

128. Blindt R, Bosserhoff AK, Zeiffer U, Krott N, Hanrath P, vom Dahl J. Abciximab inhibits the migration and invasion potential of human coronary artery smooth muscle cells. J Mol Cell Cardiol 2000;32:2195–2206.

129. Patterson C, Stouffer GA, Madamanchi N, Runge MS. New tricks for old dogs: nonthrombotic effects of thrombin in vessel wall biology. Circ Res 2001;88:987–997.

130. Clowes AW, Karnowsky MJ. Suppression by heparin of smooth muscle cell proliferation in injured arteries. Nature 1977; 265:625–626.

131. Guyton JR, Rosenberg RD, Clowes AW, Karnovsky MJ. Inhibition of rat arterial smooth muscle cell proliferation by heparin. In vivo studies with anticoagulant and nonanticoagulant heparin. Circ Res 1980;46:625–634.

132. Pukac LA, Castellot JJ Jr, Wright TC Jr, Caleb BL, Karnovsky MJ. Heparin inhibits c-fos and c-myc mRNA expression in vascular smooth muscle cells. Cell Regul 1990;1:435–443.

133. Ornitz DM, Herr AB, Nilsson M, Westman J, Svahn CM, Waksman G. FGF binding and FGF receptor activation by synthetic heparan-derived di- and trisaccharides. Science 1995;268:432–436.

134. Snow AD, Bolender RP, Wight TN, Clowes AW. Heparin modulates the composition of the extracellular matrix domain surrounding arterial smooth muscle cells. Am J Pathol 1990; 137:313–330.

135. Clowes AW, Clowes MM. Kinetics of cellular proliferation after arterial injury. II. Inhibition of smooth muscle growth by heparin. Lab Invest 1985;52:611–616.

136. Abendschein DR, Recchia D, Meng YY, Oltrona L, Wickline SA, Eisenberg PR. Inhibition of thrombin attenuates stenosis after arterial injury in minipigs. J Am Coll Cardiol 1996;28:1849–1855.

137. Sarembock IJ, Gertz SD, Gimple LW, Owen RM, Powers ER, Roberts WC. Effectiveness of recombinant desulphatohirudin in reducing restenosis after balloon angioplasty of atherosclerotic femoral arteries in rabbits. Circulation 1991;84:232–243.

138. Gallo R, Padurean A, Toschi V, et al. Prolonged thrombin inhibition reduces restenosis after balloon angioplasty in porcine coronary arteries. Circulation 1998;97:581–588.

139. Thome LM, Gimple LW, Bachhuber BG, et al. Early plus delayed hirudin reduces restenosis in the atherosclerotic rabbit more than early administration alone: potential implications for dosing of antithrombin agents. Circulation 1998;98:2301–2306.

140. Brack MJ, Ray S, Chauhan A, et al. The Subcutaneous Heparin and Angioplasty Restenosis Prevention (SHARP) trial. Results of a multicenter randomized trial investigating the effects of high dose unfractionated heparin on angiographic restenosis and clinical outcome. J Am Coll Cardiol 1995;26:947–954.

141. Ellis SG, Roubin GS, Wilentz J, Douglas JS Jr, King SB 3rd. Effect of 18- to 24-hour heparin administration for prevention of restenosis after uncomplicated coronary angioplasty. Am Heart J 1989;117:777–782.

142. Faxon DP, Spiro TE, Minor S, et al. Low molecular weight heparin in prevention of restenosis after angioplasty. Results of Enoxaparin Restenosis (ERA) Trial. Circulation 1994; 90:908–914.

143. Karsch KR, Preisack MB, Baildon R, et al. Low molecular weight heparin (reviparin) in percutaneous transluminal coronary angioplasty. Results of a randomized, double-blind, unfractionated heparin and placebo-controlled, multicenter trial (REDUCE trial). Reduction of Restenosis After PTCA, Early Administration of Reviparin in a Double-Blind Unfractionated Heparin and Placebo-Controlled Evaluation. J Am Coll Cardiol 1996;28:1437–1443.

144. Kiesz RS, Buszman P, Martin JL, et al. Local delivery of enoxaparin to decrease restenosis after stenting: results of initial multicenter trial: Polish-American Local Lovenox NIR Assessment study (The POLONIA study). Circulation 2001;103:26–31.

145. Bittl JA, Strony J, Brinker JA, et al. Treatment with bivalirudin (Hirulog) as compared with heparin during coronary angioplasty for unstable or postinfarction angina. Hirulog Angioplasty Study Investigators. N Engl J Med 1995;333:764–769.

146. Serruys PW, Herrman JP, Simon R, et al, for the Helvetica Investigators. A comparison of hirudin with heparin in the prevention of restenosis after coronary angioplasty. N Engl J Med 1995;333:757–763.

147. Wohrle J, Al-Khayer E, Grotzinger U, et al. Comparison of the heparin coated vs the uncoated Jostent—no influence on restenosis or clinical outcome. Eur Heart J 2001;22:1808–1816.

148. Cook JJ, Sitko GR, Bednar B, et al. An antibody against the exosite of the cloned thrombin receptor inhibits experimental arterial thrombosis in the African green monkey. Circulation 1995;91:2961–2971.

149. Takada M, Tanaka H, Yamada T, et al. Antibody to thrombin receptor inhibits neointimal smooth muscle cell accumulation without causing inhibition of platelet aggregation or altering hemostatic parameters after angioplasty in rat. Circ Res 1998; 82:980–987.

150. Cheung WM, D'Andrea MR, Andrade-Gordon P, Damiano BP. Altered vascular injury responses in mice deficient in protease-activated receptor-1. Arterioscler Thromb Vasc Biol 1999;19: 3014–3024.

151. Azevedo LC, Pedro MA, Souza LC, et al. Oxidative stress as a signaling mechanism of the vascular response to injury: the redox hypothesis of restenosis. Cardiovasc Res 2000;47:436–445.

152. Iuliano L, Pratico D, Greco C, et al. Angioplasty increases coronary sinus F2-isoprostane formation: evidence for in vivo oxidative stress during PTCA. J Am Coll Cardiol 2001; 37:76–80.

153. Ruef J, Liu SQ, Bode C, Tocchi M, Srivastava S, Runge MS, Bhatnagar A. Involvement of aldose reductase in vascular smooth muscle cell growth and lesion formation after arterial injury. Arterioscler Thromb Vasc Biol 2000;20:1745–1752.

154. Ferns GA, Forster L, Stewart-Lee A, Konneh M, Nourooz-Zadeh J, Anggard EE. Probucol inhibits neointimal thickening and macrophage accumulation after balloon injury in the cholesterol-fed rabbit. Proc Natl Acad Sci USA 1992;89: 11312–11316.

155. Freyschuss A, Stiko-Rahm A, Swedenborg J, et al. Antioxidant treatment inhibits the development of intimal thickening after balloon injury of the aorta in hypercholesterolemic rabbits. J Clin Invest 1993;91:1282–1288.

156. Nunes GL, Sgoutas DS, Redden RA, et al. Combination of vitamins C and E alters the response to coronary balloon injury in the pig. Arterioscler Thromb Vasc Biol 1995;15:156–165.

157. Schneider JE, Berk BC, Gravanis MB, et al. Probucol decreases neointimal formation in a swine model of coronary artery balloon injury. A possible role for antioxidants in restenosis. Circulation 1993;88:628–637.

158. DeMaio SJ, King SB 3rd, Lembo NJ, et al. Vitamin E supplementation, plasma lipids and incidence of restenosis after percutaneous transluminal coronary angioplasty (PTCA). J Am Coll Nutr 1992;11:68–73.

159. Setsuda M, Inden M, Hiraoka N, et al. Probucol therapy in the prevention of restenosis after successful percutaneous transluminal coronary angioplasty. Clin Ther 1993;15:374–382.

160. Watanabe K, Sekiya M, Ikeda S, Miyagawa M, Hashida K. Preventive effects of probucol on restenosis after percutaneous transluminal coronary angioplasty. Am Heart J 1996;132:23–29.

161. Tardif JC, Cote G, Lesperance J, et al, for the Multivitamins and Probucol Study Group. Probucol and multivitamins in the prevention of restenosis after coronary angioplasty. N Engl J Med 1997;337:365–372.

162. Daida H, Kuwabara Y, Yokoi H, et al. Effect of probucol on repeat revascularization rate after percutaneous transluminal coronary angioplasty (from the Probucol Angioplasty Restenosis Trial [PART]). Am J Cardiol 2000;86:550–552, A9.

163. Rodes J, Cote G, Lesperance J, et al. Prevention of restenosis after angioplasty in small coronary arteries with probucol. Circulation 1998;97:429–436.

164. Yokoi H, Daida H, Kuwabara Y, et al. Effectiveness of an antioxidant in preventing restenosis after percutaneous transluminal coronary angioplasty: the Probucol Angioplasty Restenosis Trial. J Am Coll Cardiol 1997;30:855–862.

165. Serruys PW, Foley DP, Hofling B, et al. Carvedilol for prevention of restenosis after directional coronary atherectomy: final results of the European carvedilol atherectomy restenosis (EUROCARE) trial. Circulation 2000;101:1512–1518.

166. Arora RR, Konrad K, Badhwar K, Hollman J. Restenosis after transluminal coronary angioplasty: a risk factor analysis. Cathet Cardiovasc Diagn 1990;19:17–22.

167. Jorgensen B, Simonsen S, Endresen K, et al. Luminal loss and restenosis after coronary angioplasty. The role of lipoproteins and lipids. Eur Heart J 1999;20:1407–1414.

168. Violaris AG, Melkert R, Serruys PW. Influence of serum cholesterol and cholesterol subfractions on restenosis after successful coronary angioplasty. A quantitative angiographic analysis of 3336 lesions. Circulation 1994;90:2267–2279.

169. Nakamura Y, Yamaoka O, Uchida K, et al. Pravastatin reduces restenosis after coronary angioplasty of high grade stenotic lesions: results of SHIPS (SHIga Pravastatin Study). Cardiovasc Drugs Ther 1996;10:475–483.

170. Walter DH, Schachinger V, Elsner M, Mach S, Auch-Schwelk W, Zeiher AM. Effect of statin therapy on restenosis after coronary stent implantation. Am J Cardiol 2000;85:962–968.

171. Mulder HJ, Bal ET, Jukema JW, et al. Pravastatin reduces restenosis two years after percutaneous transluminal coronary angioplasty (REGRESS trial). Am J Cardiol 2000; 86:742–746.

172. Bertrand ME, McFadden EP, Fruchart JC, et al. Effect of pravastatin on angiographic restenosis after coronary balloon angioplasty. The PREDICT Trial Investigators. Prevention of Restenosis by Elisor after Transluminal Coronary Angioplasty. J Am Coll Cardiol 1997;30:863–869.

173. Serruys PW, Foley DP, Jackson G, et al. A randomized placebo-controlled trial of fluvastatin for prevention of restenosis after successful coronary balloon angioplasty; final results of the fluvastatin angiographic restenosis (FLARE) trial. Eur Heart J 1999;20:58–69.

174. Serruys PW, Foley D, Pieper M, Kleijne J, de Feyter P, on behalf of the TRAPIST Investigators. The TRAPIST Study. A multicentre randomized placebo controlled clinical trial of trapidil for prevention of restenosis after coronary stenting, measured by 3-D intravascular ultrasound. Eur Heart J 2001;22:1938–1947.

175. Kusama H, Kikuchi S, Tazawa S, et al. Tranilast inhibits the proliferation of human coronary smooth muscle cell through the activation of p21waf1. Atherosclerosis 1999; 143:307–313.

176. SoRelle R. Late-breaking clinical trials at the American Heart Association's scientific sessions 2001. Circulation 2001; 104:E9046–E9048.

177. Gallo R, Padurean A, Jayaraman T, et al. Inhibition of intimal thickening after balloon angioplasty in porcine coronary arteries by targeting regulators of the cell cycle. Circulation 1999;99:2164–2170.

178. Herdeg C, Oberhoff M, Baumbach A, et al. Local paclitaxel delivery for the prevention of restenosis: biological effects and efficacy in vivo. J Am Coll Cardiol 2000;35:1969–1976.

179. Farb A, Heller PF, Shroff S, et al. Pathological analysis of local delivery of paclitaxel via a polymer-coated stent. Circulation 2001;104:473–479.

180. Suzuki T, Kopia G, Hayashi S, et al. Stent-based delivery of sirolimus reduces neointimal formation in a porcine coronary model. Circulation 2001;104:1188–1193.

181. Marks AR. Cellular functions of immunophilins. Physiol Rev 1996;76:631–649.

182. Heitman J, Movva NR, Hall MN. Targets for cell cycle arrest by the immunosuppressant rapamycin in yeast. Science 1991;253: 905–909.

183. Sousa JE, Costa MA, Abizaid A, et al. Lack of Neointimal Proliferation After Implantation of Sirolimus-Coated Stents in Human Coronary Arteries: A Quantitative Coronary Angiography and Three-Dimensional Intravascular Ultrasound Study. Circulation 2001;103:192–195.

184. Sousa JE, Costa MA, Abizaid AC, et al. Sustained suppression of neointimal proliferation by sirolimus-eluting stents: one-year angiographic and intravascular ultrasound follow-up. Circulation 2001;104:2007–2011.

185. Zhu NL, Wu L, Liu PX, et al. Downregulation of cyclin G1 expression by retrovirus-mediated antisense gene transfer inhibits vascular smooth muscle cell proliferation and neointima formation. Circulation 1997;96:628–635.

186. Macejak DG, Lin H, Webb S, et al. Adenovirus-mediated expression of a ribozyme to c-myb mRNA inhibits smooth muscle cell proliferation and neointima formation in vivo. J Virol 1999;73:7745–7751.

187. Chen D, Krasinski K, Sylvester A, Chen J, Nisen PD, Andres V. Downregulation of cyclin-dependent kinase 2 activity and cyclin A promoter activity in vascular smooth muscle cells by p27(KIP1), an inhibitor of neointima formation in the rat carotid artery. J Clin Invest 1997;99:2334–2341.

188. Yang ZY, Simari RD, Perkins ND, et al. Role of the p21 cyclin-dependent kinase inhibitor in limiting intimal cell proliferation in response to arterial injury. Proc Natl Acad Sci USA 1996;93:7905–7910.

189. Yonemitsu Y, Kaneda Y, Tanaka S, et al. Transfer of wild-type p53 gene effectively inhibits vascular smooth muscle cell proliferation in vitro and in vivo. Circ Res 1998;82:147–156.

190. McArthur JG, Qian H, Citron D, et al. p27-p16 Chimera: a superior antiproliferative for the prevention of neointimal hyperplasia. Mol Ther 2001;3:8–13.

191. Maillard L, Van Belle E, Tio FO, et al. Effect of percutaneous adenovirus-mediated Gax gene delivery to the arterial wall in double-injured atheromatous stented rabbit iliac arteries. Gene Ther 2000;7:1353–1361.

192. Waksman R, Rodriguez JC, Robinson KA, et al. Effect of intravascular irradiation on cell proliferation, apoptosis, and vascular remodeling after balloon overstretch injury of porcine coronary arteries. Circulation 1997;96:1944–1952.

193. Fischell TA, Kharma BK, Fischell DR, et al. Low-dose, beta-particle emission from 'stent' wire results in complete, localized inhibition of smooth muscle cell proliferation. Circulation 1994;90:2956–2963.

194. Hehrlein C, Gollan C, Donges K, et al. Low-dose radioactive endovascular stents prevent smooth muscle cell proliferation and neointimal hyperplasia in rabbits. Circulation 1995; 92:1570–1575.

195. Wiedermann JG, Marboe C, Amols H, Schwartz A, Weinberger J. Intracoronary irradiation markedly reduces restenosis after balloon angioplasty in a porcine model. J Am Coll Cardiol 1994;23:1491–1498.

196. Coussement PK, de Leon H, Ueno T, et al. Intracoronary beta-radiation exacerbates long-term neointima formation in balloon-injured pig coronary arteries. Circulation 2001;104:2459–2464.

197. King SB 3rd, Williams DO, Chougule P, et al. Endovascular beta-radiation to reduce restenosis after coronary balloon angioplasty: results of the beta energy restenosis trial (BERT). Circulation 1998;97:2025–2030.

198. Teirstein PS, Massullo V, Jani S, et al. Three-year clinical and angiographic follow-up after intracoronary radiation: results of a randomized clinical trial. Circulation 2000;101:360–365.

199. Costa MA, Sabat M, van der Giessen WJ, et al. Late coronary occlusion after intracoronary brachytherapy. Circulation 1999;100:789–792.

200. Waksman R, Ajani AE, White RL, et al. Prolonged antiplatelet therapy to prevent late thrombosis after intracoronary gamma-radiation in patients with in-stent restenosis: Washington Radiation for In-Stent Restenosis Trial plus 6 months of clopidogrel (WRIST PLUS). Circulation 2001;103:2332–2335.

201. Albiero R, Nishida T, Adamian M, et al. Edge restenosis after implantation of high activity (32)P radioactive beta-emitting stents. Circulation 2000;101:2454–2457.

202. Teirstein PS, Kuntz RE. New frontiers in interventional cardiology: intravascular radiation to prevent restenosis. Circulation 2001;104:2620–2626.

203. Rogers C, Parikh S, Seifert P, Edelman ER. Endogenous cell seeding. Remnant endothelium after stenting enhances vascular repair. Circulation 1996;94:2909–2914.

204. Asahara T, Chen D, Tsurumi Y, et al. Accelerated restitution of endothelial integrity and endothelium-dependent function after phVEGF165 gene transfer. Circulation 1996;94:3291–3302.

205. Van Belle E, Tio FO, Chen D, Maillard L, Chen D, Kearney M, Isner JM. Passivation of metallic stents after arterial gene transfer of phVEGF165 inhibits thrombus formation and intimal thickening. J Am Coll Cardiol 1997;29:1371–1379.

206. van der Giessen WJ, Lincoff AM, Schwartz RS, et al. Marked inflammatory sequelae to implantation of biodegradable and nonbiodegradable polymers in porcine coronary arteries. Circulation 1996;94:1690–1697.

207. Teirstein PS. Living the dream of no restenosis. Circulation 2001;104:1996–1998.

208. Ye YW, Landau C, Willard JE, et al. Bioresorbable microporous stents deliver recombinant adenovirus gene transfer vectors to the arterial wall. Ann Biomed Eng 1998;26:398–408.

IV ARRHYTHMIAS

18 Induction and Patterning of the Purkinje Fiber Network

Takashi Mikawa, PhD, Robert G. Gourdie, PhD,
Kimiko Takebayashi-Suzuki, PhD, Nobuyuki Kanzawa, PhD,
David J. Pennisi, PhD, Clifton P. Poma, BSc,
and Maxim Shulimovich, BSc

CONTENTS

INTRODUCTION

Our studies in the embryonic chick heart have shown that impulse-conducting Purkinje cells differentiate from myocytes during embryogenesis. This conversion of contractile myocytes into conduction cells is induced by paracrine signals, such as endothelin (ET), derived from the endocardium and developing coronary arteries. Active ET is secreted through proteolytic processing from its precursor by ET-converting enzyme-1 (ECE-1) and triggers signaling by binding to its receptors. In the embryonic heart, two ET receptors, ETA and ETB, are expressed by myocytes. ECE-1 is predominantly expressed in endothelial cells of the endocardium and coronary arteries, but not in veins or capillaries. Furthermore, retroviral co-expression of exogenous ECE-1 with ET precursor in the embryonic heart is sufficient to induce ectopic myocyte conversion to conduction cells. Thus, localized expression of ECE-1 in endocardial and arterial endothelia is a key mechanism defining the site of Purkinje fiber recruitment in the embryonic myocardium. Inhibition of endogenous ECE-1 expression via suppression of stretch-sensitive channels results in down-regulated expression of Purkinje fiber markers. This finding suggests that biophysical forces acted on, and created by, the cardiovascular system during embryogenesis may play a critical role in induction and patterning of Purkinje fibers.

The autonomous rhythm of the heart beat is coordinated by the precisely timed sequence of electrical impulses initiated and propagated through a unique set of

From: *Contemporary Cardiology: Principles of Molecular Cardiology*
Edited by: M. S. Runge and C. Patterson @ Humana Press Inc., Totowa, NJ

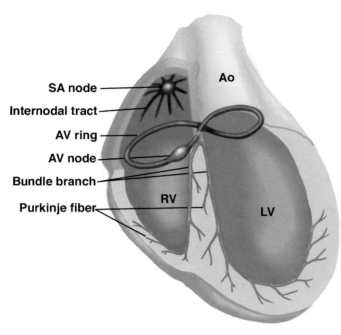

Fig. 1.

OVERVIEW OF THE DEVELOPMENT OF THE CONDUCTION SYSTEM

The conduction system begins to develop after the initial beating of the primitive heart, which comprises a double-walled tube, the outer myocardium and the inner endocardium *(12)*. At this stage of development, all epithelioid myocytes are electrically active, but pacemaking impulses are generated predominantly by myocytes in the posterior inflow tract (the presumptive sinus venosus and atrium) *(13–15)*. The impulses spread to the anterior end of the heart toward the outflow tract through gap junctions between the epithelioid myocytes (Fig. 2). This spread pattern generates a posterior-to-anterior contractile wave along the heart tube *(16)*. Although the presumptive ventricle and atrium are molecularly distinguishable at this stage *(17)*, action potentials propagate throughout a straight heart tube without any local changes in velocity. Except for the pacemaker cells, no other subcomponents of the conduction system are present at this stage.

Soon after the heart tube undergoes a right-sided looping, the pattern of impulse propagation along the myocardium changes. The speed of the impulse slows significantly at the AV junction where a morphogenic constriction begins to divide atrial and ventricular chambers (Fig. 2) *(18,19)*. This AV delay is believed to give rise to an effective peristaltic wave of myocardial contraction, thereby increasing the pumping efficiency of the embryonic heart. Although the mechanism underlying the AV delay has not been identified, myocytes at the AV junction preferentially express connexin-45 *(20)*, a high voltage-sensitive and low conductance gap junction channel that is found in the SA node and the AV node and ring system of the mature heart *(21)*.

As looping of the heart tube continues, atrial and ventricular chambers are further constricted by AV septa. This separation between chambers dissociates the direct electrical coupling of the two chambers through myocyte–myocyte gap junctions. The atrial and ventricular chambers are further divided into right and left sides by interatrial and interventricular septa. During chamber separation by septation, the propagation of pacemaking impulses in the ventricle dramatically changes from base-to-apex to apex-to-base *(19,22,23)*. This change in the impulse-propagation pathway ensures the effective pumping function of the four-chambered heart.

The dynamic, topological shift of the impulse-transmission pathway in the ventricle depends on the differentiation and patterning of the ventricular conduction system, including the AV bundle, bundle branches, and Purkinje fiber network (Fig. 1). The main function of

specialized muscle tissues called the excitation and conduction system *(1–3)*. This specialized system comprises several distinct subcomponents (Fig. 1): the sinoatrial (SA) node, the internodal tract, the atrioventricular (AV) node and ring, the AV bundle, and Purkinje fibers. The cardiac pacemaking impulse is rhythmically generated at the SA node *(4,5)* and is conducted across the atrial chambers, which induces contraction of the atria *(5–8)*. The pacemaking impulses first converge on the AV node *(1)*. After a slight delay, impulses are rapidly propagated along the AV bundle *(9)* and its branched limbs *(1)* and conducted into the working ventricular muscle via the Purkinje fiber network *(1,10,11)*.

Dysfunction of this cardiac tissue system in adults causes arrhythmias that often lead to sudden death. In addition, defects in the development of the conduction system may contribute to arrhythmias and conduction block in infants and children. Understanding the mechanisms that regulate development of the cardiac conduction system will help in developing new therapeutic approaches for repairing the pacemaking–conduction system after heart injury or in patients with congenital disease. Molecular and cellular events involved in differentiation and patterning of the conduction system network during morphogenesis of the heart have been studied extensively. Evidence indicates that communication between myocyte and non-myocyte cardiac cells is important in the induction and patterning of the integrated conduction system network in the embryonic heart.

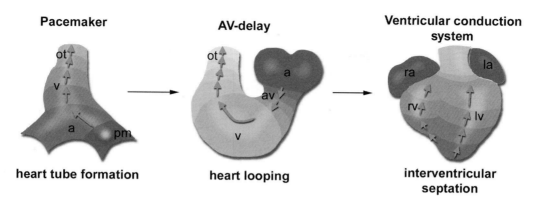

Fig. 2.

these three subcomponents is to rapidly propagate pace-making impulses to the apex of the ventricular myocardium, thereby coordinating the apex-to-base contraction of the ventricle. In addition to their faster conduction velocity, cells in the ventricular conduction system differ in morphological and/or molecular characteristics from other cardiac cells depending on species *(24–28)*.

From an evolutionary point of view, pacemaking impulses in the fish heart, which has a single ventricular chamber, propagate through preferential pathways *(29)*. In birds, all components of the mammalian ventricular conduction system persist across evolutionary borders, including Purkinje fibers, which penetrate the myocardium from the subendocardium and follow coronary artery branches *(30–32)*. Purkinje fibers vary widely in morphology between species and are classified into three broad categories *(33)*. Purkinje fibers in egg-laying (monotremes) and hoofed (ungulates) mammals, as in birds, have large diameters and are typically well differentiated. In contrast, Purkinje fibers in humans, monkeys, squirrels, cats, and dogs have smaller diameters and are difficult to distinguish from ventricular myocytes. In rodents such as bats, rats, guinea pigs, and rabbits, Purkinje fibers show little cellular differentiation but are believed to be located subendocardially; intramyocardial Purkinje fibers are not well characterized in these species.

CELLULAR ORIGIN OF THE VENTRICULAR CONDUCTION SYSTEM

The establishment of the complicated but predictable pattern of a wiring tissue network during heart development is a challenging topic. Identifying the cell types that give rise to conduction cells is essential in understanding the development of the conduction system; therefore, cellular ontogeny of conduction cells has

been extensively studied by probing for morphology and expression of marker genes and proteins. Although helpful, these techniques have not provided direct answers regarding the lineage of conduction cells and the relations between cells of the conduction system and other cardiac cell types. Both neural and muscle cell morphology and gene expression have been found in cells of the conduction system *(25,26)*. The complex phenotype of conduction cells suggests that specialized conduction tissue arises from two different cell types: myogenic *(16,34)* and neural crest *(35–37)*. Recent retroviral cell lineage studies in the embryonic chick heart *(24,32,38–41)* have helped to clarify the issue of cell origin of the conduction system.

SINGLE CELL FATE TRACING IN THE EMBRYONIC HEART

Classic fate map studies of cells in the chick embryo have shown that the heart is composed of cells from three distinct embryonic origins: cardiogenic mesoderm, neural crest, and proepicardial organ *(42)*. Mesodermal cells bilateral to Hensen's node, which become committed to cardiac lineages just after gastrulation begins, form the double-walled tubular heart during neurula stages. Cardiac neural crest cells migrate from the embryonic hind brain to the beating heart tube to form great vessel smooth muscle and cardiac ganglia *(43,44)*. Before cardiac neural crest cells migrate to the heart, cells of the proepicardial organ migrate from the mesothelium toward the looping beating heart tube and form the epicardium *(45–48)* and coronary vessels *(49–52)*.

The cell lineage relations among cardiac cell types derived from the three embryonic sources have been examined by retroviral single-cell tagging and tracing studies in the embryonic chick heart *(40,41)*. The use of replication-defective, retrovirus-mediated genetic tags for analyzing

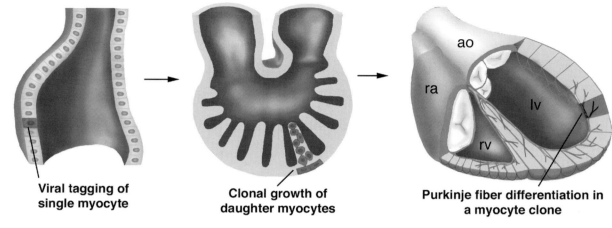

Fig. 3.

cell lineages was first shown in pioneering studies on neuronal cells of the eye *(53)* and the central nervous system. Replication-defective retroviruses stably integrate their genetic material into the infected host cell, and this genetic information is inherited by every descendant of that initially infected cell without horizontal transmission from primary infected cells. Therefore, retroviral-mediated gene transfer is one of the most reliable methods for introducing a genetic tag into the desired cell type at a particular time in the developing heart.

Retroviral single-cell fate studies on cardiogenic mesoderm and heart tubes *(32,38,39,54)*, cardiac neural crest *(32,54)*, and epicardial and coronary progenitors *(49,51)* have shown unequivocally that conduction tissues originate from cardiomyocytes and not from any other cardiac cell types. Individual myocyte precursor cells give rise to a series of progeny that migrate more vertically than horizontally to form clones that usually span the full thickness of the myocardium (i.e., from epicardial to endocardial surfaces of the muscle wall) (Fig. 3) *(24,38–41,55,56)*.

Purkinje fibers are found exclusively and frequently in myocyte clones. In contrast, no conduction cells are produced from cardiac neural crest or epicardial primordial cells. Independent evidence for the non-neurogenic origin of the conduction system has recently been provided by studies on neural crest derivatives in the mouse embryo *(57,58)*. The results from these studies show that Purkinje fibers are differentiated from a subset of contractile myocytes and not from neural crest as previously suggested (Fig. 4). The finding of Purkinje fiber differentiation within individual myocyte clones has provided new insight into the mechanism by which the Purkinje system grows and is patterned during heart development.

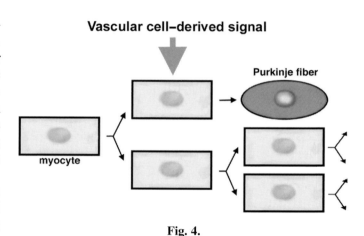

Fig. 4.

MECHANISM OF PURKINJE SYSTEM DEVELOPMENT

Two models have been proposed for development of the Purkinje system network in the ventricular myocardium (Fig. 4): the outgrowth model *(23,26,42,59,60)* and the ingrowth model *(24,28,40,61)*. The outgrowth model is based on progression of expression of conduction cell markers in the ventricle during heart development. When the looping heart tube initiates formation of the interventricular septum, conduction cell markers become detectable in a ring-like cluster of cells called the "primary conduction ring" *(62)* at the junction of the presumptive right and left ventricles *(23,60,63)*. As heart development proceeds, marker genes are eventually expressed within the entire Purkinje system. Based on the proximal–distal wave of marker expression, the outgrowth model (Fig. 4) proposes that the entire conduction network is established by proliferative outgrowth of daughter cells derived from a precursor cell population such as primary ring cells *(23,26,42,59,60)*.

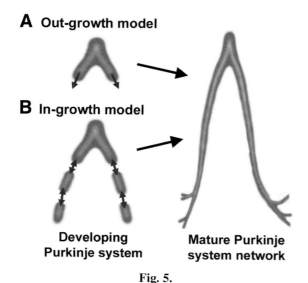

A Out-growth model

B In-growth model

Developing Purkinje system   Mature Purkinje system network

Fig. 5.

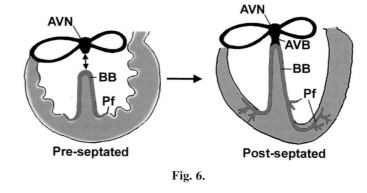

Fig. 6.

An obvious problem of the outgrowth model is that non–DNA-synthesizing cells and cells with low proliferative capacity in the embryonic heart map to primitive conduction tissues *(54,64–66)*. Another problem with the outgrowth model is that conduction cells differentiate within individual myocyte clones that occupy only a segment of the myocardium (Fig. 3). This clone-based differentiation is common in both central conduction fascicles, such as the His bundle *(54)*, and in the peripheral Purkinje system *(32)*. Thus, clonally related conduction cells form only a segment of the Purkinje network.

The second proposed model, the ingrowth model, can explain the proximal–distal wave of development of the conduction system *(24,28,40,61)*. In this model, conduction cells are recruited locally within each clonal domain and are linked together *in situ* to establish the Purkinje system network (Fig. 5). The ingrowth model is supported by birthdating studies in the chick that indicate that differentiation of the proximal conduction system, such as the AV rings, His bundle, and bundle branches, ends soon after formation of the ventricular septum is complete *(54,67)*, whereas recruitment of cells to the peripheral conduction network continues up until hatching *(66,68)*.

In addition, the ingrowth model is supported by recent studies on two linkage sites critical for conduction network formation: (1) the connection site between the AV bundle (a proximal component derived from the primary conduction ring) and the bundle branches (a distal conduction component derived from the interventricular septum) (Fig. 6); and (2) the linkage site between subendocardial and intramural Purkinje fibers. In the chick heart, electrical coupling between the AV bundle and

bundle branches occurs concomitantly with completion of fusion of the interventricular septum *(22,69)*. In a pre-septated heart, the bundle branches differentiate at the tip and along the sides of the primitive interventricular septum (Fig. 6). When the interventricular septum fuses, the anterior tip of the differentiating bundle branches is covered on the superior aspect by cells of the posterior end of the AV bundle. Unlike the complex coupling between the AV bundle and bundle branches, the subendocardial and periarterial Purkinje fiber networks appear to be linked by a simple mechanism. The two distal conduction components are coupled invariably at the sites where the interventricular arteries and arterioles juxtapose the subendocardial conduction cells *(61)*.

MECHANISMS OF CONDUCTION CELL DIFFERENTIATION

Because conduction cells have been identified as originating from myocytes, determining the mechanisms that convert working myocytes from a muscle to a conducting phenotype should contribute to our understanding of Purkinje fiber differentiation. The unique location of Purkinje fiber recruitment within individual myocyte clones has provided important insight into the cellular and molecular factors involved in this inductive event in the embryonic heart. Paracrine interactions between embryonic myocytes and cardiac endothelial cells may be important in the local recruitment of conduction cells from beating myocytes.

INTERACTIONS BETWEEN CARDIAC ENDOTHELIAL CELLS AND MYOCYTES

Although the presence of the peripheral intramyocardial component of the ventricular conduction system varies among species *(26,27)*, the proximal components of the conduction system run subendocardially in all species. In avian hearts in which both proximal and peripheral components of the Purkinje fiber network persist, intramyocardial Purkinje fibers penetrate from the subendocardium into the myocardium following coronary artery branches, but not venous to capillary networks (30–32,61,70). Differentiation of Purkinje fibers within individual myocyte clones (32,54) suggests that the subendocardial and periarterial location of Purkinje fibers does not result from migration or proliferative invasion of conduction cells into these two regions. Instead, Purkinje fibers are found in these two restricted sites of the myocardium by the local conversion of myocytes into conducting cells in the periarterial and subendocardial regions. Therefore, paracrine interactions of myocytes with endocardial and arterial cells may induce the differentiation of conduction cells (24,32,41).

This hypothesis has been tested by two complementary approaches: inhibition or activation of coronary arterial branching (71). Suppression of coronary vessel development resulted in a significant loss of intramural Purkinje fiber differentiation, which indicates the necessity of coronary arterial beds for intramural differentiation of conduction cells. Purkinje fibers developed along arteries that were ectopically induced in the myocardium (71); therefore, coronary arterial beds are not only necessary but also sufficient for recruiting adjacent myocytes to differentiate into conduction cells. Because endothelial cells are the only cell type usually found in the endocardium and the arteries where adjacent myocytes differentiate into Purkinje fibers, endothelial cell–derived signal(s) may induce recruitment of conduction cells. In support of this idea, Pennisi et al. (72) reported that the expression of a conduction cell marker gene in presumptive ventricular conduction cells in the mouse embryonic heart depends on the presence of cardiac endothelial cells. These studies have provided a basis for the progress in searching for the molecular mechanism(s) involved in this inductive event in the myocyte lineage.

ENDOTHELIAL CELL–DERIVED FACTORS IN PURKINJE FIBER DIFFERENTIATION

Purkinje fibers differentiate subendocardially and periarterially but never adjacent to the venous system or the capillary network (32,70). The endothelial cell population, with the expression of endothelial cell markers, is significantly heterogeneous (73–76). Vascular bed–specific phenotypes of endothelial cells are regulated by environmental factors (77–79). Shear-stress, which can differ with the vascular bed, regulates the expression and secretion of vascular cytokines (80). Endothelial cells of the

endocardium and arterial branches are exposed to higher shear stress than those of venous and capillary networks. Cultured embryonic myocytes can be induced to express conduction cell makers by endothelin (ET)-1, which is induced by shear stress (81–83). This ET-1-dependent conversion of myocytes is dose-dependent and inhibited by specific antagonists of ET receptors. Furthermore, this myocyte conversion is not seen after treatment with other cytokines that are important in vascular development, including fibroblast growth factor, vascular endothelial growth factor, and platelet-derived growth factor.

ET was originally identified as a potent vasoconstrictor derived from endothelial cells (82). Paracrine secretion of ET ligands depends on two steps of post-translational processing of the ET precursor, preproET (84). First, preproET is cleaved by furin proteases into bigET. In the second step, ET-specific metalloprotease, ECE-1, processes bigET into the biologically active ET (84,85). Activation of ET-signaling begins with the binding of ET to G protein–coupled receptors (86,87). In the embryonic heart, ET receptors are expressed by all myocytes and absent from cardiac endothelial cells (70,88). In contrast, ECE-1 is expressed in a portion of the endocardium and coronary arterial endothelium, and is absent from myocytes and the endothelium of cardiac veins and capillaries (70,89). Because the expression pattern of ECE-1 in the embryonic heart coincides with the timing and location of endogenous Purkinje fiber differentiation, localized ET-dependent induction of embryonic myocytes in vivo may be explained by the distribution of endogenous ECE-1. Studies of viral-mediated expression of ECE-1 and preproET-1 in the chick embryonic heart support the role of endogenous ECE-1 in Purkinje fiber differentiation (70). Exogenous co-expression of ECE-1 and preproET-1 in the embryonic ventricular myocardium resulted in the ectopic and precocious differentiation of Purkinje fibers. These results are consistent with the model (Fig. 7) that induction of conduction cells is localized in the ventricular myocardium by the site-specific cleavage of bigET-1 by ECE-1 (70).

This model for ET-dependent Purkinje fiber differentiation is based on the finding that ET stimulates expression of many Purkinje fiber marker genes and downregulates genes specific for heart muscle both in vitro and in vivo (70,81). However, in a recent study (90) the expression of a subset of genes, which are upregulated in Purkinje fibers in vivo, was not significantly increased by ET in vitro. These results are the first to show marker genes for Purkinje fibers that do not respond to ET, a finding that suggests conduction cells may not undergo complete differentiation in culture. In addition, an ET-independent pathway may play a role in regulation of a unique gene

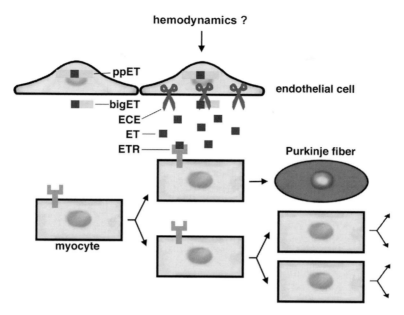

Fig. 7.

expression pattern in Purkinje fibers *(90)*. Although ET has been the only factor shown to induce embryonic cardiomyocytes to differentiate into Purkinje fibers, other paracrine interactions such as the interaction of neuregulin and its receptor tyrosine kinases, erbB2 and erbB4, with the endocardium and the myocardium may be involved *(26)*. In the heart, expression of neuregulin is confined to the endocardium, whereas erbB2 and erbB4 are expressed in the myocardium. A loss-of-function mutation in the neuregulin or erbB gene in the mouse results in the loss of trabeculae formation, but the compact zone of the myocardium is normal *(91–93)*. These mutant embryos have irregular heart beats and eventually die. Although the cause of death of these mutant embryos is unknown, conduction disturbances may be associated with insufficient contractile capacity *(26)*. Neuregulin expression is regulated by ET, and further study of the interactions between different paracrine signaling cascades will contribute to our understanding of molecular mechanisms involved in conduction cell differentiation.

GENE EXPRESSION IN THE CONDUCTION SYSTEM

The pattern of gene expression in cells of the conduction system is complex. Although the mechanisms of transcriptional regulation of conduction cell differentiation are largely unknown, several transcription factors expressed in the conduction system and a potential *cis*-element in Purkinje fibers have been recently identified.

CIS-ELEMENT FUNCTION IN PURKINJE FIBERS

Purkinje fibers have a unique pattern of gene expression *(25–28,40)*, and many of these genes are found in either neuronal or skeletal muscle cells. Although the mechanisms underlying neuronal cell–type gene expression in conduction cells are unknown, a muscle-specific enhancer/promoter of the desmin gene is involved in expression in Purkinje fibers *(94)*. Desmin, which belongs to the family of intermediate filaments *(95)*, is expressed in all myogenic cell lineages: skeletal, cardiac, and smooth muscle *(96–98)*. A 1 kb 5′ region of the desmin gene encodes several *cis*-acting elements *(99)*, including the E-box for binding of the basic/helix-loop-helix family of muscle determination transcription factors *(100)* and the CArG-box of the serum response element *(101)*. The proximal 280 bp of the 5′ regulatory sequence (DES1) fused to a reporter gene, β-galactosidase (β-gal), directs gene expression in skeletal muscle but not in smooth muscle or the working myocardium of the heart *(94)*. In addition, the DES1 enhancer/promoter directs β-gal expression in the Purkinje system through embryonic development and after birth. These findings indicate that the 280 bp noncoding region of the desmin gene can direct skeletal muscle-specific expression in vivo, and other *cis*-elements in the 5′ regulatory region direct expression for cardiac and smooth muscle.

TRANSACTIVATORS

Msx-2, a homeobox domain gene homologous to the *Drosophila* muscle segment homeobox gene *(msh)*, is the first transcription factor identified in the conduction system. In the developing chick heart, Msx-2 is expressed transiently in progenitors of the proximal conduction system, such as the AV ring, but it is never expressed in subendocardial and periarterial Purkinje fibers *(60)*. In the developing human heart, TBX5, a T-box transcription factor, is present in the AV node at higher levels than in the ventricular myocardium of the human embryonic heart *(102)*. The role of Msx-2 and TBX5 in the formation and patterning of the conduction system is unknown. Another homeobox transcription factor Csx/Nkx2.5 *(103,104)*, the mammalian homologue of the *tinman* gene in *Drosophila (105)*, has been linked to the conduction system. In humans, mutations in the CSX/NKX2.5 gene result in an autosomal dominant congenital heart disease characterized by an atrial septal defect and AV conduction delays *(106)*. In the mouse, Csx/Nkx-2.5 is expressed in the myocardium of embryonic and adult hearts *(103)*, and knockout of the gene for Csx/Nkx-2.5 results in embryonic death at the tubular heart stage *(104)*. Csx/Nkx2.5 can bind to GATA4, a zinc-finger-domain protein *(107)*, and these two transcription factors cooperatively activate the expression of atrial natriuretic factor *(108,109)*, which is found in high levels in both the atrium and the ventricular conduction system *(110,111)*. Expression of Csx/Nkx and GATA4 is increased in differentiating conduction cells of the chick embryo *(90,112)*. These data on the four cardiac-type transcription factors do not explain how ventricular muscle-specific genes are downregulated in Purkinje fibers or how genes usually found in neuronal or skeletal muscle lineages are upregulated in conduction cells.

In addition to the studies showing that an E-box-containing skeletal muscle-specific enhancer/promoter of the desmin gene functions in the Purkinje system *(94)*, studies have been conducted in a transgenic mouse model to assess the ability of skeletal muscle transcription factors to activate a skeletal muscle program in the embryonic heart. The ectopic expression of myoD in the developing mouse heart *(113)* induces several skeletal muscle proteins in late stage embryonic hearts. However, ectopic myoD does not activate Myf-5 or MRF-4 *(113)*. The only myogenic counterpart induced in the transgenic mouse by myoD is myogenin. Low levels of myoD, but not myogenin or MRF4, are expressed in the frog heart, but the cell type that expresses myoD has not been determined *(114)*. In the embryonic chick heart, both non-manipulated and ET-induced Purkinje fibers express myoD, whereas expression of Myf5 or MRF4 is undetectable *(90)*. These findings suggest that the transcriptional mechanisms for inducing skeletal muscle type-genes in conduction cells may differ from those used in skeletal muscle.

CONCLUSION

Lineage studies in cardiac cells have determined the time and location of the differentiation and patterning of cells of the cardiac conduction system. The plasticity of embryonic myocytes in committing to lineage and in terminally differentiating into conduction cells allows for the study of the molecular mechanisms involved in these processes. The following questions need to be addressed: (1) What factors recruit embryonic myocytes to differentiate into the proximal conduction system, such as the AV node and ring? (2) What mechanisms control linkage of the Purkinje fiber network to the proximal conduction system? (3) What mechanisms cause the cardiac endothelium to produce an inductive signal? (4) Which mechanism defines the sites of electrical coupling between Purkinjefibers and contractile myocytes? (5) What transcriptional factors and *cis*-elements regulate the expression of the unique set of genes in conduction cells? A clarification of these questions will contribute significantly to our understanding of the development and integrated function of the cardiac conduction system.

ACKNOWLEDGMENT

This work was supported by a grant from the National Institutes of Health.

REFERENCES

1. Tawara S. Das reizleitungssystem des Säugetierherzens. Gustav Fischer. Jena, 1906.
2. Goldenberg M, Rothberger CJ. Über des Elektrogramm der spezifischen Herz muskulature. Pflügers Arch 1936;237: 295–306.
3. Botzler E. The initiation of impulses in cardiac muscle. Am J Physiol 1942;138:273–282.
4. Keith A, Flack M. The form and nature of the muscular connections between the primary divisions of the vertebrate heart. J Anat Physiol 1907;41:172–189.
5. Brooks C, Mc C, Lu HH. The sinoatrial pacemaker of the heart. Springfield: Charles C. Thomas, 1972.
6. Wenckebach KF. Beiträge zur Kenntnis der menschlichen Hetztätigkeit. Arch Anat Physiol 1906;1-2:297–354.
7. Thörel C. Vorläufige Mitteilung über eine besondere Muskelverbindung zwischen der Cava superior und dem His'schen Bündlel. Münch Med Wschr 1909;56:2159.
8. Robb JS, Petri R. Expansions of the atrio-ventricular system in the atria. In: Paes de Carvalho A, De Mello WC, Hoffman BS, eds. The Specialized Tissue of the Heart. Amsterdam: Elsevier, 1961:1–18.
9. His W Jr. Die Tätigkeit des embryonalen Herzens und deren Bedeutung für die Lehre von der Herzbewegung beim Erwachsenen. Arb Med Klin Leipzig 1893;14.
10. Purkinje J. Mikroskopisch-neurologische Beobachtungen. Arch Anat Physiol Wiss Med 1845;12:281–295.
11. Kölliker A. Gewebeslehre. 6 Aufl Lpz 1902.

12. Manasek FJ. Embryonic development of the heart: I. A light and electron microscopic study of myocardial development in the early chick embryo. J Morphol 1968;125:329–365.

13. Kamino K, Hirota A, Fujii S. Localization of pacemaking activity in early embryonic heart monitored using voltage-sensitive dye. Nature 1981;290:595–597.

14. Yada T, Sakai T, Komuro H, Hirota A, Kamino K. Development of electrical rhythmic activity in early embryonic cultured chick double-heart monitored optically with a voltage-sensitive dye. Dev Biol 1985;110:455–466.

15. Kamino K. Optical approaches to ontogeny of electrical activity and related functional organization during early heart development. Physiol Rev 1991;71:53-91.

16. Patten BM, Kramer TC. The initiation of contraction in the embryonic chick heart. Am J Anat 1933;53:349–375.

17. Yutzey KE, Rhee JT, Bader D. Expression of the atrial-specific myosin heavy chain AMHC1 and the establishment of antero-posterior polarity in the developing chicken heart. Development 1994;120:871–883.

18. Lieberman M, Paes de Carvalho A. The electrophysiological organization of the embryonic chick heart. J Gen Physiol 1965; 49:351–363.

19. de Jong F, Opthof T, Wilde AA, et al. Persisting zones of slow impulse conduction in developing chicken hearts. Circ Res 1992;71:240–250.

20. Alcolea S, Theveniau-Ruissy M, Jarry-Guichard T, et al. Downregulation of connexin 45 gene products during mouse heart development. Circ Res 1999;841:1365–1379.

21. Coppen SR, Severs NJ, Gourdie RG. Connexin45 (alpha 6) expression delineates and extended conduction system in the embryonic and adult rodent heart. Dev Genet 1999;24:82–90.

22. Chuck ET, Freeman DM, Watanabe M, Rosenbaum DS. Changing activation sequence in the embryonic chick heart. Implications for the development of the His-Purkinje system. Circ Res 1997;81:470–476.

23. Rentschler S, Vaidya DM, Tamaddon H, et al. Visualization and functional characterization of the developing murine cardiac conduction system. Development 2001;128:1785–1792.

24. Mikawa T, Fischman DA. The polyclonal origin of myocyte lineages. Annu Rev Physiol 1996;58:509–521.

25. Schiaffino S. Protean patterns of gene expression in the heart conduction system. Circ Res 1997;80:749–750.

26. Moorman AF, de Jong F, Denyn MM, Lamers WH. Development of the cardiac conduction system. Circ Res 1998; 82:629–644.

27. Welikson RD, Mikawa T. Cytoskeletal gene expression in the developing cardiac conduction system. In: Dube DK, ed. Myofibrillogenesis. New York: Springer, 2002:153–177.

28. Gourdie RG, Kubalak S, O'Brien T, Chien KR, Mikawa T. Development of cardiac myocyte and conduction system lineages. In: Chien KR, ed. The Molecular Basis of Cardiovascular Disease, 2nd Ed. Philadelphia: Saunders, 2004:279–281.

29. Randall DJ. The circulatory system. In: Hoar WS, Randall DJ, eds. Fish Physiology. New York: Academic Press, 1970:133–172.

30. Davies F. The conducting system of the bird's heart. J Anat 1930;64:129–146.

31. Vassall-Adams PR. The development of the atrioventricular bundle and its branches in the avian heart. J Anat 1982;134: 169–183.

32. Gourdie RG, Mima T, Thompson RP, Mikawa, T. Terminal diversification of the myocyte lineage generates Purkinje fibers of the cardiac conduction system. Development 1995;121:1423–1431.

33. Truex RC, Smythe MQ. Comparative morphology of the cardiac conduction tissue in animals. Ann N Y Acad Sci 1965; 127:19–33.

34. Patten BM. The development of the sinoventricular conduction system. Med Bull (Ann Arbor) 1956;22:1–21.

35. Gorza L, Schiaffino S, Vitadello M. Heart conduction system: a neural crest derivative? Brain Res 1988;457:360–366.

36. Gorza L, Vettore S, Vitadello M. Molecular and cellular diversity of heart conduction system myocytes. Trends in Cardiovasc Med 1994;4:153–159.

37. Vitadello M, Matteoli M, Gorza L. Neurofilament proteins are co-expressed with desmin in heart conduction system myocytes. J Cell Sci 1990;97:11–21.

38. Mikawa, T, Borisov A, Brown AM, Fischman DA. Clonal analysis of cardiac morphogenesis in the chicken embryo using a replication-defective retrovirus: I. Formation of the ventricular myocardium. Dev Dyn 1992;193:11–23.

39. Mikawa T, Cohen-Gould L, Fischman DA. Clonal analysis of cardiac morphogenesis in the chicken embryo using a replication-defective retrovirus. III: Polyclonal origin of adjacent ventricular myocytes. Dev Dyn 1992;195:133–141.

40. Mikawa T. Cardiac lineages. In: Harvey RP, Rosenthal N., eds. Heart Development. New York: Academic Press, 1998:19–33.

41. Mikawa T. Determination of heart cell lineages. In: Moody SA, ed. Cell Fate Determination. New York: Academic Press, 1998: 449–460.

42. Fishman MC, Chien KR. Fashioning the vertebrate heart: earliest embryonic decisions. Development 1997;124:2099–2117.

43. Kirby ML. Cellular and molecular contributions of the cardiac neural crest to cardiovascular development. Trends Cardiovasc Med 1993;3:18–23.

44. Noden DM, Poelmann RE, Gittenberger-de Groot AC. Cell origins and tissue boundaries during outflow tract development. Trends Cardiovas Med 1995;5:69–75.

45. Viragh SZ, Challice CE. The development of the conduction system in the mouse embryo heart. Dev Biol 1982;89:25–40.

46. Ho E, Shimada Y. Formation of the epicardium studied with the scanning electron microscope. Dev Biol 1978;66:579–585.

47. Hiruma T, Hirakow R. Epicardial formation in embryonic chick heart: computer-aided reconstruction, scanning, and transmission electron microscopic studies. Am J Anat 1989;184:129–138.

48. Manner J. Experimental study on the formation of the epicardium in chick embryos. Anat Embryol 1993;187:281–289.

49. Mikawa T, Fischman DA. Retroviral analysis of cardiac morphogenesis: discontinuous formation of coronary vessels. Proc Natl Acad Sci USA 1992;89:9504–9508.

50. Poelmann RE, Gittenberger-de Groot AC, Mentink MT, Bokenkamp R, Hogers B. Development of the cardiac coronary vascular endothelium, studied with antiendothelial antibodies, in chicken-quail chimeras. Circ Res 1993;73:559–568.

51. Mikawa T, Gourdie RG. Pericardial mesoderm generates a population of coronary smooth muscle cells migrating into the heart along with ingrowth of the epicardial organ. Dev Biol 1996;173:221–232.

52. Dettman RW, Denetclaw W Jr, Ordahl CP, Bristow J. Common epicardial origin of coronary vascular smooth muscle, perivascular fibroblasts, and intermyocardial fibroblasts in the avian heart. Dev Biol 1998;193:169–181.

53. Cepko C. Retrovirus vectors and their application in neurobiology. Neuron 1988;1:345–353.

54. Cheng G, Litchenberg WH, Cole GJ, Mikawa T, Thompson RP, Gourdie RG. Development of the cardiac conduction system

involves recruitment within a multipotent cardiomyogenic lineage. Development 1999;126:5041–5049.

55. Mikawa T, Hyer J, Itoh N, Wei Y. Retroviral vectors to study cardiovascular development. Trends Cardiovasc Med 1996;6:79–86.

56. Mikawa T. Retroviral targeting of FGF and FGFR in cardiomyocytes and coronary vascular cells during heart development. Ann N Y Acad Sci 1995;752:506–516.

57. Jiang X, Rowitch DH, Soriano P, McMahon AP, Sucov HM. Fate of the mammalian cardiac neural crest. Development 2000;127:1607–1616.

58. Epstein JA, Li J, Lang D, et al. Migration of cardiac neural crest cells in Splotch embryos. Development 2000;127:1869–1878.

59. Lamers WH, De Jong F, De Groot IJ, Moorman AF. The development of the avian conduction system, a review. Eur J Morphol 1991;29:233–253.

60. Chan-Thomas PS, Thompson RP, Robert B, Yacoub MH, Barton PJ. Expression of homeobox genes Msx-1 (Hox-7) and Msx-2 (Hox-8) during cardiac development in the chick. Dev Dyn 1993;197:203–216.

61. Mikawa T, Gourdie RG, Hyer J, Takebayashi-Suzuki K. Cardiac conduction system development. In: Tomanek RJ, Runyan RR, eds. Formation of the Heart and its Regulation. New York: Springer, 2001:121–135.

62. Anderson RH, Davies MJ, Becker AE. Atrio-ventricular ring specialized tissue in the normal heart. Eur J Cardiol 1974;2: 219–230.

63. Wessels A, Vermeulen JL, Verbeek FJ, et al. Spatial distribution of "tissue-specific" antigens in the developing human heart and skeletal muscle. III. An immunohistochemical analysis of the distribution of the neural tissue antigen G1N2 in the embryonic heart; implications fro the development of the atrioventricular conduction system. Anat Rec 1992;232:97–111.

64. Rumiantsev PP. DNA synthesis and mitotic division of myocytes of the ventricles, atria and conduction system of the heart during the myocardial development in mammals. Tsitologiia 1978;20:132–141.

65. Thompson RP, Lindroth JR, Wong YMM. Regional differences in DNA synthetic activity in the preseptation myocardium of the chick. In: Clark E, Takao A, eds. Developmental Cardiology; Morphogenesis and Function. New York: Futura Publishing Co., 1990:219–234.

66. Litchenberg WH, Gang C, Klatt SC, Mikawa T, Thompson RP, Gourdie RG. Adenoviral and retroviral gene targeting of the cardiac conduction system. In: Clark E, et al., eds. Etiology and Morphogenesis of Congenital Heart Disease. Oxford: Blackwell, 2000:241–246.

67. Thompson RP, Kanai T, Gourdie RG, et al. Organization and function of early specialized myocardium. In: Clark EB, Markwald RR, Takao A, eds. Developmental Mechanisms of Congenital Heart Disease. New York: Futura Publishing Co., 1995:269–279.

68. Thompson RP, Rosenthal P, Cheng G. Origin and fate of cardiac conduction tissue. In: Clark EB, Takao A, Nakazawa M, eds. Etiology and Morphogenesis of Congenital Heart Disease. Tokyo: Sankei Press, 2000:247–251.

69. Chuck ET, Watanabe M. Differential expression of PSA-NCAM and HNK-1 epitopes in the developing cardiac conduction system of the chick. Dev Dyn 1997;209:182–195.

70. Takebayashi-Suzuki K, Yanagisawa M, Gourdie RG, Kanzawa N, Mikawa, T. In vivo induction of cardiac Purkinje fiber differentiation by coexpression of preproendothelin-1 and endothelin converting enzyme-1. Development 2000;127:3523–3532.

71. Hyer J, Johansen M, Prasad A, et al. Induction of Purkinje fiber differentiaiton by coronary arterialization. Proc Natl Acad Sci USA 1999;96:13214–13218.

72. Pennisi DJ, Rentchler S, Gourdie RG, et al. Induction and patterning of the cardiac conduction system. Int J Dev Biol 2002;46:765–775.

73. Cines DB, Pollak ES, Buck CA, et al. Endothelial cells in physiology and in the pathophysiology of vascular disorders. Blood 1998;91:3527–3561.

74. Gerritsen ME. Functional heterogeneity of vascular endothelial cells. Biochem Pharmacol 1987;36:2701–2711.

75. Page C, Rose M, Yacoub M, Pigott R. Antigenic heterogeneity of vascular endothelium. Am J Pathol 1992;141:673–683.

76. Rajotte D, Arap W, Hagedorn M, Koivunen E, Pasqualini R, Ruoslahti E. Molecular heterogeneity of the vascular endothelium revealed by in vivo phage display. J Clin Invest 1998;102:430–437.

77. Aird WC, Jahroudi N, Weiler-Guettler H, Rayburn HB, Rosenberg RD. Human von Willebrand factor gene sequences target expression to a subpopulation of endothelial cells in transgenic mice. Proc Natl Acad Sci USA 1995;92: 4567–4571.

78. Aird WC, Edelberg JM, Weiler-Guettler H, Simmons WW, Smith TW, Rosenberg RD. Vascular bed-specific expression of an endothelial cell gene is programmed by the tissue microenvironment. J Cell Biol 1997;138:1117–1124.

79. Guillot PV, Guan J, Liu L, et al. A vascular bed-specific pathway. J Clin Invest 1999;103:799–805.

80. McCormick SM, Eskin SG, McIntire LV, et al. DNA microarray reveals changes in gene expression of shear stressed human umbilical vein endothelial cells. Proc Natl Acad Sci USA 2001;98:8955–8960.

81. Gourdie RG, Wei Y, Kim D, Klatt SC, Mikawa T. Endothelin-induced conversion of embryonic heart muscle cells into impulse-conducting Purkinje fibers. Proc Natl Acad Sci USA 1998;95:6815–6818.

82. Yanagisawa M, Kurihara H, Kimura S, et al. A novel potent vasoconstrictor peptide produced by vascular endothelial cells. Nature 1988;332:411–415.

83. Yoshizumi M, Kurihara H, Sugiyama T, et al. Hemodynamic shear stress stimulates endothelin production by cultured endothelial cells. Biochem Biophys Res Commun 1989;161:859–864.

84. Xu D, Emoto N, Giaid A, et al. ECE-1: a membrane-bound metalloprotease that catalyzes the proteolytic activation of big endothelin-1. Cell 1994;78:473–485.

85. Emoto N, Yanagisawa M. Endothelin-converting enzyme-2 is a membrane-bound, phosphoramidon-sensitive metalloprotease with acidic pH optimum. J Biol Chem 1995;270: 15262–15268.

86. Arai H, Hori S, Aramori I, Ohkubo H, Nakanishi S. Cloning and expression of a cDNA encoding an endothelin receptor. Nature 1990;348:730–732.

87. Sakurai T, Yanagisawa M, Takuwa Y, et al. Cloning of a cDNA encoding a non-isopeptide-selective subtype of the endothelin receptor. Nature 1990;348:732–735.

88. Clouthier DE, Hosoda K, Richardson JA, et al. Cranial and cardiac neural crest defects in endothelin-A receptor-deficient mice. Development 1998;125:813–824.

89. Yanagisawa H, Yanagisawa M, Kapur RP, et al. Dual genetic pathways of endothelin-mediated intercellular signaling revealed by targeted disruption of endothelin converting enzyme-1 gene. Development 1998;125:825–836.

90. Takebayashi-Suzuki K, Pauliks BL, Eltsefon Y, Mikawa T. Purkinje fibers of the avian heart express a myogenic transcription factor program distinct from cardiac and skeletal muscle. Dev Biol 2001;234:390–401.

91. Meyer D, Birchmeier C. Multiple essential functions of neuregulin in development. Nature 1995;78:378:753.

92. Lee KF, Simon H, Chen H, Bates B, Hung MC, Hauser C. Requirement for neuregulin receptor erbB2 in neural and cardiac development. Nature 1995;378:394–398.

93. Gassmann M, Casagranda F, Orioli D, et al. Aberrant neural and cardiac development in mice lacking the ErbB4 neuregulin receptor. Nature 1995;378:390–394.

94. Li Z, Marchand P, Humbert J, Babinet C, Paulin D. Desmin sequence elements regulating muscle-specific expression in transgenic mice. Development 1993;117:947–959.

95. Lazarides E. Intermediate filaments: a chemically heterogeneous, developmentally regulated class of proteins. Ann Rev Biochem 1982;51:219–250.

96. Babai F, Musevi-Aghdam J, Schurch W, Royal A, Gabbiani G. Coexpression of alpha-sarcomeric actin, alpha-smooth muscle actin and desmin during myogenesis in rat and mouse embryos I. Skeletal muscle. Differentiation 1990;44:132–142.

97. Furst DO, Osborn M, Weber, K. Myogenesis in the mouse embryo: differential onset of expression of myogenic proteins and the involvement of titin in myofibril assembly. J Cell Biol 1989;109:517–527.

98. Hill CS, Duran S, Lin ZX, Weber K, Holtzer H. Titin and myosin, but not desmin, are linked during myofibrillogenesis in postmitotic mononucleated myoblasts. J Cell Biol 1986;103:2185–2196.

99. Li ZL, Paulin D. High level desmin expression depends on a muscle-specific enhancer. J Biol Chem 1991;266:6562–6570.

100. Buckingham ME. Muscle: the regulation of myogenesis. Curr Opin Genet Dev 1994;4:745–751.

101. Treisman R. The serum response element. Trends Biochem Sci 1992;17:423–426.

102. Hatcher CJ, Goldstein MM, Mah CS, Delia CS, Basson CT. Identification and localization of TBX5 transcription factor during human cardiac morphogenesis. Dev Dyn 2000;219:90–95.

103. Komuro I, Izumo S. Csx: a murine homeobox-containing gene specifically expressed in the developing heart. Proc Natl Acad Sci USA 1993;90:8145–8149.

104. Lyons I, Parsons LM, Hartley L, et al. Myogenic and morphogenetic defects in the heart tubes of murine embryos lacking the homeo box gene Nkx2-5. Genes Dev 1995;9:1654–1666.

105. Bodmer R. The gene tinman is required for specification of the heart and visceral muscles in Drosophila. Development 1993;118:719–729.

106. Schott JJ, Benson DW, Basson CT, et al. Congenital heart disease caused by mutations in the transcription factor NKX2-5. Science 1998;281:108–111.

107. Molkentin JD, Kalvakolanu DV, Markham BE. Transcription factor GATA-4 regulates cardiac muscle-specific expression of the alpha-myosin heavy-chain gene. Mol Cell Biol 1994;14:4947–4957.

108. Durocher D, Charron F, Warren R, Schwartz RJ, Nemer M. The cardiac transcription factors Nkx2-5 and GATA-4 are mutual cofactors. EMBO J 1997;16:5687–5696.

109. Lee Y, Shioi T, Kasahara H, et al. The cardiac tissue-restricted homeobox protein Csx/Nkx2.5 physically associates with the zinc finger protein GATA4 and cooperatively activates atrial natriuretic factor gene expression. Mol Cell Biol 1998;18:3120–3129.

110. Wharton J, Anderson RH, Springall D, et al. Localisation of atrial natriuretic peptide immunoreactivity in the ventricular myocardium and conduction system of the human fetal and adult heart. Br Heart J 1988;60:267–274.

111. Hansson M, Forsgren S. Presence of immunoreactive atrial natriuretic peptide in nerve fibres and conduction cells in the conduction system of the bovine heart. Anat Embryol 1993;188:331–337.

112. Thomas PS, Kasahara H, Edmonson AM, et al. Elevated expression of Nkx-2.5 in developing myocardial conduction cells. Anat Rec 2001;263:307–313.

113. Miner JH, Miller JB, Wold BJ. Skeletal muscle phenotypes initiated by ectopic MyoD in transgenic mouse heart. Development 1992;114:853–860.

114. Jennings CG. Expression of the myogenic gene MRF4 during Xenopus development. Dev Biol 1992;151:319–332.

19   Mechanisms of Sudden Cardiac Death

Wayne E. Cascio, MD

CONTENTS

INTRODUCTION

Sudden cardiac death (SCD) accounts for more that half of all cardiovascular deaths in the United States. The mechanisms of SCD are diverse and include arrhythmic and nonarrhythmic causes. Ventricular fibrillation (VF), ventricular tachycardia (VT), and asystole account for most episodes of SCD; nonarrhythmic causes such as pulmonary embolism, aortic dissection, pericardial tamponade, and stroke also contribute. Because ventricular arrhythmias represent the predominant cause of SCD, this chapter emphasizes the molecular and cellular processes that determine risk for life-threatening ventricular arrhythmia.

Most individuals who experience SCD have preexisting cardiac disease, whereas approx 5% have normal hearts *(1)*. Conditions such as hypertension, diabetes, cardiomyopathy, valvular heart disease, and congestive heart failure are all associated with higher rates of SCD. In particular, more than half of SCD cases occur in the setting of myocardial ischemia or infarction.

SCD is associated with several clinical conditions having a genetic basis. These include primary electrical abnormalities and cardiomyopathies. Some of the specific gene mutations of these conditions are known and provide the molecular basis for these diseases. Yet, much remains unknown regarding the risk determinants for SCD. For example, epidemiological studies indicate that a paternal history of SCD imparts a risk of dying suddenly during myocardial infarction (MI) *(2,3)*. This association is intriguing, because it goes beyond the known inherited abnormalities and risk factors and suggests that certain individuals are predisposed to life-threatening arrhythmias due to a genetically determined factor exposed by ischemia. The increasing prevalence of coronary artery disease (CAD), diabetes, and obesity combined with an aging population makes it imperative to understand the molecular mechanisms of SCD.

HISTORICAL PERSPECTIVE

Study of the mechanisms accounting for the clinical syndrome of SCD is entering its third century. During the latter part of the 19th century, physiologists identified VF as the cause of SCD in animal models. Drawing upon this experimental experience, MacWilliam proposed in 1889 that VF caused SCD in humans *(4,5)*. His reasoning proved correct, as the 20th century saw the maturation of basic and clinical sciences and the identification of VF as the predominant cause of SCD. The investigative method of electrocardiography proved this conclusion. Cellular mechanisms explaining arrhythmia emerged later from studies utilizing

From: *Contemporary Cardiology: Principles of Molecular Cardiology*
Edited by: M. S. Runge and C. Patterson © Humana Press Inc., Totowa, NJ

cellular electrodes and membrane voltage–clamping techniques permitting the study of impulse formation and propagation and the electrical currents responsible for these phenomena. An understanding of the electrophysiological mechanisms benefited from the characterization of the encoding genes, structure, and biophysical properties of channel proteins, exchangers, and transporters, as well as the regulation and signaling processes determining their expression, interaction, and function. Studies are now exploring the integration of membrane and signaling components as an interactive system modified by intrinsic and external stresses or disease through gene regulation, protein trafficking, and post-translational protein modification. Hence, a model of SCD risk is emerging from genetically determined cellular responses of myocytes and their neighboring cells in response to external stresses and autocrine and paracrine effectors that result in changes in electrical and structural properties of the myocardium.

DEFINITION AND MAGNITUDE OF THE PROBLEM

SCD is defined as an unexpected natural death from a cardiac cause occurring within a short period. Generally, a death is considered sudden when it happens within 1 h of the onset of symptoms and occurs in an individual without any other condition considered fatal (6,7). SCD results from hemodynamically significant arrhythmias, including VF, VT, bradycardia, and asystole, and represents a final common pathway for many cardiac diseases. SCD accounts for 1–2 deaths per 1000 adults over the age of 35 years in the United States each year (7), and approx 12.5 deaths per 1000 adults in individuals at high risk for SCD (8).

The most recent data on SCD are reflected in U.S. vital statistics mortality data maintained by the National Center for Health Statistics at the Centers for Disease Control and Prevention (9). In 1998, SCD occurred in 456,076 people older than 35 years of age. This represents approx 63% of the total number of cardiac deaths. Thus, the majority of cardiac deaths are sudden when the definition includes those dying out of the hospital, enroute to the hospital, or in the emergency department shortly after collapse. The proportion of SCD was greatest for the youngest age group, 35–44 years (74%) and decreased with age reaching 58% for individuals aged 75–84 years. Overall, the proportions of SCD did not differ between men and women; however, the mean age of SCD was 70 years in men and 82 years in women. Age-specific death rates were greater for men until the age of

85 years. Overall age-adjusted death rates for men and women differed about 50%—411 and 275 deaths per 100,000 population, respectively. African Americans had the highest age-adjusted death rate from SCD, followed by Caucasian, Native American, and Asian. Such differences in the age-specific death rates related to gender and race suggest the potential for a molecular basis to these observations.

The rate of arrhythmic SCD varies widely, depending on the definition used and available clinical information. For example, in a large cohort of 834 patients having implantable cardiac defibrillators (ICDs), 109 patients died during follow-up. Seventeen of these deaths (16%) were categorized as SCD, i.e., "death of cardiac origin that occurred unexpectedly within 1 hour of the onset of new symptoms or a death that was unexpected and not witnessed" (8). Yet, of the 17 individuals presumed to have SCD caused by an arrhythmia, seven other causes were discovered at autopsy, i.e., MI, pulmonary embolism, cerebral infarction, and ruptured thoracic and abdominal aortic aneurysms. Only seven individuals had an ICD discharge temporally related to the time of death. Each of these cases would have been categorized as SCD according to the criteria applied by National Center for Health Statistics at the Centers for Disease Control and Prevention. Because of these important observations, SCD cannot be assumed to represent arrhythmic deaths. SCD rates are likely to vary substantially, particularly when clinical information and autopsy data are limited or absent, as generally encountered in public health surveillance statistics.

Despite these limitations, a broad definition of SCD as a death occurring out of hospital, in the emergency room, or dead on arrival remains useful. It provides a reasonable estimate of SCD in the population (10–12) and is appropriate for compiling public health statistics and population-based genomic studies.

MOLECULAR DETERMINANTS OF ELECTRICAL PROPERTIES

Impulse formation and propagation in the heart are determined by the electrical characteristics of the cardiac cell membrane, cellular ion regulation, and the structural characteristics of the individual cells and tissues (see review, 13). The electrical properties of the sarcolemmal membrane are mainly determined by the specialized transmembrane proteins that carry current, transport ions, transduce mechanical stress, and respond to oxidative stress, extracellular and intracellular signaling molecules, and the energetic state. A schematic model of the relation

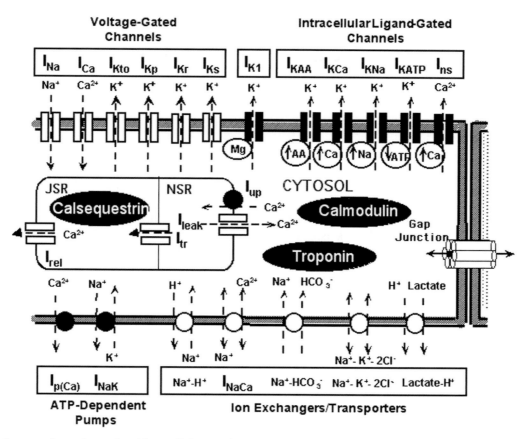

Fig. 1. Schematic diagram of sarcolemmal and intracellular membrane channels, pumps, and exchangers generating the action potential and determining the electrophysiologic properties of excitable cardiac cells. The sarcolemmal proteins are separated into four distinct groups: voltage-gated channels, intracellular ligand-gated channels, ATP-dependent pumps, and ion exchangers or transporters. The ligands that alter the conductance of the outward K+ currents are shown in the circles adjacent to the channel. These include Mg^{2+}, arachidonic acid (AA), Na^+ ATP and Ca. The sarcoplasmic reticulum contains an ATP-dependent Ca^{2+}-pump and the Ca^{2+}–release channels. Intracellular interaction occurs through aqueous pores formed by gap junctions. I_{Na} = fast Na current; $I_{Ca(L)}$ = Ca current through L-type Ca channels; I_{Kto} = transient outward K current; I_{Kp} = plateau K current, I_{Kr} = fast component of the delayed rectifier K current; I_{Ks} = slow component of the delayed rectifier K current; I_{K1} = inward rectifier K current; I_{KAA} = arachidonic acid activated K current, I_{KCa} = calcium activated K current, I_{KNa} = sodium activated K current, I_{KATP} = ATP sensitive K current; I_{NS} = nonspecific repolarizing current; $I_{p(Ca)}$ = Ca pump in the sarcolemma; I_{NaK} = Na–K pump current; Na^+-H^+ = sodium–hydrogen exchanger; I_{NaCa} = Na-Ca exchange current; Na^+-HCO_3^- = sodium–bicarbonate co-transporter; Na^+–K^+–$2Cl^-$ = sodium–potassium–chloride co-transporter; Lactate-H^+ = monocarboxylic acid monotransporter. In the sarcoplasmic reticulum, calcium uptake and release are regulated by specialized channel proteins. I_{up} = Ca uptake for the myoplasm to network sarcoplasmic reticulum (NSR); I_{rel} = Ca release from junctional sarcoplasmic reticulum (JSR); I_{leak} = Ca leakage from NSR to myoplasm; I_{tr} = Ca translocation from NSR to JSR. Calmodulin, troponin and calsequestrin are Ca buffers.

between these membrane channels and exchangers is shown in (Fig. 1) *(14)*. Excitatory currents carried by the voltage-dependent Na^+ and L-type Ca^{2+} channels and transferred between cells through gap junctions determine the speed of impulse propagation, whereas the type and distribution of a large and diverse family of K^+ channels and Cl^- channels determine the time course of repolarization and refractoriness.

In general, the transmembrane currents result in a time-dependent change in the transmembrane voltage, i.e., the action potential. Intracellular Ca^{2+} loading occurs during the action potential causing the Ca^{2+}-induced Ca^{2+} release from the sarcoplasmic reticulum (SR) via an interaction with the cardiac ryanodine receptor (RyR2), culminating in the activation of the contractile apparatus. Yet, the action potential characteristics for a given type of cardiac tissue are determined by the patterns of gene and protein expression unique to the heart's specialized tissues. The diversity of channels and their unique biophysical properties impart the particular electrical properties of the sinus node, atrium, atrioventricular (AV) node, specialized conduction system, and the ventricular myocardium.

This concept has been illustrated in the canine heart *(15)* in a study that attributed the molecular basis for marked differences in action potential characteristics between different cardiac tissues to the differences in the expression of genes encoding ionic channels and their respective proteins. In comparison to ventricular myocytes, Purkinje fibers demonstrate spontaneous depolarization, a prominent transient outward current, and a longer action potential. HCN genes are believed to encode subunits that determine the nonselective cation current, α_2, and contribute to spontaneous depolarization and pacemaker activity. Consistent with the presence of automaticity in Purkinje fibers and its absence in ventricular muscles, mRNA expression for HCN4 and the corresponding proteins for HCH2 and HCN4 was greater in Purkinje fibers *(15)*. The transient outward K^+ current, IK_{to}, is increased in Purkinje cells compared with ventricular myoctyes and results in a prominent notch immediately after the action potential upstroke. The K channel protein subunits Kv1.4 and Kv4.2 determine IK_{to}. Although Kv1.4 and Kv4.2 were expressed to the same extent in Purkinje fibers and ventricular muscle, decreased expression of KChIP2, a K channel accessory protein that accelerates the reactivation of I_{to} in Purkinje fibers, might account for the differences in Purkinje fibers relative to ventricular muscle *(15)*. Decreased IK_r and IK_s lengthen the action potential of Purkinje fibers when compared with ventricular muscle. As anticipated, expression of the channel subunits responsible for IK_r and IK_s, ERG, KvLQT1, and minK was decreased in the Purkinje fiber relative to ventricular muscle.

Action potential characteristics vary among heart regions. Such regional differences are also determined by the spatial heterogeneity of the expression of specific channel proteins. Because the expression of these proteins is a dynamic process with a relatively short time constant, environmental stresses or disease is likely to modify gene expression, contributing to differences in channel type, number, and density—a concept known as electrical remodeling.

Molecular Determinants of Conduction

Normal electrical impulses of the myocardium, driven by inward Na^+ current, propagate rapidly along the cardiac cell and across gap junctions, activating the adjacent cell. Because cells are more tightly coupled by gap junctions at the terminal ends of the adjoining cells relative to their lateral connections, the speed of conduction is faster along the long axis of the fibers than in the transverse direction; impulse propagation is anisotropic. The intercellular conduction delay imposed by the higher electrical resistance of the gap junction is not perceptible at the macroscopic scale of the tissue, so propagation appears continuous. By contrast, under pathological conditions of structural alterations or modulation of gap junctional conductance, cell-to-cell electrical coupling decreases the delay in action potential transfer between neighboring cells and discontinuous conduction increases. As the delay between cell-to-cell propagation increases, the rapidly inactivating Na^+ current no longer contributes sufficient excitatory current. Under these conditions, inward Ca^{2+} current maintains conduction, but at a reduced speed. The slow inward current can be maintained by extending the duration of the action potential plateau by drugs or by channelopathies, i.e., mutations of the genes encoding membrane channels prolonging repolarization.

Mechanisms of Arrhythmia

Life-threatening ventricular arrhythmias occur secondary to abnormal automaticity or reentrant circuits. Abnormal automaticity is usually ascribed to triggered activity characterized by spontaneous beats, originating either during the action potential plateau or during the terminal phase of repolarization. Spontaneous activity during the plateau is referred to as early after-depolarizations (EADs) and is related to reactivation of inward currents during the action potential. Spontaneous activity occurring during or soon after the terminal part of repolarization is called delayed after-depolarizations (DADs) and is thought to relate to cellular Ca^{2+} overload and spontaneous Ca^{2+} release from the SR.

Reentrant arrhythmias require two functional conducting pathways with transient unidirectional block in one of those pathways. Such reentrant pathways are known to exist on different spatial scales, including the whole heart, localized tissue, or groups of cells. Spach *(16)* summarized the factors determining the electrical substrate accounting for these different types of reentry in myocardium. Reentry is predicted to occur consequent to alterations of membrane current kinetics, resistive discontinuities, or the geometry of the propagating wavefront. Changes in inward ionic currents, pumps, and exchangers can contribute to slowing of impulse propagation on the microscopic scale or between different regions of the heart. Discontinuities in impulse propagation can also occur on the cellular scale secondary to gap junctional properties and tissue structure. Finally, the curvature of the excitatory wavefront may also contribute to the characteristics of the reentrant circuit and the development of spiral waves in two dimensions or scroll waves in three dimensions. Thus, it is conceivable that genetically determined changes in channel proteins will alter membrane current kinetics, resistive discontinuities,

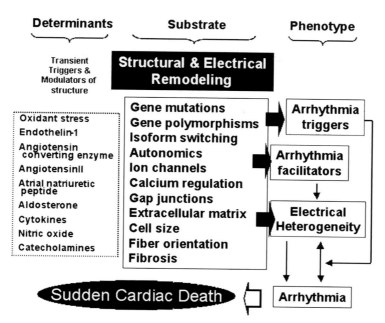

Fig. 2. Genetic and environmental conditions. Intrinsic biological stressors induce structural and electrical remodeling of cardiac tissue via numerous cellular mechanisms. Changes in the heterogeneity of channel density, distribution and biophysical properties as well as changes in the structural characteristics of the cardiac tissue create an electrophysiological substrate that supports the triggering and facilitation of arrhythmia. Sustained arrhythmia decreasing blood pressure with attendant impairment of heart and brain perfusion can be rapidly fatal.

or the geometry of the propagating wavefront, thereby increasing the likelihood of arrhythmia formation—a concept further developed in (Fig. 2).

Genetic factors and environmental conditions interact to increase the risk of arrhythmia. These factors lead to structural, electrical, and neurohumoral remodeling of the excitable tissue. Arrhythmia can result from changes in the electrophysiological tissue properties, which occur in association with disease processes that remodel the distribution, density, and function of channels or the tissue's architecture. Alternatively, inherited or spontaneous mutations of cardiac channels can lead directly to an increased risk of serious ventricular arrhythmia and SCD.

Remodeling affects electrical properties by changing numerous membrane proteins. For example in response to chronically elevated heart rates, I_{to} and I_{K1} decrease, resulting in a prolongation of the action potential consistent with decreased outward currents (17). Analogously, slow heart rhythms can contribute to remodeling of the heart. Complete AV block in the rabbit heart results in a prolonged QT interval, left ventricular hypertrophy (LVH), and polymorphic ventricular tachycardia (PVT). The ionic mechanism of these changes relates to a decrease in the delayed rectifier K^+ currents, IK_r and IK_s, an increase in IK_1, and a shift of the activation curve of the L-type Ca^+ channel in the

negative direction (18). Because impulse propagation requires the efficient transfer of excitatory current between cells involving gap junctions and their constituent protein connexins, current flow through gap junctions modulates the speed and microscopic continuity of conduction. As described previously, decreased current flow secondary to a decreased number or conductance of gap junctions slows conduction and increases the discontinuity of microscopic conduction on the cellular scale. Decreased expression of connexins in failing heart is believed to contribute to abnormal conduction (19).

The general molecular components responsible for abnormal heart rhythms are shown in Table 1. As outlined by Marban (20), mechanisms underlying rhythm disorders can be classified on the scale of groups of myocytes or as the result of interactions of the excitatory currents, cell-to-cell electrical coupling, and the network properties of the tissue. The scheme presented in Table 1 aids in conceptualizing the mechanisms responsible for syndromes associated with SCD that result from hereditary or acquired functional changes in a single protein.

(Table 1) represents a simplified approach to a description of potential mechanisms accounting for arrhythmias that cause SCD. It emphasizes the concept that arrhythmias generally originate within a complex and spatially heterogeneous cellular network that integrates changes in

Table 1
Cellular and Molecular Mechanisms of Arrhythmia

Scale of integration	Site of molecular target	Proposed arrhythmic mechanism	Clinical or experimental arrhythmias	Relevant disease associations
Myocyte Level				
Impulse initiation	Pacemaker current T-type Ca^{2+} channels	Suppression or acceleration of the physiologic pacemaker	Sinus tachycardia or sinus bradycardia	
	Not known	Abnormal automaticity	Ectopic atrial tachycardia	
	Na$^+$–Ca^{2+} exchange Ca$^+$-activated Cl$^-$ channel Ca$^+$-activated nonspecific cation channel	Triggered diastolic activity (DADs)	VT	Digoxin toxicity Reperfusion arrhythmias?
Excitation	Na$^+$ channels ATP-sensitive channels	Conduction slowing or block in atria or ventricles	Heart block VT VF	Ischemic arrhythmias with slow conduction resulting from interstitial K$^+$ accumulation
	L-type Ca^{2+} channels	Conduction or conduction block in the AV node	Heart block	Iatrogenic caused by Ca^{2+} channel blockers
Repolarization	Voltage-dependent K$^+$ channels L-type calcium channels Na–Ca exchange RyR2 receptors	Action potential prolongation EADs EADs	Torsades de pointe Polymorphic VT Polymorphic VT	Congenital LQT Drug-induced LQT Reperfusion arrhythmias?
Multicellular Level				
Cell-cell coupling	Connexins	Conduction delay or block caused by cellular uncoupling	VT and VF AF (?)	LVH, myocardial ischemia Atrial disease, ARVD
Tissue properties	Extracellular matrix proteins	Reentry Impedance mismatch Discontinuous conduction	Monomorphic VT around an infarct AV reciprocating tachycardia	LVH, Healed infarction Inherited: WPW syndrome

DAD, delayed afterdepolarization; ATP, adenosine triphosphate; AV, atrioventricular; ARVD, arrhythmogenic right ventricular dysplasia; EAD, early afterdepolarizaton; LVH, left ventricular hypertrophy; RyR2, cardiac ryanodine receptor channels; VF, ventricular fibrillation; VT, ventricular tachycardia. Modified from Marban *(20)*.

gene expression, ion channel, ion exchanger function, and cell-to-cell electrical coupling occurring in response to comorbid conditions, e.g., hypertension, diabetes, ischemia, healed infarction, hypertrophy, cardiomyopathy, and heart failure.

Mathematical Models and Molecular Mechanisms of Arrhythmia

Mathematical models of biological systems and computer simulations are useful for exploring the interrelations of cellular properties determining physiological characteristics over a broad range of spatial scales, i.e., the biological membranes, the whole cell, a tissue, or the heart. In particular, mathematical models having the unique biophysical properties associated with particular mutant channel proteins can now be use to study the relation between a specific genetic defect and the resultant cellular phenotype. Such models provide insight into the mechanism of arrhythmia and possibly SCD associated with particular genotypes.

Changes in the properties of such membrane-bound proteins or their associated proteins caused by gene mutations result in differences in excitability and impulse propagation, and consequently increase or decrease the likelihood of arrhythmia. Chapter 21 provides the details of the molecular causes of arrhythmias mediated by channelopathies. A mathematical model of the long QT3 (LQT3) syndrome incorporating a mutation of the SCN5A gene encoding the α-subunit of the Na^+ channel illustrates the usefulness of mathematical modeling and computer simulations to elucidate possible cellular mechanisms of arrhythmia. Clancy and Rudy (21) modeled the most severe from the LQT3 syndrome—the ΔKPQ mutation, a three-amino acid deletion of lysine 1505, proline 1506, and glutamine 1507. The absence of these amino acids in the II–IV linker decreases the rate of fast inactivation of the Na^+ current, leading to lengthening of the action potential, the prolongation of the QT interval on the surface electrocardiogram, and an increased risk for SCD secondary to PVT.

Previously Luo and Rudy (22) developed a mathematical model of the cardiac action potential incorporating numerous membrane channels, pumps, and exchangers that simulate action potential generation and propagation. In it, the excitatory Na^+ current is modeled by equations having variables scaled by values measured in physiological experiments. In order to study the role of a specific gene mutation, i.e., the ΔKPQ mutation, the biophysical properties were modified and include a burst mode and background mode of operation (21). With this modification, the Na^+ current characteristics of the model correlated closely to currents measured directly in cardiac cells expressing the SCN5A mutant. As shown in (Fig. 3), the ΔKPQ mutant was associated with a persistent inward Na^+ current that lengthened the action potential at fast rates and generated EADs at slower rates. The lower panels of Fig. 3 show that the incidence of EADs was enhanced by an increased proportion of the mutant channel, documenting the EAD as a potential source of premature beats in this syndrome (21).

As the computational capabilities of the computer increase, the complexity of mathematical models will likewise increase, yielding more realistic representations

of the complex interaction of the electrical and structural properties of the heart. Such mathematical models and computer simulations will be useful for testing hypotheses related to the role of specific gene mutations and the attendant changes in protein structure, biophysical properties for modifying membrane excitability, impulse propagation, triggered activity, and reentry in heart.

Risk Factors Associated with Sudden Cardiac Death and the Development of the Conditional Substrate for Sudden Cardiac Death

Acute and chronic ischemic heart disease are the greatest contributors to SCD (Table 2) (9). Other important conditions include primary electrophysiological abnormalities, hypertensive heart disease, cardiomyopathy, valvular heart disease, and congenital heart disease. These conditions are modified by other factors such as age, gender, race, autonomic modulation, and physical activity.

VENTRICULAR HYPERTROPHY

Left ventricular mass is induced by age, obesity, hypertension, and diabetes and is predictive of cardiovascular morbidity and mortality (23). The presence of left ventricular hypertrophy (LVH), whether identified by electrocardiographic criteria (23–25) or echocardiographic criteria (26,27), increases the risk for adverse cardiovascular events. Many studies have confirmed these early observations and further linked LVH to cardiovascular mortality. Haider and colleagues (28) showed a strong association between the presence of LVH and SCD in a general adult population. By using the Framingham Offspring Study database, the study enrolled 5124 men and women who were offspring or spouses of offspring from the original Framingham Heart study subjects. M-mode echochardiography determined LV dimensions and parameters of LVH. A group of 1634 men and 2027 women were monitored for an average of 10 years. The unadjusted hazard ratio for the presence of LVH was 2.16 after adjustment for age, gender, and the usual risk factors associated with adverse cardiovascular events. The effect of LVH was greater in men: the hazard ratio was 2.89 after adjustment for age and other risk factors.

LVH is associated with changes in cellular metabolism, energy utilization, and electrical remodeling modifying mechanical and electrical properties. Hypertrophic myocardium is associated with changes in channel function, the density and distribution of channel proteins, and cellular architecture affecting electrophysiological properties, in particular the changes in channel function in the L-type Ca^{2+} channel, Na^+/Ca^{2+} exchanger, RyR2, K^+ channels, and gap junctions, which give rise

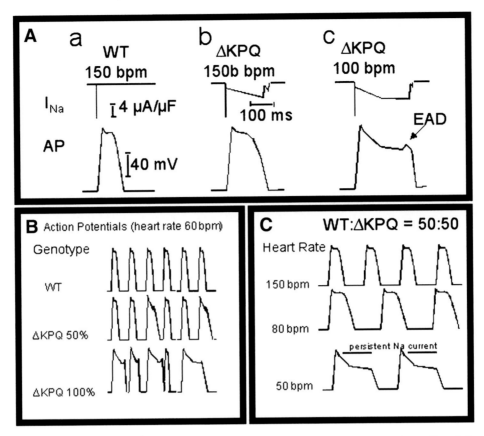

Fig. 3. Effect of the sodium channel ΔKPQ mutation on the action potential contour of the cardiac cell and the development of early after-depolarizations (EADs). **(A)** Persistent sodium current (I_{Na}) (upper panel) prolongs the action potential duration (compare to WT in a). These mathematically modeled and computer simulated currents closely resemble those measured experimentally in ref. *230*. Slowing the rate (b and c) results in APD prolongation (b) and EAD development at a heart rate of 100 bpm in c. **(B)** At a fixed heart rate of 60 bpm EADs form when the WT: ΔKPQ channel stoichiometry within a single cell increases to 50%. **(C)** Effect of pacing cycle length of EAD development. The mutant channel population contained 50% of the ΔKPQ cells. As the heart rate slows, persistent inward sodium current prolongs the action potential duration.

to membrane depolarization, action potential prolongation, conduction slowing, dispersion of refractoriness, and EADs.

Electrical remodeling accompanying LVH increases the risk of ventricular arrhythmia in the setting of myocardial ischemia *(29)*, antiarrhythmic drugs *(30)*, serum ion abnormalities and, possibly, with autonomic imbalance. Using a canine model of LVH, Kozhevnikov et al. *(31)* showed that transmural dispersion of refractoriness was increased by LVH and increased the susceptibility to PVT in the presence of a class III antiarrhythmic drug. Increased dispersion of refractoriness, suggested by an increased dispersion of the QT interval is increased among individuals who have hypertension and arrhythmias when compared with individuals without arrhythmias *(32)*.

The susceptibility of hypertrophied ventricular myocardium to electrical instability and VF is not a feature shared by all hypertrophic myocardium. The hearts of highly trained athletes undergo remodeling in response to the stresses of their training, producing both eccentric and concentric hypertrophy *(33)*. Such remodeling gives rise to increased voltage and a strain pattern on the ECG and may explain the higher prevalence of ventricular ectopy identified among trained athletes who have exercise-induced increases in LV mass *(34)*. The possible benign nature of this increase in LV mass and ectopy in this population is supported by the observation that even frequent and complex ventricular arrhythmias do not confer an increased long-term risk for SCD in athletes *(35)*. Genetic factors such as a polymorphism of the angiotensinogen gene (M235T) may determine ventricular remodeling in athletes *(36)*.

INFLAMMATION

Inflammation is thought to have a role in the initiation and progression of atherosclerosis *(37)*, plaque rupture

Table 2
Distribution of Underlying Cause of Death Among Sudden Cardiac Death Decedents Aged ≥35 yr According to Age Group:
United States, 1998

Type of Cardiac Disease	35–64 yr (n = 78,356)	≥ 65 yr (n = 377,720)	Total (n = 456,076)
	%	%	%
Acute ischemic heart disease	32.9	25.7	26.9
Chronic ischemic heart disease	26.0	37.2	35.3
Cardiovascular disease, unspecified	14.3	11.7	12.1
Cardiomyopathy and dysrhythmias	11.6	8.8	9.3
Hypertensive heart diseases	7.7	4.6	5.1
Heart failure	2.0	7.7	6.7
All others	5.5	4.3	4.6

Modified from Zheng et al. (9).

(38), and thrombosis (39). Consequently, it follows that plasma markers of inflammation such as C-reactive protein (CRP) and interleukin 6 predict cardiovascular events (40) and stroke (41,42). One study has further defined the role of inflammation on cardiovascular events and specifically identified an association between CRP and the risk for SCD (43). Yet, the mechanism is not known.

CRP is elevated in individuals with atrial arrhythmias (44), suggesting that inflammation is probably involved in the structural and electrical remodeling process. As a paradigm of the host's response to extrinsic factors, it is consistent with the concept outlined for the development of the substrate for electrical instability. Genetic polymorphisms of proinflammatory genes or their receptors might affect the cellular response to inflammation and modify electrical and structural remodeling of myocardium. Whether inflammation and cytokines directly remodel the electrical properties of the ventricular myocardium is not known.

DISEASES ASSOCIATED WITH SUDDEN CARDIAC DEATH

Primary Electrophysiologic Abnormalities (Channelopathies)

Primary electrical abnormalities secondary to mutations of cardiac proteins involved in excitation, repolarization, and intracellular Ca^{2+} regulation are related to a variety of congenital and acquired ventricular arrhythmias that are associated with SCD. These clinical syndromes and their underlying genetic basis are provided in Chapters 20 and 21 and in several reviews (14,45). (Table 3) shows an abbreviated brief list of established mutations accounting for arrhythmias and SCD.

SODIUM CHANNELS

Mutations of SCN5A gene encoding for the voltage-gated Na^+ channel produce clinical phenotypes that include LQT3, Brugada syndrome, and conduction defects including heart block (46,47). In general, mutations of the SCN5A gene produce a biophysical phenotype consistent with the clinical syndrome. Alternatively, mutations of an associated gene may result in an accessory protein that modifies the biophysical properties of a normal voltage-gated channel such that the resultant properties produce disease. Chauhan and colleagues (48) characterized such an interaction in the biophysical properties of Na^+ channels in a mouse lacking ankyrin$_B$. In the absence of ankyrin$_B$, the Na^+ current density was decreased, although inward current persisted due to slower inactivation, longer opening times, and late-openings of the channel, resulting in a longer time to repolarization. Interestingly, the genes for ankyrin$_B$ and the unknown gene responsible for LQT syndrome 4 (LQT4) are both located on chromosome 4 in humans. Based on this coincidence, it is speculated that LQT4 is related to an abnormality of ankyrin$_B$, i.e., a cytoskeleton mutation modifying the biophysical properties of the Na^+ channel.

CARDIAC RYANODINE RECEPTOR GENE

The RyR2 channel is a large protein in the SR that couples excitation to contraction through the release of Ca^{2+} from the SR stimulated by the L-type Ca current, i.e., Ca^{2+} induce Ca^{2+} release. Mutations of the RyR2 gene and calsequestrin 2 are associated with catecholaminergic polymorphic ventricular tachycardia (CPVT), whereas mutations of the RyR2 gene are associated with familial polymorphic ventricular tachycardia (FPVT) and arrhythmogenic ventricular dysplasia type 2 (ARVD2).

Table 3
Genetic Basis of Channelopathies

Disease	Gene [alternate name]	Protein	Mechanisms
LQTS			
Autosomal dominant	SCN5A	IN$_a$ channel α subunit	Repolarization
	HERG [KCNH2]	IK$_r$ channel α subunit	Repolarization
	KvLQT1 [KCNQ1]	IK$_s$ channel α subunit	Repolarization
	minK [KCNE1]	IK$_s$ channel α subunit	Repolarization
LQTS			
Autosomal recessive	KvLQT1 [KCNQ1]	IK$_s$ channel α subunit	Repolarization
	minK [KCNE1]	IK$_s$ channel β subunit	Repolarization
Drug-induced	MiRP1 [KCNE2]	IK$_r$ channel β subunit	Repolarization
FPVT			
Autosomal dominant	SCN5A	IN$_a$ channel α subunit	Repolarization
CPVT			
Autosomal dominant	RyR2	Ryanodine receptor	Ca^{2+} overload
Autosomal dominant(?)	CASQ2	Calsequestrin 2	Ca^{2+} overload
Autosomal recessive	CASQ2	Calsequestrin 2	Ca^{2+} overload

FPVT, familial polymorphic ventricular tachycardia; CPVT, catechecholaminergic polymorphic ventricular tachycardia; LQTS, long QT syndrome.

Molecular studies of the clinical syndrome CPVT (49,50) indicate that it is linked to chromosome 1q42-q43 (51). Priori et al. (52) reported a mutation of the gene coding for the human RyR2 (hRyR2) among 12 individuals having this syndrome. The hRyR2 mutation, which probably accounts for CPVT because RyR2 maps to chromosome 1q42-q43, occurred de novo in three of the four probans and was found in four affected family members and in none of three unaffected family members of the fourth proband. The mutations were not found in any of the control subjects. The hRyR2 mutations consisted of four different single nucleotide substitutions causing missense mutations, i.e., nonconservative amino acid changes. In one family, the Leu was substituted for serine at position 2246 (exon 44). In another proband, serine was substituted for arginine at position 2474 (exon 49). In another, lysine was substituted for asparagine at position 4104 (exon 90), and cystine was substituted for arginine at position 4497 (exon 93) (52). The CPVT phenotype was also identified in an inbred Bedouin tribe in Israel (53). This autosomal recessive condition was linked to chromosome 1p13-21, although the specific mutated gene was not identified.

FPVT is an autosomal-dominant inherited disorder characterized by biventricular tachycardia, PVT, syncope, and SCD in the young triggered by adrenergic stimulation in a structurally normal heart (54). The genetic basis of FPVT in a Finnish family was determined to be caused by a mutation of the RyR2 gene on chromosome 1q42-q43 (55). In affected individuals from three of the families, three different missense mutations of the RyR2 gene were identified. These include P2328S as part of the amino-terminal domain, whereas the other two mutations, Q4201R and V4653F, are part of the transmembrane segment of the carboxy-terminal region (55). These three mutations were not identified in 100 control subjects or any of the unaffected family members.

Mechanistically, a mutation of the RyR2 receptor is likely to contribute to cellular Ca^{2+} overload and gives rise to arrhythmias triggered by abnormal automaticity such as EADs. Circumstantial evidence linking cellular Ca^{2+} overload and the VT associated with RyR2 receptor mutations relates to the observation of biventricular tachycardia also occurring with cellular Ca^{2+} overload caused by digitalis glycoside toxicity.

Hyperphosphorylation of RyR2 has been implicated in the formation of arrhythmia in cardiomyopathy and heart failure (56) that may affect the diastolic release of Ca^{2+} giving rise to after depolarizations (57). The mechanism underlying the increased risk of catacholamine-induced VT was studied in a mouse model in which a mutation R4496C is present in the RyR2 (58). The mouse mutation increased the basal RyR2 channel activity, and showed frequent spontaneous Ca^{2+} oscillations when expressed in a mammalian cell line.

Marks *(59,60)* has suggested that the sympathetic nervous system activates the β-adrenergic signaling pathway, resulting in the hyperphosphorylation of the RyR2 that is more sensitive to protein kinase A (PKA) phosphorylation due to the structural change induced by the mutation RyR2. A similar mechanism of arrhythmia is suggested in failing ventricles where PKA phosphorylation of RyR2 is thought to dissociate the FK binding protein 12.6, causing a Ca^{2+} leak, augmenting Na^+/Ca^{2+} exchange currents, and triggering ventricular arrhythmias *(60)*. In this way, the molecular pathophysiology of SCD among individuals with CPVT may be the same as that associated with congestive heart failure. The changes in the biophysical properties of the ryanodine receptor caused by mutations to RyR2 are not known.

ARRHYTHMOGENIC RIGHT VENTRICULAR CARDIOMYOPATHY/DYSPLASIA

The arrhythmogenic right ventricular cardiomyopathy or dysplasia (ARVC/D) was described in 1977 and referred to as "arrhythmogenic right ventricular dysplasia" *(61)*. ARVC/D is a primary myocardial disease defined by the World Health Organization as a progressive fibrofatty replacement of right ventricular myocardium *(62,63)*. The fibrofatty infiltration begins as focal or regional areas in the RV and then progresses to include much of the RV and eventually some part of the LV, while sparing the septum. These pathological changes result in severe dilation and decreased RV ejection fraction, localized RV aneurysms, left bundle branch block, and ventricular arrhythmias, and can result in SCD *(64)*, although the disease can be mild or without symptoms *(65)*.

Autosomal-dominant *(66–71)* and autosomal-recessive forms of ARVC/D are described. The autosomal-dominant form of the disease is localized to chromosomes 1 (1q42-q43) *(67)*, 2 (2q32.1-q32.2) *(68)*, 3 (3p23) *(70)*, 10 (10p12-p14) *(71)*, and 14 (14q23-q24 [66], and 14q12-q22) *(69)*. The gene coding for plakoglobin has been implicated in the origins of the autosomal-recessive condition associated with palmoplantar keratodema, known as Naxos disease *(64,72)*. The loss of plakoglobin, a protein involved in cell-to-cell coupling, is thought to contribute to apoptotic cell death and fatty infiltration and fibrosis. Alternatively, mutations of the cardiac ryanodine receptor gene are associated with ARVC/D type 2 *(73)*. In addition to apoptotic cell death, other proposed mechanisms for ARVC/D development include infection or inflammation possibly due to a viral pathogen, a degenerative process similar to muscular dystrophy or the transdifferentiation of myocytes into adipose cells. A

specific subgroup of ARVC/D, ARVD2, maps to chromosome 1q42-q43 and has similarities to FPVT.

Sudden Infant Death Syndrome

Sudden infant death syndrome (SIDS) occurs in approx 1 in 500 infants *(74)*, and is likely to have multiple mechanisms, including abnormalities of the cardiorespiratory system, the central nervous system, primary electrical abnormalities, and inborn errors in metabolism. The possibility that SIDS may relate to a genetic disorder of repolarization has been considered for more than 30 years. Molecular screening is now providing new insights into the causes of SIDS. In 1976, Maron et al. *(75)* identified an increased prevalence of prolonged QT interval among the parents of infants that died of SIDS. Some infants do appear to have abnormal repolarization as indicated by a prolonged QT interval *(75–77)*. The link between abnormal repolarization and SIDS was strengthened by the observation in 1998 that infants having a heart rate–corrected QT interval >440 ms measured in the first week of life had a 41-fold increased risk of SIDS *(78)*. Moreover, these investigators found a prolonged QT interval in 50% of the infants dying of SIDS. A direct molecular link between spontaneous mutations of SCN5A in infants and PVT *(79)* and SIDS *(80)* is now established. However, the proportion of deaths that can be attributed to primary electrical abnormalities secondary to cardiac channel mutations is unknown. Ackerman and colleagues *(81)* used the term "molecular autopsy" to describe the postmortem diagnosis of channelopathies that might explain SCD. Thus, the ability to perform molecular autopsies on archived necropsy material undoubtedly will transform the forensic evaluation of SIDS when suitable tissue specimens are available.

Supraventricular Tachycardias

In one small series of patients, supraventricular arrhythmias accounted for about 5% of patients referred for electrophysiological evaluation after aborted SCD *(82)*. Accessory conduction was present in 46% of these patients, in association with either atrial fibrillation or atrioventricular nodal reentrant tachycardia. In each case, the rapid supraventricular tachycardia degenerated into VF. Alternatively, atrial fibrillation and atrioventricular nodal reentrant tachycardia with rapid ventricular response were sufficient to initiate VF.

Wolff–Parkinson–White Syndrome

Among patients with an accessory pathway linking the atria and ventricles, Wolff–Parkinson–White (WPW) syndrome is characterized by preexcitation of the ventricles and predisposition to reentrant atrioventricular reciprocating tachycardia, atrial fibrillation, and SCD. In the adult population, the incidence of SCD is about 3–4% among patients having symptoms of tachycardia (83,84). An autosomal-dominant inheritance pattern of disease transmission with incomplete penetrance has been suggested by Öhnell (85), Vidaillet et al. (86), and Gillette et al. (87). In most individuals with WPW syndrome, no other cardiac abnormalities are present, yet some have associated congenital heart disease such as Epstein's anomaly. In a subset of individuals Gollob et al. (88,89) reported the association of WPW with cardiac disease, namely atrial arrhythmias and conduction system disease associated with a mutation in the AMP-activated protein kinase γ-2 subunit (PRKAG2) gene in the presence and absence of ventricular hypertrophy.

In an Italian study (90), 3.6% of young people (<35 years of age) were found to have preexcitation prior to death. Of these cases, 40% were asymptomatic before dying suddenly. The remainder had experienced symptoms of presyncope and syncope. The finding of atrial myocarditis in some suggests that myocardial inflammation may be a trigger for SCD among children and young adults with WPW.

Atrial Fibrillation or Flutter with Rapid Atrioventricular Conduction

Atrial tachycardias such as atrial fibrillation or flutter with a rapid ventricular response are associated with increased rates of hospitalization and cardiovascular morbidity. Prolonged episodes of increased heart rate can lead to tachycardia-induced cardiomyopathy. In response to the rapid rate, the atrial and ventricular myocardium undergoes a remodeling process characterized by a change in the expression of membrane proteins (91).

Cell-to-cell coupling provides the syncytial properties of myocardium by adjacent myocytes via the gap junctional connexin protein. In atria.the predominant connexins are 43 (Cx43) and 40 (Cx40). The distribution, density, and their relative abundance contribute to the electrical properties of the tissue. Atrial tissue obtained at the time of cardiac surgery from humans with a history of atrial fibrillation showed 2.7-fold greater Cx40 expression than individuals in sinus rhythm. No differences were detected in Cx43, although the spatial distribution of both connexins was modified by atrial fibrillation (92). Increased expression of Cx40 has also been identified in individuals with postoperative atrial fibrillation (93). In an experimental animal model of atrial fibrillation in the goat, the time course of the remodeling of atrial cell-to-cell coupling mediated by the differential expression of connexins indicated that the remodeling of gap junctions in the fibrillating atrium con-

tributes to the stabilization of atrial fibrillation (94). The rate and activation sequence–induced change in the expression of connexins might serve as a model of electrical remodeling in heart that may result in other electrophysiological changes associated with other stresses.

The signaling mechanisms and the regulation of transcriptional factors underlying these changes in Cx43 expression are not known in fibrillating atria. Studies have shown that increased Wnt signaling resulted in increased Cx43 expression and enhanced cell-to-cell coupling (95).

Coronary Heart Disease
MYOCARDIAL ISCHEMIA

Coronary heart disease is the leading cause of death in the industrialized world (96). Acute coronary syndromes are most commonly caused by disruption of an atherosclerotic plaque or thrombosis resulting in ischemia, ventricular arrhythmia, and SCD (97,98). Ischemia-related SCD also occurs secondary to coronary artery spasm (99). In normal myocardium, ischemia can directly induce VF or PVT that degenerates into VF. Because CAD and ischemia play such important roles in the occurrence of SCD, it follows that the risk factors for SCD and CAD are the same.

The electrophysiological changes associated with ischemia and their relation to the induction of VF have been extensively reviewed (100–102). In acute ischemia, the onset of VF within the first 45 min. after coronary occlusion can be attributed to the heterogeneous metabolic, ionic, and neurogenic changes resulting from interrupted arterial inflow (103–105). Membrane depolarization and rate-dependent conduction slowing and block are characteristic of the myocardium at this time. The electrophysiological changes reflect the hydrolysis of high-energy phosphates, the development of intracellular acidosis, the efflux of K^+ from the intracellular to the extracellular space, and changes in intracellular Na^+ and Ca^{2+} concentrations occurring as a result of Na^+/K^+, Na^+/H^+ and Na^+/Ca^{2+} exchange mechanisms (101,106). The absence of venous washout leads to the accumulation of the end products of anaerobic metabolism, particularly protons, lactate, K^+, CO_2, adenosine, and lysophosphoglycerides in the interstitial and extracellular spaces of the ischemic myocardium. The production, diffusion, and accumulation of CO_2, K^+, and other metabolic products of anaerobic metabolism, lipolysis, and purine metabolism and the diffusion of O_2 determine the characteristics of the ischemic borderzone. In addition, heterogeneity exists within the ischemic zone itself, representing the normal transmyocardial differences in high-energy phosphate content and the different rates at which these high-energy phosphates are hydrolyzed during

Table 4
Adjusted RRs Associated with Sudden Death and Fatal Myocardial Infarction in the Paris Prospective Study I
by Multivariate Analysis

Variables	Sudden death		Fatal myocardial infarction	
	RR (95% CI)	p	RR (95% CI)	p
Body mass index	1.21 (1.03–1.87)	0.03	0.97 (0.84–1.14)	NS
Tobacco consumption	1.34 (1.11–1.51)	0.0001	1.25 (1.13–1.36)	0.0001
Diabetic status	2.21 (1.10–4.44)	0.02	1.18 (0.55–2.52)	NS
Heart rate	1.22 (1.12–1.49)	0.007	1.25 (1.11–1.35)	0.006
Systolic blood pressure	1.23 (1.02–1.46)	0.02	1.37 (1.19–1.56)	0.0001
Cholesterol	1.23 (1.13–1.72)	0.0001	1.18 (1.09–1.53)	0.009
Parental MI	1.16 (0.60–2.25)	NS	2.30 (1.47–3.60)	0.0003
Parental sudden death	1.80 (1.11–2.88)	0.01	0.85 (0.52–1.39)	NS

Tobacco consumption is the average consumption (g/d) in the 5 yr preceding the screening. Increased risk of an event for 1 SD increase in variables, including age (SD = 1.9 yrs), body mass index (SD = 3.3 kg/m^2), tobacco consumption (210.5 g/d), heart rate (SD = 10.2 bpm), systolic blood pressure (SD = 20 mm Hg), cholesterol (SD = 42 mg/dL), and triglycerides (SD = 112 mg/dL). Modified from Jouven et al. (2).

ischemia (107). Heterogeneity of these metabolites and ions across the ischemic borderzone contributes to heterogeneous changes in conduction and refractoriness that predispose to local reentry and ultimately VF (108).

The heterogeneous changes in ionic, metabolic, and electrical properties induced by ischemia are present in all ischemic hearts, yet only a minority of individuals experience SCD. Consequently, other unknown factors, possibly genetically determined, are likely to contribute. Epidemiological evidence of an undiscovered genetically determined factor or factors is suggested in two studies. A population-based case control study, designed to examine the relation between primary cardiac arrest and a family history of primary cardiac arrest or MI, identified a positive association between a family history of MI or primary cardiac arrest in a first-degree relative and primary cardiac arrest (3). Importantly, a positive family history was identified as an independent predictor of primary cardiac arrest and provided predictive value like diabetes, blood pressure, smoking, or physical activity. Yet, statistical analysis of the data indicated that the effect of the family history could not be explained on the basis of the familial patterns in other risk factors. This result implicates an additional inherited factor, as yet unknown, which imparted an additional risk.

The Paris Prospective Study I also examined the association between a parental history of SCD to SCD in a cohort of middle-aged men (2). In this study 7746 native French men, aged 43–52 years, entered a longitudinal study between 1967 and 1972 while employed by the Paris Civil Service. They were monitored for the occur-

rence of death until 1994. During the study period, 118 individuals died of SCD and 192 individuals had a fatal MI. Univariate statistical analysis showed that SCD and fatal MI were associated with factors typically ascribed to cardiac risk such as age, tobacco use, heart rate, blood pressure, and lipids. Interestingly, a positive parental history of MI was associated with fatal MI, whereas a positive parental history of SCD was associated with SCD. As shown in (Table 4), the relative risk for SCD for an individual with a positive parental history of SCD was 1.8 and ranged from 1.11 to 2.88 when a multivariate statistical method was applied. The relative risk for SCD increased impressively to 9.44 for individuals of which both parents had died of SCD.

A variety of genetic factors have been suggested, including interactions between genotypes at different loci and levels of apolipoprotein A-I and HDL-C. Such an interaction might occur between genes coding for apolipoprotein A-I and cholesteryl ester transfer protein (109). An association was identified between SAH, an acyl-CoA synthetase gene, and hypertriglyceridemia, obesity, and hypertension (110). Because of the strong association between coronary artery thrombosis, ischemia, and SCD, factors that contribute to plaque disruption and platelet aggregation are likely to be important in SCD. Alternatively, the DD polymorphism in the alpha$_{2B}$-adrenoceptor is associated with an increased risk for SCD during MI (111). Consequently, an understanding of the molecular processes that contribute to these properties of the endothelium, the plaque, platelets, and adrenergic receptor function may contribute directly to our understanding of SCD.

Table 5
Sources of Molecular Diversity in Acute Susceptibility

Mediators of infarction and ischemia
  Facilitators of atherosclerosis, plaque vulnerability, and rupture
  Activators of thrombosis, inhibition of fibrinolysis, coagulation and platelets
  Modulators of restenosis
  Modulators of endothelial function and vascular tone
Mediators of neural excitation
  Activation of central pathways
  Neural transmitters and peptides
  Autonomic balance and parasympathetic and adrenergic pathways
Mediators of membrane excitability and tissue conduction
  Determinants of cellular K loss during ischemia
  Intracellular ionic, metabolic and peptide modifiers
  Subunit permutations, channel and transporter interactions
  Redox and energetic metabolites
  Factors affecting coupling and cell-to-cell conduction

Modified from Spooner et al. *(117)*.

Molecular methods were shown to identify the differential expression of genes present in ruptured atherosclerotic plaques when compared with intact plaques *(112)*. Of 500 randomly chosen genes, 9% showed differential expression in ruptured plaques, when compared to those with intact plaques, utilizing gene microarray technology. Some of these clones were homologous to known genes; others did not relate to sequences of DNA coding for proteins with known function. Consequently, this study identified possible candidate genes that might modulate factors contributing to plaque instability.

One possible trigger for MI is increased platelet aggregation. The heritability of platelet aggregation may be evidenced by genotyping the *Pl*[A2] polymorphisms of the glycoprotein *IIIa* gene, and the Hind *III* β-148 polymorphism of the β-fibrinogen gene and relating the genotyping to measured platelet aggregability *(113)*.

The identification of eight patients who developed prolonged QT and a pause-dependent PVT during an evolving MI may prove important *(114)*. In this case-controlled study, these eight patients represented 1.8% of the screened individuals with acute MI. Because there was no history of long QT syndrome (LQTS), drug use associated with the syndrome, or family history of SCD, it is unlikely that these cases represent LQTS. However, this observation raises the possibility that these cases may represent occult "minor mutations" *(115)* and genetic polymorphism *(116)* that manifest under conditions that modify repolarizing currents, e.g., a healing infarction.

Specific genes are associated with MI and SCD. (Table 5) summarizes a variety of sources of molecular diversity for SCD in humans *(117)*. Future investigation is needed to better define the sources of this susceptibility.

PREVIOUS MYOCARDIAL INFARCTION AND CONGESTIVE HEART FAILURE

Individuals with a history of MI, particularly those with LV dysfunction, are at higher risk for SCD. These individuals have an altered electrophysiological substrate favoring the initiation and maintenance of arrhythmia. Many animal studies confirm the risk of spontaneous VF when ischemia is superimposed on a ventricle previously injured by infarction. This electrophysiological substrate is formed through remodeling of the heart's electrical properties.

The observation that use of angiotensin-converting enzyme (ACE) inhibitors and angiotensin receptor blockers increase survival and decrease the incidence of SCD in post-MI patients suggests that a more favorable remodeling process might contribute to improved electrical characteristics and improved survival. One such parameter of electrical remodeling is dispersion of ventricular repolarization as measured by the QT interval. Previous studies have identified increased QT dispersion as an independent risk factor for SCD after MI. Interestingly, the D-allele of the ACE polymorphism was related to increased QT dispersion in a group of patients following MI but not in healthy subjects *(118)*. This observation suggests an interaction between myocardial damage and genetic predisposition that both enhances the activity of the renin angiotensin system and increases the heterogeneity repolarization of the heart, thereby leading to an arrhythmogenic substrate. The observation that ACE inhibitors reduce QT dispersion may provide insight into the potential mechanism that accounts for the benefit of ACE inhibitors after infarction.

Interaction of chronic ventricular disease with superimposed ischemia contributes to the initiation of VT (119). Remodeled ventricular myocardium is more susceptible to VF when the ionic, metabolic, and energetic changes associated with ischemia are superimposed. However, the frequency with which the ischemia directly initiates a lethal arrhythmia in hearts with healed infarction remains controversial. In some individuals, revascularization of coronary lesions prevented subsequent arrhythmia, thereby supporting the hypothesis that ischemia generates VF in diseased ventricles (120). Yet, when all patients with previous infarction, documented spontaneous, and inducible sustained ventricular arrhythmias are considered, the majority remain inducible after revascularization; in one study, approx 30% had serious ventricular arrhythmias during the subsequent 33 mo (121). Therefore, based on the experience of Brugada and others (122), the role of ischemia appears to be limited as a trigger of ventricular arrhythmia in ventricles injured previously by ischemia. Instead, the underlying remodeled myocardium appears to be sufficient to initiate and support VT and VF.

Congestive heart failure is associated with an increased risk of arrhythmia and SCD. The increased risk of arrhythmia is associated with electrophysiological remodeling of the ventricle as determined by altered cellular architecture, Ca^{2+} regulation, ion exchangers and pumps, β-adrenergic signaling, and repolarization (123). In the postinfarction rat heart, voltage-gated K channel genes, Kv2.1, Kv4.2, and Kv4.3, are down-regulated, decreasing I_{to} and I_K and prolonging the action potential (124). Decreased I_{to} was measured in hypertrophied human hearts (125). In failing, heart cardiac cells have increased cell capacitance due to larger cell size and increased fibrosis. Cellular Ca^{2+} regulation is influenced by alternations in the L-type Ca^{2+} channel, increased Na^+-Ca^{2+} exchange, and decreased activity of the SR Ca^{2+} ATPase. Taken together these cellular ionic and electrical changes increase the likelihood of triggered activity secondary to EADs, DADs, and reentry.

Cardiomyopathy

DILATED CARDIOMYOPATHY

The genetic basis of the familial dilated cardiomyopathies (DCM) is presented in Chapter 15. In general,

morphological changes in the myocardium and fibrosis contribute substantially to the maintenance of VF in dilated cardiomyoapthy (126).

HYPERTROPHIC CARDIOMYOPATHY

Hypertrophic cardiomyopathy (HCM), the most common cause of SCD in young adults, is characterized by a nondilated, hypertrophic, and poorly compliant left ventricle (127). Primary and familial forms of HCM are prevalent and are caused by mutations of genes coding for contractile proteins, including β-cardiac myosin heavy chain, troponin T, α-tropomyosin, and cardiac myosin-binding protein C (128,129). The diversity of clinical phenotypes likely relates to the specific gene mutations. For example, more severe hypertrophy is encountered in protein truncation mutations of the myosin-binding protein C gene when compared with the clinical phenotype associated with missense mutations or in-frame deletions (130). However, the severity of the hypertrophy does not necessarily relate to prognosis, as certain mutations of the T-troponin (131) and α-tropomyosin (V95A) (132) genes have a mild cardiac phenotype but have a high risk for SCD.

An epidemiogical survey of a large cohort of individuals with HCM identified three principal modes of death: SCD, progressive heart failure, and stroke associated with atrial fibrillation (133). SCD occurred more commonly in the young, although it was observed throughout all age groups, and 20% of the deaths occurred after age 65. Importantly, 71% of those dying suddenly had minimal or no symptoms prior to death, and 16% of these deaths occurred in association with moderate to severe exertion (133), emphasizing the importance of accurate identification and risk assessment of individuals.

As in the case of DCM, the mechanism of the associated arrhythmia is likely to relate to the structural changes in the myocardium associated with cellular hypertrophy and fibrosis (134). Changes in cardiac electrophysiology include sinus and AV node dysfunction, abnormal His–Purkinje conduction, and atrial and ventricular tachycardia (135). Among individuals with HCM, the risk for SCD is increased by a history of nonsustained VT or syncope, a family history of SCD, or a hypotensive blood pressure response during exercise (136). LV wall thickness was associated with increased risk in one study (136) but not in another (137).

Troponin T mutations cause disarray of myocardial fibers and may confer a particularly high risk for SCD in the young (131), even though these hearts may have lower weights, less fibrosis, and more cellular disorganization than those of other individuals with HCM (138).

These mutations show a marked difference in the clinical phenotype vis-à-vis SCD when compared to HCM of the elderly *(139)*.

Familial HCM has been described in a Spanish American cohort associated with LV dysfunction, symptomatic bradycardia, and cardiac arrest *(132)*. Of the 26 family members reviewed, 11 (42%) experienced SCD. Physical activity was associated with the occurrence of four of these SCDs. Importantly, SCD occurred in two individuals with mild or no LVH. This condition is characterized by hypertrophy of the posterior basal wall, anterolateral free wall, the apex, or a combination of these areas without evidence of LV outflow tract obstruction *(132)*. Linkage analysis identified an association of this HCM with the α-tropomyosin (TPM1) gene. Subsequent sequencing and restriction digestion analysis showed that a TPM1 mutation V95A cosegregated with the HCM.

Differentially expressed genes in HCM have been studied to assess mutations underlying the physiological, metabolic, and anatomical consequences of HCM *(140)*. This study provided a unique view of the relationship between the response cardiac genes and found a commonality between the expression of markers of secondary hypertrophy associated with acquired forms of HCM. A number of genes were found to have increased expression; however, the genes encoding for channel protein subunits in the heart were not included in this study.

An understanding of the mechanisms underlying the increased susceptibility of hearts having certain sarcomeric gene mutations will likely be enhanced by the development of transgenic mice expressing mutant proteins. For example, a mouse heterozygote for an Arg403Gln missense mutation of the α-myosin heavy chain gene (α-MHC$^{403/+}$) *(141)* was notable for the development of HCM and electrophysiologic changes including prolonged repolarization and electrogram fractionation. These electrophysiological changes were associated with increased spontaneous and inducible ventricular arrhythmias and correlated reasonably well with the cardiac phenotype present in humans *(142)*.

MYOTONIC DYSTROPHY

Myotonic dystrophy is an autosomal-dominant neuromuscluar disease associated with myotonia and degeneration of skeletal muscle, cataract formation, gonadal atrophy, frontal baldness, and mental impairment. Associated conditions include cataracts, diabetes mellitus, and premature aging. Cardiac involvement includes the initiation of abnormal impulses and abnormalities of the conduction system and cardiac myotonia, causing decreased systolic and diastolic function *(143)*. Specific arrhythmias include sinus bradycardia, sick sinus syndrome, atrial tachycardia, atrial flutter, atrial fibrillation, and premature ventricular beats. Anecdotal reports of ventricular arrhythmia and SCD secondary to these electrical abnormalities *(144,145)* include a case of torsade de pointes VT associated with prolonged QT interval *(146)*. Autopsy findings included CAD, mitral valve prolapse, myocardial fibrosis and vacuolization, and focal fatty infiltration of the conduction system *(144,147)*.

The molecular basis for myotonic dystrophy appears to be related to the expansion of the CTG trinucleotide repeat in the 3′ untranslated region of a protein kinase gene *(148,149)*. In some individuals with myotonic dystrophy, the CTG trinucleotide repeat is amplified 3000 times and represents a marked increase compared to 5 to 37 times in normal individuals *(150)*. The expansion of the CTG trinucleotide repeat from generation to generation correlates to the disease severity, although there is no consensus regarding the relation between the amplification of the CTG trinucleotide repeat and cardiac involvement *(150,151)*.

Other muscular dystrophies with cardiac involvement and SCD include Duchenne's *(152)*, Becker's, X-linked Emery–Dreifuss *(153)*, and facioscapulohumeral muscular dystrophy *(154)*.

RISK FACTORS MODIFYING THE UNDERLYING DISEASE

Gender

SCD occurs more commonly in men than in women. The age-specific death rates are higher for men and increase with age *(9)*, and men are more likely to die of MI before hospitalization *(155)*. As shown in (Table 6), the ratio of age-specific death rates for men and women is approx 3 for individuals aged 35 to 65 years. After 65 years, the preponderance of deaths in men decreases and the ratio reaches unity after 85 years of age. Much of the excess SCD in men is likely related to gender-related differences in cardiac risk factors and coronary heart disease *(156)*. A protective effect of estrogen is suggested and may relate to enhanced tolerance to ischemia or electrophysiological changes induced by estrogen-induced activation of the myocardial ATP-sensitive K$^+$ channel and an attendant "preconditioning" effect. Preconditioning has been measured in patients undergoing balloon angioplasty following intracoronary administration of estrogen *(157)*. In addition, both Kir6.2 and SUR2A, the protein subunits forming the ATP-sensitive K$^+$ channel, are increased in female guinea pigs relative to males, thereby increasing the number of functional channels in females *(158)*.

Table 6
Number and Death Rates for Sudden Cardiac Death Among Adults Aged >35 yr by Gender and Racial Characteristics

Characteristic	Male		Female		Male/female age-specific death rate
	n	per 100,000	n	per 100,000	
Age-specific rate					
35–44 yr	7,533	34	2,584	11	3.0
45–54 yr	19,575	116	5,931	33	3.5
55–64 yr	30,680	284	12,006	101	2.8
65–74 yr	49,508	600	28,874	285	2.1
75–84 yr	64,863	1,363	66,727	928	1.5
≥85 yr	48,332	4,073	119,416	4,172	1.0
Age-adjusted rate[a]					
White	193,174	407	209,219	270	1.5
Black	23,780	503	23,762	336	1.5
American Indian/Alaska	801	259	600	153	1.7
Native Asian/Pacific Islander	2,736	213	1,957	130	1.6
Total US population (≥35 yr)	220,523	411	235,553	275	1.5
Hispanic	7,160	230	5,943	147	1.6
Non-Hispanic	212,409	419	228,770	280	1.5

[a]Standardized to the 2000 projected US population. Modified from Zheng et al. (9).

Treatment of heart-derived H9c2 cells with 17β-estradiol increases the Kir6.2 and SUR2A protein in the cell membrane and enhances tolerance to hypoxia-reoxygenation (159). During hypoxia-reoxygenation, 17β-estradiol slows the increase in intracellular Ca^{2+}. This effect is blocked by HMR 1098, an inhibitor of the sarcolemmal K_{ATP} channel, but not by 5-hydroxydecanoate, an inhibitor of the mitochondrial K_{ATP} channel, suggesting that the protective effect of 17β-estradiol is mediated by its effect on the sarcolemmal K_{ATP} channel. A reduction of cellular Ca^{2+} has also been measured in female rat hearts in response to a β-adrenergic stimulation, which is associated with a decreased risk of spontaneous arrhythmia (160). Taken together these data provide circumstantial evidence that estrogen-induced changes in the K_{ATP} channel might mediate the decreased risk in women.

The records of out-of-hospital cardiac arrest in Seattle and suburban King County from 1990–1998 were used to address the relationship between gender, rates of cardiac arrest, and survival (161). This large study found that rates of cardiac arrest in women were half that occurring in men. Yet, overall survival rates were lower for women than men. This paradox appears to be resolved by the fact that VF is a treatable rhythm and, consequently, prompt treatment of VF in men improves outcome. When the data are adjusted for VF, the survival rates for men and women are

equivalent, implying that the mechanism of cardiac arrest in women is more likely to produce pulseless electrical activity or asystole—conditions associated with a poorer prognosis. The cause of these differences is not known although a variety of hypotheses have been proposed related to effects of sex hormones on autonomic function, differences in sensitivity to ischemia, responses to defibrillation and social stresses.

During myocardial ischemia, increased sympathetic activity increases the risk for SCD whereas increased parasympathetic activity decreases that risk. Estrogen increases parasympathetic tone in the cardiovascular system and decreases circulating noradrenaline (162). For this reason, the decreased risk for SCD in females may relate to modulation of the autonomic nervous system (162). Baroreflex sensitivity (BRS) and heart rate variability (HRV) are useful to measure dynamic changes in autonomic function and autonomic tone, respectively. Women have increased heart rate dynamics and high frequency heart rate power when compared with men (163). Estrogen enhances BRS, whereas progesterone antagonizes the effect of estrogen, a phenomenon measurable during the menstrual cycle in young women (164). Postmenopausal women treated with estrogen have higher BRS and HRV (165,166). Although the effect of estrogen appears to be confined to the sympathetic arm of the BRS (164,167), the observation supports a mechanistic link between estrogen and an effect on the modulation of the autonomic nervous system.

The incidence of atrial fibrillation is twice higher in men than in women. The mechanism of this difference may relate to estrogen-induced remodeling of the atrium. Previous studies show that 17β-estradiol decreases the action potential duration *(168)*, a reponse that is possibly related to inhibition of the L-type Ca^{2+} current *(169)*. Tse et al. *(170)* showed that premenopausal women have shorter effective refractory periods and less rate-dependent shortening of the effective refractory period when compared with postmenopausal women or age-matched men.

An apparent contradictory observation is that women are at greater risk of drug-induced PVT *(171)*. Women have a greater heart rate–adjusted QT interval, i.e., the QTc is longer in women than in men. This difference emerges during puberty and appears to be related to sex hormones. The complications of membrane-active drugs appear to be linked to women's increased sensitivity to the drugs, resulting in greater prolongation of the corrected QT interval *(172)*. Despite the clinical importance of this observation, the responsible cellular or molecular mechanism remains unknown. The density of IK_r appears to be lower in the female rabbit ventricle *(173)*, a finding that would prolong ventricular repolarization. Interestingly, 5α-dihydrotestosterone lessened the sensitivity of female rabbits to drugs that block IK_r *(174)*, suggesting that testosterone lengthens the QT in female mice by increasing IK_r density, although the mechanism is unknown.

The influence of gender on drug-induced PVT in mice hearts exposed to halothane has been assessed *(175)*. The induced PVT lasted 14 times longer in female mice. Despite this dramatic functional difference in susceptibility to PVT, no differences were detected in measured electrophysiological properties, including heart rate, electrocardiographic intervals, action potential durations, dispersion of refractory periods, or conduction velocities. The only measured difference was a two- to threefold higher level of the message for KCNE1, the gene coding for the auxiliary K^+ channel subunits MinK contributing to IK_r.

Another example of gender-associated differences in SCD risk is the male predominance of the clinical phenotype of the Brugada syndrome (see Chapter 21). The SCN5A gene mutation causing the Brugada syndrome is autosomal dominant with low penetrence. Consequently, the SCN5A mutation is transmitted equally to males and females, yet the clinical phenotype is present 8–10 times more frequently in males *(176)*. The possible explanation was described in a canine model, where there was an enhanced transient outward K^+ current (IK_{to}) in the right

ventricles of male dogs compared with female dogs, providing insight into a possible mechanism underlying gender-related difference in disease expression *(177)*. In that study, the density and inactivation kinetics of IK_{to} differed, resulting in an increase in IK_{to} in the right ventricles of the male dogs. No gender-related differences were measured in IK_{to} in the left ventricle. The change in IK_{to} is likely related to a change in the expression of one of the channel protein subunits forming the IK_{to} channel. Data assessing the effect of sex hormones on the expression and function of cardiac voltage-gated K channels are limited. However, it is interesting that Kv4.3, a subunit forming the IK_{to} channel, in rats is down-regulated under the influence of estrogen *(178)*. Such an effect would explain the enhanced IK_{to} current and the enhanced notch on the action potential of the right ventricle of the male canine heart and the increased susceptibility to drugs that block Na^+ and Ca^{2+} currents. If such effects of estrogen occur in humans with the Brugada-type SCN5A mutation, it may explain the preponderance of males with the clinical phenotype.

Racial Differences

Rates of SCD are greater for blacks than for whites *(11,179–183)*. A retrospective case-control study sought to confirm previous observations of racial differences in SCD rates, to establish the age dependence of this phenomenon, and to define the mechanisms accounting for the disparity in death rates between African Americans and white Americans *(182)*. This involved the evaluation and analysis of autopsied cases at the Office of the Chief Medical Examiner of the State of Maryland. From 1994 through 1999, hearts from 1025 cases were selected for further analysis. Of these, 457 met the definition of SCD, and the remainder (568 cases) were non-sudden deaths and served as the control group. The control group consisted of both cardiac and noncardiac causes of death. The underlying causes of death in this group were diverse: cardiomyopathy, nonatherosclerotic coronary heart disease, valvular heart disease, aortic dissection, cerebral bleed, congenital heart disease, pulmonary embolism, drug overdoses, trauma, seizure disorders, asthma, and others. Among those cases with SCD and acute thrombosis, the hearts were further categorized by the status of the plaque, i.e., ruptured or eroded. Cases without thrombosis were categorized as stable plaque. Plaque burden was assessed and reported as the sum of the maximal percentage narrowing of the left main, left anterior descending, left circumflex, and right coronary arteries.

The population-adjusted rate of SCD increased as age increased and was greater in African Americans in the 6th and 7th decades of life *(182)*. Rates of SCD for men were greater than those for women; however, the rates of SCD were greater for African American women than for white women. No differences were detected between white and African Americans with respect to heart weight, overall plaque burden, and incidence of healed infarction. Surprisingly, the frequency of acute thrombosis decreased with advancing age and did not differ between the races. However, rate of death with stable plaque was higher in African Americans *(182)*.

Based on these data, African Americans have a relative increase in the incidence of SCD compared with whites after the age of 50. The mechanism appears to be related in part to the prevalence of LVH *(179)*. The conclusions of this study implicate hypertension and LVH as significant risk factors for SCD in African Americans. Another study suggested that a high prevalence of LVH and severe hypertension explains the increased incidence of SCD among African Americans *(184)*.

Premature ventricular beats among a group of middle-aged individuals correlated to increasing age, the presence of heart disease, faster sinus heart rates, African American ethnicity, male gender, lower education attainment, and lower serum Mg^{2+} or K^+ concentrations. Importantly, hypertension was strongly associated with the prevalence of PVCs *(185)*, suggesting that racially determined genetic factors might modify electrical remodeling in response to hypertension and increase the risk of arrhythmia and SCD.

Membrane Active Drugs, Ionic and Metabolic Effects

The details of inherited disorders of cardiac channel structure and function responsible for the LQTS and SCD are discussed in Chapters 20 and 21. Yet, acquired LQTS secondary to drugs, electrolyte disturbances and autonomic imbalance is more common and is presented here in the context of the interaction of extrinsic factors, e.g., membrane active drugs or electrolyte disturbances with preexisting channel modifications increasing the risk of serious ventricular arrhythmia and SCD. Certain antiarrhythmic and nonarrhythmic drugs and congenital LQTS cause SCD as the result of PVT. Intramural reentry triggered and enhanced by the heterogeneity of repolarization in the ventricle accounts for both congenital and acquired LQTS. The repolarization characteristics are determined by the biophysical properties of Na and K channels. It has long been established that hypokalemia increases the risk of VT among individuals treated with antiarrhythmic drugs and those with LQTS, although the molecular basis for these clinical observations is not established. Because asymptomatic mutations of channels are present in the population, individuals with these mutations may be at risk for developing abnormal repolarization when the balance of currents that repolarize the membrane is affected, either by the use of an antiarrhythmic drug or by electrolyte disturbances. Two studies provide a mechanism by which asymptomatic individuals with silent channelopathy become symptomatic with the superimposition of an antiarrhythmic agent or electrolyte disturbance *(186,187)*. Some mutations in K and Na channels are not associated with an apparent prolongation of the QT interval and under normal conditions are asymptomatic. Yet such individuals are at risk of developing overt prolongation of the QT interval, torsades de pointe PVT, and SCD in the presence of membrane-active drugs or electrolyte abnormalities.

K channels formed with specific mutations of *MiRP1* (T8A and Q9E) *(116,186)* and KvLQT1 (Y315C) *(187)* are more sensitive to K^+ channel-blocking drugs and are associated with drug-induced arrhythmia. In a survey of the genes encoding the pore-forming channel proteins, KvLQT1 (KCNQ1), HERG (KCNH2), and SCN5A, five of 92 individuals were identified with a history of acquired LQTS with a missense mutation of LvLQT1 and HERG *(188)*. Polymorphisms in other subunits forming K channels such as *minK* (D85N) might confer increased risk for acquired LQTS *(189)*. In a survey of individuals with a history of drug-induced long QT arrhythmia, polymorphisms of SCN5A gene coding for the α-subunit of the voltage-dependent Na^+ channel that related to acquired LQTS were not identified *(188)*. However, a mutation of SCN5A has been identified with such a history. DNA from individuals with nonfamilial cardiac arrhythmias was screened for polymorphisms of the SCN5A gene *(190)*. In one subject, prolongation of cardiac repolarization evidenced by increased corrected QT interval and torsade de pointes PVT was found in response to the combination of hypokalemia and the antiarrhythmic drug amiodarone. DNA analysis of this African American woman with a history of DCM showed a heterozygous transversion of C to A in codon 1102 of *SCN5A*, resulting in a substitution of serine (S1102) for tyrosine (Y1102) *(190)*.

The functional significance of this polymorphism is that the Y1102 polymorphism increases the rate of cardiac Na^+ channel activation, increasing both the peak Na^+ current and the sustained Na^+ current. The Y1102 polymorphism was identified in 19.2% of people originating from West Africa and the Caribbean, 13.2% of African Americans, and 0.8% of Hispanics, and was absent in Caucasians and Asians. Based on these proportions, Splawski et al. *(190)*

estimate that 4.6 million African Americans carry the Y1102 polymorphism of *SCN5A* gene.

In another case, an individual was identified when she developed a prolonged QT interval prolongation and PVT after administration of cisapride, an I_{Kr} blocker (191). In this case, DNA sequencing identified a T to C transition causing the substitution of proline for leucine1825 (L1825P) located in the C-terminal cytosolic tail of the Na channel gene, *SCN5A*. Subsequently, the L1825P SCN5A mutation was expressed heterologously in a human cell line. Electrophysiological assessment of the Na^+ currents in the cells containing the recombinant L1825P was compared with wild-type channels. The L1825P mutation showed increased late Na^+ current, decreased current density, and a negative shift of the steady-state inactivation curve when compared with the wild-type channel (191).

Thus, pharmacological agents and electrolyte abnormalities can interact with the underlying molecular and cellular architecture to modify electrophysiological properties and increase the risk for SCD. Other polymorphisms will undoubtedly be identified that also have subtle electrophysiological effects enhancing the risk of life-threatening arrhythmias in the presence of membrane active drugs, electrolyte abnormalities, or both. Data do not exist at a population level to support such speculation, yet three large studies have identified diuretic-induced hypokalemia as a risk factor for SCD.

Epidemiological data obtained from the Multiple Risk Factor Intervention Trial Research Group (MRFIT) (192), the Group Health Cooperative of Puget Sound (193), and Studies Of Left Ventricular Dysfunction (SOLVD) (194) show that the use of non–K^+-sparing diuretics is associated with an increased risk for SCD. In the MRFIT study, the relative risk for SCD was increased to 3.34 by the use of a thiazide diuretic in individuals with an abnormal electrocardiogram (192). Even among a population of individuals without overt heart disease, the Group Health Cooperative of Puget Sound between 1977 and 1990 provided circumstantial evidence that K^+-wasting diuretics were associated with an increased risk for SCD (193). In this study, the risk of primary cardiac arrest among patients taking K^+-wasting diuretics was increased (193). The addition of a K^+-sparing diuretic decreased the relative risk for SCD to 0.3, thereby implicating the loss of serum K^+ as an important determinant of risk.

The concept that K^+ loss confers increased risk for SCD was further investigated in a retrospective analysis of SOLVD, in a clinical trial assessing the role of ACE inhibitors in the treatment of patients with and without symptomatic heart failure. In this study non–K^+-sparing

diuretic use (194) was associated with increased risk of arrhythmic death. Non–K^+-sparing diuretic use remained independently associated with arrhythmic death even after adjusting for other arrhythmia risk factors such as disease severity, comorbid illness, and contemporaneous medication use. Importantly, like another study (193), K^+-sparing diuretics were not associated with increased arrhythmic death. Perhaps polymorphisms of membrane proteins determining electrical properties account for some measure of these adverse affects.

Autonomic Effects

The autonomic nervous system is highly integrated into the control system of normal heart rhythm and plays an important role in the initiation, modification, and termination of arrhythmia (195). Clinical conditions such as hereditary LQTS, neurocardiogenic hypotension, and bradycardia-dependent atrial fibrillation are all initiated by the autonomic nervous system. In addition, activation of the sympathetic or parasympathetic system modifies the characteristics of arrhythmia. Congenital LQTS is a classic example of a life-threatening arrhythmia mediated by cardiac neural input. In this condition, the dispersion of refractoriness is accentuated by catecholamines resulting in PVT. Treatments have included β-adrenergic blockade or left stellate ganglion ablation to reduce the effect of the sympathetic system. Ambulatory ECGs recorded during episodes of SCD generally show an increase in heart rate preceding the onset of VT and VF. Analysis of these tracings from patients with CAD implicates sudden changes in the neural input to the heart just before the onset of the arrhythmia (196). The effects of autonomic influences of arrhythmia formation are not limited to the ventricle or to humans. Heterogeneous electrophysiological properties, which may be due in part to autonomic innervation, are important in the maintenance of atrial fibrillation (197). Heterogeneous sympathetic innervation is thought to be the underlying cause of an inherited disorder of ventricular arrhythmias and SCD in German shepherd dogs (198).

The concept of "sympathetic imbalance" as trigger for the initiation and maintenance of serious ventricular arrhythmia was proposed in 1984 (199). Such imbalance may be generated by inherent differences in cardiac innervation. Investigations into the autonomic nervous system are focusing on development and application of end-points predicting risk to identify individuals at high risk (200). Techniques such as HRV and BRS provide prognostic information after MI, for those with CHF, and identify individuals at higher risk for SCD. Yet, consideration should be given to using such techniques to prospectively assess human responses to cognitive and mental stress to determine the genetic determinants of these responses that contribute to fatal ventricular arrhythmia.

Animal studies show that blockade of the adrenergic receptors, stimulation of the vagus nerve, or both, significantly reduce the incidence of spontaneous VF during exercise-induced myocardial ischemia in dogs with healed infarctions (201). During the convalescent phase of MI, dogs are susceptible to VF when myocardial ischemia is superimposed during an exercise test. Stimulation of the right cervical vagus nerve during the superimposed ischemia reduced the incidence of VF during exercise from 56% to 10% (202). Thus, the electrophysiological effects secondary to the vagally mediated antagonism of the sympathetic activity on the heart protects the heart from VF during ischemia.

The most likely mechanism for the increased risk of VF during ischemia in the presence of autonomic imbalance is the heterogeneous effect of autonomic innervation within and around ischemic myocardium and secondary effects on the spatial heterogeneity of cellular K^+ loss and repolarization (203). Increased dispersion of repolarization contributes to reentry and ventricular arrhythmia in a transgenic mouse model in which a dominant negative protein was expressed for one of the repolarizing K^+ channels. Optical mapping confirmed previous studies that increased dispersion of repolarization is sufficient to cause arrhythmia. A general concept of how the autonomic nervous system can influence dispersion of repolarization results in arrhythmia is discussed below.

Nitric oxide (NO) is formed in the endothelium and modulates the autonomic activity of cardiac nodal tissue and ventricles. In general, NO synthase inhibition serves to enhance the effects of sympathetic stimulation while decreasing the effects of vagal stimulation (204). There is a known link between NO and modulation of the autonomic activity in the ventricle (205). The NO donor L-arginine limited the shortening of effective refractory period on the epicardial surface of the heart during sympathetic stimulation, an effect that was inhibited by the NO synthase inhibitor L-NMMA. During coronary occlusion, sympathetic stimulation increases ventricular arrhythmia. By contrast, NO donor infusion reduces ischemia-induced arrhythmia (205).

The modulation of cardiac neural input can now be clinically assessed noninvasively with HRV and BRS testing, while simultaneously assessing the effects on dispersion of repolarization with assessment of QT intervals and t-wave alternans on the surface ECG. HRV describes the small beat-to-beat variability of the RR interval present in the normal cardiac rhythm. This variability in RR interval is influenced by many factors, including cardiac neural input. HRV is reported in both the time-domain and frequency-domain. Time-domain parameters include the standard deviation of normal NN intervals, the standard deviation of the averages of NN intervals in all 5-min segments of the record, the square root of the mean of squared differences between adjacent NN intervals, and the percentage of RR intervals greater than 50 ms. The frequency-domain parameters relate to the power spectrum of the RR intervals over specific frequency ranges obtained using fast Fourier or autoregressive methods. High-frequency power between 0.15 and 0.40 Hz relates to the input of the parasympathetic system, whereas the low-frequency power between 0.04 and 0.15 Hz relates to a contribution from both limbs of the autonomic system. Thus, HRV in both the time and frequency domain provides information about the modulation of cardiac neural input. The frequency range characteristic for each limb of the autonomic nervous system results directly from the time course of the heart's cellular response to either acetylcholine in the case of the parasympathetic system or to norepinephrine for the sympathetic system. Acetylcholine activates a G protein–mediated process that opens a membrane-bound K^+ channel, leading to an immediate cellular response. By contrast, the effect of norepinephrine is mediated by the accumulation of intracellular cyclic AMP, which takes seconds to occur. Thus, the parasympathetic system initiates high-frequency responses, whereas the sympathetic system imparts low-frequency responses. HRV is believed to represent a measure of the parasympathetic modulation of the heart rate rather than the absolute magnitude of parasympathetic tone (206).

Decreased HRV is associated with cardiovascular risk factors such as age, gender, hypertension, obesity, lipid abnormalities and diabetes, and increased mortality. The aging process is associated with a loss of HRV (207,208) and loss of vasodilation, including NO synthesis (209). In a large clinical epidemiological study HRV was measured in 2359 men and women aged 45–64 years from the biracial, population-based Atherosclerosis Risk in Communities Study. HRV was reduced in people with hypertension, diabetes, and dyslipidemia (210). These findings suggest that these disorders adversely affect cardiac autonomic control; reduced autonomic control may contribute to the increased risk for subsequent cardiovascular events. Plasma total cholesterol and low-density lipoprotein-cholesterol correlate inversely with 24-h HRV, and this relationship is independent of prevalent CAD (211). The potential relation between reduced HRV and the progression of CAD was studied prospectively (212). Heart rate and HRV were analyzed in ambulatory ECG recordings from 265 patients participating in a multicenter study to evaluate the progression of CAD in patients with prior coronary artery bypass surgery and low high-density lipoprotein cholesterol concentrations. Reduced HRV predicted more rapid progression of CAD.

During convalescence from an MI, patients with reduced HRV are at a higher risk for SCD, suggesting that reduced HRV may identify an arrhythmogenic substrate. Insight into this phenomenon emerges from human and animal studies where increased sympathetic or decreased parasympathetic activation increases the risk of spontaneous VF and that associated with ischemia. For example, the spectral power of HRV increases just before the onset of VT, although a mechanistic link between changes in the spectral characteristics of HRV and arrhythmia remains controversial (213). Nevertheless, there is a consensus that short-term changes in neurohormonal activity contribute to some arrhythmia.

The state of sleep influences autonomic input to the heart and may contribute to the increased incidence of MI, SCD, and discharge of implanted cardioverter-defibrillators (214). Although generally assumed to be a quiet restful time, sleep is characterized by extremes in autonomic behavior (215). During slow-wave sleep, parasympathetic tone and BRS increase with a slowing of the heart rate. By contrast, sympathetic activity increases and BRS decreases during REM sleep. Dreams are associated with increased autonomic activity that reaches its greatest peak during night terrors and nightmares. Yet, the proof that dreams are associated with SCD remains circumstantial. Sleep can also induce intense vagal activity, slowing the heart rate and causing asystole. Such events may be particularly adverse for individuals with bradycardia-dependent ventricular arrhythmia, for example, those with channelopathies such as SCN5A linked to chromosome 3, individuals having a drug-induced LQT, or those with acquired heterogeneity of cardiac repolarization.

Dietary Fatty Acids

Dietary fish intake is associated with decreased risk for coronary heart disease (216) and fatal cardiac events (217). A prospective study of a cohort of U.S. male physicians showed that dietary intake of fish and ω-3 fatty acid decreased the risk for SCD, but did not decrease the risk for MI or nonsudden cardiac death (217). In a subsequent study, the serum levels of ω-3 fatty acids were associated with decreased risk for SCD (218). The finding that fish and n-3 fatty acid intake decrease SCD while having no significant effect on MI or nonsudden cardiac death implicates a specific effect of dietary fish and n-3 fatty acid intake on arrhythmia formation.

The role of n-3 polyunsaturated fatty acids in influencing mortality among survivors of MI was studied in the Gruppo Italiano per lo Studio della Sopravvivenza nell'Infarto Miocardioco-Prevenzione trial (219). Supplementation of n-3 polyunsaturated fatty acids (1 g/d) decreased the incidence of SCD by 4 mo after MI. The mechanism may relate to an antifibrillatory effect of the polyunsaturated fatty acid in ischemic heart, as suggested in a canine model of myocardial ischemia in which ω-3 fatty acids administered intravenously decreased the incidence of ischemia-induced VF (220). At the cellular level the antiarrhythmic effect of ω-3 fatty acids may relate to hastening the loss of excitability in ischemic myocardium and suppressing DADs by inhibiting the L-type Ca^+ channel and the Na^+ channel (221,222).

In contrast to ω-3 fatty acids, nonesterified fatty acids are associated with increases in arrhythmia and risk for SCD (223–226). In particular, nonesterified fatty acids (227) and trans-fatty acids (228) increase the incidence of SCD. The relationship of trans-fatty acids to the incidence of primary cardiac arrest was specifically investigated in a population-based case-control study in Seattle, WA (228), which measured red blood cell trans-fatty acid as a biomarker of dietary intake of trans-fatty acids. The measured concentration of trans isomers of linoleic acid (trans-18:2) in the red blood cells correlated with the dietary intake of total trans-fatty acid and was associated with an increased risk for SCD.

The increased risk for SCD is believed to relate to an increased risk of VF based on animal studies implicating the interaction of free fatty acids with the sarcolemmal membrane, with attendant conformational changes in channel proteins and electrophysiological properties of the tissue. Electrophysiological consequences of nonesterified fatty acids are likely to relate to cellular Ca^{2+} loading during ischemia, resulting from effects on ATP-sensitive and insensitive channels and the Na^+/K^+ pump. Such interactions are suggested to lower the VF threshold (229).

FUTURE DIRECTIONS OF RESEARCH

Because SCD often occurs as the first sign of a channelopathy, structural heart disease, or ischemia, the most effective approach to decrease the incidence of SCD will be to establish primary measures to prevent disease and identify those at risk. The education of the public in the early signs and symptoms of ischemic heart disease and the effective treatment of ischemia are also likely to decrease SCD. Future research must seek to define the mechanisms of cellular remodeling in heart disease, the modification of the cardiac currents and electrophysiological properties, and their subsequent interaction with neurogenic factors, ischemia, drugs, toxins, electrolyte abnormalities, and environmental factors. Such information will be essential for the development of genetic therapy and pharmacological approaches to prevent or reverse electrical and structural remodeling and decrease ischemia-induced VF and arrhythmias associated with cardiomyopathy and congenital and acquired PVT. These investigations will require unprecedented cooperation between clinicians and scientists specializing in public health, epidemiology, genetics, informatics, biomedical engineering, and the basic medical sciences.

Investigations are beginning this century into the genetic and molecular causes of SCD. Novel proteomic and genomic studies at the population level will likely identify the proteins and genes associated with SCD, while cellular studies will delineate the signaling pathways accounting for the physiological changes predisposing to SCD. Elucidation of the molecular mechanisms will translate into novel approaches to alter the excitability of cardiac tissue or the cellular responses to stress, thereby decreasing the likelihood of SCD.

ACKNOWLEDGMENTS

This study was supported by grant P01 HL27430 from the National Heart, Lung and Blood Institute, National Institutes of Health, Bethesda, MD, USA, and cooperative agreement CR-829522 to the University of North Carolina at Chapel Hill, NC, from the U.S. Environmental Protection Agency. Although the literature review described in this article has been funded in part by the U.S. Environmental Protection Agency through cooperative agreement CR829522 with the Center for Environmental Medicine, Asthma, and Lung Biology at the University of North Carolina at Chapel Hill, it has not been subjected to the Agency's required peer and policy review; therefore, it does not necessarily reflect the views of the Agency, and no official endorsement should be inferred. Mention of trade names or commercial products does not constitute endorsement or recommendation for use.

REFERENCES

1. Chugh SS, Kelly KL, Titus JL. Sudden cardiac death with apparently normal heart. Circulation 2000;102:649–654.
2. Jouven X, Besnos M, Guerot C, Ducimetiére P. Predicting sudden death in the population. The Paris Prospective Study I. Circulation 1999;99:1978–1983.
3. Friedlander Y, Siscovick DS, Weinmann S, et al. Family history as a risk factor for primary cardiac arrest. Circulation 1998; 97:55–160.
4. MacWilliam JA. Cardiac failure and sudden death. Br Med J 1889;1:6–8.
5. de Silva RA. John MacWilliam, evolutionary biology and sudden cardiac death. J Am Coll Cardiol 1989;14:1843–1849.
6. Zipes DP, Wellens HJJ. Sudden cardiac death. Circulation 1998;98:2334–2351.
7. Myerburg RJ, Castellanos A. Cardiac arrest and sudden cardiac death. In: Braunwald EA, ed. Heart Disease: A Texbook of Cardiovascular Medicine. 6th ed. Philadelphia: Saunders, 2001:890–931.
8. Pratt CM, Greenway PS, Schoenfeld MH, Hibben ML, Reiffel JA. Exploration of the precision of classifying sudden cardiac death. Implications for the interpretation of clinical trials. Circulation 1996;93:519–524.
9. Zheng Z-J, Croft JB, Giles WH, Mensah GA. Sudden cardiac death in the United States; 1989-1998. Circulation 2001; 104:2158–2163.
10. Gillum RF. Sudden coronary death in the United States: 1980–1985. Circulation 1989;79:756–765.
11. Gillum RF. Sudden cardiac death in Hispanic Americans and African Americans. Am J Public Health 1997;87:1461–1466.
12. Gillum RF, Folsom A, Luepker RV, et al. Sudden cardiac death and acute myocardial infarction in a metropolitian area, 1970–1980: the Minnesota Heart Survey. N Engl J Med 1983;309:1353–1358.
13. Kléber AG, Janse MJ, Fast VG. Normal and abnormal conduction in the heart. In: Page E, ed. Handbook of Physiology: Oxford University Press, 2001:455–530.
14. Priori SG, Barhanin J, Hauer RNW, et al. Genetic and molecular basis of cardiac arrhythmias. Impact on clinical management. Eur Heart J 1999;20:174–195.
15. Han W, Bao W, Wang Z, Nattel S. Comparison of ion-channel subunit expression in canine cardiac Purkinje fibers and ventricular muscle. Circ Res 2002;91:790–797.
16. Spach MS. Mechanisms of the dynamic of reentry in a fibrillating myocardium. Developing a genes-to-rotors paradigm. Circ Res 2001;88:753–755.
17. Kaab S, Nuss BB, Chiamvimonvat N, et al. Ionic mechanism of action potential prolongation in ventricuar myocytes from dogs with pacing-induced heart failure. Circ Res 1996;78: 262–273.
18. Tsuji Y, Opthof T, Yasui K, et al. Ionic mechanisms of acquired QT prolongation and torsades de pointes in rabbits with chronic complete atrioventricular block. Circulation 2002;106:2012–2018.
19. Peters NS. New insights into myocardial arrhythmogenesis distribution of gap-junctional coupling in normal, ischemic and hypertrophied human hearts. Clin Sci 1996;90:447–452.
20. Marban E. Molecular approaches to arrhythmogenesis. In: Chien KR, ed. Molecular Basis of Cardiovascular Disease. Philadelphia: Saunders, 1999:313–328.
21. Clancy CE, Rudy Y. Linking a genetic defect to its cellular phenotype in a cardiac arrhythmia. Nature 1999;400:566–569.
22. Luo C-H, Rudy Y. A dynamic model of the cardiac ventricular action potential. I. Simulations of ionic currents and concentration changes. Circ Res 1994;74:1071–1096.
23. Kuperstein R, Hanly P, Niroumand M, Sasson Z. The importance of age and obesity on the relation between diabetes and left ventricular mass. J Am Coll Cardiol 2001;37:1957–1962.
24. Kannel WE, Grodon T, Offutt D. Left ventricular hypertrophy by electrocardiogram: prevalence, incidence and mortality in the Framingham Study. Ann Intern Med 1969;71:99–105.
25. Kannel WE, Gordon T, Castelli WP, Margolis JR. Electrocardiographic left ventricular hypertrophy and risk of coronary heart

disease, the Framingham Heart Study. Ann Intern Med 1970;72:813–822.

26. Levy D, Garrison R, Savage D, Kannel W, Castelli W. Prognostic implications of echocardiographically determined left ventricular mass in the Framingham Heart Study. N Engl J Med 1990; 322:1561–1566.

27. Verdecchia P, Carini G, Circo A, et al. Left ventricular mass and cardiovascular morbidity in essential hypertension: The MAVI study. J Am Coll Cardiol 2001;38:1829–1835.

28. Haider AW, Larson MG, Benjamin EJ, Levy D. Increased left ventricular mass and hypertrophy are associated with increased risk of sudden death. J Am Coll Cardiol 1998;32:1454–1459.

29. Kohya T, Kimura S, Myerburg RJ, Bassett AL. Susceptibility of hypertrophied rat hearts to ventricular fibrillation during acute ischemia. J Mol Cell Cardiol. 1988;20:159–168.

30. Volders PG, Sipido KR, Vos MA, et al. Cellular basis of biventricular hypertrophy and arrhythmogenesis in dogs with chronic complete atrioventricular block and acquired torsade de points. Circulation 1998;98:1136–1147.

31. Kozhevnikov DO, Yanamoto K, Robotis D, Restivo M, El-Sherif N. Electrophysiological mechanism of enhanced susceptibility of hypertrophied heart to acquired Torsade de Pointes arrhythmias. Tridimensional mapping of activation and recovery patterns. Circulation 2002;105:1128–1134.

32. Facchini M, Malfatto G, Ciambellotti F, et al. Markers of electrical instability in hypertensive patients with and without ventricular arrhythmias. Are they useful in identifying patients with different risk profiles? J Hypertens 2000;18:763–768.

33. Pluim BM, Zwinderman AH, van de Laarse A, van der Wall EE. The athlete's heart: A meta-analysis of cardiac structure and function. Circulation 1999;100:336–344.

34. Palatini P, Maraglino G, Sperti G, et al. Prevalence and possible mechanisms of ventricular arrhythmias in athletes. Am Heart J 1985;110:560–567.

35. Biffi A, Pelliccia A, Verdile L, et al. Long-term clinical significance of frequent and complex ventricular tacyarrhythmias in trained athletes. J Am Coll Cardiol 2002;40:446–452.

36. Karjalainen J, Kujala UM, Stolt A, et al. Angiotensinogen gene M235T polymorphism predicts left ventricular hypertrophy in endurance athletes. J Am Coll Cardiol 1999;34:494–499.

37. Libby P, Ridker PM, Maseri A. Inflammation and atherosclerosis. Circulation 2002;105:1135–1143.

38. Van der Wal AC, Becker AE, van der Loos CM, Das PK. Site of intimal rupture or erosion of thrombosed coronary atherosclerotic plaques is characterized by an inflammatory process irrespective of the dominant plaque morphology. Circulation 1994;89:36–44.

39. Libby P, Simon DI. Inflammation and thrombosis: the clot thickens. Circulation 2001;103:1718–1720.

40. Ridker PM, Cushman M, Stampfer MJ, Tracy RP, Hennekens CH. Inflammation, aspirin, and the risk of cardiovascular disease in apparently healthy men. N Engl J Med 1997;336:973–979.

41. Gussekloo J, Schaap MC, Frölich M, Blauw GJ, Westendorp RGJ. C-reactive protein is a strong but nonspecific risk factor of fatal stroke in elderly persons. Arterioscler Thromb Vasc Biol 2000;20:1047–1051.

42. Engström G, Lind P, Hedblad B, et al. Effects of cholesterol and inflammation-sensitive plasma proteins on incidence of myocardial infarction and stroke in men. Circulation 2002; 105:2632–2637.

43. Albert CM, Ma J, Rifai N, Stampfer MJ, Ridker PM. Prospective study of C-reactive protein, homocysteine, and plasma lipid levels as predictors of sudden cardiac death. Circulation 2002;105:2595–2599.

44. Chung MK, Martin DO, Sprecher D, et al. C-reactive protein elevation in patients with atrial arrhythmias. Inflammatory mechanisms and persistence of atrial fibrillation. Circulation 2001;104:2886–2891.

45. Marban E. Cardiac channelopathies. Nature 2002;415:213–218.

46. Grant AO. Molecular biology of sodium channels and their role in cardiac arrhythmias. Am J Med 2001;110:296–305.

47. Bezzina CR, Rook MB, Wilde AAM. Cardiac sodium channel and inherited arrhythmia syndromes. Cardiovasc Res 2001;49:257–271.

48. Chauhan VS, Tuvia S, Buhusi M, Bennett V, Grant AO. Abnormal cardiac Na$^+$ channel properties and QT heart rate adaptation in neonatal ankyrinB knockout mice. Circ Res 2000;86:441–447.

49. Coumel P, Fidelle J, Lucet V, Attuel P, Bouvrain Y. Catecholamine-induced severe ventricular arrhythmias with Adams-Stokes syndrome in children: report of four cases. Br Heart J 1978;40:28–37.

50. Leenhardt A, Lucet V, Denjoy I, et al. Catecholaminergic polymorphic ventricular tachycardia in children: a 7-year follow-up of 21 patients. Circulation 1995;91:1512–1519.

51. Swan H, Piippo K, Viitasalo M, et al. Arrhythmic disorder mapped to chromosome1q42-q43 causes malignant polymorphic ventricular tachycardia in structurally normal hearts. J Am Coll Cardiol 1999;34:2035–2045.

52. Priori SG, Napolitano C, Tiso N, et al. Mutation in the cardiac ryanodine receptor gene (hRyR2) underlie catecholaminergic polymorphic ventricular tachycardia. Circulation 2001;103:196–200.

53. Lahat H, Eldar M, Levy-Nissenbaum E, et al. Autosomal recessive catecholamine- or exercise-induced polymorphic ventricular tachycardia. Clinical features and assignment of the disease gene to chromosome 11p13-21. Circulation 2001; 103:2822–2827.

54. Fisher JD, Krikler D, Hallidie-Smith KA. Familial polymorphic ventricular arrhythmias: a quarter century of successful medical treatment based on serial exercise-pharmacologic testing. J Am Coll Cardiol 1999;34:2015–2022.

55. Laitinen PJ, Brown KM, Piippo K, et al. Mutations of the cardiac ryanodine receptor (RyR2) gene in familial polymorphic ventricular tachycardia. Circulation 2001;103:485–490.

56. Marx SO, Reiken S, Hisamatsu Y, et al. PKA phosphorylation dissociates FKBP12.6 from the calcium release channel (ryanodine receptor): defective regulation in failing hearts. Cell 2000;101:365–376.

57. Schlotthauer K, Bers DM. Sarcoplasmic reticulum Ca^{2+} release causes myocyte depolarization. Underlying mechanism and threshold for triggered action potentials. Circ Res 2000;87:774–780.

58. Jiang D, Xiao B, Zhang L, Chen SRW. Enhanced basal activity of a cardiac Ca^{2+} release channel (ryanodine receptor) mutant associated with ventricular tachycardia and sudden death. Circ Res 2002;91:218–225.

59. Marks AR, Reiken S, Marx SO. Progression of heart failure: is protein kinase a hyperphosphorylation of the ryanodine receptor a contributing factor. Circulation 2002;105:272 –275.

60. Marks AR. Ryanodine receptors/calcium release channels in heart failure and sudden cardiac death. J Mol Cell Cardiol 2001;33:615–624.

61. Fontaine G, Guiraudon G, Frank R, et al. Stimulation studies and epicardial mapping in ventricular tachycardia. Study of mechanisms and selection for surgery. In: Kulbertus HE, ed. Reentrant Arrhythmias: Mechanisms and Treatment. Lancaster: MTP Press Limited, 1977:334–350.

62. Richardson P, McKenna WJ, Bristow M, et al. Report of the 1995 WHO/ISFC Task Force on the definition and classification of cardiomyopathies. Circulation 1996;93:841–842.

63. Gemayel C, Pelliccia A, Thompson PD. Arrhythmogenic right ventricular cardiomyopathy. J Am Coll Cardiol 2001; 38:1773–1781.

64. Protonotarios N, Tsatsopoulou A, Anastasakis A, et al. Genotype-phenotype assessment in autosomal recessive arrhythmogenic right venticular cardiomyopathy (Naxos Disease) caused by a deletion in plakoglobin. J Am Coll Cardiol 2001; 38:1477–1484.

65. Nava A, Bauce B, Basso C, et al. Clinical profile and long-term follow-up of 37 families with arrhythmogenic right ventricular cardiomyopathy. J Am Coll Cardiol 2000;36:226–233.

66. Rampazzo A, Nava A, Danieli G, et al. The gene for arrhythmogenic right ventricular cardiomyopathy maps to chromosome 14q23-q24. Hum Mol Genet 1994;12:959–962.

67. Rampazzo A, Nava A, Erne P, et al. A new locus for arrhythmogenic right ventiruclar cardiomyopathy (ARVD2) maps to chromosome 1q42-q43. Hum Mol Genet 1995; 4:2151–2154.

68. Rampazzo A, Nava A, Miorin M, et al. ARVD 4, a new locus for arrhythmogenic right ventricular cardiomyopathy, maps to chromosome 2 long arm. Genomics 1997;45:259–263.

69. Severini GM, Krajinovic M, Pinamonti B, et al. A new locus for arrhyhmogenic right ventricular dysplasia on the long arm of chromosome 14. Genomics 1996;31:193–200.

70. Ahmad F, Li D, Karibe A, et al. Localization of a gene responsible for arrhythmogenic right ventricular dysplasia to chromosome 3p23. Circulation 1998;98:2791–2795.

71. Li D, Ahmad F, Gardner MJ, et al. The locus of a novel gene responsible for arrhythmogenic right ventricular dysplasia characterized by early onset and high penetrance maps to chromosome 10p12-p14. Am J Hum Genet 2000;66:148–156.

72. McKoy G, Protonotarios N, Crosby A, et al. Identification of a deletion of plakoglobin in arrhythmogenic right ventricular cardiomyopathy with palmoplantar keratoderma and woolly hair (Naxos disease). Lancet 2000;355:2119–2124.

73. Tiso N, Stephan DA, Nava A, et al. Identification of mutations in the cardiac ryanodine receptor gene in families affected with arrhythmogentic right ventricular cardiomyopathy type 2 (ARVD2). Hum Mol Genet 2001;10:189–194.

74. Shannon DC, Kelly DH. SIDS and near-SIDS. N Engl J Med 1982;306:959–965.

75. Maron BJ, Clark CE, Goldstein RE, Epstein SE. Potential role of QT interval prolongation in sudden infant death syndrome. Circulation 1976;54:423–430.

76. Southall DP. QT interval and SIDS. Circulation 1983;67:707–708.

77. Kelly DH, Shannon DC, Liberthson RR. The role of the QT interval in the sudden infant death syndrome. Circulation 1977;55:633–635.

78. Schwartz PJ, Stramba-Badiale M, Segantini A, et al. Prolongation of the QT interval and the sudden infant death syndrome. N Engl J Med 1998;338:1709–1714.

79. Schwartz PJ, Priori SG, Dumaine R, et al. A molecular link between the sudden infant death syndrome and the long-QT syndrome. N Engl J Med 2000;343:262–267.

80. Wedekind H, Smits JPP, Schulze-Bahr E, et al. De novo mutation in the SCN5A gene associated with early onset of sudden infant death. Circulation 2001;104:1158–1164.

81. Ackerman MJ, Tester DJ, Driscoll DJ. Molecular autopsy of sudden unexplained death in the young. Am J Forensic Med Pathol 2001;22:105–111.

82. Wang Y, Scheinman MM, Chien WW, et al. Patients with supraventricular tachycardia present with aborted sudden death: Incidence, mechanism and long-term follow-up. J Am Coll Cardiol 1991;18:1711–1719.

83. Munger TM, Packer DL, Hammill SC, et al. A population study of natural history of Wolff-Parkinson-White syndrome in Olmsted County, Minnesota, 1953-1989. Circulation 1993; 87:866–873.

84. Flensted-Jensen E. Wolff-Parkinson-White syndrome: a long-term follow-up of 47 cases. Acta Med Scand 1969;186:65–74.

85. Öhnell RF. Preexcitation: a cardiac abnormality. Acta Med Scand 1944;52:1–167.

86. Vidaillet HJ, Pressley JC, Henke E, Harrell FE, German LD. Familial occurrence of accessory atrioventricular pathways (preexcitation syndrome). N Engl J Med 1987;317:65–69.

87. Gillette PC, Freed D, McNamara DG. A proposed autosomal dominant method of inheritance of the Wolff–Parkinson–White syndrome and supraventricular tachycardia. J Pediatr 1978;93: 257–258.

88. Gollob MH, Seger JJ, Gollob TN, et al. Novel PRKAG2 mutation responsible for the genetic syndrome of ventricular preexcitation and conduction system disease with childhood onset and absence of cardiac hypertrophy. Circulation 2001;104:3030–3033.

89. Gollob MH, Green MS, Tang ASL, et al. Identification of a gene responsible for familial Wolff-Parkinson-White Syndrome. N Engl J Med 2001;344:1823–1831.

90. Basso C, Corrado D, Rossi L, Thiene G. Ventricular preexcitation in children and young adults. Atrial myocarditis as a possible trigger of sudden death. Circulation 2001;103:269–275.

91. Shinagawa K, Li D, Leung TK, Nattel S. Consequences of atrial tachycardia-induced remodeling depend on the preexisting atrial substrate. Circulation 2002;105:251–257.

92. Polontchouk L, Haefliger J-A, Ebelt B, et al. Effects of chronic atrial fibrillation on gap junction distribution in human and rat atria. J Am Coll Cardiol 2001;38:883–891.

93. Dupont E, Ko Y-S, Rothery S, et al. The gap-junctional protein connexin40 is elevated in patients susceptible to postoperative atrial fibrillation. Circulation 2001;103:842–849.

94. van der Velden HMW, Ausma J, Rook MB, et al. Gap junctional remodeling in relation to stabilization of atrial fibrillation in the goat. Cardiovasc Res 2000;46:476–486.

95. Ai Z, Fischer A, Spray DC, Brown AMC, Fischman GI. Wnt-1 regulation of connexin43 in cardiac myocytes. J Clin Invest 2001;105:161–171.

96. Murray CJ, Lopez AD. Alternative projections of mortality and disability by cause 1990-2020: Global Burden of Diseases Study. Lancet 1997;349:1498–1504.

97. Davies MJ, Thomas A. Thrombosis and acute coronary-artery lesions in sudden cardiac ischemic death. N Engl J Med 1984;310:1137–1140.

98. Burke AP, Kolodgie FD, Farb A, et al. Healed plaque ruptures and sudden coronary death. Evidence that subclinical rupture has a role in plaque progression. Circulation 2001; 103:934–940.

99. Chevalier P, Dacosta A, Defaye P, et al. Arrhythmic cardiac arrest due to isolated coronary artery spasm: Long-term outcome of seven resuscitated patients. J Am Coll Cardiol 1998; 31:57–61.

100. Janse MJ, Wit AL. Electrophysiological mechanism of ventricular arrhythmias resulting from myocardial ischemia and infarction. Physiol Rev 1989;69:1049–1169.

101. Carmeliet E. Cardiac ionic currents and acute ischemia: From channels to arrhythmias. Physiol Rev 1999;79:917–1017.

102. Gettes LS, Cascio WE. Effect of ischemia on cardiac electrophysiology. In: Fozzard HA, Haber E, Jennings RB, Katz AM, Morgan HE, eds. The Heart and Cardiovascular System. Scientific Foundations. 2nd Edition ed. New York, NY: Raven Press, 1991:2021–2054.

103. Janse MJ, Cinca J, Moréna H, et al. The "border zone" in myocardial ischemia: An electrophysiological, metabolic, and histochemical correlation in the pig heart. Circ Res 1979; 44:576–588.

104. Coronel R, Fiolet JWT, Wilms-Schopman FJG, et al. Distribution of extracellular potassium and its relation to electrophysiologic changes during acute myocardial ischemia in the isolated perfused porcine heart. Circulation 1988; 77:1125–1138.

105. Johnson TA, Engle CL, Boyd LM, et alS. Magnitude and time course of extracellular potassium inhomogeneities during acute ischemia in pigs. Effect of verapamil. Circulation 1991; 83:622–634.

106. Cascio WE, Johnson TA, Gettes LS. Electrophysiologic changes of ischemic ventricular myocardium: I. Influence of energetic, ionic and metabolic changes. J Cardiovasc Electrophysiol 1995; 6:1039–1062.

107. Reimer KA, Jennings RB. In: Fozzard H, ed. The Heart and Cardiovascular System: Scientific Foundations. New York, NY: Raven Press, 1986.

108. Pogwizd SM, Corr PB. Reentrant and nonreentrant mechanisms contribute to arrhythmogenesis during early myocardial ischemia: Results using three-dimensional mapping. Circ Res 1987;61:352–371.

109. Kondo I, Berg K, Drayna D, Lawn R. DNA polymorphism at the locus for human cholesteryl ester transfer protein (CETP) is associated with high density lipoprotein cholesterol and apolipoprotein levels. Clin Genet 1989;35:49–56.

110. Iwai N, Katsuya T, Mannami T, et al. Association between SAH, an acyl-CoA synthetase gene, and hypertriglyceridemia, obestiy and hypertension. Circulation 2002;105:41–47.

111. Snapir A, Mikkelsson J, Perola M, et al. Variation in the alpha2B-adrenergic gene as a risk factor for prehospital fatal myocaridal infarction and suden cardiac death. J Am Coll Cardiol 2003;41:190–194.

112. Faber BCG, Cleutjens KBJM, Niessn RLJ, et al. Identfification of genes potentially involved in rupture of human atherosclerotic plaques. Circ Res 2001;89:547–554.

113. O'Donnell CJ, Larson MG, Feng D, et al. Genetic and environmental contributions to platelet aggregation. The Framingham Heart Study. Circulation 2001;103:3051–3056.

114. Halkin A, Roth A, Lurie I, et al. Pause-dependent torsade de pointes following myocardial infarction. J Am Coll Cardiol 2001;38:1168–1174.

115. Donger C, Denjoy I, Berthet M, et al. KVLQT1 C-terminal missense mutation causes a forme fruste long QT syndrome. Circulation 1997;96:2778–2781.

116. Sesti F, Abbott GW, Wei J, et al. A common polymorphism associated with antibiotic-induced cardiac arrhythmia. Proc Natl Acad Sci USA 2000;12:10613–10618.

117. Spooner PM, Albert C, Benjamin EJ, et al. Sudden cardiac death, genes, and arrhythmogenesis. Consideration of new population and mechanistic approaches from a National Heart, Lung, and Blood Institute Wowrkshop, Part II. Circulation 2001;103:2447–2452.

118. Jeron A, Hengstenberg C, Engle S, et al. The D-allele of the ACE polymorphism is related to increased QT dispersion in 609 patients after myocardial infarction. Eur Heart J 2001;22:663–668.

119. Uretsky BF, Thygesen K, Armstrong PW, et al. Acute coronary findings at autopsy in heart failure patients with sudden death. Results from the assessment of treatment with Lisinopril and survival (ATLA) trial. Circulation 2000;102:611–616.

120. Berntsen RF, Gunnes P, Lie M, Rasmussen K. Surgical revascularization in the treatment of ventricular tachycardia and fibrillation exposed by exercise-induced ischemia. Eur Heart J 1993;14:1297–1303.

121. Brugada J, Aguinaga L, Mont L, et al. Coronary artery revascularization in patitents with sustained ventricular arrhythmias in the chronic phase of a myocardial infarction: Effects on the electrophysiologic substrate and outcome. J Am Coll Cardiol 2001;37:529–533.

122. Gomes JA, Alexopoulos D, Winters SL, et al. The role of silent ischemia, the arrhythmic substrate and the short-long sequence in the genesis of sudden cardiac death. J Am Coll Cardiol 1989;14:1618–1625.

123. Tomaselli GF, Marbán E. Electrophysiological remodeling in hypertorphy and heart failure. Cardiovasc Res 1999;42:270–283.

124. Huang B, Qin D, El-Sherif N. Early down-regulation of K^+ channel genes and currents in the postinfarction heart. J Cardiovasc Electrophysiol 2000;11:1252–1261.

125. Bailly P, Benitah JP, Mouchoniere M, Vassort G, Lorente P. Regional alteration of the transient outward current in human left ventricular septum during compensated hypertrophy. Circulation 1997;96:1266–1274.

126. Wu T-J, Ong JJC, Hwang C, et al. Characteristics of wave fronts during ventricular fibrillation in human hearts with dilated cardiomyopathy: Role of increased fibrosis in the generation reentry. J Am Coll Cardiol 1998;32:187–196.

127. Liberthson RR. Sudden death from cardiac causes in children and young adults. N Engl J Med 1996;334:1039–1044.

128. Roberts R, Sigwart U. New concepts in hypertrophic cardiomyopathies, Part 1. Circulation 2001;104:2113–2116.

129. Roberts R, Sigwart U. New concepts in hypertrophic cardiomyopathies, Part II. Circulation 2001;104:2249–2252.

130. Erdmann J, Raible J, Maki-Abadi J, et al. Spectrum of clinical phenotypes and gene variants in cardiac myosin-binding protein C mutations carriers with hypertrophic cardiomyopathy. J Am Coll Cardiol 2001;38:322–330.

131. Moolman JC, Corfield VA, Posen B, et al. Sudden death due to troponin T mutations. J Am Coll Cardiol 1997;29:549–555.

132. Karibe A, Tobacman LS, Strand J, et al. Hypertrophic cardiomyopathy caused by a novel α-tropomyosin mutation (V95A) is associated with mild cardiac phenotype, abnormal calcium binding to troponin, abnormal myosin cycling, and proor prognosis. Circulation 2001;103:65–71.

133. Maron BJ, Olivotto I, Spirito P, et al. Epidemiology of hypertrophic cardiomyopathy-related death. Revisited in a large non-referral-based patient population. Circulation 2000; 102:858–864.

134. Shirani J, Rick R, Roberts WC, Maron BJ. Morphology and significance of the left ventricular collagen network in young patients with hypertrophic cardiomyopathy and sudden cardiac death. J Am Coll Cardiol 2000;35:36–44.

135. De Rose Jr JJ, Banas Jr JS, Winters SL. Current perspectives on sudden cardiac death in hypertrophic cardiomyopathy. Prog Cardiovasc Dis 1994;36:475–484.

136. Elliott PM, Poloniecki J, Dickie S, et al. Sudden death in hypertrophic cardiomyopathy: Identification of high risk patients. J Am Coll Cardiol 2000;36:2212–2218.

137. Olivotto I, Gistri R, Petrone P, et al. Maximum left ventricular thickness and risk of sudden death in patients with hypertrophic cardiomyopathy. J Am Coll Cardiol 2003;41:315–321.

138. Varnava AM, Elliott PM, Baboonian C, et al. Hypertrophic cardiomyopathy: Histopathological features of sudden death in cardiac troponin T disease. Circulation 2001; 104:1380–1384.

139. Niimura H, Patton KK, McKenna WJ, et al. Sarcomere protein gene mutations in hypertrophic cardiomyopathy of the elderly. Circulation 2002;105:446–451.

140. Lim D-S, Roberts R, Marian AJ. Expression profiling of cardiac genes in human hypertrophic cardiomyopathy: Insight into the pathogenesis of phenotypes. J Am Coll Cardiol 2001; 38:1175–1180.

141. Berul CI, Christe ME, Aronovitz MJ, et al. Electrophysioiical abnormalities and arrhythmias in aMHC mutant familial hypertrophic cardiomyopathy mice. J Clin Invest 1997;99:570–576.

142. Watkins H, Rosenzweig A, Hwang D, et al. Characteristics and prognostic implications of myosin missense mutations in familial hypertrophic cardiomyopathy. N Engl J Med 1992; 326:1108–1114.

143. Child JS, Perloff JK. Myocardial myotonia in myotonic muscular dystrophy. Am Heart J 1995;129:982–990.

144. Grigg LE, Chan W, Mond HG, Vohra JK, Downey WF. Ventricular tachycardia and sudden death in myotonic dystrophy: clinical, electrophysiologic and pathologic features. J Am Coll Cardiol 1985;6:254–256.

145. Hiromasa S, Ikeda T, Kubota K, et al. Ventricular tachycardia and sudden death in myotonic dystrophy. Am Heart J 1988; 115:914–917.

146. Umeda Y, Ikeda U, Yamamoto J, et al. Myotonic dystrophy associated with QT prolongation and torsade de points. Clin Cardiol 1999;22:136–138.

147. Moorman JR, Coleman RE, Packer DL, et al. Cardiac involvement in myotonic muscular dystrophy. Medicine 1984; 64:371–387.

148. Buxton J, Shelbourne P, Davies J, et al. Detection of an unstable fragment of DNA specific to individuals with myotonic dystrophy. Nature 1992;355:547–548.

149. Harley HG, Brook JD, Rundle SA, et al. Expansion of an unstable DNA region and phenotypic variation in myotonic dystrophy. Nature 1992;535:545–546.

150. Hayasji Y, Ikeda U, Kojo T, et al. Cardiac abnormalities and cytosine-thymine-guanine trinucleotide repeats in myotonic dystrophy. Am Heart J 1997;134:292–297.

151. Brunner HG, Nillesen W, van Oost BA, et al. Presymptomatic diagnosis of myotonic dystorphy. J Med Genet 1992;29:780–784.

152. Muntoni F, Cau M, Ganau A, Conjiu R, Arvedi G, Mateddu A, Marrosu MG, Cianchetti C, Realdi G, Cao A, et., al. Deletion of the dystrophin muscle-promoter region associated with X-linked dilated cardiomyopathy. N Engl J Med 1993;329: 921–931.

153. Fishbein MC, Siegel RJ, Thompson CE, Hopkins LC. Sudden death of a carrier of x-linded Emery-Dreifuss Muscular Dystrophy. Ann Intern Med 1993;119:900–905.

154. Woelfel AK, Cascio WE, Smith SW. Cerebral embolization in two young patients with fascioscapulohumeral muscular dystrophy and atrial dysrhythmias. Am Heart J 1989;118:632–633.

155. MacIntyre K, Stewart S, Capewell S, et al. Gender and survival: A population-based study of 201,114 men and women following a first acute myocardial infarction. J Am Coll Cardiol 2001; 38:729–735.

156. Jousilahti P, Vartianinen E, Tuomilehto J, Puska P. Sex, age cardiovascular risk factors, and coronary heart disease. A prospective follow-up study of 14,786 middle-aged men and women in Finland. Circulation 1999;99:1165–1172.

157. Lee T-M, Su S-F, Chou T-F, Tsai C-H. Pharmacologic preconditioning of estrogen by activation of the myocardial adenosine triphosphate-sensitive potassium channel in patients undergoing coronary angioplasty. J Am Coll Cardiol 2002;39:871–877.

158. Ranki HJ, Budas GR, Crawford RM, Jovanovi A. Gender-specific difference in cardiac ATP-sensitive K^+ channels. J Am Coll Cardiol 2001;38:906–915.

159. Ranki HJ, Budas GR, Crawford RM, Davies AM, Jovanovic A. 17b-estradiol regulates expression of KATP channels in heart-derived H9c2 cells. J Am Coll Cardiol 2002;40:367–374.

160. Curl CL, Went IR, Kotsanas G. Effects of gender on intracellular $[Ca^{2+}]$ in rat cardiac myocytes. Pflügers Arch 2001;441:709–716.

161. Kim C, Fahrenbruch CE, Cobb LA, Eisenberg MS. Out-of-hospital cardiac arrest in men and women. Circulation 2001;104:2699–2703.

162. Du X-J, Riemersma RA, Dart AM. Cardiovascular protection by oestrogen is partly mediated through modulation of autonomic nervous function. Cardiovasc Res 1995; 30:161–165.

163. Ryan SM, Goldberger AL, Pincus SM, Mietus J, Lipsitz LA. Gender- and age-related differences in heart rate dynamics: Are women more complex than men? J Am Coll Cardiol 1994; 24:1700–1707.

164. Minson CT, Halliwill JR, Young TM, Joyner MJ. Influence of the menstrual cycle on sympathetic activity baroreflex sensitivity, and vascular transduction in young women. Circulation 2000;101:862–868.

165. Yildirir A, Kabakci G, Yarali H, et al. Effects of hormone replacement therapy on heart rate variability in postmenopausal women. Ann Noninvasive Electrocardiol 2001;6:280–284.

166. Huikur HV, Pikkujämsä SM, Airaksinen J, et al. Sex-related differences in autonomic modulation of heart rate in middle-aged subjects. Circulation 1996;94:122–125.

167. Hunt BE, Taylor JA, Hamner JW, Gagnon M, Lipsitz LA. Estrogen replacement therapy improves baroreflex regulation of vascular sympathetic outflow in postmenopausal women. Circulation 2001;103:2909–2914.

168. De Beer EL, Keizer HA. Direct action of estradiol-17 beta on the atrial action potential. Steroids 1982;40:223–231.

169. Tanabe S, Hata T, Hiraoka M. Effects of estrogen on action potential and membrane currents in guinea pig ventricular myoctyes. Am J Physiol 1999;277:H826–H833.

170. Tse H-F, Oral H, Pelosi F, et al. Effect of gender on atrial electrophysiologic changes induced by rapid atrial pacing and elevation of atrial pressure. J Cardiovasc Electrophysiol 2001;12:986–989.

171. Drici MD, Clément N. Is gender a risk factor for adverse drug reactions? Drug Saf 2001;24:1–24.

172. Drici MD, Knollmann BC, Wang WX, Woosley RL. Cardiac actions of erythromycin: influence of female sex. JAMA 1998;280:1774–1776.

173. Liu XK, Katchman A, Drici MD, et al. Gender difference in the cycle length-dependent qT and potassium currents in rabbits. J Pharmacol Exp Ther 1998;285:672–679.

174. Pham TV, Sosunov EA, Anyukhovsky EP, Danilo P, Rosen M. Testosterone diminishes the proarrhythmic effects of dofetilide in normal female rabbits. Circulation 2002;106:2132–2136.

175. Drici M-D, Baker L, Plan P, et al. Mice display sex differences in halothane-induced polymorphic ventricular tachycardia. Circulation 2002;106:497–503.

176. Antzelevitch C, Brugada P, Brugada J, et al. The Brugada Syndrome. Armonk, NY: Futura Publishing Co, 1999.

177. Di Deigo JM, Cordeiro JM, Goodrow RJ, et al. Ionic and cellular basis for the predominance of the Brugada Syndrome phenotype in males. Circulation 2002;106:2004–2011.

178. Song M, Helguera G, Eghbali M, et al. Remodeling of Kv4.3 potassium channel gene expression under the control of sex hormones. J Biol Chem 2001;276:31883–31890.

179. Liao Y, Cooper RS, McGee DL, Mensah GA, Ghali JK. The relative effects of left ventricular hypertrophy, coronary artery disease, and ventricular dyfunction on survival among black adults. JAMA 1995;273:1592–1597.

180. Thomas J, Thomas DJ, Pearson T, Klag M, Mead L. Cardiovascular disease in African American and white physicians: the Meharry cohort and Meharry-Hopkins cohort studies. J Health Care Poor Underserved 1997;8:270–284.

181. Becker LB, Han BH, Mayer PM, et al. Racial differences in the incidence of cardiac arrest and subsequent survival. The CPR Chicago Project. N Engl J Med 1993;329:600–606.

182. Burke AP, Farb A, Pestaner J, et al. Traditional risk factors and the incidence of sudden coronary death with and without coronary thrombosis in blacks. Circulation 2002;105:419–424.

183. Traven ND, Kuller LH, Ivers DG, Rutan GH, Perper JA. Coronary heart disease mortality and sudden death among the 35 - 44 year age group in Allegheny County, Pennsylvania. Ann Epidemiol 1996;6:130–136.

184. Doherty TM, Tang W, Detrano RC. Racial differences in the significance of coronary calcium in asymptomatic black and white subjects with coronary risk factors. J Am Coll Cardiol 1999;34:787–794.

185. Simpson RJJ, Cascio WE, Schreiner PJ, et al. Prevalence of premature ventricular contractions in a population of African American and white men and women: The Atherosclerosis Risk in Communities [ARIC] Study. Am Heart J 2002;143:535–540.

186. Abbott GW, Sesti F, Splawski I, et al. MiRP1 forms IKr potassium channels with HERG and is associated with cardiac arrhythmia. Cell 1999;97:175–187.

187. Napolitano C, Schwartz PJ, Brown AM, et al. Evidence for a cardiac ion channel mutation underlying drug-induced QT prolongation and life-threatening arrhythmias. J Cardiovasc Electrophysiol 2000;11:691–696.

188. Yang P, Kanki H, Drolet B, et al. Allelic variants in long-QT disease genes in patients with drug-associated torsades de pointes. Circulation 2002;105:1943–1948.

189. Wei J, Yang IC, Tapper AR, et al. KCNE1 polymorphism confers risk of drug-induced long QT syndrome by altering kinetic properties of IKs potassium channels. Circulation 1999; :I-495.

190. Splawski I, Timothy KW, Tateyama M, et al. Variant of SCN5A sodium channels implicated in risk of cardiac arrhythmia. Science 2002;297:1333–1336.

191. Makita N, Horie M, Nakamura T, et al. Drug-induced long-QT syndrome associated with a subclinical SCN5a mutation. Circulation 2002;106:1269–1274.

192. Group MRFITR. Baseline rest electrocardiographic abnormalities, antihypertensive treatment, and mortality in the Multiple Risk Factor Intervention Trial. Am J Cardiol 1985;55:1–15.

193. Siscovick DS, Raghunathan TE, Psaty BM, et al. Diuretic therapy for hypertension and the risk of primary cardiac arrest. N Engl J Med 1994;330:1852–1857.

194. Cooper HA, Dries DL, Davis CE, Shen YL, Domanski MJ. Diuretics and risk of arrhythmic death in patients with left ventricular dysfunction. Circulation 1999;100:1311–1315.

195. Tai CT, Chiou CW, Chen SA. Interaction between the autonomic nervous system and atrial tachyarrhythmias. J Cardiovasc Electrophysiol 2002;13:83–87.

196. Huikuri HV, Seppanen T, Koistinen MJ. Abnormalities in beat to beat dynamics of heart rate before the spontaneous onset of the life threatening ventricular tachyarrhythmias in patients with prior myocardial infarction. Circulation 1996;93:1839–1844.

197. Olgin JE, Sih HJ, Hanish S, et al. Heterogeneous atrial denervation creates substrate for sustained atrial fibrillation. Circulation 1998; 98:2608–2614.

198. Dae MW, Lee RJ, Ursell PC, et al. Heterogeneous sympathetic innervation in German Shepherd dogs with inherited ventricular arrhythmia and sudden cardiac death. Circulation 1997;96:1337–1342.

199. Schwartz PJ. Sympathetic imbalance and cardiac arrhythmias. In: Randall WE, ed. Nervous Control of Cardiovascular Function. New York Oxford University Press, 1984:225–251.

200. Barron HV, Lesh MD. Autonomic nervous system and sudden cardiac death. J Am Coll Cardiol 1996;27:1053–1060.

201. De Ferrai GM, Vanoli E, Stramba-Badiale M, et al. Vagal reflexes and survival during acute myocardial ischemia in conscious dogs with a healed myocardial infarction. Am J Physiol 1991;261:H63–H69.

202. Vanoli E, De Ferrari GM, Stramba-Badiale M, et al. Vagal stimulation and prevention of sudden death in conscious dogs with a healed myocardial infarction. Circ Res 1991; 68:1471–1481.

203. Warner MR. Autonomic neural modulation of extracellular concentration during myocardial ischemia. In: Zipes DP, Jalife J, eds. Cardiac Electrophysiology: From Cell to the Bedside. Philadelphia: Saunders, 1995:460–466.

204. Elvan A, Rubart M, Zipes DP. Nitric oxide modulates autonomic effects on spontaneous sinus discharge rate and atrioventricular nodal conduction in open chest anesthetized dogs. Am J Physiol 1997;272:H263–H271.

205. Fei L, Baron A, Henry DP, Zipes DP. Intrapericardial delivery of L-arginine reduces the increased severity of ventricular arrhythmias in dogs with acute coronary occlusion. Nitric oxide modulates sympathetic effects on ventricular electrophysiologic properties. Circulation 1997;96:4044–4049.

206. Challapalli S, Kadish AH, Horvath G, Goldberger JJ. Differential effects of parasympathetic blockade and parasympathetic withdrawal on heart rate variability. J Cardiovasc Electrophysiol 1999;10:1192–1199.

207. Umetani K, Singer DH, McCraty R, Atkinson M. Twenty-four hour time domain heart rate variability and heart rate: relations to age and gender over nine decades. J Am Coll Cardiol 1998; 31:593–601.

208. Fluckiger L, Boivin JM, Quilliot D, Jeandel C, Zannad F. Differential effects of aging on heart rate variability and blood pressure variability. J Gerontol 1999;54:B219–224.

209. Luscher TF, Dohi Y, Tschudi M. Endothelium-dependent regulation of resistance arteries: alterations with aging and hypertension. J Cardiovasc Pharmacol 1992;5:S34–42.

210. Liao D, Sloan RP, Cascio WE, et al. Multiple metabolic syndrome is associated with lower heart rate variability. The Atherosclerosis Risk in Communities Study. Diabetes Care 1998;21:2116–2122.

211. Christensen JH, Toft E, Christensen MS, Schmidt EB. Heart rate variability and plasma lipids in men with and without ischaemic heart disease. Atherosclerosis 1999;145:181–186.

212. Huikuri HV, Jokinen V, Syvanne M, et al. Heart rate variability and progression of coronary atherosclerosis. Arteriosclerosis Thromb Vasc Biol 1999;19:1979–1985.

213. Anderson KP, Shusterman V, Aysin B, et al. dynamics preceding two modes of onset of spontaneous sustained ventricular tachycardia. (ESVEM) Investigators. Electrophysiologic Study Versus Electrocardiographic Monitoring. J Cardiovasc Electrophysiol 1999;10:897–904.

214. Lavery CE, Mittleman MA, Cohen MC, Muller JE, Verrier RL. Nonuniform nighttime distribution of acute cardiac events. A possible effect sleep states. Circulation 1997; 96:3321–3327.

215. Verrier RL, Muller JE, Hobson JA. Sleep, dreams, and sudden death: the case for sleep as an autonomic stress test for the heart. Cardiovasc Res 1996;31:181–211.

216. Hu FB, Bronner L, Willett WC, et al. Fish and omega-3 fatty acid intake and risk of coronary heart disease in women. JAMA 2002;287:1815–1821.

217. Albert CM, Hennekens CH, O'Donnell C, et al. Fish consumption and risk of sudden cardiac death. JAMA 1998;279: 23–28.

218. Albert CM, Campos H, Stampfer MJ, et al. Blood levels of long-chain n-3 fatty acids and the risk of sudden death. N Engl J Med 2002;346:1113–1118.

219. Marchioli R, Barzi F, Bomba E, et al. Early protection against sudden death by n-3 polyunsaturated fatty acids after myocardial infarction. Gruppo Italiano per lo Studio della Sopravvivenza nell'Infarto Miocardioco (GISSI)-Prevenzione. Circulation 2002;105:1897–1903.

220. Billman GE, Kang JX, Leaf A. Prevention of sudden cardiac death of dietary pure w–3 polyunsaturated fatty acids in dogs. Circulation 1999;99:2452–2457.

221. Xiao YF, Kang JX, Morgan JP, Leaf A. Blocking effects of polyunsaturated fatty acids on Na+ channels of neonatal rat ventricular myocytes. Proc Natl Acad Sci USA 1995;92: 11000–11004.

222. Xiao YF, Gomez AM, Morgan JP, Lederer WJ, Leaf A. Suppression of voltage-gated L-type Ca2+ currents by polyunsatured fatty acids in adult and neonatal rat ventricular myocytes. Proc Natl Acad Sci USA 1997;94::4182–4187.

223. Tansey MJ, Opie LH. Relation between plasma free fatty acids and arrhythmias within the first twelve hours of acute myocardial infarction. Lancet 1983;20:419–422.

224. Greene HL. Sudden arrhythmic cardiac death: mechanisms, resuscitation and classification: the Seattle perspective. Am J Cardiol 1990;65:4B–12B.

225. Tansey MJ, Opie LH. Relation between plasma free fatty acids and arrhythmias within the first twelve hours of acute myocardial infarction. Lancet 1983;20:419–422.

226. Oliver MF, Kurein VA, Greenwood TW. Relation between serum-free-fatty acids and arrhythmias and death after acute myocardial infarction. Lancet 1968;1:710–715.

227. Jouven X, Charles M-A, Desnos M, Ducimetiére P. Circulating nonesterified fatty acid levels as a predictive risk factor for sudden death in the population. Circulation 2001;104: 756–761.

228. Lemaitre RN, King IB, Raghunathan TE, et al. Cell membrane trans-fatty acids and the risk of primary cardiac arrest. Circulation 2002;105:697–701.

229. Murnaghan MF. Effect of fatty acids on the ventricular arrhythmia threshold in the isolated heart of the rabbit. Br J Pharmacol 1981;73:909–915.

230. Wang DW, Yazawa K, Makita N, George Jr AL, Bennett PB. Pharmacological targeting of long QT mutant sodium channels. J Clin Invest 1997;99:1714–1720.

20 Gene Therapy for Cardiac Arrhythmias

J. Kevin Donahue, MD and Eduardo Marbán, MD, PhD

Contents

INTRODUCTION

Despite recent advances in the treatment of atherosclerosis and congestive heart failure, morbidity and mortality from cardiac disease continue to be a significant problem in the developed world. Cardiac rhythm disorders contribute substantially to this problem. In the United States, cardiac arrest accounts for at least 220,000 deaths per year, more than 10% of the total deaths for the entire country *(1)*. Atrial fibrillation affects more than 2 million people in the United States, including 5–10% of people over the age of 65 and 10–35% of the 5 million patients with congestive heart failure *(2)*. Furthermore, other types of arrhythmias account for thousands of emergency room visits and hospital admissions each year.

The lack of effective treatment options for common arrhythmias contributes to the continued prevalence of arrhythmic disease. Modern treatment of cardiac arrhythmias is limited to pharmacotherapy, radiofrequency ablation, and implantable devices. Although effective at reducing some arrhythmic events, antiarrhythmic medications often have adverse systemic effects, and their proarrhythmic tendencies may increase mortality in many situations *(3)*. Radiofrequency ablation cures a limited number of arrhythmias and has become standard treatment for patients with atrioventricular (AV) node reentry tachycardia, accessory pathway–mediated tachycardia, and atrial flutter. Recent advances in technology have expanded the indications for ablation; however, the most problematic arrhythmias, atrial fibrillation and infarct-related ventricular tachycardia, are not effectively managed with ablation. Device-based therapies (pacemakers and defibrillators) correct bradyarrhythmias and can be lifesaving for patients with tachyarrhythmias; however, devices do not completely emulate normal sinus nodal function for patients with bradyarrhythmias, and they do not prevent tachyarrhythmias. In addition, devices are associated with a lifetime commitment to repeated procedures, significant expense, and potentially catastrophic complications such as infection, cardiac perforation, and lead failure.

Over the last several decades, tremendous advances have been made in understanding the pathophysiologic and genetic bases of cardiac arrhythmias. These advances, coupled with the inadequacies of current treatment options for cardiac arrhythmias, have prompted the search for genetic strategies to treat these common diseases. In this review, we will discuss the underlying pathophysiology of arrhythmias and the current status of gene therapy for the treatment of arrhythmias.

NORMAL CARDIAC ELECTROPHYSIOLOGY

The cellular basis for all cardiac electrical activity is the action potential (AP). The AP is usually divided into five phases *(0–4)* (Fig. 1). Each phase is defined by the cellular membrane potential and the activity of ion

From: *Contemporary Cardiology: Principles of Molecular Cardiology*
Edited by: M. S. Runge and C. Patterson © Humana Press Inc., Totowa, NJ

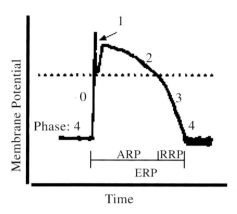

Fig. 1. Morphology of the ventricular action potential showing the different phases of the action potential. ARP, absolute refractory period; ERP, effective refractory period; RRP, relative refractory period.

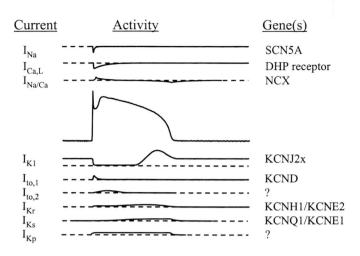

Fig. 2. Ionic current names, activities, and the gene associated with the different phases of the action potential. The dotted line is the zero-current marker. Deflections above the line are outward currents and deflections below the line are inward currents. Modified with permission from Tomaselli and Marban *(11)*.

channels that affect that potential. Phase 4 is the resting baseline. During this phase, the dominant ionic current is the inward rectifier potassium current, I_{K1}. Phase 0 is the initial membrane depolarization initiated by activation of the sodium current, I_{NA}. Phase 1 is a quick dip in the potential from the peak achieved at the end of phase 0. Activation of transient outward potassium (I_{to1}) and chloride (I_{to2}) currents and inactivation of the sodium current are responsible for phase 1 of the AP. During phase 2, the plateau period, the L-type calcium current ($I_{Ca,L}$) maintains the positive depolarization, and the rapid and slow components of the delayed rectifier potassium current (I_{Kr} and I_{Ks}) try to force repolarization. In phase 3, the potassium current ultimately dominates; the calcium current is inactivated; and the membrane potential returns to the baseline of phase 4. The membrane potential during each phase of the AP is an unsteady equilibrium between positive and negative currents, and any slight perturbation of this balance can affect the shape of the AP and potentially cause an arrhythmia. The genes responsible for most of the currents participating in the AP have been identified (Fig. 2), and mutations of these genes cause several inherited arrhythmias.

In the later stages of phase 4, normal atrial and ventricular cells are quiescent but can generate an AP if stimulated by an adjacent cell. Specialized conducting tissue in the sinoatrial (SA) node, the AV node, and the His–Purkinje system has intrinsic automaticity; therefore, these cells gradually depolarize during phase 4 until they reach a membrane potential that activates I_{NA}, at which point an AP is started. Because the cells in the SA node usually depolarize at a faster rate, the normal cardiac impulse radiates from the SA node. All cells are refractory to stimulation during phases 1–3 of the AP (Fig. 1).

In the later part of phase 3, a stronger than normal pulse can generate an AP, so this portion of the cardiac cycle is called the relative refractory period. Because cells are impervious to excitation during phases 1 and 2 and the early part of phase 3, this part of the cycle is called the absolute refractory period. The effective refractory period comprises the entire period during which the generation of an AP is impaired.

The AP is transmitted from one cell to the next via gap junctions. Within cardiac tissue, the direction of current flow is anisotropic (e.g., current flow in a longitudinal direction is faster than flow in a transverse direction) because of the distribution of gap junctions. Of the gap junction connections, about 20% are side-to-side, 33% are end-to-end, and the remaining 47% are end-to-side *(4)*. The average myocyte is connected to about 10 neighboring myocytes.

PATHOPHYSIOLOGY OF INHERITED ARRHYTHMIAS

The Long QT Syndrome

The long QT syndrome was the first arrhythmic disorder characterized at the genetic level. In genetic studies of the long QT syndrome, several potassium channel subunits have been identified, and the interactions of components of the AP are now better understood. The syndrome has been associated with mutations of the sodium channel a-subunit gene and mutations of the genes for several potassium channel subunits (Table 1). The underlying

Table 1
Long QT Syndrome Genes and Channels

Subtype (Ref)	Chr	Gene	Channel	Incidence
LQT1 (24)	11	KCNQ1	I_{Ks} α subunit	Approx 50%
LQT2 (25)	7	KCNH1	I_{Kr} α subunit	30–40%
LQT3 (26)	3	SCN5A	I_{Na} α subunit	5–10%
LQT4* (27)	4	Ankyrin-B	Structural protein	rare
LQT5 (28)	21	KCNE1	I_{Ks} β subunit	rare
LQT6 (29)	21	KCNE2	I_{Kr} β subunit	rare
LQT7*	—	—	—	rare

*Neither gene nor protein for LQT4 or LQT7 has been described.

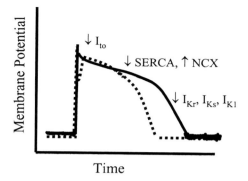

Fig. 3. Schematic of changes in the ventricular action potential in heart failure. A decrease in several potassium currents causes a loss of the notch (phase 1) and a prolongation of the action potential duration. The broken line is a normal ventricular action potential and the solid line is the altered action potential seen in heart failure. NCX, Na^{2+}/Ca^{2+} exchange; SERCA, sarcoendoplasmic reticulum calcium ATPase.

physiological defect associated with all of these mutations is an extension of the plateau phase (phase 2) of the AP. Depolarization is extended in the plateau phase because there is either a reduction in one of the potassium currents or an absence of inactivation of the sodium current. The end result is an increase in the propensity for ventricular arrhythmias from after-depolarizations or heterogeneous repolarization. Priori et al. (5) have reviewed the genetics and pathophysiology of the long QT syndrome.

The Brugada Syndrome

The Brugada syndrome, an inherited arrhythmia, is characterized by idiopathic ventricular fibrillation in patients with structurally normal hearts but with right bundle branch block pattern and ST-segment elevation in ECG leads V1–3 (6). The Brugada syndrome, like one variant of the long QT syndrome, is associated with mutations in the cardiac sodium channel gene; however, the sodium channel mutations in the Brugada syndrome are associated with a loss of sodium channel function, whereas the mutations in the long QT syndrome cause a gain of sodium channel function. The reduction in sodium current prolongs conduction time from the bundle of His to the ventricle (7). In addition, the changes in sodium current alter the balance of depolarizing and repolarizing forces. This shift is most apparent in the epicardial layer where the transient outward potassium current is relatively robust. The heterogeneity in repolarization leads to the characteristic ST-segment changes seen in the Brugada syndrome and presumably underlies the risk of ventricular fibrillation in these patients (8).

Other Inherited Arrhythmia Syndromes

Mutations in the gene for the cardiac ryanodine receptor have been described and characterized in patients with catecholaminergic polymorphic ventricular tachycardia

(VT) (9). In addition, Andersen's syndrome, a rare condition that includes periodic paralysis, cardiac arrhythmias, and several dysmorphic features, is caused by mutations in the gene for the inward rectifier channel, Kir2.1. These mutations cause loss of function and dominant negative effects on the inward rectifier current (I_{K1}) (10). Patients with catecholaminergic polymorphic VT frequently present with stress-related syncope, and VT induced with exercise or catecholamine stimulation is often seen on evaluation. The effects of the ryanodine receptor defects on function have not been studied.

PATHOPHYSIOLOGY OF COMMON CARDIAC ARRHYTHMIAS

Sudden Death in Congestive Heart Failure

Sudden death in patients with congestive heart failure is common. The associated arrhythmia is often polymorphic VT, which leads to ventricular fibrillation and death. When observable, the type of VT seen in these patients is similar to that observed in patients with the congenital long QT syndrome. Animal studies have shown similarities between these two diseases on a tissue and cellular level. In both conditions, heterogeneous increases in the action potential duration (APD) are consistently seen (Fig. 3). In heart failure, prolongation of the APD correlates with downregulation of several potassium currents: the transient outward current I_{to}, the inward rectifier current I_{K1}, and the delayed rectifier currents I_{Ks} and I_{Kr}. The plateau of the cardiac AP is an unstable equilibrium; even small changes in inward or outward currents can markedly delay repolarization. The reduction in potassium current

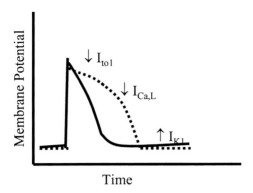

Fig. 4. Schematic of changes in the atrial action potential after prolonged atrial fibrillation. Reduction in the transient outward current, I_{to}, and the l-type calcium current, $I_{Ca,L}$, result in a decreased notch and plateau. The broken line is a normal atrial action potential, and the solid line is the action potential after prolonged atrial fibrillation.

seen in heart failure could explain the prolongation of the APD and the increase in surface ECG repolarization time. The similarities between heart failure and the long QT syndrome suggest that alterations in the potassium current underlie the arrhythmic risk; therefore, correcting the potassium channel deficit may reduce the incidence of sudden death. Ion channel alterations in heart failure are discussed in the review by Tomaselli and Marban *(11)*.

Atrial Fibrillation

Unlike the rapid hemodynamic instability and death associated with VT in heart failure, atrial fibrillation (AF) can be sustained for long periods of time since the cellular adaptive processes that occur with AF differ from those seen with heart failure. During sustained AF, the APD and refractory period shorten (Fig. 4). Clinical and experimental studies of changes in AP morphology have shown a 70% downregulation of the L-type Ca^{2+} and transient outward currents and an upregulation of the inward rectifier and adenosine/acetylcholine activated potassium currents *(12–14)*. These changes improve the ability of the atrial myocytes to sustain the rapid and chaotic impulses characteristic of AF. This situation creates a cycle in which the rapid rate causes a shortened refractory period that allows the rapid rate to continue. This process has been called "AF begets AF." The maladaptive nature of the ion channel alterations suggests that interrupting these changes on a molecular level may be a potential treatment for AF. A comprehensive discussion of the molecular changes in atrial fibrillation can be found in the review by Nattel and Li *(15)*.

GENE THERAPY FOR THE TREATMENT OF CARDIAC ARRHYTHMIAS

The study of gene therapy in the treatment of cardiac arrhythmias is in its infancy, and only one report on the in vivo use of gene therapy has been published *(16)*. Furthermore, the number of reports of in vitro gene transfer to study the cellular mechanisms of arrhythmia is limited. The general premise of gene therapy for arrhythmias is that an understanding of the basic principles of cellular electrophysiology can be used to develop therapy to target specific genes. Initial studies in isolated cardiac ventricular myocytes have shown that AP morphology can be altered *(17)*. Early efforts were directed toward the I_{to} current, which is reduced in heart failure, but overexpression of this current caused an unusual and overly shortened AP. Overexpressing the I_{Kr} current led to a more normal-appearing AP *(18)*; the kinetics of I_{Kr} include a later onset of action, which allows more time for normal phases 1–3 of the AP than is possible with the early acting I_{to} current. These studies have shown that the kinetics of the ion channels may be more important than replacing specific downregulated currents. The strategy of replacing downregulated currents may be feasible if gene expression levels can be sufficiently controlled to replicate the normal level of current.

In the only report of the in vivo use of gene transfer for treatment of an arrhythmia, $G\alpha_{i2}$ (the α-subunit of an inhibitory G protein) was targeted for overexpression in the AV node in a porcine model. The ventricular rate decreased by 15–20% during AF, both in the drug-free state and after administration of epinephrine (1 mg, intravenously) (Fig. 5). In this porcine model of acute AF, we infused the adenoviruses Adβgal and AdGi into the AV nodal artery. Adβgal, an adenovirus encoding *Escherichia coli* β-galactosidase, was used as a reporter to document the extent of gene transfer. In addition, Adβgal was used as a control to identify nonspecific effects of adenovirus infection and gene transfer in the AV node. AdGi, which encodes Gα, was the therapeutic virus. Vascular endothelial growth factor and nitroglycerin were infused into the AV nodal artery before administration of the virus to increase the efficiency of gene transfer *(19,20)*. In Adβgal-infected hearts, gene transfer to AV nodal myocytes was 45%, and no effects on AV nodal function were seen; however, a limited mononuclear inflammatory infiltrate was noted. Infection with AdGi slowed conduction through the AV node and ultimately reduced the heart rate during acute AF.

The current problems associated with gene therapy for arrhythmias relate to homogeneous delivery of the vector

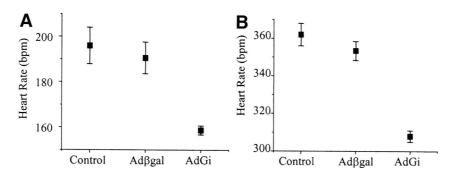

Fig. 5. Ventricular rate after acute induction of atrial fibrillation in a porcine model of gene therapy. Adenovirus was perfused into the atrioventricular nodal artery at baseline. Heart rate was measured after burst-pacing induction of atrial fibrillation at baseline and 7 d later during (**A**) the drug-free state and (**B**) after intravenous administration of 1 mg epinephrine.

to the target tissue, control of gene expression, evaluation of potentially toxic effects of the vector or the transgene, elimination of non-target organ gene transfer, and control of host immune responses. Studies in multiple areas are being conducted to address these problems. Recent studies in vector design have documented the ability of adeno-associated virus and helper–dependent adenovirus vectors to sustain long-term gene expression and to reduce host immune responses *(21,22)*. Methods used to increase microvascular permeability to vectors have improved efficacy and homogeneity of gene delivery *(20)*. Situation-specific promoters or response elements that become activated in response to hypoxia, temperature, and steroid or drug exposure have been identified *(23)* and suggest that the timing and amount of gene expression can be controlled.

CONCLUSIONS

Cardiac arrhythmias are a significant cause of morbidity and mortality in the developed world. The cellular and subcellular mechanisms involved in arrhythmias are being defined, but much is still unknown. The use of gene therapy for treating arrhythmias is promising, but concentrated efforts to solve well-documented problems are necessary. The pathophysiology of arrhythmias and the mechanics of gene therapy must be well understood before gene therapy becomes a viable option for the treatment of arrhythmias.

REFERENCES

1. American Heart Association. 2001 Heart and Stroke Statistical Update. Dallas, TX: American Heart Association, 2000.
2. Chugh SS, Blackshear JL, Shen WK, Hammill SC, Gersh BJ. Epidemiology and natural history of atrial fibrillation: clinical implications. J Am Coll Cardiol 2001;37:371–378.
3. Echt DS, Liebson PR, Mitchell LB, et al. Mortality and morbidity in patients receiving encainide, flecainide, or placebo.

The Cardiac Arrhythmia Suppression Trial. N Engl J Med 1991;324:781–788.
4. Beyer E, Veenstra R, Kanter H, et al. Molecular structure and patterns of expression of cardiac gap junction proteins. In: Zipes D, Jalife J, eds. Cardiac Electrophysiology: From cell to bedside. 2 ed. Philadelphia: W.B. Saunders Co., 1995:31–37.
5. Priori SG, Bloise R, Crotti L. The long QT syndrome. Europace 2001;3:16–27.
6. Brugada P, Brugada J. Right bundle branch block, persistent ST segment elevation and sudden cardiac death: a distinct clinical and electrocardiographic syndrome. A multicenter report. J Am Coll Cardiol 1992;20:1391–1396.
7. Alings M, Wilde A. "Brugada" syndrome: clinical data and suggested pathophysiological mechanism. Circulation 1999;99: 666–673.
8. Yan GX, Antzelevitch C. Cellular basis for the Brugada syndrome and other mechanisms of arrhythmogenesis associated with ST-segment elevation. Circulation 1999;100: 1660–1666.
9. Priori SG, Napolitano C, Tiso N, et al. Mutations in the cardiac ryanodine receptor gene (hRyR2) underlie catecholaminergic polymorphic ventricular tachycardia. Circulation 2001;103: 196–200.
10. Plaster NM, Tawil R, Tristani-Firouzi M, et al. Mutations in Kir2.1 cause the developmental and episodic electrical phenotypes of Andersen's syndrome. Cell 2001;105:511–519.
11. Tomaselli GF, Marban E. Electrophysiological remodeling in hypertrophy and heart failure. Cardiovasc Res 1999;42: 270–283.
12. Bosch RF, Zeng X, Grammer JB, Popovic K, Mewis C, Kuhlkamp V. Ionic mechanisms of electrical remodeling in human atrial fibrillation. Cardiovasc Res 1999;44:121–131.
13. Workman AJ, Kane KA, Rankin AC. The contribution of ionic currents to changes in refractoriness of human atrial myocytes associated with chronic atrial fibrillation. Cardiovasc Res 2001; 52:226–235.
14. Yue L, Feng J, Gaspo R, Li GR, Wang Z, Nattel S. Ionic remodeling underlying action potential changes in a canine model of atrial fibrillation. Circ Res 1997;81:512–525.
15. Nattel S, Li D. Ionic remodeling in the heart: pathophysiological significance and new therapeutic opportunities for atrial fibrillation. Circ Res 2000;87:440–447.
16. Donahue JK, Heldman AW, Fraser H, et al. Focal modification of electrical conduction in the heart by viral gene transfer. Nat Med 2000;6:1395–1398.

17. Nuss HB, Johns DC, Kaab S, et al. Reversal of potassium channel deficiency in cells from failing hearts by adenoviral gene transfer: a prototype for gene therapy for disorders of cardiac excitability and contractility. Gene Ther 1996; 3:900–912.

18. Nuss HB, Marban E, Johns DC. Overexpression of a human potassium channel suppresses cardiac hyperexcitability in rabbit ventricular myocytes. J Clin Invest 1999;103:889–896.

19. Nagata K, Marban E, Lawrence JH, Donahue JK. Phosphodiesterase inhibitor-mediated potentiation of adenovirus delivery to myocardium. J Mol Cell Cardiol 2001; 33:575–580.

20. Donahue JK, Kikkawa K, Thomas AD, Marban E, Lawrence H. Acceleration of widespread adenoviral gene transfer to intact rabbit hearts by coronary perfusion with low calcium and serotonin. Gene Ther 1998;5:630–634.

21. Monahan PE, Samulski RJ. AAV vectors: is clinical success on the horizon? Gene Ther 2000;7:24–30.

22. Chen HH, Mack LM, Kelly R, Ontell M, Kochanek S, Clemens PR. Persistence in muscle of an adenoviral vector that lacks all viral genes. Proc Natl Acad Sci USA 1997;94:1645–1650.

23. Fussenegger M. The impact of mammalian gene regulation concepts on functional genomic research, metabolic engineering, and advanced gene therapies. Biotechnol Prog 2001;17:1–51.

24. Wang J, Ma Y, Knechtle SJ. Adenovirus-mediated gene transfer into rat cardiac allografts: comparison of direct injection and perfusion. Transplantation 1996;61:1726–1729.

25. Curran ME, Splawski I, Timothy KW, Vincent GM, Green ED, Keating MT. A molecular basis for cardiac arrhythmia: HERG mutations cause long QT syndrome. Cell 1995;80:795–803.

26. Wang Q, Shen J, Splawski I. SCN5A mutations associated with an inherited cardiac arrhythmia, long QT syndrome. Cell 1995; 80:805–811.

27. Mohler PJ, Schott JJ, Gramolino AO, et al. Ankyrin-B mutation causes type 4 long QT cardiac arrhythmia and sudden death. Nature 2003; 421: 634–639.

28. Schulze-Bahr E, Wang Q, Wedekind H, et al. KCNE1 mutations cause jervell and Lange-Nielsen syndrome. Nat Genet 1997;17: 267–268.

29. Abbott G, Sesti F, Splawski I, et al. MiRP1 forms IKR potassium channels with HERG and is associated with cardiac arrhythmia. Cell 1999;97:175–187.

21 Genetics and Arrhythmias

Kui Hong, MD, PhD and Ramon Brugada, MD

CONTENTS

INTRODUCTION

During the last 50 yr, we have been able to prolong survival and improve the quality of life of patients with cardiac disease through innovations in technology and pharmacology and improvements in preventive and diagnostic medicine. However, most cardiac diseases are structural in origin and will progress to their ultimate outcome. Curative therapies are not available in part because of our lack of understanding of the basic mechanisms responsible for many cardiac diseases. Developments in molecular genetics and biology are likely to change the medical approach to a cardiac patient. The identification of molecular mechanisms involved in cardiac diseases provides new possibilities not only for therapeutic and diagnostic measures but also for prevention of disease.

GENETICS AND ARRHYTHMIAS

Genetically determined cardiac diseases that predispose patients to arrhythmias, both with and without structural abnormalities, have been identified (Tables 1–2). These cardiac diseases result primarily from abnormalities in the codification of three families of proteins: the sarcomeric proteins, the cytoskeletal proteins, and the ion channel proteins. Hypertrophic cardiomyopathy is associated with abnormalities in the sarcomeric proteins, which are responsible for the generation of force for the mechanical contraction of myocytes *(1)*. Dilated cardiomyopathy is associated with abnormalities in the cytoskeletal proteins, which transmit the force to neighboring cells for a coordinated contraction *(2)*. Abnormalities in ion channel proteins, which

maintain the ionic balance to generate electrical activity in the myocyte, are responsible for familial arrhythmias *(3)*. Despite the seeming simplicity of this scheme, the etiology is more complex, and there is overlap between diseases. For example, abnormal sarcomeric proteins may also cause dilated cardiomyopathy *(4)*, and mutations in the gene for sodium channel SCN5A have been associated with long QT syndrome, Brugada syndrome, and familial conduction disease *(5)*. Furthermore, research has shown that the relation between genetic mutations and prognosis is not clear-cut *(4)*. Nevertheless, this simplistic classification scheme has allowed for a better understanding of the mechanisms responsible for these three diseases, and the identification of genetic factors has contributed to an understanding of the arrhythmogenic triggers and determinants of sudden death. The data are preliminary, and the key genetic factors identified for use in risk assessment for sudden death or arrhythmias are the result of research in only a few families. Although further studies are required to confirm preliminary data, technology is evolving rapidly, and findings from genetic studies will soon be used to improve diagnosis and treatment of cardiac diseases.

ION CHANNELOPATHIES

Coordinated cardiac activity depends on ion currents, ion channels, structural proteins, and gap junctions, all of which help in transmitting the electrical and mechanical impulse across the cardiac myocyte The complexity of this process has limited our understanding of arrhythmogenesis. However, the use of molecular techniques in the field of

From: *Contemporary Cardiology: Principles of Molecular Cardiology*
Edited by: M. S. Runge and C. Patterson © Humana Press Inc., Totowa, NJ

Table 1
Genetic Disorders Causing Primary Cardiac Arrhythmias with No Structural Heart Disease

	Rhythm	Inheritance pattern[a]	Chromosome	Gene
Supraventricular				
Atrial fibrillation	Atrial fibrillation	Dominant	10	—
Atrial standstill	Atrial fibrillation	Dominant	—	—
	Sinus node dysfunction			
Absent sinus rhythm	Atrial fibrillation	Dominant	—	—
	Sinus node dysfunction			
Wolff–Parkinson–White Syndrome	AVRT	Dominant	—	—
Familial PJRT	AVRT	Dominant	—	—
Conduction disorders				
Atrioventricular block	Atrioventricular block	Dominant	19	—
Familial bundle branch block	Right bundle branch block	—	—	—
Ventricular				
Long QT syndrome (RW)	Torsade de pointes	Dominant	7	hERG
			21	minK
			21	MiRP1
			3	SCN5A
			11	KVLQT1
			4	—
Long QT syndrome (JLN)	Torsade de pointes	Recessive	11	KVLQT1
			21	minK
Familial VT	VT	Dominant	—	—
Bidirectional VT	VT	Dominant	—	—
Brugada syndrome	VT/VF	Dominant	3	SCN5A

[a]All patterns of inheritance are autosomal.

AVRT, atrioventricular reentrant tachycardia; JLN, Jervell and Lange–Nielsen; PJRT, permanent junctional reentrant tachycardia; RW, Romano–Ward; VF, ventricular fibrillation; VT, ventricular tachycardia.

cardiology has led to the discovery of the structure, function, and pathophysiology of the ion channels, which, in turn, has helped identify the role of different ionic currents in the electrical activity and electromechanical coupling of muscle contraction. The functional analysis of the ion channels involved in the generation of the cardiac action potential has provided basic information on the mechanisms of arrhythmias; however, the application of this information to clinical medicine has been facilitated by genetic studies and the identification of mutations that cause familial disease. Studies in genetics and molecular biology have contributed significantly to our knowledge base for cardiac arrhythmias such as long QT syndrome and Brugada syndrome that predispose to sudden death. Although uncommon, these familial diseases that are caused by a single gene allow for the study of cardiac disease in which a single abnormal protein triggers the arrhythmia. In addition to contributing valuable information on inherited cardiac diseases, genetic studies have provided insight into how the arrhythmias are triggered in acquired forms of the disease.

Long QT Syndrome

Long QT syndrome, a disease of repolarization, is characterized by syncopal episodes, malignant ventricular arrhythmias, and ventricular fibrillation identified by prolongation of the QT interval on electrocardiogram (ECG) (3). The usual form of ventricular arrhythmia is torsade de pointes. Both acquired and congenital forms of long QT syndrome have been identified. Acquired disease is often iatrogenic and related primarily to medications

Table 2

Genetic Disorders Causing Cardiac Arrhythmias with Structural Heart Disease

	Rhythm	Inheritance pattern	Chromosome	Gene
Supraventricular				
Familial amyloidosis	Atrial fibrillation	Dominant	—	—
Ventricular				
Hypertrophic cardiomyopathy	Atrial fibrillation & VT	Dominant	1	Troponin T
			3	Essential myosin
			11	Myosin-binding protein C
			12	Regulat myosin
			14	β-myosin
			15	Tropomyosin
			19	Troponin I
Hypertrophic cardiomyopathy/WPW	Atrial fibrillation & VT	Dominant	7	PRKAG2
Naxos disease	VT	Recessive	17	Plakoglobin
Dilated cardiomyopathy	VT	Dominant	1,2,4,10	
			3	Desmin
			14	Actin
		X-linked	X	Dystrophin, G4,5
		AR	—	—
		Mitochondrial	—	—
Mitral valve prolapse	Atrial fibrillation & SAD	AD	—	—
Conduction disorders	AV block	Dominant	—	—
Restrictive cardiomyopathy	AV block	Dominant	—	Prealbumin
Familial amyloidosis	AV block	Dominant	—	—
Holt–Oran syndrome	AV block/AT	Dominant	—	—
Atrial septal defect	AV block & atrial fibrillation	Dominant	—	—
Leopard syndrome	AV block/BBB	Dominant	—	—
Kugelbert–Welander	Atrial standstill	Recessive	—	—

ARVD, arrhythmogenic right ventricular dysplasia; AT, atrial tachycardia; AV, atrioventricular; BBB, bundle branch block; SAD, sudden arrhythmic death; VT, ventricular tachycardia, WPW, Wolff–Parkinson–White syndrome.

such as antiarrhythmics, antidepressants, and phenotiazides. In addition, acquired disease can result from an electrolyte imbalance such as hypokalemia, hypomagnesemia, or hypocalcemia, especially when associated with the above-mentioned medications. Both autosomal dominant and autosomal recessive patterns of inheritance have been described in congenital long QT syndrome (6–8). Autosomal recessive disease, first described in 1957 (6), is associated with deafness whereas the more common autosomal dominant disease is not.

The first genetic locus associated with the autosomal dominant disease was mapped to chromosome 11 in 1991 (9). Since then, six loci and five genes have been found to be associated with the autosomal dominant disease (Table 1). All the genes encode for proteins that are responsible for the automaticity of electrical activity in cardiac cells. Mutations in the DNA disrupt the formation of these proteins and alter the cardiac action potential. This situation creates a voltage gradient, especially at the ventricular level, which causes reentrant arrhythmias (3). The specific genes that have been described with autosomal dominant disease are those that encode for potassium channels KVLQT1 and minK, which interact to form the cardiac IKs current *(10)*; human ether-a-go-go (hERG) and mink-related peptide 1 (MiRP1), which integrate to form the I_{Kr} current *(11)*; and the sodium channel SCN5A *(12)*, which has also been linked to Brugada syndrome *(13)* and familial conduction disease *(14)*. The gene product for one gene on chromosome 4, LQT4, has not been identified *(15)*. The autosomal recessive forms of long QT syndrome have been linked to mutations in the genes that encode for the I_{Ks} current: KVLQT1 and minK *(16)*.

GENE-BASED THERAPY

Because of our increased understanding of the different ion channels and their function in cardiac activity, therapy may be aimed at a specific defective channel. Sodium channel blockers have been used to decrease repolarization abnormalities in patients with long QT syndrome. In two small studies, the QT interval improved on ECG after treatment with mexiletine in patients with sodium channel mutations *(17)* and after treatment with intravenous potassium in patients with mutations in the potassium channel hERG *(18)*. However, the studies are too small to assess the effect of improving the QT interval on the risk of sudden death in this disease. Nevertheless, these studies are an important step toward applying gene therapy to the treatment of arrhythmias.

Brugada Syndrome

Originally described in 1992 *(18)*, the Brugada syndrome is characterized by right bundle branch block, ST segment elevation in V1 to V3, and sudden death *(19)* (Fig. 1). The diagnosis, based on clinical and electrocardiographic data, is usually made in patients with a structurally normal heart with the characteristic ECG pattern who have had syncopal or sudden death (aborted) episodes caused by fast polymorphic ventricular tachycardia.

The incidence of sudden death in some countries in Southeast Asia is abnormally high *(20)*. The fatal event usually occurs at night and only affects males. This form of sudden death, known as sudden unexpected death syndrome (SUDS), affects between 26 and 38 per 100,000 people per year worldwide. In Thailand, SUDS is second only to car accidents in the causes of death in individuals younger than 50 yr. The recent discovery that SUDS and Brugada syndrome share defects in the same gene indicates they are allelic diseases or possibly the same disease *(21)*.

Although the average age of sudden death is 40 yr, it can strike at any age. In the original published description

of the Brugada syndrome, the first patient was 2 yr old at the time of the first cardiac arrest, and his sister who had the same ECG pattern had died at the same age a few years earlier *(19)*. Recently, other investigators have confirmed that Brugada syndrome can cause sudden death in very young children *(22)*.

Some cases of Brugada syndrome have been genetically determined, with an autosomal dominant pattern of transmission. Defects have been described in the gene for cardiac sodium channel SCN5A *(13)*, which is the same gene that causes the LQT3 variant 6 (long QT syndrome). Many mutations have been identified and, as with other familial cardiac diseases, some of the families with Brugada syndrome have not been linked to the gene, indicating the syndrome is genetically heterogeneous. Studies in *Xenopus laevis* oocytes have shown that the functional defect in the sodium channel in LQT3 is the lack of complete inactivation, which allows a continuous leak of Na^{2+} ions into the cellular interior, whereas in Brugada syndrome the inactivation of the Na^{2+} channel is rapid and leaves the potassium current Ito unopposed in phase 1 of the action potential *(23)*. Nevertheless, the end result in both LQT3 and Brugada syndrome is the same: the creation of a voltage gradient and the substrate for reentrant arrhythmias. Electrophysiologic studies have shown that the function of the mutated channel worsens at temperatures approaching the physiologic range *(24)*. This finding has clinical implications because many patients suffer cardiac arrest during febrile episodes.

The processes of identifying patients at risk and estimating the prevalence of the disease are complicated by the variability of the ECG, which can normalize over time *(25)*. The use of modulators has improved the diagnosis of Brugada syndrome. For example, intravenous injection of ajmaline, flecainide, or procainamide can identify patients who have normal ECG readings but are heterozygous for a mutation in the SCN5A gene *(26)*.

Since the initial description of patients with sudden death, changes characteristic of the Brugada syndrome have been recognized on ECG in symptomatic and asymptomatic family members and in patients with a persistent or variable ECG. Clinical observations suggest that the prognosis is better in patients in whom electrophysiologic testing does not elicit ECG changes or in patients who require intravenous antiarrhythmic medications to elicit the changes *(27)*; however, this conclusion is premature and requires further study.

Pharmacological therapy is not useful in preventing sudden death in patients with Brugada syndrome. Only implantable defibrillators have been beneficial.

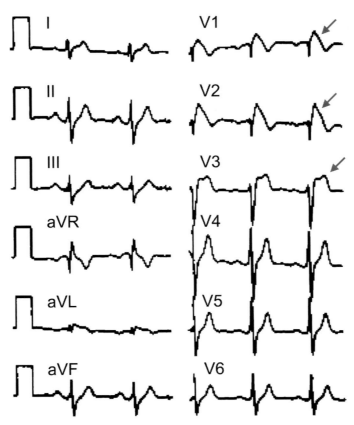

Fig. 1. Typical ECG of Brugada syndrome. Note the characteristic pattern of right bundle branch block, PR prolongation, and ST segment elevation in leads V1–V3.

Familial Polymorphic Ventricular Tachycardia

Calcium channels are critical to normal cardiac function. Because calcium channels are involved in the generation of the action potential and in myocyte contraction, calcium is a key ion in excitation–contraction coupling. Calcium intervenes in the depolarizing current and creates the plateau or phase 2 of the action potential, which triggers the release of calcium from the sarcoplasmic reticulum (SR) and activates the cardiac contractile apparatus. The SR serves primarily as an intracellular store of calcium in skeletal muscle cells.

Based on studies of other ion channel diseases, investigators have hypothesized that defects in proteins that interact with calcium may impair the electrical and contractile function of the heart. The contraction process starts in the cell membrane, where few calcium ions enter the cell through the voltage-gated, L-type calcium channels during phase 2 of the action potential. Located near the calcium-release channels of the SR, the L-type calcium channels are also called ryanodine receptors and are activated by incoming calcium, which binds to troponin C and initiates the contraction in the sarcomere. The ryanodine receptor in the SR of most muscle cells (smooth, cardiac, and skeletal) is a Ca^{2+}-activated Ca^{2+}

channel. In other words, the Ca^{2+} that enters through the voltage-gated Ca^{2+} channel from the exterior of the cell triggers the opening of the Ca^{2+} release channel, which results in an efflux of Ca^{2+} from the SR into the cytoplasm.

Mutations in the cardiac ryanodine receptor (RYR2) gene are associated with two different diseases: arrhythmogenic right ventricular dysplasia type 2 (ARVD2) *(28)* and familial polymorphic ventricular tachycardia (FPVT) *(29)*. FPVT has an autosomal dominant inheritance pattern and a mortality rate of about 30% by the age of 30 yr. Bidirectional and polymorphic ventricular tachycardias occur in response to vigorous exercise in patients with FPVT, but no structural evidence of myocardial disease is seen. In contrast, ARVD2, which is caused by a defect in the same gene associated with FPVT, is accompanied by structural abnormalities. Whether this difference is caused by the effect of the mutation, the genetic background of the patient, or an environmental factor is unknown.

Is Atrial Fibrillation a Channelopathy?

In order for the electromechanical impulse to propagate uniformly across myocardial cells, a balance

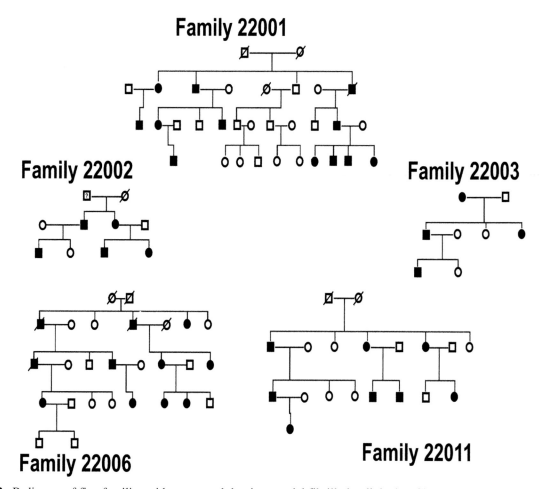

Fig. 2. Pedigrees of five families with autosomal dominant atrial fibrillation linked to Chromosome 10q22.

between structural and ionic components is required. When structural heart disease or genetic or iatrogenic factors modify this interaction, chaotic electrical activity or fibrillation that can affect the atria or the ventricles can occur. The atrial chaos or atrial fibrillation (AF) is defined as an erratic activation of the atria that causes an irregular heart rhythm at the ventricular level. AF is the Achilles' heel of cardiac rhythmology. Despite advances in the treatment of cardiac dysrhythmias, such as the introduction of radiofrequency ablation, therapeutic options for AF have remained unchanged, and treatment involves controlling the heart rate and administering anti-coagulants. Promising new surgical and ablation techniques are being developed but are labor-intensive and are available to only a small percentage of patients.

Genetic Background

The study of the molecular basis of AF in humans has focused on three main areas: (1) genetic defects that cause the familial forms of the disease, (2) a patient's genetic background which might predispose to the dis-

ease, and (3) changes in gene expression of ion channel currents involved in the formation of the atrial action potential. The third area may provide an understanding of the molecular changes associated with AF and may explain how chronic arrhythmia develops. However, assessing whether the molecular changes in the atria cause the disease or are a consequence of the disease will be difficult. This issue could be clarified by identifying the genetic defects that cause the familial form of the disease. In familial disease, the genetic defect triggers development of the pathology and provides insight into the etiology of the disease.

Atrial Fibrillation as a Monogenic Disease

The familial nature of AF, first reported in 1943, has not been well accepted. In 1996, we identified five families with AF inherited with an autosomal dominant pattern of transmission (30) (Fig. 2). Of the 103 members of these families, 42 presented with AF. The age of diagnosis ranged from 1 to 45 yr. The penetrance of the disease was high; in latter generations, three patients were diagnosed in the first month of life.

By using linkage analysis, we identified an area of 28 centimorgans (cM) in chromosome 10q22 that segregated with affected individuals. Analysis of additional families from the same geographical area confirmed the linkage and allowed the chromosomal region to be narrowed to about 800,000 base pairs. Positional cloning has been used to identify eight genes in the area, which are currently being characterized. We have collected more than 100 probands from patients with familial AF, and we have phenotypically characterized 32 families. Our conclusion is that AF is a heterogenous disease associated with more than one gene *(31)*.

CONCLUSIONS

The first gene associated with a cardiac disease was identified only 10 yr ago. Since then, we have learned much about the pathophysiological mechanisms in monogenic diseases. With the completion of the Human Genome Project, several new lines of research are being developed, and molecular interactions will be used to improve therapy in many fields of clinical medicine.

REFERENCES

1. Marian AJ, Roberts R. Recent advances in the molecular genetics of hypertrophic cardiomyopathy. Circulation 1995;92:1336–1347.
2. Olson TM, Michels VV, Thibodeau SN, et al. Actin mutations in dilated cardiomyopathy, a heritable form of heart failure. Science 1998;280:750–752.
3. Roden DM, Lazzara R, Rosen M, et al. Multiple mechanisms in the long-QT syndrome. Current knowledge, gaps and future directions. Circulation 1996;94:1996–2012.
4. Li D, Czernuszewicz GZ, Gonzalez O, et al. Novel cardiac troponin T mutation as a cause of familial dilated cardiomyopathy. Circulation 2001;104:2188–2193.
5. Brugada R, Roberts R. Brugada syndrome: why are there multiple answers to a simple question? Circulation 2001;104:3017–3019.
6. Jervell A, Lange-Nielsen F. Congenital deaf-mutism, function heart disease with prolongation of the Q-T interval and sudden death. Am Heart J 1957;54:59–68.
7. Romano C, Gemme G, Pongiglione R. Antmie cardiache rare in eta pediatrica. Clin Pediatr 1963;45:656–683.
8. Ward OC. A new familial cardiac syndrome in children. J Ir Med Assoc 1964;54:103–106.
9. Keating MT, Atkinson D, Dunn C, et al. Linkage of a cardiac arrhythmia, the long QT syndrome, and the Harvey ras-1 gene. Science 1991;252:704–706.
10. Barhanin J, Lesage F, Guillemare E, et al. KVLQT1 and IsK (minK) proteins associate to form the I_{ks} cardiac potassium current. Nature 1996;384:78–80.
11. Sanguinetti MC, Jiang C, Curran ME, et al. A mechanistic link between an inherited and an acquired cardiac arrhythmia: HERG encodes the I_{Kr} potassium channel. Cell 1995;81:299–307.
12. Wang Q, Shen J, Splawski I, et al. SCN5A mutations associated with an inherited cardiac arrhythmia, long QT syndrome. Cell 1995;80:805–811.
13. Chen Q, Kirsch GE, Zhang D, et al. Genetic basis and molecular mechanisms for idiopathic ventricular fibrillation. Nature 1998;392:293–296.
14. Probst V, Hoorntje TM, Hulsbeek M, et al. Cardiac conduction defects associate with mutations in SCN5A. Nature Genetics 1999;23:20–21.
15. Schott J, Charpentier F, Peltier S, et al. Mapping of a gene for long QT syndrome to chromosome 4q25-27. Am J Hum Genet 1995;57:1114–1122.
16. Neyroud N, Tesson F, Denjoy I, et al. A novel mutation on the potassium channel gene KVLQT1 causes the Jervell and Lange-Nielsen cardioauditory syndrome. Nature Genet 1997;15:186–189.
17. Schwartz PJ, Priori SG, Locati E, et al. Long QT syndrome patients with mutations of the SCN5A and HERG genes have differential responses to Na channel blockade and to increases in heart rate. Circulation 1995;92:3381–3386.
18. Compton SJ, Lux RL, Ramsey MR. Genetically defined therapy of inherited long-QT syndrome. Circulation 1996;94:1018–1022.
19. Brugada P, Brugada J. Right bundle branch block, persistent ST segment elevation and sudden cardiac death: A distinct clinical and electrocardiographic syndrome. J Am Coll Cardiol 1992;20:1391–1396.
20. Baron RC, Thacker SB, Gorelkin L. et al. Sudden death among Southeast Asian refugees: an unexplained nocturnal phenomenon. JAMA 1983;250:2947–2951.
21. Vatta M, Dumaine R, Varghese G, et al. Genetic and biophysical basis of sudden unexplained nocturnal death syndrome (SUNDS), a disease allelic to Brugada syndrome. Hum Mol Genet. 2002; 11:337–345.
22. Priori S, Napolitano C, Giordano U, et al. Brugada syndrome and sudden cardiac death in children. Lancet 2000;355:808–809.
23. Antzelevitch CH. The Brugada syndrome: ionic basis and arrhythmia mechanisms. J Cardiovasc Electrophysiol 2001;12:268–272.
24. Dumaine R, Towbin J, Brugada P, et al. Ionic mechanisms responsible for the electrocardiographic phenotype of the Brugada syndrome are temperature dependent. Circ Res 1999; 85:803–809.
25. Brugada J, Brugada R, Brugada P. Right bundle branch block and ST segment elevation in leads V1-V3: A marker for sudden death in patients with no demonstrable structural heart disease. Circulation 1998;97:457–460.
26. Brugada R, Brugada J, Antzelevitch A, et al. Sodium channel blockers identify risk for sudden death in patients with ST segment elevation and right bundle branch block but structurally normal hearts. Circulation 2000;101:510–515.
27. Brugada P, Geelen P, Brugada R, et al. The prognostic value of electrophysiologic investigation in Brugada syndrome. J Cardiovasc Electrophysiol 2001;12:1004–1007
28. Tiso N, Stephan DA, Nava A, et al. Identification of mutations in the cardiac ryanodine receptor gene in families affected with arrhythmogenic right ventricular cardiomyopathy type 2 (ARVD2). Hum Mol Genet 2001;10:189–194.
29. Laitinen PJ, Brown KM, Piippo K, et al. Mutations of the cardiac ryanodine receptor (RyR2) gene in familial polymorphic ventricular tachycardia. Circulation 2001;103:485–490.
30. Brugada R, Tapscott T, Czernuszewicz GZ, et al. Identification of a genetic locus for familial atrial fibrillation. N Engl J Med 1997;336:905–911.
31. Brugada R, Bachinski L, Hill R, Roberts R. Familial atrial fibrillation is a genetically heterogeneous disease. J Am Coll Cardiol 1998;31:349A.

V   Vascular Diseases

22   Therapeutic Angiogenesis for Ischemic Vascular Disease

Jai Pal Singh, PhD *and J. Anthony Ware,* MD

CONTENTS

INTRODUCTION

Until recently, it was thought that physiological angiogenesis, the formation of small capillary blood vessels from existing ones, was confined in adults solely to wound healing and development of the endometrium, corpus luteum, and placenta. But angiogenesis and arteriogenesis, the formation of larger collateral vessels with surrounding muscle-derived cells, are now recognized as part of the physiological response to ischemia or injury. Development of collaterals in response to chronic ischemia helps maintain blood flow and oxygenation and therefore is a beneficial angiogenesis. Pathological angiogenesis is commonly associated with tumor growth, retinopathy, psoriasis, hemangiomas, and rheumatoid arthritis.

Recent studies have also shown that preexisting vessels are not the only source of endothelial cells for new vessel formation in adults. Endothelial progenitor cells, derived from bone marrow or other tissues, also contribute to vessel formation following ischemia *(1–4)* and to pathological processes *(5)*. Whether bone marrow cells contribute to vasculogenesis (*in situ* formation of blood vessels from angioblasts) *(6)* in adults is not yet clear.

Angiogenesis is a highly regulated process that requires coordinated action between the extracellular matrix (ECM) and several cell types and soluble mediators. Although many aspects of the underlying biology of angiogenesis, vasculogenesis, and arteriogenesis are common, each distinct stage of these processes requires specialized cellular responses and mediators. Furthermore, depending on the functional requirements of the organ and the tissue microenvironment, different types of vessels are produced in different tissues or pathologies. For example, the vessels produced in response to inflammation appear to differ from those formed in response to hypoxia. Treatment of vessels with vascular endothelial growth factor (VEGF) alone produces capillaries, whereas treatment with monocyte chemoattractant protein-1 (MCP-1) induces arterioles *(7)*. Enlargement of preexisting vessels occurs in psoriasis, whereas sprouting leads to new vessels in patients with diabetic retinopathy. Similarly, fenestrated vessels are present only in specialized organs (e.g., endocrine glands). Thus, therapeutic modulation of angiogenesis ideally would entail a selective alteration in the inhibitors or stimuli and their receptors, signaling pathways, or transcription factors at the desired site. Many studies using a variety of animal models have demonstrated that supplemental growth factors or their genes can enhance angiogenesis *(8,9)*. In many cases, such treatments may only result in capillary formation and tissue microcirculation, because restoration of coronary or peripheral circulation requires generation of larger vessels with adequate hemodynamic properties. Thus, understanding the molecular basis of large vessel formation and acquisition of desired function is critical

From: *Contemporary Cardiology: Principles of Molecular Cardiology*
Edited by: M. S. Runge and C. Patterson © Humana Press Inc., Totowa, NJ

for the development of therapeutic strategies. In this chapter we will review the current understanding of the cell biology, molecular mediators, and signaling mechanisms of angiogenesis and their applications to developing therapies for revascularization. Specific challenges and strategies for clinical development of angiogenic agents are described.

CELLULAR AND MOLECULAR MECHANISMS OF ANGIOGENESIS
Angiogenic Triggers

Hypoxia and vascular injury are the major triggers of angiogenic responses in adults. Lack of oxygen signals the activation of hypoxia-inducible transcription factors (HIFs) 1α and 2α. HIFs regulate the expression of VEGF, also known as vascular permeability factor, and its receptors VEGF receptor (VEGFR)-1, VEGFR-2, and neuropilin (10). VEGF and the coagulation factors generated in response to increased vascular permeability initiate endothelial responses required for tube formation. VEGF also induces endothelial nitric oxide synthase (eNOS), transforming growth factor-β (TGFβ), platelet-derived growth factor (PDGF), insulin-like growth factor-1 (IGF-1), interleukin-1 (IL-1), tissue factor, and Tie-1, all of which mediate vessel assembly and maturation (11). Analogous endothelial responses are initiated during angiogenesis in response to ischemia and tissue injury. Platelets, monocytes, and other inflammatory cells recruited to the injury site are the primary source of mediators, including VEGF, fibroblast growth factor (FGF), TGFβ, interleukin-8 (IL-8), PDGF, IGF-1, and MCP-1 (11,12). Secondary factors, such as PDGF or MCP-1, are probably important for arteriogenesis but not capillary formation.

The early mediators released in response to oxygen deprivation or injury trigger endothelial cell activation, migration, proliferation, survival, and tube formation. An important early modulator of the angiogenic pathway is nitric oxide (NO). NO produced at the injury site in response to mediators such as VEGF induces vasodilation and increased permeability (13). This facilitates loosening and migration of endothelial cells. In addition, a host of ECM-degrading enzymes, which are induced by either the initial HIF-VEGF activation or the coagulation process, facilitate the dissociation of endothelial cells from the ECM and their migration to form new tubes. VEGF and FGF also induce expression of ECM-remodeling enzymes, such as urokinase-type plasminogen activator (uPA), matrix metalloproteinase (MMPs), and integrins, which are required for cell adhesion and migration (13,14). Remodeling and vessel stabilization and maturation follow

tube formation. These processes require additional cell types and mediators as listed in (Table 1).

Cellular Components of Angiogenesis

Endothelial cells are not only central to initiating and driving the formation of new blood vessels, they are also sufficient to form initial tube-like structures. In early embryogenesis, hemangioblasts give rise to angioblasts and differentiated endothelial cells that assemble into vascular tubes. Until recently, it was thought that preexisting endothelial cells are the sole source of endothelium in new blood vessels in adults. Recent discoveries have revealed the existence of endothelial precursor cells (EPCs) that circulate and are in the bone marrow (1–4). Mobilization, recruitment, and incorporation of EPCs into newly formed vessels occur in models of coronary and peripheral ischemia. EPCs can be mobilized by cytokines such as granulocyte macrophage–colony stimulating factor (GM–CSF), VEGF, and IGF-1. 3-Hydroxy-3-methylglutaryl CoA (HMGCoA) reductase inhibitors (statins), which activate Akt kinase and NO production, also increase circulating EPCs in animal models and in patients with stable coronary artery disease (15,16). Direct transplantation of bone marrow precursor cells enhances formation of new vessels and functional recovery in animal models of ischemia (17). GM–CSF, which stimulates bone marrow hematopoetic, myeloid, and stromal precursor cells, significantly increases the number of circulating EPCs and enhances neovascularization (18). Although current evidence strongly suggests that circulating and bone marrow EPCs participate in the formation of new blood vessels, the magnitude of the cells contributing to vessel composition or provision of specific mediators is not yet understood.

The formation of stable functional vessels requires cooperation and temporal participation of endothelial cells, smooth muscle cells (SMCs), pericytes, and inflammatory cells. Pericytes produce mediators and ECM that inhibit migration and proliferation of endothelial cells and enhance their survival. These activities contribute to stabilization of the vessels: a lack of SMCs or pericytes leads to vessel regression (19). Arteriogenesis requires assembly of multiple layers of SMCs, which confer vasomotor properties to the vessels (20). These SMCs arrive at their new destination by migrating from existing vessels and probably also by differentiating from endothelial cells, mesenchymal cells, bone marrow precursor cells, or macrophages. The formation of mature vessels, particularly arterioles, requires participation of not only endothelial cells, SMCs, and pericytes, but also of monocytes, which produce factors and enzymes for vascular remodeling.

Table 1
Cells and Key Mediators of Revascularization

Response	Cells[a]	Key Mediators
Hypoxia/Injury	EC	HIF1α, VEGF, FGF, BK1, Thrombin
Sprouting	EC	VEGF, NO, FGF, TF, MMPs
Tube formation	EC EPC	VEGF, FGF, HGF, SDF-1
Stabilization/maturation	EC, EPC SMC Macrophage Pericytes	Ang-1, FGF, PIGF, PDGF MCP-1, TGF-β GM–CSF
Arteriogenesis	EC, SMC Macrophage Pericytes	PDGF, MCP-1, PIGF

[a]EC, endothelial cells; EPC, endothelial progenitor cells; SMC, smooth muscle cells; BK1, bradykinin 1.

Angiogenic Mediators

A variety of soluble and ECM-associated molecules orchestrate the angiogenic activities of vascular cells. Gene deletion studies have provided substantial insights into the role of various mediators and their receptors in developmental angiogenesis. Such insights are reviewed elsewhere in this book. Several of the polypeptides described below enhance angiogenesis in models of ischemic vascular disease.

Vascular Endothelial Growth Factor

The VEGF gene family has five known members: VEGF (VEGF-A), VEGF-B, VEGF-C, VEGF-E, and placental growth factor (PIGF) (21). In addition, there are several known splice variants of VEGF: to date they include those with 121, 145, 189, and 206 amino acids. Because VEGF 121 lacks a heparin-binding domain, it is readily released into circulation. VEGF 189 and 206 bind tightly to heparan sulfate and mostly remain bound to the ECM.

VEGF is one of the major mediators of vascular development during embryogenesis and physiological and pathological angiogenesis in adults. The action of VEGF is limited largely to endothelial cells, although it does also stimulate hematopoietic cells and monocytes (22). VEGF induces a variety of early endothelial activities required for angiogenesis, including NO-induced vasodilation, vascular permeability, cell migration and proliferation, EPC recruitment, and tube formation (21). Disruption of one VEGF allele in mice produces gross abnormalities in embryonic vascular development (23). VEGF and its receptors are thought to have a critical role in angiogenesis in adults, because they are expressed in response to ischemia, and because enhancement of vessel formation follows VEGF gene or peptide delivery (8,9).

PIGF induces endothelial cell migration in vitro and angiogenesis in vivo. PIGF also induces monocyte recruitment, suggesting its potential role in vessel remodeling and maturation (24,25).

VEGF interacts with several cell surface receptors. Some are required for direct signal transduction. Others modify VEGF's responses. Three distinct signal transducing receptors for VEGF isoforms, mainly expressed in endothelial cells, have been identified (26). Angiogenic activity of VEGF is predominantly mediated by activation of VEGFR-1 and VEGFR-2. VEGFR-3 is expressed in lymphatic endothelium. VEGF signaling via VEGFR-2, also known as Flk in mice or kinase insert domain-containing region (KDR) in humans, is critical for angioblast differentiation and endothelial migration and proliferation during embryogenesis (27–34). VEGFR-2 signaling also contributes to hematopoiesis and produces EPCs and hematopoietic cells (28). VEGFR-1, known as Flt-1 in mice, is believed to mediate endothelial migration and vessel assembly (29,33). When VEGFR-1 is expressed on monocytes, it mediates their chemotaxis and expression of tissue factor. The differences in the cellular actions of VEGFR-1 and VEGFR-2 suggest that their signaling evolved to produce distinct functional outcomes in endothelial cells. For example, VEGFR-2, but not VEGFR-1, mediates endothelial cell growth (34).

In addition to interacting with its signaling receptors, VEGF also interacts with other cell surface matrix receptors, including the integrin αvβ3, vascular/endothelial (VE)-cadherin, and neuropilin (35,36). Such interactions may promote VEGF signaling and mitogenic activity (36).

Fibroblast Growth Factors

FGFs have evolved into a large gene family whose members have various tissue expression and functions. Eighteen members of the FGF gene family have been identified (37). The first isolated FGF proteins, FGF-1 and FGF-2, have been widely studied in vascular development. FGF-1 and FGF-2 exhibit pleiotropic activity, stimulating growth, differentiation, migration and survival of a variety of cell types, including fibroblast, epithelial, smooth muscle, endothelial, and neuronal cells (38). Heparin binding is important for localizing FGFs and binding to specific receptors.

Different FGF isoforms may have evolved to act in organotypic manners. For example, FGF-7 is a selective mitogen for keratinocytes, whereas FGF-8 affects neuronal cell survival and dendritic growth (39,40). Whether different FGFs could mediate endothelial responses in a tissue-specific manner has not been tested. Because FGFs also affect SMC migration and proliferation, they potentially mediate both tube formation and vessel maturation.

Like VEGF, FGFs act by binding to members of the cell-surface receptor tyrosine kinase (RTK) family. Four different genes encoding FGF receptors have been identified (41). Receptor-bound FGF is internalized, and a fraction of it is translocated to the nucleus. Some studies suggest that nuclear FGF mediates mitogenic activity (42). In vascular cells, the pleiotropic activities of FGFs are mediated by activation of multiple signaling pathways that are common to other RTKs and lead to cell growth, migration, and survival. Control of the diverse actions of FGFs occurs at multiple levels, including the expression of ligand, secretion from the cells, ECM binding, receptor expression, and signaling mechanisms that may be specific to individual cell types.

Angiopoietins

Angiopoietin proteins primarily mediate vessel stabilization and maturation through enhancing cell–cell interactions between endothelial cells and SMCs or pericytes. Angiopoietin-1 (Ang-1) acts in a paracrine manner: it is expressed in mesenchymal cells, including vascular SMCs, and it acts on endothelial cells via the Tie-2 RTK (43). Tie-2–deficient mice exhibit gross defects in vessel formation and vascular integrity (44,45). In vitro, Ang-1 is a chemoattractant and a survival factor for endothelial cells but not a mitogen for them (45). In adult vessels, Ang-1 maintains vessel integrity and prevents plasma leakage (46). Ang-2 also binds to Tie-2 but does not activate it. Instead, Ang-2 antagonizes Ang-1 activation of Tie-2 (47). The cell survival and migration activity of Ang-1 involves activation of the phosphoinositide 3 (PI3)-kinase pathway

(48,49). Ang-1 also activates signal transducer and activator of transcription 3 (STAT3), a transcription factor that mediates endothelial cell survival (50). Recently, other homologs of Ang-1 have been identified whose role in vessel development is being investigated (51).

Hepatocyte Growth Factor

Initially identified as scatter factor, hepatocyte growth factor (HGF) is also a potent modulator of endothelial function. The 92-kDa HGF precursor protein is proteolytically processed to an active form of two subunits linked by a disulfide bond. HGF has 38% amino acid sequence homology with plasminogen. In the vasculature, HGF acts in a paracrine manner: it is produced by mesenchymal cells, fibroblasts, and SMCs, and it binds to a specific RTK, c-met, expressed in heart and blood vessel endothelial cells (52–54). HGF expression in endothelium and macrophages is enhanced following myocardial infarction. Like VEGF, HGF modulates cell growth, migration, and morphogenesis in vitro and promotes angiogenesis in vivo (49).

Yet there are some striking differences in the biological activities of HGF and VEGF. For example, unlike VEGF, HGF has a delayed expression in response to ischemia (54), which may reflect the recruitment and activation of the cells expressing HGF. Furthermore, HGF does not increase vascular permeability. In blood vessels, the mitogenic action of HGF appears to be restricted to endothelial cells. HGF does not stimulate mitogenesis in SMCs. In vivo delivery of the HGF gene or protein enhances angiogenesis in ischemic or granulation tissue (55).

Organotypic Factors

A large number of growth factors produce similar effects on endothelial cells. For example, FGF-1, FGF-2, VEGF, HGF, and angiopoietins all affect one or more angiogenic activities such as cell growth, migration, and survival. The significance of this redundancy is not understood. It is possible that some of these molecules locally maintain and renew tissue microvasculature. VEGF, FGF, angiopoietins, and their receptors are broadly expressed in a variety of organs and induce angiogenesis in most tissues, whereas other growth factors may have evolved to induce organ-specific angiogenesis and specialized endothelial functions. Indeed, an organ-specific angiogenic factor was recently identified (56): endocrine gland–derived vascular endothelial cell growth factor (EG–VEGF), a novel protein with no significant homology to VEGF, is functionally similar to VEGF in its ability to induce vascular permeability and the migration and proliferation of endothelial cells from endocrine glands. The expression of EG–VEGF is restricted to steroidogenic glands, ovaries, testes, the placenta, and adrenal tissues. EG–VEGF exhibits an unexpectedly high degree of selectivity for endothelial cells derived from endocrine glands. EG–VEGF does not stimulate growth of endothelial cells derived from a variety of nonendocrine sources, nor of SMCs, pericytes, keratinocytes, or fibroblasts. Furthermore, like VEGF, EG–VEGF's expression is regulated by hypoxia in an HIF-1α–dependent manner (56). Since VEGF and EG–VEGF are coordinately expressed in response to hypoxia, the two proteins may have synergistic effects. Understanding organ-specific regulation of angiogenesis is important for developing organ-specific angiogenic therapies.

FACTORS AFFECTING PERIENDOTHELIAL CELLS

As noted above, the formation of the endothelial tube is followed by recruitment of surrounding SMCs and pericytes that stabilize the vessels. Several growth factors, including PDGF, FGF, TGFβ, MCP-1, G-CSF and GM-CSF promote the migration or proliferation of the peri-endothelial cells. These cytokines also induce expression of early mediators, and this leads to maintenance and amplification of angiogenic responses.

Platelet-Derived Growth Factor

With the exception of certain capillary endothelial cells, most endothelial cells do not express PDGF receptors (57,58), which means it is unlikely that PDGF has a direct role in endothelial tube formation. Instead, PDGF appears to help vessel maturation by recruiting SMCs and pericytes and facilitating the interactions of endothelial SMCs and pericytes (59,60). The vasculature of Patch mice (homozygous PDGF receptor a -/- mutant) contain fewer SMCs than wild type, indicating that the PDGF receptor has a role in SMC recruitment (61). In addition to being a chemoattractant for monocytes, PDGF is a potent inducer of other genes involved in angiogenesis, including MCP-1.

Monocyte Chemoattractant Protein-1

Collateral development is enhanced by monocytes (62), which are an important source of cytokines and growth factors that promote vessel formation and maturation. MCP-1 is an important inflammatory chemokine that has been implicated in monocyte recruitment and the development of atherosclerosis (63). In a rabbit hindlimb ischemia model, a comparative study showed that treatment with MCP-1, but not with VEGF, induced a significant increase in arteriogenesis (7). The growth factors and cytokines produced from activated macrophages probably support recruitment of SMCs and pericytes and remodeling of the ECM (7).

COAGULATION FACTORS

Enzymes from the coagulation pathway facilitate endothelial cell migration by degrading matrix, generating fibrin substrate via tissue factor VIIa (TF-VIIa), and activating factor X (64). Recent studies suggest that coagulation factors may mediate the induction and maintenance of angiogenic responses. Thrombin receptor (PAR-1) knock-out studies have shown that PAR-1–deficient vessels are fragile (65). PAR-1 may mediate recruitment of endothelial cells as well as SMCs and pericytes. And thrombin itself increases VEGFR expression and NO production by endothelial cells (65,66).

Tissue factor may also promote angiogenesis via production of TF-VIIa–mediated inflammatory cytokines (67). Production of inflammatory cytokines by TF-VIIa interaction can recruit macrophages and SMCs. As shown in (Fig. 1), human macrophages that express TF-FVIIa induce the angiogenic cytokine IL-8. A critical role of tissue factor in angiogenesis is confirmed by the fact that tissue factor–deficient mice form fragile vessels (68).

Integrins

Angiogenesis requires interaction between endothelial cells and the ECM. Integrins, which are cell surface ECM receptors, facilitate this interaction and influence cell adhesion, migration, proliferation, survival, and spatial organization. A number of integrins are important in both vascular development and adult angiogenesis. They include integrins αvβ3, αvβ5, α5β1, and α2β1 (69,70). Gene knock-out studies as well as antibody/antagonist studies have demonstrated that integrins play a role in vascular development (70). The anti-αvβ3 antibody inhibits FGF-induced angiogenesis in animal models in vivo, whereas anti-αvβ5 blocks VEGF-induced angiogenesis (71). Integrins are crucial to promoting endothelial cell survival: growth factors such as FGF and VEGF depend on the ECM to induce cell survival (72,73) and are ineffective in preventing apoptosis in suspended cultures of endothelial cells (73). In promoting cell survival, the integrin αvβ3's signal transduction pathway appears to require the transcription factor nuclear factor κB (NFκB) (73).

Small Molecule Angiogenic Stimuli

Several small-molecular weight compounds are being investigated for their ability to promote angiogenesis. Nicotine stimulates endothelial cell growth and tube formation in vitro and capillary and collateral growth following ischemia in vivo (74). The effects of nicotine are

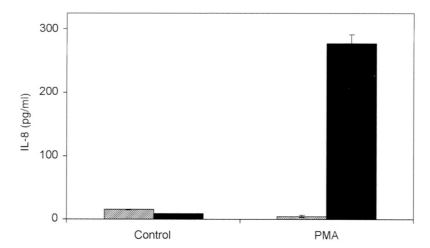

Fig. 1. IL-8 production in human macrophage THP-1 cells in response to factor VIIa. THP cells were treated with PMA for 24 h, washed, and then the control and PMA-treated cells were incubated in the absence (hatched bars) or presence of 50 n*M* factor VIIa (solid bars). After 24 h, IL-8 production in supernatant was determined by using an IL-8 ELISA.

apparently mediated by the endothelial acetylcholine receptor and involve NO, VEGF, and MCP-1 production *(75,76)*. Nicotine treatment can enhance atherosclerotic lesion development in ApoE knock-out mice *(73)*. Yet other studies have not found an adverse cardiovascular effect of chronic nicotine treatment *(77–79)*. Kinins produced at the site of injury and ischemia promote angiogenesis *(80)*. Kinin B1 binds to a G protein–coupled receptor on endothelial cells and stimulates NO synthesis and FGF-2 expression *(81)*. Since the kinin B1 receptor is not normally expressed, but is induced in response to ischemia *(82)*, a selective kinin B1 agonist may offer selective induction of angiogenesis in ischemic myocardium, thus reducing the potential for the side effects observed with growth factor delivery. Recent studies have shown that HMGCoA reductase inhibitors enhance endothelial progenitor cell mobilization and angiogenesis *(15,16)*. A critical role of the Akt kinase pathway in promoting angiogenesis via VEGF has been demonstrated as well. Compounds enhancing Akt kinase activity, such as Akt phosphatase inhibitors, could be potential small-molecular-weight angiogenic agonists. And, as described earlier, peroxisome proliferator activated receptor-γ (PPARγ) agonists induce the expression of VEGF, HGF, and angiopoietin-related proteins *(83–85)*. Potent and selective PPARγ agonists are now available and should be tested for their therapeutic use in modulating angiogenesis. Another potential approach to developing small-molecular-weight angiogenic agents involves molecular modeling of either proline rich peptide-39's (PR-39's) proteosome binding site or a selective proteosome inhibitor mimicking PR-39 activity *(86)*.

Inhibitors of Angiogenesis

Vascular homeostasis requires coordinated actions of both angiogenic stimuli and inhibitors. A number of endogenous inhibitors of angiogenesis have been identified. They include thrombospondin-1, angiostatin, endostatin, antithrombin, pigment epithelium–derived factor (PEDF), interferon β, prolactin, lif-1, platelet factor-4 (PF-4), and thromboxane A2 receptor ligands, all of which are expressed at the site of angiogenesis and inhibit endothelial cell activities (proliferation, migration, survival) in vitro as well as angiogenesis in vivo *(87,88)*. In many cases the inhibitors exist as inactive precursors until they are proteolytically processed *(89)*. The loss of an antiangiogenic signal may lead to an angiogenic phenotype *(87)*.

Angiogenic inhibitors presumably function by inducing endothelial apoptosis. The antiangiogenic activity of thrombospondin-1 (TSP-1) and PEDF is mediated by the Fas/Fas ligand pathway *(89)*. Proapoptotic angiostatin reduces Bcl-2 and Bcl-XL. Cell surface integrins promote endothelial cell survival and angiogenesis, and apoptosis is prevented when endothelial cells are in contact with ECM *(72,73)*. The "balance hypothesis" for the "angiogenic switch" postulates that inhibitors, antibodies, or antisense oligonucleotides could be a therapy for enhancing vascularization by blocking endogenous angiogenic inhibitors. For example, deletion of the thromboxane A2 receptor TP enhances angiogenesis following myocardial ischemia in mice (Patan et al. unpublished data, 2005).

Angiogenic Signal Transduction Pathways

The primary intracellular signals for angiogenesis are transduced via cell surface receptors of the RTK family.

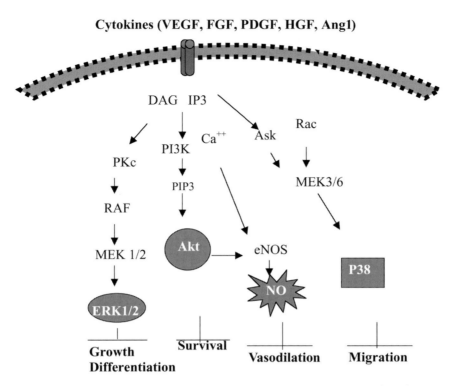

Cytokines (VEGF, FGF, PDGF, HGF, Ang1)

DAG   IP3

PKc

PI3K   Ca^{++} Ask   Rac

RAF

PIP3   MEK3/6

MEK 1/2

Akt   eNOS

P38

ERK1/2   NO

Growth   Survival   Vasodilation   Migration
Differentiation

Fig. 2. Some of the key intracellular signaling pathways mediating growth factor responses. Activation of RTK by growth factors produces activation of ERK pathway that leads to cell growth. The Akt pathway mediates cell survival, as well as modulation of eNOS leading to NO-induced vasodilation. Activation of p38 pathway provides signals for cell migration.

Mediators such as VEGF, FGF, Tie, HGF, and PDGF bind to their specific RTK and induce receptor autophosphorylation, which leads to several intracellular signaling cascades. Within these cascades, the roles of phospholipase-γ(PLCγ), PI3-kinase, protein kinase C (PKC), Akt kinase, and mitogen-activated protein kinase (MAPK) have been studied extensively. Cell proliferation in response to VEGF, FGF, PDGF, and HGF appears to involve activation of PLCγ, PI3-kinase, and PKC. Inhibiting either of two members of the PKC family, PKC-α or PKC-Θ, blocks endothelial cell migration, proliferation, and tube formation *(90,91)*. Inhibition of PKC-α with antisense oligonucleotides in vivo limits myocardial angiogenesis following myocardial infarction *(90)*. The role of Ras in VEGF signaling remains controversial. Cell migration and cytoskeletal organization involves activation of Rac and the P38 kinase pathway *(48,49,92,93)*. The Akt pathway mediates cell survival and eNOS activation and expression. A simplified signal transduction pathway leading to angiogenic activity of endothelial cells is presented in (Fig. 2).

Therapeutic Angiogenesis

Rapid progress in the study of angiogenesis, including most notably the identification of angiogenic mediators,

has led to significant optimism for the development of novel vascular therapies. Administration of the angiogenic factors VEGF, FGF, HGF, and PlGF or transfer of their genes has effectively promoted vascularization in models of myocardial ischemia in mice, rats, dogs, and pigs *(8,9)*. In many of these studies, there was also a resulting improvement in regional blood flow or left ventricular function. Similarly, delivery of growth factor proteins or genes resulted in enhanced collaterals, blood flow, and limb function in hind limb ischemia models *(9)*. VEGF gene transfer preserves motor and sensory impairment induced by ischemia *(94)*. These preclinical studies have provided proof of concept and a strong impetus to apply these findings into practical therapies for treating coronary and peripheral vascular disease. These studies have also raised a number of biological and medical issues that will need to be addressed in clinical studies. They include deciding when either arteriogenesis or angiogenesis is appropriate, measuring the extent to which vessels induced by growth factors are mature and stable, choosing a mode of delivery (local or systemic) and a delivery system, and finding any potential side effects of the therapeutic agents.

Medical Rationale for Angiogenic Therapy

There are two main types of patients who could benefit from angiogenesis therapy: those with coronary artery disease and those with peripheral vascular disease. Despite many exciting advances in recent years, current therapy for coronary artery disease is less than ideal, particularly for patients with chronic myocardial ischemia. The available medicines for chronic ischemia mostly reduce the work of the myocardium and thus the requirement for blood flow. Many affected patients require an invasive procedure to restore blood flow to areas of the heart not receiving adequate blood supply, either to improve prognosis or to relieve symptoms. Unfortunately, in many patients, especially those with diffuse disease, revascularization is not possible by catheter-based therapies such as angioplasty or by aortocoronary bypass grafting, because of either technical limitations or concomitant illnesses (95). It is estimated that there are more than 100,000 of these patients, representing 12% of people that undergo coronary angiography (96). Thus, there is a significant need for therapy for these patients at minimum. And if the therapy is effective, safe, and economical, a much larger group of patients might benefit as well.

Patients with peripheral vascular disease face similar unmet needs. Many patients who have symptoms of claudication are not treated with the available medical therapy and are referred for surgery instead. But the vast majority of these patients do not undergo surgical reconstruction. Many of them have a maximum walking capacity of less than a block or have disability so severe that it restricts them to their homes. Some patients who have symptoms of claudication are as impaired as those who have New York Heart Association class III heart failure.

Induction of angiogenesis represents a novel form of therapy for patients with coronary artery or peripheral vascular disease. As seen by angiography, these patients have a naturally occurring compensatory arteriogenesis, and angiogenesis therapy can be considered an enhancement of this process (97,98). True angiogenesis, as demonstrated either by sprouting of capillaries or intussusceptive remodeling, has also been shown to occur following ischemia but is thought to contribute less than arteriogenesis to the tissue blood supply. For reasons that are not well understood, in most patients, blood flow is not sufficiently restored to prevent symptoms and preserve function of the downstream organ (99,100).

Patients with severe congestive heart failure but without severe coronary artery obstruction may also benefit from angiogenesis therapy. This possibility is suggested by studies in VEGF-A knock-out mice, who had impaired myocardial contractility with reduced dP:dT and depressed left ventricular (LV) relaxation (101). These mice also had enlarged hearts, subendocardial ischemia, and impaired angiogenesis. The phenotype implies that in the absence of VEGF, myocardial vascularization is restricted, which leads to ischemic cardiomyopathy. This observation in mice and the knowledge that aging results in reduced angiogenic capacity suggest that replacing deleted portions of VEGF could promote microcirculatory revascularization and improve the function of a failing heart—even when the heart failure is not caused by severe atherosclerotic obstruction of major coronary vessels (102).

In testing angiogenesis therapy, clinical studies should be designed to select patients who are appropriate candidates for therapy. The majority of patients tested thus far in clinical trials of angiogenesis therapy are those who have failed multiple revascularization attempts (103). Such patients might be expected to respond poorly to angiogenic cytokines, as they have not only inadequate natural angiogenic capacity but also impaired response to revascularization. They are also likely to be taking many cardiac medicines, some of which, including spironolactone, aspirin, nitrates, and some statins, may affect angiogenesis. Also, age, hypercholesterolemia, smoking, and diabetes all impair the natural process of collateral formation following ischemia and therefore might hinder the effects of exogenous angiogenic agents as well (104). Thus, patients that are likely to be ideal candidates for therapeutic angiogenesis include those with a single longstanding occlusion, those with proximate coronary arteries feeding a viable myocardium, and those with multi-vessel diffuse disease with evidence of inducible ischemia and myocardial viability and with adequate feeder vessels and distal runoff (104).

Methods of Delivering Angiogenic Growth Factors

Successful clinical angiogenic therapy requires a practical method of growth factor delivery. Exogenous angiogenic growth factors have been administered through many routes. These include intravenous delivery, delivery through the left atrium, intracoronary delivery, transepicardial placement via thoracotomy, transendocardial intramyocardial delivery by electromechanical catheter at the time of bypass surgery or during a separate procedure, and intrapericardial delivery (105). Local delivery of recombinant protein or gene product is likely to be the method physicians accept most, because it lacks systemic exposure; however, the intramyocardial strategy of local delivery is not an ideal one unless the patient is undergoing aortic coronary bypass surgery. An attractive method for delivering growth factor locally at the time of bypass surgery is to implant heparin alginate capsules that provide a prolonged (4- to 5-wk) release of growth factor from the polymer *(104,106)*. These capsules have not been associated with an inflammatory response. Epicardial perivascular delivery has a particular appeal because it may result in arteriogenesis rather than angiogenesis, since the epicardium is the site at which arteriogenesis occurs. In recent studies, percutaneous catheters were used to transfer genes into the myocardium, and this approach could also be used to deliver recombinant proteins *(107)*. Intracoronary infusions probably involve shorter exposure of angiogenic growth factor than do intravenous infusions, although hypotension has been associated with both. Identifying agents that are specific for the targeted vasculature would obviate many of the problems with local drug delivery and would allow a simple method of administration *(108)*. But thus far no agent has been found that is both specific for a given vascular bed and successful in improving perfusion and function of the ischemic myocardial bed.

Angiogenic agents have been delivered either as recombinant proteins or through gene transfer. Thus far, no small molecular agonists have been tested in patients with ischemia. In principle, no essential differences exist between gene-transfer and protein-based therapy; with gene transfer, the goal is to have infected or transfected cells produce and release angiogenic proteins that would be similar to recombinant ones. However, gene-transfer therapy might be more favorable *(109)*, because it may provide longer protein expression than protein therapy. However, it should be noted that the optimal length of time for expression of an angiogenic protein has not been established. And in experimental models, angiogenesis can be stimulated by a short-term injection of angiogenic proteins or by means of delivery that produce a longer effect, such as slow release polymers *(106)* and adenoviral constructs encoding angiogenic proteins *(110)*. Many believe that angiogenic protein activity should last at least a week, which is similar to the length of time that adenoviral constructs express proteins. Protein-based therapy can result in a similar time course and release when slow-release polymers are delivered with newer devices such as drug-coated stents and injectible drug-impregnated matrices *(109)*. In fact, because adenoviral constructs can encounter antiadenoviral antibodies, barriers to cellular uptake, and other negative factors, the pharmokinetics achieved with gene-transfer therapy may be less predictable than those achieved with protein therapy. Thus, further studies are needed to determine the relative efficacies of both gene-transfer and protein therapies.

Adenovirus is the most commonly used vector for gene-transfer therapies, but there are a number of ways to deliver genes into cells. Naked plasmid DNA can be transfected into cells, and there are several expression vector systems that are used for preclinical and clinical testing, including replication-deficient adenovirus, retrovirus, lentivirus, and adeno-associated virus *(111)*. (For a more complete description of gene therapy, please see Chapter 4.)

Adenoviral vectors can cause inflammation at the site of injection, which leads to the formation of new capillaries there; thus, studies in which these vectors are used need to be carefully controlled. Adeno-associated viral vectors, on the other hand, appear to produce less inflammation, but it is not known whether these vectors can express growth factors that induce angiogenesis. Lentiviral vectors can stably express marker genes in hematopoietic progenitor cells *(113)*. Thus, one could envision using lentiviral vectors to alter bone marrow–derived endothelial precursor cells to release angiogenic substances following implantation. Others have raised the possibility, however, that integration of a lentiviral-mediated gene into the host genome could induce gene mutations or unregulated, continuous transgene expression, both of which can cause hemangiomas *(114,115)*.

Potential Risks of Angiogenic Therapy

Risks of angiogenic therapy can be associated with an individual therapeutic agent, the method for delivering the agent, or the angiogenesis itself *(105)*.

As noted above, bolus infusions of recombinant proteins, especially infusions of VEGF, can induce hypotension *(103,105)*. This hypotension results from the stimulation and release of NO, a powerful vasodilator, and it limits the dose of VEGF that can be infused. Thus far, hypotension has not resulted from gene-transfer experiments with VEGF *(105)*. Infusions of members of the FGF family can cause hypotension *(103)*, but to a lesser extent than VEGF can. In addition to inducing hypotension, VEGF can induce vascular permeability *(116)*. It is not clear whether vascular permeability facilitates angiogenesis. Vascular permeability may, however, have undesirable consequences: local edema has been observed in patients who received VEGF for lower extremity ischemia *(117)*. It is not clear whether this is more than a cosmetic concern for these patients, nor whether similar edema occurs with local injection into the heart, where it might be a great deal more problematic. In preclinical models, FGF-2 appears to result in renal insufficiency due to membrane nephropathy accompanied by proteinuria, although this effect has not been significant in clinical trials when FGF-2 is used as intracoronary infusion *(103)*. The mechanism that causes this nephropathy is not known.

With gene-transfer therapy, there are potential risks associated with introducing foreign genetic material into a patient's genome and with exposing patients to viral vectors. There are also concerns about the inflammatory responses that have been associated with the use of adenoviral vectors (111) and about the "angiomatas" that are composed of insufficient vessels and produced by local injection or intense gene expression in some models (114,115).

With any systemic administration of angiogenic agents, there is a potential for adverse events in both remote and targeted tissues. Pathological angiogenesis, such as retinopathies or malignancies, can occur in remote tissues, and adverse events such as angiomas can occur in targeted tissues (104). Neither VEGF nor FGF-2 has been shown to increase the risk of neoplastic growth or metastasis. This has been extensively investigated preclinically (118), and thus far short-term safety profiles for VEGF and FGF-2 therapies are promising (104,105). As judged by serial funduscopic examinations, there is no evidence that administration of angiogenic agents increases retinopathy, despite the fact that many of the patients enrolled in the clinical trial have a history of diabetes and retinopathy. The reasons why angiogenic agents do not cause malignancies or retinopathies are not clear, but they may result from the relatively short half-life of these agents (119).

There is no equivocal evidence that administering growth factors has a target organ or "bystander" effect of accelerating atherosclerosis. The vasa vasorum in the vascular wall must extend into the media if the vessel wall is thicker than 0.5 mm, which implies that thickening of the arterial wall requires new blood vessel growth. The severity of atherosclerosis and the instability of atherosclerotic plaques have been linked to the presence and exuberance of the vasa vasorum growth (120), but it is not clear whether this vessel growth is causative. Inhibitors of angiogenesis inhibit plaque progression in a hypercholesterolemic mouse model of atherosclerosis (121). Although there are limits to applying results from these models to atherosclerosis in humans, these results suggest that neovascularization is necessary for the development and progression of atherosclerotic plaque. Recent studies have shown that VEGF administration advances existing atherosclerosis in animal models (122). These studies are controversial, however, and whether VEGF would have the same effect in humans is less clear (123,124).

Furthermore, there are several studies in animals and humans that have found no evidence that administering vascular growth factors accelerates atherosclerosis—in fact, the results of some studies suggest that vascular growth factors slow atherosclerosis (105,120). Thousands of patients have been treated with angiogenic agents, and there is no evidence that the treatment contributed to further atherosclerosis. In experimental animals, angiogenic factors were added during the early stages of atherosclerosis progression. Yet the clinically most relevant question is whether these factors contribute to atherosclerosis to the extent that therapeutic angiogenesis is then needed (102). Furthermore, experimental evidence suggests that enhancing endothelial function and regrowth reduces vascular damage. The reduction in damage likely occurs because certain functions of the intact endothelium—such as regulating permeability and thrombogenicity and producing antiangiogenic substances—are critical in preventing intimal thickening.

Clinical Methods of Evaluating Therapeutic Angiogenesis

For more than 5 years, there has been considerable discussion and debate regarding how to best evaluate the efficacy of therapeutic angiogenesis in patients with coronary heart disease (99,103,105). It is not clear whether angiogenic therapy might be expected to lengthen survival or just alleviate symptoms of patients with chronic ischemia. Determining the goal of therapy would help clinicians decide when the risks and expense of the therapy are justified. If inducing angiogenesis serves only to alleviate symptoms then a substantial enhancement of the quality of life would be necessary to justify treatment (104).

For angiogenic therapy to be accepted, its physiological benefits will need to be demonstrated. Possible benefits include improved myocardial perfusion, improvement in global or regional left ventricular function, increased blood flow, and formation of collateral vessels (99). Clinical studies thus far have focused on the endpoints historically used to evaluate new antianginal drugs, including angina class, time to exercise, and quality of life (105). As noted in previous analyses, the placebo effect has confounded many of the angiogenic therapy studies to date. In addition, exercise treadmill time can be influenced by several factors, such as motivation, that are unrelated to cardiac health. Also problematic is the high variability of exercise performance on a day-to-day basis. At least part of this variability is due to the subjective nature of the indications for terminating exercise (105). Improving health-related quality of life is an important therapeutic objective (104). Tools for assessing disease-specific and generic quality of life measures have been developed and standardized and have become quite reliable and reproducible. An important limitation to this approach has been making physicians aware of the value of these tools in assessing methods of revascularization.

Nuclear imaging has been used extensively in clinical practice to provide objective estimates of relative myocardial blood flow. The major concern regarding the technology is whether single-photon-emission computed tomography (SPECT) has sufficient sensitivity and spatial resolution for detecting subtle improvements in perfusion. SPECT is highly sensitive for detecting and localizing large areas of ischemia or infarction in obstructed major coronary arteries, but there is less evidence that SPECT is effective in detecting small increases of blood flow via collaterals. Nonetheless, there is evidence from phase I clinical studies that SPECT may be able to detect improvement in myocardial blood flow (104,105).

The techniques positron emission tomography (PET), which can quantify regional coronary blood flow at rest and during vasodilation (104), and modified magnetic resonance (MR) perfusion imaging (125) have promise for assessing angiogenesis. Thus far, use of these technologies, especially MR perfusion imaging, has been limited to a small number of clinical sites (105). In recent studies, contrast echocardiography has documented improved perfusion following treatment with an angiogenic agent (126). This technique offers considerable advantages, but it has only been in use for a short period of time.

It might be assumed that angiography would be valuable in detecting evidence of neovascularization; however, that has not proved to be the case. Detection of collateral vessels by angiography has been limited by the variability that results from injecting contrast by hand and the spatial resolution of the technique. The diameter of many collaterals formed in response to arterial occlusion and/or therapeutic angiogenesis is less than 200 μm (127), which is below the limits of resolution of conventional angiography. Thus, although extensive work has been done to develop quantitative indices for angiography (128), it is not clear that it will be a suitable technique for detecting therapeutically significant angiogenesis.

Angiogenic Growth Factors in Clinical Testing

Several studies using animal models of coronary ischemia have shown that therapeutic agents can enhance collateral formation. Both FGF-1 and FGF-2 have been shown to be effective, as have several VEGF isoforms and other agents as well (99,103,105). Recently, gene transfer of FGF-5 in an adenoviral vector by a single intracoronary infusion provided relief of stress-induced myocardial ischemia, with improved collateral flow and 12 wk of documented growth factor expression (129). Intracoronary delivery of this vector was followed by 98% first pass metabolism, indicating minimal systemic exposure, which suggests most of it went to the heart.

The results of these studies mean that inducing angiogenesis with a pharmacological agent is an attractive alternative therapy for patients with severe coronary or peripheral disease who remain symptomatic despite maximal medical care. Most commonly, such patients have been administered naturally occurring growth factors prepared in purified or recombinant form. It is assumed that these growth factors promote growth of new collateral blood vessels from preexisting vascular structures. To date, FGF-2, also known as basic FGF, and VEGF have been most commonly used in clinical trials testing induction of angiogenesis. The first trial to demonstrate induction of neovascularization in ischemic myocardium was carried out by injecting FGF-1 (acidic FGF) into the myocardium of patients undergoing coronary artery bypass grafting (130). Unlike many of the early studies, this one was controlled, in that a group of patients received an inactive form of the growth factor. The endpoint tested was increased vascularity, as determined by increased contrast densities. As a result of the injections of active growth factor, vascular networks in the region of the left anterior coronary artery were enhanced. Echocardiography showed an increase in left ventricular regional wall motion in the study group and the patients had some improvement in the New York Heart Association classification. In treated patients, the dense capillary network that arose in the region into which the factor had been injected lasted for several years, as determined by angiography (131). Thus, the feasibility of inducing new blood vessels was shown; however, clinical endpoints were difficult to interpret, as all of the patients in the study had received bypass grafting. Nonetheless, this study was an important proof of principle.

Several uncontrolled clinical trials have shown that VEGF, in particular, administered either by gene transfer or as a recombinant protein, can induce angiogenesis. Early attempts to induce angiogenesis were done by intramuscular injections of plasmid DNA encoding VEGF—first the studies were done in patients with critical limb ischemia (132), and later studies were done in patients with severe myocardial ischemia (133). In these studies, ulcers healed in four of seven patients with limb ischemia, and proliferating endothelial cells could be demonstrated in tissue obtained from treated patients at 10 wk. The ankle brachial indices were also improved in the treated group.

Treatment with VEGF has not been exclusive to patients with peripheral vascular disease: in several studies during the last few years, plasmids encoding VEGF have been injected into the myocardium of patients with coronary disease. In the first of these, the VEGF plasmids were directly injected via a left anterior thoracotomy into the ischemic myocardial areas of patients with symptomatic angina in whom conventional therapy had failed *(133)*. In these patients, reduced ischemia could be demonstrated after 30 and 60 d by pharmacologic stress testing with SPECT as an endpoint. In addition, the collateral flow of these patients improved. A second study was conducted by investigators who used an adenoviral vector that encoded VEGF *(134)*. They delivered the vector to patients by direct myocardial injection into an area of ischemia, and they did so chiefly as an adjunct to conventional aorta coronary bypass grafting. These patients subsequently had reduced symptoms, improved nuclear imaging, and increased duration of exercise during stress testing. In a third study, investigators used electromechanical mapping to assess whether plasmids that encode VEGF can stimulate angiogenesis in patients with chronic or refractory angina. These patients received VEGF via a limited thoracotomy with direct injection into the myocardium *(135)*.

In a further placebo controlled study in patients with myocardial ischemia, electromechanical mapping, which can identify viable myocardium, showed that injection of VEGF C-DNA plasmid resulted in a decrease in the area of ischemic myocardium, 60 d after injection *(107)*. This decrease was confirmed by imaging with nuclear tracers. In addition, the patients experienced an increase in their exercise capacity and a decrease in anginal symptoms and in their use of antianginal medications.

Another angiogenic factor, FGF-2, was administered to patients with refractory angina by either intracoronary or intravenous injection. In these patients, myocardial perfusion abnormalities were reduced at 180 d after the injection, as determined by SPECT *(136)*.

In most of the early studies, there were no control groups. This is far from trivial, because in clinical trials of angiogenic agents, patients who receive placebo often exhibit a very significant improvement in both subjectively and objectively measured outcomes. In some cases this improvement is similar to that which has been documented with conventional therapies. Thus, before a particular angiogenic therapy can be accepted, it is essential that trials be carefully controlled and double-blinded to allow proper interpretation of the results.

A recent small study examined whether another FGF family member, FGF-4, could affect the length of time patients with chronic stable angina can exercise *(110)*. This study was carried out primarily to establish the safety of and determine the most effective dose for treating patients with FGF-4 in a replication-deficient adenoviral vector by intracoronary injection. Although the drug appeared to be safe and was tolerated well by the majority of patients, the duration of exercise time was not significantly different in the small group of patients ($n = 60$) who received the drug versus those who did not, nor was there difference in the time of exercise before angina developed. However, among a subset of patients whose pretreatment exercise times were below 10 mins, those who received FGF-4 did have 20–30% improvement in their times, and they also could exercise longer before developing angina. A transient rise in liver enzymes was seen in two treated patients and may have been caused by hepatotoxicity of the adenoviral vector. The 20–30% improvement is approximately the range seen with angioplasty or bypass surgery, and it is possible that a larger study would have resulted in significant improvement in this parameter.

The first double-blind placebo-controlled phase II trial of FGF-2 evaluated its use as an adjunct to bypass surgery in 24 patients *(106)*. All of these patients had at least one ungraftable vessel supplying ischemic but viable myocardium. They were randomly assigned to receive either 10 μg or 100 μg of FGF-2 incorporated in heparin–alginate beads. The control group received beads without the growth factor. These beads were implanted during coronary bypass surgery along the distribution of the vessel that could not be bypassed. This technique had the advantage of not increasing plasma FGF-2 levels and thus resulted in truly local delivery. All 16 patients who received FGF-2 were free of angina 90 d following surgery. Two of eight patients who received the placebo pellets continued to have angina. Remarkably, the nuclear scans demonstrated target perfusion in all of the patients who received a high dose of FGF-2, but in only 40% of the control and low-dose FGF groups combined. In patients receiving the high dose of FGF-2, MRI analysis detected some improvement in regional wall motion. This trial was small, but it provides some optimism for the prospect of using local angiogenic therapy to promote complete revascularization in patients who undergo bypass surgery *(106)*.

The first large placebo-controlled phase II study of combined intracoronary and intravenous treatment was done using recombinant VEGF-1 *(137)*. The vascular endothelial growth factor in ischemia for vascular angiogenesis (VIVA) study evaluated 178 so-called "no option" patients. Two separate doses of VEGF were given—the first was given as a single intracoronary infusion and the second was given as three separate intravenous infusions. Exercise time, the primary endpoint in the VIVA study, was not different in any of the three groups. This lack of difference could be explained by the placebo group's increase of exercise time, and it is possible that a larger study might have shown a significant difference. In support of the negative findings, at 60 d after treatment there were no differences between the groups in patients' classification of angina or quality of life measurements. Interestingly, there was a significant reduction in angina assessed at 120 d in the group that received the high dose of VEGF; the main reason for this is the reduction of the placebo effect. No differences were detected by angiography or nuclear perfusion at 120 d. It is of interest that three patients developed malignancy following enrollment in the study; all three had been randomly assigned to the placebo group.

A larger study, entitled FGF initiating revascularization trial (FIRST), was carried out by treating 337 patients with FGF-2 *(138)*. This placebo-controlled study evaluated patients at a time point 90 d after FGF-2 administration. There were no significant differences between the placebo and FGF groups in regards to the primary endpoint of exercise time. Angina was less frequent in the FGF group as determined by the Seattle Angina Questionnaire, but the difference was not statistically significant. Analysis of a subgroup chosen after the study without a prespecified endpoint revealed significant improvement in exercise time in patients older than 63 yr and improvement in symptoms of angina in patients who had moderate to severe angina at baseline. These results suggest that if an older, sicker population with severe angina had been tested, there may have been a more positive outcome for the group who received FGF.

The first phase II, double-blind, placebo-controlled study that used FGF-2 to treat patients with peripheral vascular disease was completed recently *(139)*. This study, entitled therapeutic angiogenesis with recombinant fibroblast growth factor-2 for treatment of claudication (TRAFFIC), evaluated several dosing regimens of FGF-2, including single and double infusions. The primary endpoint for this study was a change in peak walking time—that is, patients' duration of exercise at d 90 relative to their baseline time. Secondary endpoints were peak walking time at 180 d, quality of life, and other measurements standard for coronary trials. The arterial infusion of recombinant FGF-2 appeared safe. The results of this trial differed from both of the intracoronary trials described, in that treatment with the drug resulted in increased exercise times at 90 d. This difference was seen only in the group that received a single infusion. Unfortunately, at 180 d this difference was no longer seen. In addition, the quality of life and other measurements were not remarkably different between the groups at either 90 or 180 d. The lack of difference in exercise times between the groups at 180 d

was not caused by a decline in the benefit of the active drug but rather an improvement in the placebo group.

FUTURE DIRECTIONS

It has been suggested that the overall lack of success in using angiogenic agents to treat patients with heart disease is because the agents selectively act on the endothelium, and they lack the ability to coordinate the surrounding periendothelial tissues to allow for a mature, impermeable, and thus beneficial blood vessel *(140)*. A fundamental difference between capillaries and large collateral blood vessels lies in their relative abilities to produce myocardial blood flow—a single, medium-sized collateral provides more blood flow to the tissues than millions of capillaries *(141)*. Experimentally, formation of these arteriogenic vessels can be induced by regional ischemia and also by macrophage-based cytokines such as MCP-1 *(142)*. There are several approaches that might stimulate arteriogenesis in a clinical population. One approach that has been used preclinically, but for which no clinical trials have yet been reported, is administering combinations of growth factors to reproduce the cascade of factors that are required to produce vascular networks and activated in response to ischemia *(140)*. For instance, one might co-administer VEGF and the cytokine Ang-1 to stabilize endothelium or VEGF and a growth factor, such as PDGF that recruits pericytes or SMCs. A second approach is to administer a single factor that operates as a "master gene" and has pleiotropic effects on endothelial and other vascular and inflammatory cells. For instance, HIF-1α has been shown to increase expression of VEGF, Ang-1, PDGF, and other genes and is currently in clinical testing following its success in preclinical studies *(103)*. Also, the PR-39 peptide, which can induce angiogenesis *(86)*, not only affects HIF-1α degradation, but also induces expression of other genes beneficial for angiogenesis.

A growth factor that can induce both angiogenesis and arteriogenesis is hepatic growth factor (HGF). HGF can induce angiogenesis when administered by intramuscular injection into hind limbs of rat with diabetes and ischemia *(143)*. Transfecting HGF can also induce angiogenesis in a rat myocardial infarction model *(144)*. Clinical trials are underway to test whether intramuscular injections of HGF-encoding plasmid DNA can stimulate angiogenesis in patients with peripheral vascular disease.

A potential approach to stimulate arteriogenesis is to treat patients with GM–CSF. In a recent double-blind placebo-controlled study, patients with extensive coronary artery disease who were not eligible for coronary artery bypass surgery *(18)* were randomly assigned to either receive GM–CSF or not. The endpoint measured was the invasive collateral flow index (CFI), and it was recorded immediately before intracoronary injection of the growth factor and after a 2-wk period during which the growth factor was administered subcutaneously. CFI, which measures collateral flow during coronary occlusion, markedly increased in the GM–CSF group and decreased in the placebo group. This is the first clinical trial to show that treatment with a growth factor can stimulate growth of large conductive collaterals *(145)*. GM–CSF may stimulate arteriogenesis by activating macrophages, which have been shown to induce arteriogenesis *(146)*. GM–CSF could potentially activate macrophages locally or cause them to be released in precursor form from the bone marrow. Because of the small number of patients in this study, there was considerable variability and it is possible that the differences between the two groups might be greater in a study with more patients. Confirmation of these results in a larger study will help determine if this technique may be more generally applied to patients with myocardial ischemia.

REFERENCES

1. Asahara T, Masuda H, Takahashi T, et al. Bone marrow origin of endothelial progenitor cells responsible for postnatal vasculogenesis in physiological and pathological neovascularization. Circ Res 1999;85:221–228.
2. Takahashi T, Kalka C, Masuda H, et al. Ischemia- and cytokine-induced mobilization of bone marrow-derived endothelial progenitor cells for neovascularization. Nat Med 1999; 5:434–438.
3. Asahara T, Murohara T, Sullivan A, et al. Isolation of putative progenitor endothelial cells for angiogenesis. Science 1997;275:964–967.
4. Luttun A, Carmeliet G, Carmeliet P. Vascular progenitors. From biology to treatment. Trends Cardiovas Med 2002;12:88–96.
5. Lyden D, Hattori K, Dias S, et al. Impaired recruitment of bone-marrow-derived endothelial and hematopoietic precursor cells blocks tumor angiogenesis and growth. Nat Med 2001;7: 1194–1201.
6. Risau W. Mechanisms of angiogenesis. Nature 1997;386:671–674.
7. Deindl E, Buschman I, Hoefer IE, et al. Role of ischemia and of hypoxia-inducible genes in arteriogenesis after femoral artery occlusion in the rabbit. Circ Res 2001;89:779–786.
8. Freedman SB, Isner JM. Therapeutic angiogenesis for coronary artery disease. Ann Intern Med 2002;136:54–71.
9. Manninen HI, Makinen K. Gene therapy techniques for peripheral arterial disease. Cardiovasc Intervent Radiol 2002;25:98–108.
10. Semenza GL. Hypoxia-inducible factor 1: master regulator of O2 homeostasis. Curr Opin Genet Dev 1998;8:588–594.
11. Oh H, Takagi H, Suzuma K, Otani A, Matsumura M, Honda Y. Hypoxia and vascular endothelial growth factor selectively up-regulate angiopoietin-2 in bovine microvascular endothelial cells. J Biol Chem 1999;274:15732–15739.
12. Sunderkotter C, Steinbrink K, Goebeler M, Bhardwaj R, Sorg C. Macrophages and angiogenesis. J Leukoc Biol 1994;55:410–422.
13. Fukumura D, Gohongi T, Kadambi A, et al. Predominant role of endothelial nitric oxide synthase in vascular endothelial growth factor-induced angiogenesis and vascular permeability. Proc Natl Acad Sci USA 2001;98:2604–2609.
14. Pepper MS, Ferrara N, Orci L, Montesano R. Vascular endothelial growth factor (VEGF) induces plasminogen activators and plasminogen activator inhibitor-1 in microvascular endothelial cells. Biochem Biophys Res Commun 1991;181:902–906.
15. Dimmeler S, Aicher A, Vasa M, et al. HMG-CoA reductase inhibitors (statins) increase endothelial progenitor cells via the PI 3-kinase/Akt pathway. J Clin Invest 2001;108:391–397.
16. Llevadot J, Murasawa S, Kureishi Y, et al. HMG-CoA reductase inhibitor mobilizes bone marrow—derived endothelial progenitor cells. J Clin Invest 2001;108:399–405.
17. Kamihata H, Matsubara H, Nishiue T, et al. Implantation of bone marrow mononuclear cells into ischemic myocardium enhances collateral perfusion and regional function via side supply of angioblasts, angiogenic ligands, and cytokines. Circulation 2001;104:1046–1052.
18. Seiler C, Pohl T, Wustmann K, et al. Promotion of collateral growth by granulocyte-macrophage colony-stimulating factor in patients with coronary artery disease. Circulation 2001; 104:2012–2017.
19. Benjamin LE, Hemo I, Keshet E. A plasticity window for blood vessel remodelling is defined by pericyte coverage of the preformed endothelial network and is regulated by PDGF-B and VEGF. Development 1998;125:1591–1598.
20. Schaper W, Ito WD. Molecular mechanisms of coronary collateral vessel growth. Circ Res 1996;79:911–919.
21. Ferrara N, Houck K, Jakeman L, Leung DW. Molecular and biological properties of the vascular endothelial growth factor family of proteins. Endocr Rev 1992;13:18–32.
22. Partanen TA, Makinen T, Arola J, Suda T, Weich HA, Alitalo K. Endothelial growth factor receptors in human fetal heart. Circulation 1999;100:583–586.
23. Carmeliet P, Ferreira V, Breier G, et al. Abnormal blood vessel development and lethality in embryos lacking a single VEGF allele. Nature 1996;380:435–439.
24. Park JE, Chen HH, Winer J, Houck KA, Ferrara N. Placenta growth factor. Potentiation of vascular endothelial growth factor bioactivity, in vitro and in vivo, and high affinity binding to FLT-1 but not to FLK-1/KDR. J Biol Chem 1994;269:25646–25654.
25. Carmeliet P, Moons L, Luttun A, et al. Synergism between vascular endothelial growth factor and placental growth factor contributes to angiogenesis and plasma extravasation in pathological conditions. Nat Med 2001;7:575–583.
26. Barleon B, Hauser S, Schollmann C, et al. Differential expression of the two VEGF receptors flt and KDR in placenta and vascular endothelial cells. J Cell Biochem 1994; 54:56–66.
27. Clauss M, Gerlach M, Gerlach H, et al. Vascular permeability factor: a tumor-derived polypeptide that induces endothelial cell and monocyte procoagulant activity, and promotes monocyte migration. J Exp Med 1990;172:1535–1545.
28. Shalaby F, Ho J, Stanford WL, et al. A requirement for Flk1 in primitive and definitive hematopoiesis and vasculogenesis. Cell 1997;89:981–990.
29. Ferrara N. Role of vascular endothelial growth factor in the regulation of angiogenesis. Kidney International 1999;56:794–814.
30. Ferrara N, Carver-Moore K, Chen H, et al. Heterozygous embryonic lethality induced by targeted inactivation of the VEGF gene. Nature 1996;380:439–442.

31. Shalaby F, Rossant J, Yamaguchi TP, et al. Failure of blood-island formation and vasculogenesis in FLK-1- deficient mice. Nature 1995;376:62–66.

32. Fong GH, Rossant J, Gertsenstein M, Breitman ML. Role of the FLT-1 receptor tyrosine kinase in regulating the assembly of vascular endothelium. Nature 1995;376:66–70.

33. Clauss M, Weich H, Breier G, et al. The vascular endothelial growth factor receptor Flt-1 mediates biological activities. Implications for a functional role of placenta growth factor in monocyte activation and chemotaxis. J Biol Chem 1996; 271:17629–17634.

34. Waltenberger J, Claesson-Welsh L, Siegbahn A, Shibuya M, Heldin CH. Different signal transduction properties of KDR and Flt1, two receptors for vascular endothelial growth factor. J Biol Chem 1994;269:26988–26995.

35. Soker S, Takashima S, Miao HQ, Neufeld G, Klagsbrun M. Neuropilin-1 is expressed by endothelial and tumor cells as an isoform-specific receptor for vascular endothelial growth factor. Cell 1998;92:735–745.

36. Soldi R, Mitola S, Strasly M, Defilippi P, Tarone G, Bussolino F. Role of alphavbeta3 integrin in the activation of vascular endothelial growth factor receptor-2. Embo J 1999;18:882–892.

37. Hu MC, Qiu WR, Wang YP, et al. FGF-18, a novel member of the fibroblast growth factor family, stimulates hepatic and intestinal proliferation. Mol Cell Biol 1998;18:6063–6074.

38. Mason IJ. The ins and outs of fibroblast growth factors. Cell 1994;78:547–552.

39. Crossley PH, Martin GR. The mouse FGF8 gene encodes a family of polypeptides and is expressed in regions that direct outgrowth and patterning in the developing embryo. Development 1995;121:439–451.

40. Finch PW, Rubin JS, Miki T, Ron D, Aaronson SA. Human KGF is FGF-related with properties of a paracrine effector of epithelial cell growth. Science 1989;245:752–755.

41. John D, Williams T. Structional and functional diversity in the FGF receptor multi gene family. Adv Cancer Res 1993;60:1L–4L.

42. Wiedlocha A, Falnes PO, Rapak A, Munoz R, Klingenberg O, Olsnes S. Stimulation of proliferation of a human osteosarcoma cell line by exogenous acidic fibroblast growth factor requires both activation of receptor tyrosine kinase and growth factor internalization. Mol Cell Biol 1996;16:270–280.

43. Davis S, Aldrich TH, Jones PF, et al. Isolation of angiopoietin-1, a ligand for the TIE2 receptor, by secretion-trap expression cloning. Cell 1996;87:1161–1169.

44. Dumont DJ, Gradwohl G, Fong GH, et al. Dominant-negative and targeted null mutations in the endothelial receptor tyrosine kinase, tek, reveal a critical role in vasculogenesis of the embryo. Genes Dev 1994;8:1897–1909.

45. Puri MC, Rossant J, Alitalo K, Bernstein A, Partanen J. The receptor tyrosine kinase TIE is required for integrity and survival of vascular endothelial cells. Embo J 1995;14:5884–5891.

46. Thurston G, Rudge JS, Ioffe E, et al. Angiopoietin-1 protects the adult vasculature against plasma leakage. Nat Med 2000;6:460–463.

47. Maisonpierre PC, Suri C, Jones PF, et al. Angiopoietin-2, a natural antagonist for Tie2 that disrupts in vivo angiogenesis. Science 1997;277:55–60.

48. Papapetropoulos A, Fulton D, Mahboubi K, et al. Angiopoietin-1 inhibits endothelial cell apoptosis via the Akt/survivin pathway. J Biol Chem 2000;275:9102–9105.

49. Fujikawa K, de Aos Scherpenseel I, Jain SK, Presman E, Christensen RA, Varticovski L. Role of PI 3-kinase in angiopoietin-1-mediated migration and attachment-dependent survival of endothelial cells. Exp Cell Res 1999;253:663–672.

50. Korpelainen EI, Karkkainen M, Gunji Y, Vikkula M, Alitalo K. Endothelial receptor tyrosine kinases activate the STAT signaling pathway: mutant Tie-2 causing venous malformations signals a distinct STAT activation response. Oncogene 1999;18:1–8.

51. Yoon JC, Chickering TW, Rosen ED, et al. Peroxisome proliferator-activated receptor gamma target gene encoding a novel angiopoietin-related protein associated with adipose differentiation. Mol Cell Biol 2000;20:5343–5349.

52. Nakamura Y, Morishita R, Higaki J, et al. Expression of local hepatocyte growth factor system in vascular tissues. Biochem Biophys Res Commun 1995;215:483–488.

53. Aoki M, Morishita R, Taniyama Y, et al. Angiogenesis induced by hepatocyte growth factor in non-infarcted myocardium and infarcted myocardium: up-regulation of essential transcription factor for angiogenesis, ets. Gene Ther 2000;7:417–427.

54. Ono K, Matsumori A, Shioi T, Furukawa Y, Sasayama S. Enhanced expression of hepatocyte growth factor/c-Met by myocardial ischemia and reperfusion in a rat model. Circulation 1997;95:2552–2558.

55. Taniyama Y, Morishita R, Hiraoka K, et al. Therapeutic angiogenesis induced by human hepatocyte growth factor gene in rat diabetic hind limb ischemia model. Circulation 2001;104:2344–2350.

56. LeCouter J, Kowalski J, Foster J, et al. Identification of an angiogenic mitogen selective for endocrine gland endothelium. Nature 2001;412:877–884.

57. Shinbrot E, Peters KG, Williams LT. Expression of the platelet-derived growth factor beta receptor during organogenesis and tissue differentiation in the mouse embryo. Dev Dyn 1994; 199:169–175.

58. Dumont DJ, Fong GH, Puri MC, Gradwohl G, Alitalo K, Breitman ML. Vascularization of the mouse embryo: a study of FLK-1, tek, tie, and vascular endothelial growth factor expression during development. Dev Dyn 1995;203:80–92.

59. Leveen P, Pekny M, Gebre-Medhin S, Swolin B, Larsson E, Betsholtz C. Mice deficient for PDGF B show renal, cardiovascular, and hematological abnormalities. Genes Dev 1994; 8:1875–1887.

60. Lindahl P, Johansson BR, Leveen P, Betsholtz C. Pericyte loss and microaneurysm formation in PDGF-B-deficient mice. Science 1997;277:242–245.

61. Schatteman GC, Motley ST, Effmann EL, Bowen-Pope DF. Platelet-derived growth factor receptor alpha subunit deleted Patch mouse exhibits severe cardiovascular dysmorphogenesis. Teratology 1995;51:351–366.

62. Arras M, Ito WD, Scholz D, Winkler B, Schaper J, Schaper W. Monocyte activation in angiogenesis and collateral growth in the rabbit hindlimb. J Clin Invest 1998;101:40–50.

63. Aiello RJ, Bourassa PA, Lindsey S, et al. Monocyte chemoattractant protein-1 accelerates atherosclerosis in apolipoprotein E-deficient mice. Arterioscler Thromb Vasc Biol 1999;19:1518–1525.

64. Johnsen M, Lund LR, Romer J, Almholt K, Dano K. Cancer invasion and tissue remodeling: common themes in proteolytic matrix degradation. Curr Opin Cell Biol 1998;10:667–671.

65. Coughlin SR. Thrombin signalling and protease-activated receptors. Nature 2000;407:258–264.

66. Griffin CT, Srinivasan Y, Zheng YW, Huang W, Coughlin SR. A role for thrombin receptor signaling in endothelial cells during embryonic development. Science 2001;293:1666–1670.

67. Siegbahn A. Cellular consequences upon factor VIIa binding to tissue factor. Haemostasis 2000;30:S41–S47.

68. Carmeliet P, Mackman N, Moons L, et al. Role of tissue factor in embryonic blood vessel development. Nature 1996;383:73–75.

69. Shattil SJ, Ginsberg MH. Integrin signaling in vascular biology. J Clin Invest 1997;100:S91–S95.

70. Rupp PA, Little CD. Integrins in vascular development. Circ Res 2001;89:566–572.

71. Brooks PC, Clark RA, Cheresh DA. Requirement of vascular integrin alpha v beta 3 for angiogenesis. Science 1994;264:569–571.

72. Maeshima Y, Yerramalla UL, Dhanabal M, et al. Extracellular matrix-derived peptide binds to v3 integrin and inhibits angiogenesis. J Biol Chem 2001;276:31959–31968.

73. Scatena M, Giachelli C. The alpha(v)beta3 integrin, NF-kappaB, osteoprotegerin endothelial cell survival pathway. Potential role in angiogenesis. Trends Cardiovas Med 2002;12:83–88.

74. Heeschen C, Jang JJ, Weis M, et al. Nicotine stimulates angiogenesis and promotes tumor growth and atherosclerosis. Nat Med 2001;7:833-839.

75. Conklin BS, Zhao W, Zhong D-S, Chen C. Nicotine and cotinine up-regulate vascular endothelial growth factor expression in endothelial cells. Am J Pathol 2002;160:413–418.

76. Cucina A, Corvino V, Sapienza P, et al. Nicotine regulates basic fibroblastic growth factor and transforming growth factor beta1 production in endothelial cells. Biochem Biophys Res Commun 1999;257:306–312.

77. Joseph AM, Norman SM, Ferry LH, et al. The safety of transdermal nicotine as an aid to smoking cessation in patients with cardiac disease. N Engl J Med 1996;335:1792–1798.

78. Waldum HL, Nilsen OG, Nilsen T, et al. Long-term effects of inhaled nicotine. Life Sci 1996;58:1339–1346.

79. Li Z, Barrios V, Buchholz JN, Glenn TC, Duckles SP. Chronic nicotine administration does not affect peripheral vascular reactivity in the rat. J Pharmacol Exp Ther 1994;271:1135–1142.

80. Emanueli C, Bonaria Salis M, Stacca T, et al. Targeting kinin B(1) receptor for therapeutic neovascularization. Circulation 2002;105:360–366.

81. Parenti A, Morbidelli L, Ledda F, Granger HJ, Ziche M. The bradykinin/B1 receptor promotes angiogenesis by up-regulation of endogenous FGF-2 in endothelium via the nitric oxide synthase pathway. FASEB 2001;15:1487–1489.

82. Tschope C, Heringer-Walther S, Koch M, et al. Upregulation of bradykinin B1-receptor expression after myocardial infarction. Br J Pharmacol 2000;129:1537–1538.

83. Jiang JG, Johnson C, Zarnegar R. Peroxisome proliferator-activated receptor gamma-mediated transcriptional up-regulation of the hepatocyte growth factor gene promoter via a novel composite cis-acting element. J Biol Chem 2001;276:25049–25056.

84. Xin X, Yang S, Kowalski J, Gerritsen ME. Peroxisome proliferator-activated receptor gamma ligands are potent inhibitors of angiogenesis in vitro and in vivo. J Biol Chem 1999;274:9116–9121.

85. Yue Tl TL, Chen J, Bao W, et al. In vivo myocardial protection from ischemia/reperfusion injury by the peroxisome proliferator-activated receptor-gamma agonist rosiglitazone. Circulation 2001;104:2588–2594.

86. Li J, Post M, Volk R, et al. PR39, a peptide regulator of angiogenesis. Nat Med 2000;6:49–55.

87. Hanahan D, Folkman J. Patterns and emerging mechanisms of the angiogenic switch during tumorigenesis. Cell 1996;86:353–364.

88. Stellmach V, Crawford SE, Zhou W, Bouck N. Prevention of ischemia-induced retinopathy by the natural ocular antiangiogenic agent pigment epithelium-derived factor. Proc Natl Acad Sci USA 2001;98:2593–2597.

89. Singh J, Mendelsohn LG. Angiogenesis inhibition. In: Bikafelvi A, ed. Vascular Biology and Pathology: Springer Press, 1999:8–15.

90. Wang A, Nomura M, Patan S, Ware JA. Inhibition of protein kinase Ca prevents endothelial cell migration and vascular tube formation in vitro and myocardial neovascularization in vivo. Circ Res 2002;90:609–616.

91. Tang S, Morgan KG, Parker C, Ware JA. Requirement for protein kinase C theta for cell cycle progression and formation of actin stress fibers and filopodia in vascular endothelial cells. J Biol Chem 1997;272:28704–28711.

92. Rousseau S, Houle F, Landry J, Huot J. P38 MAP kinase activation by vascular endothelial growth factor mediates actin reorganization and cell migration in human endothelial cells. Oncogene 1997;15:2169–2177.

93. Kontos CD, Stauffer TP, Yang WP, et al. Tyrosine 1101 of Tie2 is the major site of association of p85 and is required for activation of phosphatidylinositol 3-kinase and Akt. Mol Cell Biol 1998;18:4131–4140.

94. Schratzberger P, Schratzberger G, Silver M, et al. Favorable effect of VEGF gene transfer on ischemic peripheral neuropathy . Nat Med 2000;6:405–413.

95. Kim MC, Kini A, Sharma KK. Refractory angina pectoris. J Am Coll Cardiol 2002;39:923–934.

96. Mukherjee D, Bhatt DL, Roe MT, Patel V, Ellis SG. Direct myocardial revascularization and angiogenesis—how many patients might be eligible? Am J Cardiol 1999;84:598–600.

97. Carmeliet P. Mechanisms of angiogenesis and arteriogenesis. Nat Med 2000;6:389–395.

98. Buschmann I, Schaper W. The pathophysiology of the collateral circulation (arteriogenesis). J Pathol 2000;190:338–342.

99. Ware JA, Simons M. Angiogenesis in ischemic heart disease. Nat Med 1997;3:158–164.

100. Helisch A, Ware JA. Therapeutic angiogenesis for ischemic heart disease. In: Maragoudakis KA, ed. Angiogenesis: From the Molecular to Integrative Pharmacology. New York: Plenum Publishers, 2000.

101. Carmeliet P, Ng YS, Nuyens D, et al. Impaired myocardial angiogenesis and ischemic cardiomyopathy in mice lacking the vascular endothelial growth factor isoforms VEGF164 and VEGF188. Nat Med 1999;5:495–502.

102. Isner JM, Losordo DW. Therapeutic angiogenesis for heart failure. Nat Med 1999;5:491–492.

103. Simons M. Therapeutic coronary angiogenesis: a fronte praecipitium a tergo lupi? Am J Heart Circ Physiol 2001;280:H1923–H1927.

104. Simons M, Bonow RO, Chronos N, et al. Clinical trials in coronary angiogenesis: issues, problems, consensus: an expert panel summary. Circulation 2000;102:e73–e86.

105. Freedman SB, Isner JM. Therapeutic angiogenesis for ischemic cardiovascular disease. J Mol Cell Cardiol 2001;33:379–393.

106. Laham RJ, Sellke FW, Edelman ER, et al. Local perivascular delivery of basic fibroblast growth factor in patients undergoing coronary bypass surgery: results of a phase I randomized, double-blind, placebo-controlled trial. Circulation 1999;100:1865–1871.

107. Vale PJ, Losordo DW, Milliken CE, et al. Randomized, single-blind, placebo-conrolled pilot study of catheter-based myocardial gene transfer for therapeutic angiogenesis using left ventricular electromechanical mapping in patients with chronic myocardial ischemia. Circulation 2001;103:2138–2143.

108. Carmeliet P. Creating unique blood vessels. Nature 2001; 412:868–869.

109. Post MJ, Simons M. Gene therapy versus protein-based therapy: a matter of pharmacokinetics. Drugs Discovery Today 2001; 6:769–770.

110. Grines CL, Watkins MW, Helmer G, et al. Angiogenic gene therapy (AGENT) trial in patients with stable angina pectoris. Circulation 2002;105:1291–1297.

111. Emanueli C, Madeddu P. Angiogenesis gene therapy to rescue ischaemic tissue: achievements and future directions. Br J Pharmacol 2001;133:951–958.

112. Emanueli C, Zacheo A, Minasi A, et al. Adenovirus-mediated human tissue kallikrein gene delivery induces angiogenesis in normoperfused skeletal muscle. Arterioscler Thromb Vasc Biol 2000;20:2379–2385.

113. Kay MA, Gloriosco JC, Naldini L. Viral vectors for gene therapy: the art of turning infectious agents into vehicles of therapeutics. Nat Med 2001;7:33–40.

114. Lee RJ, Springer ML, Blanco-Bose WE, Shaw R, Ursell PC, Blau HM. VEGF gene delivery to myocardium: deleterious effects of unregulated expression. Circulation 2000;102:898–901.

115. Carmeliet P. VEGF gene therapy: stimulating angiogenesis or angioma-genesis? Nat Med 2000;6:1102–1103.

116. Epstein SE, Kornowski R, Fuchs S, Dvorak HF. Angiogenesis therapy: amidst the hype, the neglected potential for serious side effects. Circulation 2001;104:115–119.

117. Baumgartner I, Rauh G, Pieczek A, et al. Lower-extremity edema associated with gene transfer of naked DNA encoding vascular endothelial growth factor. Ann Intern Med 2000;132:880–884.

118. Folkman J. Therapeutic angiogenesis in ischemic limbs Circulation 1998;97:1108–1110.

119. Patterson C, Runge MS. Therapeutic myocardial angiogenesis via vascular endothelial growth factor gene therapy: moving on down the road. Circulation 2000;102:940.

120. Post MJ, Ware JA. Angiogenesis in atherosclerosis and restenosis. In: Ware JA, Simons M, eds. Cardiovascular Disease. New York: Oxford University Press, 1999:143–158.

121. Moulton KS, Heller E, Konerding MA, Flynn E, Palinski W, Folkman J. Angiogenesis inhibitors endostatin or TNP-470 reduce intimal neovascularization and plaque growth in apolipoprotein E-deficient mice. Circulation 1999;99:1726–1732.

122. Celletti FL, Waugh JM, Amabile PG, Brendolan A, Hilfiker PR, Dake MD. Vascular endothelial growth factor enhances atherosclerotic plaque progression. Nat Med 2001;7:425–429.

123. Ware JA. Too many vessels? Not enough? The wrong kind? The VEGF debate continues. Nat Med 2001;7:403–404.

124. Losordo DW, Isner JM. Vascular endothelial growth factor-induced angiogenesis: crouching tiger or hidden dragon? J Am Coll Cardiol 2001;37:2131–2135.

125. Pearlman JD, Gertz ZM, Wu Y, Simons M, Post MJ. Serial motion assessment by reference tracking (SMART): application to detection of local functional impact of chronic myocardial ischemia. J Comput Assist Tomogr 2001;25:558–562.

126. Villanueva FS, Abraham JA, Schreiner GF, et al. Myocardial contrast echocardiography can be used to assess the microvascular response to vascular endothelial growth factor-121. Circulation 2002;105:759–765.

127. White FC, Carroll SM, Magnet A, Bloor CM. Coronary collateral development in swine after coronary artery occlusion. Circ Res 1992;71:1490–1500.

128. Gibson CM, Ryan K, Sparano A, et al. Angiographic methods to assess human coronary angiogenesis. Am Heart Journal 1999;137:169–179.

129. Giordano FJ, Ping P, McKirnan MD, et al. Intracoronary gene transfer of fibroblast growth factor-5 increases blood flow and contractile function in an ischemic region of the heart. Nat Med 1996;2:534–539.

130. Schumacher B, Pecher P, von Specht BU, Stegmann T. Induction of neoangiogenesis in ischemic myocardium by human growth factors: first clinical results of a new treatment of coronary heart disease. Circulation 1998;97:645–650.

131. Pecher P, Schumacher BA. Angiogenesis in ischemic human myocardium: clinical results after 3 years. Ann Thorac Surg 2000;69:1414–1419.

132. Baumgartner I, Pieczek A, Manor O, et al. Constitutive expression of phVEGF165 after intramuscular gene transfer promotes collateral vessel development in patients with critical limb ischemia. Circulation 1998;97:1114–1123.

133. Losordo DW, Vale PR, Symes JF, et al. Gene therapy for myocardial angiogenesis: initial clinical results with direct myocardial injection of phVEGF165 as sole therapy for myocardial ischemia. Circulation 1998;98:2800–2804.

134. Rosengart TK, Lee LY, Patel SR, et al. Angiogenesis gene therapy: phase I assessment of direct intramyocardial administration of an adenovirus vector expressing VEGF121 cDNA to individuals with clinically significant severe coronary artery disease. Circulation 1999;100:468–474.

135. Vale PR et al. Left ventricular electromechanical mapping to assess efficacy of phVEGF165 gene transfer for therepeutic angiogenesis in chronic myocardial ischemia. Circulation 102: 965, 2000.

136. Udelson JE, Dilsizian V, Laham R, et al. Therapeutic angiogenesis with recombinant fibroblast growth factor-2 improves stress and rest myocardial perfusion abnormalities in patients with severe symptomatic chronic coronary artery disease. Circulation 2000;102:1605–1610.

137. Henry T, Annex BH, Azrin MA, et al. Final results of the VIVA trial of rhVEGF human therapeutic angiogenesis. Circulation 1999;100:I–476.

138. Kleiman NS, Califf RM. Results from late-breaking clinical trials sessions at ACCIS 2000 and ACC 2000. American College of Cardiology. J Am Coll Cardiol 2000;36:310–325.

139. Lederman RJ, Mendelsohn FO, Anderson RD, et al. Therapeutic angiogenesis with recombinant fibroblast growth factor-2 for intermittent claudication: The TRAFFIC study. Lancet 2002: In Press.

140. Blau H, Banfi A. The well-tempered vessel. Nat Med 2001; 7:532–534.

141. Schaper W, Piek JJ, Munoz-Chapuli R, Wolf C, Ito WD. Collateral circulation of the heart. In: Ware JA, Simons M, eds. Cardiovas Dis. New York: Oxford University Press, 1999:159–198.

142. Ito WD, Arras M, Winkler B, Scholz D, Schaper J, Schaper W. Monocyte chemotactic protein-1 increases collateral and peripheral conductance after femoral artery occlusion. Circ Res 1997;80:829–837.

143. Taniyama Y, Morishita R, Nakagami H, et al. Potential contribution of a novel antifibrotic factor, hepatocyte growth factor, to prevention of myocardial fibrosis by angiotensin II blockade in cardiomyopathic hamsters. Circulation 2000;102:246–252.

144. Aoki M, Morishita R, Taniyama K, Ogihara T. Therapeutic angiogenesis induced by hepatocyte growth factor: potential gene therapy for ishcemic diseases. J Athero Thrombosis 2000;7:71–76.

145. Schaper W. Therapeutic arteriogenesis has arrived. Circulation 2001;104:1994–1995.

146. Polverini PJ, Cotran PS, Gimbrone MA, Unanue ER. Activated macrophages induce vascular proliferation. Nature 1977; 269:804–806.

23 Nitric Oxide in Cardiovascular Biology and Pathophysiology

Marshall A. Corson, MD

CONTENTS

INTRODUCTION

During the past 2 decades, our understanding of the role of endothelium-derived nitric oxide (NO) in maintaining cardiovascular homeostasis has increased significantly. The physiologic synthesis, secretion, and function of NO form the basis for healthy endothelial function. The endothelium is usually a quiescent monolayer of cells that lines the luminal surface of blood vessels and the heart. Because of its location at the interface between flowing blood and the vascular wall, the endothelium is ideally situated to sense changes in hemodynamic forces and humoral mediators and to respond in a way that maintains structural and functional stability of the vessel. Although endothelial cells secrete several constriction and dilation factors, NO is the most important, particularly in areas of high laminar shear stress such as arterial endothelial beds. However, over time and in the presence of risk factors for atherosclerosis, NO function may become impaired, a feature common to most major cardiovascular disease states in contemporary Western civilization. Dysregulation of NO has been proposed as both cause and consequence of the pathophysiology that accompanies cardiovascular disease. In recent drug intervention studies in humans, therapy targeted toward restoring NO function to normal levels has yielded favorable results, including stabilizing the disease state and reducing events.

This chapter will describe the molecular mechanisms that regulate synthesis and function of NO within the cardiovascular system and the importance of NO in maintaining cardiovascular homeostasis. In addition, the processes by which NO function becomes impaired and the established and new interventions for restoring NO function in cardiovascular pathology will be reviewed.

CHARACTERIZING THE CARDIOVASCULAR NITRIC OXIDE/ENDOTHELIAL NITRIC OXIDE SYNTHASE SYSTEM

The existence of an important endothelium-derived relaxing factor (EDRF) was first indicated by the observation that an intact endothelium was required for blood vessels to relax in response to acetylcholine *(1)*. Perfusion of a preconstricted normal vessel with acetylcholine, which is a cholinergic receptor agonist, stimulated the

From: *Contemporary Cardiology: Principles of Molecular Cardiology*
Edited by: M. S. Runge and C. Patterson © Humana Press Inc., Totowa, NJ

release of a factor that could relax a detector muscle ring placed in series. In subsequent studies, this EDRF had identical physical and chemical properties as authentic NO gas, including marked instability (biological half-life of 2 to 4 s), inactivation by superoxide anion, stabilization by superoxide dismutase, and reaction with hemoglobin to yield nitrosylhemoglobin (2). In studies of aortic endothelial cells stimulated with agonists such as thrombin, bradykinin, or ATP, EDRF/NO synthesis required extracellular Ca^{2+} and transmembrane capacitative entry sufficient to increase free cytoplasmic Ca^{2+} levels from <100 nM to the 1 μM range. Analysis of cell extracts showed that most of the NO synthetic activity was found in the particulate fraction and that synthesis of NO and L-citrulline required L-arginine and nicotinamide adenine dinucleotide phosphate (NADPH) (3). NO synthase (NOS) was purified from both brain and cultured endothelial cells with the use of 2′, 5′-ADP sepharose chromatography and elution with NADPH. The requirement for Ca^{2+}-complexed calmodulin for enzyme activation was consistent with the Ca^{2+} sensitivity of NOS. In contrast, a cytosolic form of NOS that did not require Ca^{2+} for activation was purified from leukocytes stimulated with bacterial endotoxin (4), which indicates a heterogenous NOS superfamily.

Subsequent studies have identified three separate NOS gene products (cDNAs) with both common conserved and individually divergent regions. The NOS family has been classified both by tissue origin and by a numerical system as neuronal NOS (nNOS, type I), inducible NOS (iNOS, type II), and endothelial NOS (eNOS, type III). eNOS and nNOS, expressed constitutively in many cell types, are low-capacity NO generators that produce tightly regulated amounts of NO (nanomolar concentrations). eNOS- and nNOS-derived NO functions as a signal molecule and a sink for reactive oxygen species and thereby mediates homeostasis within the cardiovascular and nervous systems. iNOS, however, is a functionally distinct, high-capacity NO generator (micromolar concentrations) that produces NO as a cytotoxic agent in inflammatory states (5).

Based on the sequence of eNOS cDNAs cloned from aortic endothelial cells, eNOS is a protein of about 133 kDa, with about 60% amino acid homology to rat brain nNOS and about 50% homology to mouse macrophage iNOS (6). All NOS isoforms share a bidomain structure that comprises amino-terminal oxygenase and carboxyl-terminal reductase domains, linked by the calmodulin-binding region. In addition, all NOS isoforms produce NO homodimers in the activated state that are stabilized by the binding of heme, L-arginine, and tetrahydrobiopterin (BH_4). Sequence analysis has shown regions of homology within the reductase domain of NOS isoforms to known

binding motifs for electron donors NADPH, flavin adenine dinucleotide (FAD), and flavin mononucleotide (FMN) and regions of homology within the oxygenase domain for binding of L-arginine, heme, and BH_4. Although binding of calmodulin to eNOS and nNOS is reversible and stimulated by intracellular Ca^{2+} concentrations greater than those present in resting cells (<100 nM), binding of calmodulin to iNOS occurs independently of Ca^{2+}, rendering it fully active upon synthesis. eNOS and nNOS share a 52 to 55 amino acid sequence in the FMN-binding region that functions as an "autoinhibitory" domain (7) to stabilize these species in an inactive, non–calmodulin-bound state (Fig. 1).

eNOS is unique because it is cotranslationally modified by irreversible myristoylation at glycine 2 and reversible palmitoylation at cysteines 15 and 26. Although myristoylation anchors eNOS to cell membranes, palmitoylation directs eNOS to specialized membrane domains. eNOS is found in two major cell regions; it is complexed with caveolin-1 and other important signal transduction molecules in cholesterol-rich surface membrane caveolae/lipid rafts, and it is located with β-COP (coat protein) within the Golgi (perinuclear) membranes (8). Mutated forms of eNOS lacking acylation sites cannot be physiologically activated, which indicates the necessity of these anchoring moieties. Localized in these two cell regions, eNOS can associate with multiple regulatory proteins, such as receptors, kinases, phosphatases, G proteins, and chaperones. Direct binding of eNOS to caveolins (caveolin 1 in endothelial cells and caveolin 3 in the myocardium) and phosphorylation of eNOS at threonine 495 or 497 (depending on the species) help to maintain eNOS in an inhibited state (9).

Other major pathways for activating eNOS have been identified since the original reports of Ca^{2+}-dependent agonist activation of eNOS. Important physiologic agonists such as vascular endothelial growth factor (VEGF), insulin, and corticosteroids activate eNOS by activating phosphatidylinositol 3-kinase (PI 3-kinase) and the protein serine kinase Akt. Activated Akt phosphorylates eNOS on serine 1177 or 1179, near the carboxyl-terminus in the reductase domain (10). This phosphorylation may activate eNOS allosterically, causing it to assume the activated conformation (Fig. 1). A common chaperone protein, heat shock protein 90 (HSP90), provides interacting domains for both Akt and eNOS and facilitates eNOS phosphorylation (11). The domain of eNOS that interacts with HSP90 overlaps the eNOS domain that binds caveolins, and it has been demonstrated that activated Akt/HSP90 can displace caveolin from this binding site, as is the case for Ca^{2+}/calmodulin. Dephosphorylation of basally phosphorylated threonine 495/497, probably by the serine–threonine

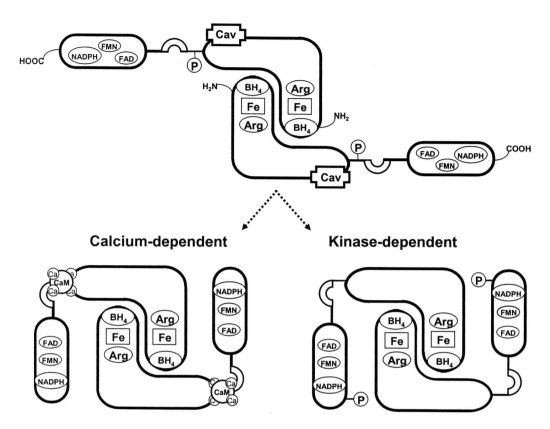

Fig. 1. Endothelial nitric oxide synthase (eNOS) structural domain and activation mechanisms. eNOS in the enzymatically inactive (open) conformation comprises interactive antiparallel oxidase domains (with binding sites for tetrahydrobiopterin [BH$_4$], heme iron [Fe], L-arginine [Arg], and caveolin [Cav]) and linked reductase domains (with threonine 495/7 phosphorylation site [P], autoinhibitory domain [semicircle], and binding sites for flavin adenine dinucleotide [FAD], flavin mononucleotide [FMN], and nicotinamide adenine dinucleotide phosphate [NADPH]). Calcium-dependent activation through binding of Ca^{2+}-bound calmodulin (CaM) requires displacement of caveolin and dephosphorylation of threonine 495/7 and results in assumption of the active (closed) conformation (lower left). Alternatively, activation of the phosphotidylinositol 3 (PI 3)-kinase/Akt pathway results in C-terminal phosphorylation at serine 1177/9 and activation through an allosterically mediated conformational change (lower right).

phosphatase PP1 (protein phosphatase 1), appears to facilitate the activating phosphorylation of serine 1177/79. In addition, phosphorylation by Akt and enzymatic activation of eNOS is stimulated by increased fluid shear stress caused by the viscous drag exerted by blood elements tangential to the direction of flow *(12)*. When cells under constant low shear stress are suddenly exposed to higher shear stress, intracellular Ca^{2+} levels do not increase, indicating that fluid shear stress, like VEGF and insulin, activates eNOS in a Ca^{2+}-independent manner *(13)* (Fig. 2). Recent work indicates that some agonists stimulate cAMP-dependent protein kinase to phosphorylate eNOS at serines 635/637, with enhancement of eNOS' enzymatic activity of an equivalent magnitude to that observed with serine 1177/1179 phosphorylation by Akt. In the same study, phosphorylation at serine 617/619 was also shown to increase the sensitivity of eNOS for Ca^{2+}-CaM binding *(14)*.

NO is formed in endothelial cells as a consequence of oxidation of the guanidino nitrogen atom of L-arginine within the active site of eNOS. Ca^{2+}–calmodulin binding or phosphorylation of eNOS initiates the flow of NADPH-derived electrons from the reductase to the oxygenase domain *(15)*. As a consequence, the heme iron is reduced and forms a transient ferrous–dioxygen complex. In the presence of adequate local concentrations of L-arginine and reduced BH$_4$, the ferrous–dioxygen complex is further reduced to form water and a hydroxylating heme–oxo species, which oxidizes L-arginine to NO and L-citrulline. Circulating levels of L-arginine are determined by dietary intake and, to a lesser extent, by metabolism of urea. The transport of L-arginine across the membrane into the endothelial cell is mediated by high-affinity cationic amino acid transporters (CATs). At physiologic circulating levels of L-arginine, the transport rate of CAT should be sufficient

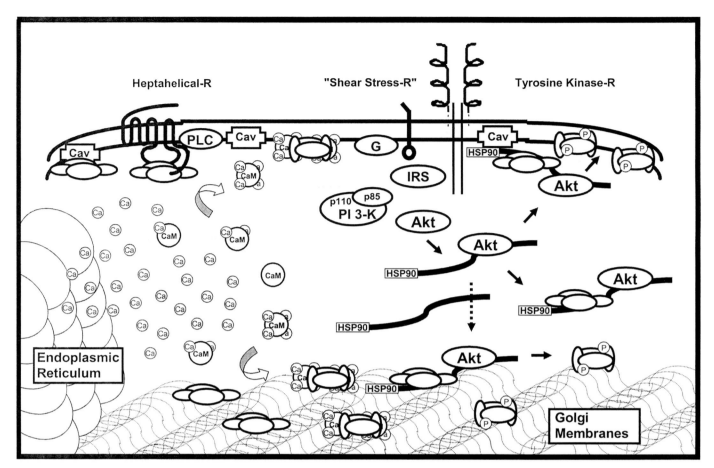

Fig. 2. Schematic for endothelial nitric oxide synthas (eNOS) activation. In resting cells eNOS is associated with caveolin (Cav) in cell membrane caveolae, which are specialized regions where signal transduction molecules are located, or is found intracellularly in Golgi membranes. Binding of agonists to heptahelical receptors (such as bradykinin BK_2) results in activation of phospholipase C (PLC) and mobilization of Ca^{2+} via transmembrane entry and release from the endoplasmic reticulum. Ca^{2+}–calmodulin (CaM) binds to eNOS (curved arrows, left) and causes it to adopt an active conformation. Alternatively, ligand binding to tyrosine kinase receptors (such as insulin) or an increase in fluid shear stress recruits a signal complex that activates insulin receptor substrate (IRS) protein(s), phosphotidylinositol 3 (PI 3)-kinase, and Akt (dark arrows, right). Heat shock protein 90 (HSP90) provides a template for Akt-eNOS interactions resulting in eNOS release from caveolin, dephosphorylation of threonine 495/7, and phosphorylation of serine 1177/9. The putative cytoplasmic HSP90–eNOS–Akt complex shown has not been reported in vivo.

to provide intracellular concentrations of L-arginine that fully saturate eNOS. However, the regulation of L-arginine appears to be more complex. As is discussed belows, proper intracellular trafficking of L-arginine appears to be critical for physiologic synthesis of NO by eNOS.

An additional negative modulator of eNOS, NOS inhibitory protein (NOSIP), has been recently identified by yeast two-hybrid screening in which the eNOS oxygenase domain is "bait" *(16)*. A cDNA was isolated that encodes a 34-kDa protein with striking homology to CG125, a *Caenorhabditis elegans* protein of unknown function. Anti-NOSIP serum showed binding of eNOS and NOSIP in both cotransfected chinese hamster ovary (CHO) and cultured human umbilical vein endothelial cells. Overexpression of

NOSIP decreased eNOS activity in an arginine-to-citrulline conversion assay and resulted in a redistribution of eNOS from caveolin-rich to caveolin-poor cytoskeletal-associated cell microdomains as shown by immunofluorescence microscopy. Additional studies with intact physiologic endothelial cells will be required to fully establish the role of NOSIP in eNOS regulation.

HOMEOSTATIC MECHANISMS OF NITRIC OXIDE IN THE NORMAL CARDIOVASCULAR SYSTEM

NO mediates vasodilation and tonically regulates ambient blood pressure. The antihypertensive role of NO is indicated by increased blood pressures (15–30 mmHg) in transgenic mice that are homozygous null for eNOS *(17)*. Nitric oxide has high reactivity and an attendant short half-life (ms to 2 s, estimated in vivo). The primary molecular target of NO in subjacent vascular smooth muscle cells (VSMC) is guanylate cyclase, a heme-containing protein. NO reacts with the iron center of guanylate cyclase resulting in the production of cyclic guanosine monophosphate (cGMP). cGMP activates VSMC cGMP-dependent protein kinase to phosphorylate cell substrates such as the vasodilator-stimulated phosphoprotein (VASP), leading to Ca^{2+} extrusion and VSMC relaxation *(18)*.

NO regulates vessel architecture as an antagonist to growth-factor-dependent VSMC growth and extracellular matrix synthesis. These antagonistic effects, which may also result from nitrosylation of guanylate cyclase, may be mediated by inhibition of phosphorylation of the cytoskeletal protein paxillin *(19)*. In addition, NO modulates endothelial cells in other ways; NO operates as an anti-apoptotic factor, responds to the flow of blood components, and maintains a low cell turnover rate in normal vessels. In vascular injury or remodeling, VEGF stimulates endothelial cell proliferation and migration in an eNOS-dependent manner *(20)* and appears to depend on the inhibition of protein kinase C and the activation of the mitogen activated protein (MAP) kinase superfamily and Akt. After the aortas of rats have been scratch wounded, eNOS expression is increased at the leading edge of regenerating endothelial cells. The increased expression of eNOS may serve as an autocrine–paracrine mechanism to accelerate coverage of exposed subendothelial matrix *(21)*.

The antithrombotic effect of NO includes inhibition of platelet adherence and aggregation, which appears to be mediated, at least in part, by platelet cGMP-dependent protein kinase. Platelets contain small amounts of NOS and can generate NO, which may prevent platelet activation through an autocrine mechanism *(22)*.

The antioxidant effects of NO are mediated through multiple mechanisms, including inhibition of the expression of oxidative enzymes and direct scavenging of superoxide anion. The product of the latter reaction, peroxynitrite, may nitrosylate protein sulfhydryl groups to form S-nitrosothiols, which can mediate vasodilation and inhibit platelet aggregation and monocyte adhesion *(23)*. In addition, NO may terminate the autocatalytic chain of lipid peroxidation that is initiated by oxidized low-density lipoproteins (LDLs) and may directly suppress the generation of oxygen-derived radicals by nitrosylating and inactivating enzymes such as NADPH oxidase. Furthermore, evidence indicates NO can directly

inhibit transcription by targeting specific transcriptional activators such as nuclear factor κB (NF-κB). NO stabilizes the inactive NF-κB/inhibitor of κB (IκB) complex to inhibit the transcription of oxidative enzymes and adhesive glycoproteins, such as vascular cell adhesion molecule and monocyte chemoattractant protein 1, which would otherwise recruit activated macrophages to the vascular wall. In contrast, inhibition of eNOS upregulates these pro-atherogenic mediators *(24)*.

Chronic exposure to low, physiologic concentrations of eNOS-derived NO induces adaptive cytoprotective responses such as the production of heme oxygenase-1 and Mn superoxide dismutase. By regulating critical mitochondrial functions such as respiration, membrane potential, and release of cytochrome *c*, NO protects against cell death induced by apoptotic stimuli. Evidence indicates that these effects are mediated by a functionally distinct compartmentalized mitochondrial eNOS fraction *(25)*. Through these pathways, NO may be able to couple metabolic function in the mitochondria with cytoprotection instead of oxidative stress.

Cardiac myocytes constitutively express moderate amounts of eNOS and may express significant levels of iNOS in the presence of inflammatory cytokines. Studies of NOS inhibitors or eNOS knockout mice indicate that baseline activity of eNOS results in mild to moderate improvement in heart rate and myocardial contraction *(26)*. Contractile improvement, or positive inotropism, is mediated via guanylate cyclase activation, cGMP formation, and cGMP-inhibited cAMP-phosphodiesterase (PDE III) activation, all of which lead to accumulation of cAMP. At higher concentrations of NO, negative inotropic effects begin to predominate, as shown by inhibition of mitochondrial electron transport, ATP synthesis, and voltage-dependent Ca^{2+} channels. eNOS may have a cytoprotective role, as suggested by the increased myocardial injury seen in eNOS knockout mice subjected to ischemia-reperfusion. Cardiodepressive effects of NO are mediated by induction of iNOS and by local myocardial accumulations of micromolar to submillimolar concentrations of NO. These effects are probably important in chronic heart failure and sepsis.

MECHANISMS OF NITRIC OXIDE/ENDOTHELIAL NITRIC OXIDE SYNTHASE DYSFUNCTION IN CARDIOVASCULAR DISEASE

The recognition of endothelial dysfunction in clinical medicine began with reports of paradoxical vasoconstrictor responses to infusion of endothelium-dependent vasodilators. These vasodilators normally stimulate the release of NO from endothelial cells, which offsets the contractile effects of the agonist on subjacent vascular myocytes, and the net response is relaxation. In an early report, the intracoronary injection of acetylcholine in patients with coronary atherosclerosis resulted in coronary constriction, even when the vessels relaxed fully in response to infused endothelium-independent vasodilators such as the NO donors, nitroglycerin, or sodium nitroprusside (27). The abnormal responses of epicardial (conductance) and arteriolar (resistance) vessels under different conditions can be delineated with the use of quantitative coronary angiographic techniques and direct catheter-based measurement of coronary blood flow, respectively.

Furthermore, the development of noninvasive techniques such as impedance plethysmography and brachial ultrasound has facilitated identification of an increased number of patients having abnormalities in endothelial function.

Abnormal epicardial constrictor responses, which indicate abnormal NO/eNOS function, have been observed in patients with hypertension, hypercholesterolemia, and diabetes and in patients with cardiac risk factors that characterize a preclinical disease state. In this section, the mechanisms by which NO/eNOS becomes dysfunctional will be reviewed.

Proximal defects in endothelial receptor or postreceptor signal events can result in acquired dysfunction in the above-mentioned diseases. Although hyporesponsiveness to acetylcholine has been most commonly documented, the response to substance P, bradykinin, or serotonergic stimulation may also be affected. Evidence linking a particular disease state with a defined receptor abnormality is lacking, and the molecular mechanisms are diverse. For example, coupling of acetylcholine, substance P, or serotonin receptors to signal responses may become impaired at the level of the heterotrimeric G proteins (28). Under normal conditions, bradykinin binding to its BK_2 receptor causes eNOS to be released from a direct inhibitory interaction with the receptor, thereby allowing the receptor to interact with phospholipase C, resulting in Ca^{2+} mobilization and eNOS activation (29). Abnormal flow-dependent, NO-mediated vasodilation in individuals with endothelial dysfunction may be manifest as a blunted increase in flow after a period of vessel occlusion (reactive hyperemia). Because the proximal receptors of an increase in fluid shear stress are unknown, the locus of this abnormality has not been identified, but cell surface glycoproteins or other adhesion receptors such as the β1-integrins may be involved.

Changes in the level of eNOS expression may reduce the NO response in cardiovascular disease. Although considered a "constitutive" isoform, eNOS expression can vary greatly. Several binding domains for transcription factors have been identified for the eNOS promoter, which suggests complex transcriptional regulation. Cell culture experiments have shown that hemodynamic changes and soluble mediators can upregulate expression of eNOS. Increased fluid shear stress, high cyclic strain, and increased levels of transforming growth factor-β1, estrogens, glucose, and histamine stimulate eNOS mRNA and protein expression. Glucocorticoids and inflammatory cytokines such as tumor necrosis factor-α downregulate expression of eNOS. A recently described protein that binds to the 3′-untranslated region of eNOS and accelerates its degradation has been proposed as a regulator of eNOS mRNA stability (30). Evidence suggests that exercise increases eNOS mRNA and protein levels in vivo, presumably by a sustained increase in shear stress and that inactivity decreases levels by a decrease in shear stress; however, the physiologic significance of other mechanisms that regulate expression is unknown.

Abnormal NO/eNOS function may be caused by intrinsic alterations in eNOS function that result from genetic variation (31). Population studies have identified polymorphisms in the eNOS gene that have pathophysiological implications. In one polymorphism, the substitution of a glutamate for aspartate at eNOS position 298 correlates with increased vascular reactivity, hypertension, and susceptibility to coronary artery disease in some ethnic groups. Another polymorphism (eNOS4) has a low allelic frequency distribution, but patients with diabetes who are homozygous for the abnormal allele have a significantly increased risk of diabetic microvascular diseases, such as retinopathy. A third polymorphism, a cysteine to threonine substitution at position 786, is associated with increased oxidative stress and risk of cerebrovascular events.

Circulating levels of L-arginine exceed the Michaelis constant (k_m) of eNOS in vitro for L-arginine by at least an order of magnitude, and without other regulatory mechanisms, the level of L-arginine would not be expected to limit NO production. Thus, any functional limitation within the intact cell should result from altered intracellular transport or distribution of L-arginine or from competition for uptake with a related but inactive substance(s). The uptake of L-arginine into endothelial cells is regulated by CAT, and the intracellular trafficking of L-arginine into caveolae for interaction with eNOS is actively regulated. When measured experimentally, the levels of L-arginine required to saturate eNOS in the intact cell are about 30-fold greater than those required in vitro. Thus, changes in uptake and transport of L-arginine could lead to a reduction in the fraction available at the active site of the enzyme (32). Under these conditions, the mass action consequences of increased levels of extracellular L-arginine and the intrinsic activity of CAT-1 become important determinants of the adequacy of biologically available L-arginine. Hypoxia-induced membrane depolarization, oxidized LDL, and longstanding hyperglycemia downregulate CAT-1 activity, which is accompanied by a reduction in the transport of L-arginine. In contrast, adenosine, endotoxin, and inflammatory cytokines stimulate the transport of L-arginine into vascular cells. A family of constitutive and inducible arginases regulates not only the intracellular transport of L-arginine but also the metabolism of L-arginine to ornithine. Increased levels of serum arginase have been found in patients with heart failure and with sickle cell disease. This increase in serum arginase may be significant because cell surface adhesion receptors normally suppressed by NO are also upregulated. A potential mechanism for changes in L-arginine levels has arisen based on results from a study in smokers showing an association between reduced levels of L-arginine and increased formation of cyanomethyl-L-arginine, which is a direct antagonist of eNOS function (33).

The NO pathway may also be disrupted through changes in the affinity of eNOS for L-arginine. These changes may be mediated by a conformational change in the eNOS enzyme structure that results from covalent modification or reduced levels of required cofactors. eNOS requires adequate local concentrations of L-arginine, reduced BH_4, and HSP90 to complete the complex five-electron transfer necessary for the complete oxidation of L-arginine to NO and L-citrulline. In the absence of any of these cofactors, the ferrous-dioxygen complex may dissociate to form superoxide and iron (III) heme. This conversion of eNOS from an NO generator to a superoxide generator is called "uncoupling" (34) and may be an important mediator of adverse vascular outcomes in conditions where cofactors are limited.

An example of a condition with a limiting cofactor is ischemia-reperfusion. Huk and colleagues (35) assessed the role of acute L-arginine depletion in a rabbit hindlimb model in which blood flow was stopped for 2.5 h by femoral artery occlusion, and then normal perfusion was reestablished. In control animals the levels of NO increased following occlusion but then declined to undetectable levels with prolonged tissue ischemia. In animals pretreated with the NOS inhibitor L-N^G-monomethyL-arginine (L-NMMA), pre-occlusion NO levels were lower than in control animals, did not rise as much following occlusion but were not obliterated by reperfusion. These experiments are consistent with a burst of NO production with ischemia onset, followed by consumption with prolonged ischemia and quantitative destruction with oxidative

radical release upon reperfusion. In another group of animals, L-arginine pretreatment was associated with a similar abrupt increase in NO levels after vessel occlusion, but the plateau was near baseline level after 150 min. L-arginine infusion prevented the precipitous decline in NO levels seen without supplementation, which suggests that L-arginine was depleted under control conditions. In the same ischemia-reperfusion model, the production of superoxide was measured by lucigenin chemiluminescence in freshly excised tissue from each experimental group. In control animals, superoxide levels were opposite those of NO, nearly doubling with reperfusion. In contrast, in the L-arginine–supplemented animals the increase in superoxide with reperfusion was half of that seen with NO. Together, these studies show that tissue ischemia in vivo is a potent stimulus for L-arginine- and eNOS-dependent NO production. With massive and prolonged organ ischemia, normal tissue reserves of L-arginine are depleted, and eNOS uncoupling results in potent superoxide production.

Physiologic function of eNOS is susceptible to inhibition by analogs of L-arginine such as cyanomethyl-L-arginine in smokers and methylated L-arginine derivatives in patients with cardiovascular diseases. In particular, an endogenously produced L-arginine derivative, asymmetric dimethyl-L-arginine (ADMA) competitively inhibits NO synthesis and antagonizes endothelium-dependent vasodilation (36). Methylated L-arginine results from degradation of proteins internally methylated by S-adenosylmethionine during cell metabloism, such as protein N-methyltransferase, yielding N^G-monomethyl-L-arginine, ADMA, and a symmetric dimethyl-L-arginine. Of these, ADMA has the highest concentration, with plasma levels averaging about 1 µmol/L. Aging, glucose intolerance, hypercholesterolemia, and established atherosclerosis are associated with two- to five-fold increases in ADMA. The most dramatic increases, possibly 10-fold, may occur in patients on hemodialysis. ADMA levels correlate negatively with urinary nitrate excretion (as a measure of endothelial NO production) and are associated with constrictor responses to endothelium-dependent vasodilators by forearm impedance plethysmography. ADMA is degraded by hydrolysis to citrulline by a family of dimethylarginine dimethylaminohydrolases (DDAHs), which are dynamically regulated. Oxidized LDLs decrease the activity of DDAHs and lead to pathologically increased ADMA levels and endothelial dysfunction. In patients with insulin resistance, treatment with the peroxisome proliferator-activated receptor-γ (PPARγ) agonist rosiglitazone reduces ADMA levels and improves insulin sensitivity, which suggests rosiglitazone is beneficial. Supplementation with oral L-arginine may increase circulating levels of L-arginine to compete with ADMA for NOS utilization and reverse endothelial dysfunction, but the efficacy of this approach has not been confirmed (37).

Endothelium-dependent vasodilation is impaired in both micro- and macrocirculation during acute hyperglycemia in normal volunteers and in patients with diabetes. Furthermore, diabetic patients have a disproportionate incidence of macrovascular pathology than can be accounted for by coexistent risk factors, and the pathology progresses even with long-term modest increases in glycohemoglobin. A newly postulated mechanism for NO/eNOS dysfunction in diabetic hyperglycemia involves posttranslational modification of eNOS at the serine residue phosphorylated by Akt (38). This modification may result from activation of the hexosamine pathway and excessive levels of glucosamine caused by glucose overload in endothelial cells and increased production of superoxide in the mitochondria. In tissue culture and in diabetic rat aorta, the transfer of glucosamine to eNOS serine 1177 blocked the Akt phosphorylation site by modification with O-linked N-acetylglucosamine. This finding suggests there is an additional mechanism of interference with eNOS function and a specific target for therapy in diabetes that could improve endothelial dysfunction.

The rate of NO destruction increases with oxidative stress. The production of free radicals increases with higher levels of activity of vascular wall enzymes such as 15-lipoxygenase, xanthine oxidase, or NADPH oxidase. NO is highly reactive with superoxide or hydrogen peroxide and yields peroxynitrite, which may subsequently release the highly reactive hydroxyl radical. All of these species can damage cell membranes, membrane lipids, and free thiol groups. Moreover, homocysteine and high levels of glucose can increase the rate of NO destruction. In addition to reacting directly with NO, glucose can be modified through a series of intially reversible reactions followed by conversion to irreversible advanced glycation end products.

THERAPIES TO RESTORE NORMAL NITRIC OXIDE/ENDOTHELIAL NITRIC OXIDE SYNTHASE FUNCTION

Organic nitrate and nitrite esters have been used for more than 100 yr as cardiovascular therapeutics to treat ischemic heart disease, hypertension, and heart failure. However, the efficacy of these agents is limited by short biological half-lives, potential adverse hemodynamic effects caused by systemic absorption, and the development of

tolerance. Commonly used preparations including nitroglylcerin, isosorbide 5-mononitrate, isosorbide dinitrate, and nicorandil are metabolized by enzymes such as NADPH-cytochrome P450 reductase and glutathione-S-transferase located within the microsomal membranes (39). In humans treated continuously with nitrate preparations for more than 8 h, responsiveness to continued administration decreases, and cross-tolerance to endogenous endothelium-derived NO develops. When the agents are administered intermittently with a "nitrate-free interval," drug efficacy is restored. The mediators of tolerance are being identified, and evidence suggests that increased production of superoxide from NADPH oxidase and uncoupling of eNOS may contribute to the tolerance (40). Superoxide generated in this way reacts with NO derived from the NO donor to form peroxynitrite and results in increased production of urinary 3-nitrotyrosine in nitrate-tolerant patients. The VSMC phosphodiesterase PDE_{1A1}, which degrades cGMP, is upregulated during the development of nitrate tolerance (41) and is associated with decreased cGMP-dependent protein kinase activity, which is manifested as reduced phosphorylation of VASP serine 239 (42). Nitrate tolerance may be prevented or reduced by several agents, such as ascorbate, L-arginine, BH_4, hydralazine, angiotensin-converting enzyme (ACE) inhibitors, folate, and low-molecular-weight thiols; however, none of these agents has been routinely used for this purpose in clinical practice.

Direct NO donors spontaneously release NO from a nitroso or anitrosyl group. Sodium nitroprusside, the prototypical NO donor, is often administered intravenously to reduce systemic blood pressure and afterload in heart failure. Therapy with inhaled NO gas has yielded some benefit for pulmonary vascular disorders, but the efficacy of NO gas is limited by its short half-life and its reactivity toward molecular oxygen. In limited studies, newer direct NO donors including the diazeniumdiolates (or NONO-ates), the sydnonimines, and the S-nitrosothiols have shown promise for wider applications. The S-nitrosothiols have particularly favorable features, such as a limited capacity for inducing tolerance and increasing vascular oxidant stress. The creation of bifunctional donors, such as nitro-aspirin or nitro-nonsteroidal anti-inflammatory drugs, combines the primary therapeutic benefit of the parent compound with the cytoprotective effects of simultaneous NO release. NO-releasing aspirin is more effective than aspirin alone in suppressing neointimal formation after rat carotid balloon injury; the benefit correlates with the production of bioactive NO levels (43).

Several evidence-based cardiovascular therapies that target NO and/or elements of the eNOS activation pathways have been developed. Of these therapies, the ACE inhibitors and statins are the most important. ACE inhibitors inhibit the formation of angiotensin II and the degradation of bradykinin. Increased bradykinin levels result in direct release of NO from the endothelium, and ACE inhibitors improve endothelial function, as seen by improved response to endothelium-dependent agonists in many vascular beds. In humans, chronic treatment with the vessel wall–avid ACE inhibitor quinapril improves flow-mediated dilation in the peripheral circulation and agonist-dependent vasodilation in the coronary circulation. This benefit of ACE inhibitors in high-risk cardiovascular patients, not seen with angiotensin II receptor blockers (ARB), may involve a bradykinin-induced increase in NO, a mechanism that is not seen with ARB. Functional antagonism of the renin–angiotensin–aldosterone system by either class improves the balance of NO and superoxide by reducing the angiotensin II–dependent production of superoxide by NAD(P)H oxidase(s). The importance of NO in mediating cardiovascular benefits of renin–angiotensin–aldosterone system antagonists has been shown in a study in knockout mice rendered homozygous null for eNOS (44). After coronary artery ligation, adverse cardiac remodeling and ventricular systolic dysfunction were seen in both eNOS-null and wild-type mice. Treatment with an ACE inhibitor or an ARB prevented the time-dependent deterioration in left ventricular systolic function and caused a reduction in myocyte size, cross-sectional and interstitial collagen fraction in wild-type mice but not in eNOS knockout mice. These findings indicate the absence of eNOS does not alter the development of heart failure after coronary ligation and myocardial infarction but does markedly reduce the cardioprotective benefits of agents that affect the renin–angiotensin–aldosterone system when given post-infarction.

During the past decade, a series of randomized, placebo-controlled clinical trials has shown that 3-hydroxy-3-methylglutaryl-coenzyme A reductase inhibitors (statins) reduce recurrent cardiovascular events and death in humans with atherosclerosis. Although treated groups initially included patients with prior myocardial infarction and markedly increased levels of LDL, recent studies have shown similar benefits in individuals with pre-clinical disease (multiple cardiac risk factors) and LDL levels previously classifed as risk neutral (unpublished data, Heart Protection Study). Reduction of LDL levels in high-risk patients by diet, exercise, or non-statin drugs is also beneficial, which suggests the mechanism may involve a direct reduction in LDL such as decreased lipid egress into the vessel wall, reduced levels of substrate for LDL oxidation,

and reduced activation of inflammatory mediators (macrophages and cytokines). However, several additional, non–LDL-dependent mechanisms of benefit with statins have recently been identified. Statins inhibit the synthesis of several isoprenoid intermediates such as geranylgeranyl pyrophosphate, farnesyl pyrophosphate, and isopentyl pyrophosphate that serve as lipid anchors for many membrane-associated proteins, and geranylgeranyl pyrophosphate serves as an anchor for the small G protein rho. Activation of rho destabilizes eNOS mRNA, which results in a decrease in eNOS protein expression and thus a reduction in NO production. Statins downregulate the activity of rho via this inhibitory effect on geranylgeranyl pyrophosphate synthesis (45). Statin treatment also leads to reduced superoxide production in endothelial cells, which is mediated by a reduction in isoprenylation of p21-rac, another small G protein involved in the assembly and function of the NAD(P)H oxidase. In a recent study statins inhibited expression of caveolin-1, an eNOS inhibitory factor, which suggests another possible mechanism of how statins are beneficial (46). Exposure of cultured aortic endothelial cells to concentrations of LDL that are pathogenetic in vivo (150–200 mg/dL) increases the expression of caveolin-1, whereas treatment with atorvastatin reduces expression of caveolin-1. In this study, statin treatment increased the fraction of non–caveolin-bound eNOS, favoring its activation by Ca^{2+}/calmodulin and Akt phosphorylation. Regional heterogeneity in the percent of caveolin-1–bound eNOS has been reported, so this mechanism may not apply to all vascular beds.

Many other agents affect eNOS expression. Dihydropyridine Ca^{2+} channel blockers improve endothelial function, possibly by upregulating eNOS expression, modulating endothelial membrane potential, or increasing the activation of superoxide dismutase (39). Both estrogen and glucocorticoids activate eNOS through non-transcriptional mechanisms not related to traditional cytoplasmic steroid-receptor activation. For example, dexamethasone activates the PI 3-kinase pathway with eNOS activation by Akt phosphorylation. Estrogen may increase eNOS activity via a caveolae-localized heterotrimeric G protein (Gα), the PI 3-kinase/Akt pathway, or both.

The use of gene therapy directed at NOS is being studied in animal models. Several studies have shown that beneficial effects of NO can be achieved with currently available techniques. Overexpression of wild-type eNOS in balloon-injured rat carotid arteries with the use of fusigenic liposomes restored NO production within the vessel wall and significantly improved agonist-dependent vessel relaxation (47). In addition, expression of the eNOS transgene was associated with a 70% inhibition of neointima formation. Similar findings have been obtained in other animal models with different gene-transduction strategies, including direct instillation of adenovirus into isolated vessel segments or the use of interventional drug delivery devices. The reconstitution of VEGF-regulated vasorelaxation in the carotid arteries of eNOS knockout mice was recently accomplished by luminal delivery of adenovirus encoding a constitutively active (serine 1179 aspartate) form of eNOS *(48)*.

Developing methods for manipulating other eNOS regulatory mechanisms within the endothelial cell is important for several reasons. The complexity of eNOS regulatory mechanisms is illustrated by the need for co- and post-translational modification for optimal cell localization and the interaction of eNOS with its many "partners." In addition, dysregulated, uncoupled eNOS may synthesize superoxide with harmful rather than palliative consequences. These complex issues were recently assessed in a recent study comparing overexpression of wild type or constitutively activated (S1179D) eNOS constructs in canine cerebral vessels maintained ex vivo in organ culture *(49)*. Transgene expression was seen mainly in the adventitia 24 h after adenoviral transfection, but the content and reactivity differed significantly in vessels transfected with the constitutively active S1179D mutant compared with those transfected with wild type eNOS. Basal (unstimulated) levels of cGMP were higher in S1179D eNOS–transfected vessels in an L-N^G-Nitroarginine methyl ester (L-NAME)-dependent manner than in control (empty vector-transfected) and wild type eNOS-transfected cells. Relaxation to bradykinin was higher in wild type eNOS-transfected vessels than in control vessels; however, relaxation was the same in S1179D eNOS-transfected vessels and in control empty vector-transfected vessels. Several explanations are possible for this result. The S1179D eNOS transfection may have created a state of tolerance through the production of tonically increased NO, or an increased production of superoxide with S1179D eNOS transfection may have competed with bradykinin-dependent NO for guanylate cyclase. Nevertheless, the specific regulators of eNOS function must be defined and the ability to modulate these regulators in the target vessel(s) must be achieved before eNOS gene therapy will become a feasible therapeutic option.

SUMMARY

During the past 2 decades, we have learned much about the physiologic and pathophysiologic role of NO in the cardiovascular system. The many actions of NO in the vasculature and heart are tightly regulated by a panoply of mechanisms that we have briefly mentioned. Within just the past few years, the benefits of several major classes of cardiovascular therapeutics have been critically linked to their effects on the NO/eNOS system. Further progress will likely depend on our ability to target selectively the deranged mechanisms in specific endothelial pathologies.

ACKNOWLEDGMENTS

Support for the study of eNOS function in the author's laboratory, through funding from the American Heart Association and the National Institutes of Health, is gratefully acknowledged. Numerous colleagues have made contributions to the work, and those of Byron Gallis and Francis Kim are particularly valued by the author.

REFERENCES

1. Furchgott RF, Zawadzki JV. The obligatory role of endothelial cells in the relaxation of arterial smooth muscle by acetylcholine. Nature 1980;288:373–376.
2. Ignarro LJ, Buga GM, Wood KS, Byrns RE, Chaudhuri G. Endothelium-derived relaxing factor produced and released from artery and vein is nitric oxide. Proc Natl Acad Sci USA 1987;84:9265–9269.
3. Forstermann U, Pollock JS, Schmidt HH, Heller M, Murad F. Calmodulin-dependent endothelium-derived relaxing factor/nitric oxide synthase activity is present in the particulate and cytosolic fractions of bovine aortic endothelial cells. Proc Natl Acad Sci USA 1991;88:1788–1792.
4. Stuehr DJ, Cho HJ, Kwon NS, Weise MF, Nathan CF. Purification and characterization of the cytokine-induced macrophage nitric oxide synthase: an FAD- and FMN-containing flavoprotein. Proc Natl Acad Sci USA 1991;88:7773–7777.
5. Schwentker A, Billiar TR. Inducible nitric oxide synthase: from cloning to therapeutic applications. World J Surg 2002;26:7.
6. Nishida K, Harrison DG, Navas JP, et al. Molecular cloning and characterization of the constitutive bovine aortic endothelial cell nitric oxide synthase. J Clin Invest 1992;90:2092–2096.
7. Nishida CR, Ortiz de Montellano PR. Autoinhibition of endothelial nitric-oxide synthase. Identification of an electron transfer control element. J Biol Chem 1999;274:14692–14698.
8. Fulton D, Fontana J, Sowa G, et al. Localization of endothelial nitric-oxide synthase phosphorylated on serine 1179 and nitric oxide in Golgi and plasma membrane defines the existence of two pools of active enzyme. J Biol Chem 2002;277:4277–4284.
9. Harris MB, Ju H, Venema VJ, et al. Reciprocal phosphorylation and regulation of endothelial nitric-oxide synthase in response to bradykinin stimulation. J Biol Chem 2001;276:16587–16591.
10. Fulton D, Gratton JP, McCabe TJ, et al. Regulation of endothelium-derived nitric oxide production by the protein kinase Akt. Nature 1999;399:597–601.
11. Balligand JL. Heat shock protein 90 in endothelial nitric oxide synthase signaling: following the lead(er)? Circ Res 2002;90:838–841.
12. Gallis B, Corthals GL, Goodlett DR, et al. Identification of flow-dependent endothelial nitric-oxide synthase phosphorylation sites by mass spectrometry and regulation of phosphorylation and nitric oxide production by the phosphatidylinositol 3-kinase inhibitor LY294002. J Biol Chem 1999;274:30101–30108.

13. Corson MA, James NL, Latta SE, Nerem RM, Berk BC, Harrison DG. Phosphorylation of endothelial nitric oxide synthase in response to fluid shear stress. Circ Res 1996;79:984–991.
14. Michell BJ, Harris MB, Chen ZP. Identification of regulatory sites of phosphorylation of the bovine endothelial nitrix-oxide synthase at serine 617 and serine 635. J Biol Chem 2002;277:42344–51.
15. McCabe TJ, Fulton D, Roman LJ, Sessa WC. Enhanced electron flux and reduced calmodulin dissociation may explain "calcium-independent" eNOS activation by phosphorylation. J Biol Chem 2000;275:6123–6128.
16. Dedio J, Konig P, Wohlfart P, Schroeder C, Kummer W, Muller-Esterl W. NOSIP, a novel modulator of endothelial nitric oxide synthase activity. Faseb J 2001;15:79–89.
17. Huang PL, Huang Z, Mashimo H, et al. Hypertension in mice lacking the gene for endothelial nitric oxide synthase. Nature 1995;377:239–242.
18. Ibarra-Alvarado C, Galle J, Melichar VO, Mameghani A, Schmidt HH. Phosphorylation of blood vessel vasodilator-stimulated phosphoprotein at serine 239 as a functional biochemical marker of endothelial nitric oxide/cyclic GMP signaling. Mol Pharmacol 2002;61:312–319.
19. Fang S, Sharma RV, Bhalla RC. Enhanced recovery of injury-caused downregulation of paxillin protein by eNOS gene expression in rat carotid artery. Mechanism of NO inhibition of intimal hyperplasia? Arterioscler Thromb Vasc Biol 1999;19:147–152.
20. Rudic RD, Shesely EG, Maeda N, Smithies O, Segal SS, Sessa WC. Direct evidence for the importance of endothelium-derived nitric oxide in vascular remodeling. J Clin Invest 1998;101:731–736.
21. Poppa V, Miyashiro JK, Corson MA, Berk BC. Endothelial NO synthase is increased in regenerating endothelium after denuding injury of the rat aorta. Arterioscler Thromb Vasc Biol 1998;18:1312–1321.
22. Mehta JL, Chen LY, Kone BC, Mehta P, Turner P. Identification of constitutive and inducible forms of nitric oxide synthase in human platelets. J Lab Clin Med 1995;125:370–377.
23. Stamler JS, Simon DI, Osborne JA, et al. S-nitrosylation of proteins with NO: synthesis and characterization of biologically active compounds. Proc Natl Acad Sci USA 1992;89:444–448.
24. Marui N, Offermann MK, Swerlick R, et al. Vascular cell adhesion molecule-1 (VCAM-1) gene transcription and expression are regulated through an antioxidant-sensitive mechanism in human vascular endothelial cells. J Clin Invest 1993;92:1866–1874.
25. Paxinou E, Weisse M, Chen Q, et al. Dynamic regulation of metabolism and respiration by endogenously produced nitric oxide protects against oxidative stress. Proc Natl Acad Sci USA 2001;98:11575–11580.
26. Kojda G, Kottenberg K. Regulation of basal myocardial function by NO. Cardiovasc Res 1999;41:514–523.
27. Ludmer PL, Selwyn AP, Shook TL, et al. Paradoxical vasoconstriction induced by acetylcholine in atherosclerotic coronary arteries. N Engl J Med 1986;315:1046–1051.
28. Maxwell AJ. Mechanisms of dysfunction of the nitric oxide pathway in vascular diseases. Nitric Oxide 2002;6:101–124.
29. Golser R, Gorren AC, Leber A, et al. Interaction of endothelial and neuronal nitric-oxide synthases with the bradykinin B2 receptor. Binding of an inhibitory peptide to the oxygenase domain blocks uncoupled NADPH oxidation. J Biol Chem 2000;275:5291–5296.
30. Searles CD, Miwa Y, Harrison DG, Ramasamy S. Posttranscriptional regulation of endothelial nitric oxide synthase during cell growth. Circ Res 1999;85:588–595.
31. Wattanapitayakul SK, Mihm MJ, Young AP, Bauer JA. Therapeutic implications of human endothelial nitric oxide synthase gene polymorphisms. Trends Pharmacol Sci 2001;22:361–368.
32. McDonald KK, Zharikov S, Block ER, Kilberg MS. A caveolar complex between the cationic amino acid transporter 1 and endothelial nitric-oxide synthase may explain the "arginine paradox". J Biol Chem 1997;272:31213–31216.
33. Wong PC, and Van der Vliet A. Inhibition of nitric oxide synthesis by cigarette smoke. Nitric Oxide 2000;4:241–244.
34. Xia Y, Tsai AL, Berka V, Zweier JL. Superoxide generation from endothelial nitric-oxide synthase. A Ca^{2+}/calmodulin-dependent and tetrahydrobiopterin regulatory process. J Biol Chem 1998;273:25804–25808.
35. Huk I, Nanobashvili J, Neumayer C, et al. L-arginine treatment alters the kinetics of nitric oxide and superoxide release and reduces ischemia/reperfusion injury in skeletal muscle. Circulation 1997;96:667–675.
36. Vallance P, Leone A, Calver A, Collier J, Moncada S. Endogenous dimethylarginine as an inhibitor of nitric oxide synthesis. J Cardiovasc Pharmacol 1992;20:S60–S62.
37. Blum A, Hathaway L, Mincemoyer R, et al. Oral L-arginine in patients with coronary artery disease on medical management. Circulation 2000;101:2160–2164.
38. Du XL, Edelstein D, Dimmeler S, Ju Q, Sui C, Brownlee M. Hyperglycemia inhibits eNOS activity by posttranslational modification at the Akt site. J Clin Invest 2001;108:1341–1348.
39. Ignarro LJ, Napoli C, Loscalzo J. Nitric oxide donors and cardiovascular agents modulating the bioactivity of nitric oxide: an overview. Circ Res 2002;90:21–28.
40. Kurz MA, Boyer TD, Whalen R, Peterson TE, Harrison DG. Nitroglycerin metabolism in vascular tissue: role of glutathione S- transferases and relationship between NO. and NO2-formation. Biochem J 1993;292:545–550.
41. Kim D, Rybalkin SD, Pi X, et al. Upregulation of phosphodiesterase 1A1 expression is associated with the development of nitrate tolerance. Circulation 2001;104:2338–2343.
42. Schulz E, Tsilimingas N, Rinze R, et al. Functional and biochemical analysis of endothelial (dys)function and NO/cGMP signaling in human blood vessels with and without nitroglycerin pretreatment. Circulation 2002;105:1170–1175.
43. Napoli C, Aldini G, Wallace JL, et al. Efficacy and age-related effects of nitric oxide-releasing aspirin on experimental restenosis. Proc Natl Acad Sci USA 2002;99:1689–1694.
44. Liu YH, Xu J, Yang XP, Yang F, Shesely E, Carretero OA. Effect of ACE inhibitors and angiotensin II type 1 receptor antagonists on endothelial NO synthase knockout mice with heart failure. Hypertension 2002;39:375–381.
45. Laufs U, Liao JK. Direct vascular effects of HMG-CoA reductase inhibitors. Trends Cardiovasc Med 2000;10:143–148.
46. Brouet A, Sonveaux P, Dessy C, Moniotte S, Balligand JL, Feron O. Hsp90 and caveolin are key targets for the proangiogenic nitric oxide-mediated effects of statins. Circ Res 2001;89:866–873.
47. von der Leyen HE, Dzau VJ. Therapeutic potential of nitric oxide synthase gene manipulation. Circulation 2001;103:2760–2765.
48. Scotland RS, Morales-Ruiz M, Chen Y, et al. Functional reconstitution of eNOS reveals the importance of serine 1179 in endothelium-dependent vasomotion. Circ Res 2002;90:904–910.
49. Akiyama M, Eguchi D, Weiler D, et al. Expression and function of recombinant S1179D endothelial nitric oxide synthase in canine cerebral arteries. Stroke 2002;33:1071–1076.

24 Vasculitis

Ronald J. Falk, MD and J. Charles Jennette, MD

Contents

INTRODUCTION

Vasculitis is an inflammatory disorder of the blood vessel wall that can affect vessels of all sizes, ranging from capillaries to large vessels such as the aorta (Fig. 1) *(1)*. Vasculitides have been classified by the size and type of vessel involved and, to a certain degree, by the distribution of injured organs (e.g., renal limited vasculitis, limited Wegener's granulomatosis). The pathogenesis of vasculitis has been studied both in vitro and in vivo; however, the causes of many types of vasculitis remain unknown. In fact, the number of etiologic agents involved in most types of vasculitis is unknown. Many forms of vasculitis probably require several synergistic "hits"; multiple factors must act together to alter the endothelium to allow activated leukocytes to adhere to and penetrate the vessel wall.

Several classification schemes have been proposed for vasculitis over the past 150 yr; therefore, the history of nomenclature is rich with various names and descriptions *(2–8)*. In this chapter, we use the Chapel Hill nomenclature system, which has been agreed upon by an international group of clinicians and pathologists with special interest in vasculitis (Table 1) *(9)*. This system has been widely adopted throughout the Americas, Europe, and Asia.

In this chapter, we will discuss the types of vasculitides and the potential pathogenic factors that contribute to vascular inflammation in each major vasculitic disease.

LARGE VESSEL VASCULITIS

Giant cell arteritis and Takayasu's arteritis, which are the two major forms of large vessel vasculitis, primarily affect the aorta and its major branches, including arteries to the extremities, head, and neck *(10–13)*. No definitive diagnostic test is available to differentiate the two conditions; therefore, presumptive rather than definitive diagnoses are usually made in patients with large vessel vasculitis. Because giant cell and Takayasu's arteritis are so clinically and pathologically similar, patient age is the most reliable discriminator. Most patients with giant cell arteritis are more than 50 yr old, whereas Takayasu's arteritis is usually seen in patients who are less than 50 yr of age *(14–16)*.

Owing to the lack of definitive diagnosis for these disorders, the incidence and prevalence of the vasculitides are unknown; however, general observations can be made *(17,18)*. Although incidence rates vary, giant cell arteritis is more common in northern climates *(19–21)*. The highest incidence rates are reported in Northern Europe and the United States. In Iceland, the rate is 50 cases per 100,000 of those over the age of 50. The Mayo Clinic studies over a 42-yr period ranged from 6.2 to 19.1 cases. The geographic distribution of Takayasu's arteritis differs significantly from that of giant cell arteritis. Takayasu's arteritis is prevalent in Asian populations. In Japan, about 150 new cases are diagnosed each year, whereas in Olmstead County, Minnesota, the incidence is

From: *Contemporary Cardiology: Principles of Molecular Cardiology*
Edited by: M. S. Runge and C. Patterson © Humana Press Inc., Totowa, NJ

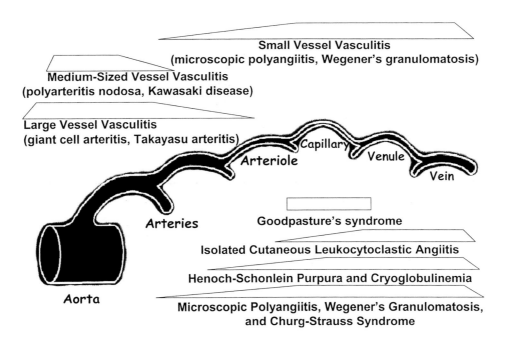

Fig. 1. This diagram depicts the relation between the names of specific vasculitides and the blood vessels that are involved by each entity.

only 2.6 cases per million per year *(22)*. In addition, the incidence of Takayasu's arteritis is high in Americans of Japanese descent.

Large vessel vasculitis is characterized by constitutional symptoms, including fatigue, anorexia, and malaise *(11,23)*. These symptoms are common to most vasculitides and suggest the possibility of an antecedent infection. More than half of patients with giant cell arteritis have low-grade fever, and some patients are diagnosed with "fever of unknown origin." Most symptoms of giant cell arteritis are caused by damage to the organs supplied by the affected arteries. Headache, the most common symptom, is present in at least two thirds of giant cell patients and is often described as "the worst headache of my life." The pain is usually localized to temporal areas, but may be diffuse, frontal, or occipital.

Loss of vision is a serious complication of giant cell arteritis that can result from ischemia to the optic nerve caused by occlusion of the branches of either the ophthalmic or the posterior ciliary arteries *(24,25)*. The visual loss may initially be temporary, mimicking amaurosis fugax, but may eventually become a fixed visual field defect. As the severity of vascular inflammation increases, the vascular lumen becomes reduced and thrombosed, which results in infarction of the tissue supplied by the involved vessel.

Most patients with Takayasu's arteritis present with neurological symptoms related to occlusion of cerebral blood vessels *(22)*. Ophthalmological symptoms similar to those of giant cell are found in one fourth of patients. Almost half of patients with Takayasu's arteritis have hypertension and pain in the extremities. Although patient age is the best way to differentiate between giant cell and Takayasu's arteritis, other differences in presentation may be helpful. Valve dilatation or aortic valve regurgitation caused by aortitis may develop in 40–50% of patients with Takayasu's arteritis. Coronary arteritis may cause symptoms of ischemic heart disease or congestive heart failure or the development of arrhythmias. In contrast, giant cell arteritis rarely causes cardiovascular symptoms. Thoracic aortic aneurysms and dissection of the aorta are late complications of giant cell arteritis. These observations suggest that some factor must alter the cardiac endothelium early in Takayasu's and even giant cell arteritis.

Vascular injury associated with giant cell arteritis results from inflammation in the arterial wall. Lymphocytes and macrophages appear to be involved in the development of giant cell arteritis, and the inflammation may be initiated by an immune response to an unidentified antigen *(26)*. Infiltrates of T lymphocytes, monocytes, and macrophages are present in the intima, media, and adventitia of vessels affected by giant cell arteritis. The inflammatory cells can damage the vessel wall by direct activation and by production of granzymes, which result in apoptotsis of target cells. Activated macrophages damage the arterial wall directly or by the release of toxic substances, including reactive oxygen species and metalloproteinase. The

Table 1
Chapel Hill Nomenclature System

Large Vessel Vasculitis[*]

Giant cell (temporal arteritis)	Granulomatous arteritis of the aorta and its major branches, with a predilection for the extracranial branches of the carotid artery. *Often involves the temporal artery. Usually occurs in patients older than 50 and often is associated with polymyalgia rheumatica.*
Takayasu's arteritis	Granulomatous inflammation of the aorta and its major branches. *Usually occurs in patients younger than 50.*

Medium-Sized Vessel Vasculitis[*]

Polyarteritis nodosa (classic polyarteritis nodosa)	Necrotizing inflammation of medium-sized or small arteries without glomerulonephritis or vasculitis in arterioles, capillaries, or venules.
Kawasaki's disease	Arteritis involving large, medium-sized, and small arteries and associated with mucocutaneous lymph node syndrome. *Coronary arteries are often involved. Aorta and veins may be involved. Usually occurs in children.*

Small Vessel Vasculitis[*]

Wegener's granulomatosis[†,‡]	Granulomatous inflammation involving the respiratory tract and necrotizing vasculitis affecting small to medium-sized vessels, e.g., capillaries, venules, arterioles, and arteries. *Necrotizing glomerulonephritis is common.*
Churg–Strauss syndrome[†,‡]	Eosinophil-rich and granulomatous inflammation involving the respiratory tract and necrotizing vasculitis affecting small to medium-sized vessels and associated with asthma and blood eosinophilia.
Microscopic polyangiitis (microscopic polyarteritis)[†,‡]	Necrotizing vasculitis with few or no immune deposits affecting small vessels, i.e., capillaries, venules, or arterioles. *Necrotizing arteritis involving small and medium-sized arteries may be present. Necrotizing glomerulonephritis is very common. Pulmonary capillaritis often occurs.*
Henoch–Schönlein purpura[‡]	Vasculitis with IgA-dominant immune deposits affecting small vessels, i.e., capillaries, venules, or arterioles. *Typically involves the skin, gut, and glomeruli and is associated with arthralgias or arthritis.*
Essential cryoglobulinemic vasculitis[‡]	Vasculitis with cryoglobulin immune deposits affecting small vessels, i.e., capillaries, venules, or arterioles, and associated with cryoglobulins in serum. Skin and glomeruli are often involved.
Cutaneous leukocytoclastic angiitis	Isolated cutaneous leukocytoclastic angiitis without systemic vasculitis or glomerulonephritis.

[*]Large artery refers to the aorta and the largest branches directed toward major body regions (e.g., to the extremities and the head and neck); medium-sized artery refers to the main visceral arteries (e.g., renal, hepatic, coronary, and mesenteric arteries); and small artery refers to the distal arterial radials that connect with arterioles (e.g., renal arcuate and interlobular arteries). Note that some small and large vessel vasculitides may involve medium-sized arteries; but large and medium-sized vessel vasculitides do not involve vessels smaller than arteries.
[†]Strongly associated with anti-neutrophil cytoplasmic autoantibodies (ANCA).
[‡]May be accompanied by glomerulonephritis and can manifest as nephritis or pulmonary–renal vasculitic syndrome.
Modified from Jennette JC, Falk RJ, Andrassy K, et al. *(9).*

inflammatory process causes smooth muscle cells within the vascular wall to migrate into the intima and proliferate, resulting in obstruction of the vascular lumen. During the active phases of disease, giant cells are found in the inflammatory infiltrates. As the process becomes more chronic, vascular sclerosis occurs, with little or no active inflammation.

Several lines of evidence indicate that T lymphocytes are important in the pathogenesis of large vessel vasculitis *(27,28)*. First, T lymphocytes are found in the inflammatory infiltrates, as well as in and around the blood vessel walls. Second, T lymphocytes found at the site of the lesion express activation markers, including interleukin (IL)-2 receptors and major histocompatibility complex (MHC) class II molecules. Third, T lymphocytes disappear as tissue function improves. Finally, the pattern of cytokine release suggests a TH-1 or TH-2 type of lymphocyte response. To be an effector cell in an immune response, T lymphocytes must have antigen presented to them in the context of an MHC molecule by antigen-presenting cells such as dendritic cells. MHC molecules, which are involved in T lymphocyte regulation, are encoded by the MHC genes that display allelic polymorphisms within normal human populations. HLA polymorphisms, variants of MHC class II antigens in particular, determine the binding of the T cell receptor with antigenic peptides.

Takayasu's arteritis and giant cell arteritis are associated with particular MHC polymorphisms. Takayasu's arteritis is associated with polymorphisms in class I molecules encoded at the HLA-B locus, which indicate stimulation of CD-8 positive T cells by antigenic peptides (29). In contrast, giant cell arteritis is associated with polymorphisms in MHC II-HLA-DR loci, which indicate a role for CD-4 positive T cells in the immune response (30,31). These findings suggest different pathogenetic mechanisms for large vessel disease. Stimulation of cytotoxic CD-8 positive T cells could directly damage the wall of the blood vessel, whereas stimulation of CD-4 positive T cells activates macrophages, which then effect an immune response that results in arterial wall injury.

The pathogenesis of giant cell arteritis is closely related to the syndrome of polymyalgia rheumatica. Characterized by the presence of morning stiffness and pain in proximal joints, polymyalgia rheumatica limits patient activity and occasionally requires confinement to bed. Criteria for the diagnosis of polymyalgia rheumatica include the presence of morning stiffness lasting for at least 30 min; aching and pain in the shoulder girdle, hip girdle, and neck or torso; and an increase in the erythrocyte sedimentation rate or the level of C reactive protein. Polymyalgia rheumatica is not attributable to a vasculitis per se, but may provide clues to the pathogenesis of giant cell arteritis. Monocytes from patients with polymyalgia rheumatica produce increased levels of IL-6, which is a potent inducer of an acute phase response and is associated with muscle aches (32).

Epidemiological data suggest that giant cell arteritis and Takayasu's arteritis may be a consequence of infection. Both diseases have seasonal and annual variations, and urban and rural differences suggest that environmental pressures such as infectious disease may be involved. In addition, several human and animal viruses can infect endothelial cells, both in vivo and in vitro (33). The list of viral agents associated with vasculitides includes the hepatitis virus, retroviruses, human immunodeficiency virus, and herpesvirus. Enteroviruses that have been associated with vasculitides include echovirus, poliovirus, Coxsackievirus, parvovirus B19, rubella, and the influenza virus. In addition, common bacteria, fungi, and spirochetes, including Borrelia burgdorferi and Treponema palladum, can contribute to vasculitic disease. Specifically, parvovirus B19 and cytomegalovirus have been associated with the development of giant cell arteritis (34). Takayasu's arteritis has been associated with mycobacterial, streptococcal,

and spirochetal infections. However, a causal relationship has not been established for these associations.

Viruses may induce vasculitis either by direct invasion of the vessel wall or by initiation of an immune complex response. Activation and destruction of the endothelium are a result of the cytopathic effect of viruses or the deposition of immune reactants within the vessel wall. Vasculitis secondary to a bacterial or fungal infection may result in direct extension of infection into the vessel wall, or organisms may infect the endothelium via hematogenous dissemination. Even if a pathogen does not directly invade the endothelium, infections may still contribute to vasculitis. Infections often precede the onset or relapse of vasculitis. The mechanism by which an infectious agent causes vascular inflammation is not known. Molecular mimicry may be involved; pathogens may share epitopes with host proteins, thereby causing an autoimmune response. Another possibility is that the upregulation of viral proteins results in an alteration of host proteins (35). Bacterial components, such as lipopolysaccharides and peptidoglycans, and CpG motifs present in bacterial DNA can directly stimulate T and B lymphocytes (36,37).

MEDIUM-SIZED VESSEL VASCULITIS

Polyarteritis nodosa and Kawasaki's disease are two of the most significant medium-sized vessel vasculitides (8,38,39). Kawasaki's disease affects young children, especially those of Asian ancestry. In Japan, the incidence rate is about 50–200 cases per 100,000 children, whereas in the United States the incidence rate ranges from 6–15 cases per 100,000 children less than 5 yr of age (39). The epidemiology of polyarteritis nodosa varies, depending on the location, the population, and the distribution of suspected pathogens. For example, polyarteritis nodosa has been associated with hepatitis B infection in adults and with hemolytic group A streptococcal infection in children (40–42).

Kawasaki's disease and polyarteritis nodosa are necrotizing arteritides that affect arteries leading to major viscera and their initial branches within the viscera. Both diseases are characterized in the acute phase by a fibrinoid necrosis caused by transmural invasion of neutrophils and monocytes. Neutrophils predominate in polyarteritis nodosa, and cells of the monocyte/macrophage lineage are more common in Kawasaki's disease. Necrotizing inflammation erodes completely through the arterial wall into the perivascular tissue, resulting in the formation of pseudoaneurysms. This necrotizing process results in thrombosis, infarction, and hemorrhage. Arterial injury in Kawasaki's disease and polyarteritis nodosa occurs at arterial branch points, where shear stress is increased and activation of endothelial inflammatory factors such as intercellular adhesion molecule-1 (ICAM-1) and transcription factors such as NFκB are increased (43–48). Medium-sized vessel vasculitis may affect only arteries because shear stress is important in initiating the pathogenetic lesion.

Kawasaki's disease, which is associated with mucocutaneous lymph node syndrome, is an acute febrile illness of young children characterized by systemic arteritis, non-suppurative lymphadenopathy, polymorphous or edematous rash, erythema of the oropharyngeal mucosa, conjunctivitis, erythema of the palms and soles, and edema and desquamation of extremities (39,49). Cardiovascular manifestations of Kawasaki's syndrome are prominent, especially in the acute phase; myocarditis is common, and pericardial effusion is seen in 30% of patients. Morbidity and mortality are high when the coronary arteries are involved. Coronary artery aneurysms, which range in size from small to large, are more often proximal than distal and may result in coronary ischemia.

The mechanisms involved with Kawasaki's disease and its associated mucocutaneous lymph node syndrome are unknown. Activated leukocytes may secrete a cytokine that inflames the skin and mucosa. The epidemic and endemic nature of Kawasaki's disease suggest that either an infectious agent or an environmental toxin contributes to the pathogenesis. Substantial epidemiological data suggest that the primary cause is infectious (50). In addition, enterotoxins and exotoxins of staphylococci and streptococci have been identified in cultures from patients. These toxins could produce the inflamed strawberry tongue and skin lesions characteristic of Kawasaki's disease.

The earliest lesion of Kawasaki's disease is best described as an accumulation of neutrophils and monocytes beneath the endothelial cell layer. Over time, the lesion progresses to a transmural accumulation of mononuclear leukocytes, with subsequent edema and smooth muscle degeneration in the media (Fig. 2). The infiltrating cells are predominantly monocytes, macrophages, and T lymphocytes, especially CD-8 T lymphocytes (51).

Although neutrophils may play a role in the early acute stages of Kawasaki's disease, most evidence indicates that monocytes are the primary contributor to this form of vasculitis (52–58). Monocyte-derived products have been found in the circulation of patients with Kawasaki's disease, and ultrastructural and immunocytochemical studies have identified monocytes in the affected tissue. Furthermore, activated monocytes and macrophages are present within coronary artery lesions (59). The expression of monocyte chemotactic protein 1 (MCP-1) correlates with the degree of acute inflammation, especially early in coronary vasculitis. Intravenous treatment with gamma globulin decreases the circulating levels of MCP-1 but not cytokine IL-8 or tumor necrosis factor-α (TNF-α) (58). Moreover, expression levels of CD-14, a receptor for endotoxin found on monocytes and neutrophils, and its soluble form are higher in patients with Kawasaki's disease than in patients with infectious diseases. Specifically, circulating levels of CD-14 were higher in patients with Kawasaki's disease than in patients with Gram-negative bacterial infections. In addition, CD-14 receptor expression on neutrophils was higher during the acute phase of Kawasaki's disease than during the convalescent phases, but CD-14 expression on monocytes decreased during the acute phase. These findings suggest that monocytes shed the CD-14 receptor during the course of the disease (60). Another presumptive conclusion may be that a factor derived from an activated monocyte results in the toxic features of the mucocutaneous lymph node system.

Anti-endothelial cell antibodies are found in the circulation of patients with several types of systemic vasculitis, including those with Kawasaki's disease (61–63). The role of these antibodies in the pathogenesis of Kawasaki's disease is unclear because anti-endothelial cell antibodies are also found in other febrile patients. Because these antibodies may share antigenic epitopes with lysosomal membrane proteins and membrane proteins of endothelial cells, they may cross-react with endothelial cells and cause damage to the endothelium.

Like Kawasaki's disease, polyarteritis nodosa is a systemic necrotizing arteritis; however, unlike Kawasaki's disease, polyarteritis nodosa does not occur primarily in children and is not accompanied by mucocutaneous lymph node syndrome. In addition, the pathology of polyarteritis nodosa differs from that of Kawasaki's disease. In the acute phase, polyarteritis nodosa is characterized by an intense infiltration of neutrophils in the artery wall and by extensive fibrinoid necrosis (Fig. 2), whereas Kawasaki's disease is characterized by marked infiltration of monocytes, macrophages, and T lymphocytes, without prominent fibrinoid necrosis. These differences suggest that the etiology of polyarteritis nodosa and Kawasaki's disease arteritis differs. The cause of polyarteritis nodosa is unknown; however, there is evidence in some patients for an infectious etiology, possibly mediated through the formation of immune complexes in artery walls (40–42).

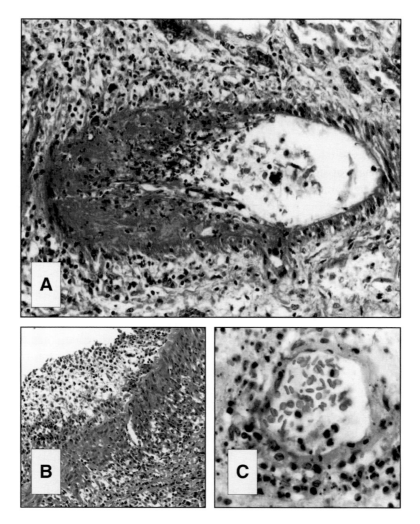

Fig. 2. Light microscopy of acute necrotizing arteritis. **(a)** A medium-sized artery affected by polyarteritis nodosa showing an intact artery wall to the right and transmural fibrinoid with infiltration of predominantly neutrophils on the left. **(b)** A medium-sized artery affected by Kawasaki's disease arteritis showing the lumen in the upper left and adventitia in the lower right. There is transmural infiltration by mononuclear leukocytes that include lymphocytes, monocytes, and macrophages. The intima is markedly thickened by the inflammation. **(c)** A small artery affected by microscopic polyangiitis showing segmental acute inflammation with neutrophil infiltration and leukocytoclasia

SMALL VESSEL VASCULITIS

Small vessel vasculitides are characterized by necrotizing inflammation of capillaries and postcapillary venules; veins, arterioles, and arteries may also be involved (Fig. 1). The small vessel vasculitides can be divided into two groups. In the first group, immune complexes are found within or along the vessel wall. Many types of immune complex vasculitides have been identified (Table 2). The second group, the pauci-immune vasculitides, is characterized by a sparse deposition of immune reactants in the vessel wall. The pauci-immune group is often associated with anti-neutrophil cytoplasmic autoantibodies (ANCA),

which are autoantibodies directed against normal constituents of neutrophils and monocytes.

Lupus Nephritis and Vasculitis

Systemic lupus erythematosus (SLE) is the prototype of an immune complex–induced small vessel vasculitis. Many clinical and pathological abnormalities are associated with SLE, but the pathogenesis remains unknown despite much investigation. Nevertheless, immune complexes present in the circulation and in tissue are pathogenetic factors *(64,65)*. Where the immune complexes form is under debate; however, whether formed in the circulation or *in situ*, immune

Table 2
Immune Complex Small Vessel Vasculitis

Lupus

Henoch–Schönlein purpura

Cryoglobulinemia

Serum sickness

Rheumatoid

Drug-induced immune complex

Infection-induced immune complex diseases

Goodpasture's syndrome

complexes activate the complement cascade, resulting in the consumption of complement components, especially C4 and C3. Normal immune clearance mechanisms, such as C3b and Fc receptors on phagocytes, are inadequate to clear these immune complexes. Immune complexes are generated by autoantibodies against a variety of nuclear antigens and tissue antigens on other cell types, including red blood cells, lymphocytes, platelets, and clotting factors. Rheumatoid factor, an antibody reactive to a portion of an antibody, and cryoglobulin, an abnormal plasma protein, are found in SLE patients. In addition to lymphopenia, T lymphocyte function is reduced, with a decrease in the generation of cytotoxic and suppressor T lymphocytes.

In most immune complex forms of vascular injury, the antibody–antigen deposits activate the complement system, which is the major effector of the humoral branch of the immune response designed to facilitate antigen clearance and generate an inflammatory response. The terminal sequence of complement activation results in formation of the membrane attack complex, which causes osmotic lysis of target cells. In addition, complement activation releases anaphylatoxins such as C3a and C5a. The Fc receptor on the immunoglobulin molecule itself activates neutrophils, monocytes, and macrophages, resulting in the production of oxygen radicals and the release of tissue-damaging proteases. Macrophages have the unique ability to produce coagulant tissue factors that help form fibrin deposits and that stimulate transforming growth factor-β, which results in extracellular matrix production and scar formation.

Lupus vasculitis, which may be found in any organ system, is caused by the localization of immune complexes in tissue and the resultant inflammatory lesions characterized by the presence of neutrophils, lymphocytes, and monocytes in the vessel wall. Arteriolar thrombi may be observed because of an aggressive vasculitis and in lupus may be due to the presence of anti-phospholipid antibodies. Vascular-damaging immune complexes arise from autoantibodies to epitopes present on DNA or on portions of the chromatin itself.

Henoch–Schönlein Purpura

Henoch–Schönlein purpura (HSP), a small vessel vasculitis caused by IgA-dominant immune complexes, affects the skin, joints, kidneys, and gastrointestinal tract, usually before the age of 20. Immunofluorescence microscopy of small vessels in affected organs shows granular immune complex deposits containing primarily IgA and C3. Circulating IgA immune complexes are found in some patients. Abnormal glycosylation of IgA may contribute to the formation of immune complexes. Studies suggest that the alternative pathway of complement plays a pathogenic role in HSP. The membrane attack complex, like that seen in patients with lupus, is seen in patients with HSP and contributes to vascular injury in addition to the monocytes and macrophages present at the site of inflammation.

Anti-Glomerular Basement Membrane Antibody Disease and Goodpasture's Syndrome

Anti-glomerular basement membrane (anti-GBM) antibodies cause inflammatory injury to glomerular capillaries and pulmonary alveolar capillaries. Anti-GBM disease, when accompanied by pulmonary and renal disease, is known as Goodpasture's syndrome. Of patients with anti-GBM antibodies, about half have Goodpasture's syndrome and half have anti-GBM glomerulonephritits. Anti-GBM pulmonary disease without glomerulonephritis is rare.

The major antigen recognized by anti-GBM antibodies is located in the noncollagenous domain of type IV collagen (66). Type IV collagen forms the backbone of the glomerular basement membrane and comprises three α chains that form a triple helix. The antigen bound by anti-GBM antibodies is found in the α-3 chain of type IV collagen; nine discontinuous amino acids in the internal region of this α chain are critical for the epitope formation (67). Animal models based entirely on the passive transfer of anti-GBM antibodies have provided valuable information on the pathogenesis of Goodpasture's syndrome. Glomerular injury results from the binding of antibody to the basement membrane and the subsequent activation of the complement cascade, which is accompanied by an influx of effector cells including neutrophils, monocytes, and macrophages. Studies in animal models suggest that T lymphocytes are important in the development of disease, and crescentic glomerulonephritis involves CD-4 positive T cells in contrast to CD-8 positive T cells.

Pauci-Immune Small Vessel Vasculitis

The three major types of pauci-immune small vessel vasculitis are Wegener's granulomatosis, Churg–Strauss syndrome, and microscopic polyangiitis (MPA) *(1,68)*. Each type has a histologically identical necrotizing vasculitis that affects arteries, arterioles, venules, and capillaries, especially glomerular and pulmonary alveolar capillaries. Pauci-immune small vessel vasculitides have little or no localization of immunoglobulins in the vascular wall, and necrotizing and crescentic glomerulonephritis are often an integral part of the systemic vasculitis. The acute lesion is characterized by segmental necrosis with perivascular and mural fibrinoid material and may be accompanied by thrombosis in the vascular lumen. The initial acute inflammatory infiltrate is marked by the conspicuous infiltration of neutrophils that undergo leukocytoclasis (Fig. 2). Over time, the composition of the infiltrate transforms from neutrophils to predominantly mononuclear leukocytes *(69)*.

The overall frequency of vasculitis is approx 42 cases per million among whites. The incidence of MPA in Norwich, England is approx 5.2 cases per million. Found more commonly among whites, MPA is relatively infrequent in blacks or Indians. In our study of more than 300 patients with pauci-immune small vessel vasculitis from the southeast United States, 88% of patients were white, despite the fact that one third of our patients who undergo renal biopsy are black. The incidence of Wegener's granulomatosis may be increasing from the 0.7 per million found in the mid 1980s to more recent observations of 5–12.5 cases per million over the last several years *(70,71)*. Churg–Strauss syndrome is rare, with an annual incidence of only 2.4 cases per million inhabitants in the United Kingdom from 1988 to 1994 *(72)*. But in this population, 5.1 million inhabit rural areas compared with 1.8 million in urban areas. Part of the increased incidence of Wegener's granulomatosis may be attributed, in part, to an increase in the diagnosis of small vessel vasculitis after the introduction of ANCA assays in the late 1980s *(17,72)*.

Patients with pauci-immune small vessel vasculitis have a high incidence of exposure to environmental agents, particularly to inhalants, compared with the general population. In a case control study in the southeast United States, the odds ratio of developing pauci-immune disease was 4.4 with silica exposure in patients with pauci-immune small vessel vasculitis when compared with a control population of patients with lupus nephritis or other renal disease *(73–76)*. In addition, inhalation of silica and grain particles may increase the risk of developing Wegener's granulomatosis. These findings suggest that silica may act as an adjuvant in promoting an immune response.

One of the most common environmental stimulants associated with ANCA small vessel vasculitis is pharmaceutical agents, including propylthiouracil, hydralazine, colony stimulating factors and d-penicillamine, phenytoin, and various antibiotics. The interval between drug exposure and the appearance of symptoms varies, ranging from hours to days. Vasculitis may occur at first exposure to a drug or after an increase in the dosage. Drug-associated vasculitis often occurs after the agent has been discontinued and the patient is re-challenged with another regimen of the same drug. Most vasculitides resolve after the drug is discontinued; however, some patients develop severe life-threatening manifestations requiring treatment with glucocorticoids and alkylating agents. Several pathogenetic mechanisms have been postulated for this type of vasculitis. Certain drugs may cause the deposition of immune complexes by altering the complement cascade or by acting as a hapten. Alternatively, the drug may stimulate T lymphocytes directly or through a metabolite. Drugs or their metabolites may cause changes in cells by altering the structure of the cell membrane or by changing macromolecules within the cell *(77)*. ANCA vasculitis is often associated with the use of propylthiouracil in the treatment of hyperthyroidism and with the use of aminoguanidine in the experimental treatment of diabetes.

Infection may play a role in small vessel vasculitis. Staphylococcal infection has been associated with vasculitis in Wegener's granulomatosis. The incidence of relapse is increased in patients who are nasal carriers of *Staphylococcus aureus (78,79)*. Staphylococcal strains that carry superantigen genes are found more often than superantigen-negative staphylococcal strains in patients who relapse with Wegener's granulomatosis. Prophylactic treatment with sulfamethoxazole and trimethoprim decreased the relapse rate of patients with Wegener's granulomatosis when compared with placebo controls; relapses were almost exclusively associated with infection of the upper respiratory tract, especially the nasal passages *(80)*.

The immune response may be initiated by superantigens in ANCA small vessel vasculitis and other vasculitides *(81,82)*. Superantigens can stimulate naïve lymphocytes without the use of specific antigen receptors. Two types of superantigens have been identified: those that directly activate autoreactive T cells and those that stimulate autoreactive B cells through either T cell–dependent or T cell–independent pathways *(81)*. Superantigens that activate autoreactive T lymphocytes could mediate autoimmune-induced destruction of the vessel wall through cell-mediated pathways, whereas autoreactive B lymphocytes could produce pathogenetic antibodies. These mechanisms have been implicated in pauci-immune small vessel vasculitis and in arteritis associated with Kawasaki's disease.

The pathogenesis of ANCA-associated small vessel vasculitis has been examined in clinical and pathological studies (83,84). Although almost all vascular beds can be affected by vasculitis, the kidney, lung, skin, and upper and lower respiratory tracts are most commonly affected. Small vessel disease can take a rapidly progressive fulminant course, resulting in massive pulmonary hemorrhage and renal failure. In contrast, in some patients the course may be indolent, characterized by relapsing and remitting episodes of hematuria and proteinuria. Variation in the clinical expression of vasculitic injury presumably results from an interplay of pathogenetic factors and host responses. Small vessel vasculitis usually is focal; adjacent vascular beds may be severely damaged or entirely spared. For example, in the kidney, focal areas of glomerular necrosis may be adjacent to normal glomerular segments. Similarly, petechiae in the skin appear as clusters of leukocytoclastic vasculitis separated by areas of normal skin. Small vessel disease can affect any part of the lower respiratory tract, from the subglottis to the alveolar sac. Patients with microscopic polyangiitis or Goodpasture's syndrome present with transient pulmonary infiltrates that may initially be diagnosed as an infectious process. When hemoptysis develops, the infiltrates persist and cause dyspnea and hypoxemia. Widespread pulmonary capillaritis results in massive pulmonary hemorrhage. In contrast, the course of Wegener's granulomatosis is more indolent. The hallmark lesion of Wegener's granulomatosis is necrotizing granulomatous inflammation that may wax and wane.

Churg–Strauss syndrome, another variant of ANCA-associated pulmonary vasculitis, is characterized by the presence of eosinophilia in the circulation and within the pulmonary parenchyma. Otherwise, lesions are similar to those seen in microscopic polyangiitis or Wegener's granulomatosis. Although eosinophils appear to play a role in the pathogenesis of this disorder, the mechanism is unknown and therefore no explanation is available for this difference between Churg–Strauss syndrome and the other pauci-immune small vessel vasculitides.

The role of ANCA in pauci-immune small vessel vasculitis has been studied extensively (68,85–87). The two target antigens recognized by ANCA are myeloperoxidase and a serine protease known as proteinase 3. When ANCA bind myeloperoxidase, a perinuclear pattern is noted on indirect immunofluorescence of ethanol-fixed neutrophils. Cytoplasmic positive sera is detected when ANCA bind proteinase 3. Most patients with pauci-immune vasculitis have circulating ANCA to either myeloperoxidase or proteinase 3. ANCA-activated, primed neutrophils and monocytes produce reactive oxygen metabolites and proteolytic

enzymes (88). Several techniques have been used to show activation of neutrophils and monocytes by ANCA (89–96) (Fig. 3). Neutrophils and monocytes are primed by proinflammatory cytokines such as tumor necrosis factor and interleukin-1β to express target antigens on the cell surface (91,92,97,98). The binding of ANCA to these cell surface target antigens activates leukocytes. Whether this activation is caused by direct binding of Fab′2 receptors to antigen or by activation of the Fc receptors is controversial. Current data suggest that both mechanisms of leukocyte stimulation are important. ANCA-induced leukocyte activation may occur in the circulation or when cells are attached to the endothelial surface. The induction of endothelial damage by ANCA-activated neutrophils requires β integrin ligation by the antibody. Cultured endothelial cells are killed by exposure to neutrophils that have been activated by ANCA.

An alternative theory for the pathogenetic mechanism of ANCA-induced endothelial damage is that ANCA antigens planted along the endothelium at the time of leukocyte activation interact with ANCA and form immune complexes in situ. Both ANCA antigens, myeloperoxidase and proteinase 3, are cationic proteins that bind to cell surfaces and could be recognized in situ by ANCA. Studies in animal models support this hypothesis (99). Administration of myeloperoxidase with hydrogen peroxidase and other granular enzymes into the renal artery in rats preimmunized with human ANCA results in the deposition of immune complexes and the development of renal diseases. This mechanism is probably not the primary cause of small vessel vasculitis in humans because of the lack of immune complex deposition in human disease.

Both ANCA antigens can be taken up by endothelial cells. Proteinase 3 causes apoptosis in endothelial cells in a time- and dose-dependent manner; however, the mechanism is unknown (100). Similarly, myeloperoxidase can enter endothelial cells and create reactive oxygen species in the presence of oxygen radicals.

Animal models have been developed for studying small vessel vasculitis. Several autoimmune strains of mice have polyclonal B cell activation and an anti-myeloperoxidase response (101). Crescentic glomerulonephritis and vasculitis develop in several of these mouse models, including SCG/Kj mice (102). A rat model has been developed in which anti-GBM nephritis develops and is aggravated by anti-rat myeloperoxidase antibodies (103). Rats previously immunized with myeloperoxidase and injected with sub-nephritogenic doses of anti-GBM antibodies develop glomerulonephritis characterized by hematuria and proteinuria (104). Myeloperoxidase-immunized rats injected with anti-GBM antibodies developed fibrinoid

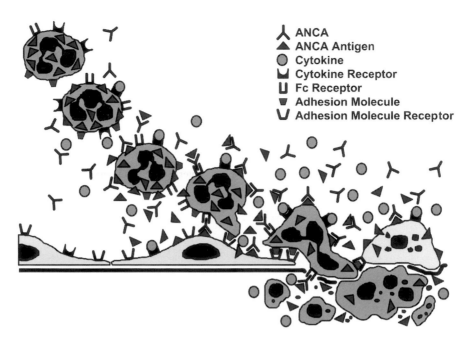

Fig. 3. The diagram depicts pathogenic events that are consistent with in vitro observations about the interactions between ANCA, ANCA antigens, neutrophils, and endothelial cells. Beginning in the upper left, cytokines stimulate neutrophils to express ANCA antigens at the cell surface. Binding of ANCA to antigens at the cell surface and in the microenvironment around neutrophils results in neutrophil activation by direct binding of Fab receptors to antigens on the surface of neutrophils and by engagement of Fc receptors by ANCA bound to antigens. ANCA antigens released by neutrophils also bind to endothelial cell surfaces and may result in low-level *in situ* immune complex formation. ANCA antigens enter endothelial cells and have toxic effects. Activated neutrophils bind to endothelial cells via adhesion molecules and release toxic and lytic enzymes and oxygen metabolites, resulting in vascular necrosis. From Jennette JC, Falk RJ (107), with permission.

necrosis of glomerular capillaries and crescent formation, whereas rats that received only the anti-GBM antibodies developed only mild glomerulonephritis.

We recently developed a model of ANCA injury in which myeloperoxidase deficient mice were immunized with murine myeloperoxidase and developed necrosis and crescentic glomerulonephritis. Transfer of splenocytes to immunodeficient recombinase activating gene-2 deficient (RAG2−/−) mice resulted in necrotizing and crescentic glomerulonephritis and a small vessel vasculitis. Transfer of anti-myeloperoxidase antibodies derived from myeloperoxidase-immunized myeloperoxidase knockout mice into RAG2−/− mice resulted in a pauci-immune form of necrotizing glomerulonephritis. These data indicate that ANCA cause a necrotizing capillaritis and that splenocytes amplify the vascular injury (105,106).

SUMMARY

In this chapter, we have described current concepts about the pathogenesis of several types of vasculitis. Several

factors must come together to cause inflammation in the vascular wall. The initial pathogenetic factors are unknown but may result from infection or environmental pressures. Once the inflammatory injury has begun, the nature of the lesion depends on several factors, including autoantibodies, antigens, leukocytes, genetic factors, and environmental pressures. A complex interplay is seen between factors that perpetuate inflammation and the host responses designed to eliminate or resolve the inflammation.

A very exciting yet essentially unexplored area is the role of the endothelium in vasculitis. Most vasculitides are focal in nature. For instance, in giant cell arteritis, lesions in the temporal artery may skip from one region of the artery to another. In ANCA small vessel vasculitis, one area of the glomerulus may be inflamed, whereas an adjacent segment may be entirely unaffected. Neither the mechanism of selective endothelial injury nor the derivation of the immune response is well understood. Using the techniques of molecular immunology, we may be able to dissect the origin of these responses and unlock one of the basic mysteries of autoimmunity.

REFERENCES

1. Jennette JC, Falk RJ. Small-vessel vasculitis. N Engl J Med 1997;337:1512–1523.

2. Kussmaul A, Maier R. Uber eine bisher nicht beschreibene eigenthumliche Arterienerkrankung (Periarteritis nodosa), die mit Morbus Brightii und rapid fortschreitender allgemeiner Muskellahmung einhergeht. Dtsch Arch Klin Med 1866;1: 484–518

3. Ferrari E. Ueber Polyarteritis actua nodosa (sogenannte Periarteriitis nodosa), und ihre Beziehungen zur Polymyositis and Polyneuritis acuta. Beitr Pathol Anat 1903;34:350–386.

4. Davson J, Ball J, Platt R. The kidney in periarteritis nodosa. Q J Med 1948;17:175–202.

5. Klinger H. Grenzformen der Periarteritis nodosa. Frankf Ztschr Pathol 1931;42:455–480.

6. Zeek PM. Periarteritis nodosa: a critical review. Am J Clin Pathol 1952;22:777–790.

7. Godman GC, Churg J. Wegener's granulomatosis. Pathology and review of the literature. Arch Pathol Lab Med 1954;58:533–553.

8. Shackelford PG, Strauss AW. Kawasaki's syndrome. N Engl J Med 1991;324:1664–1666.

9. Jennette JC, Falk RJ, Andrassy K, et al. Nomenclature of systemic vasculitides. Proposal of an international consensus conference. Arthritis Rheum 1994;37:187–192.

10. Caselli RJ, Hunder GG. Giant cell (temporal) arteritis. Neurol Clin 1997;15:893–902.

11. Hunder GG. Giant cell arteritis in polymyalgia rheumatica. Am J Med 1997;102:514–516.

12. Hunder GG. Clinical features of GCA/PMR. Clin Exp Rheumatol 2000;18:S6–S8.

13. Hunder GG, Valente RM. Giant cell arteritis: clinical aspects. In: Hoffman GS, Weyand CM, eds. Inflammatory Diseases of Blood Vessels. New York: Marcel Dekker, Inc., 2002:425–441.

14. Wilke WS. Large vessel vasculitis (giant cell arteritis, Takayasu arteritis). Baillieres Clin Rheumatol 1997;11:285–313.

15. Emmerich J, Fiessinger JN. [Epidemiology and etiological factors in giant cell arteritis (Horton's disease and Takayasu's disease)]. Ann Med Interne (Paris) 1998;149:425–432.

16. Planchon B, Cassagnau E, Pottier P, Pistorius M. [Systemic vasculitis]. J Mal Vasc 2000;25:166–174.

17. Watts RA, Jolliffe VA, Carruthers DM, Lockwood M, Scott DG. Effect of classification on the incidence of polyarteritis nodosa and microscopic polyangiitis. Arthritis Rheum 1996; 39:1208–1212.

18. Watts RA, Scott DG. Epidemiology of vasculitis. In: Ball GV, Bridges SL, Ball EV, eds. Vasculitis. Oxford University Press, 2000:176–201.

19. Salvarani C, Gabriel SE, O'Fallon WM, Hunder GG. The incidence of giant cell arteritis in Olmsted County, Minnesota: apparent fluctuations in a cyclic pattern. Ann Intern Med 1995; 123:192–194.

20. Baldursson O, Steinsson K, Bjornsson J, Lie JT. Giant cell arteritis in Iceland. An epidemiologic and histopathologic analysis. Arthritis Rheum 1994;37:1007–1012.

21. Salvarani C, Gabriel SE, O'Fallon WM, Hunder GG. Epidemiology of polymyalgia rheumatica in Olmsted County, Minnesota, 1970–1991. Arthritis Rheum 1995;38: 369–373.

22. Numano F. Differences in clinical presentation and outcome in different countries for Takayasu's arteritis. Curr Opin Rheumatol 1997;9:12–15.

23. Bahlas S, Ramos-Remus C, Davis P. Clinical outcome of 149 patients with polymyalgia rheumatica and giant cell arteritis. J Rheumatol 1998;25:99–104.

24. Aiello PD, Trautmann JC, McPhee TJ, Kunselman AR, Hunder GG. Visual prognosis in giant cell arteritis. Ophthalmology 1993;100:550–555.

25. Hayreh SS, Podhajsky PA, Zimmerman B. Ocular manifestations of giant cell arteritis. Am J Ophthalmol 1998;125:509–520.

26. Weyand CM, Goronzy JJ. Arterial wall injury in giant cell arteritis. Arthritis Rheum 1999;42:844–853.

27. Wagner AD, Bjornsson J, Bartley GB, Goronzy JJ, Weyand CM. Interferon-gamma-producing T cells in giant cell vasculitis represent a minority of tissue-infiltrating cells and are located distant from the site of pathology. Am J Pathol 1996;148:1925–1933.

28. Brack A, Geisler A, Martinez-Taboada VM, Younge BR, Goronzy JJ, Weyand CM. Giant cell vasculitis is a T cell-dependent disease. Mol Med 1997;3:530–543.

29. Yoshida M, Kimura A, Katsuragi K, Numano F, Sasazuki T. DNA typing of HLA-B gene in Takayasu's arteritis. Tissue Antigens 1993;42:87–90.

30. Weyand CM, Hicok KC, Hunder GG, Goronzy JJ. The HLA-DRB1 locus as a genetic component in giant cell arteritis. Mapping of a disease-linked sequence motif to the antigen binding site of the HLA-DR molecule. J Clin Invest 1992;90:2355–2361.

31. Weyand CM, Hunder NN, Hicok KC, Hunder GG, Goronzy JJ. HLA-DRB1 alleles in polymyalgia rheumatica, giant cell arteritis, and rheumatoid arthritis. Arthritis Rheum 1994;37: 514–520.

32. Roche NE, Fulbright JW, Wagner AD, Hunder GG, Goronzy JJ, Weyand CM. Correlation of interleukin-6 production and disease activity in polymyalgia rheumatica and giant cell arteritis. Arthritis Rheum 1993;36:1286–1294.

33. Misiani R. Virus-associated vasculitides: pathogenesis. In: Hoffman GS, Weyand CM, eds. Inflammatory Diseases of Blood Vessels. New York: Marcel Dekker, Inc., 2002:553–563.

34. Hunder GG. Epidemiology of giant-cell arteritis. Cleve Clin J Med 2002;69(Suppl 2):SII79–SII82.

35. Cohen IR. Autoimmunity to chaperonins in the pathogenesis of arthritis and diabetes. Annu Rev Immunol 1991;9:567–589.

36. Dziarski R. Preferential induction of autoantibody secretion in polyclonal activation by peptidoglycan and lipopolysaccharide. I. In vitro studies. J Immunol 1982;128:1018–1025.

37. Krieg AM, Yi AK, Matson S, et al. CpG motifs in bacterial DNA trigger direct B-cell activation. Nature 1995;374:546–549.

38. Amano S, Hazama F, Hamashima Y. Pathology of Kawasaki's disease: II. Distribution and incidence of the vascular lesions. Jpn Circ J 1979;43:741–748.

39. Barron KS, Shulman ST, Rowley A, et al. Report of the National Institutes of Health Workshop on Kawasaki's Disease. J Rheumatol 1999;26:170–190.

40. Godeau P, Guillevin L, Bletry O, Wechsler B. [Periarteritis nodosa associated with hepatitis B virus. 42 cases (author's transl)]. Nouv Presse Med 1981;10:1289–1292.

41. Guillevin L, Lhote F, Cohen P, et al. Polyarteritis nodosa related to hepatitis B virus. A prospective study with long-term observation of 41 patients. Medicine (Baltimore) 1995;74:238–253.

42. Tervaert JW. Infections in primary vasculitides. Cleve Clin J Med 2002;69(Suppl 2):SII24–SII26.

43. Zeek PM, Smith CC, Weeter JC. Studies on periarteritis nodosa. III. The differentiation between the vascular lesions of periarteritis nodosa and of hypersensitivity. Am J Pathol 1948;24: 889–917.

44. Naoe S, Takahashi K, Masuda H, Tanaka N. Kawasaki's disease. With particular emphasis on arterial lesions. Acta Pathol Jpn 1991;41:785–797.

45. Morigi M, Zoja C, Figliuzzi M, et al. Fluid shear stress modulates surface expression of adhesion molecules by endothelial cells. Blood 1995;85:1696–1703.

46. Nagel T, Resnick N, Dewey CF Jr, Gimbrone MA Jr. Vascular endothelial cells respond to spatial gradients in fluid shear stress by enhanced activation of transcription factors. Arterioscler Thromb Vasc Biol 1999;19:1825–1834.

47. Iiyama K, Hajra L, Iiyama M, et al. Patterns of vascular cell adhesion molecule-1 and intercellular adhesion molecule-1 expression in rabbit and mouse atherosclerotic lesions and at sites predisposed to lesion formation. Circ Res 1999;85:199–207.

48. Cybulsky MI, Lichtman AH, Hajra L, Iiyama K. Leukocyte adhesion molecules in atherogenesis. Clin Chim Acta 1999;286:207–218.

49. Kawasaki's T. [Acute febrile mucocutaneous syndrome with lymphoid involvement with specific desquamation of the fingers and toes in children]. Arerugi 1967;16:178–222.

50. Curtis N, Zheng R, Lamb JR, Levin M. Evidence for a superantigen mediated process in Kawasaki's disease. Arch Dis Child 1995;72:308–311.

51. Jennette JC, Sciarrotta J, Takahashi K, Naoe S. Predominance of monocytes and macrophages in the inflammatory infiltrates of acute Kawasaki's disease arteritis. Pediatr Res. In press.

52. Hamamichi Y, Ichida F, Yu X, et al. Neutrophils and mononuclear cells express vascular endothelial growth factor in acute Kawasaki's disease: its possible role in progression of coronary artery lesions. Pediatr Res 2001;49:74–80.

53. Meroni PL, Pappa ND, Raschi E, Tinvani A, Balestrieri G, Youinou P. Antiendothelial cell antibodies (AECA): From laboratory curiosity to another useful autoantibody. In: Shoenfeld Y, ed. The Decade of Autoimmunity. Amsterdam: Elsevier Health Sciences, 1999:227–251.

54. Furukawa S, Matsubara T, Jujoh K, et al. Peripheral blood monocyte/macrophages and serum tumor necrosis factor in Kawasaki's disease. Clin Immunol Immunopathol 1988;48:247–251.

55. Ichiyama T, Yoshitomi T, Nishikawa M, et al. NF-kappaB activation in peripheral blood monocytes/macrophages and T cells during acute Kawasaki's disease. Clin Immunol 2001;99:373–377.

56. Kim HY, Lee HG, Kim DS. Apoptosis of peripheral blood mononuclear cells in Kawasaki's disease. J Rheumatol 2000;27:801–806.

57. Nakatani K, Takeshita S, Tsujimoto H, Kawamura Y, Kawase H, Sekine I. Regulation of the expression of Fc gamma receptor on circulating neutrophils and monocytes in Kawasaki's disease. Clin Exp Immunol 1999;117:418–422.

58. Suzuki H, Uemura S, Tone S, et al. Effects of immunoglobulin and gamma-interferon on the production of tumour necrosis factor-alpha and interleukin-1 beta by peripheral blood monocytes in the acute phase of Kawasaki's disease. Eur J Pediatr 1996;155:291–296.

59. Ariga S, Koga M, Takahashi M, Ishihara T, Matsubara T, Furukawa S. Maturation of macrophages from peripheral blood monocytes in Kawasaki's disease: immunocytochemical and immunoelectron microscopic study. Pathol Int 2001;51:257–263.

60. Takeshita S, Nakatani K, Tsujimoto H, Kawamura Y, Kawase H, Sekine I. Increased levels of circulating soluble CD14 in Kawasaki's disease. Clin Exp Immunol 2000;119:376–381.

61. Praprotnik S, Rozman B, Blank M, Shoenfeld Y. Pathogenic role of anti-endothelial cell antibodies in systemic vasculitis. Wien Klin Wochenschr 2000;112:660–664.

62. Kaneko K, Savage CO, Pottinger BE, Shah V, Pearson JD, Dillon MJ. Antiendothelial cell antibodies can be cytotoxic to endothelial cells without cytokine pre-stimulation and correlate with ELISA antibody measurement in Kawasaki's disease. Clin Exp Immunol 1994;98:264–269.

63. Carvalho D, Savage CO, Isenberg D, Pearson JD. IgG antiendothelial cell autoantibodies from patients with systemic lupus erythematosus or systemic vasculitis stimulate the release of two endothelial cell-derived mediators, which enhance adhesion molecule expression and leukocyte adhesion in an autocrine manner. Arthritis Rheum 1999;42:631–640.

64. Cameron JS. Systemic lupus erythematosus. In: Neilson EG, Couser WG, eds. Immunologic Renal Diseases. Philadelphia: Lippincott Williams & Wilkins, 2001:1057–1104.

65. Couser WG, Baker PJ, Adler S. Complement and the direct mediation of immune glomerular injury: a new perspective. Kidney Int 1985;28:879–890.

66. Neilson EG, Kalluri R, Sun MJ, et al. Specificity of Goodpasture autoantibodies for the recombinant noncollagenous domains of human type IV collagen. J Biol Chem 1993;268:8402–8405.

67. Hellmark T, Burkhardt H, Wieslander J. Goodpasture disease. Characterization of a single conformational epitope as the target of pathogenic autoantibodies. J Biol Chem 1999;274:25862–25868.

68. Kallenberg CG, Brouwer E, Weening JJ, Tervaert JW. Anti-neutrophil cytoplasmic antibodies: current diagnostic and pathophysiological potential. Kidney Int 1994;46:1–15.

69. Jennette JC, Falk RJ. The pathology of vasculitis involving the kidney. Am J Kidney Dis 1994;24:130–141.

70. Andrews M, Edmunds M, Campbell A, Walls J, Feehally J. Systemic vasculitis in the 1980s—is there an increasing incidence of Wegener's granulomatosis and microscopic polyarteritis? J R Coll Physicians Lond 1990;24:284–288.

71. Watts RA, Scott DG, Lane SE. Epidemiology of Wegener's granulomatosis, microscopic polyangiitis, and Churg-Strauss syndrome. Cleve Clin J Med 2002;69(Suppl 2):SII84–SII86.

72. Watts RA, Carruthers DM, Scott DG. Epidemiology of systemic vasculitis: changing incidence or definition? Semin Arthritis Rheum 1995;25:28–34.

73. Gregorini G, Tira P, Frizza J, et al. ANCA-associated diseases and silica exposure. Clin Rev Allergy Immunol 1997;15:21–40.

74. Nuyts GD, Van Vlem E, De Vos A, et al. Wegener granulomatosis is associated to exposure to silicon compounds: a case-control study. Nephrol Dial Transplant 1995;10:1162–1165.

75. Hogan SL, Satterly KK, Dooley MA, Nachman PH, Jennette JC, Falk RJ. Silica exposure in anti-neutrophil cytoplasmic autoantibody-associated glomerulonephritis and lupus nephritis. J Am Soc Nephrol 2001;12:134–142.

76. Stratta P, Canavese C, Messuerotti A, Fenoglio I, Fubini B. Silica and renal diseases: no longer a problem in the 21st century? J Nephrol 2001;14:228–247.

77. ten Holder SM, Joy MS, Falk RJ. Cutaneous and systemic manifestations of drug-induced vasculitis. Ann Pharmacother 2002;36:130–147.

78. Stegeman CA, Tervaert JW, Sluiter WJ, Manson WL, de Jong PE, Kallenberg CG. Association of chronic nasal carriage of Staphylococcus aureus and higher relapse rates in Wegener granulomatosis. Ann Intern Med 1994;120:12–17.

79. Reinhold-Keller E, De Groot K, Rudert H, Nolle B, Heller M, Gross WL. Response to trimethoprim/sulfamethoxazole in Wegener's granulomatosis depends on the phase of disease. QJM 1996;89:15–23.

80. Stegeman CA, Tervaert JW, de Jong PE, Kallenberg CG. Trimethoprim-sulfamethoxazole (co-trimoxazole) for the

prevention of relapses of Wegener's granulomatosis. Dutch Co-Trimoxazole Wegener Study Group. N Engl J Med 1996; 335:16–20.

81. Tervaert JW, Popa ER, Bos NA. The role of superantigens in vasculitis. Curr Opin Rheumatol 1999;11:24–33.

82. Friedman SM, Tumang JR, Crow MK. Microbial superantigens as etiopathogenic agents in autoimmunity. Rheum Dis Clin North Am 1993;19:207–222.

83. Falk RJ, Hogan S, Carey TS, Jennette JC. Clinical course of anti-neutrophil cytoplasmic autoantibody-associated glomerulonephritis and systemic vasculitis. The Glomerular Disease Collaborative Network. Ann Intern Med 1990;113: 656–663.

84. Pusey CD, Gaskin G. Disease associations with anti-neutrophil cytoplasmic antibodies. Adv Exp Med Biol 1993;336:145–155.

85. Hagen EC, Ballieux BE, van Es LA, Daha MR, van der Woude FJ. Antineutrophil cytoplasmic autoantibodies: a review of the antigens involved, the assays, and the clinical and possible pathogenetic consequences. Blood 1993;81:1996–2002.

86. Niles JL, Pan GL, Collins AB, et al. Antigen-specific radioimmunoassays for anti-neutrophil cytoplasmic antibodies in the diagnosis of rapidly progressive glomerulonephritis. J Am Soc Nephrol 1991;2:27–36.

87. Falk RJ, Jennette JC. Anti-neutrophil cytoplasmic autoantibodies with specificity for myeloperoxidase in patients with systemic vasculitis and idiopathic necrotizing and crescentic glomerulonephritis. N Engl J Med 1988;318:1651–1657.

88. Falk RJ, Terrell RS, Charles LA, Jennette JC. Anti-neutrophil cytoplasmic autoantibodies induce neutrophils to degranulate and produce oxygen radicals in vitro. Proc Natl Acad Sci USA 1990;87:4115–4119.

89. Charles LA, Caldas ML, Falk RJ, Terrell RS, Jennette JC. Antibodies against granule proteins activate neutrophils in vitro. J Leukoc Biol 1991;50:539–546.

90. Brouwer E, Huitema MG, Mulder AH, et al. Neutrophil activation in vitro and in vivo in Wegener's granulomatosis. Kidney Int 1994;45:1120–1131.

91. Porges AJ, Redecha PB, Kimberly WT, Csernok E, Gross WL, Kimberly RP. Anti-neutrophil cytoplasmic antibodies engage and activate human neutrophils via Fc gamma RIIa. J Immunol 1994;153:1271–1280.

92. Mulder AH, Heeringa P, Brouwer E, Limburg PC, Kallenberg CG. Activation of granulocytes by anti-neutrophil cytoplasmic antibodies (ANCA): a Fc gamma RII-dependent process. Clin Exp Immunol 1994;98:270–278.

93. Savage CO, Pottinger BE, Gaskin G, Pusey CD, Pearson JD. Autoantibodies developing to myeloperoxidase and proteinase 3 in systemic vasculitis stimulate neutrophil cytotoxicity toward cultured endothelial cells. Am J Pathol 1992;141:335–342.

94. Ewert BH, Jennette JC, Falk RJ. Anti-myeloperoxidase antibodies stimulate neutrophils to damage human endothelial cells. Kidney Int 1992;41:375–383.

95. Brouwer E, Huitema MG, Klok PA, et al. Antimyeloperoxidase-associated proliferative glomerulonephritis: an animal model. J Exp Med 1993;177:905–914.

96. Yang JJ, Jennette JC, Falk RJ. Immune complex glomerulonephritis is induced in rats immunized with heterologous myeloperoxidase. Clin Exp Immunol 1994;97:466–473.

97. Kocher M, Edberg JC, Fleit HB, Kimberly RP. Antineutrophil cytoplasmic antibodies preferentially engage Fc gammaRIIIb on human neutrophils. J Immunol 1998;161:6909–6914.

98. Kettritz R, Jennette JC, Falk RJ. Crosslinking of ANCA-antigens stimulates superoxide release by human neutrophils. J Am Soc Nephrol 1997;8:386–394.

99. Heeringa P, Brouwer E, Tervaert JW, Weening JJ, Kallenberg CG. Animal models of anti-neutrophil cytoplasmic antibody associated vasculitis. Kidney Int 1998;53:253–263.

100. Yang JJ, Kettritz R, Falk RJ, Jennette JC, Gaido ML. Apoptosis of endothelial cells induced by the neutrophil serine proteases proteinase 3 and elastase. Am J Pathol 1996;149:1617–1626.

101. Esnault VL, Mathieson PW, Thiru S, Oliveira DB, Martin-Lockwood C. Autoantibodies to myeloperoxidase in brown Norway rats treated with mercuric chloride. Lab Invest 1992; 67:114–120.

102. Kinjoh K, Kyogoku M, Good RA. Genetic selection for crescent formation yields mouse strain with rapidly progressive glomerulonephritis and small vessel vasculitis. Proc Natl Acad Sci USA 1993;90:3413–3417.

103. Kobayashi K, Shibata T, Sugisaki T. Aggravation of rat nephrotoxic serum nephritis by anti-myeloperoxidase antibodies. Kidney Int 1995;47:454–463.

104. Heeringa P, Brouwer E, Klok PA, et al. Autoantibodies to myeloperoxidase aggravate mild anti-glomerular-basement-membrane-mediated glomerular injury in the rat. Am J Pathol 1996;149:1695–1706.

105. Jennette JC, Xiao H, Heeringa P, et al. Induction of pauci-immune necrotizing and crescentic glomerulonephritis (NCGN) by intravenous administration of anti-myeloperoxidase (anti-MPO) antibodies to recombinase activating gene-2 deficient (RAG-2 −/−) mice. Cleve Clin J Med 2002;69(Suppl 2);SII–13.

106. Xiao H, Heeringa P, Liu Z, et al. Induction of necrotizing and crescentic glomerulonephritis (NCGN) and small-vessel vasculitis (SVV) by adoptive transfer of anti-myeloperoxidase (anti-MPO) lymphocytes into recombinase activating gene-2 deficient (RAG-2 −/−) mice. Cleve Clin J Med 2002;69(Suppl 2);SII–13.

107. Jennette JC, Falk RJ. Pathogenesis of the vascular and glomerular damage in ANCA-positive vasculitis. Nephrol Dial Transplant 1998;13 (Suppl 1):16–20.

25 Primary Pulmonary Hypertension

Evangelos D. Michelakis, MD and Stephen L. Archer, MD

CONTENTS

INTRODUCTION
HISTOPATHOLOGY
MECHANISMS AND GENETICS
VASCULAR BIOLOGY
ETIOLOGY OF PRIMARY PULMONARY HYPERTENSION
CLINICAL ASPECTS OF PRIMARY PULMONARY HYPERTENSION
FUTURE DIRECTIONS
COMPREHENSIVE PROGRAMS FOR PRIMARY PULMONARY HYPERTENSION
ACKNOWLEDGMENTS
REFERENCES

INTRODUCTION

Primary pulmonary hypertension (PPH) is a disease of the pulmonary vasculature defined by an increase in pulmonary vascular resistance (PVR) that eventually leads to heart failure and premature death. Fifty years after the original antemortem description of PPH *(1)*, the cause remains unknown, and no cure is available.

Several challenges are associated with the search for the cause of PPH and its cure. First, PPH is rare, with an annual incidence of about 1 per 1,000,000, making randomized clinical trials difficult to conduct. Second, the syndrome of PPH is not homogeneous. Both idiopathic sporadic and familial forms of PPH have been identified (Table 1). Other cases known as pulmonary arterial hypertension (PAH) appear to be triggered by or associated with diverse environmental stimuli such as anorexigen drugs or infection. In addition to its inhomogeneity, PPH is characterized by nonspecific symptoms and signs. Because the disease evolves slowly and the symptoms, such as shortness of breath and fatigue, are nonspecific, early diagnosis is difficult.

Another obstacle in searching for the cause of PPH is identifying the primary lesion. PPH is associated with diverse abnormalities in the vascular lumen and the arterial wall. The components of the pulmonary vasculature, including endothelial cells, smooth muscle cells (SMC), the vascular extracellular matrix, and platelets, are often abnormal in patients with PPH. Finally, studying PPH is complicated by the lack of a suitable animal model for human disease. The models of chronic hypoxic pulmonary hypertension *(2,3)*, monocrotaline-induced pulmonary hypertension *(4–6)*, and the fawn-hooded rat *(7,8)* recapitulate only limited aspects of PAH. For example, plexiform lesions are not seen in any of these models.

Prompted by an epidemic of PPH linked to the use of anorexigens (diet pills), the World Health Organization (WHO) sponsored a meeting in 1973 to assess PPH. WHO defined pulmonary hypertension as a mean pulmonary artery (PA) pressure of greater than 25 mm Hg at rest or greater than 30 mm Hg with exercise. The National Registry on Primary Pulmonary Hypertension was created by the National Institutes of Health in 1981. The PPH registry, which comprised an epidemiologic core, a pathology core, and 32 clinical facilities, sponsored important studies, defined the natural history of PPH, and created a valuable collection of pathology specimens *(9)*.

During the past decade, several important molecular discoveries have been made in the study of PPH, including the recent identification of mutations in the gene for bone morphogenetic protein receptor II (BMPR-II) that

From: Contemporary Cardiology: Principles of Molecular Cardiology
Edited by: M. S. Runge and C. Patterson © Humana Press Inc., Totowa, NJ

413

Table 1
WHO Classification of Causes of Pulmonary Hypertension

I. Pulmonary Arterial Hypertension

    A. Primary pulmonary hypertension

       sporadic

       familial

    B. PAH related to:

       collagen vascular disease

       congenital systemic to pulmonary shunts

       portal hypertension

       HIV infection

       drugs/toxins

       persistent pulmonary hypertension of the newborn

       other

II. Pulmonary Venous Hypertension

    A. Left-sided atrial or ventricular heart disease

    B. Left-sided valvular disease

    C. Extrinsic compression of central pulmonary veins

       fibrosing mediastinitis

       adenopathy/tumors

    D. Pulmonary veno-occlusive disease

    E. Other

III. Pulmonary Hypertension Associated with Disorders of the Respiratory System or Hypoxemia

    A. Chronic obstructive lung disease

    B. Interstitial lung disease

    C. Sleep disorder breathing

    D. Alveolar hypoventilation disorders

    E. Chronic exposure to high altitude

    F. Neonatal lung disease

    G. Alveolar-capillary dysplasia

    H. Other

IV. Pulmonary Hypertension due to Chronic Thrombotic and/or Embolic Disease

    A. Thromboembolic obstruction of proximal pulmonary arteries

    B. Obstruction of distal pulmonary arteries

       pulmonary embolism (thrombus, tumor ova/parasites, foreign material)

    C. *in situ* thrombosis

    D. Sickle cell disease

V. Pulmonary Hypertension due to Disorders Directly Affecting the Pulmonary Vasculature

    A. Inflammatory

       schistosomiasis

       sarcoidosis

       other

    B. Pulmonary capillary hemangiomatosis

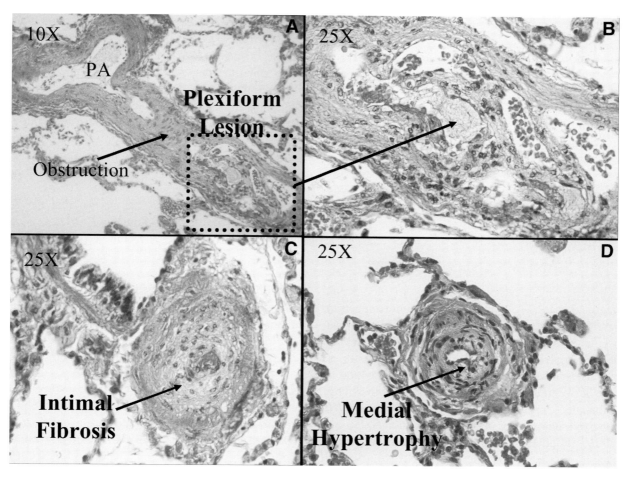

Fig. 1. Histology of PPH. **Panel A**: Plexiform lesion (Original magnification × 10). Note the plexiform lesion occurs distal to the vascular obstruction. PA, pulmonary artery. **Panel B**: Magnification of plexiform lesion occurring distal to vascular obstruction (Original magnification × 25). **Panel C**: Intimal fibrosis of small pulmonary artery causing vascular obstruction (Original × 25). **Panel D**: Medial hypertrophy (Original × 25).

are associated with PPH *(10,11)*. Several abnormalities that may cause or sustain PPH have been identified, including decreased expression and function of specific SMC potassium (K^+) channels, abnormal regulation of the pulmonary vascular extracellular matrix, endothelial dysfunction, and excessive production of serotonin and endothelin-1 (ET-1) *(12)*.

In a second meeting 25 yr after the original meeting, the WHO adopted a new classification scheme for pulmonary hypertension syndromes *(13)*. PAH refers to several distinct diseases that result in high pulmonary artery pressure (PAP) through unknown mechanisms. PPH (both sporadic and familial) and several other forms of pulmonary hypertension with known associations such as the use of anorectics, collagen vascular disease, infection with human immunodeficiency virus (HIV), congenital systemic to pulmonary shunts, and persistent pulmonary hypertension of the newborn were classified as PAH (Table 1). This

classification scheme reflects the fact that the clinical presentation and histologic profile of different forms of PAH are indistinguishable, which suggests common pathogenetic mechanisms, regardless of the initial cause. This scheme also allows physicians to consider the use of a therapy proven beneficial for PPH in patients with other forms of PAH. In this chapter, we discuss the vascular biology of PPH and the management of patients with PPH.

HISTOPATHOLOGY

Pulmonary arteries in PPH are characterized by intimal fibrosis, medial hypertrophy, adventitial proliferation, obliteration of small arteries, and *in situ* thrombosis. Vasculitis or changes in the walls of the pulmonary veins are sometimes seen *(14)* (Fig. 1), and plexiform lesions, which are focal vascular structures, are found in many cases of PPH. Plexiform lesions are not pathognomonic of PPH and are found in some cases of severe, secondary pulmonary hypertension, such as those related to congenital heart disease (e.g., Eisenmenger's syndrome). Similar to the renal glomerulus, the plexiform lesion in PPH has many vascular channels lined with endothelial cells rich in type 3 nitric oxide synthase (NOS) *(15)*, factor VIII, vimentin *(16)*, and the receptor for vascular endothelial growth factor (VEGF) *(17)*. Plexiform lesions may be part of an angiogenic response to local ischemia or hypoxia, such as occurs when collateral vessels develop in other vascular beds with obstructed arteries. Computerized three-dimensional reconstruction of vessels in PPH have shown that plexogenic lesions occur distal to vascular obstructive lesions *(17)* (Fig. 1).

MECHANISMS AND GENETICS

The challenge in developing a theory for the mechanisms involved in PPH is to account for the entire spectrum of the syndrome, including pulmonary artery vasoconstriction, vascular remodeling, and thrombosis *in situ*. Several abnormalities described in PPH can explain some or all aspects of the syndrome. These abnormalities include an imbalance between endothelial production of constrictor/dilator substances, excessive production of serotonin *(18)*, potassium channelopathy of pulmonary vascular SMCs and platelets *(19)*, monoclonal proliferation of endothelial cells *(20)*, and abnormal matrix production *(21)*. Only one or two of these abnormalities are primary, whereas most are secondary to the pulmonary hypertension and shear stress. In a recent study, a gene chip was used to compare gene expression in the lungs from patients with PAH and controls (*n* = 6, each group). The results showed upregulation of certain oncogenes such as *v-myc* and *jun D* in patients with PAH and suppression of other genes such as those for apoptosis or voltage-gated K$^+$ channels (Kv). New genetic techniques show the complexity of genetic changes in the development of PPH and the difficulties in identifying primary and secondary abnormalities in the pathogenesis of PPH. Despite the appeal of mass screening approaches, gene expression does not always indicate function. Because of the large number of pathways involved in PAH, a translational, multidisciplinary approach will be required to find the cause of PPH.

Although most cases of PPH are sporadic, about 6–12% are inherited in an autosomal-dominant manner with incomplete penetrance *(22)*. The disease may skip generations and may not affect all siblings in a generation; therefore, the proportion of familial cases may be underestimated. Although clinical and pathological features are the same in both forms, familial PPH displays genetic anticipation (i.e., it onsets at decreasing ages in subsequent generations). In a study of one family with familial PPH, Loyd et al. *(23)* reported that the

age of death decreased successively over three generations from 46 ± 15 yr to 36 ± 13 yr to 24 ± 11 yr. This phenomenon has been seen in fragile X syndrome and several dominantly inherited diseases such as myotonic dystrophy and Huntington's disease. The occurrence of genetic anticipation suggests that the molecular basis of familial PPH, like that seen in myotonic dystrophy, may be trinucleotide repeat expansion *(24)*. Although a GGC$_{8-16}$ trinucleotide repeat has been described in the 5' regulatory region of the PPH gene *(25)*, no evidence of expansion of the repeat has been observed *(26)*.

Genetic linkage analysis has shown that the gene for familial PPH, previously known as PPH1, is located on chromosome 2q33 *(22,27,28)*. In a positional candidate approach, the gene for BMPR-II has been identified as a cause of familial PPH *(10,11)*. Heterogeneous germline mutations have been identified in BMPR-II in multiple family members (60%) of patients with familial PPH. Moreover, mutations in this gene have been seen in several patients with PPH who have no family history of the disease, suggesting a genetic basis for sporadic PPH *(29)*.

Bone morphogenetic proteins (BMPs), a family of secreted growth factors, are part of the transforming growth factor (TGF)-β superfamily. Originally described as proteins that induce ectopic bone and cartilage formation when implanted subcutaneously *(30)*, BMPs are now known to be important regulators of mammalian development *(31)*. For example, targeted misexpression studies indicate that BMP-4 is important in embryonic lung development *(32)*. TGF-β superfamily members interact with two classes of transmembrane receptor serine–threonine kinases, type I and II receptors *(33)*. Type II receptors have constitutively active cytoplasmic kinase domains but are unable to activate downstream signals in the absence of a type I receptor. Furthermore, several TGF-β family members use the same receptors as the BMPs, which increases the plasticity of the regulation of downstream responses *(33)*. This plasticity is further increased by the cell-specific activation of several downstream signaling pathways after the binding of BMPs to BMP receptors I and II *(33)*. The Smad family, an important signaling system, includes the BMPR-activated Smads (Smad-1, 5, and 8) and the common mediator Smad (Smad-4) *(34)*. In the nucleus, the activated Smad-1,5,8–Smad-4 complex regulates several DNA binding transcription factors and cofactors that are required to initiate specific positive and negative transcriptional responses *(34)*. The Smads were originally named after a gene in *Drosophila melanogaster* called "mothers against decapentaplegic (dpp)" *(35)*, which encodes a growth factor of the TGF-β superfamily that is important in multiple cell–cell signaling events throughout development. Activation of the BMPR-II pathway leads to suppression of several transcription factors, which favors apoptosis. BMPR-II is heavily expressed in the human pulmonary artery (Fig. 2A).

Homozygous deletion of the BMPR-II in vivo is associated with embryonic death (36). More than 40 different germline mutations in the BMPR-II gene have been described in both familial and sporadic PPH and include missense and frameshift mutations (33). Most of the mutations result in loss of function of the BMPR-II gene product (26), but how this loss of function leads to the development of PPH is unknown. Pulmonary artery smooth muscle cells (PASMCs) from patients with PPH, but not secondary pulmonary hypertension, were recently shown to have increased growth responses to TGF-β1 and BMPs (37). The existence of complex, cell–specific signaling systems downstream of BMPR-II might explain why mutations in a ubiquitously expressed receptor result in the highly restricted pattern of disease seen in patients with PPH. Whether BMPR-II mutations result in disease by inhibiting a normal rate of apoptosis, or whether something else stimulates a need for apoptosis (a process that cannot be supported when BMPR-II is dysfunctional) is unknown. Although, because BMPR-II mutations affect many transcription factors, multiple mechanisms may be at work, each relating to altered transcription of relevant genes, such as genes for Kv channels, ET-1, or the 5-HTT.

PPH occurs three times more frequently in women than in men (23,38). This gender imbalance, which is an unsolved clue to the genetics of PPH, is not seen before puberty and is not directly related to the use of oral contraceptives or to childbirth.

VASCULAR BIOLOGY

The Endothelium

Whether endothelial dysfunction is an early primary lesion in PPH is unknown; however, the PA endothelium is highly abnormal in later stages of the disease. Because PPH is usually detected only in the late stages of the disease, knowledge of endothelial function in patients with early PPH is lacking. Endothelial dysfunction causes an imbalance in endothelial-derived vasoactive factors, with an overall increase toward vasoconstriction.

Endothelial abnormalities contribute to the abnormal production of vasoactive mediators and to the formation of plexiform lesions. Plexiform lesions, which are seen in both PPH and PAH (but not in secondary forms of pulmonary hypertension), are characterized by the abnormal proliferation of endothelial cells. In a study of the clonal origin of the proliferation of endothelial cells in plexiform lesions in PPH, Lee et al. (20) examined the methylation

pattern of the human androgen receptor gene by polymerase chain reaction in endothelial cells from plexiform lesions. They reported that 77% of endothelial lesions were monoclonal in PPH, whereas 100% of the endothelial lesions were polyclonal in secondary pulmonary hypertension. In contrast, SMCs in both PPH and secondary pulmonary hypertension were polyclonal in all but one case (20,39). These findings suggest that PPH has a "neoplastic" aspect; however, the number of samples studied was small, and the technique applied only to females and independent confirmation is required.

VASODILATOR/VASOCONSTRICTOR IMBALANCE

In both PPH and secondary pulmonary hypertension, patients excrete increased levels of a thromboxane A2 metabolite and reduced amounts of prostacyclin (40). Thromboxane A2 is a potent vasoconstrictor and stimulus for platelet aggregation, whereas prostacyclin is an antiproliferative, antiaggregatory, vasodilator product of the endothelium. Although this platelet–endothelial abnormality, which occurs in both PPH and secondary pulmonary hypertension, is probably not casual, the finding has had significant therapeutic value.

The vasoconstrictor ET-1 may be increased and nitric oxide (NO) may be decreased in PPH. Using immunohistochemistry techniques, Giaid and Saleh (41) found that expression of endothelial nitric oxide synthase (eNOS) is lower in the lungs of PPH patients than in control subjects, but NOS function was not measured in this study. In contrast, lung production of NO, which may not reflect pulmonary vascular NO production, is increased (42) or maintained in PPH (43). PPH patients also have higher urinary concentrations of cyclic guanosine monophosphate (cGMP) than asthmatic patients or healthy controls (44). Although PPH may appear to result from a deficiency of NO, this hypothesis is unlikely because most blood vessels respond to increased tone with a homeostatic increase in NO production (45). NO deficiency in PPH may represent a late failure of this pathway. Alternatively, patients with abnormal endothelium or eNOS may be predisposed to certain forms of PAH, such as that caused by ingesting anorexigens (42).

Levels of ET-1, a potent vasoconstrictor and mitogen, are increased in experimental (46,47) and human (48–54) pulmonary hypertension. The presence of higher levels of ET-1 in arterial than in venous plasma in PPH is consistent with the pulmonary production of ET-1, suggesting that ET-1 may contribute to an increase in PVR (54). However, ET-1 is increased in many other diseases such as congestive heart failure. Nevertheless, Giaid et al. (55) found that expression of ET-1 in vascular endothelial cells was increased in pulmonary hypertension, suggesting

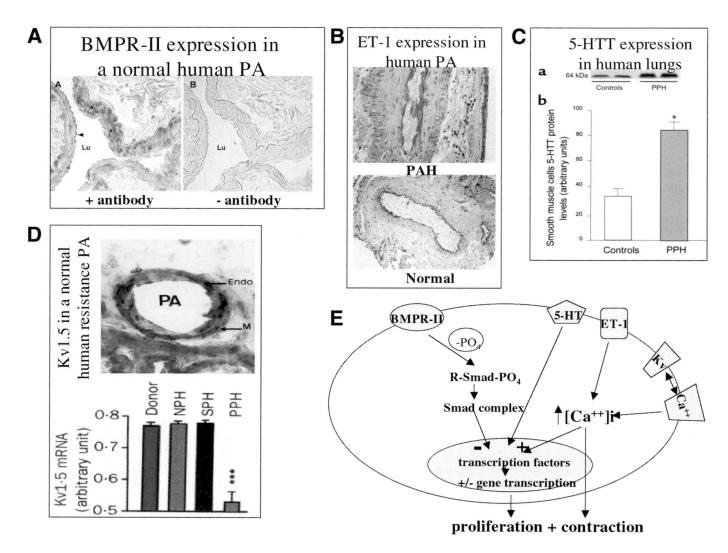

Fig. 2. PPH mechanisms. Panel A: Immunohistochemistry shows that BPMR-II is expressed in both endothelial (arrow) and smooth muscle cells (*) in normal pulmonary arteries (PA). BMPR-II, bone morphogenetic protein receptor-II; Lu,lumen. (Adapted with permission from ref. *33*). **Panel B**: Immunohistochemistry shows that expression of endothelin-1 (ET-1) is higher in the pulmonary artery (PA) of a patient with PPH than in a patient without pulmonary hypertension. (Adapted with permission from ref. *55*). **Panel C: (top)** Immunohistochemistry of pulmonary arteries from a rat shows the Kv1.5 channel in the smooth muscle cells of pulmonary arteries (PA). Kv1.5 is also present in the endothelium, but is not seen because the slide is double-stained with an antibody to endothelial nitric oxide synthase. M, media; Endo, endothelium. **(bottom)** Reverse transcriptase polymerase chain reaction shows that PPH patients have less messenger RNA for Kv1.5 than normal patients, patients with chronic lung disease and normal PVR (NPH), or patients with secondary pulmonary hypertension (SPH). Expression of other proteins, including β-actin and the Kvβ1.1 subunit were unaffected. (Reproduced with permission from ref. *60*). **Panel D**: Immunoblotting analysis of the serotonin receptor (5-HTT) protein in smooth muscle cells in pulmonary arteries from patients with PPH and controls. **(a)** 5-HTT immunoreactivity detected in cells from two controls and from two patients with PPH. **(b)** Quantification of the 5-HTT signal in each group ($p<0.05$). (Adapted with permission from ref. *71*). **Panel E**: A proposed link between the abnormalities in the pathogenesis of PPH. Increased serotonin (5-HT) and endothelin-1 (ET-1) signaling and decreased Kv channel activity and expression (and the secondary depolarization and activation of the L-type Ca^{2+} channels) lead to increased levels of intracellular Ca^{2+}. The increased Ca^{2+} and K^+ levels lead to vasoconstriction and activation of several genes involved in cell proliferation and apoptosis. In contrast, downstream signaling from the bone morphogenetic protein receptors (BMPR), via several systems including the Smads, inhibits genes involved in proliferation and activates genes involved in apoptosis. Therefore, the loss of function mutations in the BMPR-II, combined with 5-HT, ET-1 and Kv abnormalities, may act synergistically in the development of PPH *(83)*.

that local production of ET-1 may contribute to the pathogenesis of PPH (Fig. 2B). PPH has been associated with increased levels of endothelin-converting enzyme, but enzyme function has not been assessed (56).

The Smooth Muscle Cell

POTASSIUM CHANNEL DYSREGULATION

K^+ channels are transmembrane-spanning proteins that contain a K^+-selective pore. Tonically active in vascular SMCs, K^+ channels allow a slow efflux of K^+ along its intracellular/extracellular concentration gradient of 145/5 mM. Several types of K^+ channels have been identified: voltage-gated (Kv), inward rectifier (Kir), and calcium-sensitive (K_{Ca}). Kv channels, with a voltage sensor, respond to and contribute to determining membrane potential. Inhibition of Kv channels results in accumulation of positively charged K^+ ions within the cell and increases the membrane potential to more positive levels (depolarization), which activates the voltage-gated, L-type calcium channel (57). Calcium then enters the cell and activates the contractile apparatus, which leads to vasoconstriction. In acute hypoxia, hypoxic pulmonary vasoconstriction is initiated by inhibition of Kv channel in the PASMC (57,58).

Nine families of Kv channels have been identified (Kv1-9), and each family has many members (Kv1.1–Kv1.7) (59). Kv1.5 is heavily expressed in PASMCs (Fig. 2C). In patients with PPH, mRNA levels for Kv1.5 are decreased in PASMCs (Fig. 2C), and this decrease has been associated with membrane depolarization and increased cytosolic Ca^{2+} (60). Thus, decreased expression or function of K^+ channels in PASMCs in PPH patients may initiate and maintain pulmonary vasoconstriction, thereby contributing to the pathogenesis of PPH (60).

Less is known about Kv2.1, which is involved in setting E_M in rat PASMCs (61). Both Kv1.5 (62) and Kv2.1 (63) are directly inhibited by the anorexigen, dexfenfluramine, and expression of both Kv1.5 and Kv2.1 is selectively downregulated in experimental pulmonary hypertension (64,65). A causal role for K^+ channel deficiency in PPH has been postulated (19), but questions remain, including which K^+ channels are involved and whether the loss of specific K^+ channels is a cause or a response to pulmonary hypertension. There is a precedence for ion channelopathies causing human disease, for example, chloride channel mutations causing cystic fibrosis and mutation of K^+ and Na^+ channels cause the long QT syndrome.

The Extracellular Matrix

Vascular remodeling, a prominent feature of PPH, is characterized by muscularization of normally nonmuscular peripheral arteries (related to differentiation of pericytes), medial hypertrophy, and intimal proliferation. These changes occur because of hypertrophy, proliferation, and migration of PASMCs and increased production of extracellular matrix (collagen, elastin, fibronectin, and tenascin-C). Altered mitogenesis, like the procoagulant state, appears to be a secondary response to an initial injury.

Rabinovitch and colleagues (21,66) have suggested that endothelial abnormalities early in PPH permit extravasation of blood factors that stimulate production of a vascular serine elastase by SMCs. Production of elastase liberates matrix-bound SMC mitogens, such as basic fibroblast growth factor, and increases matrix degradation by activating other MMPs. MMPs stimulate production of a mitogenic cofactor, tenascin. The binding of tenascin to its α-β_3 integrin receptors leads to phosphorylation of growth factor receptors and proliferation of SMCs. Inhibition of MMPs reduces tenascin levels, which leads to apoptosis (21). Cowan et al. (21) recently showed that inhibition of MMP-2 and serine elastases leads to regression of PA hypertrophy. Although originally thought to function only in remodeling, MMPs are now known to affect vascular tone. MMP-2 and MMP-9 activate platelets (67), whereas intravascular MMP-2 stimulates production of vasoconstrictors, including a novel form of endothelin, and inhibits the action of endogenous vasodilators (68). Therapy for PPH may eventually be directed at modulating MMPs or elastases to restore normal vascular architecture.

Platelet/Serotonin

Several groups have proposed that serotonin is important in the development of pulmonary hypertension (18,69,70). Evidence to support this hypothesis comes from the finding that plasma levels of serotonin are higher in PPH patients than in controls, whereas platelets from PPH patients have decreased serotonin concentrations (18). In addition, serotonin released during in vitro platelet aggregation is higher in PPH patients than in controls. These abnormalities in PPH patients persist after heart–lung transplantation, suggesting that platelet abnormality is not secondary to pulmonary hypertension (18).

Most circulating serotonin is stored and released by the platelet-dense granule. In platelet delta storage pool disease, the number and content of the granules are reduced. In a patient with platelet delta storage pool disease who developed PPH, the plasma concentration of serotonin was 15 times higher than normal levels (18). The anorexigens that caused several epidemics of PPH not only inhibit K^+ channels but also prevent the reuptake of serotonin. These anorexigens are substrates for the serotonin transporter (5-HTT) and thus are actively transported into the cells.

When stimulated with serotonin or serum, PASMCs from patients with PPH grow faster than PASMCs from controls; these effects are caused by increased expression of 5-HTT *(71)*. The expression of 5-HTT in cultured PASMCs and in platelets and lungs is higher in PPH patients than in controls (Fig. 2D) *(71)*. 5-HTT expression is increased in PPH and is predominantly expressed in the media of the thickened pulmonary arteries *(71)*. The L-allelic variant of the 5-HTT gene promoter, which is associated with 5-HTT overexpression and increased PASMC growth, was found in homozygous form in 65% of PPH patients but in only 27% of controls. This finding suggests that 5-HTT activity is important in the pathogenesis of PASMC proliferation in PPH and that a 5-HTT polymorphism may confer susceptibility to PPH *(71)*. These data indicate another possible susceptible genotype for PPH in addition to mutations in the BMPR-II gene.

THROMBOSIS IN SITU

Patients with PPH have several prothrombotic abnormalities, including increased platelet aggregation, high levels of serotonin and plasminogen-activator inhibitor, and decreased levels of thrombomodulin *(72)*. The importance of a prothrombotic diathesis in the progression of PPH is supported by the finding that thrombosis *in situ* is common and that anticoagulation may improve survival *(73,74)*. Prothrombotic abnormalities are also common in patients with secondary pulmonary hypertension, but the specific abnormalities (increased levels of von Willebrand factor and fibrinogen and decreased fibrinolytic activity) are different from those found in PPH *(75)*. Hypercoaguability may occur in response to pulmonary hypertension and may be related to endothelial injury, though abnormal coagulation may initiate PPH in some patients.

Animal Models

Although an ideal model of PPH is lacking, the PAH caused by injection of normal rats with monocrotaline, an alkaloid derived from the plant *Crotalaria spectabilis (4,5)*, and the spontaneous PAH in fawn-hooded rats resemble PPH in humans. PAH in the fawn-hooded rat is associated with an inherited defect in platelet serotonin-storage *(7,8)* but its etiology is unknown. Pulmonary vascular endothelial dysfunction is also seen in the fawn-hooded rat. Nevertheless, the pathophysiology of chronic hypoxic pulmonary hypertension *(2,3)* is distinct from PPH, and the rat model may not be directly applicable to PPH in humans. For example, Tyler et al. *(76)* compared the NO system in rats with three types of experimental pulmonary hypertension (chronically hypoxic, monocrotaline-induced, and fawn-hooded). NOS products and eNOS expression were

decreased in fawn-hooded and monocrotaline rats but were increased in CH-pulmonary hypertension *(76)*. eNOS knockout mice *(77)* and rats fed a NOS inhibitor *(78)* develop a mild increase in PVR but do not have the extensive, obstructive vascular remodeling or severe pulmonary hypertension seen in PPH.

ETIOLOGY OF PRIMARY PULMONARY HYPERTENSION

Whether a link exists between the different theories of etiology of PPH is unknown. K^+ channels may be the possible connection between the abnormalities seen in platelets and endothelial cells and in serotonin handling and the vascular tone in PPH. K^+ channels have a common role in controlling membrane potential and, thus, can modulate ionic flux and function in platelets, SMCs, and possibly endothelial cells. Although speculative, this link is supported by well-substantiated individual observations.

Spontaneous PPH and anorexigen-induced PPH both involve a decrease in Kv current in PASMCs and possibly in platelets. Dexfenfluramine inhibits Kv channels in the megakaryocyte, which is the progenitor cell for platelets *(19)*. Furthermore, the Kv channel inhibitor, 4-aminopyridine, mimics dexfenfluramine in causing release of serotonin from platelets and in markedly reducing serotonin reuptake *(79)*. Thus, the loss or inhibition of Kv channels that occurs in PPH may account for the decrease in platelet serotonin stores and the increase in plasma levels of serotonin. Increased serotonin, in the presence of endothelial dysfunction, acts as a vasoconstrictor *(80)*, particularly during PASMC membrane depolarization and when levels of cytosolic Ca^{2+} are high. Indeed, serotonin and evolothein both inhibit Kv channels by a protein kinase C-dependent mechanism. In anorexigen-induced PPH, the Kv channel may be directly inhibited by the drug *(62,63,81)*. In spontaneous PPH, a predisposing genetic channelopathy or an acquired loss of Kv channels may similarly lead to membrane depolarization.

The relation between this K^+ channel hypothesis and the MMP and prothrombotic hypotheses is unknown. We do not know whether PPH, once initiated, is sustained and exacerbated by elastase and MMP-induced matrix remodeling and a prothrombotic diathesis. In contrast, MMP abnormalities could be causal and could result in pulmonary hypertension with a secondary inhibition of Kv channel expression. As seen from recent studies in dilated cardiomyopathy, several molecular mechanisms may result in a final common phenotype or disease *(82)*.

Whether primary or secondary, the loss of K^+ channels and the increased levels of endothelin and serotonin eventually increase intracellular Ca^{2+} levels in PASMC (Fig. 2E). This change results in vasoconstriction and activation of genes that lead to cell proliferation. Under normal circumstances, the BMPR-II, via the Smad pathway, has negative tonic control of gene transcription and promotes apoptosis rather than proliferation (Fig. 2E). The "loss of function" mutations in the BMPR-II along with one or more other abnormalities (Kv channels, endothelin, or serotonin), creates an imbalance that favors vasoconstriction and proliferation (83) (Fig. 2E).

Environmental Stimuli

Epidemics of vascular disease caused by environmental toxins happen fairly frequently (84). Much has been learned about the etiology of PPH from three outbreaks that occurred in the latter half of the 20th century caused by ingestion of anorexigens, infection with HIV, and consumption of adulterated rapeseed oil.

ANOREXIGENS

The anorexigens aminorex, fenfluramine, and dexfenfluramine are modified amphetamines that increase serotonin release and inhibit serotonin reuptake in the brain, which results in appetite suppression and a 5–10% weight loss. Between 1967 and 1972, an outbreak of PPH related to the anorectic agent aminorex occurred in Europe (85). Although 61% of the 582 PPH patients had taken aminorex, only 0.1% of those who took aminorex manifested PPH. In the 1980s and 1990s, a similar PPH epidemic was associated with the use of fenfluramine and dexfenfluramine. Although use of these appetite suppressants for 3 mo was associated with a 23-fold increase in the risk of developing PPH, the annual incidence of PPH in the population as a whole remained very low (1.7 per million) (86). Thus, only a small proportion of the patients exposed to the anorexigens aminorex or dexfenfluramine developed PPH, suggesting a requirement for one or more predisposing conditions.

Several predisposing factors in anorexigen-induced PPH have been suggested. Many of the anorexigens are also 5-HTT substrates (87) and, thus, are translocated into pulmonary vascular cells where the intrinsic toxicity is amplified, depending on the degree of drug retention. Endothelial dysfunction, either acquired or genetic, is probably a predisposing factor for developing PPH. Patients with anorexigen-induced PPH tended to be older and frequently had known risk factors for endothelial dysfunction such as cigarette use or obesity (42). Patients with anorexigen-associated PAH have lower lung NO production than do patients with PPH (42).

A strong link exists between the anorexigens, Kv channels, and the endothelium in PPH. Kv channel inhibition and membrane depolarization partially account for the pulmonary (19) and systemic vasoconstriction induced by anorexigens (80). Recent studies show that Kv1.5 and Kv2.1 are directly inhibited by anorexigens, even when the channels are studied in heterologous expression systems (62,63). For Kv1.5, channel inhibition occurs by means of open channel block, which would favor channel inhibition when the SMC is depolarized (88). In addition to their effects on SMCs, anorexigens promote vasoconstriction by increasing Ca^{2+} release from the sarcoplasmic reticulum (89). The anorexigens block Kv channels in platelet progenitor cells, or megakaryocytes (19), and Kv channel inhibition in platelets leads to serotonin release (19). Furthermore, fenfluramine reduces levels of Kv1.5 mRNA by 50% in PASMCs from normotensive patients (90), which suggests that inhibited gene transcription and expression of Kv channels may be important in anorexigen-induced PPH.

Several animal studies indicate that endothelial dysfunction and Kv channel inhibition or downregulation may be predisposing factors in anorexigen-associated PPH. In isolated rat lungs, aminorex, dexfenfluramine, and fenfluramine cause small but consistent increases in PVR at doses higher than those used clinically. However, in the presence of both a cycloxygenase and NOS inhibitors, the anorexigens dramatically increase PVR at relevant doses (81). Anorexigens may be Kv channel blockers that cause their intended effects (appetite suppression and alteration of serotonin levels) and their unintended effects (altered platelet function and increased vascular tone) by controlling membrane potential and cytosolic Ca^{2+} levels (19,80). The newer anorexigens/ antidepressants, fluoxetine and venlafaxine, do not inhibit Kv current at the resting membrane potential (88) and, therefore, may present less risk of inducing PPH. Phentermine, an anorexigen that has not been shown to cause PPH, does not inhibit Kv current in PASMC (88).

HUMAN IMMUNODEFICIENCY VIRUS (HIV)

Another environmental stimuli that results in PPH is infection with HIV. About 90 cases of HIV-associated PPH have been reported as of 2002 (91). Of these patients, 61% were male and 83% had no additional factors predisposing to PPH. HIV-associated PPH progresses more rapidly than spontaneous PPH, and the prognosis may be worse (only 51% of patients with HIV have a 1-year survival rate vs 68% for patients with non–HIV-associated PPH) (92). However, the pathology

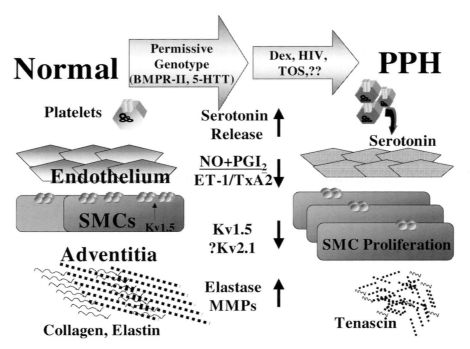

Fig. 3. The "multiple hit hypothesis" for PPH. In this "three strike model" a patient with a permissive genotype develops PPH on exposure to a stimulus. The three strikes are an abnormal genotype, dysfunctional endothelium and/or K+ channels, and a triggering stimulus. Trigger stimuli include anorexigens, such as dexfenfluramine (Dex), human immunodeficiency virus (HIV), toxic oil (TOS), or other unidentified stimuli. The abnormalities outlined that are associated with PPH may contribute to the cause or the progression of the disease. However, in some individuals, all three strikes may not be necessary to cause disease; one of sufficient intensity (abnormal gene) may be enough. Because PPH may not be one disease, multiple molecular mechanisms may cause the syndrome. BMPR, bone morphogenetic protein receptor; ET-1, endothelin-1; 5-HTT, serotonin receptor; MMPs, matrix metalloproteinases; NO, nitric oxide; PGI_2, prostaglandin; SMC, smooth muscle cell; and TxA2, thromboxane.

is similar to that seen in spontaneous PPH, with plexiform lesions noted in 85% of cases (92). Expression of Kv1.3, an important molecular target for immunosuppressive agents in T lymphocytes, is inhibited via a PKC-dependent mechanism in HIV–PPH (93), which suggests a link between cellular electrophysiology, immunity, and PPH (94).

TOXIC OIL SYNDROME (TOS)

In 1981, 20,000 people were poisoned by aniline dye–contaminated rapeseed oil that was intended for industrial use and sold illegally in Spain (95,96). The acute clinical manifestations included a respiratory distress syndrome, myalgias, eosinophilia, and widespread vascular and neural lesions. Pulmonary hypertension developed in 20% of the patients and spontaneously regressed in many; however, in a few patients, pulmonary hypertension progressed to a fatal form of PAH (97). Examination of the contaminated oils suggests the pathogenic products of this dye include fatty acid oleyl anilides and the mono- and diester of 3-phenylamino-1,2-propanediol (96,98). TOS–PPH, like spontaneous PPH, is characterized by endothelial damage (99). TOS–PPH has been associated

with a genotype and human leukocyte antigen (HLA) profile; it is found more in females and the HLA profile is the HLA-A24, DR4-DQ8 genotype (100).

We have learned from these toxic PPH outbreaks that PPH may be a "three strike" syndrome (Fig. 3). A permissive genotype (abnormal genes for BMPR-II, 5HTT, and/or Kv channels), a susceptible phenotype (genetic or acquired, such as endothelial dysfunction), and an environmental stimulus (HIV, toxic oil, or dexfenfluramine) combine to promote PPH. The low likelihood that this triad would occur is consistent with the low incidence of PPH. However, when the stimulus is unusually potent or ubiquitous, the susceptible members of the population are at risk. Some subjects may require all three strikes to manifest PPH, whereas PPH may result as a consequence of a single devastating strike in others.

CLINICAL ASPECTS OF PRIMARY PULMONARY HYPERTENSION

Prognosis and Natural History

The NIH Registry (1981–1987), which established the natural history and prognosis of PPH (101), serves as an important reference because it was conducted before the use of current conventional therapies such as prostacyclin and Bosevtan. The median survival of enrolled patients was 2.8 yr from diagnosis. The independent predictors of prognosis, such as mean right atrial pressure, cardiac output, and mean pulmonary arterial pressure, reflect right ventricular (RV) function; therefore, the prognosis of a patient with PPH may be linked to the adaptive response of the RV to the chronic pressure overload state. The thin-walled (3 mm) RV is much less capable of adapting to increases in afterload than the thick-walled (11 mm) left ventricle (Fig. 4).

The natural history of patients who present with secondary forms of pulmonary hypertension, such as congenital heart disease or collagen vascular disease, is less well characterized. Prognosis in these patients is related both to the severity of the pulmonary hypertension and the underlying illness. The best-characterized group of patients with secondary pulmonary hypertension are those with congenital heart disease (102). These patients seem to live longer with severe pulmonary hypertension than patients with PPH. This increased survival time may relate to a more efficient adaptation of the RV, resulting from increased expression of embryonic genes that regulate fetal contractile proteins of the RV from the time of birth (103).

The role of RV dysfunction and RV ischemia (caused by a supply/demand mismatch) has not been adequately defined in PPH. Right heart failure underlies many of the signs and symptoms (Table 2) of PPH (syncope and exercise intolerance), and almost half of PPH patients develop angina pectoris despite having normal coronary arteries (104). A finding that may indicate the degree of importance of RV and/or lung ischemia in PPH is that PPH patients have increased blood levels of uric acid, and the uric acid level strongly correlates with right atrial pressure (105). Uric acid levels are sometimes reduced by therapy (105), and some investigators have suggested that PPH patients, although not hypoxemic or polycythemic, may have relative RV ischemia caused by excessive uric acid production (105). Hyperuricemia is seen in myeloproliferative disorders, and an alternative explanation for the hyperuricemia in PPH may relate to excessive cell turnover in the pulmonary circulation.

The addition of continuous epoprostenol infusion to the treatment regimen of patients with PPH may significantly alter prognosis. Although randomized controlled trial data are incomplete, epoprostenol has been shown to improve survival and quality of life (106). Nonetheless, this expensive treatment, which costs over $100,000/year, has not cured PAH, and many patients remain in New York Heart Association functional class II or III.

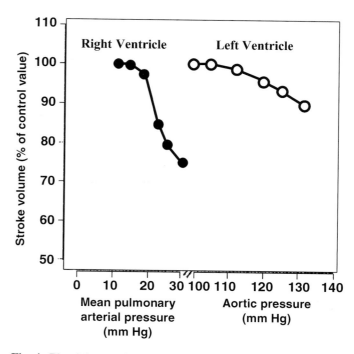

Fig. 4. The right ventricle responds to an increase in right ventricular afterload with a significant decrease in the right ventricular stroke volume compared with the left ventricle. (Adapted with permission from the American College of Cardiology, Adult Clinical Cardiology Self Assessment Program CD-ROM [ACCSAP 1999®].)

Diagnostic Approach

Because pulmonary hypertension is uncommon and has nonspecific symptoms, patients often have symptoms for months or years before diagnosis. Although symptoms of pulmonary hypertension do not directly reflect PAP, patients are usually asymptomatic until PAP has doubled. Most symptoms (Table 2) reflect the decreased cardiac output that results from either RV failure at rest or impaired functional reserve that prevents an increase in cardiac output with exercise or in response to systemic vasodilation. Similarly, the most important physical signs (Table 2) essentially reflect RV failure and thus lack sensitivity for early PAH specificity for advanced PAH. The most specific physical sign for pulmonary hypertension is a loud pulmonic component of the second heart sound in the apex, where it is normally not audible. A chest radiograph and an ECG should complete the initial assessment of the patient suspected to have PAH (Fig. 5).

Although often considered a diagnosis of exclusion, PPH has unique clinical features that allow diagnosis with a reasonable level of certainty without exhaustive testing to rule out rare, improbable conditions. In contrast, some conditions that cause or affect the severity of pulmonary hypertension can be diagnosed only through

Table 2
Mechanisms Associated with the Signs and Symptoms of Pulmonary Hypertension

Sign	Mechanism
Accentuated pulmonic component of S2	Increased force of P valve closure
Early systolic click of the pulmonary valve	Sudden interruption of P valve closure
Midsystolic ejection murmur	Turbulance in P valve outflow
Diastolic murmur	P valve regurgitation
Holosystolic right parasternal murmur increasing with inspiration	Tricuspid regurgitation
Increased jugular a wave	Increased RV filling pressure
Edema, ascites, hepatomegaly	RV failure

Symptom in severe disease	Mechanism
Dyspnea, fatigue	Decreased cardiac output
Chest pain	RV ischemia, PA dilatation
Syncope	Decreased cardiac output, arrhythmias
Hoarseness (Ortner syndrome)	Laryngeal nerve compression caused by the dilated PA
Nausea	Right heart failure, GI submucosal edema

GI, gastrointestinal; PA, pulmonary artery; RV, right ventricular; P, pulmonic.

medical testing. The most important of these conditions is underlying chronic thromboembolic disease, which can have an insidious onset and present with clinical symptoms and findings indistinguishable from those of PPH (107). Chronic thromboembolic pulmonary hypertension is readily treated with excellent results by surgical thromboendarterectomy, placement of a caval filter, and anticoagulation; therefore, the diagnosis should be considered in the patient evaluation. Perfusion lung scanning or spiral CT scanning is essential in assessing these patients (Fig. 5). The strategic approach toward treating patients with pulmonary hypertension is affected by the status of left ventricular end-diastolic pressure, which can be determined accurately only from cardiac catheterization. Underlying conditions such as congenital heart disease, collagen vascular disease, and interstitial lung disease should be suspected when the appropriate clinical clues are present.

An echocardiogram can exclude several secondary causes of pulmonary hypertension, including left ventricular dysfunction, valvular and congenital heart disease. Furthermore, an echocardiogram can directly confirm the presence of pulmonary hypertension, RVH, and RV dysfunction (Fig. 5) and quantify the severity of each condition. With appropriate image and quality of the Doppler signals, the assessment of RV systolic pressure correlates well with that obtained from right heart catheterization (r=0.96) (108). Because of its simplicity and noninvasiveness, echocardiography is important not only in diagnosing PAH but also in assessing the response to treatment. Nevertheless, most

patients with suspected PPH should undergo right heart catheterization in addition to echocardiography (Fig. 5). Right heart catheterization is the best way to measure of PVR, and it is the only method that can reliably assess the response to acute vasodilator challenge, which is an important predictor of prognosis and guide to therapy.

The use of vasodilators to treat pulmonary hypertension is based on the premise that pulmonary vasoconstriction contributes significantly to the vascular disease and that small reductions in RV afterload will substantially improve RV function (Fig. 4). Although varying degrees of pulmonary vasoconstriction are present in some forms of pulmonary hypertension, other forms are predominantly characterized by vascular obstruction or obliteration. In the latter setting, vasodilators would probably not be beneficial and may produce serious adverse effects. Therefore, the use of vasodilators should be based on establishment of the etiology of pulmonary vascular disease and assessment of the potential for reversible vasoreactivity in each patient.

In about one fourth of patients with PPH, PAP is significantly reduced (≥20%) and cardiac output is increased in response to vasodilator administration (74). In the other 80% of patients, vasodilators have no substantial hemodynamic effect or they produce deleterious effects, such as systemic hypotension. The use of inhaled NO (iNO) is the gold standard for acute vasodilator trials in evaluating patients for PPH. Incremental doses of iNO (10–80 ppm) are delivered, and more than a 20% reduction in PVR is considered a

A PAH case history

A 32 year old woman presents with fatigue and dyspnea on exertion of one years duration. Her JVP is 11cm H_2O, there is a loud P_2 and pulmonic flow murmur. There is mild peripheral edema.

Her ECG shows right axis deviation and right ventricular hypertrophy.

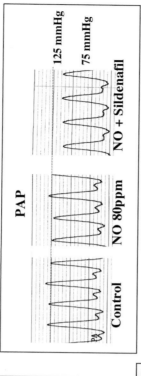

Given the JVP, the estimated PAP is $92+11=103$mmHg. A right heart catheterization confirms this value. There is no decrease in the PAP (or PVR) with a maximal dose of inhaled nitric oxide (iNO, 80ppm); however, there is significant decrease in the PAP and PVR with the combination of NO and a single oral dose of sildenafil (75mg). Because the PVR decreased by 20%, this patient is considered a "responder".

PAP

Control   NO 80ppm   NO + Sildenafil

125 mmHg
75 mmHg

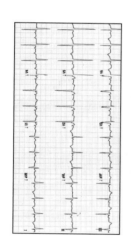

Her CXR shows cardiomegaly and no evidence of pulmonary venous hypertension. There is evidence of proximal pulmonary artery dilatation (arrow) and pruning of the peripheral pulmonary arteries

A ventilation/perfusion (V/Q) scan is low probability for pulmonary embolism but shows a characteristic "moth-eaten" abnormality in the perfusion image

An transthoracic echocardiogram excludes left ventricular and valvular disease. A contrast study rules out intracardiac shunts but does show right ventricular dilatation. The systolic flattening of the system is diagnostic of right ventricular pressure overload. Doppler interrogation across the tricuspid valve shows a gradient of 92mmHg.

The patient is started on Ca^{++} blockers but she cannot tolerate even moderate doses of nifedipine because of severe peripheral edema, dizziness and hypotension. She is started on Bosentan 125mg P.O. bid. She continues to deteriorate and 6 months later she is started on continuous intravenous epoprostenol. A workup for heart/lung transplantation is initiated at the same time. Her condition is stable for the following 2 years (Class II). She has yearly right heart catheterizations and cardiac ultrasound as well as treadmill exercise tests.

She attends the Multidisciplinary Pulmonary Hypertension clinic as well as the bimonthly PAH support group where she also sees a dietician and a psychologist.

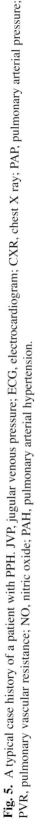

Fig. 5. A typical case history of a patient with PPH. JVP, jugular venous pressure; ECG, electrocardiogram; CXR, chest X ray; PAP, pulmonary arterial pressure; PVR, pulmonary vascular resistance; NO, nitric oxide; PAH, pulmonary arterial hypertension.

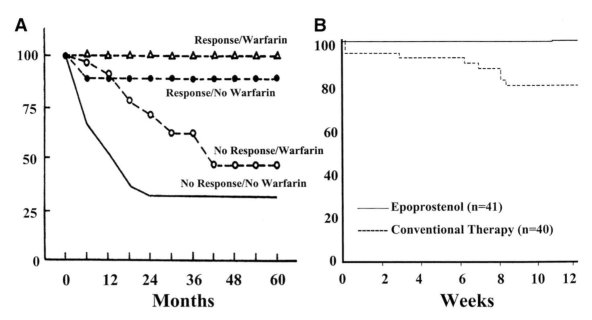

Fig. 6. Calcium channel blockers, warfarin, and prostacyclin improve survival in PPH. **Panel A**: Survival was greater in PPH patients who had an acute, favorable response to vasodilators (about a 20% reduction in pulmonary vascular resistance) than in those who did not show acute pulmonary vasodilatation. Warfarin was beneficial in both responders and nonresponders. (Reproduced with permission from ref. *74*). **Panel B**: Prognosis is better in patients with PPH treated with prostacyclin (epoprostenol) than in those treated with conventional therapy (calcium channel blockers and warfarin). (Reproduced with permission from ref. *106*).

positive response (Fig. 5). In some centers, intravenous prostacyclin or adenosine is used.

Although an open lung biopsy was once considered essential for the confirmation of the diagnosis of PPH, the NIH Registry has confirmed that an accurate diagnosis of PPH can be made without a lung biopsy *(109)*. Lung biopsies should be performed in patients in whom a concern over a parenchymal lung process requires a diagnosis. The morbidity of an open lung biopsy is markedly increased in patients with severe pulmonary hypertension.

Treatment

Understanding the molecular disorders in PAH provides a clear rationale for many of the therapies used in clinical medicine. More important, as new mechanisms are defined, new therapies will be suggested.

ANTICOAGULANTS

Warfarin has been used in the treatment of patients with pulmonary hypertension for many years. Patients with PPH have features of a hypercoagulable state that may predispose to the development of thrombosis *in situ* in the pulmonary arteriolar bed *(110)*. Even a small pulmonary embolus can be life threatening in PPH patients because of compromised pulmonary vasculature beds and the reduced ability to dilate or recruit new vessels.

In retrospective and prospective series, chronic use of warfarin anticoagulation has improved survival (Fig. 6A). Because histological studies in patients with most forms of secondary pulmonary hypertension (congenital heart disease and collagen vascular disease) show similar evidence of *in situ* thrombosis, patients with secondary pulmonary hypertension may also benefit from chronic anticoagulation. The current recommendation targets an INR of 2–2.5 times control levels, which should provide effective anticoagulation with minimal risk of bleeding. Anticoagulation is well tolerated in patients with PPH, despite their predisposition to hemoptysis.

The use of unfractionated or low-molecular-weight heparins should provide similar benefits as warfarin therapy with the added beneficial effects on endothelial and SMC growth *(111,112)*, but no reports have been published on their chronic use in PPH patients.

CALCIUM CHANNEL BLOCKERS

Ca^{2+} channel blockers were the first class of drugs to have dramatic beneficial long-term effects in selected PPH patients *(74)* (Fig. 6B). Ca^{2+} channel blockers provide benefits primarily through vasodilatation, as seen by the rapid decrease in mean PAP that occurs with treatment.

Ca^{2+} channel blockers should be offered to patients who respond positively (with a 20% reduction in PAP or PVR,

Fig. 6) to an acute pulmonary vasodilator trial with a short-acting agent such as iNO or prostacyclin. This vasodilator trial is the only method that can accurately identify patients for Ca^{2+}-channel blocker therapy and should be conducted in a coronary care unit or cardiac catheterization laboratory. Patients who respond positively to the trial tend to have less advanced disease and more recent onset of symptoms. These patients may be a subset in whom PPH has been triggered by increased Ca^{2+} levels in PASMCs caused by abnormalities in the Kv channel (113). High doses of Ca^{2+} channel blockers are often, but not always, necessary to achieve the maximum beneficial effect; this dose requirement may relate in part to impaired absorption and to increased requirement for calcium in the pulmonary vascular bed (114). The duration of the beneficial effect is unclear.

However, the indiscriminate use of Ca^{2+} channel blockers in patients with PPH is potentially harmful. Systemic hypotension is an adverse effect of Ca^{2+} channel blockers and can produce reflex tachycardia, sympathetic stimulation, and RV ischemia, which may lead to hemodynamic collapse and death. Reports of adverse responses to Ca^{2+} channel blockers in some patients, particularly those with overt RV failure, underscore the need to initiate oral therapy only after an acute trial of a short-acting vasodilator has confirmed reversible vasoconstriction (115). The use of these drugs requires close follow-up and documentation of beneficial effects.

PROSTAGLANDINS

The use of sodium epoprostenol (Flolan®) in NYHA class III–IV patients with PPH and secondary pulmonary hypertension has been studied extensively over the past decade. Prostacyclin, a local vasodilator, helps regulate local vasomotor tone in all vascular beds (116). When administered intravenously to pulmonary hypertension patients, prostacyclin is a potent but nonselective vasodilator. It minimally lowers systemic blood pressure and modestly reduces PAP. Prostacyclin is a positive inotrope and increases cardiac output in patients with pulmonary hypertension (117). Epoprostenol reduces resting heart rate and lowering mean right atrial pressure (118,119). PPH is not primarily a disease of vasoconstriction, but rather one of cell proliferation; therefore, chronic infusion of prostacyclin may be beneficial, even in patients who lack an acute vasodilator response on initial testing (120).

Continuous use of intravenous prostacyclin, like the Ca^{2+} channel blockers, has potentially harmful effects. The optimal dose is usually established by dose titration. Patients rapidly develop tachyphylaxis to the vasodilator side effects of prostacyclin (121). Long-term use of high doses of prostacyclin can be associated with high-output cardiac failure and severe side effects such as marked flushing, diarrhea, thrombocytopenia, and unremitting foot pain (117). Non-specific alveolitis may develop, and the onset of diastolic RV failure, which can be refractory to treatment (122), has been reported. Moreover, continuous infusion of prostacyclin requires the placement of a permanent indwelling venous catheter, which is associated with the risk of potentially life-threatening infections. For reasons of convenience, safety, and cost (more than $100,000/patient/year) related to prostacyclin, new therapies are needed.

The dramatic success of long-term intravenous prostacyclin has led to the development of prostacyclin analogues and new drug delivery systems. Uniprost (treprostinil), an analogue of prostacyclin that has better stability at room temperature and a longer half-life, is administered subcutaneously via an insulin pump that allows the patient to remain ambulatory. In preliminary studies, intravenous uniprost has similar properties as intravenous prostacyclin and, when administered long-term, uniprost improves exercise tolerance and hemodynamics similarly to prostacyclin (123). Pain, induration, and erythema at the local injection site may be serious in many patients and often prevents administration of adequate doses. However, uniprost offers the beneficial effects of prostacyclin without the morbidity of central line infection.

Iloprost, another analog of prostacyclin, can be inhaled and is currently being evaluated in an international multicenter trial (124). With inhalation, lower doses of the drug can be used and still achieve a therapeutic effect on the pulmonary vascular bed with only minimal systemic side effects (125). The drawback is that the short half-life of the drug necessitates frequent inhalations (every 2 h) during waking hours. Whether this type of "pulsed therapy" will yield similar long-term effects as infusion therapies is unknown.

Beraprost is an oral prostacyclin analog that is reasonably well absorbed and produces both acute and short-term beneficial effects in patients with pulmonary hypertension (126). Although not yet evaluated in a prospective randomized trial, beraprost has produced favorable hemodynamic changes and has improved exercise tolerance in preliminary studies. Because beraprost has a relatively short half-life, frequent dosing is required, and side effects could limit the ability of a patient to receive adequate doses. A multicenter randomized clinical trial of beraprost in patients with pulmonary hypertension is currently underway.

NITRIC OXIDE AND PHOSPHODIESTERASE TYPE 5 INHIBITORS

NO helps regulate local vasomotor tone in the pulmonary circulation and is a potentially effective pulmonary

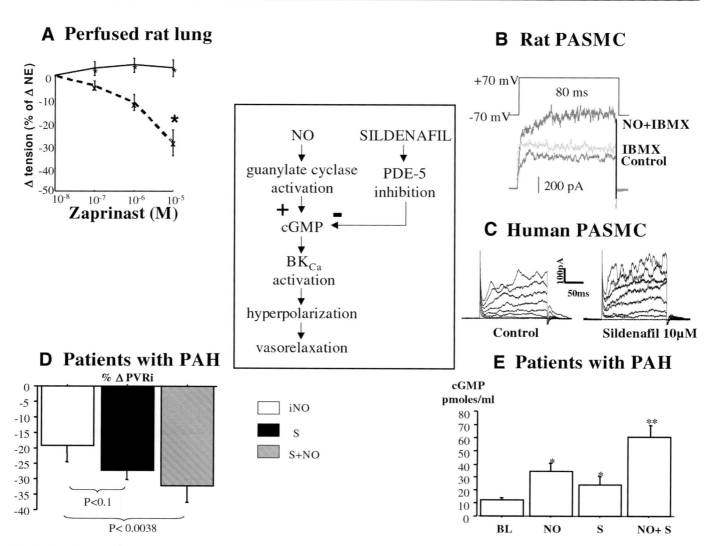

Fig. 7. The NO and phospodiesterase-5 inhibitors "synergism" in the pulmonary circulation. The mechanisms of vasodilatation caused by nitric oxide (NO) and sildenafil are shown in the inset. **Panel A**. The phosphodiesterase (PDE)-5 blocker zaprinast dilates the pulmonary vasculature in the isolated perfused rat lung. The dotted line represents the tetraethyl ammonium treatment group, and the solid line represents the control group. NE, norepinephrine (Adapted with permission from ref. *127*). **Panel B**. The nonspecific phosphodiesterase inhibitor isobutyl-methylxanthine (IBMX) and exogenous nitric oxide (NO) increase the outward K^+ current in freshly isolated rat pulmonary arterial smooth muscle cells (PASMC) as assessed by standard whole cell patch clamping technique. (Adapted with permission from ref. *127*). **Panel C**. Sildenafil increases the outward K^+ current in freshly isolated human pulmonary arterial smooth muscle cells (PASMC) taken from the pulmonary artery of a heart transplant donor. The morphology and the characteristics of the current are compatible with a BK_{Ca} current. **Panel D**. A single dose (75 mg) of oral sildenafil (S) decreases the pulmonary vascular resistance (PVR) in patients with pulmonary arterial hypertension as much as the maximal dose of inhaled nitric oxide (iNO, 80ppm) Adapted with permission *(132)*. The combination of sildenafil and inhaled nitric oxide (iNO) decreases PVR more than iNO alone. **Panel E**. In the same study presented in panel D, the combination of iNO and sildenafil synergistically increases serum levels of cyclic-guanosine monophosphate (cGMP) *(132)*. Adapted with permission *(132)*. BL, baseline.

vasodilator in some patients with chronic pulmonary hypertension. The mechanism by which NO causes relaxation involves activation of guanylate cyclase, and an increase in cGMP levels, which can cause vasodilatation by several means, including the opening of K^+ channels *(59)* (Fig. 7). In the pulmonary circulation, NO causes vasodilatation in part by the opening of large conductance, Ca^{2+}-sensitive K^+ channels, called BK_{Ca} channels, via

cGMP-dependent kinase *(127)*. cGMP levels in the PASMC reflect the balance between production (caused by the tonic effects of endothelium-derived or exogenous NO and particulate guanylate cyclase) and breakdown of cGMP (by phosphodiesterase [PDE]-5, which is most abundantly expressed in the pulmonary and penile circulation). Therefore, synergism is found between both endogenous and exogenous NO and the PDE inhibitors, and this synergism occurs at all levels of the cGMP pathway, from the electrophysiology (opening of BK_{Ca} channels) to the final vasodilatation (Fig. 7).

iNO is approved by the U.S. Food and Drug Administration (FDA) for treatment of neonatal pulmonary hypertension associated with hypoxia (128). However, because of recent enforcement of a patent, the cost of this once inexpensive therapy has increased to $15,000 (Canadian dollars)/week at the University of Alberta Hospital. In addition to being widely used as an acute test of vasodilator response in patients with chronic pulmonary hypertension, iNO has been used as short-term treatment of patients with pulmonary hypertension caused by a variety of conditions (129). Patients that respond acutely to iNO may be responsive to oral therapy with Ca^{2+} channel blockers, and the acute test is safe and easy to perform during cardiac catheterization (130). Experience with the chronic use of iNO as a treatment for pulmonary hypertension is limited (131). Because NO is short-lived, chronic iNO therapy is cumbersome, expensive, and requires a fairly sophisticated delivery system; patient mobility is limited by the need for a canister to deliver the gas at all times. Nevertheless, iNO dilates the pulmonary circulation without systemic vasodilatation and has been successful in short-term therapy in critically ill patients, particularly in patients who have undergone cardiac surgery or transplantation.

The synergism between NO and PDE inhibitors is being studied in clinical medicine. The oral PDE-5 inhibitor sildenafil (Viagra®, Pfizer) is a good candidate drug for testing because it is has been used extensively in the clinical setting and its most important side effect (potential systemic hypotension) is seen primarily in patients that use systemic nitrates for angina. The use of sildenafil to treat conditions other than erectile dysfunction is not complicated by inappropriate erections because the drug does not cause spontaneous erections but only facilitates erection subsequent to sexual stimulation when the levels of penile NO secreted from nerve endings increase. In 13 patients with PAH, a single dose of sildenafil (75 mg) decreased PVR to a similar extent as the maximal doses of iNO (80 ppm, Fig. 7D) (132). More important, sildenafil significantly increased cardiac output and, in contrast to iNO, decreased pulmonary artery wedge pressure (132). Like iNO, sildenafil does not decrease systemic arterial pressure. Finally, the combination of iNO and sildenafil is well tolerated acutely and is superior to iNO used alone in reducing PVR. This finding suggests that PDE-5 inhibitors may be a safe alternative to iNO in patients with PAH (Fig. 5). However, the long-term effects of sildenafil in patients with PAH need to be studied.

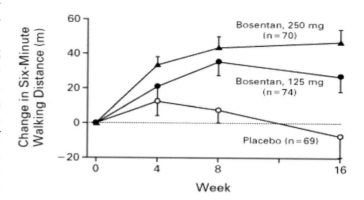

Fig. 8. The nonselective endothelin-1 receptor blocker, bosentan, improves the functional capacity of patients with pulmonary arterial hypertension more than placebo as early as 8 wk after the initiation of treatment ($p < 0.05$). (Adapted with permission from ref. 136).

ENDOTHELIN ANTAGONISTS

The role of an increased production of endothelin (ET) in the etiology of the disease in some patients is unclear; however, the role of endothelin as a mediator is unquestioned (54). Non-selective antagonists such as bosentan that block both ET-A and B receptors and ET-A-receptor selective antagonists such as sitaxsentan are being evaluated in clinical trials. The superiority of one antagonist over the other has not been determined. Blockade of the ET-A receptor, which is involved in the development of vasoconstriction and SMC hypertrophy, should be helpful (133). The role of ET-B receptors is less clear. They may be involved in the clearance of ET-1 across the pulmonary circulation and, thus, leaving the ET-B receptor unblocked might be of clinical value. Moreover, studies suggest that the ET-B receptor may be involved in nitric oxide induced vasodilatation, in which case leaving it unblocked could be beneficial.

Sitaxsentan acutely decreases PAP in patients with pulmonary hypertension associated with severe congestive heart failure (134). In a preliminary 12-wk, open-label study in patients with PAH, sitaxsentan moderately decreased PAP, but patient performance in a 6-min walk improved only minimally (135). Bosentan, which blocks both the ET-A and -B receptors, has been studied more extensively. In a recent double-blind placebo-controlled study, 213 patients with PAH (primary or associated with scleroderma) were randomly assigned to bosentan (125 or 250 mg twice daily) or placebo for a minimum of 12 wk (136). Bosentan caused a significant but modest 34 m improvement in patient performance on the 6-min walk (primary end point, Fig. 8) compared with the placebo group. At the dose used in this study, liver function abnormalities, reported as severe in larger doses in patients with

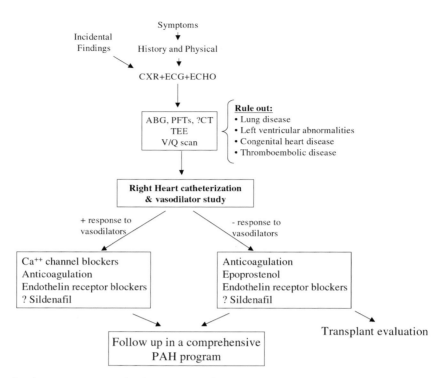

Fig. 9. A simplified algorithm for the management of pulmonary arterial hypertension (PAH). ABG, arterial blood gas; CT, computed tomography scan; CXR, chest X-ray; ECG, electrocardiogram; ECHO, echocardiography; PFTs, pulmonary function tests; TEE, transesophageal echocardiography; V/Q, ventilation/perfusion.

congestive heart failure, were rare, mild, and reversible. After this study, bosentan (Tracleer®, at the dose of 125 mg po twice a day) was approved by the FDA (November 2001) as the first oral therapy for the treatment of PPH. Bosentan is expensive, and the possibility of adverse effects on liver function requires further study in clinical trials. Moreover, patients treated with bosentan should be carefully monitored, and liver function tests are recommended. The effect of bosentan, either alone or combined with prostacyclin, on survival in patients with PPH is unknown. The effect of bosentan treatment early in the disease has not been assessed. A simplified algorithm summarizing the major steps in the evaluation and treatment of patients with PPH is shown in (Fig. 9).

FUTURE DIRECTIONS

Because of the recent recognition of the role of Kv channels in the pathogenesis of PPH, new therapies will focus on activation or replacement of the inhibited or downregulated Kv channels. Dichloroacetate (a metabolic modulator) reverses chronic hypoxic pulmonary hypertension by activating and upregulating Kv2.1 (65). Although not well defined, the mechanism of action of dichloroacetate may involve both redox actions because

dichloroacetate inhibits pyruvate dehydrogenase kinase and non-redox actions involving tyrosine kinase. Dichloroacetate has been used in patients to treat coronary disease and heart failure and has an excellent safety profile. Elastase inhibitors reverse monocrotaline-induced pulmonary hypertension (21) and will be tested in clinical trials.

Finally, gene therapy shows great potential for use in patients with pulmonary vascular disease. Proteins have been identified that could be targets for use in gene therapy. Adenoviral vectors have been used successfully to transfect genes into the airways and small pulmonary arteries via airway nebulization. Genes for prostacyclin synthase and NOS have been transiently overexpressed in animals (137,138). However, significant problems need to be addressed before gene therapy can be successfully used in humans. For example, a site-specific delivery system must be developed that would allow preferential concentration of the virus in the pulmonary circulation. Furthermore, sustained expression of the gene has not been achieved in vivo, and inflammatory reactions to the vector are a concern. New vectors, such as adenoviral-associated viruses, that integrate the transgene stably into the genome and allow prolonged gene expression and non-adenoviral vectors may be useful. Defining the vascular pathobiology of

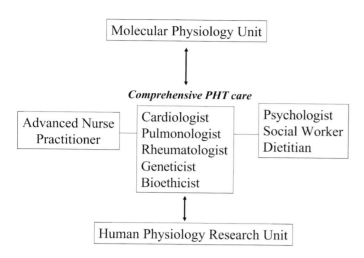

Fig. 10. The structure of modern comprehensive pulmonary arterial hypertension (PAH) programs.

pulmonary vascular disease will lead to the development of specific gene therapies. Potential targets for gene therapy, such as Kv1.5, Kv2.1, BMPR-II receptors, and 5-HTT, are suggested as abnormal pathways involved in PPH.

COMPREHENSIVE PROGRAMS FOR PRIMARY PULMONARY HYPERTENSION

PAH is a model disease in vascular biology. The pathogenesis of PAH, which involves all elements of the vasculature (Fig. 3), is characterized by complex interactions between a predisposing genome, a permissive phenotype, and environmental stimuli. The pathogenesis of the disease is multifactorial, and several different mechanisms may result in a common disease phenotype. The maladies associated with PPH span the expertise of several conventional medical specialties; therefore, the approach to the patient should be multifactorial and comprehensive and should include the coordinated care of cardiologists, pulmonologists, and rheumatologists. The discovery of the PPH gene indicates that more patients have gene mutations and polymorphisms than previously thought. Adding a geneticist to the team of caregivers is advisable. The ability to test for a genetic disease that lacks a definitive treatment will bring new bioethical challenges to the PPH teams. Recently approved treatments are expensive, requiring specialized monitoring, and have limited efficacy which suggests that management of these patients should be restricted to specialized tertiary care centers in dedicated PPH programs (Fig. 10).

Fewer than a dozen PPH programs exist in North America, and more are needed. Several programs include advanced nurse practitioners, sociologists, dieticians, and psychologists. With the addition of prostacyclin to the treatment regimen, patients live longer and face the problems associated with having a severe chronic disease such as depression, malnutrition, and social issues. PPH support groups are integral components of some PPH programs. The recent increase in our knowledge of vascular molecular biology and physiology and the emphasis in translational research reveal a need for the addition of comprehensive basic and human research laboratories to modern PPH programs (Fig.10).

ACKNOWLEDGMENTS

Doctors Michelakis and Archer are both supported by the Canadian Institutes for Health Research, The Heart and Stroke Foundation of Canada, and the Alberta Heritage Foundation for Medical Research.

REFERENCES

1. Dresdale DT, Schultz M, Mitchom RJ. Primary pulmonary hypertension. 1. Clinical and hemodynamic study. Am J Med 1951;11:686–673.
2. Tucker A, McMurtry IF, Reeves JT, et al. Lung vascular smooth muscle as a determinant of pulmonary hypertension at high altitude. Am J Physiol 1975;228:762–767.
3. Vender RL. Chronic hypoxic pulmonary hypertension. Cell biology to pathophysiology. Chest 1994;106:236–243.
4. Hayashi Y, Lalich JJ. Renal and pulmonary alterations induced in rats by a single injection of monocrotaline. Proc Soc Exp Biol Med 1967;124:392–396.
5. Wilson DW, Segall HJ, Pan LC, et al. Mechanisms and pathology of monocrotaline pulmonary toxicity. Crit Rev Toxicol 1992;22:307–325.
6. Altiere RJ, Olson JW, Gillespie MN. Altered pulmonary vascular smooth muscle responsiveness in monocrotaline-induced pulmonary hypertension. J Pharmacol Exp Ther 1986;236:390–395.
7. Sato K, Webb S, Tucker A, et al. Factors influencing the idiopathic development of pulmonary hypertension in the fawn hooded rat. Am Rev Respir Dis 1992;145:793–797.
8. Le Cras TD, Kim DH, Markham NE, et al. Early abnormalities of pulmonary vascular development in the Fawn-Hooded rat raised at Denver's altitude. Am J Physiol Lung Cell Mol Physiol 2000;279:L283–L291.
9. Fishman A. Introduction to the National Registry on Primary Pulmonary Hypertension. In: (ed) FA, ed. The Pulmonary Circulation: Normal and Abnormal. Philadelphia: University of Pensylvania Press; 1990:437–439.
10. Lane KB, Machado RD, Pauciulo MW, et al. Heterozygous germline mutations in BMPR2, encoding a TGF-beta receptor, cause familial primary pulmonary hypertension. The International PPH Consortium. Nat Genet 2000;26:81–84.
11. Machado RD, Pauciulo MW, Thomson JR, et al. BMPR2 haploinsufficiency as the inherited molecular mechanism for primary pulmonary hypertension. Am J Hum Genet 2001;68:92–102.
12. Archer S, Rich S. Primary pulmonary hypertension: a vascular biology and translational research "Work in progress". Circulation 2000;102:2781–2791.
13. Fishman A. Clinical classification of pulmonary hypertension. Clin Chest Med 2001;22:385–391.

14. Chazova I, Loyd JE, Zhdanov VS, et al. Pulmonary artery adventitial changes and venous involvement in primary pulmonary hypertension. Am J Pathol 1995;146:389–397.

15. Mason NA, Springall DR, Burke M, et al. High expression of endothelial nitric oxide synthase in plexiform lesions of pulmonary hypertension. J Pathol 1998;185:313–318.

16. Tuder RM, Groves B, Badesch DB, et al. Exuberant endothelial cell growth and elements of inflammation are present in plexiform lesions of pulmonary hypertension. Am J Pathol 1994; 144:275–285.

17. Cool CD, Stewart JS, Werahera P, et al. Three-dimensional reconstruction of pulmonary arteries in plexiform pulmonary hypertension using cell-specific markers. Evidence for a dynamic and heterogeneous process of pulmonary endothelial cell growth. Am J Pathol 1999;155:411–419.

18. Herve P, Launay JM, Scrobohaci ML, et al. Increased plasma serotonin in primary pulmonary hypertension. Am J Med 1995; 99:249–254.

19. Weir EK, Reeve HL, Johnson G, et al. A role for potassium channels in smooth muscle cells and platelets in the etiology of primary pulmonary hypertension. Chest 1998;114:200S–204S.

20. Lee SD, Shroyer KR, Markham NE, et al. Monoclonal endothelial cell proliferation is present in primary but not secondary pulmonary hypertension. J Clin Invest 1998;101:927–934.

21. Cowan KN, Jones PL, Rabinovitch M. Elastase and matrix metalloproteinase inhibitors induce regression, and tenascin-C antisense prevents progression, of vascular disease. J Clin Invest 2000;105:21–34.

22. Nichols WC, Koller DL, Slovis B, et al. Localization of the gene for familial primary pulmonary hypertension to chromosome 2q31-32. Nat Genet 1997;15:277–280.

23. Loyd JE, Butler MG, Foroud TM, et al. Genetic anticipation and abnormal gender ratio at birth in familial primary pulmonary hypertension. Am J Respir Crit Care Med 1995;152:93–97.

24. Loyd JE, Slovis B, Phillips JA, 3rd, et al. The presence of genetic anticipation suggests that the molecular basis of familial primary pulmonary hypertension may be trinucleotide repeat expansion. Chest 1997;111:82S–83S.

25. Deng Z, Morse JH, Slager SL, et al. Familial primary pulmonary hypertension (gene PPH1) is caused by mutations in the bone morphogenetic protein receptor-II gene. Am J Hum Genet 2000;67:737–744.

26. Thomas A, Gaddipati R, Newman J, et al. Genetics of primary pulmonary hypertension. Clin Chest Med 2001;22:477–491.

27. Deng Z, Haghighi F, Helleby L, et al. Fine mapping of PPH1, a gene for familial primary pulmonary hypertension, to a 3-cM region on chromosome 2q33. Am J Respir Crit Care Med 2000; 161:1055–1059.

28. Morse JH, Jones AC, Barst RJ, et al. Mapping of familial primary pulmonary hypertension locus (PPH1) to chromosome 2q31-q32. Circulation 1997;95:2603–2606.

29. Thomson JR, Machado RD, Pauciulo MW, et al. Sporadic primary pulmonary hypertension is associated with germline mutations of the gene encoding BMPR-II, a receptor member of the TGF- beta family. J Med Genet 2000;37:741–745.

30. Wozney JM, Rosen V, Celeste AJ, et al. Novel regulators of bone formation: molecular clones and activities. Science 1988; 242:1528–1534.

31. Hogan BL. Bone morphogenetic proteins: multifunctional regulators of vertebrate development. Genes Dev 1996;10:1580–1594.

32. Bellusci S, Henderson R, Winnier G, et al. Evidence from normal expression and targeted misexpression that bone morphogenetic protein (Bmp-4) plays a role in mouse embryonic lung morphogenesis. Development 1996;122:1693–1702.

33. De Caestecker M, Meyrick B. Bone morphogenetic proteins, genetics and the pathophysiology of primary pulmonary hypertension. Respir Res 2001;2:193–197.

34. Massague J, Wotton D. Transcriptional control by the TGF-beta/Smad signaling system. Embo J 2000;19:1745–1754.

35. Sekelsky JJ, Newfeld SJ, Raftery LA, et al. Genetic characterization and cloning of mothers against dpp, a gene required for decapentaplegic function in Drosophila melanogaster. Genetics 1995;139:1347–1358.

36. Beppu H, Kawabata M, Hamamoto T, et al. BMP type II receptor is required for gastrulation and early development of mouse embryos. Dev Biol 2000;221:249–258.

37. Morrell NW, Yang X, Upton PD, et al. Altered growth responses of pulmonary artery smooth muscle cells from patients with primary pulmonary hypertension to transforming growth factor-beta(1) and bone morphogenetic proteins. Circulation 2001;104:790–795.

38. Morse JH, Horn EM, Barst RJ. Hormone replacement therapy: a possible risk factor in carriers of familial primary pulmonary hypertension. Chest 1999;116:847.

39. Voelkel NF, Cool C, Lee SD, et al. Primary pulmonary hypertension between inflammation and cancer. Chest 1998; 114:225S–230S.

40. Christman BW, McPherson CD, Newman JH, et al. An imbalance between the excretion of thromboxane and prostacyclin metabolites in pulmonary hypertension. N Engl J Med. 1992; 327:70–75.

41. Giaid A, Saleh D. Reduced expression of endothelial nitric oxide synthase in the lungs of patients with pulmonary hypertension. N Engl J Med 1995;333:214–221.

42. Archer SL, Djaballah K, Humbert M, et al. Nitric oxide deficiency in fenfluramine- and dexfenfluramine-induced pulmonary hypertension. Am J Respir Crit Care Med 1998; 158:1061–1067.

43. Forrest IA, Small T, Corris PA. Effect of nebulized epoprostenol (prostacyclin) on exhaled nitric oxide in patients with pulmonary hypertension due to congenital heart disease and in normal controls. Clin Sci (Colch) 1999;97:99–102.

44. Bogdan M, Humbert M, Francoual J, et al. Urinary cGMP concentrations in severe primary pulmonary hypertension. Thorax 1998;53:1059–1062.

45. Resta TC, Gonzales RJ, Dail WG, et al. Selective upregulation of arterial endothelial nitric oxide synthase in pulmonary hypertension. Am J Physiol 1997;272:H806–H813.

46. Frasch HF, Marshall C, Marshall BE. Endothelin-1 is elevated in monocrotaline pulmonary hypertension. Am J Physiol 1999; 276:L304–L310.

47. Stelzner TJ, O'Brien RF, Yanagisawa M, et al. Increased lung endothelin-1 production in rats with idiopathic pulmonary hypertension. Am J Physiol 1992;262:L614–L620.

48. Cacoub P, Dorent R, Nataf P, et al. Endothelin-1 in the lungs of patients with pulmonary hypertension. Cardiovasc Res 1997;33:196–200.

49. Kumar P, Kazzi NJ, Shankaran S. Plasma immunoreactive endothelin–1 concentrations in infants with persistent pulmonary hypertension of the newborn. Am J Perinatol 1996; 13:335–341.

50. Ishikawa S, Miyauchi T, Sakai S, et al. Elevated levels of plasma endothelin-1 in young patients with pulmonary hypertension caused by congenital heart disease are decreased after

successful surgical repair. J Thorac Cardiovasc Surg 1995; 110:271–273.

51. Allen SW, Chatfield BA, Koppenhafer SA, et al. Circulating immunoreactive endothelin-1 in children with pulmonary hypertension. Association with acute hypoxic pulmonary vasoreactivity. Am Rev Respir Dis 1993;148:519–522.

52. Yoshibayashi M, Nishioka K, Nakao K, et al. Plasma endothelin concentrations in patients with pulmonary hypertension associated with congenital heart defects. Evidence for increased production of endothelin in pulmonary circulation. Circulation 1991;84:2280–2285.

53. Cody RJ, Haas GJ, Binkley PF, et al. Plasma endothelin correlates with the extent of pulmonary hypertension in patients with chronic congestive heart failure. Circulation 1992;85:504–509.

54. Stewart DJ, Levy RD, Cernacek P, et al. Increased plasma endothelin-1 in pulmonary hypertension: marker or mediator of disease? Ann Intern Med 1991;114:464–469.

55. Giaid A, Yanagisawa M, Langleben D, et al. Expression of endothelin-1 in the lungs of patients with pulmonary hypertension. N Engl J Med 1993;328:1732–1739.

56. Giaid A. Nitric oxide and endothelin-1 in pulmonary hypertension. Chest 1998;114:208S–212S.

57. Weir EK, Archer SL. The mechanism of acute hypoxic pulmonary vasoconstriction: the tale of two channels. FASEB 1995;9:183–189.

58. Post J, Hume J, Archer S, et al. Direct role for potassium channel inhibition in hypoxic pulmonary vasoconstriction. Am J Physiol 1992;262:C882–C890.

59. Archer S, Rusch N. Potassium Channels in Cardiovascular Biology. Norwell, MA: Kluwer/Plenum Publishing Corporation; 2000.

60. Yuan XJ, Wang J, Juhaszova M, et al. Attenuated K+ channel gene transcription in primary pulmonary hypertension. Lancet 1998;351:726–727.

61. Archer SL, Souil E, Dinh-Xuan AT, et al. Molecular identification of the role of voltage-gated K+ channels, Kv1.5 and Kv2.1, in hypoxic pulmonary vasoconstriction and control of resting membrane potential in rat pulmonary artery myocytes. J Clin Invest 1998;101:2319–2330.

62. Perchenet L, Hilfiger L, Mizrahi J, et al. Effects of anorexinogen agents on cloned voltage-gated K(+) channel hKv1.5. J Pharmacol Exp Ther 2001;298:1108–1119.

63. Patel AJ, Lazdunski M, Honore E. Kv2.1/Kv9.3, a novel ATP-dependent delayed-rectifier K+ channel in oxygen-sensitive pulmonary artery myocytes. Embo J 1997;16:6615–6625.

64. Platoshyn O, Yu Y, Golovina VA, et al. Chronic hypoxia decreases K(V) channel expression and function in pulmonary artery myocytes. Am J Physiol Lung Cell Mol Physiol 2001; 280:L801–L812.

65. Michelakis ED, McMurtry MS, Wu XC, et al. Dichloroacetate, a metabolic modulator, prevents and reverses chronic hypoxic pulmonary hypertension in rats: role of increased expression and activity of voltage-gated potassium channels. Circulation 2002;105:244–250.

66. Rabinovitch M. It all begins with EVE (endogenous vascular elastase). Isr J Med Sci 1996;32:803–808.

67. Fernandez-Patron C, Martinez-Cuesta MA, Salas E, et al. Differential regulation of platelet aggregation by matrix metalloproteinases-9 and -2. Thromb Haemost 1999;82:1730–1735.

68. Fernandez-Patron C, Radomski M, Davidge S. Vascular matrix metalloproteinase-2 cleaves big endothelin-1 yielding a novel vasoconstrictor. Circ Res 1999;85:906–911.

69. Egermayer P, Town GI, Peacock AJ. Role of serotonin in the pathogenesis of acute and chronic pulmonary hypertension. Thorax 1999;54:161–168.

70. MacLean MR. Endothelin-1 and serotonin: mediators of primary and secondary pulmonary hypertension? J Lab Clin Med 1999;134:105–114.

71. Eddahibi S, Humbert M, Fadel E, et al. Serotonin transporter overexpression is responsible for pulmonary artery smooth muscle hyperplasia in primary pulmonary hypertension. J Clin Invest 2001;108:1141–1150.

72. Frank H, Mlczoch J, Huber K, et al. The effect of anticoagulant therapy in primary and anorectic drug- induced pulmonary hypertension. Chest 1997;112:714–721.

73. Fuster V, Steele PM, Edwards WD, et al. Primary pulmonary hypertension: natural history and the importance of thrombosis. Circulation 1984;70:580–587.

74. Rich S, Kaufmann E, Levy PS. The effect of high doses of calcium-channel blockers on survival in primary pulmonary hypertension. N Engl J Med 1992;327:76–81.

75. Welsh CH, Hassell KL, Badesch DB, et al. Coagulation and fibrinolytic profiles in patients with severe pulmonary hypertension. Chest 1996;110:710–717.

76. Tyler RC, Muramatsu M, Abman SH, et al. Variable expression of endothelial NO synthase in three forms of rat pulmonary hypertension. Am J Physiol 1999;276:L297–L303.

77. Steudel W, Ichinose F, Huang PL, et al. Pulmonary vasoconstriction and hypertension in mice with targeted disruption of the endothelial nitric oxide synthase (NOS 3) gene. Circ Res 1997;81:34–41.

78. Hampl V, Archer SL, Nelson DP, et al. Chronic EDRF inhibition and hypoxia: effects on the pulmonary circulation and systemic blood pressure. J Appl Physiol 1993;75:1748–1757.

79. Michelakis E, Johnson G, Leis L, et al. Dexfenfluramine and 4-aminopyridine (an inhibitor of voltage gated potassium channels) increase serotonin release from human platelets. Am J Resp Crit Care Med 1998;157:A588.

80. Michelakis ED, Weir EK, Nelson DP, et al. Dexfenfluramine elevates systemic blood pressure by inhibiting potassium currents in vascular smooth muscle cells. J Pharmacol Exp Ther 1999;291:1143–1149.

81. Weir EK, Reeve HL, Huang JMC, et al. The anorexic agents, aminorex, fenfluramine, and dexfenfluramine inhibit potassium current in rat pulmonary vascular smooth muscle and cause pulmonary vasoconstriction. Circulation 1996;94:2216–2220.

82. Graham RM, Owens WA. Pathogenesis of inherited forms of dilated cardiomyopathy. N Engl J Med 1999;341:1759–1762.

83. Rabinovitch M. Linking a serotonin transporter polymorphism to vascular smooth muscle proliferation in patients with primary pulmonary hypertension. J Clin Invest 2001;108:1109–1111.

84. Egermayer P. Epidemics of vascular toxicity and pulmonary hypertension: what can be learned? J Intern Med 2000;247:11–17.

85. Gurtner HP. Pulmonary hypertension, "plexogenic pulmonary artericopathy" and the appetite depressant drug aminorex: post or propter. Bull Eur Physiopath Res 1979;15:897–923.

86. Abenhaim L, Moride Y, Brenot F, et al. Appetite-suppressant drugs and the risk of primary pulmonary hypertension. International Primary Pulmonary Hypertension Study Group. N Engl J Med 1996;335:609–616.

87. Rothman RB, Ayestas MA, Dersch CM, et al. Aminorex, fenfluramine, and chlorphentermine are serotonin transporter substrates. Implications for primary pulmonary hypertension. Circulation 1999;100:869–875.

88. Reeve HL, Nelson DP, Archer SL, et al. Effects of fluoxetine, phentermine, and venlafaxine on pulmonary arterial pressure and electrophysiology. Am J Physiol 1999;276:L213–L219.

89. Reeve HL, Archer SL, Soper M, et al. Dexfenfluramine increases pulmonary artery smooth muscle intracellular Ca2+, independent of membrane potential. Am J Physiol 1999; 277:L662–L666.

90. Wang J, Juhaszova M, Conte JV, Jr, et al. Action of fenfluramine on voltage-gated K+ channels in human pulmonary-artery smooth-muscle cells. Lancet 1998;352:290.

91. Golpe R, Fernandez-Infante B, Fernandez-Rozas S. Primary pulmonary hypertension associated with human immunodeficiency virus infection. Postgrad Med J 1998;74:400–404.

92. Mesa RA, Edell ES, Dunn WF, et al. Human immunodeficiency virus infection and pulmonary hypertension: two new cases and a review of 86 reported cases. Mayo Clin Proc 1998;73:37–45.

93. Dellis O, Bouteau F, Guenounou M, et al. HIV-1 gp160 decreases the K+ voltage-gated current from Jurkat E6.1 T cells by up-phosphorylation. FEBS Lett 1999;443:187–191.

94. Kalman K, Pennington MW, Lanigan MD, et al. ShK-Dap22, a potent Kv1.3-specific immunosuppressive polypeptide. J Biol Chem 1998;273:32697–32707.

95. James TN. The toxic oil syndrome. Clin Cardiol 1994; 17:463–470.

96. Posada de la Paz M, RM P, Abaitua Borda I, et al. Factors associated with pathogenicity of oils related to the toxic oil syndrome epidemic in Spain. Epidemiology 1994;5:404–409.

97. Gomez-Sanchez M, Saenz de la Calzada C, Gomez-Pajuelo C, et al. Clinical and pathologic manifestations of pulmonary vascular disease in the toxic oil syndrome. J Am Coll Cardiol 1991;18:1539–1545.

98. Bell SA, Sander C, Kuntze I, et al. The acute pathology of fatty acid anilides and linoleic diester of 3-phenylamino-1,2-propanediol in mice: possible implication as aetiologic agents for the toxic oil syndrome. Arch Toxicol 1999;73:493–495.

99. Gomez Pajuelo C, Gomez Sanchez MA, Alonso Gutierrez M, et al. Acute effect of intrapulmonary enalaprilat in ten patients with severe pulmonary hypertension due to toxic oil syndrome. Cor Vasa 1990;32:225–230.

100. Arnaiz-Villena A, Martinez-Laso J, Corell A, et al. Frequencies of HLA-A24 and HLA-DR4-DQ8 are increased and that of HLA-B blank is decreased in chronic toxic oil syndrome. Eur J Immunogenet 1996;23:211–219.

101. D'Alonzo GE, Barst RJ, Ayres SM, et al. Survival in patients with primary pulmonary hypertension. Results from a national prospective registry. Ann Intern Med 1991;115:343–349.

102. Hopkins WE, Ochoa LL, Richardson GW, et al. Comparison of the hemodynamics and survival of adults with severe primary pulmonary hypertension or Eisenmenger syndrome. J Heart Lung Transplant 1996;15:100–105.

103. Hunter JJ, Chien KR. Signaling pathways for cardiac hypertrophy and failure. N Engl J Med 1999;341:1276–1283.

104. Bristow MR, Zisman LS, Lowes BD, et al. The pressure-overloaded right ventricle in pulmonary hypertension. Chest 1998;114:101S–106S.

105. Voelkel MA, Wynne KM, Badesch DB, et al. Hyperuricemia in severe pulmonary hypertension. Chest 2000;117:19–24.

106. Barst RJ, Rubin LJ, Long WA, et al. A comparison of continuous intravenous epoprostenol (prostacyclin) with conventional therapy for primary pulmonary hypertension. The Primary Pulmonary Hypertension Study Group. N Engl J Med 1996; 334:296–302.

107. Archibald CJ, Auger WR, Fedullo PF, et al. Long-term outcome after pulmonary thromboendarterectomy. Am J Respir Crit Care Med 1999;160:523–528.

108. Currie PJ, Seward JB, Chan KL, et al. Continuous wave Doppler determination of right ventricular pressure: a simultaneous Doppler-catheterization study in 127 patients. J Am Coll Cardiol 1985;6:750–756.

109. Pietra GG, Edwards WD, Kay JM, et al. Histopathology of primary pulmonary hypertension. A qualitative and quantitative study of pulmonary blood vessels from 58 patients in the National Heart, Lung, and Blood Institute, Primary Pulmonary Hypertension Registry. Circulation 1989;80:1198–1206.

110. Hassell KL. Altered hemostasis in pulmonary hypertension. Blood Coagul Fibrinolysis 1998;9:107–117.

111. Hassoun PM, Thompson BT, Hales CA. Partial reversal of hypoxic pulmonary hypertension by heparin. Am Rev Respir Dis 1992;145:193–196.

112. Thompson BT, Spence CR, Janssens SP, et al. Inhibition of hypoxic pulmonary hypertension by heparins of differing in vitro antiproliferative potency. Am J Respir Crit Care Med 1994;149:1512–1517.

113. Yuan JX, Aldinger AM, Juhaszova M, et al. Dysfunctional voltage-gated K+ channels in pulmonary artery smooth muscle cells of patients with primary pulmonary hypertension. Circulation 1998;98:1400–1406.

114. Phillips BG, Bauman JL, Schoen MD, et al. Serum nifedipine concentrations and response of patients with pulmonary hypertension. Am J Cardiol 1996;77:996–999.

115. Packer M, Medina N, Yushak M. Adverse hemodynamic and clinical effects of calcium channel blockade in pulmonary hypertension secondary to obliterative pulmonary vascular disease. J Am Coll Cardiol 1984;4:890–901.

116. Moncada S. Prostacyclin, from discovery to clinical application. J Pharmacol 1985;16:71–88.

117. Rich S, McLaughlin VV. The effects of chronic prostacyclin therapy on cardiac output and symptoms in primary pulmonary hypertension. J Am Coll Cardiol 1999;34:1184–1187.

118. Barst RJ, Rubin LJ, McGoon MD, et al. Survival in primary pulmonary hypertension with long-term continuous intravenous prostacyclin. Ann Intern Med 1994;121:409–415.

119. Saadjian A, Philip-Joet F, Paganelli F, et al. Long-term effects of cicletanine on secondary pulmonary hypertension. J Cardiovasc Pharmacol 1998;31:364–371.

120. McLaughlin VV, Genthner DE, Panella MM, et al. Reduction in pulmonary vascular resistance with long-term epoprostenol (prostacyclin) therapy in primary pulmonary hypertension. N Engl J Med 1998;338:273–277.

121. Archer SL, Mike D, Crow J, et al. A placebo-controlled trial of prostacyclin in acute respiratory failure in COPD. Chest 1996; 109:750–755.

122. Kesten S, Dainauskas J, McLaughlin V, et al. Development of nonspecific interstitial pneumonitis associated with long-term treatment of primary pulmonary hypertension with prostacyclin. Chest 1999;116:566–569.

123. McLaughlin V, Barst R, Rich S, et al. Efficacy and safety of UT-15, a prostacyclin analog, for primary pulmonary hypertension. Eur J Cardiol 1999;20:486.

124. Olschewski H, Walmrath D, Schermuly R, et al. Aerosolized prostacyclin and iloprost in severe pulmonary hypertension. Ann Intern Med 1996;124:820–824.

125. Hoeper MM, Olschewski H, Ghofrani HA, et al. A comparison of the acute hemodynamic effects of inhaled nitric oxide and

aerosolized iloprost in primary pulmonary hypertension. German PPH study group. J Am Coll Cardiol 2000;35:176–182.

126. Nagaya N, Uematsu M, Okano Y, et al. Effect of orally active prostacyclin analogue on survival of outpatients with primary pulmonary hypertension. J Am Coll Cardiol 1999; 34:1188–1192.

127. Archer SL, Huang JM, Hampl V, et al. Nitric oxide and cGMP cause vasorelaxation by activation of a charybdotoxin-sensitive K channel by cGMP-dependent protein kinase. Proc Natl Acad Sci USA 1994;91:7583–7587.

128. Clark RH, Kueser TJ, Walker MW, et al. Low-dose nitric oxide therapy for persistent pulmonary hypertension of the newborn. Clinical Inhaled Nitric Oxide Research Group. N Engl J Med 2000;342:469–474.

129. Snell GI, Salamonsen RF, Bergin P, et al. Inhaled nitric oxide used as a bridge to heart-lung transplantation in a patient with end-stage pulmonary hypertension. Am J Respir Crit Care Med 1995;151:1263–1266.

130. Ricciardi MJ, Knight BP, Martinez FJ, et al. Inhaled nitric oxide in primary pulmonary hypertension: a safe and effective agent for predicting response to nifedipine. J Am Coll Cardiol 1998; 32:1068–1073.

131. Perez-Penate G, Julia-Serda G, Pulido-Duque JM, et al. One-year continuous inhaled nitric oxide for primary pulmonary hypertension. Chest 2001;119:970–973.

132. Michelakis E, Tymchak W, Lien D, et al. Oral sildenafil is an effective and specific pulmonary vasodilator in patients with pulmonary arterial hypertension: comparison with inhaled nitric oxide. Circulation 2002;105:2398–2403.

133. Langleben D, Barst RJ, Badesch D, et al. Continuous infusion of epoprostenol improves the net balance between pulmonary endothelin-1 clearance and release in primary pulmonary hypertension. Circulation 1999;99:3266–3271.

134. Givertz MM, Colucci WS, LeJemtel TH, et al. Acute endothelin A receptor blockade causes selective pulmonary vasodilation in patients with chronic heart failure. Circulation 2000; 101:2922–2927.

135. Barst R, Horn E, Widlitz A. Circulation 2000;102:II–716.

136. Rubin SR, Bodesch DB, Borst RJ, et al. Bosentan therapy for pulmonary arterial hypertension. N Engl J Med 2002;346:896–903.

137. Champion HC, Bivalacqua TJ, D'Souza FM, et al. Gene transfer of endothelial nitric oxide synthase to the lung of the mouse in vivo. Effect on agonist-induced and flow-mediated vascular responses. Circ Res 1999;84:1422–1432.

138. Champion HC, Bivalacqua TJ, Toyoda K, et al. In vivo gene transfer of prepro-calcitonin gene-related peptide to the lung attenuates chronic hypoxia-induced pulmonary hypertension in the mouse. Circulation 2000;101:923–930.

26

The Molecular Basis of Cerebrovascular Malformations

Douglas A. Marchuk, PhD

CONTENTS

INTRODUCTION
ARTERIOVENOUS MALFORMATIONS
CONCLUSIONS
REFERENCES

INTRODUCTION

Four categories of cerebrovascular lesions have been identified: telangiectasias, venous malformations, arteriovenous malformations, and cavernous malformations. Telangiectasias are vascular lesions composed of small vessels separated by normal brain tissue. Small (0.3–1.0 cm) and rarely symptomatic, telangiectasias are usually identified as an incidental finding upon autopsy. Venous malformations, also usually benign, appear to be a normal variant of veins separated by normal brain tissue. With no definitive arterial input, venous malformations rarely cause hemorrhage or seizures.

In contrast to telangiectasias and venous malformations, arteriovenous and cavernous malformations are clinically significant and will be the focus of this chapter. In both cases, genetic studies of the inherited form of the disease have contributed significantly to our understanding of the underlying pathology of the lesion, which is inherited as a simple Mendelian trait. Molecular analyses can be used to locate the chromosomal region with the genetic defect, leading ultimately to the identification of mutations in the causative gene. In turn, the nature of the causative gene can shed light on the pathogenesis of the inherited form of the disease, and possibly, the more common sporadically occurring forms. The genes responsible for these syndromes often encode proteins that act at critical points in the pathways that control fundamental biological processes such as cell division, differentiation, and cell death;

these processes are disrupted in disease states. Gene products identified as contributing factors in the inherited form of the disease may also be involved in the common form of the disease.

ARTERIOVENOUS MALFORMATIONS

Arteriovenous malformations consist of a large tangle of dilated blood vessels characterized by rapid blood flow and early draining veins. The lesion forms early during embryonic life through the direct communication of an artery with a vein, without an intervening capillary bed. The feeding arteries progressively enlarge during fetal development and after birth, leading to a concomitant dilation of the draining veins. The veins in particular may appear grossly dilated because of the lack of supporting connective tissue and smooth muscle. Because the entire lesion eventually consists of the dilated feeding arteries and draining veins, the nidus, which is the site of the direct arteriovenous communication, may be difficult to identify radiologically.

During fetal development, the concurrent formation of the cerebral arteriovenous malformation and the brain results in the presence of neural tissue between the dilated arteries and veins. The brain tissue can become atrophic, gliotic, and even calcified. Arteriovenous malformations can be identified with several imaging techniques. The lesion appears as a tangle of dense tubular structures on a computed tomography (CT) scan and as a tangle of serpentine curvilinear hypointensities on

From: *Contemporary Cardiology: Principles of Molecular Cardiology*
Edited by: M. S. Runge and C. Patterson © Humana Press Inc., Totowa, NJ

magnetic resonance imaging (MRI). With angiography, the arteriovenous malformation often presents as multiple dilated feeding arteries and large early draining veins.

Clinical Presentation

The arteriovenous malformation is the hallmark vascular lesion of hereditary hemorrhagic telangiectasia (HHT), which is also known as Rendu–Osler–Weber syndrome. An autosomal dominant condition, HHT is characterized by multisystemic arteriovenous malformations and hemorrhage from the associated vascular lesions. The diagnosis of HHT requires the presence of three of four criteria: spontaneous recurrent epistaxis, telangiectasias at characteristic sites, a visceral manifestation, and a family history of HHT (1). Because various organs and tissues may contain vascular lesions, HHT has a wide range of clinical features.

Telangiectasias are red to violet lesions that appear on the digits; the facial, nasal, and buccal mucosa; and the gastrointestinal tract. The lesions are dilated venules that connect directly to several arterioles without intervening capillaries; this arrangement results in bleeding. Telangiectasias may be the direct precursor to arteriovenous malformations, which are seen most commonly in the lung. In pulmonary arteriovenous malformations, a branch of a pulmonary artery connects directly with a pulmonary vein through a thin-walled aneurysm. A direct right-to-left shunt can form, particularly when multiple lesions are present, and can lead to profound dyspnea, fatigue, cyanosis, and polycythemia. Stroke is a common and serious complication because pulmonary arteriovenous malformations allow blood clots to traverse the region and enter the brain (2). In addition, pulmonary lesions allow bacteria to pass into the brain, thus causing brain abscesses (2). In patients with HHT, pregnancy is a serious risk factor for the formation of pulmonary arteriovenous malformations, especially in the third trimester (3–6) when recurrent hemoptysis and hemothorax can occur.

Gastrointestinal bleeding is found in 10–30% of patients with HHT (7–10), usually in the fourth or fifth decade of life (11). Vascular lesions occur most frequently in the upper gastrointestinal tract, predominantly in the stomach and duodenum (11). Gastrointestinal lesions are nodular on endoscopy and do not differ significantly from cutaneous telangiectasias.

The presence of multiple arteriovenous malformations in the liver or atypical cirrhosis is an important manifestation of HHT (12,13). In retrospective studies, an estimated 8–31% of patients with HHT have liver involvement (14,15). Liver involvement in HHT can be assessed with Doppler ultrasound angiography, CT with contrast enhancement, and MRI. Sonography shows increased blood flow within the dilated hepatic artery, which is a sensitive diagnostic indicator for hepatic involvement in HHT. Typical features on angiographic and CT analyses are the presence of dilated hepatic artery and veins, multiple aneurysms of the intraparenchymal branches of the hepatic artery, and both hepatoportal and hepatohepatic arteriovenous fistulae (17). Cholestasis is often the clinical sign that correlates with the severity of hepatic vascular abnormalities (16). High cardiac output caused by left-to-right shunting within the liver can lead to heart failure (13).

Neurological symptoms of HHT include migraine headache, brain abscess, transient ischemic attack, stroke, seizure, and intracerebral and subarachnoid hemorrhage. Brain abscess, transient ischemic attack, and ischemic stroke occur as neurologic sequelae of pulmonary arteriovenous malformations. Cerebral or spinal lesions can cause subarachnoid hemorrhage, and less commonly, paraparesis. Cerebral vascular lesions were originally thought to affect only 5–10% of patients with HHT (18); however, the use of new, more sensitive screening techniques in HHT families indicates the frequency of cerebral vascular lesions is much greater (19).

Vascular lesions seen in HHT patients range from small cutaneous and mucocutaneous telangiectasias to larger visceral arteriovenous malformations. Early histologic studies of HHT-associated telangiectasias showed thin-walled, dilated vessels comprising a single layer of endothelium without a connective or muscular tissue layer. The hallmark feature of the HHT-associated lesion is direct arteriovenous communication. This direct shunting of arterial blood suggests that increased blood flow through the lesion may increase the likelihood of hemorrhage.

Three studies have examined the microscopic structure of skin lesions. In the most recent systematic study, microscopy of a series of biopsy specimens of skin lesions (20) showed lesion development over time (Fig. 1). Very early lesions showed dilatation of the postcapillary venule with preservation of the capillary bed. As the lesions increased in size, the capillary segments disappeared, leaving a direct arteriovenous connection that enlarged under pressure. The lesions were associated with a perivascular cell infiltrate comprising a mixture of lymphocytes and monocytic cells.

As seen via electron microscopy, mucosal and cutaneous telangiectasias have small venules that are dilated and have thin endothelial cell walls (21). The junctions between endothelial cells show evidence of weakness. Dilatation often results in cavernous spaces filled with fibrin and erythrocytes. Abnormal regions are not associated with smooth muscle cells or fibroblasts. The presence of dilated postcapillary venules has been confirmed by another study

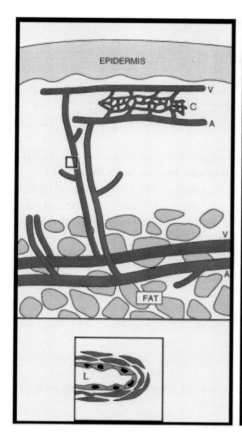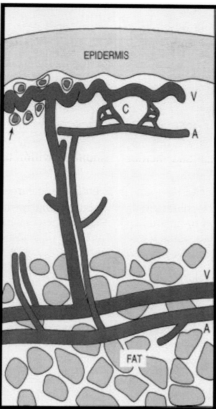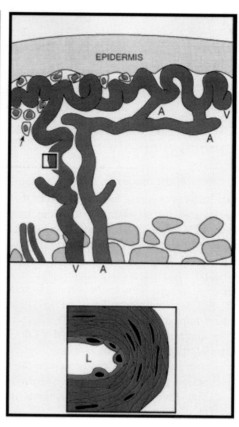

Fig. 1. Development of cutaneous vascular malformations in hereditary hemorrhagic telangiectasia (HHT). In normal skin, arterioles (A) in the papillary dermis connect to venules (V) through multiple capillaries (C). A normal postcapillary venule (shown in cross section in the inset) consists of a lumen (L), a single layer of endothelial cells, and two to three layers of pericytes. In the early stage of telangiectasia, a single venule becomes dilated, but it remains connected to an arteriole through one or more capillaries. A perivascular lymphocytic infiltrate is present. In the fully developed lesion, the venule and its branches become markedly dilated, elongated, and convoluted throughout the dermis. In addition, the connecting arterioles become dilated and communicate directly with the venules without an intervening capillary bed. The perivascular infiltrate is still present. The dilated descending venule is markedly thickened with as many as 11 layers of smooth muscle cells. Adapted from *(20)*.

that also reported that the basal lamina in mucosal and cutaneous telangiectasias is often duplicated and thickened *(22)*. These findings suggest considerable endothelial cell death and regeneration or abnormal turnover of old basal membrane. Extravasation of blood was seen and included erythrocytes and fibrin deposition, which could form the basis for new capillary sprouts, although no such sprouts were noted. The factor that initiates formation of a telangiectasia is unknown. Moreover, the reasons why only specific areas of skin and mucous membranes are affected are unclear. Thermal insult, ultraviolet light, or a second genetic mutation may initiate lesion formation.

Genetics of Hereditary Hemorrhagic Telangiectasia

Genetic studies in families have linked HHT to markers on human chromosome 9q33-q34 *(23,24)*. Mutations in the gene for endoglin, which is a homodimeric integral membrane protein, have been identified in family members *(25,26)*. Expressed at high levels on vascular endothelial cells of all blood vessels in humans *(26)*, endoglin is the most abundant transforming growth factor β (TGF-β) binding protein on endothelial cells *(27)*.

The 90-kDa endoglin protein contains 658 amino acids. Endoglin has a single transmembrane domain, a short cytoplasmic domain of 47 amino acids, and an extracellular domain of 586 amino acids, including the signal peptide (Fig. 2A). The endoglin gene comprises 15 exons *(28,29)*. A splice variant called S-endoglin (for short endoglin) has been identified that encodes an 85-kDa protein *(30)*. The extracellular and transmembrane domains of S-endoglin and the longer endoglin (L-endoglin) are identical; however, S-endoglin has a novel, 14-amino-acid residue in the cytoplasmic domain. Although the

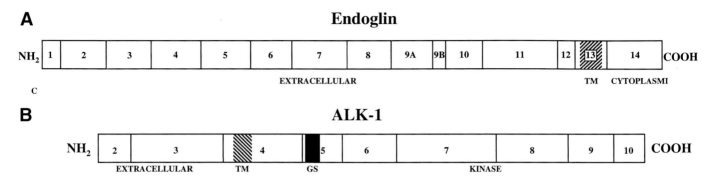

Fig. 2. (A) Schematic representation of the endoglin gene. Endoglin is encoded by a gene consisting of 15 exons mapping to human chromosome 9q34. Most of the coding region corresponds to the extracellular, ligand-binding domain. Exon 13 encodes a transmembrane (TM) domain, and exon 14 encodes a short cytoplasmic tail. The transmembrane region and cytoplasmic tail of endoglin show significant homology (71% identity) to the corresponding regions of the type III transforming growth factor β (TGF-β) receptor, also known as betaglycan. This homology suggests that endoglin, like betaglycan, may be a cell-surface receptor for TGF-β. Mutations identified throughout the endoglin gene in hereditary hemorrhagic telangiectasia (HHT) 1 kindreds include missense mutations, nonsense mutations, frameshifts, and deletion mutations. Mutation data suggest that the mutations lead to the loss of function of endoglin. (B) Schematic representation of the activin receptor-like kinase 1 (ALK-1) gene. ALK-1 is encoded by a gene consisting of 9 exons mapping to human chromosome 12q13, with at least one additional noncoding exon contributing to the 5' untranslated region. ALK-1 is a type I transforming growth factor β (TGF-β) receptor, a member of the serine/threonine kinase family. The coding region corresponds to the extracellular ligand-binding domain, a short transmembrane (TM) domain, and the kinase domain. A glycine and serine rich (GS) region, present in all type I TGF-β receptors, is the site of autoregulatory phosphorylation at serine residues. Mutations in ALK-1 in hereditary hemorrhagic telangiectasia (HHT) 2 kindreds have been identified throughout the gene and include missense mutations, nonsense mutations, frameshifts, and deletion mutations. Mutation data suggest that the mutations lead to loss of function of ALK-1.

two isoforms are coexpressed in different cell types, most transcripts code for L-endoglin.

More than 50 mutations have been identified in the endoglin gene in HHT families. The types of mutations include missense mutations, nonsense mutations, large genomic deletions, splice site changes, and small nucleotide insertions and deletions that lead to shifts in the reading frame and premature stop codons. Each mutation in the endoglin gene may decrease levels of functional endoglin at the endothelial cell surface.

Not all families with HHT have mutations that are linked to chromosome 9q3 (24,31,32). A second HHT locus (HHT2) has been identified in the pericentromeric region of chromosome 12 (33,34). The gene for activin receptor-like kinase 1 (ALK-1) maps within this interval, and mutations have been identified in this gene in HHT2 families (35).

ALK-1, a type I cell-surface receptor for the TGF-β superfamily of ligands, is expressed primarily on endothelial cells and in highly vascularized tissues (34) and has a molecular weight of 60–70 kDa, depending on its glycosylation status. The ALK-1 gene (Fig. 2B) contains 10 exons, 9 of which encode the protein sequence (36). ALK-1 (also called TSR1, R3) has been cloned independently by three different groups (34,35,37). More than 20 mutations, including nonsense and missense mutations and frameshifts, have been identified throughout the

ALK-1 gene in HHT2 families. Genetic and biochemical analyses of missense mutations suggest that most of them create null alleles, meaning such mutations in the ALK-1 receptor would likely reduce its signaling capacity.

Endoglin and ALK-1

Endoglin and ALK-1 are receptors for members of the TGF-β superfamily of ligands. TGF-β, which has three isoforms (β1, β2, and β3), is the prototypical member of this family of ligands that includes activins, bone morphogenetic proteins, and mullerian inhibitory substance. This group of cytokines regulates many aspects of cellular function, such as proliferation, differentiation, adhesion, migration, and extracellular matrix (ECM) formation (38–40).

Signaling through TGF-β occurs via different ligand-induced heteromeric receptor complexes consisting of type I and type II transmembrane serine/threonine kinase receptors. Several models for TGF-β and activin signaling have been proposed (39,41,42). First, TGF-β or activin binds the constitutively phosphorylated type II receptor, which recruits the type I receptor into the ligand/type II receptor complex. Then, the type II receptor phosphorylates the type I receptor's serine and threonine residues in its cytoplasmic juxtamembrane GS domain (43). The type I receptor then phosphorylates downstream signaling mediators such as members of the recently identified Smad family, which translocate to the nucleus to modify gene expression (44–46).

Initially identified as a surface antigen of acute lymphoblastic leukemia cells (47,48), endoglin, also called CD105, is also expressed on endothelial cells from all blood vessels, including capillaries, arterioles, small arteries, venules, high endothelial venules, and in umbilical cord veins (49). Endoglin is classified as a TGF-β type III receptor based on its sequence homology to the proteoglycan betaglycan (50–52). Betaglycan binds all three TGF-β isoforms and presents the ligands to the signaling receptors TβR-II and TβR-I, which increases the signaling activity of the type I receptor (53). Endoglin, the most abundant TGF-β binding protein on endothelial cells (27), binds the β1 and β3 isoforms, but not the β2 isoform. Despite its sequence similarities with betaglycan, endoglin inhibits TGF-β signaling (54,55).

Studies of sequence homology have shown that ALK-1, which is expressed primarily on endothelial cells, is a member of the type I receptors for the TGF-β family of ligands. Studies of a chimeric ALK-1 receptor comprising the extracellular ligand-binding domain of ALK-1 fused to the intracellular signaling domain of TβRI showed that ALK-1 binds TGF-β1 and -β3, but not -β2 (56). This ligand specificity is similar to that of endoglin (27).

Pathogenesis of Arteriovenous Formation

The mechanisms by which mutations affect the function of endoglin and ALK-1 are being elucidated; however, the factor(s) responsible for the formation of vascular lesions are unknown. If levels of endoglin or ALK-1 are reduced by 50%, there is no effect on the development of a normal vascular system *in utero,* because the incidence of miscarriage is not increased in HHT families. However, 100% of HHT patients who have a mutation in endoglin or ALK-1 develop vascular lesions. The congenital nature of the lesion, which is a critical aspect of lesion development, has yet to be determined. The lesions may be congenital but microscopic at birth and may increase in size over time; however, the presence of the cutaneous lesion suggests the contrary. Studies of pulmonary arteriovenous malformations suggest that several factors can affect the growth and development of vascular lesions, regardless of the mechanism of development.

Hormones may play a role in HHT pathogenesis. Epistaxis is increased in women with HHT when circulating levels of endogenous estrogen are low, such as during menopause, after ovariectomy, and at the end of menstruation (57). Estrogen–progesterone therapy reduces gastrointestinal hemorrhage and epistaxis, although this may relate more to hemorrhage than lesion development. The increased risk for developing pulmonary arteriovenous malformations associated with pregnancy suggests a direct influence of hormones on lesion development. Hemodynamic status may contribute to the pathogenesis of HHT. Pregnancy induces profound changes in hemodynamic flow that might affect the development or exacerbation of pulmonary lesions, especially during the third trimester.

Genetic studies in mice have assessed the role of the endoglin and ALK-1 genes in vascular development. The absence of the endoglin gene as seen in homozygous knockout mice results in embryonic death caused by arrested endothelial remodeling (58–60). In knockout mice, the primitive vascular plexus of the yolk sac does not mature into defined vessels, leading to channel dilation and rupture. Embryos show distended yolk sac blood vessels by E9.5 and a lack of vascular organization by E10.5, and embryos are resorbed by E11.5. In addition, the differentiation of smooth muscle cells and their recruitment to blood vessels is defective. Heart defects, such as abnormal cardiac looping and enlarged cardiac ventricles and pericardical sac, have been reported. The formation of heart valves is disrupted, and the size and organization of the atrioventricular endocardial cushions is reduced. These findings indicate the importance of endoglin in the development of the heart.

ALK-1 homozygous null embryos also die because of defects in vascular development (61,62). Mature blood vessels in the yolk sac are not developed by E9.5, and the embryos are resorbed by E10.5. Histological analyses of the mutant embryos show excessive fusion of capillary plexes into cavernous vessels. In addition, large vessels are hyperdilated, and differentiation and recruitment of smooth muscle cells are lacking. Moreover, the endocardium and myocardium are immature, which suggests ALK-1 has a role in heart development.

The vascular abnormalities seen in ALK-1 knockout mice may relate to the role of TGF-β in angiogenesis. During angiogenesis, endothelial cells are found either in an activation phase or a resolution phase (Fig. 3). The activation phase is characterized by endothelial cell invasion and migration into the extracellular space, followed by proliferation and capillary tube formation. Proteolytic degradation of the basement membrane is required to initiate the activation phase. The resolution phase is characterized by the cessation of migration and proliferation and the reestablishment of the basement membrane. Studies of the TGF-β response of endothelial cells in which ALK-1 or ALK-5 receptors have been removed by antisense RNA

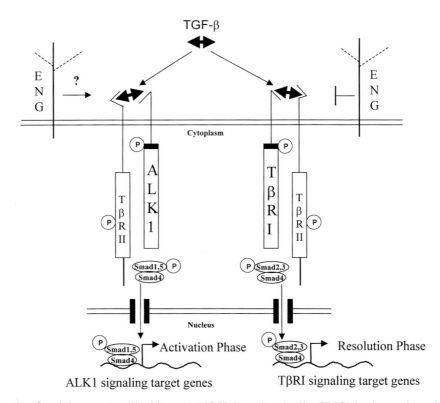

Fig. 3. A model for the role of activin receptor-like kinase 1 (ALK-1) and endoglin (ENG) in the angiogenic switch observed during capillary morphogenesis. Transforming growth factor β (TGF-β) can signal via two distinct receptor-mediated pathways in endothelial cells. TβRI is a ubiquitously expressed type I receptor that in concert with ligand binding with TβRII (type II receptor) activates a pathway that includes Smad2/3 and Smad4 complexes. This pathway leads to transcriptional activation of genes involved in the activation phase of angiogenesis. ALK-1 is an endothelial-specific type I receptor for TGF-β that in concert with ligand binding with TβRII signals through a pathway that includes Smad1/5 and Smad4. This pathway leads to transcriptional activation of genes involved in the resolution phase of angiogenesis. Endoglin is a negative modulator of TGF-β signaling through the TβRI receptor, although its role in signaling via the ALK-1 receptor is less clear. Modulation of TGF-β concentrations in the surrounding tissue would favor signaling through one or the other receptor, thus promoting the activation or resolution phases.

suggest that the two receptors are involved in the balance between the activation and resolution phase of angiogenesis (63). Infection of endothelial cells with constitutively active ALK-1 increases cell migration and proliferation. In contrast, the presence of constitutively active ALK-5 decreases migration and proliferation. In addition, activated ALK-5 induces plasminogen activator-inhibitor-1, suggesting a role for ALK-5 in vessel maturation.

Biochemical data and mouse knockout studies suggest a model for the roles of endoglin and ALK-1 in angiogenesis and the pathogenesis of HHT (Fig. 4). Vascular abnormalities in the ALK-1 null mice may result from the inappropriate persistence of the resolution phase of angiogenesis. ALK-1 may regulate the transition of endothelial cells from the activation to the resolution phase of angiogenesis. The biphasic effect of TGF-β on endothelial cells may be part of this transition (64). Low concentrations of TGF-β may favor binding to the higher affinity TβR-I

receptor, which may modulate genes involved in the resolution phase of angiogenesis. Higher concentrations of the TGF-β ligand may be required for binding to the lower affinity ALK-1 receptor, which inhibits the TβRI pathway, and thus may shift the gene expression profile to favor the activation phase of angiogenesis.

Mutations in the ALK-1 gene may reduce signaling through the ALK-1 receptor, thereby favoring signaling through the TβRI receptor and thus the resolution phase of angiogenesis. Mutations in endoglin may have a similar effect; endoglin mutations may remove the negative modulation of TGF-β through the TβRI receptor, thereby shifting the balance of signal to favor the activation phase. This model assumes that endoglin increases (or at least does not inhibit) ALK-1 receptor-mediated signaling.

There is no obvious phenotype in preliminary analyses of knockout mice that are heterozygous for both ALK-1

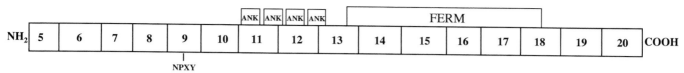

Fig. 4. A schematic representation of the KRIT1 (krev interaction trapped 1) gene. KRIT1 is encoded by 16 exons mapping to human chromosome 7q21, with at least 4 additional exons encoding the 5' untranslated region (not shown). Domains identified from the KRIT1 sequence include 4 putative ankryin (ANK) repeats and a FERM domain (FERM stands for the proteins Band 4.1, Ezrin, Radixin, and Moesin). Although FERM domains are observed in several proteins, KRIT1 is unique in that its FERM domain is at the carboxyl terminus. Mutations identified throughout the gene in CCM (cerebral cavernous malformations) 1 kindreds include small insertions and deletions, splice-site mutations, and nonsense mutations. No missense mutations have been identified; those that appeared to be missense mutations were subsequently shown to activate a cryptic splice site. The combined mutation data suggest that the CCM1 mutations lead to loss of function of KRIT1.

and endoglin, which are the best genetic models for assessing HHT phenotype. No phenotype has been reported for the ALK-1 heterozygotes. In a study of endoglin heterozygotes, a subtle phenotype of vessel dilation under the abdominal skin was noted *(60)*. In another study, a phenotype of epistaxis and cutaneous telangiectasias was apparent in a minority of endoglin heterozygotes when crossed into the inbred mouse strain background, 129/Ola *(59)*. As previously described, strain-specific phenotypes are seen with TGF-β1–deficient mice *(65)*. Other genes may modify the mouse phenotypes. Because the phenotype can vary widely in humans with HHT even in the same family, other genetic and environmental factors may modify the phenotype. The identification of modifier genes in the mouse may eventually lead to the discovery of human homologues in HHT kindreds.

The vascular lesions in HHT are localized to discrete regions within the affected tissue; evidence of abnormal vascular structure or pathology is not seen outside the lesions. This finding suggests that some genetic, physiologic, or mechanical event initiates the formation of each vascular lesion. The pathobiology of the disease may be related to remodeling of the vascular endothelium after an unknown initiating event. TGF-β1 mediates vascular remodeling by modifying the production of ECM by endothelial cells, stromal interstitial cells, smooth muscle cells, and pericytes. In HHT, perturbations in the TGF-β signaling pathway may alter repair of vascular endothelium and remodeling of the vascular tissue via changes in the expression of ECM proteins.

Cerebral Cavernous Malformations

Cerebral cavernous malformations (CCMs), also called cavernous angiomas or cavernous hemangiomas, are congenital vascular anomalies of the brain that comprise closely packed, grossly enlarged capillary-like vessels (caverns). Lesions, which are lined by a single layer of endothelium, are focal and may be single or multiple, ranging in size from a few millimeters to a few centimeters. Histopathological studies show focal, well-circumscribed, thin-walled vascular spaces that are often encapsulated. The vascular spaces can vary between capillaries, sinusoids, and larger cavernous spaces. The closely clustered vessels of the lesion are devoid of elastic, smooth muscle, and mature vessel wall elements *(66–68)* and usually lack neural parenchyma. Calcification and hemosiderin (iron) deposition in and around the lesions may represent recurrent occult hemorrhage. Lesions are most common in the cerebral hemispheres of the brain (70–90%) *(69)* but may affect any part of the central nervous system.

Sometimes referred to as a blood sponge, a CCM is a slow-flow vascular lesion, not a shunt. Because of the slow flow, these lesions are not usually identified on routine angiography and are often referred to as "occult" or "cryptic" malformations. Asymptomatic cases can be detected with MRI, which is the diagnostic method of choice for CCM *(67)*. The T1 weighted image shows foci of hyperintensity in areas of hemorrhage, whereas the T2 weighted image shows a black halo surrounding the lesion caused by hemosiderin deposition.

In two recent reports, tight junctions were lacking at endothelial interfaces of the CCM *(70,71)*. In several cases, gaps between adjacent endothelial cells allowed direct contact between the vessel lumen of the vascular sinusoid and the basal lamina *(71)*. Hemosiderin deposits underlying the vascular channels were found, without evidence of a ruptured vessel. The lack of tight junctions suggests a defect in the blood–brain barrier at the site of the lesion, which might cause slow, chronic leakage of red blood cells into the brain.

Clinical Presentation

CCMs account for 5–15% of all cerebrovascular malformations. Large retrospective reviews of autopsy and MRI studies have suggested that the incidence rate for CCM in the general population is 0.4–0.5% (72–75). Although CCMs have been reported in infants and children, most patients present with symptoms between the second and fifth decades (72,73,76); therefore, many people are unaware of their disease status early in life. Lesions are an incidental finding, often found during work-up for headache, in 15–20% of patients (72,73). Symptoms are absent in 40% of patients, even in those with familial CCM or multiple lesions (76).

Patients often present with seizures, intracerebral hemorrhage, recurrent headaches, and focal neurological deficits (68,77). Cerebrovascular accidents are the second most common clinical presentation in familial cases. Hemorrhagic stroke caused by massive intracerebral hemorrhage of the vascular lesion can be fatal and may be the first presenting symptom (78). Retrospective and prospective studies show that stroke occurs in 9–40% of all symptomatic patients. The overall lifetime risk of at least one bleeding episode is 30–40%, depending on the size of the lesion and the history of hemorrhage. Patients with a previous bleed have a 4.5% chance of recurrent bleeding, and hemorrhagic stroke occurs at a frequency of 0.25–0.7% per lesion-year. Intracerebral hemorrhage of the vascular lesion can be fatal and may be the only clinical presentation of the disorder (78). Surgical excision of isolated lesions is curative in most patients.

Genetics

CCM is found in familial and sporadic forms; 50% of cases are familial (66). Together, familial and sporadic forms of CCM are diagnosed in 0.1–0.5% of the general population and account for 10–20% of all vascular abnormalities of the central nervous system (66,68). Patients with the sporadic form usually present with one or two lesions and no family history of neurologic disease. In the familial form, patients often present with multiple lesions and a strong family history of seizures (69). However, a recent report suggests that up to 75% of patients with the sporadic form are members of an affected family; in these patients, asymptomatic vascular lesions in relatives masked the familial segregation (79). Careful imaging analyses of family members of affected patients without a clear family history of CCM have shown the hereditary segregation, particularly in small families. Because of the common occurrence of asymptomatic vascular lesions, the autosomal dominant segregation pattern may often be hidden, particularly in smaller families. If so, the incidence of familial CCM has been underestimated.

Genetic linkage studies have shown that an autosomal dominant form of the disease, CCM1, maps to chromosome 7q (69,80,81). A second locus, CCM2, maps to chromosome 7p and a third, CCM3, to chromosome 3q (82). The common occurrence of CCM in Hispanic Americans and the indication of a founder mutation in affected members of this population (83,84) helped identify the gene responsible for CCM1.

Mutations in the gene encoding KRIT1 (krev interaction trapped 1) have recently been identified as causing CCM1 (85,86) (Fig. 5). Mutations in affected patients include frameshift mutations, nonsense mutations, and mutations in invariant splice-site sequences; these mutations are likely to result in a loss of function. The founder effect in Hispanic Americans has been confirmed by mutation analysis. The identical mutation, C742T, which leads to a premature termination codon, Q248X, is seen in 75% of family members of Hispanic patients, which makes presymptomatic DNA testing especially effective in family members (86).

KRIT1

KRIT1 was initially identified by yeast two-hybrid screening of a HeLa cell cDNA library with the use of Rap1a (also known as KREV-1), a Ras-family GTPase, as bait (87). The strong interaction between KRIT1 and Rap suggested that KRIT1 was involved in Rap1a signal transduction. Rap1a was initially identified by its ability to revert the Ras-transformed phenotype of cells transformed by Kirsten murine sarcoma virus that carried a Ras oncogene (88). In addition, Rap1a and Ras have nearly identical effector domains, suggesting that Rap1a and Ras may compete for effector molecules (89). Rap1a interacts with downstream effectors of Ras such as Raf-1. The ability of Rap1a to revert the Ras-transformed phenotype might result from Rap1a competitively sequestering components of the Ras signal transduction pathway, namely downstream effector molecules such as Raf-1. KRIT1 may be involved in this process, and the loss of KRIT1 in CCM1 might alter the ability of Rap1a to sequester effector molecules, which would result in excessive Ras-mediated cell proliferation and the development of CCM1 lesions.

Alternatively, the ability of Rap1a to revert the Ras-transformed phenotype may be an artifact of Rap1a overexpression (90). Another model of KRIT1 function involves a Rap1a-specific cell proliferation pathway. In this alternative model, KRIT1 is a negative regulator of Rap1a-dependent cell proliferation. Loss of KRIT1

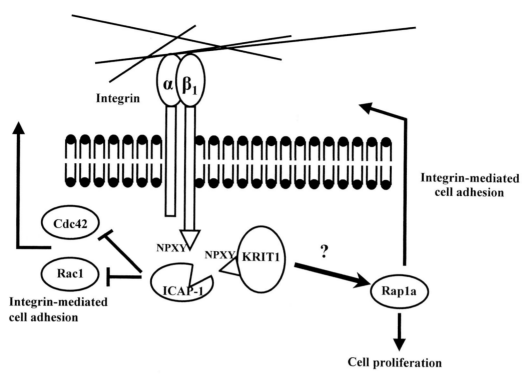

Fig. 5. A model for KRIT1 (krev interaction trapped 1) involvement in integrin signaling. KRIT1 interacts with integrin cytoplasmic domain–associated protein 1 (ICAP-1), an integrin binding protein. Integrins span the cell membrane and attach to extracellular matrix proteins such as laminin and fibronectin. ICAP-1 interacts with both KRIT1 and β1 integrin through their NPXY amino acid motifs; therefore, β1 integrin and KRIT1 may compete for ICAP-1 binding. Loss of KRIT1 may shift the balance toward integrin binding. Signaling via ICAP-1 negatively regulates Cdc42 and Rac1 effectors that may influence cell adhesion *(114)*. Interaction of KRIT1 with Rap1a, if shown to be authentic, may affect cell proliferation and integrin-mediated cell adhesion.

function in CCM1 would lead to excessive Rap1a-driven cell proliferation. An analogous scenario has been confirmed in another autosomal dominant disorder involving the formation of focal lesions. A mutation in the tuberin gene (Tsc-2) causes tuberous sclerosis type 2, which is characterized by hamartomas in multiple organs *(91)*. Tuberin has GTPase activating protein (GAP) activity for Rap1a, and loss of tuberin activity in tuberous sclerosis type 2 results in constitutive activation of Rap1a, which in turn causes uncontrolled cell proliferation *(92)*. KRIT1 may possess analogous GAP activity for Rap1a, and loss of KRIT1 activity in CCM1 may result in uncontrolled Rap1a-driven cell proliferation.

The structure of KRIT1 provides speculation about the protein's cellular function. KRIT1 structural elements include a carboxyl-terminal FERM domain (FERM stands for the proteins Band 4.1, Ezrin, Radixin, and Moesin), which is found in a superfamily of proteins including the ERM (Ezrin, Radixin, and Moesin) protein family that regulates the interaction between actin in the cytoskeleton and the plasma membrane *(93)*. The FERM domain helps maintain cell integrity, differentiation, and

motility. The presence of a carboxyl-terminal FERM domain in KRIT1 is rare; most members of the FERM superfamily have amino-terminal FERM domains. A series of four putative ankyrin repeats is located on the amino-terminal side of the predicted FERM domain. The ankyrin repeats are found in more than 400 proteins and are involved in many biological functions, including regulating protein–protein interactions. The presence of the FERM domain and the ankyrin repeat domains indicates that KRIT1 has multiple binding partners. Identifying binding partners specific for these well-characterized domains is essential to understanding KRIT1 function, which likely involves biochemical pathways.

Pathogenesis of Cerebral Cavernous Malformation

To study the role of KRIT1 in CCM1 pathogenesis, protein binding partners were identified by using KRIT1 as bait in yeast two-hybrid screens *(95,96)*. KRIT1 interacted specifically with integrin cytoplasmic domain–associated protein-1 (ICAP-1). Mutations in the amino-terminal KRIT1 NPXY amino acid sequence, a motif critical for ICAP-1 binding to β_1 integrin molecules, completely abolish the KRIT1/ICAP-1 interaction. Identifying ICAP-1 as a KRIT1 binding protein indicates a new role for KRIT1 in CCM1 pathogenesis—that of cell adhesion processes and ECM interactions mediated by integrin signaling.

Integrin molecules are heterodimeric transmembrane receptors that mediate cell–cell and cell–ECM interactions. Integrin signaling is bidirectional; binding to ECM ligands such as fibronectin, laminin, vitronectin, and collagen is affected by intracellular signaling events ("inside–out" signaling), whereas binding a particular ECM ligand generates a signal that is transmitted into the cell ("outside–in" signaling) (97). Ultrastructural analysis of lesions from patients with CCM has shown an abnormal basal lamina underlying the endothelial cells (71), a finding that supports the role of integrin and the ECM in CCM1 pathogenesis. Abnormalities in the basal lamina may indicate a disturbance in inside–out integrin signaling, possibly caused by a reduction of the KRIT1/ICAP-1 interaction by CCM1 mutations.

The cytoplasmic tails of integrin molecules lack intrinsic enzymatic activity (97); therefore, regulation of the inside–out and outside–in integrin signaling depends on adaptor proteins that have enzymatic activity or serve as linkers connecting the integrin tail and the actin cytoskeleton. ICAP-1 is an example of an integrin adaptor protein. ICAP-1 is a 200-amino-acid phosphoprotein identified as a yeast two-hybrid binding partner for the β_1 integrin cytoplasmic tail (98,99). Like KRIT1 (85,87), ICAP-1 transcripts have a relatively broad tissue distribution as seen on Northern analysis. However, the putative murine ortholog of ICAP-1, bodenin, has a more restricted expression of a gene trap LacZ insertion, which includes the visual system, the heart, and specific regions of the forebrain and cerebellum of newborn and adult mice, which is relevant to CCM1 pathogenesis (100).

ICAP-1 binds specifically with the β1 integrin cytoplasmic tail and does not interact with other β integrin and α cytoplasmic tails (98,99). Other proteins that bind the β1 integrin cytoplasmic tail include protein kinases such as integrin-linked kinase (101) and focal adhesion kinase (102) and the cytoskeletal proteins filamin (103), α-actinin (104), paxillin (105), and talin (106). These molecules participate in integrin-mediated signaling either as signal transducers or as cytoskeletal linkers. Because of the lack of similarity with these β_1 integrin cytoplasmic tail-binding proteins (99), ICAP-1 is not grouped with either the kinase or cytoskeletal proteins. ICAP-1 is phosphorylated after binding the β_1 integrin cytoplasmic tail (98,99) and may participate in cell migration mediated by β1 integrins (99). Thus, phosphorylation of ICAP-1 and its subsequent interaction with KRIT1 may be important in regulating integrin-mediated adhesion or cell migration processes. Mutational analyses show that the NPXY binding motif in KRIT1, as with β_1 integrins, is critical for ICAP-1 interaction. Sharing of the ICAP-1 binding motif by KRIT1 and β_1 integrins suggests the molecules functionally compete, perhaps through a phosphorylation-dependent or ECM-dependent mechanism.

Integrin cytoplasmic tails not only connect integrin to the cytoskeleton, they are also involved in multiple signal transduction pathways, including those that drive apoptosis and the cell cycle (97). In addition, integrins are associated with receptor pathways for growth factors and are necessary for optimal activation of growth factor receptors (97). For example, the receptor for vascular endothelial growth factor requires integrins for appropriate cell adhesion conditions and proper ligand activation (107). Thus, the KRIT1/ICAP-1 interaction may affect signaling cascades for cell cycle progression, apoptotic pathways, or growth factor receptor crosstalk events. Any of the above pathways might be affected by mutations in the KRIT1 gene.

These diverse signaling pathways may lead back to the Ras family member, Rap1a. Although KRIT1 was originally isolated as a binding partner for Rap1a (87), the role of KRIT1 in Rap1a signaling has not been determined. The KRIT1/Rap1a interaction has not been verified by direct biochemical binding assays except in the yeast two-hybrid system. In addition, KRIT1 and Rap1a in the opposite bait–prey orientation from the original screen (87) does not yield a two-hybrid interaction (95,96).

However, the interaction of KRIT-1 and ICAP-1 is a potential connection between integrin and Rap1a signaling. KRIT1 may be a Rap1a effector, thereby linking integrin signaling and Rap1a signaling and placing the KRIT1/Rap1a interaction in a new paradigm. Rap1a activates integrin molecules and contributes to integrin-mediated cell adhesion (108–110). Specifically, Rap1a is involved in inside–out integrin signaling because it mediates the activation of integrins by stimulating cell surface receptors. For example, CD31 (platelet endothelial cell adhesion molecule)–induced adhesion is blocked by inactive Rap1a (Rap1N17) (108). In addition, Rap1a may be involved in outside–in signaling (111), where cell adhesion events affect Rap1a activity. Moreover, Rap1a-associated molecules regulate integrin adhesive events. Evidence indicates that a GAP for Rap1a, SPA-1, affects the regulation of integrin-mediated cell adhesion (112). Thus, CCM1 mutations in KRIT1 may disrupt its function as a Rap1a effector molecule and therefore disrupt a link between integrin-mediated cell adhesion and downstream Rap1a signaling. The interaction between ICAP-1 and KRIT1 and the presence of a FERM domain in KRIT1 suggest that KRIT1 may be involved in bidirectional signaling between integrin molecules and the cytoskeleton. Furthermore, KRIT1 may affect cell adhesion processes via integrin signaling in CCM1 pathogenesis.

Defects identified in ultrastructural analyses of CCM lesions suggest that integrin signaling may be involved in the pathogenesis of CCM. The lack of a competent blood–brain barrier *(70,71)* may result from defects in integrin signaling. Moreover, evidence suggests that β_1 integrin interacts with claudin-11, which is a tight junction protein *(113)*. Thus, mutation of KRIT-1 may alter integrin signaling involved in the formation of the tight junction of endothelial cells, which would lead to a defect in the blood–brain barrier.

CONCLUSIONS

Cerebrovascular malformations are clinically significant vascular anomalies of the brain that cause considerable morbidity and mortality. Despite the importance of these malformations, little information is available concerning the underlying molecular etiology. The study of inherited forms of these vascular lesions, such as HHT and familial CCM, has contributed significantly to the understanding of the genetic processes involved in disease pathogenesis.

HHT is an autosomal dominant disorder characterized by multisystemic arteriovenous malformations. The study of HHT and the microanatomy of the associated vascular lesions has provided important information about vascular morphogenesis. The study of HHT began with the identification of mutations in two genes that correspond to type I and type II HHT. The mutations identified in the endoglin and ALK-1 genes indicate that the underlying pathogenesis of HHT involves perturbation of TGF-β signaling in vascular endothelial cells. Results from biochemical analyses and mouse studies suggest that the two genes are critical members of the angiogenic switch, regulating the shift from the activation phase to the resolution phase of blood vessel formation. Studying the role of these proteins in the development of these lesions will help in understanding the pathogenesis of arteriovenous malformations.

Genetic studies of familial CCM, another autosomal dominant disorder, have yielded the three loci, but so far only one has an associated gene that has been identified. The CCM1 gene, KRIT1, encodes a protein identified as a Krev-1/Rap1a binding partner. Although its role in Rap1a signaling is unknown, KRIT1 binds ICAP-1, an integrin binding protein; therefore, CCM pathogenesis may

be controlled by integrin signaling. Cellular functions controlled by integrin signaling include cell migration and cell adhesion. Recent evidence suggests that CCM lesions lack tight junctions between endothelial cells, which suggests that KRIT1 may be involved in junctional maturation of vessels. Further study of KRIT1 and identification of the CCM2 and CCM3 loci will increase our understanding of CCM pathogenesis.

REFERENCES

1. Shovlin CL, Guttmacher AE, Buscarini E, et al. Diagnostic criteria for hereditary hemorrhagic telangiectasia (Rendu-Osler-Weber syndrome). Am J Med Genet 2000;91:66–67.
2. White RI, Jr., Lynch-Nyhan A, Terry P, et al. Pulmonary arteriovenous malformations: techniques and long-term outcome of embolotherapy. Radiology 1988;169:663–669.
3. Gammon RB, Miksa AK, Keller FS. Osler-Weber-Rendu disease and pulmonary arteriovenous fistulas. Deterioration and embolotherapy during pregnancy. Chest 1990; 98:1522–1524.
4. Swinburne AJ, Fedullo AJ, Gangemi R, Mijangos JA. Hereditary telangiectasia and multiple pulmonary arteriovenous fistulas. Clinical deterioration during pregnancy. Chest 1986; 89:459–460.
5. Laroche CM, Wells F, Shneerson J. Massive hemothorax due to enlarging arteriovenous fistula in pregnancy. Chest 1992; 101:1452–1454.
6. Shovlin CL, Winstock AR, Peters AM, Jackson JE, Hughes JM. Medical complications of pregnancy in hereditary haemorrhagic telangiectasia. QJM 1995;88:879–887.
7. Smith C, Bartholomew L, Cain J. Hereditary hemorrhagic telangiectasia and gastrointestinal hemorrhage. Gastroenterology 1963; 44:1–6.
8. Cachin Y, Sauvage JP, Schwaab G. Rendu-Osler disease: apropos of 50 cases followed at the Gustave- Roussy Institute. Ann Otolaryngol Chir Cervicofac 1976;93:103–108.
9. Driscoll J, Rabe M. Hemorrhagic telangiectasis of the gastrointestinal tract, an obscure source of gastrointestinal bleeding. Am Surg 1954;20:1281–1290.
10. Vase P, Holm M, Arendrup H. Pulmonary arteriovenous fistulas in hereditary hemorrhagic telangiectasia. Acta Med Scand 1985;218:105–109.
11. Vase P, Grove O. Gastrointestinal lesions in hereditary hemorrhagic telangiectasia. Gastroenterology 1986;91:1079–1083.
12. Martini GA. The liver in hereditary haemorrhagic teleangiectasia: an inborn error of vascular structure with multiple manifestations: a reappraisal. Gut 1978;19:531–537.
13. Bernard G, Mion F, Henry L, Plauchu H, Paliard P. Hepatic involvement in hereditary hemorrhagic telangiectasia: clinical, radiological, and hemodynamic studies of 11 cases. Gastroenterology 1993;105:482–487.
14. Cloogman HM, DiCapo RD. Hereditary hemorrhagic telangiectasia: sonographic findings in the liver. Radiology 1984;150:521–522.
15. Goes E, Van Tussenbroeck F, Cottenie F, Hulstaert J, Osteaux M. Osler's disease diagnosed by ultrasound. JCU J Clin Ultrasound 1987;15:129–131.
16. Buscarini E, Buscarini L, Danesino C, et al. Hepatic vascular malformations in hereditary hemorrhagic telangiectasia:

Doppler sonographic screening in a large family. J Hepatol 1997;26:111–118.

17. Rapaccini GL, Pompili M, Caturelli E, et al. Ultrasound-guided fine-needle biopsy of hepatocellular carcinoma: comparison between smear cytology and microhistology. Am J Gastroenterol 1994;89:898–902.

18. Roman G, Fisher M, Perl DP, Poser CM. Neurological manifestations of hereditary hemorrhagic telangiectasia (Rendu-Osler-Weber disease): report of 2 cases and review of the literature. Ann Neurol 1978;4:130–144.

19. Fulbright RK, Chaloupka JC, Putman CM, et al. MR of hereditary hemorrhagic telangiectasia: prevalence and spectrum of cerebrovascular malformations. AJNR Am J Neuroradiol 1998;19:477–484.

20. Braverman IM, Keh A, Jacobson BS. Ultrastructure and three-dimensional organization of the telangiectases of hereditary hemorrhagic telangiectasia. J Invest Dermatol 1990;95:422–427.

21. Hashimoto K, Pritzker MS. Hereditary hemorrhagic telangiectasia. An electron microscopic study. Oral Surg Oral Med Oral Pathol 1972;34:751–768.

22. Menefee MG, Flessa HC, Glueck HI, Hogg SP. Hereditary hemorrhagic telangiectasia (Osler-Weber-Rendu disease). An electron microscopic study of the vascular lesions before and after therapy with hormones. Arch Otolaryngol 1975;101:246–251.

23. McDonald MT, Papenberg KA, Ghosh S, et al. A disease locus for hereditary haemorrhagic telangiectasia maps to chromosome 9q33-34. Nat Genet 1994;6:197–204.

24. Shovlin CL, Hughes JM, Tuddenham EG, et al. A gene for hereditary haemorrhagic telangiectasia maps to chromosome 9q3. Nat Genet 1994;6:205–209.

25. McAllister KA, Grogg KM, Johnson DW, et al. Endoglin, a TGF-beta binding protein of endothelial cells, is the gene for hereditary haemorrhagic telangiectasia type 1. Nat Genet 1994;8:345–351.

26. Gougos A, Letarte M. Primary structure of endoglin, an RGD-containing glycoprotein of human endothelial cells. J Biol Chem 1990;265:8361–8364.

27. Cheifetz S, Bellon T, Cales C, et al. Endoglin is a component of the transforming growth factor-beta receptor system in human endothelial cells. J Biol Chem 1992;267:19027–19030.

28. Shovlin CL, Hughes JM, Scott J, Seidman CE, Seidman JG. Characterization of endoglin and identification of novel mutations in hereditary hemorrhagic telangiectasia. Am J Hum Genet 1997;61:68–79.

29. Gallione CJ, Klaus DJ, Yeh EY, et al. Mutation and expression analysis of the endoglin gene in hereditary hemorrhagic telangiectasia reveals null alleles. Hum Mutat 1998;11:286–294.

30. Bellon T, Corbi A, Lastres P, et al. Identification and expression of two forms of the human transforming growth factor-beta-binding protein endoglin with distinct cytoplasmic regions. Eur J Immunol 1993;23:2340–2345.

31. Heutink P, Haitjema T, Breedveld GJ, et al. Linkage of hereditary haemorrhagic telangiectasia to chromosome 9q34 and evidence for locus heterogeneity. J Med Genet 1994;31:933–936.

32. McAllister KA, Lennon F, Bowles-Biesecker B, et al. Genetic heterogeneity in hereditary haemorrhagic telangiectasia: possible correlation with clinical phenotype. J Med Genet 1994; 31:927–932.

33. Johnson DW, Berg JN, Baldwin MA, et al. Mutations in the activin receptor-like kinase 1 gene in hereditary haemorrhagic telangiectasia type 2. Nat Genet 1996;13:189–195.

34. Attisano L, Carcamo J, Ventura F, Weis FM, Massague J, Wrana JL. Identification of human activin and TGF beta type I

receptors that form heteromeric kinase complexes with type II receptors. Cell 1993;75:671–680.

35. ten Dijke P, Ichijo H, Franzen P, et al. Activin receptor-like kinases: a novel subclass of cell-surface receptors with predicted serine/threonine kinase activity. Oncogene 1993;8:2879–2887.

36. Berg JN, Gallione CJ, Stenzel TT, et al. The activin receptor-like kinase 1 gene: genomic structure and mutations in hereditary hemorrhagic telangiectasia type 2. Am J Hum Genet 1997; 61:60–67.

37. He WW, Gustafson ML, Hirobe S, Donahoe PK. Developmental expression of four novel serine/threonine kinase receptors homologous to the activin/transforming growth factor-beta type II receptor family. Dev Dyn 1993; 196: 133–142.

38. Kingsley DM. The TGF-beta superfamily: new members, new receptors, and new genetic tests of function in different organisms. Genes Dev 1994;8:133–146.

39. Massague J. TGF-beta signal transduction. Annu Rev Biochem 1998;67:753–791.

40. Sporn MB, Roberts AB. Autocrine secretion—10 years later. Ann Intern Med 1992;117:408–414.

41. Wrana JL, Attisano L, Wieser R, Ventura F, Massague J. Mechanism of activation of the TGF-beta receptor. Nature 1994; 370:341–347.

42. Piek E, Westermark U, Kastemar M, et al. Expression of transforming-growth-factor (TGF)-beta receptors and Smad proteins in glioblastoma cell lines with distinct responses to TGF- beta1. Int J Cancer 1999;80:756–763.

43. Wieser R, Wrana JL, Massague J. GS domain mutations that constitutively activate T beta R-I, the downstream signaling component in the TGF-beta receptor complex. Embo J 1995; 14:2199–2208.

44. Heldin CH, Miyazono K, ten Dijke P. TGF-beta signalling from cell membrane to nucleus through SMAD proteins. Nature 1997;390:465–471.

45. Attisano L, Wrana JL. Mads and Smads in TGF beta signalling. Curr Opin Cell Biol 1998;10:188–194.

46. Kretzschmar M, Massague J. SMADs: mediators and regulators of TGF-beta signaling. Curr Opin Genet Dev 1998;8:103–111.

47. Quackenbush EJ, Letarte M. Identification of several cell surface proteins of non-T, non-B acute lymphoblastic leukemia by using monoclonal antibodies. J Immunol 1985; 134:1276–1285.

48. Haruta Y, Seon BK. Distinct human leukemia-associated cell surface glycoprotein GP160 defined by monoclonal antibody SN6. Proc Natl Acad Sci USA 1986;83:7898–7902.

49. Gougos A, Letarte M. Identification of a human endothelial cell antigen with monoclonal antibody 44G4 produced against a pre-B leukemic cell line. J Immunol 1988;141: 1925–1933.

50. Lopez-Casillas F, Cheifetz S, Doody J, Andres JL, Lane WS, Massague J. Structure and expression of the membrane proteoglycan betaglycan, a component of the TGF-beta receptor system. Cell 1991;67:785–795.

51. Wang XF, Lin HY, Ng-Eaton E, Downward J, Lodish HF, Weinberg RA. Expression cloning and characterization of the TGF-beta type III receptor. Cell 1991;67:797–805.

52. Moren A, Ichijo H, Miyazono K. Molecular cloning and characterization of the human and porcine transforming growth factor-beta type III receptors. Biochem Biophys Res Commun 1992;189:356–362.

53. Lopez-Casillas F, Wrana JL, Massague J. Betaglycan presents ligand to the TGF beta signaling receptor. Cell 1993;73:1435–1444.

54. Letamendia A, Lastres P, Botella LM, et al. Role of endoglin in cellular responses to transforming growth factor- beta. A comparative study with betaglycan. J Biol Chem 1998;273:33011–33019.

55. Lastres P, Letamendia A, Zhang H, et al. Endoglin modulates cellular responses to TGF-beta 1. J Cell Biol 1996; 133:1109–1121.

56. Lux A, Attisano L, Marchuk DA. Assignment of transforming growth factor beta1 and beta3 and a third new ligand to the type I receptor ALK-1. J Biol Chem 1999;274:9984–9992.

57. Koch H, Escher G, Lewis J. Hormonal management of hereditary haemorrhagic telangiectasis. JAMA 1952;149:1376–1380.

58. Li DY, Sorensen LK, Brooke BS, et al. Defective angiogenesis in mice lacking endoglin. Science 1999;284:1534–1537.

59. Bourdeau A, Dumont DJ, Letarte M. A murine model of hereditary hemorrhagic telangiectasia. J Clin Invest 1999;104: 1343–1351.

60. Arthur HM, Ure J, Smith AJ, et al. Endoglin, an ancillary TGFbeta receptor, is required for extraembryonic angiogenesis and plays a key role in heart development. Dev Biol 2000;217: 42–53.

61. Oh SP, Seki T, Goss KA, et al. Activin receptor-like kinase 1 modulates transforming growth factor-beta 1 signaling in the regulation of angiogenesis. Proc Natl Acad Sci USA 2000;97: 2626–2631.

62. Li C, Hampson IN, Hampson L, Kumar P, Bernabeu C, Kumar S. CD105 antagonizes the inhibitory signaling of transforming growth factor beta1 on human vascular endothelial cells. Faseb J 2000;14:55–64.

63. Goumans MJ, Valdimarsdottir G, Itoh S, Rosendahl A, Sideras P, ten Dijke P. Balancing the activation state of the endothelium via two distinct TGF-beta type I receptors. Embo J 2002;21: 1743–1753.

64. Pepper MS. Transforming growth factor-beta: vasculogenesis, angiogenesis, and vessel wall integrity. Cytokine Growth Factor Rev 1997;8:21–43.

65. Bonyadi M, Rusholme SA, Cousins FM, et al. Mapping of a major genetic modifier of embryonic lethality in TGF beta 1 knockout mice. Nat Genet 1997;15:207–211.

66. Rigamonti D, Hadley MN, Drayer BP, et al. Cerebral cavernous malformations. Incidence and familial occurrence. N Engl J Med 1988;319:343–347.

67. Tomlinson FH, Houser OW, Scheithauer BW, Sundt TM, Jr., Okazaki H, Parisi JE. Angiographically occult vascular malformations: a correlative study of features on magnetic resonance imaging and histological examination. Neurosurgery 1994;34: 792–799.

68. Gil-Nagel A, Wilcox KJ, Stewart JM, Anderson VE, Leppik IE, Rich SS. Familial cerebral cavernous angioma: clinical analysis of a family and phenotypic classification. Epilepsy Res 1995; 21:27–36.

69. Dubovsky J, Zabramski JM, Kurth J, et al. A gene responsible for cavernous malformations of the brain maps to chromosome 7q. Hum Mol Genet 1995;4:453–458.

70. Wong JH, Awad IA, Kim JH. Ultrastructural pathological features of cerebrovascular malformations: a preliminary report. Neurosurgery 2000;46:1454–1459.

71. Clatterbuck RE, Eberhart CG, Crain BJ, Rigamonti D. Ultrastructural and immunocytochemical evidence that an incompetent blood-brain barrier is related to the pathophysiology of cavernous malformations. J Neurol Neurosurg Psychiatry 2001;71:188–192.

72. Curling ODJ, Kelly DLJ, Elster AD, Craven TE. An analysis of the natural history of cavernous angiomas. J Neurosurg 1991;75:702–708.

73. Robinson JR, Awad IA, Little JR. Natural history of the cavernous angioma. J Neurosurg 1991;75:709–714.

74. McCormick WF. Pathology of Vascular Malformarions. In: Wilson CB, Stein BM, eds. Intracranial Arteriovenous Malformations. Baltimore: Williams and Wilkins, 1984.

75. Otten P, Pizzolato GP, Rilliet B, Berney J. 131 cases of cavernous angioma (cavernomas) of the CNS, discovered by retrospective analysis of 24,535 autopsies. Neurochirurgie 1989;35:82–83.

76. Zabramski JM, Wascher TM, Spetzler RF, et al. The natural history of familial cavernous malformations: results of an ongoing study. J Neurosurg 1994;80:422–432.

77. Kondziolka D, Lunsford LD, Kestle JR. The natural history of cerebral cavernous malformations. J Neurosurg 1995;83:820–824.

78. Maraire JN, Awad IA. Intracranial cavernous malformations: lesion behavior and management strategies. Neurosurgery 1995;37: 591–605.

79. Labauge P, Laberge S, Brunereau L, Levy C, Tournier-Lasserve E, Neurochirurgie SFd. Hereditary cerebral cavernous angiomas: clinical and genetic features in 57 French families. Lancet 1998;352:1892–1897.

80. Gunel M, Awad IA, Anson J, Lifton RP. Mapping a gene causing cerebral cavernous malformation to 7q11.2-q21. Proc Natl Acad Sci USA 1995;92:6620–6624.

81. Marchuk DA, Gallione CJ, Morrison LA, et al. A locus for cerebral cavernous malformations maps to chromosome 7q in two families. Genomics 1995;28:311–314.

82. Craig HD, Gunel M, Cepeda O, et al. Multilocus linkage identifies two new loci for a mendelian form of stroke, cerebral cavernous malformation, at 7p15-13 and 3q25.2-27. Hum Mol Genet 1998;7:1851–1858.

83. Johnson EW, Iyer LM, Rich SS, et al. Refined localization of the cerebral cavernous malformation gene (CCM1) to a 4-cM interval of chromosome 7q contained in a well-defined YAC contig. Genome Res 1995;5:368–380.

84. Gunel M, Awad IA, Finberg K, et al. A founder mutation as a cause of cerebral cavernous malformation in Hispanic Americans. N Engl J Med 1996;334:946–951.

85. Laberge-le Couteulx XS, Jung HH, Labauge P, et al. Truncating mutations in CCM1, encoding KRIT1, cause hereditary cavernous angiomas. Nat Genet 1999a;23:189–193.

86. Sahoo T, Johnson EW, Thomas JW, et al. Mutations in the gene encoding KRIT1, a Krev-1/rap1a binding protein, cause cerebral cavernous malformations. Mol Genet 1999;8:2325–2333.

87. Serebriiskii I, Estojak J, Sonoda G, Testa JR, Golemis EA. Association of Krev-1/rap1a with Krit1, a novel ankyrin repeat-containing protein encoded by a gene mapping to 7q21-22. Oncogene 1997;15:1043–1049.

88. Kitayama H, Sugimoto Y, Matsuzaki T, Ikawa Y, Noda M. A ras-related gene with transformation suppressor activity. Cell 1989;56:77–84.

89. Bos JL. All in the family? New insights and questions regarding interconnectivity of Ras, Rap1 and Ral. Embo J 1998;17: 6776–6782.

90. Zwartkruis FJ, Wolthuis RM, Nabben NM, Franke B, Bos JL. Extracellular signal-regulated activation of Rap1 fails to interfere in Ras effector signalling. Embo J 1998;17:5905–5912.

91. Wienecke R, Konig A, DeClue JE. Identification of tuberin, the tuberous sclerosis-2 product. J Biol Chem 1995;270: 16407–16414.

92. Soucek T, Pusch O, Wienecke R, DeClue JE, Hengstschlager M. Role of the tuberous sclerosis gene-2 product in cell cycle control. Loss of the tuberous sclerosis gene-2 induces quiescent cells to enter S phase. J Biol Chem 1997;272: 29301–20308.

93. Chishti AH, Kim AC, Marfatia SM, et al. The FERM domain: a unique module involved in the linkage of cytoplasmic proteins to the membrane. Trends Biochem Sci 1998;23: 281–281.

94. Sedgwick SG, Smerdon SJ. The ankyrin repeat: a diversity of interactions on a common structural framework. Trends Biochem Sci 1999;24:311–316.

95. Zhang J, Clatterbuck RE, Rigamonti D, Chang DD, Dietz HC. Interaction between krit1 and icap1alpha infers perturbation of integrin beta1-mediated angiogenesis in the pathogenesis of cerebral cavernous malformation. Hum Mol Genet 2001;10: 2953–2960.

96. Zawistowski JS, Serebriiskii IG, Lee MF, Golemis EA, Marchuk DA. KRIT1 association with the integrin-binding protein ICAP-1: a new direction in the elucidation of cerebral cavernous malformations (CCM1) pathogenesis. Hum Mol Genet 2002;11:389–396.

97. Giancotti FG, Ruoslahti E. Integrin signaling. Science 1999;285:1028–1032.

98. Chang DD, Wong C, Smith H, Liu J. ICAP-1, a novel B1 integrin cytoplasmic domain-associated protein, binds to a conserved and functionally important NPXY sequence motif of B1. J Cell Biol 1997;138:1149–1147.

99. Zhang XA, Hemler ME. Interaction of the integrin beta1 cytoplasmic domain with ICAP-1 protein. J Biol Chem 1999;274: 11–19.

100. Faisst AM, Gruss P. Bodenin: a novel murine gene expressed in restricted areas of the brain. Dev Dyn 1998;212:293–303.

101. Hannigan GE, Leung-Hagesteijn C, Fitz-Gibbon L, et al. Regulation of cell adhesion and anchorage-dependent growth by a new beta 1-integrin-linked protein kinase. Nature 1996; 379: z91–96.

102. Schaller MD, Otey CA, Hildebrand JD, Parsons JT. Focal adhesion kinase and paxillin bind to peptides mimicking beta integrin cytoplasmic domains. J Cell Biol 1995; 130: 1181–1187.

103. Pfaff M, Liu S, Erle DJ, Ginsberg MH. Integrin beta cytoplasmic domains differentially bind to cytoskeletal proteins. J Biol Chem 1998;273:6104–6109.

104. Otey CA, Vasquez GB, Burridge K, Erickson BW. Mapping of the alpha-actinin binding site within the beta 1 integrin cytoplasmic domain. J Biol Chem 1993;268:21193–21197.

105. Tanaka T, Yamaguchi R, Sabe H, Sekiguchi K, Healy JM. Paxillin association in vitro with integrin cytoplasmic domain peptides. FEBS Lett 1996;399:53–58.

106. Horwitz A, Duggan K, Buck C, Beckerle MC, Burridge K. Interaction of plasma membrane fibronectin receptor with talin—a transmembrane linkage. Nature 1986;320:531–533.

107. Soldi R, Mitola S, Strasly M, Defilippi P, Tarone G, Bussolino F. Role of alphavbeta3 integrin in the activation of vascular endothelial growth factor receptor-2. Embo J 1999; 18:882–892.

108. Reedquist KA, Ross E, Koop EA, et al. The small GTPase, Rap1, mediates CD31-induced integrin adhesion. J Cell Biol 2000;148:1151–1158.

109. Katagiri K, Hattori M, Minato N, Irie S, Takatsu K, Kinashi T. Rap1 is a potent activation signal for leukocyte function-associated antigen 1 distinct from protein kinase C and phosphatidylinositol-3-OH kinase. Mol Cell Biol 2000;20: 1956–1969.

110. Caron E, Self AJ, Hall A. The GTPase Rap1 controls functional activation of macrophage integrin alphaMbeta2 by LPS and other inflammatory mediators. Curr Biol 2000;10:974–978.

111. Bos JL, de Rooij J, Reedquist KA. Rap1 signalling: adhering to new models. Nat Rev Mol Cell Biol 2001;2:369–377.

112. Tsukamoto N, Hattori M, Yang H, Bos JL, Minato N. Rap1 GTPase-activating protein SPA-1 negatively regulates cell adhesion. J Biol Chem 1999;274:18463–18469.

113. Tiwari-Woodruff SK, Buznikov AG, Vu TQ, et al. OSP/claudin-11 forms a complex with a novel member of the tetraspanin super family and beta1 integrin and regulates proliferation and migration of oligodendrocytes. J Cell Biol 2001;153:295–305.

114. Degani S, Balzac F, Brancaccio M, et al. The integrin cytoplasmic domain-associated protein ICAP-1 binds and regulates Rho family GTPases during cell spreading. J Cell Biol 2002;156: 377–387.

27 Thrombotic Vascular Disease

Stephan Moll, MD and Gilbert C. White II, MD

CONTENTS

PHYSIOLOGY OF COAGULATION

When vascular integrity is interrupted, the coagulation process is initiated by the contact of plasma factor VIIa with tissue factor expressed on extravascular cells, mainly fibroblasts and monocytes. Thrombus formation is complex and involves four major systems: (1) activation of coagulation factors in several steps (initiation, amplification, propagation) *(1,2)*; (2) participation of platelets; (3) limitation of clot extension via the natural anticoagulant system; and (4) dissolution of thrombus through the fibrinolytic system.

Initiation of Coagulation

Low concentrations of activated factor VII (VIIa) normally circulate in the bloodstream. Disruption of vascular integrity brings plasma factor VIIa in contact with tissue factor expressed on extravascular cells. Although free factor VIIa is a weak enzyme, the enzymatic activity of factor VIIa markedly increases upon binding to tissue factor. The membrane-bound complex of tissue factor and factor VIIa (TF:VIIa complex) initiates coagulation (Fig. 1A). Factor X binds to this complex and becomes activated to factor Xa. When factor Xa leaves the protected environment of the cell surface, it is rapidly inactivated by antithrombin or tissue factor pathway inhibitor, but the factor Xa that remains on the tissue factor–bearing cell surface leads to limited proteolysis of inactive factor V, thus generating factor Va. The factor Xa:factor Va complex on the tissue factor–bearing cell leads to cleavage of prothrombin and the production of small amounts of

From: *Contemporary Cardiology: Principles of Molecular Cardiology*
Edited by: M. S. Runge and C. Patterson © Humana Press Inc., Totowa, NJ

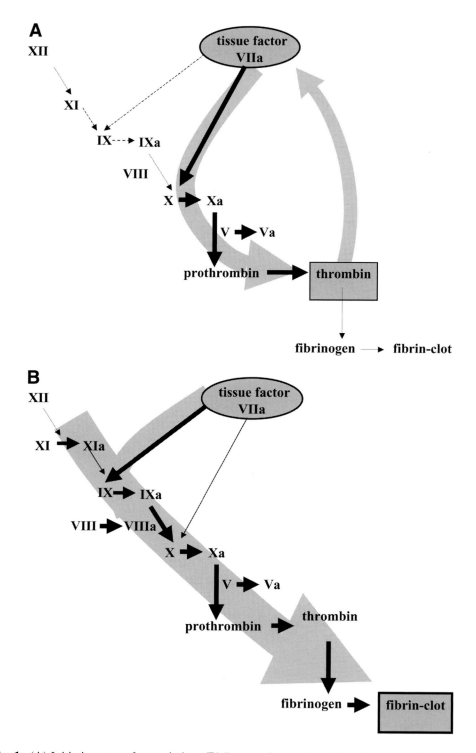

Fig. 1. **(A)** Initiation step of coagulation. **(B)** Propagation and amplification steps of coagulation.

thrombin. Amplification and propagation steps are needed to generate sufficient amounts of thrombin for thrombus formation. Another event that occurs in the initiation phase is the activation of factor IX to IXa by the TF:VIIa complex. However, factor IXa cannot activate factor X to factor Xa because factor VIIIa, a necessary cofactor, has not yet been formed. Factor VIIIa becomes available only after the initial small amount of thrombin has been generated and has enzymatically cleaved factor VIII to factor VIIIa.

Amplification

The small amount of thrombin generated on the surface of the tissue factor–bearing subendothelial cells during the initiation phase activates platelets that have adhered to the subendothelial matrix via von Willebrand factor at the site of injury (3). In addition, this phase includes the activation of platelet-bound factor VIII to factor VIIIa, activation of factor V to factor Va, activation of inactive TF:VII complex to TF:VIIa complex, activation of factor XI to factor XIa (4), and further activation of factor IX to factor IXa (Fig. 1B).

Propagation

During the propagation phase, the activated coagulation factors generated during the amplification phase combine with their cofactors on the activated platelet surface and form the "tenase" and "prothrombinase" complexes. This combination results in large-scale thrombin generation, or the so-called "thrombin burst," which leads to fibrinogen cleavage and fibrin polymerization. The main pathway for the thrombin burst is via TF:VIIa complex–induced activation of factor IX to factor IXa. The direct activation of factor X to factor Xa by the TF:VIIa complex plays a minor role in this propagation step.

Platelet Participation

The initial response of platelets in the coagulation process is to adhere to the extravascular matrix at the site of vascular injury. The interaction of the platelet glycoprotein (GP) Ib/IX/V receptor complex with collagen through the binding of von Willebrand factor mediates platelet adherence to the matrix. The platelet surface provides the phospholipids for binding of coagulation factors so that the platelet membrane–based coagulation reactions leading to the thrombin burst can occur. The thrombin burst during the propagation phase of coagulation further activates platelets, which causes a conformational change of the glycoprotein IIb/IIIa receptors. Fibrinogen and other adhesive molecules can then bind to these altered receptors. The bivalent fibrinogen molecules bridge two glycoprotein IIb/IIIa receptors of adjacent platelets, thus forming platelet aggregates and stabilizing the clot.

Clot Stabilization

Once the platelet-fibrin clot has formed, fibrin is stabilized by factor XIII. In the presence of fibrin, thrombin converts factor XIII to the enzyme factor XIIIa. Factor XIIIa catalyzes the formation of intermolecular ε-(γ-glutamyl) lysine bonds between various protein substrates such as fibrinogen monomers, α_2 antiplasmin, fibronectin, and collagen. These intermolecular cross-linking reactions contribute to hemostasis and to wound healing.

Natural Anticoagulant System

When thrombin is generated and a thrombus forms at the site of vascular injury, a system of natural anticoagulants is activated that inhibits extension of the thrombus by several containment mechanisms.

TISSUE FACTOR PATHWAY INHIBITOR

Tissue factor pathway inhibitor, a 276-amino-acid glycoprotein produced by endothelial cells, is the main inhibitor of the tissue factor pathway. It inhibits the tissue factor:factor VIIa/factor Xa complex by binding to both tissue factor:factor VIIa and factor Xa.

ACTIVATED PROTEIN C

Activated protein C (APC) inhibits thrombin generation by regulating levels of factor Va and VIIIa, which are cofactors in the reactions leading to generation of thrombin and factor Xa. In an autoregulatory mechanism, thrombin activates protein C in a reaction localized to the vessel wall. Thrombin binds to thrombomodulin, which is expressed on the endothelial cells adjacent to the site of vascular injury. Thrombomodulin is a cofactor for the conversion of protein C to APC by thrombin. Together with its cofactor protein S, APC inactivates factor Va and factor VIIIa (5). Factor Va is cleaved by proteolytic degradation at amino acid positions 506 and 306, and factor VIII is cleaved at positions 562 and 336.

ANTITHROMBIN

Antithrombin, formerly antithrombin III, inhibits thrombin, factor Xa, and other serine proteinases, such as factors IXa, XIa, XIIa, and kallikrein. Because antithrombin inhibits free thrombin and free factor Xa more efficiently than thrombin and factor Xa bound to platelet surfaces or clots, its main role may be to control low-level basal activation of the coagulation system that occurs in the normal circulation. Alone, antithrombin is not a very effective anticoagulant, unless given in high doses. The inhibitory action of antithrombin is markedly potentiated by heparin.

HEPARIN COFACTOR II

Heparin cofactor II (HcII) is a 480-amino-acid glycoprotein produced in hepatocytes that circulates in plasma. Although it inhibits thrombin, HcII does not inhibit factor Xa or other coagulation factors. Unlike antithrombin, HcII has the advantage of inhibiting surface-bound thrombin. HcII probably participates in the in vivo inhibition of thrombin as indicated by the presence of low levels of thrombin-HcII complexes in normal plasma samples. Binding of heparin potentiates HcII thrombin inhibitory activity about 1000-fold.

Fibrinolytic System

Once formed, clots can be lysed by the action of plasmin on fibrin. Plasmin is the primary enzyme of the fibrinolytic system and is generated by the activation of the precursor protein plasminogen to plasmin. Plasminogen, which circulates as an inactive zymogen in plasma, is incorporated throughout the thrombus by binding to lysine-binding sites on the polymerizing fibrin molecule. In response to poorly understood stimuli, possibly via thrombin, tissue plasminogen activator (tPA) is released from endothelial cells (6). tPA converts plasminogen, especially plasminogen bound to fibrin, to the active serine protease plasmin. Under physiologic conditions, α_2 antiplasmin rapidly and irreversibly inactivates plasmin. Because free plasmin is more rapidly and efficiently inhibited than fibrin-bound enzyme, fibrin-bound plasmin can actively degrade fibrin (7). The primary role of the plasminogen–plasmin system is not to dissolve large clots, but to prevent excessive fibrin and clot formation.

PATHOPHYSIOLOGY OF THROMBUS FORMATION

Venous thrombosis is usually caused by disturbances in the plasma coagulation system, with minimal platelet participation. In contrast, platelets play a major role in arterial thrombosis, with some participation of the plasma coagulation system. This paradigm helps explain why coagulation protein abnormalities, such as factor V Leiden or deficiencies of protein C, protein S, and antithrombin, usually lead to venous thromboembolism. In addition, this scenario explains why antiplatelet drugs prevent arterial thrombosis, but are less effective on venous disease. Thrombus formation in the cardiac ventricles and atria is often attributed to stagnant blood flow in akinetic, dyskinetic, or aneurysmal parts of the heart chambers or in fibrillating atria. Arising in a slow-flow environment, these thrombi are more likely caused by mechanisms similar to the ones that lead to venous thrombosis.

Arterial clots usually form in areas of atherosclerotic vascular damage. The events leading to atherosclerosis, mainly lipid disturbances, oxidative stress, and inflammation, are discussed elsewhere. The composition and vulnerability of plaque, rather than its volume, and the severity of stenosis are the most important determinants for the development of arterial ischemic syndromes (8). Monocytes and macrophages in plaque express high levels

of tissue factor (9). When the fibrous cap or endothelium overlying an atheromatous plaque is disrupted, collagen and tissue factor are exposed, which causes platelets to adhere and aggregate and thrombus to form (10). Recent understanding of the events leading to arterial thrombosis has led to the development of treatment strategies that are directed against the local vascular prothrombotic milieu. These strategies include the following: (1) topical application of anticoagulants (11–13); (2) placement of stents or grafts with virus-transduced confluent endothelial cells that secrete anticoagulants (14); and (3) locally applied gene therapy to express inhibitors of tissue factor (15,16) or to manipulate function of vascular smooth muscle cells or local inflammatory processes (17,18).

Stasis of blood is a well-known trigger factor for venous thrombosis. However, the events that trigger an episode of spontaneous (often called "idiopathic") venous thromboembolism in a specific location and at a certain time are not well understood. The lack of understanding of the initiating events of spontaneous venous thrombosis makes it impossible to develop locally active antithrombotic strategies.

Although the events leading to arterial thromboembolism are better understood than those leading to venous thromboembolism, the thrombophilic abnormalities predisposing to arterial events are less understood. Multiple inherited abnormalities that increase a patient's risk for venous thromboembolism are known, but few are known that predispose to arterial events. The defects involving the protein C anticoagulant pathway, mainly protein C and S deficiency, factor V Leiden, and APC resistance, have been well studied and have been associated with venous thromboembolism. Scientists are beginning to understand how a specific genotype leads to a certain phenotype and to disease for several of the polymorphisms, such as the fibrinogen and platelet glycoprotein receptor molecules (Table 1). However, results have been conflicting with regard to the association of many polymorphisms with arterial thrombotic disease.

FIBRINOGEN

Fibrinogen is a complex glycoprotein that consists of two disulfide-linked monomers. Each monomer is 1482 amino acids long and comprises three different polypeptide chains: an α-, β-, and γ-chain. The complete amino acid sequence for human fibrinogen has been determined (19). The complex assembly of the three polypeptide chains that form the trinodular fibrinogen structure has been partially defined (20). Fibrinogen is synthesized, processed, and assembled primarily in hepatocytes. The synthesis of

Table 1
Summary of Genetic and Molecular Properties of Blood Coagulation Proteins

	Chromosome location	Gene symbol	DNA base pairs	Number of exons	Amino acid length	Molecular weight (kDa)	Plasma concentration	Function
Antithrombin	1q23–q25	AT3	14 kb	6	432	62	290 µg/mL	Serine protease inhibitor
Protein C	2q13–q14	PROC	11 kb	9	461	62	5 µg/mL	Serine protease
Protein S	3p11.1–q11.2	PROS1	>80 kb	15	635	69	25 µg/mL	Cofactor for APC
Fibrinogen	4q23–q32	FGA	10	5	625	340	2000–4000 µg/mL	Substrate for thrombin
		FGB	10	8	461			
		FGC	10	10	411			
Prothrombin (Factor II)	11p11–q12	F2	~21 kb	14	579	72	100 µg/mL	Serine protease
Factor V	1q23	F5	70 kb	25	2,196	330	10 µg/mL	Cofactor
Factor VII	13q34	F7	12 kb	9	416	50	0.5 µg/mL	Serine protease
Factor VIII	Xq28	F8C	190 kb	26	2,330	330	0.1 µg/mL	Cofactor
Factor IX	Xq27	F9	8 kb	33	415	55	5 µg/mL	Serine protease
Factor XI	4q34–q35	F11	23 kb	15	608	80	5 µg/mL	Serine protease
Factor XIII (A$_2$B$_2$)						320	10 µg/mL	Clot stabilizer
Factor XIIIA	6p24–p25	F13A1	>200 kb	15	731			
Factor XIIIB	1q31–q32.1	F13B	28 kb	12	641			
Plasminogen	6q26–q27	PLG	52.5	19	791	88	200 µg/mL	Serine protease
PAI-1	7q22.1–q22.3	PLANH1	12 kb	9	379	50	10 µg/mL	Serine protease inhibitor
tPA	8q12–q11.2	PLAT	33 kb	14	527	68	0.005 µg/mL	Serine protease

fibrinogen is markedly increased during an acute-phase state caused by inflammation, tissue damage, or stress. Production of interleukin-6 by inflammatory cells stimulates hepatocytes to increase the production of hepatocyte nuclear factor, which increases transcription of fibrinogen (21). Fibrinogen is transformed to fibrin after thrombin proteolytically removes fibrinopeptide A from the amino terminus of the α chain and fibrinopeptide B from the β chain. Removal of these peptides exposes sites on the fibrinogen molecule that allow for polymerization or for intermolecular reactions between fibrinogen dimers, thereby forming a fibrin network.

High levels of plasma fibrinogen, an important risk factor for arterial disease, are associated with the development of ischemic heart disease (22–24), stroke (25), and peripheral vascular disease complications (26). The relative risk for most of these associations is up to twofold when comparing patients in the top 10% of the distribution of fibrinogen levels with the remainder (24). Several mechanisms for this increased risk have been postulated: (1) increased blood viscosity, (2) increased fibrin formation, and (3) increased availability of fibrinogen for platelet aggregation (27). However, an alternative explanation for this association is that fibrinogen levels increase as atherosclerotic disease progresses. The association may therefore reflect a reactive rather than a causative process (28).

Genetic variation in the fibrinogen genes may contribute to the rate of synthesis of fibrinogen, such as an increased basal rate of transcription of the β fibrinogen gene (29). Several polymorphisms have been identified in the three genes coding for fibrinogen, including –455G/A, –854G/A, C148T, and BclI in the β chain gene, and TaqI and Thr312Ala in the α chain gene (30). However, results of studies of the association of these polymorphisms with increased fibrinogen levels and vascular disease have been conflicting.

The –455G/A polymorphism, which defines a recognition site for the restriction enzyme HaeIII, has been of particular interest (31). The A allele of –455G/A has distinct nuclear protein binding properties and is associated with a higher basal rate of transcription of the β fibrinogen gene (29). This allele could increase the risk of vascular disease, and some studies have shown an association between the polymorphism and arterial occlusive disease (peripheral, coronary, or cerebrovascular) (32,33); however, other studies have not (34–36). Studies of the –455G/A polymorphism and a critical review of the relations between genotype, phenotype, and disease within clinical studies have been published (31). Even though a small effect cannot be excluded, –455G/A does not appear to be an important genetic determinant of arterial vascular disease.

High fibrinogen levels are a risk factor for venous thromboembolism, and the increase in risk of thrombosis is four times higher in patients with plasma fibrinogen levels greater than 5 g/L than in those with low levels (37). Fibrinogen gene polymorphisms have been less extensively studied in venous thromboembolism. No association was found between the C148T (38), the –455G/A, or the BclI polymorphisms (39) and venous thromboembolism. The Thr312Ala polymorphism was associated with pulmonary embolism, but not deep vein thrombosis (40).

Several fibrinogen gene mutations have been identified that lead to dysfibrinogenemias. The clinical presentation varies. About half of patients are asymptomatic; the other half has either a bleeding or clotting tendency (41). Venous thrombosis predominates over arterial thrombosis (41).

FACTOR VII

Factor VII is a vitamin K–dependent, 416-amino-acid single-chain glycoprotein that is produced in the liver and circulates in plasma as a zymogen. Factor VII is converted to the serine protease factor VIIa by limited proteolysis in the presence of thrombin, factor IXa, factor Xa, and factor XIIa. The TF:VIIa complex further activates factor X to factor Xa and factor IX to factor IXa and initiates subsequent thrombin formation.

High levels of factor VII activity were associated with an increased risk of ischemic heart disease in the Northwick Park study (22). However, in several follow-up studies, such as the Prospective Cardiovascular Munster (PROCAM) study (42), the Edinburgh Artery study (43), and the Etude Cas Temoin sur l'Infarctus du Myocarde (ECTIM) study (44), no association was found. Small amounts of activated factor VIIa circulate in plasma under physiologic conditions. However, increased factor VIIa levels are not associated with an increased risk of coronary artery disease or previous myocardial infarction (45,46). Increased factor VII levels are not associated with venous thromboembolism (37).

Several polymorphic sites have been identified in the factor VII gene. These sites are associated with plasma factor VII levels and together may account for up to 40% of the fluctuations in factor VII plasma levels (47). However, the relation between these polymorphisms and ischemic vascular disease has not been consistently shown. The most extensively studied polymorphism is Arg353Gln (31). Homozygosity for the Gln allele appears to lower plasma factor VII levels (44,48–51). Although decreased factor VII levels were associated with a lower risk of myocardial infarction in individuals with the Gln allele of the Arg353Gln polymorphism in one study *(50)*, these findings were not confirmed in several large studies *(44,48)*. Moreover, the Gln allele was associated with an increased risk of myocardial infarction in the Survival of Myocardial Infarction Long-term Evaluation (SMILE) study *(49)*. A recent study indicates that the Gln allele of the Arg353Gln polymorphism with its associated lower factor VII plasma levels protects against myocardial infarction only in patients with preexisting coronary artery disease *(51)*. No association has been found between factor VII polymorphisms and stroke *(52)* or venous thromboembolism *(39)*.

FACTOR VIII AND VON WILLEBRAND FACTOR

Factor VIII

Factor VIII, a 2330-amino-acid glycoprotein, is one of the largest coagulation proteins. Activated factor VIIIa is a cofactor in the tenase complex for the activation of factor X to factor Xa by factor IXa. Factor VIIIa increases by 200,000-fold the rate of activation of factor X to Xa *(53)*. Primarily synthesized by hepatic sinusoidal endothelial cells and Kupffer cells and to a lesser degree by hepatocytes *(54)*, factor VIII is an acute phase protein that is transcriptionally responsive to interleukin-6.

High factor VIII levels have been associated in several large studies with an increased risk of ischemic heart disease *(55–57)* and stroke *(58,59)*. However, high levels were not an independent risk factor for coronary heart disease in the Atherosclerosis Risk in Communities (ARIC) study *(60)*.

When measured at a time separate from the acute thrombotic event, high factor VIII levels are the single most common abnormality detected in patients with unexplained venous thromboembolism, occurring in 25.4% of patients *(61)*. High factor VIII levels are associated with a fivefold risk for venous thromboembolism *(62)* and are a risk factor for recurrence *(63)*. The mechanisms that cause high factor VIII levels are unclear.

von Willebrand Factor

von Willebrand factor is synthesized primarily in endothelial cells and has three functions: (1) binding to exposed subendothelial collagen at a site of vascular injury, (2) promoting platelet adhesion via the glycoprotein Ib/IX/V receptor, and *(3)* binding and stabilizing factor VIII, which prolongs its half-life in plasma. Factor VIII and von Willebrand factor circulate in plasma bound to one another. These factors therefore have similar associations with cardiovascular disease. Evidence suggests, albeit inconsistently, that von Willebrand factor is an independent risk factor for cardiovascular disease.

Several studies reported an association between high levels of von Willebrand factor and cardiovascular disease *(55,56,60)*; however, no independent association with coronary heart disease or stroke was found in two studies *(43,64)*. von Willebrand factor is not an independent risk factor for venous thromboembolism *(65)*.

FACTOR IX AND FACTOR XI

Factor IX is a vitamin K–dependent glycoprotein, which, when activated by factor VIIa-tissue factor or factor XIa, converts factor X to factor Xa. The formation of factor Xa leads to the formation of the fibrin clot. Increased factor IX levels are a risk factor for venous thromboembolism *(66)*. The risk of venous thrombosis is two to three times higher in patients with factor IX levels above the 90th percentile of control subjects than in those below the 90th percentile *(66)*.

Factor XI is activated to factor XIa by thrombin. Factor XIa participates in the coagulation process and thrombin formation. High levels of factor XI are a risk factor for deep vein thrombosis, and the risk is doubled at the highest levels present in 10% of the population *(67)*.

FACTOR V

Factor V, a 2196-amino-acid protein with a molecular weight of 33 kDa, is activated to factor Va in the initiation step of coagulation by factor Xa and in the subsequent amplification and propagation steps by thrombin. Factor Va participates as a cofactor in the prothrombinase complex formation that leads to the generation of thrombin. APC inactivates factor Va at two primary cleavage sites, Arg 506 and Arg 306. Two mechanisms for this cleavage have been proposed. In one view, initial cleavage at Arg 506 promotes a more rapid cleavage at Arg 306, which is the main inactivation step *(68)*. The second hypothesis is that cleavage at both sites is random but is much slower at Arg 306 *(69)*.

Factor V Leiden

A common polymorphism, G1691A, leads to an Arg506Gln mutation (also called R506Q) and is referred to as factor V Leiden *(70,71)*. The expressed mutant is resistant to APC because it lacks the APC cleavage site at Arg506 *(72)*. Factor V Leiden, discovered in 1994 by a group of researchers in Leiden outside of Amsterdam *(70)*, is a mutation that arose in Europe and is predominately found in Caucasians and, to a lesser degree, in populations that have some Caucasian ancestry. The carrier frequency is 8.8% in Europeans, 5.3% in Caucasian Americans, 2.2% in Hispanic Americans, 1.25% in Native Americans, 1.2% in African Americans, and 0.45% in Asian Americans

(73,74). Haplotype analysis of factor V gene polymorphisms indicates that the factor V Leiden mutation arose 21,000–34,000yr ago and originated from a single Caucasoid ancestor *(75)*. The mutation does not occur in native Africans and native Asians.

Factor V Leiden is the most common inherited risk factor for venous thrombosis. The risk of thrombosis is seven times higher for heterozygous patients and 80 times higher for homozygous patients than for those without this mutation *(76)*. This risk is further amplified by other genetic and environmental thrombosis risk factors *(77,78)*. The absolute annual incidence of spontaneous venous thromboembolism in asymptomatic carriers of the factor V Leiden mutation is low (0.26% per year) *(79)*. Although some studies indicated that the risk for recurrent venous thromboembolism may not be higher in carriers of factor V Leiden than in those without it, a meta-analysis of these studies indicated a slightly higher recurrence risk in carriers *(80)*. However, current recommendations for length of oral anticoagulation after a first thrombotic event are the same for carriers and non-carriers *(81)*.

The role of factor V Leiden in arterial disease has been studied with inconsistent findings. In most studies, factor V Leiden was not associated with arterial disease *(82–88)*. However, an occasional study has shown a slightly increased risk for arterial thrombotic disease with factor V Leiden *(89)* or reported a positive association in highly selected populations, such as women younger than 45 yr old who smoke *(90)*. Most investigators conclude that factor V Leiden does not affect ischemic heart disease or stroke, except for in highly selected subgroups of patients in the presence of other arterial risk factors.

The diagnosis of factor V Leiden is made either by genetic testing or by the functional coagulation test called the APC resistance assay. The sensitivity of the assay varies, depending on the test kit and the APC ratio cut-off used *(91,92)* and can be as high as 97.1% *(91)*. Depending on the APC resistance assay used and the population studied, up to 37% of patients with an abnormal APC resistance test do not have factor V Leiden *(93)*. An abnormal APC resistance test should always be followed by genetic testing because other conditions, such as a lupus anticoagulant, can cause an abnormal result *(92)*.

Factor V HR2 Haplotype

An HR2 haplotype of factor V has been described, which includes a 4070A→G polymorphism in exon 13 of the factor V gene, replacing His (R1 allele) by Arg (R2 allele) at position 1299 of the B domain *(94)*. Because the HR2 haplotype was associated with decreased plasma factor V levels, this haplotype was suspected to increase the

risk of thrombosis if factor V Leiden was also present (i.e., if a patient was double heterozygous) *(94)*. The findings of several case-control studies have been conflicting on whether the HR2 haplotype increases the risk of venous thrombosis, either by itself or in combination with factor V Leiden *(95–97)*. A recent large prospective study found that homozygosity for the HR2 haplotype is rare but may be a risk factor for venous thrombosis *(98)*. Although the heterozygous HR2 haplotype is not a risk factor for venous thrombosis, patients who are double heterozygous for HR2 and factor V Leiden have a higher risk of venous thrombosis than those with factor V Leiden alone *(98)*. The HR2 haplotype is not associated with an increased risk of myocardial infarction *(99)*.

Factor V Cambridge

A G1091C factor V polymorphism leading to an Arg306Thr substitution is referred to as factor V Cambridge and has been associated with APC resistance in one report *(100)*. In a study of 104 patients with venous thromboembolism and 208 controls without thrombosis, factor V Cambridge was found in only one control participant *(101)*. These limited data suggest that factor V Cambridge may not be a risk factor for venous thromboembolism.

Factor V Hong-Kong

A polymorphism in the factor V gene (A1090G) results in an Arg306Gly substitution and is referred to as factor V Hong-Kong *(102)*. In one report, factor V Hong-Kong was not associated with APC resistance *(102)*. In a small study of 43 Chinese patients with venous thromboembolism and 40 controls without thromboembolism, factor V Hong-Kong was found in 4.7% of thromboembolic patients and 2.5% of controls *(102)*. The data are too few to assess whether this polymorphism is a risk factor for venous thromboembolism in Chinese patients. However, because of its rarity in Caucasians, this polymorphism is not an epidemiologically important risk factor in that group *(101)*.

PROTHROMBIN (FACTOR II)

Prothrombin is a 579 amino acid glycoprotein that circulates in plasma as a zymogen. During the final stages of the blood coagulation process, prothrombin is converted to thrombin by the cleavage of an internal Arg-271-Thr peptide bond. This reaction is catalyzed by factor Xa in the presence of factor Va, calcium ions, and phospholipids. A complex of these components is called the prothrombinase complex.

A G to A substitution at nucleotide position 20210 in the 3′ untranslated end of the prothrombin gene is common *(104)*. Individuals who are heterozygous for this polymorphism have slightly higher levels of circulating prothrombin and are at a 2.8-fold increased risk for venous thromboembolism over those who are homozygous for the wild type *(104)*. The overall prevalence of heterozygous II20210 is 2% in Caucasians, 3% in southern Europeans, and 1.7% in northern Europeans *(105)*. The prothrombin variant is rare in individuals of Asian and African descent and in African-Americans, of whom 0.3% are heterozygous for the prothrombin 20201 mutation *(106)*. The homozygous prothrombin 20210 mutation is uncommon, occurring in approx 1 in 10,000 individuals, and fewer than 50 cases have been reported *(107)*. Several homozygous individuals had venous thromboses and several were asymptomatic; however, the small number of reported cases precludes a solid risk assessment.

The prothrombin 20210 mutation has not been associated with arterial thrombotic disease in most studies *(86,88,108,109)*. However, some studies have shown an association in selected subgroups, such as patients with premature atherosclerotic disease who have had a myocardial infarction or who have major cardiovascular risk factors *(110,111)*.

PROTEIN S

Protein S, first isolated and characterized from human plasma in 1977 *(112)*, is a vitamin K-dependent, 635 amino acid single-chain glycoprotein *(113)*. "S" stands for Seattle, where the discovery was made *(112)*. Forty percent of protein S is found in a free form and the remaining 60% in a complex with C4b-binding protein *(114)*. Only free protein S functions as a cofactor of APC in the inactivation of factor Va and VIIIa. Protein S can be cleaved by thrombin, which inactivates protein S cofactor activity *(115)*.

Protein S deficiency, an autosomal dominant disorder, was first described in 1984 *(116–118)*. A database of protein S gene mutations comprising 131 different mutations that cause protein S deficiency has been published *(119,120)*. Severe protein S deficiency caused by homozygous or double heterozygous mutations leads to severe neonatal purpura fulminans and death *(121)*.

Three types of protein S deficiency have been identified. Type I, a quantitative deficiency, is characterized by decreased levels of both free and total protein S antigens. In type II deficiency, which is a qualitative defect caused by a dysfunctional protein, protein S activity is low, but free and total antigen levels are normal. In type III deficiency, another quantitative defect, free protein S antigen levels are low, but the total antigen level is normal. Type III deficiency reflects either a high concentration of C4b-binding

protein in plasma or an abnormal binding of protein S to this carrier protein. Most mutations (about 93%) lead to a quantitative deficiency, either type I or type III.

The prevalence of inherited protein S deficiency in the general population varies between 0.03% and 0.13% *(122)*; however, the true prevalence is unknown because of diagnostic difficulties *(123)*. In addition, protein S deficiency occurs as an acquired condition in the setting of oral contraceptive use, pregnancy, liver disease, nephrotic syndrome, disseminated intravascular coagulation, and therapy with vitamin K antagonists *(122,124–128)*. Inherited protein S deficiency cannot be diagnosed in these circumstances until the underlying condition is corrected.

Inherited protein S deficiency predisposes mainly to venous thromboembolism *(129)*. Arterial thromboembolism has been reported *(130–132)*, but a true association has not been shown. Inherited protein S deficiency increases the risk of venous thromboembolism 2.4- to 11.5-fold *(129,133–135)*. Some investigators have not found an increased risk of thrombosis in individuals with inherited protein S deficiency *(123,136)*. The clinical phenotype of patients with protein S deficiency is clearly heterogeneous, a fact that should be considered when making decisions on anticoagulant treatment and family counseling.

The presence of free and bound protein S in plasma makes the diagnosis of protein S deficiency difficult. The most useful measurement or reference range for diagnosing this deficiency has not been identified. The diagnosis is further complicated by an overlap of protein S levels in normal and heterozygous protein S-deficient individuals and by fluctuations in protein S levels over time. Furthermore, age, sex, pregnancy, and hormonal status affect protein S levels *(123)*. A reliable test for quantitative protein S deficiency is the determination of free protein S antigen levels *(134,135)*. However, type II protein S deficiency will be missed when antigen levels alone are determined. If only activity is determined, some patients with quantitative and qualitative protein S deficiency may not be diagnosed because some activity assays give false normal results *(137)*. Therefore, both functional testing (protein S activity) and immunologic testing (free and total protein S antigen) should be conducted in the evaluation of protein S deficiency.

PROTEIN C

Protein C is a 461-amino-acid, vitamin K–dependent glycoprotein that circulates in the blood as a precursor to a serine protease. Protein C is converted to APC by the thrombin:thrombomodulin complex on endothelial cells. APC is a serine protease that acts as a natural anticoagulant.

Together with protein S as a cofactor, APC inactivates factor Va and factor VIIIa by proteolytic cleavage, rendering them incapable of acting as cofactors in the activation of factor X and prothrombin. Thus, protein C regulates the tenase and prothrombinase complexes.

Protein C deficiency as a cause of thromboembolism was first described in 1981 *(138)*. Type I deficiency is a quantitative deficiency with low functional protein C (activity) and immunologic (antigen) levels, whereas type II is a qualitative deficiency with low activity but normal antigen levels. Type II varieties include defects in activation of protein C by the thrombin:thrombomodulin complex; abnormal binding to thrombomodulin, calcium, or phospholipid; and defective protease activity against factor Va or factor VIIIa. Of the reported cases, about 85% have type I deficiency and 15% type II. A database of the more than 160 mutations causing protein C defiency is available on the Internet but the site has not been updated since 1994 *(139,140)*.

The prevalence of inherited protein C deficiency in the general population is about one in 500 to 600 *(141,142)*. Like deficiency of antithrombin and protein S, protein C deficiency is a risk factor mainly for venous thromboembolism *(143,144)*. A few cases of arterial thromboembolism have been reported in patients with protein C deficiency *(145,146)*, and one study showed that congenital protein C deficiency contributes to earlier onset of arterial occlusive diseases, especially acute myocardial infarction *(142)*. However, a causative relationship with arterial thrombosis was not found in other studies *(143)*.

The degree of risk for venous thrombosis associated with protein C deficiency varies, as with protein S deficiency. The risk of venous thromboembolism increases 3.8-fold when protein C deficiency is diagnosed by repeatedly low protein C activity and 6.5-fold when a protein C gene mutation is identified *(136)*. Homozygous protein C deficiency is associated with catastrophic thrombotic complications at birth, manifested by purpura fulminans. When testing a patient for protein C deficiency, a protein C functional (activity) test should always be performed because obtaining only antigen levels will miss type II deficiencies.

ANTITHROMBIN

Antithrombin, a 432-amino-acid, single-chain glycoprotein, is a member of a superfamily of proteins known as serine proteinase inhibitors (serpins) and is the most important natural anticoagulant and inhibitor of thrombin. Inhibition of proteinases by antithrombin involves the active site of the proteinase binding to the reactive center of antithrombin, which inactives the proteinase-inhibitor complex. In addition, antithrombin has a binding site for heparin and similar glycosaminoglycans. Binding of heparin to the latter site induces a conformational change of antithrombin that accelerates the inhibition of proteinases.

First described in 1965 *(147)*, antithrombin deficiency is inherited as an autosomal dominant trait and has an incidence in the general population of 1:500 to 1:600 *(148,149)*. Antithrombin deficiency is classified as type I when both functional and immunological levels are low or as type II when a dysfunctional protein leads to low activity but normal antigen levels. Patients with heterozygous antithrombin deficiency usually have about half the normal level of antithrombin activity. Several cases of homozygous deficiency have been described *(150)*.

Most of the many mutations that cause antithrombin deficiency have been identified in families with thrombophilia *(150,151)*, and information on these mutations is available on the Internet at www.med.ic.ac.uk/divisions/7/antithrombin. Type I deficiency can be caused by a variety of point mutations, small insertions, and partial and whole gene deletions. Type II deficiency is caused by reactive site defects, mutations in the heparin binding site, and mutations with pleiotropic effects. Some antithrombin mutations lead to increased binding of heparin to antithrombin and others to decreased binding, resulting in clinically relevant heparin sensitivity or heparin resistance *(150)*.

Antithrombin deficiency is often considered a strong risk factor for venous thrombosis but is rarely associated with arterial thrombosis, although it has been reported *(152,153)*. The occurrence of symptomatic venous thrombosis in individuals with inherited antithrombin deficiency varies significantly. Some studies report that venous thrombosis develops in about half of antithrombin-deficient individuals before the age of 30 *(154)*, whereas the risk is lower in other studies, with only 23.5% of antithrombin-deficient individuals developing a thrombosis during their lifetime *(155)*. The decision to start anticoagulation in an individual with antithrombin deficiency who has never had a clot should be made on an individual basis, as do decisions on length of anticoagulant treatment in a patient with antithrombin deficiency who has had a thrombosis. Antithrombin deficiency, a less common thrombophilia, is found in approx 1.1% of patients with a first venous thrombotic event *(136,156)*.

The following factors should be considered when diagnosing antithrombin deficiency: (1) antithrombin levels can be decreased at the time of an acute clot or during heparin therapy; (2) liver synthetic dysfunction and nephrotic syndrome can lead to low antithrombin levels; and *(3)* specific reference ranges that consider age, sex, and use of oral contraceptives should be used *(157)*. Some patients were probably mistakenly diagnosed as antithrombin-deficient because antithrombin levels were tested at the time of the acute clot or during heparin therapy.

ANTIPHOSPHOLIPID ANTIBODIES

Antiphospholipid antibodies (APLA) are acquired antibodies against phospholipids or phospholipid-binding proteins, such as β-2-glycoprotein-I (β-2-GPI) and prothrombin. APLA have been associated with arterial or venous thrombosis and spontaneous pregnancy loss *(158,159)*. The mechanisms of thrombosis are highly heterogeneous and multifactorial and include the following *(160)*: (1) interference with the protein C pathway by antibody-binding to protein C or inhibition of the activation of protein C; (2) inhibition of tissue factor pathway inhibitor; (3) interference with plasminogen activation and fibrinolysis; (4) promotion of tissue factor synthesis and exposure; (5) endothelial injury; (6) induction of apoptosis on vascular cells; (7) activation *(161)* or agglutination *(162)* of platelets; and (8) disruption of the annexin-V anticoagulant shield in the placenta *(160)*.

APLA syndrome is defined as the occurrence of thrombosis (arterial or venous) or recurrent pregnancy loss in patients with repeatedly positive APLA antibody tests (lupus anticoagulant and/or at least moderately increased IgG or IgM anticardiolipin antibodies) *(163)*. APLA syndrome can be a primary syndrome not associated with any other diseases, or a secondary syndrome associated with autoimmune diseases, malignancy, or drugs. Patients who have developed a thrombosis are at high risk for recurrence, and indefinite anticoagulation is often indicated after one episode of venous or arterial thromboembolism *(164)*. The optimal oral anticoagulation level has been debated, and the international normalized ratio is invalid in some patients on oral anticoagulants because of a lupus anticoagulant effect on the ratio *(165)*. Alternative tests, such as chromogenic or clot-based factor II or X activity, to measure the oral anticoagulant effect are indicated in these patients *(165)*. Individual treatment decisions should be made with the help of a thrombophilia specialist.

Familial clustering of increased APLA levels has been described *(166)*, but the characterization of the APLA syndrome, coexisting autoimmune diseases, and clinical complications has been heterogeneous. Genetic factors may be involved in the pathophysiology of the APLA syndrome *(167)*. In studies of the genetic variants of β-2-GPI, the valine/leucine247 polymorphism has been identified as a genetic marker for having anti-β-2-GPI antibodies and APLA syndrome *(168)*.

FACTOR XIII

Factor XIII stabilizes the fibrin clot. Thrombin activates the proenzyme factor XIII to the enzyme factor XIIIa, which catalyzes the formation of intermolecular ε-(γ-glutamyl) lysine bonds between various proteins, such as fibrin monomers, fibronectin, α_2 plasmin inhibitor, and collagen. These reactions increase the mechanical strength, elasticity, and resistance to degradation by plasmin and promote wound healing *(169)*. Factor XIII deficiency leads to a bleeding disorder and wound healing problems.

Factor XIII, with a molecular weight of 320 kDa, is a heterotetramer that comprises two A-subunits and two B-subunits (A_2B_2) *(169)* held together by noncovalent bonds. The A-subunit contains the catalytic site, whereas the B-subunit appears to protect or stabilize the A-subunit. Several factor XIII polymorphisms have been identified in the gene encoding the A-subunit. The Val34Leu polymorphism is of relevance for thrombophilia because several studies have shown that the Leu34 polymorphism is associated with a decreased risk of occlusive arterial disease such as myocardial infarction *(170–172)*, thrombotic cerebral artery occlusion *(173,174)*, and venous thromboembolism *(175,176)*. However, findings have not been consistent, and some studies did not show an association with arterial *(177–179)* or venous thrombotic disease *(179–181)*.

Val34Leu resides just three amino acids upstream of the thrombin cleavage site of the factor XIII A-subunit at Arg37-Gly38. The 34Leu allele is cleaved more rapidly and by lower doses of thrombin than 34Val *(182,183)*, which affects the structure of the cross-linked fibrin clot and produces a finer meshwork, thinner fibers, and altered permeation characteristics *(182)*. This finding supports the protective role of 34Leu polymorphism against thrombosis. However, the biochemical consequences of the 34Leu polymorphism are not fully understood, and the finding that factor XIII 34Val and factor XIII 34Leu have the same mean specific factor XIII activity in plasma *(180)* can be used to argue against an association of the polymorphism with thrombosis. Thus, the association of the Val34Leu polymorphism with arterial or venous thrombosis is not clear cut.

PLATELET MEMBRANE GLYCOPROTEINS

Membrane glycoproteins play a fundamental role in platelet adhesion and aggregation. Integrins are membrane glycoprotein heterodimers composed of noncovalently associated α and β transmembrane subunits. Several integrins have been defined on human platelets, including α_{IIb}/β_3 (also known as GP IIb/IIIa or fibrinogen receptor), α_2/β_1 (GP Ia/IIa or collagen receptor), α_5/β_1 (fibronectin receptor), and α_6/β_1 (laminin receptor). Several polymorphisms of platelet membrane glycoproteins have been described and have been identified in some studies as risk factors for arterial thrombotic events. However, findings have not been consistent, and no polymorphism has been unequivocally found to predispose to arterial thrombosis. No studies suggest that the polymorphisms are associated with venous thromboembolism.

Glycoprotein IIb/IIIa Complex

Glycoprotein IIb (integrin α_{IIb}) is a 150 kDa protein that associates with the 90 kDa protein glycoprotein IIIa (integrin β_3) to form the covalent heterodimer glycoprotein IIb/IIIa (GP IIb/IIIa), also known as integrin α_{IIb}/β_3. GP IIb/IIIa is anchored in the platelet membrane, is the most abundant glycoprotein on the platelet surface, and is abundant in platelet α granules. Platelet activation leads to (1) translocation of GP IIb/IIIa from within the platelet to the surface, increasing the receptor surface density by 30–50%, from approx 40,000 to nearly 80,000 molecules per platelet (184) and (2) a conformational change of GP IIb/IIIa that markedly increases ligand binding affinity (185). The major ligand for GP IIb/IIIa is fibrinogen, which binds to the receptor via the C-terminal 12 residues of the γ chain (H12). In addition, GP IIb/IIIa binds von Willebrand factor, fibronectin, vitronectin, and thrombospondin; all of these adhesive molecules contain the Arg-Gly-Asp (RGD) sequence, which is the minimal recognition sequence for the receptor.

A point mutation in GP IIIa results in a substitution of Leu to Pro at position 33 (31). The Leu wild type is called the Pl^{A1}, and the Pro polymorphism is the Pl^{A2}. About 85% of individuals of Northern European ancestry are homozygous for Pl^{A1}, 13% carry Pl^{A1} and Pl^{A2}, and 2% are homozygous for Pl^{A2} (186). The Pl^A polymorphism is located near the ligand-binding pocket of GP IIb/IIIa (187,188) but does not appear to affect fibrinogen binding. Pl^{A2} platelets have a lower threshold for activation, although the reason is unknown (189). This finding may suggest that individuals with the Pl^{A2} polymorphism have a higher risk for thrombotic disease; however, clinical data supporting this assumption have been inconsistent.

Although initial studies indicated that Pl^{A2} is a risk factor for acute coronary thrombosis (87,190,191), several large studies did not confirm this association (192, 193). Furthermore, a meta-analysis showed that the Pl polymorphism was not associated with an increased risk of myocardial infarction, either overall or in selected subgroups, such as patients with premature disease onset (age ≤ 60 yr), patients with a first acute myocardial infarction, male patients, female patients, and Caucasian patients (194). The data on whether the Pl^{A2} polymorphism leads to higher risk of in-stent thrombosis or restenosis after coronary stent placement are inconsistent; some studies show an association (195,196), and others do not (197,198).

Recent studies indicate that the response to antiplatelet drugs varies, depending on which Pl^A allele is present. Heterozygous Pl^A platelets are more sensitive to inhibition of aggregation by pharmacologically relevant concentrations of aspirin (189). The findings on the response to the GP IIb/IIIa antagonist abciximab have been inconsistent: increased sensitivity of heterozygous Pl^A platelets in one study (189) and decreased sensitivity in another (199).

Glycoprotein Ib/IX/V Complex

The glycoprotein Ib/IX/V complex (GP Ib/IX/V) is the platelet receptor for von Willebrand factor and mediates binding to collagen (200). The receptor comprises four gene products: GP Ibα, GP Ibβ, GP IX, and GP V.

Three polymorphisms in the GP Ibα gene are possibly associated with thrombotic disease. One is a 39 bp variable nucleotide tandem repeat (VNTR) for a 13-amino-acid repeat (201), with up to four polymorphic forms with one, two, three, or four repeats. These repeats affect the length of the extracellular domain of GP Ib, which affects the distance between the von Willebrand factor binding domain and the platelet surface. It is not known whether this influences platelet function. This hypervariable region is linked to a Thr145 Met substitution of uncertain consequences for platelet function (202). The third polymorphism, –5T/C, was reported as a determinant of the membrane levels of the GP Ib/IX/V complex in one study (203), but not in another (204). An association of these polymorphisms with cardiac or cerebral arterial thrombotic disease has not been established (31). In two studies, the 39 bp VNTR/Thr145Met polymorphisms were associated with coronary artery disease (205,206), but the association was not seen in three studies (87,204,207). The GP Ibα polymorphisms were associated with cerebrovascular disease in several studies (206,208) but not in one (204,209).

Glycoprotein Ia/IIa Complex

The glycoprotein Ia/IIa complex (GP Ia/IIa; α_2/β_1 integrin) is a major collagen receptor on platelets. The ability of platelets to adhere to collagen varies among individuals because of the wide variation in expression of GP Ia/IIa on platelets (210). A silent polymorphism at position 807

(C to T) of the α_2 gene, which does not change the sequence of GP Ia, is associated with variation in GP Ia/IIa receptor density *(211)*. Carriers of the 807 T allele express higher levels of GP Ia/IIa. The T-allele has been associated with myocardial infarction *(212)* and acute coronary syndrome *(213)* in some studies but not in all *(214,215)*.

TISSUE PLASMINOGEN ACTIVATOR

Tissue plasminogen activator (tPA) is a 68 kDa serine protease that is synthesized mainly in endothelial cells but also in many different tissues. One of two physiologic plasminogen activators, tPA (the other is urokinase) is usually found in a complex with its primary inhibitor, plasminogen activator inhibitor-1 (PAI-1). Paradoxically, increased levels of tPA are a risk factor for future arterial occlusive events *(216,217)*. This finding may be due to the fact that increased tPA levels reflect preexisting disease or because of increased PAI-1 levels, which form an inactive complex with tPA. Several polymorphisms for the tPA gene have been described. An Alu insertion/deletion within the intron between the exons 8 and 9 *(218)* has been associated with an increased risk of myocardial infarction in one study *(219)* but not in another *(220)*.

PLASMINOGEN

Plasminogen is a single-chain glycoprotein produced primarily in the liver. Cleavage of plasminogen by tPA, urokinase, and streptokinase forms the active serine protease, plasmin. Fibrin-bound plasmin degrades fibrin *(7)*.

The first case of hereditary plasminogen deficiency was published in 1978 *(221)*, followed by several hundred reports of cases. Type I plasminogen deficiency is a quantitative deficiency of both activity and antigen, whereas type II is a qualitative defect (dysplasminogenemia) with low activity but normal antigen levels. At least 11 different mutations lead to plasminogen deficiency, but whether the heterozygous presence of a mutant gene is associated with an increased risk of thromboembolism is unknown. The prevalence of familial plasminogen deficiency in the general population may be as high as 2.9/1000 *(222)*. Several studies indicate that heterozygous plasminogen deficiency is not a risk factor for thrombosis *(222–224)*, but others suggest it is a mild risk factor for venous thromboembolism *(225)*. Plasminogen deficiency is not a risk factor for arterial thromboembolic disease.

PLASMINOGEN ACTIVATOR INHIBITOR-1

Produced mainly by endothelial cells and adipocytes, PAI-1, a 52 kDa glycoprotein, may also be produced by monocytes, hepatocytes, smooth muscle cells, and megakaryocytes *(226)*. In human blood, platelets are the major pool of PAI-1, which is the main inhibitor of tPA. Diurnal variation is seen in PAI-1 plasma antigen levels. Because of significant intra- and interindividual variation, assays for PAI-1 in individual patients cannot be usefully interpreted. The concentration of PAI-1 in atheromatous plaque is high. Increased PAI-1 levels have been associated with coronary artery disease and myocardial infarction in many studies *(227)*, but statistical significance is often lost after adjustment for other risk factors. This may be due to the fact that many metabolic changes, such as those seen in the insulin resistance syndrome and diabetes, affect PAI-1 levels *(227)*. The increased risk of arterial disease associated with hyperinsulinemia may be partially mediated through increased PAI-1 levels.

Several PAI-1 polymorphisms have been described, including a 4G/5G insertion/deletion –675 bp from the start of the promoter *(31)* and a HindIII site at the 3′ region of the gene *(228)*. These polymorphisms may affect PAI-1 plasma levels, but this finding has not been consistent *(30)*. Furthermore, the impact of polymorphisms on the heritability of PAI-1 levels is small *(229)*. Although some studies have suggested an association between the 4G/5G polymorphism and cardiac and cerebrovascular ischemic disease, other well-designed studies have not. In a recent summary of all studies, PAI-1 genotype does not appear to play an important role in ischemic heart disease *(31)*. An association between the 4G/5G polymorphism and venous thromboembolic disease has been found but not consistently *(230,231)*.

CLINICAL IMPLICATIONS

Medical practitioners have not reached a consensus on the extent of laboratory work-up for thrombophilia in patients with thrombosis and on the criteria for selecting which patients and asymptomatic family members should be tested for thrombophilia. Both sides can be argued, and the importance of testing is weighed differently by individual healthcare providers, by patients, and by healthcare politicians.

Physicians may want a patient to undergo testing for thrombophilia because the results may (1) influence the decision to initiate prophylactic anticoagulant treatment, the choice of drug, or the length of treatment after an episode of thrombosis, (2) help explain why a patient developed a thrombosis, and (3) help in counseling a patient about the future risk of thrombosis. Patients may want to get tested (1) to understand why a clot developed, (2) to be encouraged to make lifestyle changes that may

Table 2
Laboratory Coagulation Workup for Thrombophilia

Arterial Thromboembolism

  Protein C activity

  Protein S activity, free and total protein S antigen

  Antithrombin activity

  Anticardiolipin IgG and IgM antibodies

  Lupus anticoagulant[a]

  Fibrinogen activity

  Factor VIII activity

  Homocysteine level

Venous Thromboembolism

  Factor V Leiden

  Factor V HR2 haplotype (in patients who have factor V Leiden)

  Prothrombin 20210 mutation

  Protein C activity

  Protein S activity, free and total protein S antigen

  Antithrombin activity

  Anticardiolipin IgG and IgM antibodies

  Lupus anticoagulant[a]

  Fibrinogen activity

  Factor VIII activity

  Factor IX activity

  Factor XI activity

  Homocysteine level

[a]Two different tests should be used (i.e., dilute Russell viper venom time, lupus-sensitive aPTT, kaolin clotting time) because of the heterogeneity of lupus anticoagulants.

decrease the risk of thrombosis, and (3) to be able to inform healthcare providers of the thrombophilia to receive better prophylaxis for thrombosis. Reasons to decide against thrombophilia testing include (1) the lack of therapeutic consequences if the result is abnormal, (2) the risk of misinterpretation of a test result by the healthcare provider and of incorrect or debatable medical advice, (3) the risk of increased costs for health or life insurance premiums or of being denied insurance, (4) the possibility that paternity may have to be questioned if the inheritance pattern is inconsistent with test results of other family members, and (5) the expense of testing.

Tests that might be considered in the work-up of patients suspected of having thrombophilia are listed in (Table 2). However, the need and extent of testing for thrombophilia should be assessed on an individual basis. In conducting tests for thrombophilia, the physician is responsible for ensuring that patients and their families are counseled about the implications of positive or negative test results and educated about the thrombophilia. Availability of a genetic counselor, a specialized thrombophilia clinic, and patient education materials is important. Although some patient education tools are available *(232,233)*, better and more widely available education materials are needed.

CONCLUSIONS

Significant progress has been made in the understanding of physiologic hemostasis and in the identification of laboratory risk factors (inherited or acquired) predisposing to arterial or venous thrombosis. The identification of these risk factors will allow differentiated approaches in the management of patients with identified thrombophilia regarding (1) prediction of the likelihood of future thrombotic events, (2) modification of thrombosis risk factors, (3) use of anticoagulation prophylaxis in thrombosis risk situations, (4) length of anticoagulant treatment in patients with thrombosis, and (5) recommendations for family screening. This type of patient management is particularly applicable for venous thromboembolism because of the identification of the factor V Leiden and the prothrombin 20210 polymorphisms. Less impressive clinical consequences have been achieved in the identification of thrombophilic abnormalities predisposing to arterial thrombotic disease. Although some coagulation abnormalities help clinicians to stratify the risk in patients with arterial disease, the studies of the associations of various polymorphisms with arterial thrombosis have not been conclusive. A meaningful use of these polymorphisms in clinical decision-making is at present not possible.

REFERENCES

1. Kjalke M, Monroe DM, Hoffman M, Oliver JA, Ezban M, Roberts HR. Active site-inactivated factors VIIa, Xa, and IXa inhibit individual steps in a cell-based model of tissue factor-initiated coagulation. Thromb Haemost 1998;80:578–584.

2. Hoffman M, Monroe DM 3rd. A cell-based model of hemostasis. Thromb Haemost 2001;85:958–965.

3. Kumar R, Beguin S, Hemker HC. The effect of fibrin clots and clot-bound thrombin on the development of platelet procoagulant activity. Thromb Haemost 1995;74:962–968.

4. Baglia FA, Walsh PN. Thrombin-mediated feedback activation of factor XI on the activated platelet surface is preferred over contact activation by factor XIIa or factor XIa. J Biol Chem 2000;275:20514–20519.

5. Mohri M, Sugimoto E, Sata M, Asano T. The inhibitory effect of recombinant human soluble thrombomodulin on initiation and extension of coagulation—a comparison with other anticoagulants. Thromb Haemost 1999;82:1687–1693.

6. Levin EG, Marzec U, Anderson J, Harker LA. Thrombin stimulates tissue plasminogen activator release from cultured human endothelial cells. J Clin Invest 1984;74:1988–1995.

7. Francis CW, Marder VJ. Physiologic regulation and pathologic disorders of fibrinolysis. In: Colman RW, Hirsh J, Marder VJ, Clowes AW, George JN, eds. Hemostasis and Thrombosis: Basic Principles and Clinical Practice. Philadelphia: Lippincott, Williams & Wilkins; 2001:975–1002.

8. Falk E, Shah PK, Fuster V. Coronary plaque disruption. Circulation 1995;92:657–671.

9. Moreno PR, Bernardi VH, Lopez-Cuellar J, et al. Macrophages, smooth muscle cells, and tissue factor in unstable angina. Implications for cell-mediated thrombogenicity in acute coronary syndromes. Circulation 1996;94:3090–3097.

10. Ardissino D, Merlini PA, Bauer KA, et al. Thrombogenic potential of human coronary atherosclerotic plaques. Blood 2001;98:2726–2729.

11. Rapp JH, Pan XM, Ghermay A, Gazetas P, Brady SE, Reilly LM. A blinded trial of local recombinant tissue factor pathway inhibitor versus either local or systemic heparin in a vein bypass model. J Vasc Surg 1997;25:726–729.

12. Arnljots B, Soderstrom T, Ezban M, Hedner U. Effect of locally-applied active site-blocked activated factor VII (ASIS) on experimental arterial thrombosis. Blood Coagul Fibrinolysis 2000;11:S145–S148.

13. Soderstrom T, Hedner U, Arnljots B. Active site-inactivated factor VIIa prevents thrombosis without increased surgical bleeding: topical and intravenous administration in a rat model of deep arterial injury. J Vasc Surg 2001;33:1072–1079.

14. Lundell A, Kelly AB, Anderson J, et al. Reduction in vascular lesion formation by hirudin secreted from retrovirus-transduced confluent endothelial cells on vascular grafts in baboons. Circulation 1999;100:2018–2024.

15. Atsuchi N, Nishida T, Marutsuka K, et al. Combination of a brief irrigation with tissue factor pathway inhibitor (TFPI) and adenovirus-mediated local TFPI gene transfer additively reduces neointima formation in balloon-injured rabbit carotid arteries. Circulation 2001;103:570–575.

16. Zoldhelyi P, Chen ZQ, Shelat HS, McNatt JM, Willerson JT. Local gene transfer of tissue factor pathway inhibitor regulates intimal hyperplasia in atherosclerotic arteries. Proc Nat Acad Scie U S A 2001;98:4078–4083.

17. Zoldhelyi P, McNatt J, Xu XM, et al. Prevention of arterial thrombosis by adenovirus-mediated transfer of cyclooxygenase gene. Circulation 1996;93:10–17.

18. Zoldhelyi P, Beck PJ, Bjercke RJ, et al. Inhibition of coronary thrombosis and local inflammation by a noncarbohydrate selectin inhibitor. Am J Physiol Heart Circ Physiol 2000;279:H3065–H3075.

19. Chung DW, Harris JE, Davie EW. Nucleotide sequences of the three genes encoding for human fibrinogen. In: Liu CY, Chien S, eds. Fibrinogen, Thrombosis, Coagulation, and Fibrinolysis (Advances in Experimental Medicine and Biology, 281). New York: Plenum; 1991:39–48.

20. Greenberg DL, Davie EW. Blood coagulation factors: their complementary DNAs, genes, and expression. In: Colman RW, Hirsh J, Marder VJ, Clowes AW, George JN, eds. Hemostasis and Thrombosis: Basic Principles and Clinical Practice. Philadelphia: Lippincott, Williams & Wilkins; 2001:21–58.

21. Hu CH, Harris JE, Davie EW, Chung DW. Characterization of the 5′-flanking region of the gene for the alpha chain of human fibrinogen. J Biol Chem 1995;270:28342–28349.

22. Meade TW, Mellows S, Brozovic M, et al. Haemostatic function and ischaemic heart disease: principal results of the Northwick Park Heart Study. Lancet 1986;2:533–537.

23. Meade TW, Ruddock V, Stirling Y, Chakrabarti R, Miller GJ. Fibrinolytic activity, clotting factors, and long-term incidence of ischaemic heart disease in the Northwick Park Heart Study. Lancet 1993;342:1076–1079.

24. Ma J, Hennekens CH, Ridker PM, Stampfer MJ. A prospective study of fibrinogen and risk of myocardial infarction in the Physicians' Health Study. J Am Coll Cardiol 1999;33:1347–1352.

25. Wilhelmsen L, Svardsudd K, Korsan-Bengtsen K, Larsson B, Welin L, Tibblin G. Fibrinogen as a risk factor for stroke and myocardial infarction. N Engl J Med 1984;311:501–505.

26. Banerjee AK, Pearson J, Gilliland EL, et al. A six year prospective study of fibrinogen and other risk factors associated with mortality in stable claudicants. Thromb Haemost 1992;68:261–263.

27. Feng D, Lindpaintner K, Larson MG, et al. Platelet glycoprotein IIIa Pl(a) polymorphism, fibrinogen, and platelet aggregability: The Framingham Heart Study. Circulation 2001;104:140–144.

28. Tracy RP. Epidemiological evidence for inflammation in cardiovascular disease. Thromb Haemost 1999;82:826–831.

29. van't Hooft FM, von Bahr SJ, Silveira A, Iliadou A, Eriksson P, Hamsten A. Two common, functional polymorphisms in the promoter region of the beta-fibrinogen gene contribute to regulation of plasma fibrinogen concentration. Arterioscler Thromb Vasc Biol 1999;19:3063–3070.

30. Lane DA, Grant PJ. Role of hemostatic gene polymorphisms in venous and arterial thrombotic disease. Blood 2000;95: 1517–1532.

31. Simmonds RE, Hermida J, Rezende SM, Lane DA. Haemostatic genetic risk factors in arterial thrombosis. Thromb Haemost 2001;86:374–385.

32. Lee AJ, Fowkes FG, Lowe GD, Connor JM, Rumley A. Fibrinogen, factor VII and PAI-1 genotypes and the risk of coronary and peripheral atherosclerosis: Edinburgh Artery Study. Thromb Haemost 1999;81:553–560.

33. de Maat MP, Kastelein JJ, Jukema JW, et al. –455G/A polymorphism of the beta-fibrinogen gene is associated with the progression of coronary atherosclerosis in symptomatic men: proposed role for an acute-phase reaction pattern of fibrinogen. REGRESS group. Arterioscler Thromb Vasc Biol 1998;18:265–271.

34. Tybjaerg-Hansen A, Agerholm-Larsen B, Humphries SE, Abildgaard S, Schnohr P, Nordestgaard BG. A common mutation (G-455—>A) in the beta-fibrinogen promoter is an independent predictor of plasma fibrinogen, but not of ischemic heart disease. A study of 9,127 individuals based on the Copenhagen City Heart Study. J Clin Invest 1997;99:3034–3039.

35. Doggen CJ, Bertina RM, Cats VM, Rosendaal FR. Fibrinogen polymorphisms are not associated with the risk of myocardial infarction. Br J Haematol 2000;110:935–938.

36. Folsom AR, Aleksic N, Ahn C, Boerwinkle E, Wu KK. Beta-fibrinogen gene –455G/A polymorphism and coronary heart disease incidence: the Atherosclerosis Risk in Communities (ARIC) Study. Ann Epidemiol 2001;11:166–170.

37. Koster T, Rosendaal FR, Reitsma PH, van der Velden PA, Briet E, Vandenbroucke JP. Factor VII and fibrinogen levels as risk factors for venous thrombosis. A case-control study of plasma levels and DNA polymorphisms—the Leiden Thrombophilia Study (LETS). Thromb Haemost 1994;71:719–722.

38. Blake GJ, Schmitz C, Lindpaintner K, Ridker PM. Mutation in the promoter region of the beta-fibrinogen gene and the risk of future myocardial infarction, stroke and venous thrombosis. Eur Heart J 2001;22:2262–2266.

39. Austin H, Hooper WC, Lally C, et al. Venous thrombosis in relation to fibrinogen and factor VII genes among African-Americans. J Clin Epidemiol 2000;53:997–1001.

40. Carter AM, Catto AJ, Kohler HP, Ariens RA, Stickland MH, Grant PJ. alpha-fibrinogen Thr312Ala polymorphism and venous thromboembolism. Blood 2000;96:1177–1179.

41. Haverkate F, Samama M. Familial dysfibrinogenemia and thrombophilia. Report on a study of the SSC Subcommittee on Fibrinogen. Thromb Haemost 1995;73:151–161.

42. Heinrich J, Balleisen L, Schulte H, Assmann G, van de Loo J. Fibrinogen and factor VII in the prediction of coronary risk. Results from the PROCAM study in healthy men. Arterioscler Thromb 1994;14:54–59.

43. Smith FB, Lee AJ, Fowkes FG, Price JF, Rumley A, Lowe GD. Hemostatic factors as predictors of ischemic heart disease and stroke in the Edinburgh Artery Study. Arterioscler Thromb Vasc Biol 1997;17:3321–3325.

44. Lane A, Green F, Scarabin PY, et al. Factor VII Arg/Gln353 polymorphism determines factor VII coagulant activity in patients with myocardial infarction (MI) and control subjects in Belfast and in France but is not a strong indicator of MI risk in the ECTIM study. Atherosclerosis 1996;119:119–127.

45. Moor E, Silveira A, van't Hooft F, et al. Coagulation factor VII mass and activity in young men with myocardial infarction at a young age. Role of plasma lipoproteins and factor VII genotype. Arterioscler Thromb Vasc Biol 1995;15:655–664.

46. Danielsen R, Onundarson PT, Thors H, Vidarsson B, Morrissey JH. Activated and total coagulation factor VII, and fibrinogen in coronary artery disease. Scand Cardiovasc J 1998;32:87–95.

47. Bernardi F, Marchetti G, Pinotti M, et al. Factor VII gene polymorphisms contribute about one third of the factor VII level variation in plasma. Arterioscler Thromb Vasc Biol 1996;16: 72–76.

48. Heywood DM, Ossei-Gerning N, Grant PJ. Association of factor VII:C levels with environmental and genetic factors in patients with ischaemic heart disease and coronary atheroma characterised by angiography. Thromb Haemost 1996;76:161–165.

49. Doggen CJ, Manger Cats V, Bertina RM, Reitsma PH, Vandenbroucke JP, Rosendaal FR. A genetic propensity to high factor VII is not associated with the risk of myocardial infarction in men. Thromb Haemost 1998;80:281–285.

50. Iacoviello L, Di Castelnuovo A, De Knijff P, et al. Polymorphisms in the coagulation factor VII gene and the risk of myocardial infarction. N Engl J Med 1998;338:79–85.

51. Girelli D, Russo C, Ferraresi P, et al. Polymorphisms in the factor VII gene and the risk of myocardial infarction in patients with coronary artery disease. N Engl J Med 2000;343:774–780.

52. Heywood DM, Carter AM, Catto AJ, Bamford JM, Grant PJ. Polymorphisms of the factor VII gene and circulating FVII:C levels in relation to acute cerebrovascular disease and post-stroke mortality. Stroke 1997;28:816–821.

53. Tuddenham EGD. Factor VIII. In: High KA, Roberts HR, eds. Molecular Basis of Thrombosis and Hemostasis. New York: Marcel Dekker;1995:167–196.

54. Hollestelle MJ, Thinnes T, Crain K, et al. Tissue distribution of factor VIII gene expression in vivo—a closer look. Thromb Haemost 2001;86:855–861.

55. Meade TW, Cooper JA, Stirling Y, Howarth DJ, Ruddock V, Miller GJ. Factor VIII, ABO blood group and the incidence of ischaemic heart disease. Br J Haematol 1994;88:601–607.

56. Rumley A, Lowe GD, Sweetnam PM, Yarnell JW, Ford RP. Factor VIII, von Willebrand factor and the risk of major ischaemic heart disease in the Caerphilly Heart Study. Br J Haematol 1999;105:110–116.

57. Tracy RP, Arnold AM, Ettinger W, Fried L, Meilahn E, Savage P. The relationship of fibrinogen and factors VII and VIII to incident cardiovascular disease and death in the elderly: results from the cardiovascular health study. Arterioscler Thromb Vasc Biol 1999;19:1776–1783.

58. Folsom AR, Rosamond WD, Shahar E, et al. Prospective study of markers of hemostatic function with risk of ischemic stroke. The Atherosclerosis Risk in Communities (ARIC) Study Investigators. Circulation 1999;100:736–742.

59. Folsom AR. Hemostatic risk factors for atherothrombotic disease: an epidemiologic view. Thromb Haemost 2001;86:366–373.

60. Folsom AR, Wu KK, Rosamond WD, Sharrett AR, Chambless LE. Prospective study of hemostatic factors and incidence of coronary heart disease: the Atherosclerosis Risk in Communities (ARIC) Study. Circulation 1997;96:1102–1108.

61. O'Donnell J, Tuddenham EG, Manning R, Kemball-Cook G, Johnson D, Laffan M. High prevalence of elevated factor VIII levels in patients referred for thrombophilia screening: role of increased synthesis and relationship to the acute phase reaction. Thromb Haemost 1997;77:825–828.

62. Kamphuisen PW, Eikenboom JC, Rosendaal FR, et al. High factor VIII antigen levels increase the risk of venous thrombosis but are not associated with polymorphisms in the von Willebrand factor and factor VIII gene. Br J Haematol 2001; 115:156–158.

63. Kyrle PA, Minar E, Hirschl M, et al. High plasma levels of factor VIII and the risk of recurrent venous thromboembolism. N Engl J Med 2000;343:457–462.

64. Thogersen AM, Jansson JH, Boman K, et al. High plasminogen activator inhibitor and tissue plasminogen activator levels in plasma precede a first acute myocardial infarction in both men and women: evidence for the fibrinolytic system as an independent primary risk factor. Circulation 1998;98:2241–2247.

65. van der Meer FJ, Koster T, Vandenbroucke JP, Briet E, Rosendaal FR. The Leiden Thrombophilia Study (LETS). Thromb Haemost 1997;78:631–635.

66. van Hylckama Vlieg A, van der Linden IK, Bertina RM, Rosendaal FR. High levels of factor IX increase the risk of venous thrombosis. Blood 2000;95:3678–3682.

67. Meijers JC, Tekelenburg WL, Bouma BN, Bertina RM, Rosendaal FR. High levels of coagulation factor XI as a risk factor for venous thrombosis. N Engl J Med 2000;342:696–701.

68. Kalafatis M, Rand MD, Mann KG. The mechanism of inactivation of human factor V and human factor Va by activated protein C. J Biol Chem 1994;269:31869–31880.

69. Nicolaes GA, Tans G, Thomassen MC, et al. Peptide bond cleavages and loss of functional activity during inactivation of factor Va and factor VaR506Q by activated protein C. J Biol Chem 1995;270:21158–21166.

70. Bertina RM, Koeleman BP, Koster T, et al. Mutation in blood coagulation factor V associated with resistance to activated protein C. Nature 1994;369:64–67.

71. Greengard JS, Sun X, Xu X, Fernandez JA, Griffin JH, Evatt B. Activated protein C resistance caused by Arg506Gln mutation in factor Va. Lancet 1994;343:1361–1362.

72. Dahlback B, Carlsson M, Svensson PJ. Familial thrombophilia due to a previously unrecognized mechanism characterized by poor anticoagulant response to activated protein C: prediction of a cofactor to activated protein C. Proc Natl Acad Sci USA 1993;90:1004–1008.

73. Rees DC, Cox M, Clegg JB. World distribution of factor V Leiden. Lancet 1995;346:1133–1134.

74. Ridker PM, Miletich JP, Hennekens CH, Buring JE. Ethnic distribution of factor V Leiden in 4047 men and women. Implications for venous thromboembolism screening. JAMA 1997;277:1305–1307.

75. Zivelin A, Griffin JH, Xu X, et al. A single genetic origin for a common Caucasian risk factor for venous thrombosis. Blood 1997;89:397–402.

76. Rosendaal FR, Koster T, Vandenbroucke JP, Reitsma PH. High risk of thrombosis in patients homozygous for factor V Leiden (activated protein C resistance). Blood 1995;85:1504–1508.

77. Ridker PM, Hennekens CH, Selhub J, Miletich JP, Malinow MR, Stampfer MJ. Interrelation of hyperhomocyst(e)inemia, factor V Leiden, and risk of future venous thromboembolism. Circulation 1997;95:1777–1782.

78. De Stefano V, Martinelli I, Mannucci PM, et al. The risk of recurrent deep venous thrombosis among heterozygous carriers of both factor V Leiden and the G20210A prothrombin mutation. N Engl J Med 1999;341:801–806.

79. Middeldorp S, Meinardi JR, Koopman MM, et al. A prospective study of asymptomatic carriers of the factor V Leiden mutation to determine the incidence of venous thromboembolism. Ann Intern Med 2001;135:322–327.

80. Marchetti M, Pistorio A, Barosi G. Extended anticoagulation for prevention of recurrent venous thromboembolism in carriers of factor V Leiden—cost-effectiveness analysis. Thromb Haemost 2000;84:752–757.

81. Hyers TM, Agnelli G, Hull RD, et al. Antithrombotic therapy for venous thromboembolic disease. Chest 2001;119:176S–193S.

82. Ridker PM, Hennekens CH, Lindpaintner K, Stampfer MJ, Eisenberg PR, Miletich JP. Mutation in the gene coding for coagulation factor V and the risk of myocardial infarction, stroke, and venous thrombosis in apparently healthy men. N Engl J Med 1995;332:912–917.

83. Emmerich J, Poirier O, Evans A, et al. Myocardial infarction, Arg 506 to Gln factor V mutation, and activated protein C resistance. Lancet 1995;345:321.

84. Catto A, Carter A, Ireland H, et al. Factor V Leiden gene mutation and thrombin generation in relation to the development of acute stroke. Arterioscler Thromb Vasc Biol 1995;15:783–785.

85. Cushman M, Rosendaal FR, Psaty BM, et al. Factor V Leiden is not a risk factor for arterial vascular disease in the elderly: results from the Cardiovascular Health Study. Thromb Haemost 1998;79:912–915.

86. Longstreth WT Jr, Rosendaal FR, Siscovick DS, et al. Risk of stroke in young women and two prothrombotic mutations: factor V Leiden and prothrombin gene variant (G20210A). Stroke 1998;29:577–580.

87. Ardissino D, Mannucci PM, Merlini PA, et al. Prothrombotic genetic risk factors in young survivors of myocardial infarction. Blood 1999;94:46–51.

88. Ridker PM, Hennekens CH, Miletich JP. G20210A mutation in prothrombin gene and risk of myocardial infarction, stroke, and venous thrombosis in a large cohort of US men. Circulation 1999;99:999–1004.

89. Doggen CJ, Cats VM, Bertina RM, Rosendaal FR. Interaction of coagulation defects and cardiovascular risk factors: increased risk of myocardial infarction associated with factor V Leiden or prothrombin 20210A. Circulation 1998;97:1037–1041.

90. Rosendaal FR, Siscovick DS, Schwartz SM, et al. Factor V Leiden (resistance to activated protein C) increases the risk of myocardial infarction in young women. Blood 1997;89:2817–2821.

91. Favaloro EJ, Mirochnik O, McDonald D. Functional activated protein C resistance assays: correlation with factor V DNA analysis is better with RVVT-than APTT-based assays. Br J Biomed Sci 1999;56:23–33.

92. Van Cott EM, Soderberg BL, Laposata M. Activated protein C resistance, the factor V Leiden mutation, and a laboratory testing algorithm. Arch Pathol Lab Med 2002;126:577–582.

93. Sampram ES, Lindblad B, Dahlback B. Activated protein C resistance in patients with peripheral vascular disease. J Vasc Surg 1998;28:624–629.

94. Lunghi B, Iacoviello L, Gemmati D, et al. Detection of new polymorphic markers in the factor V gene: association with factor V levels in plasma. Thromb Haemost 1996;75:45–48.

95. Faioni EM, Franchi F, Bucciarelli P, et al. Coinheritance of the HR2 haplotype in the factor V gene confers an increased risk of venous thromboembolism to carriers of factor V R506Q (factor V Leiden). Blood 1999;94:3062–3066.

96. Luddington R, Jackson A, Pannerselvam S, Brown K, Baglin T. The factor V R2 allele: risk of venous thromboembolism, factor V levels and resistance to activated protein C. Thromb Haemost 2000;83:204–208.

97. de Visser MC, Guasch JF, Kamphuisen PW, Vos HL, Rosendaal FR, Bertina RM. The HR2 haplotype of factor V: effects on factor V levels, normalized activated protein C sensitivity ratios and the risk of venous thrombosis. Thromb Haemost 2000;83:577–582.

98. Folsom AR, Cushman M, Tsai MY, et al. A prospective study of venous thromboembolism in relation to factor V Leiden and related factors. Blood 2002;99:2720–2725.

99. Doggen CJ, de Visser MC, Vos HL, Bertina RM, Cats VM, Rosendaal FR. The HR2 haplotype of factor V is not associated with the risk of myocardial infarction. Thromb Haemost 2000; 84:815–818.

100. Williamson D, Brown K, Luddington R, Baglin C, Baglin T. Factor V Cambridge: a new mutation (Arg306→Thr) associated with resistance to activated protein C. Blood 1998;91:1140–1144.

101. Franco RF, Maffei FH, Lourenco D, et al. Factor V Arg306→Thr (factor V Cambridge) and factor V Arg306→Gly mutations in venous thrombotic disease. Br J Haematol 1998;103:888–890.

102. Chan WP, Lee CK, Kwong YL, Lam CK, Liang R. A novel mutation of Arg306 of factor V gene in Hong Kong Chinese. Blood 1998;91:1135–1139.

103. Franco RF, Elion J, Tavella MH, Santos SE, Zago MA. The prevalence of factor V Arg306→Thr (factor V Cambridge) and factor V Arg306→Gly mutations in different human populations. Thromb Haemost 1999;81:312–313.

104. Poort SR, Rosendaal FR, Reitsma PH, Bertina RM. A common genetic variation in the 3′-untranslated region of the prothrombin gene is associated with elevated plasma prothrombin levels and an increase in venous thrombosis. Blood 1996;88:3698–3703.

105. Rosendaal FR, Doggen CJ, Zivelin A, et al. Geographic distribution of the 20210 G to A prothrombin variant. Thromb Haemost 1998;79:706–708.

106. Dilley A, Austin H, Hooper WC, et al. Prevalence of the prothrombin 20210 G-to-A variant in blacks: infants, patients with venous thrombosis, patients with myocardial infarction, and control subjects. J Lab Clin Med 1998;132:452–455.

107. Souto JC, Mateo J, Soria JM, et al. Homozygotes for prothrombin gene 20210 A allele in a thrombophilic family without clinical manifestations of venous thromboembolism. Haematologica 1999;84:627–632.

108. Eikelboom JW, Baker RI, Parsons R, Taylor RR, van Bockxmeer FM. No association between the 20210 G/A prothrombin gene mutation and premature coronary artery disease. Thromb Haemost 1998;80:878–880.

109. Croft SA, Daly ME, Steeds RP, Channer KS, Samani NJ, Hampton KK. The prothrombin 20210A allele and its association with myocardial infarction. Thromb Haemost 1999;81:861–864.

110. Franco RF, Trip MD, ten Cate H, et al. The 20210 G→A mutation in the 3′-untranslated region of the prothrombin gene and the risk for arterial thrombotic disease. Br J Haematol 1999;104:50–54.

111. Gardemann A, Arsic T, Katz N, Tillmanns H, Hehrlein FW, Haberbosch W. The factor II G20210A and factor V G1691A gene transitions and coronary heart disease. Thromb Haemost 1999;81:208–213.

112. Di Scipio RG, Hermodson MA, Yates SG, Davie EW. A comparison of human prothrombin, factor IX (Christmas factor), factor X (Stuart factor), and protein S. Biochemistry 1977;16:698–706.

113. Lundwall A, Dackowski W, Cohen E, et al. Isolation and sequence of the cDNA for human protein S, a regulator of blood coagulation. Proc Natl Acad Sci U S A 1986;83:6716–6720.

114. Dahlback B. Purification of human C4b-binding protein and formation of its complex with vitamin K-dependent protein S. Biochem J 1983;209:847–856.

115. Dahlback B, Lundwall A, Stenflo J. Localization of thrombin cleavage sites in the amino-terminal region of bovine protein S. J Biol Chem 1986;261:5111–5115.

116. Schwarz HP, Fischer M, Hopmeier P, Batard MA, Griffin JH. Plasma protein S deficiency in familial thrombotic disease. Blood 1984;64:1297–1300.

117. Comp PC, Nixon RR, Cooper MR, Esmon CT. Familial protein S deficiency is associated with recurrent thrombosis. J Clin Invest 1984;74:2082–2088.

118. Comp PC, Esmon CT. Recurrent venous thromboembolism in patients with a partial deficiency of protein S. N Engl J Med 1984;311:1525–1528.

119. Gandrille S, Borgel D, Ireland H, et al. Protein S deficiency: a database of mutations. For the Plasma Coagulation Inhibitors Subcommittee of the Scientific and Standardization Committee of the International Society on Thrombosis and Haemostasis. Thromb Haemost 1997;77:1201–1214.

120. Gandrille S, Borgel D, Sala N, et al. Protein S deficiency: a database of mutations—summary of the first update. Thromb Haemost 2000;84:918.

121. Pung-amritt P, Poort SR, Vos HL, et al. Compound heterozygosity for one novel and one recurrent mutation in a Thai patient with severe protein S deficiency. Thromb Haemost 1999;81:189–192.

122. Dykes AC, Walker ID, McMahon AD, Islam SI, Tait RC. A study of Protein S antigen levels in 3788 healthy volunteers: influence of age, sex and hormone use, and estimate for prevalence of deficiency state. Br J Haematol 2001;113:636–641.

123. Liberti G, Bertina RM, Rosendaal FR. Hormonal state rather than age influences cut-off values of protein S: reevaluation of the thrombotic risk associated with protein S deficiency. Thromb Haemost 1999;82:1093–1096.

124. Comp PC, Thurnau GR, Welsh J, Esmon CT. Functional and immunologic protein S levels are decreased during pregnancy. Blood 1986;68:881–885.

125. Vigano-D'Angelo S, D'Angelo A, Kaufman CE Jr, Sholer C, Esmon CT, Comp PC. Protein S deficiency occurs in the nephrotic syndrome. Ann Intern Med 1987;107:42–47.

126. D'Angelo A, Vigano-D'Angelo S, Esmon CT, Comp PC. Acquired deficiencies of protein S. Protein S activity during oral anticoagulation, in liver disease, and in disseminated intravascular coagulation. J Clin Invest 1988;81:1445–1454.

127. Quehenberger P, Loner U, Kapiotis S, et al. Increased levels of activated factor VII and decreased plasma protein S activity and circulating thrombomodulin during use of oral contraceptives. Thromb Haemost 1996;76:729–734.

128. Oruc S, Saruc M, Koyuncu FM, Ozdemir E. Changes in the plasma activities of protein C and protein S during pregnancy. Aust N Z J Obstet Gynaecol 2000;40:448–450.

129. Martinelli I, Mannucci PM, De Stefano V, et al. Different risks of thrombosis in four coagulation defects associated with inherited thrombophilia: a study of 150 families. Blood 1998;92:2353–2358.

130. Mannucci PM, Tripodi A, Bertina RM. Protein S deficiency associated with "juvenile" arterial and venous thromboses. Thromb Haemost 1986;55:440.

131. Girolami A, Simioni P, Lazzaro AR, Cordiano I. Severe arterial cerebral thrombosis in a patient with protein S deficiency (moderately reduced total and markedly reduced free protein S): a family study. Thromb Haemost 1989;61:144–147.

132. Allaart CF, Aronson DC, Ruys T, et al. Hereditary protein S deficiency in young adults with arterial occlusive disease. Thromb Haemost 1990;64:206–210.

133. Faioni EM, Valsecchi C, Palla A, Taioli E, Razzari C, Mannucci PM. Free protein S deficiency is a risk factor for venous thrombosis. Thromb Haemost 1997;78:1343–1346.

134. Makris M, Leach M, Beauchamp NJ, et al. Genetic analysis, phenotypic diagnosis, and risk of venous thrombosis in families with inherited deficiencies of protein S. Blood 2000;95:1935–1941.

135. Simmonds RE, Ireland H, Lane DA, Zoller B, Garcia de Frutos P, Dahlback B. Clarification of the risk for venous thrombosis associated with hereditary protein S deficiency by investigation of a large kindred with a characterized gene defect. Ann Intern Med 1998;128:8–14.

136. Koster T, Rosendaal FR, Briet E, et al. Protein C deficiency in a controlled series of unselected outpatients: an infrequent but clear risk factor for venous thrombosis (Leiden Thrombophilia Study). Blood 1995;85:2756–2761.

137. Boyer-Neumann C, Bertina RM, Tripodi A, et al. Comparison of functional assays for protein S: European collaborative study of patients with congenital and acquired deficiency. Thromb Haemost 1993;70:946–950.

138. Griffin JH, Evatt B, Zimmerman TS, Kleiss AJ, Wideman C. Deficiency of protein C in congenital thrombotic disease. J Clin Invest 1981;68:1370–1373.

139. Reitsma PH. Protein C deficiency: summary of the 1995 database update. Nucleic Acids Res 1996;24:157–159.

140. www.xs4all.nl/~reitsma/Prot_C_home.htm.

141. Tait RC, Walker ID, Reitsma PH, et al. Prevalence of protein C deficiency in the healthy population. Thromb Haemost 1995; 73:87–93.

142. Sakata T, Kario K, Katayama Y, Matsuyama T, Kato H, Miyata T. Studies on congenital protein C deficiency in Japanese: prevalence, genetic analysis, and relevance to the onset of arterial occlusive diseases. Semin Thromb Hemost 2000;26:11–16.

143. Allaart CF, Poort SR, Rosendaal FR, Reitsma PH, Bertina RM, Briet E. Increased risk of venous thrombosis in carriers of hereditary protein C deficiency defect. Lancet 1993;341:134–138.

144. Bovill EG, Bauer KA, Dickerman JD, Callas P, West B. The clinical spectrum of heterozygous protein C deficiency in a large New England kindred. Blood 1989;73:712–717.

145. Camerlingo M, Finazzi G, Casto L, Laffranchi C, Barbui T, Mamoli A. Inherited protein C deficiency and nonhemorrhagic arterial stroke in young adults. Neurology 1991;41:1371–1373.

146. Simioni P, Zanardi S, Saracino A, Girolami A. Occurrence of arterial thrombosis in a cohort of patients with hereditary deficiency of clotting inhibitors. J Med 1992;23:61–74.

147. Egeberg O. Inherited antithrombin deficiency causing thrombophilia. Thromb Diath Haemorrh 1965;13:516–530.

148. Tait RC, Walker ID, Perry DJ, et al. Prevalence of antithrombin deficiency in the healthy population. Br J Haematol 1994;87: 106–112.

149. Wells PS, Blajchman MA, Henderson P, et al. Prevalence of antithrombin deficiency in healthy blood donors: a cross-sectional study. Am J Hematol 1994;45:321–324.

150. www.med.ic.ac.uk/divisions/7/antithrombin.

151. Lane DA, Bayston T, Olds RJ, et al. Antithrombin mutation database: 2nd (1997) update. For the Plasma Coagulation Inhibitors Subcommittee of the Scientific and Standardization Committee of the International Society on Thrombosis and Haemostasis. Thromb Haemost 1997;77:197–211.

152. Coller BS, Owen J, Jesty J, et al. Deficiency of plasma protein S, protein C, or antithrombin III and arterial thrombosis. Arteriosclerosis 1987;7:456–462.

153. Johnson EJ, Prentice CR, Parapia LA. Premature arterial disease associated with familial antithrombin III deficiency. Thromb Haemost 1990;63:13–15.

154. Mateo J, Oliver A, Borrell M, Sala N, Fontcuberta J. Increased risk of venous thrombosis in carriers of natural anticoagulant deficiencies. Results of the family studies of the Spanish Multicenter Study on Thrombophilia (EMET study). Blood Coagul Fibrinolysis 1998;9:71–78.

155. Demers C, Ginsberg JS, Hirsh J, Henderson P, Blajchman MA. Thrombosis in antithrombin-III-deficient persons. Report of a large kindred and literature review. Ann Intern Med 1992;116:754–761.

156. Heijboer H, Brandjes DP, Buller HR, Sturk A, ten Cate JW. Deficiencies of coagulation-inhibiting and fibrinolytic proteins in outpatients with deep-vein thrombosis. N Engl J Med 1990;323:1512–1516.

157. Lowe GD, Rumley A, Woodward M, et al. Epidemiology of coagulation factors, inhibitors and activation markers: the Third Glasgow MONICA Survey. I. Illustrative reference ranges by age, sex and hormone use. Br J Haematol 1997;97: 775–784.

158. Wahl DG, Guillemin F, de Maistre E, Perret C, Lecompte T, Thibaut G. Risk for venous thrombosis related to antiphospholipid antibodies in systemic lupus erythematosus—a meta-analysis. Lupus 1997;6:467–473.

159. Wahl DG, Guillemin F, de Maistre E, Perret-Guillaume C, Lecompte T, Thibaut G. Meta-analysis of the risk of venous thrombosis in individuals with antiphospholipid antibodies without underlying autoimmune disease or previous thrombosis. Lupus 1998;7:15–22.

160. Rand JH, Wu XX, Andree HA, et al. Pregnancy loss in the antiphospholipid-antibody syndrome—a possible thrombogenic mechanism. N Engl J Med 1997;337:154–160.

161. Nojima J, Suehisa E, Kuratsune H, et al. Platelet activation induced by combined effects of anticardiolipin and lupus anticoagulant IgG antibodies in patients with systemic lupus erythematosus—possible association with thrombotic and thrombocytopenic complications. Thromb Haemost 1999;81:436–441.

162. Wiener MH, Burke M, Fried M, Yust I. Thromboagglutination by anticardiolipin antibody complex in the antiphospholipid syndrome: a possible mechanism of immune-mediated thrombosis. Thromb Res 2001;103:193–199.

163. Wilson WA, Gharavi AE, Koike T, et al. International consensus statement on preliminary classification criteria for definite antiphospholipid syndrome: report of an international workshop. Arthritis Rheum 1999;42:1309–1311.

164. Khamashta MA, Guadrado MJ, Mujic F, Taub NA, Hunt BJ, Hughes GR. The management of thrombosis in the antiphospholipid-antibody syndrome. N Engl J Med 1995;332: 993–997.

165. Moll S, Ortel TL. Monitoring warfarin therapy in patients with lupus anticoagulants. Ann Intern Med 1997;127:177–185.

166. Hellan M, Kuhnel E, Speiser W, Lechner K, Eichinger S. Familial lupus anticoagulant: a case report and review of the literature. Blood Coagul Fibrinolysis 1998;9:195–200.

167. Atsumi T, Bertolaccini ML, Koike T. Genetics of antiphospholipid syndrome. Rheum Dis Clin North Am 2001;27:565–572, vi.

168. Atsumi T, Tsutsumi A, Amengual O, et al. Correlation between beta2-glycoprotein I valine/leucine247 polymorphism and anti-beta2-glycoprotein I antibodies in patients with primary antiphospholipid syndrome. Rheumatology 1999;38:721–723.

169. Ichinose A. Physiopathology and regulation of factor XIII. Thromb Haemost 2001;86:57–65.

170. Kohler HP, Stickland MH, Ossei-Gerning N, Carter A, Mikkola H, Grant PJ. Association of a common polymorphism in the factor XIII gene with myocardial infarction. Thromb Haemost 1998;79:8–13.

171. Wartiovaara U, Perola M, Mikkola H, et al. Association of FXIII Val34Leu with decreased risk of myocardial infarction in Finnish males. Atherosclerosis 1999;142:295–300.

172. Franco RF, Pazin-Filho A, Tavella MH, Simoes MV, Marin-Neto JA, Zago MA. Factor XIII val34leu and the risk of myocardial infarction. Haematologica 2000;85:67–71.

173. Elbaz A, Poirier O, Canaple S, Chedru F, Cambien F, Amarenco P. The association between the Val34Leu polymorphism in the factor XIII gene and brain infarction. Blood 2000;95:586–591.

174. Reiner AP, Frank MB, Schwartz SM, et al. Coagulation factor XIII polymorphisms and the risk of myocardial infarction and ischaemic stroke in young women. Br J Haematol 2002; 116:376–382.

175. Catto AJ, Kohler HP, Coore J, Mansfield MW, Stickland MH, Grant PJ. Association of a common polymorphism in the factor XIII gene with venous thrombosis. Blood 1999;93:906–908.

176. Renner W, Koppel H, Hoffmann C, et al. Prothrombin G20210A, factor V Leiden, and factor XIII Val34Leu: common mutations of blood coagulation factors and deep vein thrombosis in Austria. Thromb Res 2000;99:35–39.

177. Aleksic N, Ahn C, Wang YW, et al. Factor XIIIA Val34Leu polymorphism does not predict risk of coronary heart disease: The Atherosclerosis Risk in Communities (ARIC) Study. Arterioscler Thromb Vasc Biol 2002;22:348–352.

178. Warner D, Mansfield MW, Grant PJ. Coagulation factor XIII and cardiovascular disease in UK Asian patients undergoing coronary angiography. Thromb Haemost 2001;85:408–411.

179. Corral J, Gonzalez-Conejero R, Iniesta JA, Rivera J, Martinez C, Vicente V. The FXIII Val34Leu polymorphism in venous and arterial thromboembolism. Haematologica 2000;85:293–297.

180. Balogh I, Szoke G, Karpati L, et al. Val34Leu polymorphism of plasma factor XIII: biochemistry and epidemiology in familial thrombophilia. Blood 2000;96:2479–2486.

181. Margaglione M, Bossone A, Brancaccio V, Ciampa A, Di Minno G. Factor XIII Val34Leu polymorphism and risk of deep vein thrombosis. Thromb Haemost 2000;84:1118–1119.

182. Ariens RA, Philippou H, Nagaswami C, Weisel JW, Lane DA, Grant PJ. The factor XIII V34L polymorphism accelerates thrombin activation of factor XIII and affects cross-linked fibrin structure. Blood 2000;96:988–995.

183. Wartiovaara U, Mikkola H, Szoke G, et al. Effect of Val34Leu polymorphism on the activation of the coagulation factor XIII-A. Thromb Haemost 2000;84:595–600.

184. Wagner CL, Mascelli MA, Neblock DS, Weisman HF, Coller BS, Jordan RE. Analysis of GPIIb/IIIa receptor number by quantification of 7E3 binding to human platelets. Blood 1996;88:907–914.

185. Shattil SJ, Kashiwagi H, Pampori N. Integrin signaling: the platelet paradigm. Blood 1998;91:2645–2657.

186. von dem Borne AE, Decary F. Nomenclature of platelet-specific antigens. Transfusion 1990;30:477.

187. Calvete JJ. Clues for understanding the structure and function of a prototypic human integrin: the platelet glycoprotein IIb/IIIa complex. Thromb Haemost 1994;72:1–15.

188. Calvete JJ. Platelet integrin GPIIb/IIIa: structure-function correlations. An update and lessons from other integrins. Proc Soc Exp Biol Med 1999;222:29–38.

189. Michelson AD, Furman MI, Goldschmidt-Clermont P, et al. Platelet GP IIIa Pl(A) polymorphisms display different sensitivities to agonists. Circulation 2000;101:1013–1018.

190. Weiss EJ, Bray PF, Tayback M, et al. A polymorphism of a platelet glycoprotein receptor as an inherited risk factor for coronary thrombosis. N Engl J Med 1996;334:1090–1094.

191. Carter AM, Ossei-Gerning N, Grant PJ. Platelet glycoprotein IIIa PlA polymorphism in young men with myocardial infarction. Lancet 1996;348:485–486.

192. Ridker PM, Hennekens CH, Schmitz C, Stampfer MJ, Lindpaintner K. PIA1/A2 polymorphism of platelet glycoprotein IIIa and risks of myocardial infarction, stroke, and venous thrombosis. Lancet 1997;349:385–388.

193. Herrmann SM, Poirier O, Marques-Vidal P, et al. The Leu33/Pro polymorphism (PlA1/PlA2) of the glycoprotein IIIa (GPIIIa) receptor is not related to myocardial infarction in the ECTIM Study. Etude Cas-Temoins de l'Infarctus du Myocarde. Thromb Haemost 1997;77:1179–1181.

194. Zhu MM, Weedon J, Clark LT. Meta-analysis of the association of platelet glycoprotein IIIa PlA1/A2 polymorphism with myocardial infarction. Am J Cardiol 2000;86:1000–1005.

195. Walter DH, Schachinger V, Elsner M, Dimmeler S, Zeiher AM. Platelet glycoprotein IIIa polymorphisms and risk of coronary stent thrombosis. Lancet 1997;350:1217–1219.

196. Kastrati A, Schomig A, Seyfarth M, et al. PlA polymorphism of platelet glycoprotein IIIa and risk of restenosis after coronary stent placement. Circulation 1999;99:1005–1010.

197. Mamotte CD, van Bockxmeer FM, Taylor RR. PIa1/a2 polymorphism of glycoprotein IIIa and risk of coronary artery disease and restenosis following coronary angioplasty. Am J Cardiol 1998;82:13–16.

198. Laule M, Cascorbi I, Stangl V, et al. A1/A2 polymorphism of glycoprotein IIIa and association with excess procedural risk for coronary catheter interventions: a case-controlled study. Lancet 1999;353:708–712.

199. Wheeler GL, Braden GA, Bray PF, Marciniak SJ, Mascelli MA, Sane DC. Reduced inhibition by abciximab in platelets with the PlA2 polymorphism. Am Heart J 2002;143:76–82.

200. Berndt MC, Shen Y, Dopheide SM, Gardiner EE, Andrews RK. The vascular biology of the glycoprotein Ib-IX-V complex. Thromb Haemost 2001;86:178–188.

201. Lopez JA, Ludwig EH, McCarthy BJ. Polymorphism of human glycoprotein Ib alpha results from a variable number of tandem repeats of a 13-amino acid sequence in the mucin-like macroglycopeptide region. Structure/function implications. J Biol Chem 1992;267:10055–10061.

202. Ishida F, Furihata K, Ishida K, et al. The largest variant of platelet glycoprotein Ib alpha has four tandem repeats of 13 amino acids in the macroglycopeptide region and a genetic linkage with methionine145. Blood 1995;86:1357–1360.

203. Afshar-Kharghan V, Li CQ, Khoshnevis-Asl M, Lopez JA. Kozak sequence polymorphism of the glycoprotein (GP) Ibalpha gene is a major determinant of the plasma membrane levels of the platelet GP Ib-IX-V complex. Blood 1999;94:186–191.

204. Corral J, Lozano ML, Gonzalez-Conejero R, et al. A common polymorphism flanking the ATG initiator codon of GPIb alpha does not affect expression and is not a major risk factor for arterial thrombosis. Thromb Haemost 2000;83:23–28.

205. Murata M, Matsubara Y, Kawano K, et al. Coronary artery disease and polymorphisms in a receptor mediating shear stress-dependent platelet activation. Circulation 1997;96: 3281–3286.

206. Gonzalez-Conejero R, Lozano ML, Rivera J, et al. Polymorphisms of platelet membrane glycoprotein Ib associated with arterial thrombotic disease. Blood 1998;92:2771–2776.

207. Mercier B, Munier S, Bertault V, Mansourati J, Blanc JJ, Ferec C. Myocardial infarction: absence of association with VNTR polymorphism of GP Ibalpha. Thromb Haemost 2000;84: 921–922.

208. Reiner AP, Kumar PN, Schwartz SM, et al. Genetic variants of platelet glycoprotein receptors and risk of stroke in young women. Stroke 2000;31:1628–1633.

209. Sonoda A, Murata M, Ikeda Y, Fukuuchi Y, Watanabe K. Stroke and platelet glycoprotein Ibalpha polymorphisms. Thromb Haemost 2001;85:573–574.

210. Kunicki TJ, Orchekowski R, Annis D, Honda Y. Variability of integrin alpha 2 beta 1 activity on human platelets. Blood 1993;82:2693–2703.

211. Kunicki TJ, Kritzik M, Annis DS, Nugent DJ. Hereditary variation in platelet integrin alpha 2 beta 1 density is associated with two silent polymorphisms in the alpha 2 gene coding sequence. Blood 1997;89:1939–1943.

212. Santoso S, Kunicki TJ, Kroll H, Haberbosch W, Gardemann A. Association of the platelet glycoprotein Ia C807T gene polymorphism with nonfatal myocardial infarction in younger patients. Blood 1999;93:2449–2453.

213. Casorelli I, De Stefano V, Leone AM, et al. The C807T/G873A polymorphism in the platelet glycoprotein Ia gene and the risk of acute coronary syndrome in the Italian population. Br J Haematol 2001;114:150–154.

214. Croft SA, Hampton KK, Sorrell JA, et al. The GPIa C807T dimorphism associated with platelet collagen receptor density is not a risk factor for myocardial infarction. Br J Haematol 1999;106:771–776.

215. Morita H, Kurihara H, Imai Y, et al. Lack of association between the platelet glycoprotein Ia C807T gene polymorphism and myocardial infarction in Japanese. An approach entailing melting curve analysis with specific fluorescent hybridization probes. Thromb Haemost 2001;85:226–230.

216. Ridker PM, Vaughan DE, Stampfer MJ, Manson JE, Hennekens CH. Endogenous tissue-type plasminogen activator and risk of myocardial infarction. Lancet 1993;341:1165–1168.

217. Thompson SG, Kienast J, Pyke SD, Haverkate F, van de Loo JC. Hemostatic factors and the risk of myocardial infarction or sudden death in patients with angina pectoris. European Concerted Action on Thrombosis and Disabilities Angina Pectoris Study Group. N Engl J Med 1995;332:635–641.

218. Ludwig M, Wohn KD, Schleuning WD, Olek K. Allelic dimorphism in the human tissue-type plasminogen activator (TPA) gene as a result of an Alu insertion/deletion event. Hum Genet 1992;88:388–392.

219. van der Bom JG, de Knijff P, Haverkate F, et al. Tissue plasminogen activator and risk of myocardial infarction. The Rotterdam Study. Circulation 1997;95:2623–2627.

220. Ridker PM, Baker MT, Hennekens CH, Stampfer MJ, Vaughan DE. Alu-repeat polymorphism in the gene coding for tissue-type plasminogen activator (t-PA) and risks of myocardial infarction among middle-aged men. Arterioscler Thromb Vasc Biol 1997;17:1687–1690.

221. Aoki N, Moroi M, Sakata Y, Yoshida N, Matsuda M. Abnormal plasminogen. A hereditary molecular abnormality found in a patient with recurrent thrombosis. J Clin Invest 1978;61:1186–1195.

222. Tait RC, Walker ID, Conkie JA, Islam SI, McCall F. Isolated familial plasminogen deficiency may not be a risk factor for thrombosis. Thromb Haemost 1996;76:1004–1008.

223. Demarmels Biasiutti F, Sulzer I, Stucki B, Wuillemin WA, Furlan M, Lammle B. Is plasminogen deficiency a thrombotic risk factor? A study on 23 thrombophilic patients and their family members. Thromb Haemost 1998;80:167–170.

224. Shigekiyo T, Kanazuka M, Aihara K, et al. No increased risk of thrombosis in heterozygous congenital dysplasminogenemia. Int J Hematol 2000;72:247–252.

225. Sartori MT, Patrassi GM, Theodoridis P, Perin A, Pietrogrande F, Girolami A. Heterozygous type I plasminogen deficiency is associated with an increased risk for thrombosis: a statistical analysis in 20 kindreds. Blood Coagul Fibrinolysis 1994;5:889–893.

226. Bachmann F. Plasminogen-plasmin enzyme system. In: Colman RW, Hirsh J, Marder VJ, Clowes AW, George JN, eds. Hemostasis and Thrombosis: Basic Principles and Clinical Practice. Philadelphia: Lippincott, Williams & Wilkins; 2001:275–320.

227. Kohler HP, Grant PJ. Plasminogen-activator inhibitor type 1 and coronary artery disease. N Engl J Med 2000;342:1792–1801.

228. Dawson S, Hamsten A, Wiman B, Henney A, Humphries S. Genetic variation at the plasminogen activator inhibitor-1 locus is associated with altered levels of plasma plasminogen activator inhibitor-1 activity. Arterioscler Thromb 1991;11:183–190.

229. Freeman MS, Mansfield MW, Barrett JH, Grant PJ. Genetic contribution to circulating levels of hemostatic factors in healthy families with effects of known genetic polymorphisms on heritability. Arterioscler Thromb Vasc Biol 2002;22:506–510.

230. Sartori MT, Wiman B, Vettore S, Dazzi F, Girolami A, Patrassi GM. 4G/5G polymorphism of PAI-1 gene promoter and fibrinolytic capacity in patients with deep vein thrombosis. Thromb Haemost 1998;80:956–960.

231. Stegnar M, Uhrin P, Peternel P, et al. The 4G/5G sequence polymorphism in the promoter of plasminogen activator inhibitor-1 (PAI-1) gene: relationship to plasma PAI-1 level in venous thromboembolism. Thromb Haemost 1998;79:975–979.

232. www.fvleiden.org.

233. www.nattinfo.org.

VI   RISK FACTORS

28 Risk Factors

Ngoc-Anh Le, PhD and W. Virgil Brown, MD

CONTENTS

INTRODUCTION

The term risk factor is defined as any clinically measurable characteristic that may be used to predict clinical events. In this chapter, we will focus on lipid-related risk factors associated with clinical events resulting from arteriosclerosis involving the major arteries. The anatomical distribution of the arteries and the function of the organs they feed define the clinical syndromes resulting from arteriosclerosis. Epidemiological and clinical trial data that have been used to define risk factors therefore relate differently to the different arterial systems of the body.

The coronary arteries have received the greatest attention because death and disease associated with this vascular area are major health issues of our time. Lipoprotein abnormalities have been related most strongly to coronary artery disease. In addition, cerebrovascular disease with stroke and dementia are important problems with characteristic risk relationships, although, with these diseases, the relationship with lipids is less clear. Higher blood cholesterol has been far less predictive of stroke than of coronary disease. However, recent trials have suggested the risk factors that apply to coronary and cerebral arteriosclerosis may also apply to diseases of the aorta and peripheral vessels.

In this chapter, we will define and discuss independent and causative risk factors. An independent factor is one for which no other clinically measurable variable is an intermediate between the risk factor in question and the disease process at the vessel wall. With a causative factor, the disease process appears to respond in a predictable manner as the factor is altered. Thus, effective treatment of an independent and causative risk factor should reduce the incidence of clinical events. Low-density lipoprotein (LDL) cholesterol is both independent and causative by these definitions. High-density lipoprotein (HDL) cholesterol is an independent risk factor, but its causative nature has not been fully documented. Triglycerides (TG) are weakly independent, but few data support TG as a causative factor. Other lipid-related risk factors may be independent and causative, but strong clinical data have not been published. We will focus on factors that are supported by clinical trials.

Many risk factors do not meet criteria for independence or causation: these include body characteristics such as height, obesity, waist size, patterns of baldness, and ear lobe creases; lifestyle issues such as a diet high in cholesterol and saturated fat, and sedentary activity patterns; and immutable characteristics such as family history or age. The latter two may be definable in genetic terms and in quantitative temporal terms, respectively, but they are not directly causative in the sense of reversibility as defined above. Although these factors may provide useful data in predicting event rates and therefore meet the broader definition of risk factors, we will not discuss them in detail.

From: *Contemporary Cardiology: Principles of Molecular Cardiology*
Edited by: M. S. Runge and C. Patterson © Humana Press Inc., Totowa, NJ

Finally, many measures of vascular disease are not clinically accessible variables that can be directly treated with an expected benefit. With further investigation, these factors, or biomarkers, may be defined as causative but they are not considered such at the present time. These biomarkers include polyunsaturated fat content of adipose tissue, high sensitivity C-reactive protein (HSCRP), plasma concentrations of cell surface adherence molecules such as vascular cell adhesion molecules (VCAM) and intercellular adhesion molecules (ICAM), the size of lipoproteins (i.e., "small, dense LDL"), vascular reactivity triggered by stimuli for nitric oxide release, vascular compliance measures, and various imaging techniques such as electron beam computed tomography (EBCT), vascular wall ultrasound measures, and magnetic resonance imaging (MRI) of vessels. Although these factors may be useful in determining event rates, they do not meet the definition of causative risk factors that require intervention.

Because of the complexity of arteriosclerosis and the confluence of many etiologic factors, predicting the specific risk for clinical events in any given patient is challenging. Probability ranking is a growing possibility because of reports from community-based studies and clinical trials. From a practical standpoint, the first issue in predicting specific risk would be to select clinical characteristics that are responsive to treatment and to set appropriate goals for each variable that confers risk. These goals should be supported by clinical trial data that show a reduction in clinical events when the goal is achieved in groups of persons at risk. Data to support this approach are available for only two risk factors: LDL cholesterol and hypertension. Smoking cessation is supported by observational data, and although it is sometimes difficult to achieve, the solution is obvious, making quantitative scientific data unnecessary. Achieving a desirable body weight, although less certain and complicated by many genetic considerations, may be viewed as similar to smoking cessation. Obesity is a major concern because of its association with type II diabetes mellitus and various manifestations of vascular disease. Predicting the specific risk associated with obesity in a patient is a challenge for the physician. Reducing TG and raising HDL cholesterol are useful for risk prediction; however, the clinical trial data are not definitive, and setting goals for the right lipid levels is not possible. Furthermore, treatment options are limited.

Theories of causation and speculation about treatment regimens have been developed from research in vascular biology and lipoprotein physiology. Encouraging sensible lifestyle changes in patients and instituting drug therapy should be based on convincing evidence that these regimens will substantially change the disease probability.

Significant time, effort, and resources can be expended in the evaluation and treatment of cardiovascular risk and the disease with little likelihood of actual benefit; therefore, the physician must develop a systematic approach that combines the seemingly conflicting characteristics of conservatism and aggressiveness. Long-term monitoring and effective treatment of risk are required to reduce the clinical event rate. These tenets have been incorporated in the National Cholesterol Education Program (1).

LIPOPROTEINS AND LIPID TRANSPORT

The Function of Lipids

Four major groups of lipids are found in the body: triglycerides, cholesterol, phospholipids, and free fatty acids. Lipids provide several functions that are essential for life. All membranes of animal cells are composed of phospholipids and free cholesterol in a ratio of approx 2:1. Cholesterol is essential for the synthesis of many hormones, including all glucocorticoids, mineralocorticoids, and both male and female sex hormones. TG functions to transport energy from the liver and intestine and for storage of energy in adipose tissue. Free fatty acids released from stored TG and those found in plasma bound to albumin transport energy from adipose tissue to other organs. Phospholipids are important intracellular signaling molecules.

Controlling the functions of lipids requires intimate and specific interactions with proteins. Among these interactions is the binding of specific transport proteins called apolipoproteins, which, when combined with various lipids, form lipoproteins that provide for much of the lipid transport in the blood plasma. The synthesis, secretion, metabolic routes and, ultimately, the clearance of lipoproteins are significantly affected by the apolipoproteins on the cell surface.

The relation between plasma lipids and vascular disease risk is related to the number and composition of plasma lipoproteins. The plasma lipoproteins serve as vehicles transporting various lipids among the organs of the body (Table 1); this transport process begins and ends in the intestinal tract. We will begin discussing those lipids entering the body in the diet and end with the delivery of newly synthesized lipids that must be excreted in the feces. The bloodstream is only an intermediary—a conduit through which the lipoproteins travel in their important transport function. Vascular disease is an unfortunate adverse effect when the transport system is forced to carry lipids in excess of the capacity inherent in the machinery provided by the genetic control of certain proteins. A small percentage of these key genes and their proteins has been defined. Although many clinical syndromes are defined by plasma

Table 1
Physical and Chemical Characteristics of Plasma Lipoproteins

	Chylomicrons	VLDL	LDL	HDL
Density (g/mL)	<1.000	1.000–1.006	1.019–1.063	1.063–1.21
Diameter (nm)	75–300	30–80	22–27	7–10
% Composition				
Protein	1–2	10	25	50
Triglycerides	90–96	60	10	5
Cholesterol	2–5	12	50	20
Phospholipids	5	18	15	25
Major Apolipoproteins	ApoA-I, ApoA-II ApoA-IV ApoB-48 ApoC-I ApoC-II,ApoC-III ApoE	ApoB-100 ApoC-I ApoC-II, ApoC-III ApoE	ApoB-100	ApoA-I, ApoA-II ApoC-I ApoC-II, ApoC-III ApoE

VLDL indicates very low density lipoproteins; LDL, low-density lipoproteins; HDL, high-density lipoproteins.

lipoprotein concentrations and appear as familial traits, only a few are explained by specific molecular mechanisms.

Chylomicrons and Lipid Transport from the Intestine

Dietary fat makes up about 35% of calories in the diet, but total fat intake varies from approx 50 to 200 grams per day, depending on body size, activity level, and dietary habits. Only a small proportion of the dietary TG and phospholipids escape into the feces; most are digested into free fatty acids and monoglycerides by intestinal enzymes and transported from micelles of lipids into the epithelial cells of the small intestine. This digestion process is aided by the bile acids delivered from the liver through the biliary system. The gallbladder stores these detergent molecules, which await delivery timed with gastric emptying. The bile acids are then reabsorbed in the distal intestine for return to the liver through the portal blood (Fig. 1).

In the epithelial cell, intestinal fats are synthesized into phospholipids and TG and packaged into chylomicrons. A 250 kDa protein called apolipoprotein (Apo)B-48 receives the lipids transported by a specific protein called the microsomal TG transport protein (MTP). Without both ApoB-48 and MTP, chylomicron is not synthesized or secreted from the intestinal cells. ApoB-48 is the product of the ApoB gene, which is capable of generating a protein twice the size of that found in the intestinal products. This larger protein is referred to as ApoB-100; however, in the intestine, the mRNA is edited by an enzyme that produces a stop codon after only approx 48% of the mes-

sage has been translated and so only this shorter version of ApoB-100 is found in the intestine. Thus the protein is shortened proportionately. In the liver, the full-length protein (ApoB-100) is produced and incorporated into a very low density lipoprotein.

Other apolipoproteins are synthesized in the intestinal cells and incorporated into the surface of the chylomicron. These include ApoA-I, ApoA-II, ApoA-IV, ApoE, ApoC-I, ApoC-II, and ApoC-III. The apolipoproteins of the ApoA series are rapidly redistributed to HDL once the chylomicron enters the blood plasma. The other apolipoproteins are important in the metabolism and clearance of the lipid in chylomicrons by other tissues of the body. In fact, a significant portion of the ApoE and ApoC proteins are transferred from HDL onto the surface of the nascent chylomicron as it enters the lymph.

Intestinal cholesterol is important in chylomicron metabolism. About 200–500 mg of cholesterol is delivered into the small intestine from dietary sources and another 800–1200 mg enters from the liver with the bile. Much of the dietary cholesterol undergoes esterification with various fatty acids and must be hydrolyzed by a cholesterol esterase secreted primarily from the pancreas. Therefore, 1–2 gr of cholesterol is available for absorption from the intestinal tract over the course of the day. Once in the intestinal cell, cholesterol is mainly re-esterified with fatty acids and incorporated into the chylomicrons and secreted into the lymph. The rate of absorption varies from as little as 10% to as much as 90%; in most people, 40–60% of available free cholesterol is absorbed.

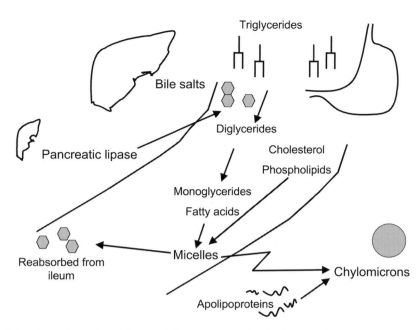

Fig. 1. Fat absorption and chylomicron formation. Dietary triglycerides reaching the intestinal lumen are hydrolyzed by pancreatic lipase into monoglycerides and free fatty acids. Bile salts synthesized from the hepatic cholesterol pool provide the ideal environment for the formation of mixed micelles to facilitate fat absorption. Absorbed fatty acids and monoglycerides are reconstituted as triglycerides and, together with dietary cholesterol and phospholipids, are assembled in the enterocytes with intestinal apolipoproteins to form chylomicrons and secreted into the circulation via the lymphatic system. The bile salts remain in the intestinal tract and are reabsorbed downstream in the ileum. Interference with the reabsorption of bile salts would result in the increased synthesis of bile salts and depletion of the hepatic cholesterol pool.

Plasma levels of cholesterol may be related in part to the percentage of dietary cholesterol absorbed (2,3). The rate of absorption is determined by two factors: (1) the function of a specific sterol transporter that is subject to inhibition and found in the apical membrane of the intestinal cell, and (2) an effluxing transport system involving the action of two proteins known as ABCG5 and ABCG8 (4). These two proteins belong to a family of proteins that contain ATP-binding cassettes (5). The major function of these specific proteins may be to rid the body of plant sterols such as sitosterol and campesterol that are partially transported with the cholesterol by the action of the influxing sterol transporter. The daily diet of persons consuming vegetable oils may contain 500 mg or more of these plant sterols. Phytosterols absorbed in large quantities promote tissue storage of cholesterol in macrophages with consequent development of xanthomata and arteriosclerosis as seen in the genetic disorder of sitosterolemia, a recessive trait caused by abnormalities in the ABCG5 or ABCG8 proteins (6,7). Although the molecular structure of the sterol transporter responsible for uptake by the intestinal cells has not been characterized, it can be inhibited by the drug ezetimibe because this sterol transporter localizes in the apical cell membrane.

The completed chylomicron is delivered through the lymph to the thoracic duct where it enters the venous blood in the neck. During this transit and later in the plasma, surface proteins rapidly equilibrate with the other plasma lipoproteins. This equilibration is mainly a function of HDL, which accepts the ApoA-I, ApoA-II, and ApoA-IV proteins, incorporating them into the structure of cholesterol- and phospholipid-rich chylomicrons. In addition, HDL gives up significant quantities of the adherent ApoC-I, ApoC-II, ApoC-III, and ApoE proteins to the surface of the chylomicron. ApoC-III significantly increases the negative surface charge of the chylomicrons, which may prevent aggregation with each other and the nonspecific interaction of chylomicron particles with cell surfaces. These TG-rich chylomicrons are thus preserved for interactions with lipoprotein lipase, a lipid ester hydrolase that lines the luminal surface of the capillaries of tissues that use the energy provided by this fat (muscle) or store it for later use (adipose tissue). Lipoprotein lipase requires the presence of ApoC-II on the surface of the chylomicron for hydrolysis of the phospholipid surface coat and the TG in the core of the particle. Fatty acids and monoglycerides then pass across the endothelium and into the adjacent parenchymal cells.

Significant impairment of the hydrolysis of chylomicrons results in two autosomal recessive disorders involving the action of lipoprotein lipase. The first disorder is caused by a deficiency in the enzyme, and many sequence abnormalities that lead to the failure to generate functional enzyme have been identified. In the second disorder, defects in this gene lead to the absence of ApoC-II. In both disorders, the TG levels may be many grams per deciliter in the blood plasma, and uptake of TG by macrophages in the spleen, bone marrow, liver, and skin may cause hepatosplenomegaly and eruptive cutaneous xanthomata. The very high levels of chylomicrons may aggregate after prolonged circulation and impair capillary blood flow with consequent ischemic symptoms in the intestinal wall, in the peripheral and central nervous systems and, most threatening, in the pancreas leading to episodes of pancreatitis. Simply removing as much fat from the diet as possible often relieves the clinical symptoms of these genetic disorders.

These metabolic defects are not associated with an increased risk of arteriosclerosis, even though the plasma lipid levels are extremely high in these patients throughout their lives. This observation implies that if chylomicrons contribute to vascular disease risk, it is a result of the particles after the action of the lipase.

Most of the TG component of chylomicrons is lost to tissues as the result of lipoprotein lipase action. In addition, a second enzyme, hepatic triglyceride lipase, may be involved in cleaving the phospholipid surface coat (8–10). A remnant particle, characterized by a relatively poor affinity for these enzymes, develops and circulates in the plasma for several minutes up to several hours, depending on the individual. These remnants are rich in TG and contain most of the cholesterol originally incorporated into the chylomicron. Chylomicron remnants are almost totally cleared by the liver, which delivers the remaining TG and the intestinally absorbed cholesterol into hepatocytes. The clearance of these remnants is greatly facilitated by the presence of ApoE on their surface. ApoE binds to the ApoB-100 receptor (LDL receptor), an LDL-receptor like protein (LRP) and other proteins on the liver cell surface. Evidence indicates that the longer the life span of these remnants, the higher the vascular risk (11–15). The molecular factors that prolong the maintenance of the remnant in the plasma are unknown.

Very Low Density Lipoprotein Metabolism and Lipid Transport from the Liver

The healthy liver secretes TG into the plasma, which provides for energy balance between the external world (diet), the major storage site of energy (adipose tissue), and those tissues that need a source of energy for continuous function (skeletal muscle, heart, kidneys, skin, brain, and most other organs of the body except the liver and bowel). Each day, approx 2000 kcal in the form of fats,

carbohydrates, and protein from the diet are converted into monoglycerides, fatty acids, simple sugars, and amino acids in the intestine, absorbed into the intestinal epithelial cells, and secreted into the portal vein and lymph system. The liver extracts a large portion of these nutrients. In addition, another 2000 kcal may enter the plasma from the adipose tissue as free fatty acids (FFA) bound by albumin, which are transported to the tissues of the body and provide the major source of calories in the fasting state. In addition, FFA are taken up by the liver in large quantities. When the energy needs of the liver have been met, the excess calories are converted to TG. Under normal circumstances, the incoming fatty acids are preferentially used as substrate for TG synthesis. This TG is transferred to newly synthesized ApoB via the microsomal TG transfer protein in the smooth endoplasmic reticulum of the liver. ApoB is required for TG packaging and synthesis of VLDL. Cholesteryl ester, free cholesterol, and phospholipids are also significant components of the VLDL. Additional apolipoproteins, including ApoE, ApoC-I, ApoC-II, and ApoC-III, are added to the surface of VLDL molecules before their secretion. Ranging in size from 30 to 80 nm as it leaves the liver, VLDL comprises about 60% TG, 12% cholesterol, 16% phospholipid, and 12% protein. One ApoB-100 molecule and variable numbers of ApoE and the ApoC proteins, depending on the lipid content and the diameter of the particle, are associated with the VLDL molecule.

In the plasma space, additional apolipoproteins are added through exchange with HDL similar to that described for chylomicrons. VLDL particles rapidly interact with capillary endothelium and undergo hydrolytic degradation of the TG component by lipoprotein lipase as activated by ApoC-II. Most of the ApoC molecules and part of the ApoE are released to HDL, and the residual particle is released from the vascular cell surface into the plasma space as a VLDL remnant. Nascent VLDL usually stays in the plasma for 1–3 h, but the VLDL remnants may have much longer half-lives of 8–16 h. Most of the plasma TG in patients with fasting TG concentrations from 150 to 400 mg/dL are probably a component of VLDL remnants. VLDL is further metabolized in the liver, where the cell surface enzyme hepatic TG lipase can hydrolyze much of the residual TG and part of the phospholipids. The remaining proteins, except for ApoB-100, are transferred to HDL, and the residual particle becomes LDL. This is the major, and perhaps only, source of LDL in human plasma. Approximately 50–70% of VLDL particles become LDL; the rest are bound tightly to the liver cell surface and are taken up for degradation in the lysosomes of the hepatocytes. Both ApoB-100 and ApoE bind to the LDL receptor, the LRP protein, or other receptors on the hepatocyte membrane. Larger VLDL remnants are more likely to be taken up with fewer surviving to become LDL.

Hypertriglyceridemic patients produce large TG-rich particles, and a minority of VLDL may be converted to LDL. These properties characterize an autosomal disorder called familial hypertriglyceridemia. Some patients produce large numbers of smaller VLDL, and the number of both VLDL and LDL particles is increased. This syndrome, also an autosomal dominant disease, is called familial combined hyperlipidemia.

In many patients with hypertriglyceridemia, VLDL remnants remain in the plasma for long periods. The accumulation of high numbers of remnants, including those of both chylomicron and VLDL origin, results from defective binding of ApoE to the liver cell surface receptors. The three common alleles for ApoE are ApoE2, ApoE3, and Apo E4. ApoE3 and ApoE4 are common and bind to the receptors with high affinity, whereas ApoE2 binds poorly because of a substitution of cysteine for arginine in a domain critical for binding to the LDL receptor. The ApoE2 allele is relatively common with single gene prevelance of approximately 15% and homozygous occurrence of 1%. In most persons this does not cause a significant problem in lipoprotein metabolism. However, if there is the superimposition of familial hypertriglyceridemia or familial combined hyperlipidemia (overproduction of VLDL) and apoE2 homozygosity, significant accumulation of VLDL and chylomicorn remnants may result. This disorder is referred to as dysbetalipoproteinemia and occurs in the general population with a prevelance of 1 in 5,000 to 1 in 10,000.

The prolonged circulation of VLDL remnants may result from saturation of the liver cell surface sites for the processing steps mentioned above. The molecular abnormalities that cause these slow processing rates have not been defined. One potential mechanism may involve an excess of the exchangeable ApoCs, particularly the most common of these: ApoC-III. These proteins can inhibit the interaction of ApoB and ApoE with ApoB/ApoE receptors and the action of hepatic triglyceride lipase (HTGL).

Other physiologic changes result from the long residence time of the remnants of TG-rich lipoproteins. These remnants interact with the cholesteryl ester transfer protein (CETP) that allows some of the TG to be exchanged for cholesteryl ester in the LDL and HDL fractions (16,17). The accumulated cholesteryl ester in the VLDL core remains with the particle until it is cleared from the plasma. LDL and HDL become TG enriched and provide a substrate for the lipolytic enzymes lining the external membranes of liver cells, particularly HTGL. As the TG is

removed, the core of these particles becomes reduced and shrinks into smaller and more dense LDL and HDL; therefore, moderate hypertriglyceridemia (150–400 mg/dL) is statistically associated with small dense LDL and HDL. During the processing of these particles in plasma, phospholipids are exchanged with other lipoproteins by the phospholipid transfer protein (PLT).

Low-Density Lipoprotein Metabolism

VLDL is degraded in human plasma to form LDL, which normally comprises about 50% cholesterol, 25% phospholipid, 20% protein, and 2–5% TG. About two thirds of the cholesterol is esterified with fatty acids. The only protein in most mature LDL particles is the 550 kDa ApoB-100, which contributes the remaining 20–25% of the particle weight. The size of LDL particles varies from approx 22–27 nm in diameter. The ApoB-100 contains a domain near the middle of the protein sequence that has stringent binding characteristics for the LDL receptor and does not bind significantly to the LRP receptor on the liver. The binding of LDL to the LDL receptor clears about 75–90% of LDL from the plasma in normal individuals, and most of this clearance results from the large population of LDL receptors on the liver cell surfaces. The liver is therefore the major uptake site for the circulating cholesterol in LDL in addition to chylomicrons and VLDL remnants.

LDL particles stay in the plasma considerably longer than VLDL or chylomicrons. In normal adults, LDL has a half-life of between 2 and 3 d and longer in patients with dysfunctional LDL receptors. The presence of a dysfunctional receptor is common, with a gene frequency of approx 1 in 500. Because the LDL receptor is the rate-limiting step in the clearance of LDL particles, a single gene abnormality produces a pattern of pseudodominant inheritance in affected families (familial hypercholesterolemia). This abnormality doubles the plasma concentration of LDLc from the usual range of 80–150 mg/dL to 190–300 mg/dL. If two genes are defective with the same sequence abnormality, the condition is called homozygous familial hypercholesterolemia (18). In most patients, the two abnormal genes result from different defects, and the condition is the result of mixed heterozygosity. In either case, little or no LDL is cleared by the normal pathway, and cholesterol levels may reach 1000 mg/dL. Clearance depends on nonspecific endocytosis by all cells of the body and on uptake through scavenger receptors by macrophages in liver, spleen, lymph nodes, and bone marrow. The half-life of LDL in these patients may approach 1 wk. Patients with these receptor defects and extremely high plasma LDL concentrations are subject to tendon and cutaneous xanthomata and to arteriosclerosis early in life. Patients with the double defect may have major clinical events secondary to vascular disease during the first decade of life.

LDL clearance by a minor but very important pathway involves the damage of these LDL particles and their recognition by macrophage scavenger receptors. Oxidation of the lipid, particularly the polyunsaturated fatty acid components of the phospholipids on the surface, can generate a variety of reactive aldehydes (i.e., malondialdehyde and 4-hydroxynonenol) that form covalent bonds with the lysine groups of the ApoB-100 protein. The amino acid side chains of the protein can be directly oxidized as in the conversion of cysteine to cysteic acid. In addition, other adducts such as glycosylation can provide for ligands that are taken up by macrophages and smooth muscle cells expressing scavenger receptors. Aggregation of the lipoproteins may provide for a similar uptake process by such cells. If the cells expressing scavenger receptors are located in the spleen, liver, or bone marrow, this type of LDL clearance has little consequence. However, if the cells are in the subendothelial layer of arteries, the accumulated lipid may lead to the expression of cytokines and enzymes that induce arteriosclerosis.

High-Density Lipoprotein Metabolism

HDL are the smallest but most heterogeneous and complex of all the lipoprotein species. They are also the most dense because of the high protein content; HDL comprises about 50% protein, 20% cholesterol (and cholesterol ester), and the rest, phospholipids. A small amount (1–3%) of TG may be present. All of the apolipoproteins mentioned above are components of HDL, with the exceptions of ApoB-48 or ApoB-100. The two major categories based on size are HDL_2 and HDL_3, with the latter being the smaller, more dense form. Using 2D gel electrophoresis, at least 9 reproducible subpopulations of HDL differing in size and charge can be identified in normal plasma.

The protein components of HDL are synthesized in the intestinal mucosa and the liver. HDL comprises about 65% ApoA-I, 25% ApoA-II, and the rest of the protein mass (5–10%) is made up of ApoA-IV, ApoE, and the ApoCs. Other proteins are present in minor quantities, including ApoD and various enzymes such as paraoxonase (see below).

HDL conducts several important functions in the plasma and extracellular space. One function is to provide a reservoir of exchangeable proteins (apoC's and apoE) that can be transferred onto the surface of newly formed TG-rich lipoproteins to induce their catabolism.

HDL can readily pass among cells in the extravascular space and help in the uptake of lipids, which is especially important for the removal of free cholesterol from extrahepatic cells. Every cell in the body can make cholesterol, but only the liver has an excretory system that can rid the body of significant quantities of cholesterol. By use of the ABCA1 transporter, cells can transfer intracellular cholesterol to the plasma membrane where HDL can adsorb the cholesterol and incorporate it into the HDL surface coat. In the plasma, an enzyme called lecithin-cholesterol acyl transferase (LCAT) transfers fatty acid from the 2-position of the phospholipid (lecithin) to the hydroxyl group of the cholesterol. The resulting cholesteryl ester is then incorporated into the lipid core of the lipoprotein, providing space for additional cholesterol to be adsorbed from the cell surfaces. This transfer of cholesterol to the larger spherical HDL particles appears to occur primarily in the peripheral cells and may involve other transfer proteins of the ATP binding cassette family, ABCG3 and ABCG4. After gaining cholesterol and cholesteryl ester in this process, the HDL particles can give up the cholesteryl ester to the liver cell through an exchange process involving another scavenger receptor protein SR-BI. This process leaves the rest of the HDL particle on the exterior of the hepatocytes and allows the cholesterol-depleted HDL to continue cycling through the extrahepatic tissues. Because HDL contains ApoE, the entire HDL particle can be taken up for degradation in the liver via either the LDL or the LRP receptors. The net result of these mechanisms is to allow for directional flow of endogenously synthesized cholesterol to enter the hepatic pool where an appropriate proportion can be excreted through the biliary ducts into the stool.

Most HDL proteins are cleared by the kidney tubule. The binding of ApoA-I by the kidney is specific, with a higher affinity for small particles. HDL particles are cleared more rapidly when there is rapid transfer of cholesterol ester from these lipoproteins. Thus, the removal of cholesteryl esters by CETP into TG remnants or into the liver by increased numbers of SR-BI receptors should lead to fewer circulating HDL—a finding that is seen in patients with high fasting TG and low HDL cholesterol and ApoA-I plasma concentrations.

HDL has other functions that may contribute to normal physiology, including the inhibition of oxidation of lipids within its own structure and in other lipoproteins. The major esterification that leads to the normal distribution of free to esterified cholesterol in human plasma is a function of LCAT, an enzyme that is activated by the ApoA-I and ApoC-I proteins of HDL.

Lipoprotein[a] Metabolism

Lipoprotein antigen (Lp[a]) was discovered by Berg, a Norwegian hematologist *(19)*, as a result of testing for antibodies in the blood of patients who had had blood transfusions. Lp[a] is a curious complex of protein and lipids formed by the addition of a second protein "little-(a)" complexed with normal LDL. This added protein has a molecular weight ranging from 300 to 800 kDa that varies among individuals. More than 30 alleles of Lp[a] with varying size and sequence have been described *(20)*. Because of this variability, there is a high probability that Lp[a] will be recognized as a foreign protein after blood transfusion, and antibodies are often induced. The lipoprotein connection is the consequence of the "little-(a)" protein binding to the surface of LDL in the plasma compartment with some specificity. This favored folding pattern presents a cysteine of the "little-a" protein at a location near a cysteine side chain of ApoB-100 with a resulting covalent bond being formed after the action of an oxidase in the plasma *(21)*. The quantity of this complex varies from person to person. In Caucasians and Orientals, the median plasma concentration is approximately 10 mg/dL, with many individuals having levels below 2 mg/dL. The distribution of concentrations in the population is markedly skewed; a small percentage have values over 100 mg/dL, and some have levels higher than 200 mg/dL. The genotype of the parents appears to be the primary determinant of plasma concentrations *(22,23)*. Diet, activity level, and other disease states have a minimal effect on Lp[a] values. The major exception is seen in women with ovarian failure; Lp[a] levels may increase 30% to 50% at menopause. This increase is partially reversible by hormone replacement therapy.

In some families, high concentrations of Lp[a] are associated with risk of vascular disease. Epidemiological data from community-based studies are not consistent, but most evidence suggests an increased risk in persons with Lp[a] concentrations higher than 30 mg/dL *(24–26)*. Although the cause of the increased risk has not been fully defined, several theories are possible. The "little-a" protein is structurally related to plasminogen, probably through a common ancestral gene. Like plasminogen, most of the protein sequence is folded and linked internally by disulfide bonds that are similar to the Danish pastry called kringles *(27)*. Some of the many alleles express structures near the carboxyl end of the molecule that, like plasminogen, bind to fibrin and could inhibit the activation of circulating plasminogen, thereby reducing its thrombolytic potential. Other functional changes have been reported in the LDL molecules involved. The binding region of the ApoB-100 for the LDL receptor is blocked, resulting in a potential buildup of LDL in plasma.

Finally, some studies suggest that this complex is more readily altered by oxidative processes and made subject to scavenger receptor activity. Any or all of these processes could contribute to the proposed sequence leading to atherosclerotic events. The heterogeneity in structure and in plasma concentrations produced by different genes for the little-a protein makes prediction of risk difficult in any given patient. The family history often provides the best clues as to the atherogenic potential of a given allele.

LIPIDS AS RISK FACTORS

Cholesterol

High cholesterol is considered a primary risk factor for atherosclerosis. The debate on the development of accelerated atherosclerosis has continued between the lipid hypothesis and the injury hypothesis. According to the lipid hypothesis, high plasma cholesterol is sufficient to cause atherosclerosis. In the injury hypothesis, the development of atherosclerosis requires not only hyperlipidemia, but also injury to the endothelium. Recent data support both hypotheses and indicate that increased plasma lipid concentrations could cause the injury to the arterial tree and thereby initiate the development of atherosclerosis. The severity of additional contributing risk factors would modulate the rate of disease progression.

Several cohort studies have shown that participants with initially high plasma cholesterol levels were more likely to develop coronary artery disease over the next 10–20 yr *(28–30)*. Results from the Multiple Risk Factor Intervention Trial (MRFIT), a landmark epidemiologic study based on a 6-yr follow-up study in more than 350,000 men *(31)*, indicate that (1) cholesterol levels between 150 and 200 mg/dL are associated with a small but significant increase in risk of CAD over concentrations less than 150 mg/dL; (2) the increase in risk is linear for cholesterol concentrations between 200 and 260 mg/dL; (3) with cholesterol concentrations greater than 260 mg/dL, the risk of coronary artery disease increases 2% for every 1% increase in total plasma cholesterol. Prospective studies worldwide have shown a strong dose-dependent relationship between plasma cholesterol and coronary artery disease (CAD), independent of gender and other risk factors *(32)*.

The evidence that cholesterol is a primary risk factor for CAD is derived from data based on three different types of interventional studies designed to reduce plasma cholesterol: diet, surgery, and pharmacological regimens. Many primary and secondary trials have studied the effects of diet on plasma cholesterol *(33,34)*. Although results from these trials have indicated that reducing cholesterol levels significantly decreases CAD deaths, other risk factors, such as smoking reduction, control of blood

Table 2
Serum LDL Cholesterol Concentrations (mg/dL) in the United States

Age (yr)		*Percentile values*		
	Mean	*10th*	*50th*	*90th*
Men				
20–34	119	87	119	156
35–44	135	91	132	186
45–54	140	95	140	188
55–64	138	90	135	182
65–74	136	92	133	182
75+	132	32	128	177
Women				
20–34	111	71	109	152
35–44	118	83	115	159
45–54	131	85	129	177
55–64	144	93	143	192
65–74	143	95	144	188
75+	145	102	128	177

LDL indicates low-density lipoprotein. From the National Health and Nutrition Survey, 1988–1994 (NHANES IV) *(44)*.

pressure, and weight loss, may have been included in these trials. A few interventional studies examined the effect of diet alone. These studies focused on the substitution of saturated fatty acids with ω6-polyunsaturated fatty acids *(35,36)* and required drastic changes in dietary habits. A P/S ratio five to six fold higher than the average western diet was used to achieve a reduction in CAD risk. Studies in women have also shown a reduction in CAD mortality by decreasing plasma cholesterol *(36)*.

For surgical studies, the Program On the Surgical Control of the Hyperlipidemias (POSCH) Study indicated that significant reductions in coronary events (including CAD deaths and nonfatal myocardial infarction) could be achieved by an increase in bile acid loss after ileal bypass surgery *(37)*. In the plasma, the intervention resulted in a 23% reduction in total cholesterol ($p < 0.00001$), a 38% reduction in LDLc ($p < 0.0001$), and a 4% increase in HDLc ($p < 0.02$) *(38)*. A 35% net reduction in coronary events ($p < 0.001$) was seen in the surgically treated group.

The first major successful pharmacologic study was the Lipid Research Clinics–Coronary Primary Prevention Trial (LRC-CPPT) *(39,40)*, which showed that a 2% reduction in CAD risk could be expected for every 1% reduction in plasma total cholesterol in participants with initially increased plasma cholesterol levels. This finding is consistent with the risk relationships seen in the screening cohort from MRFIT *(31)*. By using a different lipid-low-

ering drug, gemfibrozil, the Helsinki Heart Study showed a relationship between reduced LDLc levels and a decreased incidence of CHD *(41)*. The same conclusion was reached in the West of Scotland Coronary Prevention Study (WOSCOPS) in which an HMG CoA reductase inhibitor (statin) was used to lower plasma LDL in a primary prevention trial *(42)*.

Similar results have been reported in secondary prevention trials, including the Cholesterol Lowering and Atherosclerosis Study (CLAS), St. Thomas Atheroma Regression Study (STARS), Monitored Atherosclerosis Regression Study (MARS), Scandinavian Simvastatin Survival Study (4S), and the Cholesterol and Recurrent Events (CARE) trial. Comprehensive reviews of these interventional studies have been published *(43)*.

Low-Density Lipoprotein Cholesterol

Because 60% of the cholesterol in plasma is associated with LDL, increased concentrations of LDL are highly correlated with high cholesterol levels, and LDLc is considered a major risk factor for CAD. LDL is derived from VLDL, which is synthesized and secreted by the liver in the form of TG-rich lipoproteins. VLDL transport endogenous TG to peripheral tissues. The end-product of this process is the cholesterol-rich LDL that are removed from the circulation via interaction with specific cell surface receptors, primarily the LDL receptor.

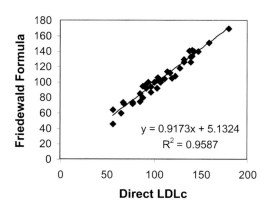
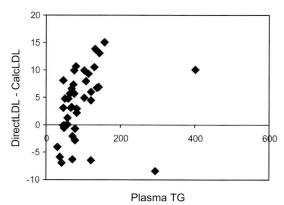

Fig. 2. (A) High correlation between the calculated value for low-density lipoprotein cholesterol (LDLc) by using the Friedewald formula and direct determination of LDLc may be misleading in patient management. High correlation can typically be obtained between the value for LDLc calculated by using the Friedewald formula and that obtained by using a homogeneous assay for direct LDLc (Equal Diagnostics, Elkton, PA). In this group of free-living volunteers, LDLc ranges from 55 to 180 mg/dL. TG, triglycerides. **(B)** On an individual basis, the two estimates for low-density lipoprotein cholesterol (LDLc) may differ by as much as 16 mg/dL, even when triglyceride concentrations (TG) are within the normal range. When individual difference in LDLc is examined for assessment of risk, it can be demonstrated that the two methods can provide values that could significantly affect the management program; differences ranged from −7 to +15 mg/dL. This difference between the two laboratory values for LDLc is not entirely due to elevated plasma triglycerides.

This receptor-mediated process is rate limiting and highly saturable. Changes in diet affect the expression of the LDL receptor and, thus, affect plasma levels of LDLc. All interventions that reduce total cholesterol will reduce LDLc and CAD risk. The distribution of LDLc in men and women based on the NHANES data set is presented in (Table 2).

The values for LDLc vary, depending on the analytical method used by the laboratory. The most common value reported for LDLc is based on a calculation using the Friedewald formula, which assumes that dividing plasma TG by 5 can approximate the cholesterol content of the TG-rich VLDL. Thus,

$$\text{Calculated LDLc} = \text{CHOL} - \text{HDLc} - \text{TG/5}$$

For lipemic plasma (TG > 400), this formula often provides an underestimate of LDLc, and sometimes a negative value for LDLc is obtained.

The Lipid Research Clinics Program (LRCP) used the ultracentrifuge to standardize the direct determination of LDLc. In this process, known as beta-quantitation or "beta-quant," TG-rich lipoproteins are removed by ultracentrifugation at density $d < 1.006$ g/mL, and the cholesterol level in the remaining more dense lipoproteins is determined directly. LDLc is defined as the difference between the cholesterol concentration in the infranate, which comprises LDL and HDL, and an independently determined estimate of HDLc. Thus,

$$\text{Beta-quant LDLc} = [\text{CHOL in } d > 1.006 \text{ density fraction}] - \text{HDLc}$$

Homogeneous enzymatic assays have been used recently to determine LDLc directly without requiring an assumption of the composition of VLDL. These assays, commonly referred to as direct LDLc, use specific polymers and/or mixtures of antibodies to precipitate HDL and VLDL, which leaves LDL in solution for the determination of LDLc. These assays, supposedly effective in patients with TG concentrations less than 750 mg/dL, work best with TG in the range of 50–500 mg/dL.

Figure 2A illustrates the relationship between calculated LDLc and direct LDLc. Although the two methods show high correlation for a group of individuals, the difference in the two values of LDLc can be as high as 1–20 mg/dL in either direction (Fig. 2B). This difference may affect patient management and, ultimately clinical outcome. Although it is commonly assumed that the difference between the two estimates of LDLc can be explained by plasma TG, Fig. 2B clearly indicates this is not the case. Current healthcare practice does not permit reimbursement for LDLc results obtained with the formula.

Increased LDLc is a primary cause of the acceleration of atherosclerosis; however, not all LDL are the same. In vitro studies have shown that human monocyte–derived macrophages do not accumulate lipids and transform into foam cells, even when exposed to concentrations of LDL several times higher than those seen in vivo. Some type of chemical modification is required to increase the uptake of LDL via the scavenger receptors *(45)* and accelerate disease progression *(46)*. In vitro studies have shown that many chemical modifications produce extensive

Table 3
Serum Triglyceride Concentrations in the United States

Age (yr)	Mean	Percentile values		
		10th	50th	90th
Men				
20–34	118	55	95	204
35–44	150	62	126	242
45–54	182	72	135	296
55–64	176	80	144	311
65–74	160	76	137	256
75+	144	71	125	220
Women				
20–34	101	49	84	177
35–44	123	53	93	170
45–54	136	59	144	239
55–64	166	72	135	313
65–74	157	76	134	253
75+	150	74	130	235

From the National Health and Nutrition Survey, 1988–1994 (NHANES IV) (44).

structural changes before the resulting modified LDL are presented as models of physiologically relevant damaged LDL. Research from the laboratories of Steinberg (46,47) and Fogelman (48) has suggested that minimal modification of LDL via enzymes involved in the oxidative stress response may be able to initiate lipid accumulation (47,49). For example, superoxide anions and thiol products released by endothelial cells and monocytes can modify circulating LDL (50,51). In addition, these cells secrete lipoxygenase, an enzyme that produces lipid oxidation products and is expressed extensively in atherosclerotic lesions. Circulating levels of oxidatively modified LDL and circulating levels of autoantibodies against these modified forms of LDL may be biomarkers for atherosclerosis (see Developing Risk Factors).

Triglycerides

Despite significant data on the relationship between hypertriglyceridemia and CAD risk, the proposition that increased TG concentration is an independent risk factor is controversial. The distribution of TG in men and women based on the NHANES data set is presented in (Table 3). One of the first studies to link hypertriglyceridemia to CAD was the report from Albrink et al. in 1959 (52). In this early study and subsequent studies, a univariate association between TG levels and incidence of CAD has been reported. After adjusting for HDLc, the relative risk

was reduced to 1.31 for men and 1.19 for women; this relative risk was no longer statistically significant (53).

In other studies, the association between TG levels and incidence of CAD remained strong after adjusting for confounding factors. In the Copenhagen Male Study, the cumulative incidence rates of ischemic heart disease in a group of 2,906 elderly men (mean age, 63 yr; range, 53–74 yr) were 2.5 times higher for those in the highest tertile for TG (11.5%) than for those in the lowest tertile (4.6%) during an 8-yr follow-up period (54). In addition, this study showed a dose-dependent increase in risk as a function of plasma TG within each level of HDLc. This relationship was significant after adjusting for total and LDL cholesterol. The Baltimore Coronary Observational Long-Term Study has redefined the appropriate plasma level of TG (55). Multiple logistic regression analysis indicated that a baseline TG greater than 100 mg/dL was one of three independent predictors of CAD events in men. Survival from CAD events was significantly lower for patients with baseline TG levels ≥100 mg/dL than for patients with TG levels <100 mg/dL. This finding raised concerns about the recommendation of the Adult Treatment Program that interventions be considered only when TG levels are greater than 200 mg/dL.

In a recent meta-analysis that combined data from 17 studies of 46,000 men and 11,000 women, an increase in plasma TG levels of 54 mg/dL was associated with a 30%

Table 4
Serum HDL Cholesterol Concentrations (mg/dl) in the United States

Age (yr)	Mean	Percentile values		
		10th	50th	90th
Men				
20–34	46	32	45	62
35–44	45	30	43	61
45–54	45	30	42	66
55–64	45	31	42	61
65–74	46	30	43	64
75+	47	31	44	66
Women				
20–34	55	38	53	74
35–44	54	38	53	72
45–54	56	38	55	77
55–64	56	37	53	78
65–74	56	37	54	76
75+	56	37	55	76

From the National Health and Nutrition Survey, 1988–1994 (NHANES IV) *(44)*.

increase in risk for men and an 80% increase for women *(56)*. However, none of these studies provided an objective measure of insulin resistance, which is a potential risk factor strongly linked to high TG levels. To define TG as an independent and causative risk factor, these studies must show a reduction in CVD events with interventions that specifically reduce plasma TG. Data from such clinical trials are not available because most interventions that reduce plasma TG usually increase HDLc. Therefore, the controversy over whether TG is an independent risk factor for CAD that deserves specific therapy remains unresolved.

The inherent biological variability of TG concentrations in individuals is a statistical problem for conducting an appropriate clinical trial. Even with modest levels of fasting TG, plasma TG can vary by as much as 30–40% 12 h after consuming a low fat load. We believe that unless the meal eaten before blood collection is standardized, this variability in the metabolism of dietary TG prevents an accurate determination of fasting TG levels. This variability in TG levels within the same individual may explain the absence of a consistent relationship between TG levels and CAD risk.

High-Density Lipoprotein Cholesterol

HDL, which accounts for 20–30% of the cholesterol in plasma, is responsible for the transport of cholesterol from peripheral tissues to the liver and kidneys. By reducing the

undesirable accumulation of cholesterol in peripheral tissues, HDL plays a key role in the reverse cholesterol transport (RCT) critical in the reduction of risk for CVD. The distribution of HDLc in men and women according to the NHANES data set is presented in (Table 4).

Eder and colleagues *(57)* used a crude electrophoretic process to show that patients with CAD have low levels of α-lipoproteins. The Tromso Heart Study *(58)* and the Honolulu Heart Study *(59)* were among the first major studies to show the clinical significance of HDLc in CAD by reporting an association between low HDL and an increased risk of myocardial infarction. This relationship has been documented in more than 25 subsequent studies. In the Helsinki Heart Study *(41)*, the use of the fibric acid derivative gemfibrozil significantly reduced CAD events when HDL was increased; however, other investigators argued that the reduced levels of LDLc and TG in this cohort may have affected the results. Results from the VA HDL Intervention Trial (VA-HIT), in which participants had normal levels of LDLc and low HDLc levels, showed a significant and dose-dependent reduction in CAD events as HDL levels increased with gemfibrozil *(60)*.

In vitro studies have shown that the interaction of the protein component of HDL, primarily ApoA-I, with the class of cell receptors ABCA1 promotes the efflux of cholesterol from cells. Much of this work related to the study of the metabolic defect associated with Tangier disease *(61)*. In Tangier disease, this active transport pathway for the efflux of cholesterol and phospholipids from cells induced by the lipid-poor HDL apolipoproteins is not active *(62,63)*, which leads to the rapid catabolism of the resulting smaller, lipid-poor HDL particles *(61)*. Patients with Tangier disease may or may not have an increased risk of atherosclerotic disease. The characterization of this receptor-mediated efflux illustrates that HDL apolipoproteins by themselves may not affect the risk of developing premature atherosclerosis.

Another pathway for the lipidation of HDL apolipoproteins is the intravascular hydrolysis of plasma TG by lipolytic enzymes. Felts et al. *(64)* have suggested that as the TG core of chylomicrons and VLDL is depleted by lipoprotein lipase, the excess surface components, comprising primarily phospholipids and unesterified cholesterol, is transferred to lipid-poor HDL apolipoproteins (Fig. 3). The transfer of these particles to circulating HDL with a larger cholesteryl ester core is completed by the action of lecithin-cholesterol acyl transferase (LCAT). The existence of this pathway supports the strong inverse relationship between plasma TG and plasma HDL cholesterol. Defects in the lipidation of HDL apolipoproteins during TG hydrolysis would result in accelerated catabolism of HDL in patients with hypertriglyceridemia *(65,66)*, which explains both the small, dense characteristic and the reduced number of HDL.

Remnant Lipoproteins

Impaired hydrolysis of endogenous TG in VLDL is linked with abnormalities in the metabolism of exogenous fats as seen in the presence of remnant lipids in fasting plasma. Intestinally derived lipoproteins are usually absent from the fasting plasma of a normal individual; however, an individual adhering to the AHA step 1 dietary recommendation who is consuming 2000 kcal/day would be transporting 600–800 mg of cholesterol and 55 g of TG in the chylomicrons. This daily supply of TG is equivalent to 10 times the total TG plasma pool of an individual with a fasting TG concentration of 150 mg/dL. In the bloodstream, chylomicrons carrying dietary fats share most of the same metabolic pathways as the hepatic VLDL carrying endogenous fats. As the rate-limiting step in the catabolism of VLDL and its products involve interactions with specific cell surface receptors, the uptake of chylomicron remnants by the chylomicron receptor is the final step in the metabolism of chylomicrons. Overproduction of hepatic VLDL would saturate these pathways resulting in delayed catabolism of chylomicrons and its remnants. Brown et al. *(14)* suggested the

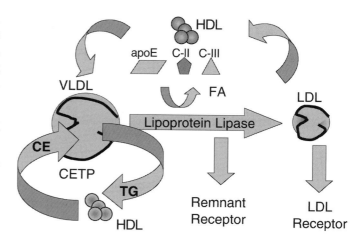

Fig. 3. Redistribution of the exchangeable apolipoproteins in the metabolism of triglyceride (TG)-rich lipoproteins. Upon entry into the circulation, triglyceride-rich lipoproteins acquire their full complement of exchangeable apolipoproteins (ApoC-II, ApoC-III, and ApoE) from plasma HDL. Interactions of triglyceride-rich lipoproteins with lipoprotein lipase that lines the endothelium result in the hydrolysis of triglycerides into monoglycerides and free fatty acids. The hydrolyzed particles can either be removed in toto by interactions with the remnant receptors or converted to smaller, more dense TG-depleted, cholesterol-rich lipoproteins. In the case of the postprandial chylomicrons, the end-product is chylomicron remnant. With hepatic very low density lipoprotein (VLDL), the end-product is low-density lipoprotein (LDL). The end-product is removed via a rate-limiting, receptor-mediated uptake process. As the triglyceride-rich lipoproteins shrink in size with the depletion of TG, the exchangeable apolipoproteins are returned to HDL. A minor component of the TG contents in the TRL can also be redistributed to other plasma lipoproteins, primarily HDL but also LDL, via the action of the enzyme cholesteryl ester transfer protein (CETP).

link between postprandial lipemia and CAD in 1961, as reviewed by Zilversmit *(12)*.

Assessing the contribution of dietary derived lipids to the population of circulating lipoproteins is challenging. Some investigators have used the concentration of a special form of ApoB, ApoB-48, unique to intestinal chylomicrons as a marker of intestinally derived lipoproteins and their remnants *(67,68)*. This intestinal form of ApoB is detected either by SDS-PAGE *(67,68)* or by using specific monoclonal antibodies that recognize epitopes on ApoB-100 but not on ApoB-48 *(69)*. Both of these methods are tedious and have poor reproducibility.

Another method for monitoring remnant lipoproteins is based on the metabolism of dietary retinol (vitamin A) *(70)*. Retinol is readily absorbed, esterified to retinyl esters, and secreted in the core of newly formed chylomicrons, similar to dietary cholesterol. In the circulation, retinyl esters seem to follow the same metabolic fate as dietary cholesterol and remain with the chylomicrons until the liver takes up these particles as chylomicron remnants. After administration of an oral dose of retinol (usually with a fat-containing mixture), the presence of a significant concentration of retinyl esters in plasma after 24 h indicates impaired catabolism of chylomicrons. Many investigators have used retinyl esters to characterize the kinetics of intestinally derived particles in various subfractions of plasma to study this abnormality in catabolism (71–74). Using this approach, Groot et al. (13) showed that the catabolism of dietary-derived retinyl esters was impaired in men with CAD as compared with men without CAD who were matched for plasma lipid levels and other traditional risk factors.

The FDA has recently approved for clinical use a new antibody-based kit for the determination of remnant cholesterol. This kit uses a combination of specific monoclonal antibodies to remove HDL, LDL, and hepatic VLDL from plasma, which allows chylomicrons and chylomicron remnants to remain in solution (75–77).

APOLIPOPROTEINS AS RISK FACTORS

Although lipid deposits in atheroma are the landmark of atherosclerotic disease, the apolipoproteins are an integral part of the system responsible for the transport and delivery of plasma lipids. Apolipoproteins modulate the rate of catabolism of the lipoproteins and target these particles to the appropriate cells. Because lipids may rapidly redistribute among other lipoproteins and tissues, apolipoprotein levels may be a more stable measure of the metabolic conditions. However, standardizing antibody-based assays for the quantitation of plasma apolipoproteins based on either immunoturbidometric or enzyme-linked immunoassays has been difficult.

Apolipoprotein B

The gene coding for ApoB has been mapped to the short arm of chromosome 2 in the p23-p24 region (78). Apolipoprotein B is a primary structural protein in chylomicrons, chylomicron remnants, VLDL, IDL, and LDL. Only one ApoB molecule is associated with each lipoprotein particle; therefore, ApoB concentrations can be used as a surrogate measure of particle numbers. However, the composition of these lipoproteins varies over a wide range from 99% lipids and 1% proteins in chylomicrons to 70% lipids and 30% protein in LDL; this variability in lipid content could affect the recognition of antigenic sites by antibodies. Furthermore, the relative concentration of the different lipoprotein classes in whole plasma may significantly affect the value obtained for plasma ApoB. In fasting plasma, VLDL may account for 5% or 50% of total plasma ApoB.

In case-control studies, ApoB is a strong discriminant for CAD (79–82). Prospective studies support this relationship, but whether ApoB is a significantly better indicator of risk than LDLc is unknown (83,84). Because of the pre-analytical factors that may affect ApoB levels and the lack of standardization for apolipoprotein measurements, the practical application of ApoB determinations for clinical use is problematic.

Molecular techniques have been used to examine ApoB polymorphisms in the diagnosis of disease. Genetic variation in the ApoB gene locus has been linked to increased cholesterol levels and dietary responsiveness to fat (85). Polymorphisms in the ApoB gene locus, however, are typically not associated with conditions that involve overproduction of ApoB. These molecular tools may potentially be used to identify individuals with familial defective ApoB who would have extreme increases in LDLc despite normal expression of the LDL receptor (86).

Apolipoprotein A-I

Apolipoprotein A-I, the primary structural protein for the α-lipoproteins, correlates significantly with plasma HDL cholesterol. The gene for ApoA-I is located on chromosome 11 (78). ApoA-I levels may be a better discriminator of CAD than HDL cholesterol (87) because intra-individual variability is less with ApoA-I levels than with HDLc. During postprandial lipemia, transient changes in HDL cholesterol but not in plasma ApoA-I can be seen in some individuals. However, the primary clinical use of ApoA-I determinations is for the diagnosis of patients with genetic disorders associated with very low levels of HDLc. Although some individuals with low HDLc and hypertriglyceridemia have normal levels of ApoA-I and accelerated clearance of HDL, ApoA-I production is decreased in individuals with isolated low HDLc levels (66). Low levels of plasma ApoA-I are seen in familial ApoA-I deficiency (88), Tangier disease (61), fish-eye disease (89), familial LCAT deficiency (90), and patients with ApoA-I$_{Milano}$ (91).

Lipoprotein[a]

Lp[a] is a special class of lipoproteins comprising one molecule of Apo(a) linked via a disulfide bridge to an LDL particle. The gene for Apo(a) is located on chromosome 6. Although data supporting the link between Lp[a] and CVD is debatable (24,25), Lp[a] can clearly be deposited in human atherosclerotic lesions (92). Because of the homology between the kringle of Apo(a) and plasminogen (93) and the in vitro data showing that Lp[a] can regulate plasminogen activator inhibitor-1 (PAI-1) expression in endothelial cells (27), Lp[a] may increase CVD risk by accelerating atherosclerosis and thrombosis (94,95). This risk may be partially independent of lipid levels (26).

One of the major problems in determining the risk associated with increased Lp[a] has been its variability in molecular weight (96,97), which makes standardization of immunoassay difficult (98). The size and concentration of Lp[a] (22) and the associated risk of developing CAD varies depending on the Apo(a) alleles (99). The relationship between size and plasma concentrations is further complicated by metabolic heterogeneity. Rader et al. (23) reported that two individuals with the same Apo(a) allele can have a 10-fold difference in plasma concentrations. In addition, variations in metabolism between ethnic groups can affect the risk of developing CAD in individuals with elevated Lp[a] (100).

Despite extensive information on the gene structure of Apo(a), the metabolism of Lp[a] is poorly understood. Specific sites on both ApoB (101) and Apo(a) (21,102) are required for the assembly of Lp[a]. Studies in transgenic mice suggest this coupling of Apo(a) to ApoB may occur in the extracellular space (103). Mice expressing human Apo(a) can secrete free Apo(a) in the circulation without the formation of Lp[a], presumably because of the difference in ApoB structure between mice and humans. Lp[a] can be detected in mouse plasma within minutes of the intravenous infusion of human LDL (103). Furthermore, mice expressing human Apo(a) can be induced to develop atherosclerotic lesions with an atherogenic diet.

Although overexpression of LDL receptors results in accelerated catabolism of Lp[a] in transgenic mice (104), therapeutic interventions that increase LDL receptor expression in humans fail to reduce Lp[a] concentrations (105,106).

Apolipoprotein E

Apolipoprotein E, a glycoprotein with a molecular weight of 34 kDa, is distributed among all plasma lipoproteins. The gene for ApoE is located on chromosome 19 (78). Newly synthesized TG-rich lipoproteins (both hepatic and intestinal) secreted into the circulation acquire ApoE from circulating plasma HDL. As TG is hydrolyzed, ApoE is either transferred back to HDL or is taken up with the partially hydrolyzed products via the LDL receptor and/or LRP located in the liver. This pathway may account for the clearance of a significant proportion of ApoB in VLDL before it can be converted to LDL. Three major isoforms of ApoE have been identi-

fied: ApoE2, E3, and E4. The ApoE3 allele is found in about 80% of the population, ApoE4 in 14%, and ApoE2 in 6% (107). Although ApoE concentrations differ as a function of the ApoE genotype, most information on risk shows it is associated with the genotype, not the plasma concentration.

Differences in the isoforms are due to substitutions of one or two amino acids within a span of 40 amino acids in the receptor-binding region. Of the ApoE isoforms, E2/2 has less than 10% binding affinity, and E4/4 has approx 120% binding affinity with the LDL receptor as compared with E3/3. This impaired binding to the receptor accounts for the presence of remnant lipoproteins enriched in cholesteryl esters in individuals with E2/2; in those with a concomitant disorder leading to overproduction of VLDL, the clinical syndrome commonly referred to as remnant disease, broad-beta disease, type III hyperlipoproteinemia, or dysbetalipoproteinemia is diagnosed.

Because of the potential impact of the ApoE phenotype on the binding and clearance of atherogenic remnant lipoproteins, the ApoE4 allele has been suggested as an independent predictor of coronary events (108–111).

Apolipoprotein C-III

ApoC-III, a small polypeptide of 9 kDa, is in dynamic equilibration with all plasma lipoproteins. The gene of ApoC-III is located on chromosome 11 within the ApoA-I, ApoC-III, ApoA-IV complex. Several regulatory elements are present within the non-coding region of the ApoC-III gene, including an insulin response element (112–114), a PPARα-regulated element (115–117), an NF-κB element (118), and others (119,120). ApoC-III is the most abundant protein on chylomicrons and is a major component of the apolipoproteins in VLDL. Because of its hydrophilic properties, ApoC-III may help modulate the metabolism of plasma lipoproteins in vivo (Fig. 4).

ApoC-III inhibits lipoprotein lipase (121–125). Transgenic mice overexpressing ApoC-III develop severe hypertriglyceridemia (126,127), whereas ApoC-III knockout mice have extremely low plasma TG and no postprandial hypertriglyceridemia (128). In a study of two sisters with ApoC-III deficiency with low plasma TG (129), production of hepatic TG was normal, and fractional clearance was higher than in normal controls (88).

ApoC-III modulates the interactions of ApoE-containing lipoproteins with receptors (130–133). Based on tracer kinetic data, we have suggested that excess ApoC-III on HDL may delay the clearance of HDL in vivo (65). Excess ApoC-III on HDL may interfere with

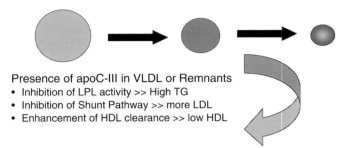

Presence of apoC-III in VLDL or Remnants
- Inhibition of LPL activity >> High TG
- Inhibition of Shunt Pathway >> more LDL
- Enhancement of HDL clearance >> low HDL

**Shunt Pathway reduces
the flux of apoB through LDL**

Fig. 4. Differential effect of ApoC-III on the metabolism of tryglyceride-rich lipoproteins and of high-density lipoprotein (HDL). The presence of ApoC-III on the tryglyceride-rich lipoproteins has been associated with impaired TG hydrolysis by lipoprotein lipase (LPL), resulting in hypertriglyceridemia. Excess accumulation of ApoC-III on triglyceride-rich lipoproteins has also been demonstrated to delay the rate of uptake of tryglyceride-rich lipoproteins by hepatic receptors. This may result in an increase flux of cholesterol into the atherogenic LDL. Furthermore, preferential association of plasma ApoC-III in the tryglyceride-rich lipoprotein fraction would leave circulating HDL unprotected, leading to the accelerated clearance of HDL and a low plasma concentration of HDLc. VLDL, very low density lipoprotein.

the interaction of the ligand with cell-surface receptors, independent of whether the ligand is ApoE or ApoB (134), as with chylomicron or VLDL remnants, or ApoA-I in the case of HDL. Polymorphisms in the ApoC-III gene have been associated with hypertriglyceridemia in several studies (113,114,135–137), and some studies have reported an association with insulin resistance and diabetes (136–138). In addition, preliminary data suggest that a specific ApoC-III haplotype may be protective against the development of hypertriglyceridemia (139). A variation in the ApoC-III gene has been associated with an increased number of ApoB-containing particles (140).

Although the role of ApoC-III in lipoprotein metabolism is unknown, it clearly regulates TG clearance from plasma. Interventional studies have suggested that the preferential association of ApoC-III with HDL and proportionally less association with VLDL is beneficial (141–143). In summary, the association of ApoC-III with plasma lipoproteins delays removal of the lipoproteins. The risk of atherosclerotic disease is increased if the particles with excess ApoC-III are the ApoB-containing lipoproteins, whereas the risk is reduced and regression is possible if the particles with excess ApoC-III are the lipoproteins containing ApoA-I.

Figure 5 summarizes the key steps in the metabolism of plasma lipoproteins in the normal individual.

DEVELOPING RISK FACTORS

Small, Dense Low-Density Lipoproteins

Small, dense LDL are seen in several metabolic abnormalities, including hypertriglyceridemia, low HDLc, impaired postprandial lipemia, obesity (central obesity), and insulin resistance (144,145). The increased flux of free fatty acids, seen in all these metabolic conditions, might be the underlying common pathway that induces the overproduction of ApoB-containing lipoproteins by the liver and secondarily leads to the predominance of small, dense LDL in plasma. This concept is consistent with the atherogenic dyslipidemia associated with the metabolic syndrome as outlined by Grundy (146).

Heterogeneity in LDL is not a new concept. Fisher et al. (147) were among the first to note that LDL has a wide range of molecular sizes. Using the ultracentrifuge to isolate the lipoprotein fraction that floats in the density range of 1.019–1.063, Sniderman et al. (148) reported that patients with a history of coronary artery disease had an increased ApoB:cholesterol ratio in the LDL fraction, despite having normal LDLc levels; they applied the term hyperapobetalipoproteinemia to these patients. Characterizing the distribution of LDL particle size in whole plasma has been simplified by the use of polyacrylamide gradient gel electrophoresis (PAGGE) (149). Other methods have been used to characterize LDL subfractions (150).

Although the actual diameter of the major electrophoretic peak of LDL ranges from 23.5 to 27.5 nm by PAGGE, most investigators have simplified the analysis by dichotomizing the LDL particle size by using the cutpoint of 24.5 nm (151), thereby introducing the concept of LDL phenotyping. Individuals whose predominant peak of LDL has a diameter greater than 24.5 nm, called the LDL phenotype A, are considered at reduced risk for heart disease. Individuals whose major peak has a diameter less than 24.5 nm, called LDL phenotype B, are considered at increased risk for heart disease (151).

In a nested case-control study, individuals with the LDL phenotype B had a threefold increase in risk of myocardial infarction, independent of age, sex, and relative weight (152). The Quebec Cardiovascular Study reported a 3.6-fold increase in risk for ischemic heart disease between the lowest and the highest tertiles of LDL particle diameter (153). Campos et al. (154) and Tornvall et al. (155) have reported similar findings in different populations. Several prospective studies in which frozen plasma samples were used showed a similar relationship between the prevalence of small, dense LDL and increased risk for CAD. The Stanford Five-City Project found that the association

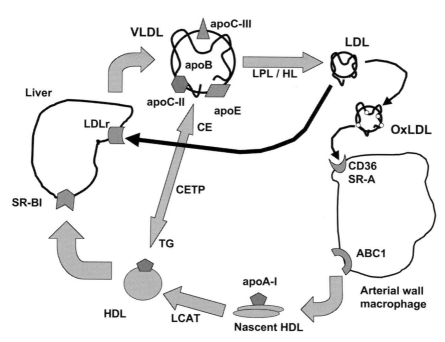

Fig. 5. Metabolism of plasma lipoproteins: Key Steps. The liver secretes very low density lipoprotein (VLDL) to deliver endogenous triglycerides (TG) as a source of energy for peripheral tissues. The end-product of this delivery process is the cholesterol-rich low-density lipoprotein (LDL), which is returned to the liver via the rate-limiting uptake process involving the LDL receptor. In the presence of inflammation and/or excess generation of reactive oxygen species, LDL can be oxidatively modified (OxLDL) and removed via the scavenger receptors (CD36, SR-A) present in monocyte-derived macrophages that may be present in the arterial wall. Nascent HDL with ApoA-I can promote the efflux of cholesterol from the macrophage via the receptor ABC1. The asserted action of the lipid transfer proteins, cholesteryl ester transfer protein (CETP) and lecithin-cholesterol acyl transferase (LCAT) promotes the formation of mature HDL for the return of cholesterol from the periphery back to the liver via the receptor SRB1 (SR-BI). Imbalance in this process resulting either from excess accumulation of OxLDL in the macrophage or low capacity of HDL for the reverse transport of cholesterol from the peripheral tissues back to the liver would promote the transformation of macrophages in the arterial wall into foam cells. A battery of inflammatory cytokines secreted by the activated macrophages can perpetuate and accelerate this vicious cycle of atherogenesis.

between reduced LDL particle diameter and increased CAD risk was graded across quintiles of LDL size *(156)*. In addition, the Physicians Health Study reported that LDL particles were significantly smaller in patients with CVD than in controls *(83)*. Adjusting for other risk factors, particularly HDLc, usually weakens this association.

The Stanford Coronary Risk Intervention Project was one of the first studies to show that LDL phenotyping may be useful in identifying the most effective management program *(157)*. The rate of luminal narrowing in patients with LDL phenotype B is decreased significantly more by aggressive multifactorial risk reduction than by usual-care programs, and patients with LDL phenotype A did not seem to gain additional benefits from the more aggressive management program. The Familial Atherosclerosis Treatment Study *(158)* combined the 4-yr follow-up data from a group of patients with documented CAD who had been randomly assigned to one of three treatment groups; their results showed that disease severity progressed the least in

patients with increased LDL buoyancy at baseline. Furthermore, the activity of hepatic lipase was inversely related to LDL buoyancy. Hepatic lipase (HTGL hepatic triglyceride lipase)is a heparin-releasable lipolytic enzyme that preferentially hydrolyzes TG and phospholipids from smaller VLDL and from TG-enriched LDL and HDL. Hepatic lipase may play a role in remodeling TG-enriched LDL resulting in the formation of an LDL subpopulation that is less lipid-enriched, and thus less buoyant.

Several genes may contribute metabolically to the predominance of small dense LDL in plasma *(159)*. As the first step in the formation and secretion of ApoB-containing lipoproteins, microsomal triglyceride transfer protein (MTP) couples the newly synthesized ApoB molecule to a lipid droplet *(160)*. Without this coupling, ApoB would be degraded intracellularly, and ApoB-containing particles would not be formed and secreted. Dreon et al. *(161–163)* suggested that although carbohydrate induction should increase hepatic TG production in all individuals, conconcomitant increase in ApoB synthesis to accomodate the increased flux of VLDL-TG occurred only in some individuals. Individuals who did not increase ApoB synthesis would presumably be able to secrete an unchanged number of particles with a larger TG core. Thus, the propensity for an individual to secrete a few large TG-rich particles or numerous smaller VLDL particles during a TG flux might be determined by MTP *(164,165)*.

In the plasma, TG-rich, ApoB-containing lipoproteins interact with lipoprotein lipase to unload their cargo of TG. Partially hydrolyzed particles can be either removed in total via interactions with specific receptors as part of the shunt pathway or converted to LDL via the action of hepatic triglyceride lipase (HTGL). The relative composition of ApoC-III and ApoE on the partially hydrolyzed particles may determine the preferred pathway for these ApoB-containing lipoproteins. Brunzell and colleagues *(158)* have suggested that the activity of HTGL may play a key role in the predominance of small, dense LDL in plasma. In addition, secretory phospholipase A2 (sPLA2), another lipolytic enzyme, and remodeling of plasma lipoproteins by the lipid transfer proteins, in particular cholesteryl ester transfer protein (CETP) and lecithin-cholesterol acyl transferase (LCAT), may contribute to the formation of small, dense LDL in vivo *(166–169)*.

High Sensitivity C-reactive Protein

In addition to being a chronic disease of lipid deposition, atherosclerosis is a state of chronic inflammation *(170–172)*. The initiating step in lipid accumulation is the adherence and subsequent infiltration of monocytes across the endothelium. This process is mediated by cellular adhesion molecules or selectins. P-selectins are stored in platelets and endothelial cells and can rapidly redistribute to the surface of these cells after stimulation by thrombin or other agonists *(173)*. E-selectins are synthesized de novo by endothelial cells that have been activated by inflammatory cytokines such as interleukin-1 (IL-1) and tumor necrosis factor α (TNFα). Both E- and P-selectins are expressed in the endothelium overlying atherosclerotic plaques.

Several markers of inflammation such as IL-6, s-ICAM-1, VCAM-1, TNFα, and high sensitivity C-reactive protein assay have been studied as possible variables that might be used to identify patients at increased risk of acute cardiovascular events *(172,174,175)*. Among these, CRP has been examined the most in clinical studies *(176,177)*. CRP is secreted by the liver and regulated by IL-6. Because of the low

levels of clinically significant CRP, a special assay, HSCRP, is required for assessment.

Baseline concentrations of CRP are a strong predictor of risk of future myocardial infarction, stroke, and peripheral vascular disease and a predictor of death from stroke and vascular disease. This measure as used in the assessment of CVD risk relates over a range of values once considered normal (1–8 mg/L). Depending on the clinical endpoint, the relative risk associated with the highest quintile of HSCRP (0.38–1.5 mg/dL) may range from 2.3 to 4.5 times greater *(177)*. In a prospective study of women, the relative risk of future cardiovascular events was 4.4 times greater for the highest quartile of CRP, followed by 3.5 times greater for the highest quartile of total:HDLc (TC/HDL) *(178)*. In multivariate analysis, only HSCRP and TC/HDL had predictive value once adjustments were made for age, smoking status, obesity, hypertension, family history, and diabetes. Similar results were reported in healthy men *(179)*. The relative risk of a future cardiovascular event for individuals in the highest quintile of HSCRP (>0.38 mg/dL or 3.8 mg/L) and TC/HDL (>6.1 for men and >5.2 for women) is estimated to be nine times greater. New guidelines for HSCRP have recently been published, suggesting that values below 1 mg/L indicate low risk and those above 3 mg/L indicate high risk. Because high levels of HSCRP may result from inflammation associated with infection and chronic conditions other than atherosclerosis, HSCRP values must be carefully interpreted within the total clinical assessment.

Several recent studies have shown that statins, in addition to reducing LDL-cholesterol, can reduce HSCRP *(180–182)*. This reduction may indicate successful treatment of the active atherosclerotic lesion and may correlate with a reduction in clinical events. However, the role of CRP levels as a marker of disease has not been confirmed.

Homocysteine

Homocysteine, a sulfur-containing amino acid, is produced during catabolism of the essential amino acid methionine. In the presence of excess methionine, homocysteine is conjugated to serine by the irreversible action of the enzyme cystathionine-β-synthase, with vitamin B6 as a required cofactor. With depletion of methionine, homocysteine is remethylated to methionine in a process involving the enzyme methionine synthase, vitamin B12, and methyltetrahydrofolate. This methionine-conserving pathway requires an adequate supply of folic acid and the enzyme methylene tetrahydrofolate reductase (MTHFR). In plasma, approximately 70% of homocysteine is found in a protein-bound form, 25% in the form of a dimer (homocystine), and 5% as mixed disulfide with other thiols or as free thiol.

McCully and Wilson *(183)* were the first investigators to suggest the "homocyst(e)ine theory of atherosclerosis." The link between hyperhomocysteinemia and atherosclerosis was suggested by the presence of premature atherothrombotic disease with the characteristic features of endothelial injury, proliferation of vascular smooth muscle cells, progressive arterial stenosis, and hemostatic changes suggestive of a prothrombotic state in patients with genetic disorders associated with high plasma concentrations of homocysteine. These rare inherited disorders include homozygous deficiency of cystathionine-β-synthase, MTHFR, or methionine synthase *(184)*.

Plasma homocysteine levels are determined by high performance liquid chromatography and represent the total concentration of homocysteine including the free and bound forms *(185)*. For accurate measurements, plasma or serum needs to be frozen immediately after collection unless analysis can be done within 24 h. Delay in the processing of whole blood before the removal of the plasma may introduce variability in the measurement. An immunoassay kit has been recently introduced for the reproducible and simple determination of plasma homocysteine *(186)*. Usually measured in the fasting state, plasma homocysteine levels range from 5–15 μmol/L in normal individuals. A range of 16–100 μmol/L is defined as mild to moderate hyperhomocysteinemia. When plasma homocysteine levels exceed 100 μmol/L, severe hyperhomocysteinemia is diagnosed. In some instances, homocysteine levels are determined with a methionine load. By determining homocysteine levels before and 4–6 h after a standard oral dose of methionine, variability in the transsulfuration pathway may be detected. Such variability may result from vitamin B6 deficiency or partial deficiency of cystathionine-β-synthase. Methionine loading may be more sensitive in identifying patients who have impaired homocysteine metabolism despite normal fasting total homocysteine *(187,188)*.

A meta-analysis of 27 studies with 4000 participants indicated that plasma levels above the 90th percentile are associated with increased risk for fatal and nonfatal atherosclerotic vascular disease in the coronary (OR 1.7), cerebral (OR 2.5), and peripheral (OR 6.8) circulation *(189)*. Using nested case-control design, the British United Provident Association reported that men who died of ischemic heart disease had higher serum homocysteine levels than age-matched controls (13.1 vs 11.8 μmol/L) *(190)*. A continuous dose-response relation was noted between CAD risk and homocysteine levels. For each 5 μmol/L increase in homocysteine level, the relative risk increased by 41%. After adjustment for other conventional risk factors, a 2.9 times increase in relative risk between the lowest and the highest quartile was seen *(190)*. A critical review of hyperhomocysteinemia and cardiovascular disease is available *(191)*.

In February 1996, the Food and Drug Administration announced a requirement for fortification of foods with folic acid (0.4–1.4 mg/lb of most enriched breads, flours, corn meals, pastas, rice, cereals and other grain products) that would be fully implemented by January 1, 1998. This change in supplementation was based on evidence that folate at this level markedly reduces neural tube defects in newborns. Based on data from a cohort of 2755 patients, a significant shift in the distribution of individuals with mild increases in homocysteine (>15 μmol/L) was noted: 43% of patients had high levels of homocysteine during the pre-announcement period (8/94–2/96); 41% had high levels during the interim period (3/96–12/97); and 28% after full implementation (1/98–10/98) *(192)*.

Paraoxonase

Paraoxonase (PON1), an enzyme found in HDL, may play an important role in vascular biology and the pathogenesis of atherosclerosis *(193,194)*. PON1 can hydrolyze nerve gases and organophosphoric pesticide metabolites, including paraoxon. Mackness et al. *(195,196)* were among the first to show that PON1 can retard the accumulation of lipid peroxides in LDL under oxidizing conditions in vitro. Watson et al. *(197)* subsequently found that the protective property of HDL against monocyte–endothelial interactions triggered by mildly oxidized LDL was a direct function of PON1. In transgenic mice, expression of human PON1 protects against atherosclerosis in a dose-dependent manner in ApoE-null mice *(198)*; HDL isolated from these mice protects LDL against oxidative modification. In contrast, HDL isolated from PON-knockout mice was unable to protect LDL from oxidative modification, and both HDL and LDL isolated from these mice were more susceptible to oxidative modification in vitro *(199,200)*.

Two major amino acid polymorphisms have been characterized in PON1, one at position 55 (methionine/leucine, M/L) and the other at position 192 (arginine/glutamine, R/Q) *(201,202)*. Paraoxon hydrolytic activity is greatest with HDL and PON1 isolated from individuals with either the PON1 192 RR genotype or the PON1 55 LL genotype. Paraoxon activity is the lowest in individuals with PON1 192 QQ and PON1 55 MM genotypes *(203,204)*. The capacity of PON1 alloenzymes to protect LDL from oxidation is inversely related to the paraoxon hydrolytic activity (202,203). A meta-analysis of case-control studies supports the hypothesis that individuals with the PON1 192 R allele are more susceptible to CHD (194). This finding is consistent with the fact that high paraoxon hydrolytic activity is associated with a reduced capacity of PON1 to protect LDL from oxidation. In fact, data suggest that the activity and concentration of PON1 may be more important than PON1 genetic polymorphism (203).

Dietary fats may affect the activity of PON1 (205–207). A cholesterol-rich diet (206) and the consumption of degraded cooking oils (207) are associated with a reduction in activity. The effects of lipid-lowering agents on PON1 activity have been varied; gemfibrozil (208) and statins (209) increase PON1 activity. Studies with other fibric acid derivatives have failed to show a change in PON1 activity (210,211).

Although PON1 provides a biochemical explanation for the antiatherogenic property of HDL other than reverse cholesterol transport, the significance of PON1 activity in predicting future cardiovascular events is unclear.

Oxidized Low-Density Lipoproteins and Autoantibodies to Oxidized Low-Density Lipoproteins

The macrophage foam cell laden with lipid deposits is a hallmark feature of atherosclerotic lesions. Although these lipids are derived from plasma LDL, incubation of macrophages in vitro with high concentrations of LDL does not lead to the accumulation of cholesteryl esters and the formation of foam cells. Brown et al. (45) provided the first hint of the missing link by showing that macrophages can take up and accumulate acetylated LDL. However, acetylation of more than 80% of the lysine residues in the protein moiety of LDL is required for effective uptake by macrophages, a step that makes this chemical modification unlikely to occur under physiologic conditions. Fogelman et al. (48) showed that modification of the lysine residues by malondialdehyde (MDA) was sufficient to cause LDL to be taken up by macrophages. This uptake was not inhibited by the presence of excess concentration of either native or acetylated LDL. Furthermore, because MDA is an end-product of lipid peroxidation, MDA-LDL could be generated in vivo. The oxidative modification of LDL in vitro by endothelial cells and smooth muscle cells has been characterized (47,49). In fact, modification of the lipid component alone is sufficient to elicit the response to oxidatively modified LDL, including the induction of monocyte chemotactic protein-1 (MCP1) to attract more monocytes (212). LDL with specific modification in the lysolecithin moiety impairs endothelium-dependent arterial relaxation (213).

Although oxidatively modified LDL is central in atherosclerosis, the model of study involves ex vivo modification of lipoprotein particles. In the presence of whole plasma, conditions necessary for the oxidative modification of LDL are not physiological. It has been suggested that LDL must be trapped in a microenvironment where it may be exposed to excess reactive oxygen radicals. Although the mechanism for the oxidative modification of LDL is not known, evidence supports the presence of oxidatively modified LDL in vivo. Negatively charged LDL with characteristics similar to those of oxidatively modified LDL has been isolated from human plasma with ion exchange chromatography (214). Antibodies to several chemically modified LDL, including MDA-LDL, 4-hydroxynonenal-conjugated (HNE) LDL, and Cu^{2+}-oxidized LDL, have been used for immunostaining of atherosclerotic lesions in rabbits (215,216). Recent reports indicate low concentrations of oxidatively modified LDL in human plasma in enzyme-linked immunoabsorbent assay (ELISA) with monoclonal antibodies against MDA-LDL (217) and Cu^{2+}-oxidized LDL (218). In the ApoE knockout mouse with accelerated atherosclerosis, naturally occurring antibodies have detected abnormal forms of LDL (219). The concentration of modified LDL was approximately 0.1 to 0.2 mg/dL in the knockout mice; levels ranging from 0.3 to 0.5 mg/dL have been reported in patients with documented cardiovascular disease (218). Whether the modified LDL was generated in the vascular space or leaked from the extracellular space is not known.

Several processes have been identified as potential candidates for the physiologic modifications of LDL. In endothelial and smooth muscle cells, oxidation of LDL may be triggered by exposure to free radicals (49). Superoxide anion and thiol products from monocytes can modify native LDL (50,51). Lipoxygenase, an enzyme seen in atherosclerotic lesions, may modify native LDL (220). Which process or combination of processes is involved in the in vivo modification of LDL has not been defined. Nevertheless, all these processes can be classified into three stages based on common features:

- Stage 1: This step involves the generation of a reactive oxygen species or other oxidants that initiate the oxidation process. Possible oxidants include superoxide radicals, nitric oxide, lipid peroxides, and hydrogen hydroperoxide. Although cells probably do not participate directly in the oxidative process, they provide the substrates that generate the extracellular oxidants.
- Stage 2: In this step, the protective antioxidants on LDL are depleted. Jessup et al. (221) have used a cell-free or a macrophage-mediated oxidation system to

Table 5
Relative Differences in Plasma Concentrations
as a Function of the ApoE Alleles

Plasma concentrations (% of normal)	E2	E3	E4
ApoE	+ 35%	−2%	−10%
ApoB	−10%	−1%	+ 5%
Total cholesterol	−7%	−1%	+ 4%
LDL cholesterol	−10%	0	+ 5%

LDL indicates low-density lipoprotein.

characterize the kinetics of vitamin E depletion of LDL. The half-life of vitamin E depletion was about 1 h in the presence of macrophages as compared with 7 h in the presence of Ham's F-10 medium only. If the donor received vitamin E supplementation (1200 mg/d for 5 d) before the isolation of LDL, the half-life was increased to 3–4 h in the presence of macrophages. When partially modified LDL was exposed to second set of fresh macrophages, degradation did not start to increase until all of the α-tocopherol had been depleted from LDL. Thus, although lipid hydroperoxides may be accumulating on LDL, their presence was not sufficient to induce uptake by macrophages. Instead, the rapid uptake of LDL by macrophages was tightly linked to the decomposition of lipid hydroperoxides that did not start until the reserve of antioxidants on the particles had been depleted.

- Stage 3: In this stage, the oxidative modification is propagated from the lipid moiety to the protein moiety. In the presence of excess vitamin E, lipid–peroxyl radicals (LOO·) may be converted to LOOH with the formation of tocopheroxyl radicals *(222)*. The subsequent decomposition of LOOH to aldehydes (e.g., MDA, HNE), which bind covalently to ApoB, may initiate fragmentation of the protein moiety. Any process that prolongs the close association of LDL with cells, such as binding with chondroitin sulfate and proteoglycans or with lipoprotein lipase, may propagate the process *(223)*.

These modified epitopes are antigenic, and antibodies are produced to oxidatively modified LDL in the vascular space *(224,225)*. Conflicting results have been reported in cross-sectional studies in humans on the protective nature of high titers of antibodies against oxidized LDL. Several studies have shown that the levels of autoantibodies against oxidatively modified LDL are lower in patients with documented CAD than in non-CAD controls *(226,227)*. These findings suggest that patients with low antibody titers were not adequately protected and were more likely to have CAD.

Considerable evidence indicates that high titers of autoantibodies against oxidatively modified LDL are anti-atherogenic. In LDL-receptor–deficient rabbits that develop spontaneous atherosclerosis, immunization with homologous MDA-LDL reduced the lesion area by 80% as compared with that in nonimmunized rabbits *(230)*. Immunization of normal New Zealand White (NZW) rabbits with either homologous or Cu^{2+}-oxidized LDL before initiation of an atherogenic diet reduced atherosclerotic lesions by 48–74% as compared with lesions in non-immunized animals *(231)*. Immunization was more beneficial with homologous LDL than with oxidized LDL. However, in this study, the use of homologous LDL isolated from animals that had been maintained on the atherogenic diet may have included a subpopulation of oxidatively modified particles.

Our environment is oxygen rich, and the generation of free radicals is a natural process associated with several normal activities, from the respiratory burst *(232)* to postprandial lipemia *(233)* and physical activity *(234)*. In fact, several lifestyle changes that have been recommended to reduce the risk of cardiovascular disease are associated with increased production of oxidative radicals, including increased intake of polyunsaturated fat (PSF) and exercise. This paradox may be explained by an imbalance, unique to patients with CAD, in the process used to respond to daily bouts of oxidative stress.

We recently reported a characteristic transient change in the level of autoantibodies against MDA-LDL during postprandial lipemia *(235)*. The acute reduction in autoantibody levels was seen only in patients with documented CAD and not in young normolipidemic individuals with normal arteries. The reduction was reproducible after an intensive regimen of caloric restriction and supervised exercise to normalize plasma lipids. Fasting levels of autoantibody titers were not affected by the reduction in plasma lipids. We believe that the interactions of TG-rich lipoproteins with lipoprotein lipase lining the arterial wall exposed the particles to free radicals from the diseased endothelium. In a follow-up study, we have reported that this acute change was specific to PSF and could not be seen with either saturated or monounsaturated fatty acids *(236)*.

CLINICAL MANIFESTATIONS AND MANAGEMENT

Patient Assessment

Medical history and physical examination should be the first step in evaluating a patient's risk of clinical events caused by cardiovascular disease. A history of myocardial infarction (MI), stroke, transient ischemic attack (TIA) of the brain, a definitive diagnostic procedure, or other notable event immediately places the patient in a high-risk category. A review of systems may show unappreciated symptoms or signs of ischemic or embolic events. A family history of early vascular catastrophes in first-degree relatives is an important factor in making decisions about risk status and treatment. In addition, current medications may be helpful in assessing symptoms such as claudication that may be related to unrecognized vascular disease.

The physical examination should begin with an evaluation of blood pressure and pulse rate. The quality of the voice, the skin, and the hair may indicate thyroid disease, which can affect cardiac and arterial function and risk of vascular disease. Xanthelasma or corneal arcus may suggest hypercholesterolemia, and retinal abnormalities associated with arterial thickening, hemorrhages, exudates, and microaneurysms may lead to the diagnosis of diabetes. In addition, hypercholesterolemia may be suspected by the presence of tendon or cutaneous xanthomata on examination of the extremities. Usually seen in the calcaneal tendons, these xanthomata may also occur in the extensor tendons of the hands and feet, the patellar tendon, and in the plantar fascia. Arterial bruits in the neck, abdomen, or groin frequently accompany generalized arterial disease. Palpation of an abdominal aortic aneurysm not only confirms the diagnosis of atherosclerosis but may also save a patient's life. Finally, reduced blood pressure or loss of pulses in the lower extremities may be definitive for peripheral vascular disease. The presence of a third heart sound, basilar rales on chest examination, or peripheral edema is a late sign of severe ischemic cardiomyopathy in many patients.

Laboratory tests should be systematic but prudent at early stages of evaluation. Patients over 20 yr of age should have a blood lipoprotein analysis, if fasting (10–12 h). If the patient is postprandial, measuring total cholesterol and HDLc is a useful screening procedure. If lipoprotein abnormalities are found, further tests of thyroid, liver, and renal function should be conducted. Measuring serum levels of thyroid stimulating hormone, alanine transferase, aspartate amino transferase, and urinary protein levels and a fasting blood glucose test is adequate in most patients. Uric acid should be measured if diabetes, hypertriglyceridemia, or gout is suspected. Creatine phosphokinase assay may provide a baseline for measuring changes in arthralgias and myalgias, which are common in older patients and may be an early sign of muscle dysfunction in statin-treated patients. Many patients have modestly increased serum levels of creatine phophokinase, which

can result in discontinuation of much-needed drug treatment for lipid levels.

Low-Density Lipoprotein Cholesterol Goal Setting

The Third Report of the National Cholesterol Education Program (NCEP) Expert Panel on Detection, Evaluation, and Treatment of High Blood Cholesterol in Adults (Adult Treatment Panel III) (1), provides valuable guidance on setting lipoprotein goals for preventing atherosclerotic vascular disease. The major focus is on reducing LDLc values to those that are appropriate for the patient based on an assessment of all relevant risk factors. According to these guidelines, patients should be classified into three levels of risk before planning a therapeutic regimen. The number of major and independent risk factors found on history, physical examination, and laboratory assessment is used to determine the risk category and therefore the LDLc goal (Table 6). Risk factors are either present or absent as determined by having met the specified criteria and are not treated as continuous functions. The action recommended is a function of the number of risk factors, not the individual characteristics.

The highest risk grouping includes patients with clinically manifest coronary heart disease, diabetes mellitus, and those with more than a 20% risk for having a myocardial infarction or coronary death during the next decade of life. This latter group includes persons with cerebrovascular disease, peripheral artery disease, arterial lesions, diabetes mellitus, and those with 20% risk predicted from the cumulative effect of several risk factors. The calculation of risk predicted from the cumulative effect is based on the predicted risk by using the mathematical relationships derived from the observations made in Framingham, Massachusetts (see below). NCEP guidelines recommend the LDLc to be maintained at less than 100 mg/dL in persons in the highest risk group.

Patients in the intermediate level of risk are those with a 10–20% risk of having an MI or CAD death over the next 10 years. Patients in this group usually have at least two major risk factors, independent of LDLc measurement, on initial assessment. Calculation of the risk with tables for the appropriate gender is recommended for all patients with two or more of the risk factors in Table 6. The LDLc goal for patients with moderately high risk should be less than 130 mg/dL.

Patients with one or none of the dichotomous risk factors will rarely have more than a 10% risk, and quantitative analysis of risk is usually not necessary, except in the elderly. Almost all men and more than half of women over 75 have more than a 10% risk. Because age is a powerful risk

Table 6
Risk Factors to consider in Initial Evaluation of Patients

Risk factor	Defination
Age	Men ≥45 years; women ≥55 years;
Cigarette smoking	Any cigaret smoking in the past month.
High blood pressure	Blood pressure ≥140/90 mm Hg, using the average of several measures as suggested by JNC VI or the current use of blood pressure lowering drugs.
Low HDL cholesterol	HDL cholesterol <40 mg/dL (averaging values on two or more occasions reduces the inherent error in the method)
Family history of CHD	Clinical CHD or CHD death documented in a first degree male relative before 55 years of age or a first degree female relative before 65 years of age.

The presence of two or more risk factors meeting these criteria in patients *without* CAD or CAD equivalent should lead to a quantitative risk assessment before setting the goal LDL cholesterol.

factor, quantitative risk assessment may be advisable for those over 65 yr. In patients with fewer than two risk factors and less than a 10% risk, the recommended goal for LDLc is less than 160 mg/dL.

The assessment of other risk factors may be relevant in some patients. In patients with a strong family history of cardiovascular events or presentation of an event at an early age, the physician should suspect genetic disease that may be seen in other measurements such as increased Lp[a] or homocysteine levels. These factors should be measured when the risk factors do not seem consistent with the history, routine laboratory results, or physical findings.

Quantitation of Risk

In patients with CAD or a CAD equivalent risk status, the risk does not need to be quantified because the goal of 100 mg/dL applies to all such patients. This approach applies mainly to those with two or more risk factors in whom the total risk is not obvious. Patients over 65 yr of age with a significant contribution from only one additional risk factor (such as high systolic pressure) may exceed the 10% risk threshold; therefore, a more complete assessment in the elderly is recommended. A single risk factor rarely places younger patients in a risk category greater than 10%, and therefore, the goal of reducing LDLc to less than 160 would apply in this group.

Mathematical functions have been derived that describe the relationships between a variety of risk factors and the event rates for myocardial infarction and coronary death observed in the Framingham Heart Study, which included more than 30 years of observations. The use of five factors—age, total cholesterol (interchangeable with LDLc), cigaret smoking, HDLc, and systolic blood pressure—was sufficient to approximate the

Table 7
Example for the Calculation of Framingham Risk Score

As an example, a 56-yr-old man (8 points) with a total cholesterol of 220 mg/dL (3 points), who smokes 20 cigarettes per day (3 points), with an HDLc of 38 mg/dL (2 points) and a systolic blood pressure of 145 mm Hg untreated (1 point) has a total score of 17 which confers a risk of ≥30% over the next decade of his life.

observed event rates *(237)*. The risk related to total cholesterol and cigarette smoking is adjusted for age and the blood pressure for treatment effect in these calculations. Because the relation between risk factors and risk of events is different for men and women, gender is an important consideration. Tables have been constucted that provide a score at each level of the given risk factor with the appropriate adjustments for men and women. The total number of points from each risk factor table is used to acquire the 10-yr risk percentage from the final table in each set for men or for women. The appropriate table must be used because the point score for a man confers a much greater percentage risk than the same score for a woman.

This example (Table 7) shows how seemingly moderate increases in several factors can create a high-risk state for a patient; therefore, quantifying risk with this method is a useful practice.

Clinical Assessment of Triglycerides

Plasma TG concentrations have predictive value in the assessment of risk. However, the relationship is more complex than that of LDL or HDL and risk. Increased levels of TG are strongly associated with obesity, lower HDLc, higher LDLc, and insulin-resistance syndromes, including type II diabetes mellitus; therefore, determining which of these factors is affecting the vascular wall is difficult. The risk of CAD increases when serum TG concentrations are at or higher than 150 mg/dL, with a maximum effect at approximately 400 mg/dL. Almost half of American men over 45 yr of age have TG concentrations above 150 mg/dL, and more than 25% of men and women in this age group have values over 200 mg/dL. Thus, treatment considerations are challenging. In the few large clinical trials in which drug treatment reduced TG levels, little or no relationship was found between a decrease in TG levels with treatment and a reduction in events. The decrease in LDL and the increase in HDL have been significant predictors in such studies. Furthermore, several trials in which LDL levels were decreased have shown a significant reduction in the risk relationship at baseline or after initiation of therapy TG levels. Thus, the independent predictive value of the cholesterol-carrying LDL and HDL may be a better guide for reducing the incidence of vascular disease. Current guidelines in the United States do not provide goals for treatment of plasma TG levels. The recommendations from the NCEP Adult Treatment Panel III for the classification of TG are presented in (Table 8).

TG concentration should be considered when planning therapy. VLDL remnants may confer risk and may contribute to lowering HDL and misleadingly lowering LDL levels because VLDL induce small and dense LDL and HDL in hypertriglyceridemic patients. Therefore, the cholesterol content of VLDL, like LDL, should be considered an indicator of risk in patients with plasma TG levels higher than 200 mg/dL. Because the only remaining cholesterol-containing lipoprotein of significance in fasting plasma is HDL, this new risk variable, called the "non-HDL cholesterol," is calculated by subtracting the HDL cholesterol from the total plasma cholesterol. The optimal TG level is below 150 mg/dL, and the ratio of the mass of TG to the mass of cholesterol in VLDL is about 5 to 1; therefore, the upper limit of an acceptable contribution of cholesterol to the plasma by VLDL is 1/5 of 150, or 30 mg/dL. Because of this reasoning, the recent NCEP (ATP III) report regarding the management of such patients recommends that for patients with TG higher than 200 mg/dL the treatment goal for "non-HDL" cholesterol is 30 mg higher than the LDL goal assigned for a given category of CHD risk (Table 9).

In some patients, hypertriglyceridemia should be treated as a specific entity. Patients with high TG levels (>500 mg/dL) are at risk of severe hypertriglyceridemia (>1000 mg/dL). TG levels can increase further in these patients with concurrent illness, weight gain, high fat

Table 8
Classification of Plasma Triglyceride Concentrations in Adults

Triglyceride category	Plasma triglyceride concentrations
Normal	<150 mg/dL
Borderline-high	150–199 mg/dL
High	200–499 mg/dL
Very high	≥500 mg/dL

Table 9
Treatment Goals Related to Risk Categories

Risk categories	LDL goal	Non-HDL goal
CHD and CHD risk equivalents	<100 mg/dL	<130 mg/dL
Two or more risk factors and/or 10 yr risk of CAD = 10–20%	<130 mg/dL	<160 mg/dL
One or fewer risk factors and/or 10 yr risk of CAD <10%	<160 mg/dL	<190 mg/dL

CHD indicates coronary heart disease; LDL, low-density lipoprotein; high-density lipoprotein; CAD, coronary artery disease.

meals, or loss of diabetic control. Plasma TG in this range can directly precipitate pancreatitis and lead to long-term disability or death. The goal in these patients is to decrease TG below 500 mg/dL, even if guidelines for vascular risk reduction have been met.

Low High-Density Lipoprotein Cholesterol

Plasma HDL cholesterol is a very powerful predictor of risk in industrialized nations in which diets are high in saturated fats and cholesterol and in which levels of LDLc are high. This relationship is weaker in individuals with an active lifestyle and a vegetable-based diet. Because few treatment regimens change only HDL levels without altering LDL and TG, proving that increasing HDL corresponds to a reduction in cardiovascular disease has not been possible. In clinical trials of agents such as niacin or fibrates, which lower LDL and increase HDL, the increase in HDL partially correlated with a reduction in clinical events. However, in the statin trials, the benefits of increasing HDL were less convincing, with greater reductions in LDL. Currently, the NCEP treatment guidelines have not set a goal for HDL cholesterol. Values of less than 40 mg/dL are defined as low, but no treatment targets are given (1). The lack of guidelines stems in part from the lack of an effective treatment regimen that consistently increases

HDL levels and by the lack of long-term studies showing that specific treatment of HDL provides benefit after LDL goals have been achieved. The Veterans Affairs HDL Intervention Trial (VA-HIT) found a 22% reduction in events in CAD patients with LDL cholesterol below 140 mg/dL (mean, 112 mg/dL) and HDL below 40 mg/dL (mean, 32 mg/dL) who were treated with gemfibrozil. However, the benefits of giving an LDL-reducing drug to achieve the current goal of <100 mg/dL in this group are unknown.

Considering the HDL, LDL, and TG levels may be wise if drug treatment is necessary; however, once the LDL and non-HDL cholesterol goals are achieved, addition of another drug specifically for increasing HDL is not recommended by available data. In evaluating HDL cholesterol in a patient, treatable causes of low HDL levels can be uncovered and can lead to significant increases in HDL if properly managed (Table 10). Genetic components, which are not well understood, may play a role in most cases. Low HDL may be a contributing factor in a patient with a family history of early CAD.

The Metabolic Syndrome

The rapid increase in obesity in industrialized nations and particularly in the United States is an underlying cause of a group of metabolic changes in adults of all ages. The expression of these changes portends a rising prevalence of type II diabetes mellitus and associated cardiovascular disease. Over the past 30 yr death rates from CAD and stroke have improved in the United States, Canada, Australia, Japan, and many European countries as healthier diets have been adopted, smoking has declined, and treatment for high blood pressure has improved. These gains may be offset by the trend of obesity. The risk related to an increase in body fat mass is caused mainly by the association of obesity with increases in insulin resistance, blood pressure, TG levels, and decreases in HDLc. The clustering of these risk factors in patients has become known as the "metabolic syndrome" (238,239). Previously, no consensus has been reached on criteria that could be used to diagnosis this disorder. The Adult Treatment Panel III has offered an approach to diagnosis that requires that patients have three of five diagnostic criteria (Table 11). Use of the non-HDL cholesterol may be particularly important in this group, and control of all risk factors should be given special emphasis. Because abdominal obesity may be a principal aggravating factor, patients should be urged to significantly reduce body fat, particularly in the waist area, by diet and exercise (240).

Table 10
Common Contributing Causes of Low HDL Cholesterol

Genetic factors

Elevated plasma triglycerides

Obesity

Type II diabetes

Physical inactivity

Cigaret smoking

Very high carbohydrate intake

TREATMENT

Therapeutic Lifestyle Changes

Although a diet high in cholesterol and saturated fat in the presence of obesity or lack of exercise are not considered in characterizing risk status by the NCEP scheme, these factors contribute significantly to several of the risk variables that are used in these calculations. Restricting dietary cholesterol to less than 300 mg/d and saturated fat to 7–10% of calories is recommended for all patients. In addition to restricting calories and increasing exercise to attain a desirable body weight, these dietary fat restrictions have been recommended for three decades to all Americans above the age of 2 yr. However, patients with high cholesterol or those in high-risk groups need to adopt a diet that is more restrictive than the recommendations for the general population.

Dietary intervention is supported by results from community-based studies that have shown that (1) the level of blood cholesterol is related to dietary fat intake, (2) the incidence of heart disease is positively related to saturated fat and cholesterol intake, and (3) the prevalence of heart disease is inversely related to polyunsaturated fat consumption. Trans fatty acids generated in the extensive hydrogenation of vegetable oils have a negative effect by increasing LDL levels and decreasing HDL (241,242). In contrast, including fish (243,244) and moderate amounts of alcohol (245) reduces the risk.

The effectiveness of cholesterol-lowering diets in reducing cardiovascular events has been assessed in long-term studies over the past 40 yr. Landmark studies include that of Dayton et al. (35) who showed that replacing saturated fat with polyunsaturated fat significantly reduced vascular disease in a domiciled group at a Veterans Administration hospital. Studies of diets with reduced animal fats and modest increases in fatty acids of vegetable origin in hypercholesterolemic Norwegian men (246) and studies in France (247) have shown significant declines in coronary disease rates with these diets.

Table 11
Guidelines for the Diagnosis of the Metabolic Syndrome

Characteristic*	Defining measure
Abdominal obesity	Waist circumference
Men	>40 in. (>102 cm)
Women	>35 in. (>88 cm)
Plasma triglycerides	>150 mg/dL
HDL cholesterol	
Men	<40 mg/dL
Women	<50 dL
Blood pressure	>130 mm Hg systolic or
	>85 mm Hg diastolic
Fasting glucose†	>110 mg/dL

Reprinted with permission *(238)*.

*The presence of any three of these characteristics confers the designation on a given patient.

†Convincing evidence of significant insulin resistance may be considered the equivalent of elevated fasting plasma glucose.

The therapeutic lifestyle changes recommended by NCEP comprise three major areas of change: (1) dietary reduction of saturated fats to less than 7% of calories and daily cholesterol intake to less than 200 mg with an increase in viscous (soluble) fiber (10–25 g/d) and plant sterols or stanol esters (2 g/d) *(248,249)*; (2) loss of excess adipose tissue, particularly in the abdominal region; and (3) increased regular physical activity. Achieving these goals frequently results in a reduction of LDLc by more than 10% and in some patients by as much as 30–40%. Failure to achieve a significant benefit usually means lack of compliance. In other patients, these recommendations may have already been met at the time of the initial evaluation. Without a dietary history, the change in dietary intake cannot be evaluated.

Therapeutic lifestyle changes are particularly important in patients with high TG levels and low HDLc in whom diet and weight loss are the most effective therapy. In addition, diet and weight loss are the best treatment for patients with insulin resistance, elevated fasting blood glucose, abdominal obesity, and for many with high blood pressure. These characteristics are found together in many patients and define the condition known as the metabolic syndrome *(238)*. For patients with the metabolic syndrome, therapeutic lifestyle changes should be the major therapeutic approach with a dietary review and counseling, and these patients should be encouraged to join support groups that will help them to maintain regular exercise habits and appropriate dietary adherence. Educating family members and encouraging the development of a positive and supportive attitude in the immediate family can be useful in

achieving long-term adherence to the recommendations for therapeutic lifestyle changes. The children often have similar risk factors and gain health benefits from being involved with therapeutic lifestyle changes.

Drug Treatment

RATIONALE AND GENERAL APPROACH

Several factors should be considered before initiating drug treatment in a patient with high blood lipids: (1) the immediate, short-term and long-term risks; (2) the potential risk reduction; (3) the expected incidence of adverse effects; (4) the achievements in adopting therapeutic lifestyle changes; and (5) the cost. In most patients, therapeutic lifestyle changes should be tried for several weeks or months before beginning drug therapy. This regimen should be followed for patients with stable vascular disease and for those who have risk less than the predicted CAD event rate of 20% that would designate CAD equivalency. Improvement in lipoproteins and blood pressure resulting from dietary changes and exercise efforts may help indicate causative issues. Documented success with diet and exercise provides long-term motivation to sustain the new habits and may help assess the efficacy of any drug regimen superimposed on the lifestyle changes. For patients with stable disease, dietary change should be maintained for 8 wk *(1)*, and if LDL or TG remains high, drug treatment may be instituted while continuing to work with TLC. If significant progress is made and the patient is highly motivated to continue, further monitoring without drug treatment would be appropriate. For patients with 10–20% risk or greater, the goal for LDL cholesterol and blood pressure should be achieved, and smoking should be stopped within 6 mo of beginning treatment *(1)*. In younger patients and those with a distant predicted onset of clinical disease, a prolonged period of lifestyle change as the only therapy is appropriate.

In patients with high short-term risk, such as those with recent occurrence of an acute coronary syndrome including unstable angina or a myocardial infarction, immediate treatment to reduce risk is required. These patients should stop smoking, reduce blood pressure, and begin a regimen of cholesterol-reducing drugs before discharge from the hospital. The incidence of a recurrence of a serious event that will require hospitalization or cause death is 12–20% in the first 4 mo after the initial hospital admission. Although not consistent, the data indicate that patients placed on cholesterol-lowering drugs have a reduced incidence of death from MI and CAD in the first year after discharge after evaluation of an acute coronary syndrome. In the only randomized trial in which this issue was studied in more than 3000 patients, all acute coronary events were reduced by 16% within 4 mo of discharge after a non-Q wave infarction or an episode of unstable angina. In addition, hospitalization for unstable angina was reduced by 24% (250).

THE RATIONALE FOR LONG-TERM DRUG TREATMENT

Many studies have assessed the benefits of LDLc-lowering drugs. The Coronary Drug Project reported a significant reduction in repeat myocardial infarction with clofibrate (251) and, in a separate cohort, with niacin therapy (252). However, neither drug significantly reduced coronary death by the end of the 5-yr observation period; however, with fewer than 1000 patients in each group, the power was insufficient to show benefit in death rates. The much larger, but flawed, World Health Organization study with clofibrate confirmed the reduction in MI (253). The first study with adequate sample size to show reductions in the sum of MI and CAD death was the Lipid Research Clinics Coronary Primary Prevention Trial (39,40) in which 3600 men without evidence of CAD but with high LDL cholesterol (>190 mg/dL) were enrolled. In this randomized, double blind trial with cholestyramine as the only therapy, cardiovascular events were reduced over a period of 7 yr. The reduction in events correlated with the change in ratio of LDL to HDLc, even though LDL was reduced by only 11% and HDL increased less than 5% (40). In almost 4000 Finish men with non-HDL cholesterol over 200 mg/dL who were randomly assigned to placebo or gemfibrozil, drug therapy reduced MI and CAD death by 34% (41,254). The combination of niacin and clofibrate in the Stockholm study of patients with recent myocardial infarction significantly reduced recurrent coronary events and provided the first evidence of a reduction in total mortality with lipid reduction (255).

With the introduction of the statins, a sustained reduction in LDLc of 25–35% or more could be achieved. In the Scandanavian Simvastatin Survival Study (4S) trial, 4444 hypercholesterolemic men and women with known heart disease were randomly assigned to simvastatin or placebo and monitored for more than 5 yr. This study showed for the first time a convincing reduction (30%) in total mortality (256), secondary to the reduction in CAD death of almost 40%. The Cholesterol and Recurrent Events (CARE) study (257) and the Long-term Intervention with Pravastatin in Ischemic Disease (LIPID) trial (258) with pravastatin and the Heart Protection Study (259) with simvastatin treatment subsequently showed significant reductions in MI and CAD death in patients with coronary heart disease and a broad range of plasma cholesterol concentrations at baseline. In the West of Scotland Coronary Prevention Study (WOSCOPS), 6600 men with high

blood cholesterol but no diagnosis of heart disease were treated for 5 yr with pravastatin with significant reductions in major coronary events (31%) and CAD death (33%); however the reduction in total mortality (22%) was of borderline statistical significance (42).

A second primary prevention study, Air Force Coronary Atherosclerosis Prevention Study/Texas Coronary Atherosclerosis Prevention Study (AFCAPS/TEXCAPS), selected men and women with average LDL (130–190 mg/dL) but below average HDLc and found that lovastatin treatment significantly reduced major CAD endpoints (37%) (260). The PROspective Study of Pravastatin in the Elderly at Risk (PROSPER) study of 6000 men and women, 70–82 yr of age, documented that statin therapy can prevent coronary disease in the elderly (261). This group of well-designed and well-conducted trials of statin therapy has provided data from more than 50,000 patients over a total exposure of more that 250,000 patient years. Statin therapy has consistently and predictably reduced LDL levels with few major adverse reactions. These findings have made statins the first-line medication for the treatment of high LDL cholesterol and the reduction of cardiovascular risk.

DRUGS FOR THE REDUCTION OF LOW-DENSITY LIPOPROTEIN CHOLESTEROL

Four classes of drugs provide primary efficacy in the reduction of LDLc: (1) statins, (2) bile acid sequestrants, (3) niacin, and (4) inhibitors of cholesterol absorption (262). Statins are the first drug of choice because of the large body of data showing efficacy and safety in altering lipoprotein levels and in reducing vascular disease events. Bile acid sequestrants, niacin, and the cholesterol absorption inhibitors, although effective, are used primarily as combination agents when additional efficacy is needed to attain the goal after statin has been tried in monotherapy (1). Fibrates are a less effective choice but can significantly reduce LDL in patients with TG under 200 mg/dL.

Statins (3-Hydroxy-3-Methylglutaryl Coenzyme A Reductase Inhibitors). Six statins are currently available for prescription use (Table 12) (263). Rosuvastatin has recently been approved in the United States and Canada. Cerivastatin has been taken off the market because of its interaction with gemfibrozil.

The approved dose ranges from 5 mg to 80 mg for most of these formulations, and the efficacy in reducing plasma concentrations of LDL cholesterol ranges from 20% to 60%. TG are reduced by 5–35%, depending on the dose and the baseline TG concentration. Higher percentage reduction is seen in patients with hypertriglyceridemia. HDLc is increased from 3% to 12%, with

Table 12
Dosages of Currently Available Statins

Drug	Initial dose	Titration regimen	Maximum Recommended dose
Atorvastatin	10mg qd	Double dose every 6 wk	80 mg qd
Fluvastatin	20–80 mg qhs	Double dose every 6 wk	80 mg (XL) qd
Lovastatin	20 mg with dinner	Double dose every 6 wk	40 mg bid
Pravastatin	10–20 mg at bedtime	Double dose every 6 wk	80 mg q PM
Rosuvastatin	5-40 mg at bedtime	Double dose every 6 wk	40 mg q PM
Simvastatin	20 mg q PM	Double dose every 6 wk	80 mg q PM

greater changes seen in patients with high TG. The individual drugs vary in efficacy because of the variability in patient responsiveness; therefore, beginning with lower doses and titrating upward is advised to achieve the goal with the lowest possible dose. The usual starting dose is 10 mg/d for atorvastatin and rosuvastatin and 20 mg for the other statins. If more than 40% reduction in LDLc is required to meet the goal, a larger starting dose may be used.

Statins work by binding directly to and competitively inhibiting HMG-CoA reductase, the rate-limiting enzyme in cholesterol synthesis (264). The reduction in intracellular cholesterol activates a sterol receptor binding protein (SRBP) that directly acts on the promoter of several proteins (265). Statins reduce LDL concentrations in the blood plasma by inducing the cell surface receptor for LDL. Because the ligands for the LDL receptor, ApoB-100 and ApoE, are found on VLDL remnants, these particles are also cleared, thereby reducing TG. The statin-induced mechanism of HDL increase is not understood but may result in part from the reduction in remnants preventing CETP from exchanging HDL cholesteryl ester for the remnant TG. Because statins are taken up primarily by the liver and most effective LDL receptors are found on the liver cell membrane, the major site of action of statins is the hepatocyte. The net result is the reduction of the half-life of LDL by as much as 50% or more.

In vitro and animal studies have suggested that statins have other effects on cellular function, including promoting the generation of nitric oxide synthase (266), reducing oxidative enzymes, and stimulating antioxidant systems. Whether functions other than the reduction of atherogenic LDL and VLDL contribute to the decrease in vascular disease is not clear.

Statins are cleared primarily through bile, although pravastatin has significant renal excretion (267). Lovastatin, simvastatin, and atorvastatin are metabolized by the action of the cytochrome P-450 enzyme CYP 3A4, but pravastatin is not affected by the cytochrome P-450 system. Fluvastatin is primarily metabolized by the CYP 2C9 enzyme. Half-life of the statins and active metabolites varies from 2–3 h to more than 48 h (atorvastatin). Drugs that are metabolized or inhibit these enzymes can reduce the clearance of statins and significantly increase plasma levels (268,269), which may contribute to adverse effects associated with statin therapy, such as myopathy (267).

A small, often transient, increase in hepatic enzymes, primarily the aminotransferases ALT and AST, is seen in some patients (270). The incidence of enzyme abnormalities increases with higher doses. An increase at three times (3 ×) the upper limit of normal (ULN) is considered significant. The incidence of a significant increase ranges from 0.2% at 10 mg/d to about 2.5% of patients treated with 80 mg/d and is usually seen within 12 wk of starting the drug or increasing the dose. Addition of other drugs may be the immediate cause. Although a modest increase between one and two times the ULN may not be significant, a repeat value should be obtained within a few days to ensure the ULN is not increasing further. In addition, relevant liver enzymes should be assessed before starting drug treatment because enzyme increases have been seen in patients on placebo treatment. When SLT and AST are increased, and not due to intrinsic liver disease (i.e., viral hepatitis and steatosis), reducing the dose or discontinuing statin therapy usually returns the enzymes to normal or pretreatment values. Evidence that statin therapy can cause permanent liver damage is not convincing (271).

Myopathy associated with statin treatment is of greater concern than liver problems. Although it is uncommon in the absence of other drugs, myopathy associated with statin use can result in severe and even fatal rhabdomyolysis (272,273). In clinical trials, the incidence of muscle symptoms with CPK elevations 10 times (10 ×) the upper limit of normal has been seen in about 1 per 1000 patients; however, patients in this situation do not have rhabdomyolysis (272,273) but rather muscle trauma or some unusual increase in exercise that will resolve without treatment and often with continuation of the drug. An increasing CPK value should be evaluated rapidly to determine if a serious and threatening myopathic syndrome is developing. The muscle symptom of greatest concern is the development of weakness with or without muscle pain. Serum CPK and a urinalysis for protein should be obtained immediately in such patients (271). The incidence of myalgia without CPK increases is higher in patients treated with statins than in patients treated with placebo, but the frequency of this symptom without other findings in large, double-blind clinical trials has been similar in treated and placebo patients. Being informed of this potentially serious muscle syndrome of myopathy may increase patient awareness of the frequent musculoskeletal pain that is common in older individuals. A recent report found that 17 of 21 statin-treated patients with myalgia without increased CPK concentrations also had myalgia with placebo treatment; however, four patients had myalgias only with statins. In three of the four patients, muscle biopsy specimens showed abnormal fibers and increased lipid droplets within the muscle cells. These changes disappeared after discontinuing statins for several weeks. Thus, a few patients with statin-associated myalgias may have a muscle disorder that does not increase CPK concentrations. Drugs that use common metabolic pathways such as the CYP 3A4 enzyme system should be avoided during statin therapy. Other causes for myopathic symptoms with CPK increases include several autoimmune disorders such as polymyositis and dermatomyositis. In addition, rhabdomyolysis may result from other causes including metabolic disorders, alcohol abuse, and infections (271).

Bile Acid Sequestrants. The oral intake of anion exchange resins such as cholestyramine, colestipol, and colesevelam results in the adsorption of bile acids onto these agents in the intestine and the increased delivery of these compounds into the stool (262). Bile acids are made in the liver through the action of several oxidative enzymes on cholesterol. Most bile acids are stored in the gallbladder, and bile acids are delivered to the gut in conjunction with the bolus of food that leaves the stomach after each meal. Bile acids are the major detergent molecules that allow the solution of dietary fats for presentation to lipolytic enzymes and the products of this lipolysis to the mucosal cells of the small intestine for absorption (274,275). Most of the enteric bile acids are then reabsorbed in the distal ileum and return to the liver via the portal blood. About 250–500 mg is lost in the stool each day, resulting in a significant loss of cho-

lesterol from the body. When bile acid sequestrants are given in doses of several grams daily, the loss of bile acids can be more than doubled, which causes the liver to use additional intrahepatic cholesterol as substrate to replace the excreted bile acids. Reducing the cholesterol content of the hepatocyte induces the synthesis of LDL receptors, which results in a reduction of plasma LDL. The efficacy is reduced because the liver also increases the activity of HMG-CoA reductase and therefore increases the *de novo* synthesis of cholesterol.

Bile acid sequestrants can reduce LDL cholesterol from 15% to 30%, with regimens of two to six doses per day. The efficacy is greater when given with meals. Cholestyramine and colestipol are provided as an insoluble powder in doses of 4 and 5 gm of active resin. In addition, colestipol is available in 1-g capsules. A minimal regimen of 8 g (cholestyramine) or 10 g at dinner may be increased to three doses twice daily. Colesevelam is supplied in 625 mg capsules, and the usual regimen is two to six capsules daily given in divided doses with meals (276).

Because bile acid sequestrants can bind negatively charged drugs, other medications should be given at least 1 h before or 4 h after the resin dosage. TG synthesis is increased modestly when the bile acid synthesis pathways are activated, which may induce a significant increase in plasma VLDL TG. This change is usually minimal in patients with fasting plasma TG concentrations of less than 300 mg/dL. Adverse effects of gastric irritation and constipation are noted by a significant number of patients. This effect is rarely seen with small doses and can be ameliorated by incorporating soluble fiber into the dosing schedule. One teaspoonful of psyllium mixed with the resin in water usually solves this problem. The "mouth-feel" of this sandy texture of psyllium is unpalatable to some patients and results in poor compliance. Mixing soluble fiber with the resin improves palatability.

Bile acid sequestrants are safe with almost no direct toxicity at recommended doses and have been part of the regimen in several studies which have shown a reduction in cardiovascular events and a decrease in the progression of lesions in the coronary arteries. Furthermore, they can be mixed with statin dosages with additive effects in lowering LDL cholesterol (277–280) and increasing HDLc (3–6%) (Fig. 6).

Niacin. The ability of niacin (nicotinic acid, Vitamin B3) to lower plasma cholesterol was discovered serendipitously almost 50 yr ago when it was used in large doses as an experimental treatment for schizophrenia (281). When given in doses of 2–3 g/d (282), niacin lowers LDL-C by 25–35%. Crystalline niacin, which is rapidly

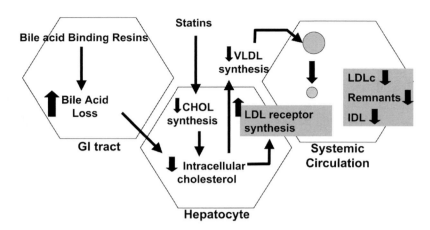

Fig. 6. Complementary action of bile acid-binding resins and statins in the control of plasma low-density lipoprotein cholesterol (LDLc). Combination therapy with a bile acid–binding resin and a statin can have an additive benefit by reducing the intracellular hepatic cholesterol pool. Bile acid-binding resins promote loss of bile salts by interfering with their reabsorption in the ileum. Intracellular cholesterol is subsequently depleted for the biosynthesis of bile salts. Inhibition of HMG CoA reductase by statins reduces the intracellular hepatic cholesterol pool by inhibition of cholesterol synthesis. Hepatocytes respond to this depletion by increasing the expression of low-density lipoprotein (LDL) receptor, resulting in a reduction in plasma LDLc, remnant lipoproteins, and intermediate-density lipoprotein (IDL). In certain instances, depletion of the intracellular cholesterol pool could lead to the reduction in the synthesis and secretion of hepatic very low density lipoprotein (VLDL), the precursor of LDL. GI, gastrointestinal.

absorbed and excreted in the urine as nicotinuric acid, has been used in most studies. Because of its short half-life, niacin must be given in divided doses two to four times daily to achieve the greatest efficacy (283). The major physiologic effect of niacin is to reduce the delivery of small VLDL into the plasma from the liver (284). In addition, niacin increases clearance of the larger VLDL. In conjunction with this effect, TG, VLDL cholesterol, and LDL cholesterol are reduced. HDLc increases in plasma by 25–35% after 8–12 wk of niacin therapy and may increase by 40% after 6–12 mo. The TG reduction is usually 20–30% in patients with baseline TG concentrations below 200 mg/dL. In severe hypertriglyceridemia (>500 mg/dL), more than a 50% reduction is common. Niacin and estrogens are the only drugs that reduce Lp[a] (285,286). In most studies, Lp[a] concentrations decrease by 25–35% with niacin doses above 2 g/d.

Niacin is available in various formulations designed to delay absorption and provide for more convenient dosing schedules of once or twice daily (287). The formulations usually involve a material that reduces the dissolution of niacin such as waxes of gel matrices. These preparations reduce the high peak plasma levels associated with crystalline niacin and consequently reduce the incidence of one of the most common adverse reactions, cutaneous vasodilation. This vasodilation may be caused by the release of prostaglandins (288), which dilate arterioles in the skin and produce a sense of heat, and may cause tachycardia and transiently reduce blood pressure.

Because of its vasodilatory effects, niacin may make inflamed tissues such as recent surgical wounds, peptic ulcers, or dermatologic conditions more painful. The incidence of these problems can be reduced by using small doses such as 50 or 100 mg tablets given with each meal and at bedtime (289). The dose can be increased at weekly intervals to 500 mg tablets given at meals and at bedtime. The extended release forms can be used two times a day or once daily in the evening. Strict adherence to the regimen is important because omission of dosing even for one day can result in the return of the dramatic vasodilation. Aspirin (one tablet two times a day) often reduces this problem and is advised during the dose escalation phase of treatment (290). The new extended release formulation "niaspan" can be started at a dose of 500 mg/d and increased to a total dose of 3000 mg/d. The usual dose is 1500–2000 mg/d. This preparation is associated with fewer symptoms of cutaneous flushing (291).

The excretion of niacin by the renal route as an acid competes with excretory pathways used by uric acid. Patients with hyperuricemia at baseline may have a significant increase in uric acid, and gouty attacks can be triggered by the use of niacin in such patients (292). Niacin has a weak effect on the cellular metabolism of insulin, and patients with significant insulin resistance may have a worsening of this condition. However, the effects on insulin resistance are less common than once thought, and most patients with type 2 diabetes and lipid disorders can be treated without significant impairment of glucose control (293). Finally, plasma levels of hepatic enzymes such as ALT and AST are increased in a significant number of patients *(294)*. This effect is primarily associated with over-the-counter preparations of niacin with delayed release properties. The incidence of liver function abnormalities is lower with crystalline niacin and extended release preparations that have been approved for prescription use. Switching from prescription preparations to delayed release over-the-counter forms of niacin with no change in daily dosage has been associated with liver failure.

In the Coronary Drug Project *(251)* niacin reduced coronary events, and when combined with bile acid sequestrants or statins, niacin reduced the size of atherosclerotic lesions and clinical events in several clinical trials *(283)*.

Fibrates. Clofibrate (p-chlor-phenoxy isobutyric acid) was discovered to lower plasma lipids when it was used as a solvent for studies of androgens as therapeutic agents *(295)*. Several fibrates are currently on the market, and clofibrate has been replaced by gemfibrozil and fenofibrate in the United States *(296)*. Bezafibrate is a fibrate used in Europe. Fibrates increase TG clearance and, thus, reduce VLDL and chylomicron lipids *(297,298)*. In addition, fibrates may reduce LDL by 20% or more in patients with high LDL but TG concentrations less than 200 mg/dL. Fibrate increases HDLc by 5–15% in such patients. In hypertriglyceridemic patients, fibrates reduce TG from 25% to 70% and increase HDLc by up to 30%; however, LDL-C may increase from below normal levels to normal or even high levels.

The lipid effects of fibrates may be caused by the activation of the so-called peroxisome proliferator-activated receptors of the alpha type (PPARα) *(299,300)*. These receptors activate a series of genes that can alter TG synthesis and secretion and the composition of VLDL and chylomicrons. One major change may be to reduce the surface coat apolipoprotein, ApoC-III *(116,117,301,302)*, which acts as a stabilizing agent and prevents TG-rich lipoproteins from coalescing and being taken up by nonspecific pathways. The TG-rich particles can then be delivered to high affinity sites such as lipoprotein lipase and remnant receptors. However, studies in transgenic mice have shown that overproduction of the ApoC molecule can produce severe hypertriglyceridemia by inhibiting the action of lipase lipoprotein. In knockout mice with no ApoC-III, TG are cleared more rapidly than in wild-type mice *(128)*. In humans with a genetic deficiency of ApoC-III, clearance of VLDL TG is accelerated *(88)*. In rodents, fibrates quickly and significantly reduce ApoC-III levels. Lipoprotein lipase increases in animals and humans treated with fibrates, possibly because of an increased clearance of TG from plasma. The mechanism

of the decrease in LDL is not fully understood but the increased loss of cholesterol in bile may activate LDL receptors *(303,304)*. HDL increases in part because of the reduction of TG and therefore the reduction in the transfer of cholesterol ester from HDL to VLDL remnants through the action of CETP. Evidence suggests that HDL may not be able to unload its cholesterol into the liver because of suppression of the SR-BI receptor *(278)*, but this finding has not been substantiated.

Fibrates have very few adverse effects. The increased cholesterol concentration in bile relative to bile acids and phospholipids converts bile into a more lithogenic composition *(305)*. In some studies cholecystectomies were more common with clofibrate, and a strong, but not statistically significant, trend to more cholecystectomies was observed in the Helsinki Heart Study with gemfibrozil *(41)*. In a very few patients (<0.5%), ALT or AST levels increased slightly, but permanent liver damage has not been associated with fibrate treatment alone. Gastric irritation has been reported in one large trial significantly more frequently with fibrate treatment than with placebo.

The combination of gemfibrozil with cerivastatin markedly increased the blood concentration of cerivastatin, and the frequency of skeletal muscle myopathy increased 30-fold higher than that with any other statin in combination with gemfibrozil. The mechanism underlying this specific interaction may be the unique metabolic alteration of gemfibrozil (among fibrates) and cerivastatin (among statins) by glucuronidation in the intestinal mucosa. The glucuronidation of cerivastatin markedly increases its uptake by the liver. When glucuronidation of cerivastatin is reduced by competition with gemfibrozil, the native compound more readily passes through the liver and increases peripheral blood concentrations, which may lead to myopathy because of the resulting muscle exposure. In addition, muscle metabolism is altered more by cerivastatin than other statins. Although other statins including atorvastatin, lovastatin, and simvastatin are glucuronidated, the change in blood levels resulting from the concurrent administration of gemfibrozil is less. Other fibrates such as fenofibrate do not alter the kinetics of cerivastatin because gemfibrozil is particularly competitive with the specific glucuronyl transferase enzymes that also modify statins *(268)*. The potential danger of this interaction has led to the voluntary withdrawal of cerivastatin by the manufacturer.

Our hypothesis for the role of oxidatively modified LDL and autoantibodies in the pathogenesis of atherosclerosis is shown in (Fig. 7).

Phytosterols. Plant sterols compete with cholesterol for the putative cholesterol transporter system in the brush bor-

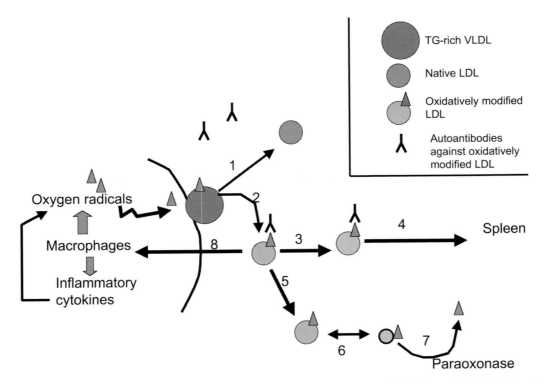

Fig. 7. Proposed hypothesis for the role of oxidatively LDL and autoantibodies against oxidatively modified LDL in atherogenesis. The presence of macrophages in the diseased endothelium is associated with excess generation of inflammatory cytokines and oxygen radicals. Interactions of TG-rich lipoproteins with LPL located along the endothelium allow the lipid-rich particles to come into close contact with a rich supply of oxygen radicals. If the TRL are enriched in highly oxidizable polyunsaturated fatty acids, the TRL can acquire the oxygen radicals. If the TRL is enriched in antioxidants the radicals are quenched and the particle is protected. (**1**) If the radicals remain attached to the partially hydrolyzed particle, it may recognized by circulating autoantibodies against oxidatively modified lipids (**2**) resulting in the formation of the circulating immune complex. (**3**) Under normal conditions, the resulting immune complex is efficiently removed via the spleen. (**4**) The oxidatively modified particle can remain minimally modified (**5**) and participate in a lipid exchange process with HDL (**6**) which result in the transfer of the oxidized epitopes to HDL. (**6**) Presence of antioxidants and/or paraoxonase on HDL may result in the cleavage of the oxidized epitopes, thus preventing irreversible damage to the lipoproteins. In the diseased state, however, the immune complex is directed toward the activated macrophages in the arterial wall (**8**) and are taken up via the scavenger receptor, leading to the formation of foam cells and atherosclerosis.

der of the intestinal epithelial cells *(306)*. Preparations of phytosterols, available for many years in doses of 3g or more daily, reduce LDLc by 5%–10% depending on the diet and the patient *(307)*. Esterification of the naturally occurring plant sterols as either phytosterols or phytostanols increases the efficacy in reducing enteric cholesterol absorption. Products such as margarines or salad dressings containing these compounds as food additives are now available *(308)*. Ingesting sufficient amounts of these compounds to provide about 2 g/d can reduce LDL by 5–10%.

Stanols are naturally occurring minor components of plant lipids that may be as effective as the plant sterols but are much less readily absorbed *(306)*. The small absorption of phytosterols is inconsequential for most people, but some have a defect in the intestinal cells that leads to an increase in plasma concentrations. This hyperabsorption of

phytosterols can produce a rare disorder called sitosterolemia *(309,310)*, which is expressed as hypercholesterolemia associated with the increased plant sterols, tendon xanthoma, and early arteriosclerosis. These patients have a defect in the efflux of sterols from the enteric cells through a transport system comprising two membrane proteins called ABCG5 and ABCG8 *(6,7)*. Whether smaller changes in plasma levels seen with supplements of phytosterols contribute to vascular disease is not clear. If so, use of stanol esters may be safer for long-term use.

Ezetimibe. Ezetimibe is the first and only representative of a new class of drugs that specifically inhibits the enteric sterol transporter responsible for uptake of both cholesterol and plant sterols by the epithelium of the small intestine *(311,312)*. Ezetimibe reduces LDLc by about 10% at a dose of 1 mg/d and by 20% at 40 mg/d *(313)*. The effect is very specific but reaches a maximum with only a moderate effect on plasma concentrations of this atherogenic lipoprotein. Only one dose size, a 10 mg tablet given once daily, is available and reduces LDLc by an average of 18% in large studies of patients with baseline plasma concentrations of LDLc between 130 and 250 mg/dL. Although the effect is confined to LDLc, ezetimibe may reduce TG by about 10% and increase HDLc by 2–4% increase (313).

Ezetimibe works even in patients consuming very low cholesterol diets because most of the cholesterol in the intestinal contents is delivered from the bile. The average dietary intake of cholesterol in the United States is approx 300 mg/d, whereas the biliary cholesterol delivers 800 to 1200 mg into the gut each day. About 40–60% of this cholesterol is absorbed into the blood as a component of chylomicrons. At the 10-mg dose, ezetimibe blocks more than 50% of this absorption (313).

After being rapidly taken up, ezetimibe enters a pool in the brush border membrane that is slowly turning over. Ezetimbe undergoes glucuronidation in the intestinal cell and is then secreted into the blood where it is tightly bound to protein (314). Most of this ezetimibe–glucuronide is cleared on first pass through the liver with minimal delivery to peripheral blood. In the glucuronide form, ezetimibe is excreted in the bile and is again rapidly absorbed. The glucuronidated drug is as effective as the native compound in reducing cholesterol absorption. Because of the enterohepatic recycling, the residence time in the intestine and liver is prolonged, and the total body half-life averages 22–24 h (315); therefore, once a day dosing is effective. The efficacy in LDLc reduction is not affected by the presence of food in the stomach or the time of day of administration.

The LDLc reduction with ezetimibe is additive with that produced by statins, and the kinetics of statins are not affected by the co-administration of ezetimibe (316–318). The efficacy of ezetimibe with other lipid-lowering agents has not been well studied. In one small study, the reduction in LDLc with ezetimibe was additive with that of fenofibrate (319). Modest increases in peripheral blood levels of ezetimibe were found with simultaneous administration of gemfibrozil (319,320) and reduced concentrations with cholestyramine. The use of cholestyramine with ezetimibe in the recommended dosing schedule (administering other drugs 2 h before or 4 h after bile acid sequestrants) has not been reported.

Vytorin is a combination of simvastatin and ezetimible that has recently been approved by the FDA for the reduction of LDLc.

Adverse effects with ezemitibe have not differed from those associated with placebo in studies of several thou-sand patients. Data on long-term safety with this agent are not available. One concern is that ezemitibe may inhibit the absorption of other molecules that are lipid soluble, and in particular, those that are derived from the sterol nucleus. However, animal studies with progestational agents, ethinyl estradiol, vitamins A and D, and bile acids have indicated no effect on absorption.

Although the increase in liver (ALT or AST) or muscle (CPK) enzymes has been no different from that seen with placebo or statins at low doses, the combination of statins with ezetimibe has been associated with slight increases in the frequency of abnormal ALT or AST (<2%). However, enzyme levels have either returned to normal during treatment or immediately after discontinuing the use of these drugs.

Ezetimibe will probably be used primarily as a second agent in patients who have not responded successfully to other drugs, particularly the statins. In about 25% of patients, ezetimibe alone reduced LDLc by more than 25%; therefore, ezetimibe may be useful as single-drug treatment in patients who cannot take statins, niacin, or bile acid sequestrants.

In homozygous familial hypercholesterolemia, an additional 25% reduction in LDLc was observed when ezetimibe, at 40- to 80-mg doses, was added to simvastatin or atorvastatin (318).

Physical Removal of Low-Density Lipoproteins. In severe hypercholesterolemia with persistent LDLc above 200 mg/dL in patients at high risk of cardiovascular events, reducing lipoprotein values to a level that offers sufficient protection may not be possible in patients with mixed heterozygous or homozygous familial hypercholesterolemia. In these patients both genes for the LDL receptor have functional defects. If the maximum drug regimen is established and the LDLc is still above 200 mg/dL in a person with CAD or CAD equivalent, physical removal of the LDL from the plasma should be considered (312,322). Procedures are available that separate cells from the blood plasma, which is then passed through columns that either bind LDL and VLDL or selectively precipitate LDL and VLDL, leaving the HDL and other plasma components intact (323–325). This treatment, which is similar to renal dialysis, is conducted on a weekly or bimonthly basis for 3 or 4 weeks. LDL can be reduced transiently below 100 mg/dL but will return to 60% to 70% of the baseline values by 2 weeks in most patients. The use of high-dose statins in conjunction with this treatment markedly delays the increase in LDL and provides for a more favorable average exposure over time (326). Several studies have shown that these dialysis-like procedures reduce the manifestations of vascular disease. However, this procedure is not widely available and is expensive and time-consuming.

REFERENCES

1. Expert Panel. Executive summary of the 3rd report of the NCEP expert panel on detection, evaluation and treatment of high blood cholesterol in adults (ATP-III). JAMA 2001;285:2486–2497.

2. Dietschy JM, Wilson JD. Regulation of cholesterol metabolism. N Engl J Med 1970;282:1128–1138.

3. Kesaniemi YA, Miettinen TA. Cholesterol absorption efficiency regulates plasma cholesterol level in the Finnish population. Eur J Clin Invest 1987;17:391–395.

4. Patel SB, Salen G, Hidaka H, et al. Mapping a gene involved in regulating dietary cholesterol absorption: The sitosterolemia locus is found at chromosome 2p21. J Clin Invest 1998;102:1041–1044.

5. Gottesman MM, Ambudkar SV. Overview: ABC transporters and human disease. J Bioenerg Biomemb 2001;33:453–458.

6. Berge KE, Tian H, Graf GA, et al. Accumulation of dietary cholesterol in sitosterolemia caused by mutations in adjacent ABC transporters. Science 2000;290:1771–1775.

7. Lee MH, Lu K, Patel SB. Genetic basis of sitosterolemia. Curr Opinion Lipidol 2001;12:141–149.

8. Datta S, Luo CC, Li WH, et al. Human hepatic lipase. Cloned cDNA sequence, restriction fragment length polymorphisms, chromosome localization, and evolutionary relationships with lipoprotein lipase and pancreatic lipase. J Biol Chem 1998; 263:1107–1110.

9. Waite M, Thuren T, Wilcox R, et al. Purification and substrate specificity of rat hepatic lipase. Meth Enzymol 1991;197:331–339.

10. Sanan DA, Fan J, Bensadoun A, Taylor JM. Hepatic lipase is abundant on both hepatocyte and endothelial surfaces in the liver. J Lipid Res 1997;38:1002–1013.

11. Zilversmit DB. A proposal linking atherogenesis to the interaction of endothelial lipase with TG-rich lipoproteins. Circ Res 1973;33:633–638.

12. Zilversmit DB. Atherogenesis: a postprandial phenomenon. Circulation 1979;60:473–485.

13. Groot PHE, van Stiphout AHJ, Krauss XH, et al. Postprandial lipoprotein metabolism in normolipidemic man with and without coronary artery disease. Arteriosl Thromb 1991; 11:653–662.

14. Brown DF, Heslin AS, Doyle JT. Postprandial lipemia in health and in ischemic heart disease. New Engl J Med 1961; 264:733–737.

15. Sharrett AR, Chambless LE, Heiss G, Paton CC, Patsch W. Association of postprandial triglyceride and retinyl palmitate responses with asymptomatic carotid artery atherosclerosis in middle-aged men and women. Arteriosl Thromb Vasc Biol 1995;15:2122–2129.

16. Lagrost L, Gandjini H, Athias A, et al. Influence of plasma CETP activity on the LDL and HDL distribution profiles in normolipidemic subjects. Arteriosl Thromb 1993;13:815–825.

17. Tall AR. Plasma cholesteryl ester transfer protein. J Lipid Res 1993;34:1255–1274.

18. Goldstein JL, Brown MS. Familial hypercholesterolemia. In the Metabolic Basis of Inherited Diseases. CR Scriver, AL Beaudet, WS Sly, and D Valle, editors. 1989.1215–1253.

19. Berg K. A new serum type system in man - the Lp system. Acta Pathol Microbiol Scand 1963;59:369–375.

20. Berg K, Dahlen G, Borresen AL. Lp(a) phenotypes, other lipoprotein parameters, and a family of coronary heart disease in middle-aged males. Clin Genet 2003;16:347–358.

21. Brunner C, Kraft HG, Utermann G, Muller HJ. Cys4057 of apolipoprotein(a) is essential for Lipoprotein(a) assembly. Proc Natl Acad Sci USA 1993;90:11643–11647.

22. Perombelon YFN, Soutar AK, Knight BL. Variation in Lp(a) concentration associated with different apo(a) alleles. J Clin Invest 1994;93:1481–1492.

23. Rader DJ, Cain W, Zech L, Usher D, Brewer HB. Variation in Lp(a) nconcentrations among individuals with the same apo(a) isoform is determined by the rate of Lp(a) production. J Clin Invest 1993;91:443–447.

24. Dahlen G, Guyton JR, Attar M, Farmer JA, Kautz JA, Gotto AM, Jr. Association of levels of Lp(a), plasma lipids and other lipoproteins with coronary artery disease documented by angiograpgy. Circulation 1986;74:758–765.

25. Rhoads GG, Dahlen G, Berg K, et al. Lp(a) lipoprotein as a risk factor for myocardial infarction. JAMA 1986;256:2540–2544.

26. Kronenberg F, Kronenberg MF, Kiechl S, et al. Role of Lp(a) and apo(a) phenotype in atherogenesis. Prospective results from the Bruneck Study. Circulation 1999;100:1154–1160.

27. Etingin OR, Hajjar DP, Hajjar KA, Harpel PC, Nachman RL. Lp(a) regulates plasminogen activator inhibitor-1 expression in endothelial cells: A potential mechanism in thrombogenesis. J Biol Chem 1991;266:2459–2465.

28. Barrett-Connor E, Suarez L, Khaw K, Criqui MH, Wingard DL. Ischemic heart disease risk factors after age 50. J Chronic Dis 1984;37:903–908.

29. Shekelle RB, Shryock AM, Paul O, et al. Diet, serum cholesterol and death from coronary heart disease. The Western Electric Study. N Engl J Med 1981;304:65–70.

30. Tyroler HA, Heyen S, Bartel A, et al. Blood pressure and cholesterol as coronary heart disease risk factors. Arch Inter Med 1971;128:907–914.

31. Stamler J, Wentworth D, Neaton JD. Is the relationship between serum cholesterol and risk of premature death from coronary heart disease continuous or graded? Findings in 356,222 primary screenees of the MRFIT. JAMA 1986;256:2823–2828.

32. Marmot MG, Mann JI. In Ischaemic Heart Disease. Fox KM, editor. MTP Press, Lancaster, UK. 1987.1–31.

33. Tyroler HA. Review of lipid-lowering clinical trials in relation to observational epidemiologic studies. Circulation 1987; 76:525–522.

34. Holme I. An analysis of randomized trials evaluating the effect of cholesterol reduction on total mortality and coronary heart disease incidence. Circulation 1990;82:1916–1924.

35. Dayton S, Pearce ML, Goldman H, et al. Controlled trial of a diet high in unsaturated fat for prevention of atherosclerotic complications. Lancet 1968;2:1060–1062.

36. Turpeinen O, Karvonen MJ, Pekkarinen M, Miettinen M, Elosuo R, Paavilainen E. Dietray prevention of coronary heart disease: the Finnish Mental Hospital Study. Intern J Epidemiol 1979;8:99–118.

37. Buchwald H, Varco RL, Matts JP, et al. Effect of partial ileal bypass surgery on mortality and morbidity from coronary heart disease in patients with hypercholesteroliemia. Report of POSCH. N Engl J Med 1990;323:946–955.

38. Buchwald H, Stoller DK, Campos CT, Matts JP, Varco RL. Partial ileal bypass for hypercholesterolemia. 20- to 26-year follow-up of he first 57 consecutive cases. Ann Surgery 1990;212:318–329.

39. LRC-CPPT Writing Group. The Lipid Research Clinics Coronary Primary Prevention Trial results: I. Reduction in incidence of coronary heart disease. JAMA 1984;251:351–364.

40. LRC-CPPT Writing Group. The Lipid Research Clinics Coronary Primary Prevention Trial results. II. The relationship of reduction in incidence of CHD to cholesterol lowering. JAMA 1984;251:365–374.

41. Frick MH, Elo O, Haapa K, et al. Helsinki Heart Study: primary prevention trial with gemfibrozil in middle-aged men with dyslipidemia. Safety of treatment, changes in risk factors, and incidence of CHD. N Engl J Med 1987;317:1237–1245.

42. Shepherd J, Cobbe SM, Ford L, et al. Prevention of CHD with pravastatin in men with hypercholesterolemia. West of Scotland Coronary Prevention Study Group. N Engl J Med 1995;333:1301–1307.

43. Kwiterovich PO. State-of-the-art update and review: Clinical trials of lipid-lowering agents. Am J Cardiol 1998;82:3U–17U.

44. National Center for Health Statistics. National Health & Nutrition Examination Survey III, 1988–1994. Washington, DC: US Dept of Health and Human Services; 1994.

45. Brown MS, Goldstein JL, Krieger M, et al. Reversible accumulation of cholesteryl ester in macrophages incubated with acetylated lipoproteins. J Biol Chem 1979;82:597–613.

46. Steinberg D, Parthasarathy S, Carew TE, Khoo JD, Witztum JL. Beyond cholesterol: modifications of LDL that increase its atherogenecity. N Engl J Med 1989;320:915–924.

47. Steinbrecher UP, Parthasarathy S, Leake DS. Modification of LDL by endothelial cells involves lipid peroxidation and degradation of LDL phospholipids. Proc Natl Acad Sci USA 1984;81:3883–3887.

48. Fogelman AM, Schechter I, Seager J. Malondialdehyde alteration of LDL leads to cholesteryl ester accumulation in human monocyte macrophages. Proc Natl Acad Sci USA 1980;77:2214–2218.

49. Morel DW, DiCorleto PE, Chisolm GM. Endothelial and smooth muscle cells alter LDL in vitro by free radical oxidation. Arteriosclerosis 1984;4:357–364.

50. Cathcart MK, McNally AK, Morel DW, DiCorleto PE, Chisolm GM. Superoxide anion participation in human monocyte-mediated oxidation of LDL and conversion of LDL to a cytotoxin. J Immunol 1989;142:1963–1969.

51. Sparrow CP, Olszewski J. Cellular oxidation of LDL is caused by thiol production in media containing transition metal ions. J Lipid Res 1993;34:1219–1228.

52. Albrink MJ, Man EB. Serum triglycerides in coronary artery disease. Arch Inter Med 1959;103:4–8.

53. Criqui MH, Heiss G, Cohn R, et al. Plasma triglyceride level and mortality from coronary heart disease. New Engl J Med 1993;328:1220–1225.

54. Jeppesen J, Hein HO, Suadicani P, Gyntelberg F. Triglyceride concentration and ischemic heart disease. An 8–year follow-up in the Copenhagen Male Study. Circulation 1998;97:1029–1036.

55. Miller M, Seidler A, Moalemi A, Pearson TA. Normal TG levels and CAD events: The Baltimore Coronary Observational Long-Term Study. J Am Coll Cardiol 1998; 31:1252–1257.

56. Hokanson JE, Austin MA. Plasma TG level is a risk factor for cardiovascular disease independent of high-density lipoprotein cholesterol: a meta-analysis of population-based prospective studies. J Cardiovasc Risk 1996;3:213–219.

57. Barr DP, Russ EM, Eder HA. Protein-lipid relationships in human plasma in atherosclerosis and related conditions. Am J Med 1951;11:480–493.

58. Miller NE, Forde OH, Thelle DS, Mjos OD. The Tromso Heart Study: HDL and CAD a prospective case-control study. Lancet 1977;1:965–967.

59. Gordon T, Castelli WP, Hjortland MC, Kannel WB, Dawber TR. HDL as a protective factor against CHD. Am J Med 1977;62:707–714.

60. Rubins HB, Robins SJ, Collins D, et al. Gemfibrozil for the secondary prevention of coronary heart disease in men with low levels of high-density lipoprotein cholesterol. New Engl J Med 1999;341:410–418.

61. Assmann G, von Eckardstein A, Brewer HB. Familial HDL deficiency. Tangier disease. In The metabolic and molecular bases of of inherited disease. Scriver CRT, Beaudet AL, Sly WS, editors. McGraw-Hill, NYC. 1995. 2053–2072.

62. Francis GA, Knopp RH, Oram JF. Defective removal of cellular cholesterol and phospholipids by apoA-I in Tangier Disease. J Clin Invest 1995;96:78–87.

63. Rogler G, Trumbach B, Klima B, Lackner KJ, Schmitz G. HDL-mediated efflux of intracellular cholesterol is impaired in fibroblasts from Tangier disease patients. Arterioscl Thromb Vasc Biol 1995;15:683–690.

64. Felts JM, Hiroshige I, Crane RT. The mechanism of assimilation of constituents of chylomicrons, VLDL and remnants - A new theory. Biochem Biophys Res Commun 1975;66:1467–1474.

65. Le NA, Gibson JC, Ginsberg HN. Independent regulation of plasma apolipoprotein C-II and C-III concentrations in very low density and high density lipoproteins: implications for the regulation of the catabolism of these lipoproteins. J Lipid Res 1988;29:669–677.

66. Le NA, Ginsberg HN Heterogeneity of apoA-I turnover in subjects with reduced concentrations of plasma HDL cholesterol. Metabolism 1988;37:614–617.

67. Kotite L, Bergeron N, Havel RJ. Quantification of apolipoproteins B-100, B48 and E in human triglyceride-rich lipoproteins. J Lipid Res 1995;36:890–900.

68. Simons LA, Dwyer T, Simons J, et al. Chylomicrons and chylomicron remnants in coronary artery disease: a case-control study. Atherosclerosis 1987;65:181–189.

69. Marcel YL, Hogue M, Theolis R, Milne RW. Mapping of antigenic determinants of human apoB using monoclonal antibodies against LDL. J Biol Chem 1982;257:13165–13168.

70. Hazzard WR Bierman EL. Delayed clearance of chylomicron remnants following vitamin-A-containing oral fat loads in broad-beta disease (type III hyperlipoproteinemia. Metabolism 1976;25:777–801.

71. Le NA, Cortner JA, Breslow JL. Metabolism of intestinal lipoproteins during the postprandial state. In Diabetes. H Rifkin, Colwell JA, Taylor SI, editors. Elsevier Science Publishers, 1991. 601–608.

72. Le NA, Coates PM, Gallagher PR, Cortner JA. Kinetics of retinyl esters during postprandial lipemia in man: A compartmental model. Metabolism 1997;46:584–594.

73. Cortner JA, Coates PM, Le NA, Cryer DR, Ragni MC, Faulkner A, Langer T. Chylomicron remnant clearance studies in normal and hypertriglyceridemic subjects. J Lipid Res 1987; 28:195–206.

74. Cortner JA, Le NA, Coates PM, Bennett MJ, Cryer DJ. Determinants of fasting plasma triglyceride levels: metabolism of hepatic and intestinal lipoproteins. Eur J Clin Invest 1992; 22:158–165.

75. Nakajima K, Okazaki M, Tanaka A, et al. Separation and determination of remnant-like particels in human serum using

monoclonal antibodies to apoB-100 and apoA-I. Clin Ligand Assay 1997;19:177–183.

76. Masuaka H, Ishikura K, Kamei S, et al. Predictive value of remnant-like aprticles cholesterol/high-density lipoprotien cholesterol ratio as a new indicator of coronary artery disease. Am Heart J 1998;136:226–230.

77. Havel RJ. Remnant lipoproteins as therapeutic agents. Current Opinion In Lipidology 2000;11:615–620.

78. Chan L, Boerwinkle E, Li W-H. Molecular Genetics of the Plasma Lipoproteins. In Molecular Biology of the Cardiovascular System. Shu Chien, editor. Lea & Febiger; Malvern, PA. 1990. 183–219.

79. Durrington PN, Hunt L, Ishola M, Kane J, Stephens WP. Serum apoA-I and apoB in middle-aged men with and without previous myocardial infacrtion. Br Heart J 1986;56: 506–512.

80. Kwiterovich PO, Coresh J, Smith HH, et al. Comparison of the plasma levels of apoB and apoA-I, and other risk factors in men and women with premature coronary artery disease. Am J Cardiol 1992;69:1015–1021.

81. Tornvall P, Baveholm P, Landou C, deFaire U, Hamsten A. Relation of plasma levels and composition of apoB containing lipoproteins to angiographically defined CAD in young patients with MI. Circulation 1993;88:180–189.

82. Lamarche B, Tchernof A, Mauriege P, et al. Fasting insulin and apoB levels and LDL particle size as risk factors for ischemic heart disease. JAMA 1998;279:1955–1961.

83. Stampfer MJ, Sacks FM, Salvani S, et al. A prospective study of cholesterol, apolipoproteins, and the risk of myocardial infarction. N Engl J Med 1991;325:378–381.

84. Sigurdsson G, Baldursdottir A, Sigvaldason H, et al. Predictive value of apolipoproteins in a prospective survey of CAD in men. Am J Cardiol 1992;69:1251–1254.

85. Talmud PJ, Boerwinkle E, Xu CF, et al. Dietary intake and gene variation influence the response of plasma lipids to dietary intervention. Genetic Epidemiology 1992;9:249–260.

86. Myant NB. Familial defective apoB: A review, including some comparisons with familial hypercholesterolemia. Atherosclerosis 1993;104:1–19.

87. Maciejko JJ, Holmes DR, Kottke BA, Zinmeister AR, DInh DM, Mao SJ. ApoA-I as a marker of angiographically assessed CAD. N Engl J Med 1983;309:385–389.

88. Ginsberg HN, Le NA, Goldberg IJ, et al. Apolipoprotein B metabolism in subjects with deficiency of apolipoproteins CIII and AI. Evidence that apolipoprotein CIII inhibits catabolism of triglyceride-rich lipoproteins by lipoprotein lipase in vivo. J Clin Invest 1986;78:1287–1295.

89. Carlson LA. Fish eye disease: A new familial condition with massive corneal opacities and dyslipoproteinemia. Eur J Clin Invest 1981;12:41–53.

90. Norum KR. Familial LCAT deficiency. In Clinical and Metabolic Aspects of HDL. Miller NE and Miller GJ, editors. Elsevier, Amsterdam. 1984. 397–432.

91. Franceschini G, Sirtori CR, Capruso A, et al. ApoA-Imilano apoprotein: decreased HDL cholesterol levels with significant lipoprotein modifications and without clinical atherosclerosis in an Intalian family. J Clin Invest 1980;66:892–900.

92. Cushing GL, Gaubatz JW, Nava ML, et al. Quantitation and localization of apo(a) and apoB in coronary artery bypass vein grafts resected at re-operation. Arteriosclerosis 1988; 9:593–603.

93. McLean JW, Tomlinson JE, Kuang W-J, et al. cDNA sequence of human apo(a) is homologous to plasminogen. Nature 1987; 330:132–137.

94. Brown MS, Goldstein JL. Teaching old dogmas new tricks. Nature 1987;330:113–114.

95. Scanu AM. Lp(a): a potential bridge between the fields of atherosclerosis and thrombosis. Arch Pathol Lab Med 1988; 112:1045–1047.

96. Gavish D, Azrolan N, Breslow JL. Plasma Lp(a) concentration is inversely correlated with the ratio of kringle IV/kringle V encoding domains in the apo(a) gene. J Clin Invest 1989;84:2021–2027.

97. Lackner C, Boerwinkle E, Leffert CC, Rahmig T, Hobbs HH. Molecular basis of apo(a) isoform size heterogeneity as revealed by pulse-field gel electrophoresis. J Clin Invest 1991; 87:2153–2161.

98. Marcovina SM, Hobbs HH, Albers JJ. Relation between number of apo(a) kringle 4 repeats and mobility in agarose gel: basis for a standardized isoform nomenclature. Clinical Chemistry 1996;42:436–439.

99. Seed M, Hoppichler F, Reaveley D, et al. Relation of serum Lp(a) concentration and apo(a) phenotype to CHD in familial hypercholesterolemia. N Engl J Med 1990;322:1494–1499.

100. Guyton JR, Dahlen GH, Patsch W, Kautz JA, Gotto AM, Jr. Relationship of plasma Lp(a) levels to race and apoB. Arteriosclerosis 1985;5:265–272.

101. Trieu VN, Olsson U, McConathy WJ. The apoB3304–3317 peptide as an inhibitor of apo(a):apoB containing lipoprotein interaction. Biochem J 1995;307:17–22.

102. Koschinsky ML, Cote GP, Gabel B, van der Hoek YY. Identification of the cysteine residue in apo(a) which mediates extracellular coupling with apoB. J Biol Chem 1993;268: 19819–19825.

103. Chiesa G, Hobbs HH, Koschinsky ML, Lawn RM, Maika SD, Hammer RE. Reconstitution of Lp(a) by infusion of human LDL into transgenic mice expressing human apo(a). J Biol Chem 1992;267:24369–24374.

104. Hofmann SL, Eaton DL, Brown MS, McConathy WJ, Goldstein JL, Hammer RE. Overexpression of human LDL receptors leads to accelerated catabolism of Lp(a) in transgenic mice. J Clin Invest 1990;85:1542–1547.

105. Vessby B, Kostner G, Lithell H, Thomis J. Diverging effects of cholesyramine on apoB and Lp(a). Atherosclerosis 1982; 44:61–71.

106. Kostner G, Gavish D, Leopold B, Bolzano K, Weintraub WS, Breslow JL. HMG CoA reductase inhibitors lower LDL cholesterol without reducing Lp(a) levels. Circulation 1989; 80:1313–1319.

107. Davignon J, Gregg RE, Sing CF. Apolipoprotein E polymorphism and atherosclerosis. Arteriosclerosis 2002;8:1–21.

108. Davignon J, Gregg RE, Singh CF. ApoE polymorphism and actherosclerosis. Arteriosclerosis 1988;8:1–21.

109. Wilson PWF, Myers RH, Larson MG, et al. ApoE alleles, dyslipidemia, and coronary heart disease: The Framingham Offspring Study. JAMA 1994;272:1666–1671.

110. Eichner JE, Kuller LH, Orchard TJ, et al. Relation of apoE phenotype to myocardial infarction and mortality from CAD. Am J Cardiol 1993;7:160–165.

111. Scuteri A, Bos AJG, Zonderman AB, Brant LJ, Lakatta AG, Fleg JL. Is the apoE4 allele an independent predictor of coronary events. Am J Med 2001;110:28–32.

112. Chen M, Breslow JL, Li W, Leff T. Transcriptional regulation of the apoC-III gene by insulin in diabetic mice: correlation with changes in plasma triglyceride levels. J Lipid Res 1994; 35:1918–1924.

113. Dallinga-Thie GM, Groenendijk M, Blom N, de Bruin TW, de Kant E. Genetic heterogeneity in the apoC-III promoter and effects of insulin. J Lipid Res 2001;42:1450–1456.

114. Groenendijk M, Cantor RM, Blom N, Rotter J, de Bruin TW, Dallinga-Thie GM. Association of plasma lipids and apolipoproteins with the insulin response element in the apoC-III promoter region in familial combined hyperlipidemia. J Lipid Res 1999;40:1036–1044.

115. Schoonjans K, Staels B, Auwerx J. The peroxisome proliferator activated receptors (PPARS) and their effects on lipid metabolism and adipocyte differentiation. Biochim Biophys Acta 1996;1302:93–109.

116. Hertz R, Bishara-Shieban J, Bar-Tana J. Mode of action of peroxisome proliferators as hypolipidemic drugs. Suppression of apolipoprotein C-III. J Biol Chem 1995;270:13470–13475.

117. Staels B, Vu-Dac N, Kosykh VA, et al. Fibrates downregulate apolipoprotein C-III expression independent of induction of peroxisomal acyl coenzyme A oxidase. A potential mechanism for the hypolipidemic action of fibrates. J Clin Invest 1995;95:705–712.

118. Gruber PJ, Torres-Rosado A, Wolak ML, Leff T. Apo CIII gene transcription is regulated by a cytokine inducible NF-kappa B element. Nucleic Acids Res 1994;22:2417–2422.

119. Leff T, Reue K, Melian A, Culver H, Breslow JL. A regulatory element in the ApoCIII promoter that directs hepatic specific transcription binds to proteins in expressing and nonexpressing cell types. J Biol Chem 1989;264:16132–16137.

120. Kardassis D, Tzameli I, Hadzopoulou-Cladaras M, Talianidis I, Zannis V. Distal apolipoprotein C-III regulatory elements F to J act as a general modular enhancer for proximal promoters that contain hormone response elements. Synergism between hepatic nuclear factor-4 molecules bound to the proximal promoter and distal enhancer sites. Arteriosl Thromb Vasc Biol 1997;17:222–232.

121. Krauss RM, HerbertPN, Levy RI, Fredrickson DS. Further observations on the activation and inhibition of LPL by apolipoproteins. Circ Res 1973;33:403–411.

122. Brown WV, Baginsky ML. Inhibition of lipoprotein lipase by an apoprotein of very-low density lipoproteins. Biochem Biophys Res Commun 1972;46:375–382.

123. Tornoci L, Scheraldi CA, Li X, Ide H, Goldberg IJ, Le NA. Abnormal activation of lipoprotein lipase by non-equilibrating apoC-II: further evidence for the presence of non-equilibrating pools of apolipoproteins C-II and C-III in plasma lipoproteins. J Lipid Res 1993;34:1793–1803.

124. McConathy WJ, Gesquiere JC, Bass H, Tartar A, Fruchart JC, Wang CS. Inhibition of lipoprotein lipase activity by synthetic peptides of apolipoprotein C-III. J Lipid Res 1992;33: 995–1003.

125. Wang C-S, McConathy WJ, Kloer HU, Alaupovic P. Modulation of lipoprotein lipase by apolipoproteins: Effect of apoC-III. J Clin Invest 1985;75:384–390.

126. Aalto-Setala K, Fisher EA, Chen X, et al. Mechanism of hypertriglyceridemia in human apolipoprotein (apo) CIII transgenic mice. Diminished very low density lipoprotein fractional catabolic rate associated with increased apo CIII and reduced apo E on the particles. J Clin Invest 1992;90:1889–1900.

127. de Silva HV, Lauer SJ, Wang J, et al. Overexpression of human apolipoprotein C-III in transgenic mice results in an accumulation of apolipoprotein B48 remnants that is corrected by excess apolipoprotein E. J Biol Chem 1994;269:2324–2335.

128. Maeda N, Li H, Lee D, Oliver P, Quarfordt SH, Osada J. Targeted disruption of the apolipoprotein C-III gene in mice

results in hypotriglyceridemia and protection from postprandial hypertriglyceridemia. J Biol Chem 1994;269:23610–23616.

129. Norum RA, Forte TM, Alaupovic P, Ginsberg HN. Clinical syndrome and lipid metabolism in hereditary deficiency of apolipoproteins A-I and C-III, variant 1. Adv Exp Med Biol 1986;201:137–149.

130. Kowal RC, Herz J, Weisgraber KH, Mahley RW, Brown MS, Goldstein JL. Opposing effects of apolipoprotein E and C on lipoprotein binding to low density lipoprotein receptor-related protein. J Biol Chem 1990;265:10771–10779.

131. Shelburne F, Hanks J, Meyers W, Quarfordt S. Effect of apoproteins on hepatic uptake of triglyceride emulsions in the rat. J Clin Invest 1980;65:652–658.

132. Windler E, Havel RJ. Inhibitory effects of C apolipoproteins from rats and humans on the uptake of triglyceride-rich lipoproteins and their remnants by the perfused rat liver. J Lipid Res 1985;26:556–565.

133. de Silva HV, Lauer SJ, Mahley RW, Weisgraber KH, Taylor JM. Apolipoproteins E and C-III have opposing roles in the clearance of lipoprotein remnants in transgenic mice. Biochem Soc Trans 1993;21:483–487.

134. Clavey V, Lestavel-Delattre S, Copin C, Bard JM, Fruchart JC. Modulation of lipoprotein B binding to the LDL receptor by exogenous lipids and apoC-I, C-II, C-III and E. Arteriosl Thromb Vasc Biol 1995;15:963–971.

135. Jansen H, Waterworth DM, Nicaud V, Ehnholm C, Talmud PJ. Interaction of the common apolipoprotein C-III (apoC3-482C>T) and hepatic lipase (LIPC-514C>T) promoter variants affects glucose tolerance in young adults. European Atherosclerosis Research Study II. Am Hum Genet 2001;65:237–243.

136. Hunter SJ, Klein RL, Le NA, et al. ApoC-III protein concentrations and gene polymorphisms in Type 1 diabetes: Effects on lipids, lipoproteins, and microvascular disease complications in the DCCT/EDIC cohort. (In press).

137. Salas J, Jansen S, Lopez-Miranda J, et al. The Sst-I polymorphism of the apoC-III gene determines the insulin response to an oral glucose tolerance test after consumption of a diet rich in saturated fats. Am J Clin Nutr 1998;68:396–401.

138. Marcais C, Bernard S, Merlin M, et al. Severe hypertriglyceridemia in type II diabetes: involvement of the apoC-III Sst-I polymorphism, LPL mutations and apoE3 deficiency. Diabetologia 2000;43:1346–1352.

139. Dammerman M, Sandkuijl LA, Halaas JL, Chung W, Breslow JL. An apolipoprotein CIII haplotype protective against hypertriglyceridemia is specified by promoter and 3' untranslated region polymorphisms. Proc Natl Acad Sci USA 1993;90: 4562–4566.

140. Ribalta J, La Ville AE, Valle JC, Humphries S, Turner PR, Masana L. A variation in the apolipoprotein C-III gene is associated with an increased number of circulating VLDL and IDL particles in familial combined hyperlipidemia. J Lipid Res 1997;38:1061–1069.

141. Blankenhorn DH, Alaupovic P, Wickham E, et al. Prediction of angiographic change in native human coronary arteries and aortocoronary bypass grafts: lipid and nonlipid factors. Circulation 1990;81:470–476.

142. Hodis HN, Mack WJ, Azen SP, et al. Triglyceride and cholesterol-rich lipoproteins have a differential effect on mild/moderate and severe lesion progression as assessed by quantitative coronary angiography in a controlled trial of lovastatin. Circulation 1994;90:42–49.

143. Sacks FM, Alaupovic P, Moye LE, et al. VLDL, apolipoproteins B, CIII, and E, and risk of recurrent events in the

Cholesterol and Recurrent Events (CARE) Trial. Circulation 2000;102:1886–1892.

144. Festa A, D'Agostino R, Jr., Mykkanen L, et al. LDL particle size in relation to insulin, proinsulin, and insulin sensitivity: The Insulin Resistance Atherosclerosis Study. Diabetes Care 1999;22:1688–1693.

145. Reaven GM, Chen YD, Jeppesen J, Maheux P, Krauss RM. Insulin resistance and hyperinsulinemia in individuals with small dense LDL particles. J Clin Invest 1993;92:141–146.

146. Grundy SM, Small LDL, atherogenic dyslipidemia, and the metabolic syndrome. Circulation 1997;95:1–4.

147. Fisher WR, Hammond MG, Warmke GL. Measurements of the molecular weight variability of plasma LDL among normals and subjects with hyper-B-lipoproteinemia. Biochem J 1972; 11:519–525.

148. Sniderman A, Shapiro S, Marpole D, Skinner B, Teng B, Kwiterovich PO. Association of coronary atherosclerosis with hyperapobetalipoproteinemia [increased protein but normal cholesterol levels in human plasma low-density (beta) lipoproteins]. Proc Natl Acad Sci USA 1980;77:604–608.

149. Krauss RM, Burke DJ. Identification of multiple subclasses of plasma LDL in normal humans. J Lipid Res 1982;23:97–104.

150. Le NA. Small, dense low-density lipoprotein: Risk or myth. Curr Atheroscler Rev 2003;5:22–28.

151. Austin MA, King MC, Vranizan KM, Newman B, Krauss RM. Inheritance of LDL subclass patterns: Results of complex segregation analysis. Am Hum Genet 1988;43:838–846.

152. Austin MA, Breslow JL, Hennekens CH, Buring JE, Willett WC, Krauss RM. LDL subclass patterns and risk of myocardial infarction. JAMA 1988;260:1917–1921.

153. Lamarche B, Tchernof A, Moorjani S, et al. Small, dense LDL particles as a predictor of the risk of ischemic heart disease in me: Prospective results from the Quebec Cardiovascular Study. Circulation 1997;95:69–75.

154. Campos H, Genest JJ, Blijlevens E, et al. LDL particle size and coronary artery disease. Arterioscl Thromb 1992;12:187–195.

155. Tornvall P, Karpe F, Carlson LA, Hamsten A. Relationships of LDL subfractions to angiographically defined coronary artery disease in young survivors of myocardial infarction. Atherosclerosis 1991;90:67–80.

156. Gardner CD, Fortmann SP, Krauss RM. Association of small LDL particles with the incidence of CAD in men and women. JAMA 1996;276:875–881.

157. Miller BD, Alderman EL, Haskell WL, Fair JM, Krauss RM. Predominance of dense LDL particles predicts angiographic benefit of therapy in the Stanford Coronary Risk Intervention Project. Circulation 1996;94:2146–2153.

158. Zambon A, Hokanson JE, Brown BG, Brunzell JD. Evidence for a new pathophysiological mechanism for CAD regression: Hepatic lipase-mediated changes in LDL density. Circulation 1999;99:1959–1964.

159. Sniderman AD, Scantlebury T, Cianflone K. Hypertriglyceridemic hyperapoB: The unappreciated atherogenic dyslipoproteinemia in type 2 Diabetes Mellitus. Ann Int Med 2001;135:447–459.

160. Davidson NO, Shelness GS. Apolipoprotein B: mRNA editing, lipoprotein assembly, and presecretory degradation. Ann Rev Nutr 2000;20:169–193.

161. Dreon DM, Fernstrom HA, Miller B, Krauss RM. LDL subclass patterns and lipoprotein response to a reduced-fat diet in men. FASEB J 1994;8:121–126.

162. Dreon DM, Fernstrom HA, Campos H, Blanche P, Williams PT, Krauss RM. Change in dietary saturated fat intake is correlated

163. with change in mass of large LDL particles in men. Am J Clin Nutr 1998;67:828–836.

163. Dreon DM, Fernstrom HA, Williams PT, Krauss RM. A very low-fat diet is not associated with improved lipoprotein profiles in men with a predominance of large LDL. Am J Clin Nutr 1999;69:411–418.

164. Lundahl B, Leren TP, Ose L, Hamsten A, Karpe F. A functional polymorphism in the promoter region of the microsomal triglyceride transfer protein (MTP -493G/T) influences lipoprotein phenotype in familial hypercholesterolemia. Arterioscl Thromb Vasc Biol 2002;20:1784–1788.

165. Juo SH, Han Z, Smith JD, Colangelo L, Liu K. Common polymorphism in promoter of MTP gene influences cholesterol, apoB and TG levels in young African American men: Results from CARDIA study. Arterioscl Thromb Vasc Biol 2000;20:1316–1322.

166. Hurt-Camejo E, Camejo G, Peilot H, Oorni K, Kovanen P. Phospholipase A2 in vascular disease. Circ Res 2001; 89:298–304.

167. Hurt-Camejo E, Camejo G, Sartipy P. Phospholipase A2 and small, dense LDL. Current Opinion In Lipidology 2000;11:465–471.

168. Carr MC, Ayyobi AF, Murdoch SJ, Deeb SS, Brunzell JD. Contribution of hepatic lipase, lipoprotein liapse, and cholesteryl ester transfer protein to LDL and HDL heterogeneity in healthy women. Arterioscl Thromb Vasc Biol 2002; 22:667–673.

169. Talmud P, Edwards KL, Turner C, et al. Linkage of the CETP gene to LDL particle size: Use of a novel tetranucleotide repeat within the CETP promoter. Circulation 1999; 101:2461–2466.

170. Ross R. Atherosclerosis: an inflammatory disease. N Engl J Med 2002;340:115–126.

171. Libby P, Ridker PM, Maseri A. Inflammation and Atherosclerosis. Circulation 2002;105:1135–1143.

172. Blake GJ, Ridker PM. Inflammatory bio-markers and cardiovascular risk prediction. J Internal Med 2002;252:283–294.

173. Sakai A, Kume N, Nishi E, Tanoue K, Mivasaka M, Kita T. P-selectin and vascular cell adhesion molecule-1 are focally expressed in aortas of hypercholesterolemic rabbits before intimal accumulation of macrophages and T lymphocytes. Arterioscl Thromb Vasc Biol 1997;17:310–316.

174. Rifai N, Ridker PM. Inflammatory markers and coronary heart disease. Curr Opinion Lipidol 2002;13:383–389.

175. Tracy R. Inflammation markers and coronary heart disease. Curr Opinion Lipidol 1999;10:435–441.

176. Folsom AR, Pankow JS, Tracy R, Arnett DK, Peacock JM, Hong Y, et al. Association of C-reactive protein with markers of prevalent atherosclerotic disease. Am J Cardiol 2001; 88:112–117.

177. Ridker PM. High-sensitivity C-reactive protein: potential adjunct for global risk assessment in the primary prevention of cardiovascular disease. Circulation 2001;103:1813–1818.

178. Ridker PM, Hennekens CH, Buring JE. C reactive protein and other markers of inflammation in the prediction of cardiovascular disease in women. N Engl J Med 2000;342:836–843.

179. Ridker PM, Cushman M, Stampfer MJ. Inflammation, aspirin, and the risk of cardiovascular disease in apparently healthy men. N Engl J Med 1997;336:973–979.

180. Albert MA, Danielson E, Rifai N, Ridker PM. Effect of statin therapy on C-reactive protein levels: the Pravastatin Inflammation/CRP Evaluation (PRINCE): a randomized trial and cohort study. JAMA 2001;286:64–70.

181. Plenge JK, Hernandez TL, Weil KM, et al. Simvastatin lowers C-reactive protein within 14 days: An effect independent of LDL-cholesterol reduction. Circulation 2002;106:1447–1452.

182. Kinlay S, Timms T, Clark M, Karam C, Bilodeau T. Comparison of effect of intensive lipid lowering with atorvastatin to less intensive lowering with lovastatin on C-reactive protein in patients with stable angina pectoris and inducible myocardial ischemia. Am J Cardiol 2002;89: 1205–1207.

183. McCully KS, Wilson RB. Homocysteine theory of atherosclerosis. Atherosclerosis 2003;22:215–227.

184. Kraus JP. Biochemistry and molecular genetics of cystathionine beta-synthase deficiency. Eur J Pediatr 1998;157:S50–S53.

185. Ueland PM. Homocysteine species as components of plasma redox thiol status. Clin Chem 1995;41:340–342.

186. Frantzen F, Faaren FL, Alfheim I, Nordhei AK. Enzyme conversion immunoassay for determining total homocysteine in plasma or serum. Clin Chem 1998;44:311–316.

187. Bostom AG, Jacques PF, Nadeau MR, Williams RR, Ellison RC, Selhub J. Post-methionine load hyperhomocysteinemia in persons with normal fasting total homocysteine: initial results from the NHLBI Family Heart Study. Atherosclerosis 1995; 116:147–151.

188. Ubbink JB, Vermaak WJ, van der Merwe A, Becker PJ. The effect of blood sampling and food consumption on plasma total homocysteine levels. Clin Chim Acta 1992;207:119–128.

189. Boushey CJ, Beresford SA, Omenn GS, Motulsky AG. A quantitative assessment of plasma homocysteine as a risk factor for vascular disease. Probable benefits of increasing folic acid intakes. JAMA 1995;274:1049–1057.

190. Wald NJ, Watt HC, Law MR, Weir DG, McPartlin J, Scott JM. Homocysteine and ischemic heart disease: results of a prospective study with implications regarding prevention. Arch Inter Med 1998;158:862–867.

191. Eikelboom JW, Lonn E, Genest J, Hankey G, Yusuf S. Homocysteine and cardiovascular disease: A critical review of the epidemiologic evidence. Ann Int Med 1999; 131:363–375.

192. Anderson JL, Horne BD, Carlquist JF, et al. Effect of implementation of folic acid fortification of food on homocysteine concentrations in subjects with coronary artery disease. Am J Cardiol 2002;90:536–539.

193. Navab M, Hama S, Hough GP, Hedrick CC, Sorenson R. High density lipoprotein associated enzymes: their role in vascular biology. Curr Opinion Lipidol 1998;9:449–456.

194. Durrington PN, Mackness B, Mackness MI. Paraoxonase and atherosclerosis. Arterioscl Thromb Vasc Biol 2001;21:473–480.

195. Mackness MI, Arrol S, Durrington PN. Paraoxonase prevents accumulation of lipoperoxides in LDL. FEBS Letters 1991; 286:152–154.

196. Mackness MI, Arrol S, Abbott, Durrington PN. Protection of LDL against oxidative modification by HDL-associated paraoxonase. Atherosclerosis 1993;104:129–135.

197. Watson AD, Berliner JA, Hama SY, et al. Protective effect of HDL-associated paraoxonase: inhibition of the biological activity of minimally oxidised LDL. J Clin Invest 1995; 96:2882–2891.

198. Tward A, Xia YR, Wang XP, et al. Decreased atherosclerotic lesion formation in human serum paraoxonase transgenic mice. Circulation 2002;106:484–490.

199. Shih DM, Gu L, Xia YR. Mice lacking serum paraoxonase are susceptible to organophosphate toxicity and atherosclerosis. Nature 1998;394:284–287.

200. Shih DM, Xia YR, Wang XP. Combined serum paraoxonase knockout/apoE knockout mice exhibit increased lipoprotein oxidation and atherosclerosis. J Biol Chem 2000; 275:17527–17535.

201. Adkins S, Gan KN, Mody M, LaDu BN. Molecular basis for the polymorphic forms of human serum paraoxonase/arylesterase: glutamine or arginine at position 191, for the respective A or B allozymes. Am J Hum Genet 1993;52:598–608.

202. Blatter-Garin MC, James RW, Dussoix P, Blanche H, Ruiz J. Paraoxonase polymorphism Met-Leu54 is associated with modified concentrations of the enzyme. J Clin Invest 1997; 99:62–66.

203. Mackness B, Mackness MI, Arrol S, Turkie W, Durrington PN. Effect of the human serum paraoxonase 55 and 192 genetic polymorphisms on the protection by HDL against LDL oxidative modification. FEBS Letters 1998;423:57–60.

204. Aviram M, Hardak E, Vava J, et al. Human serum PON1 Q and R selectively decrease lipid peroxides in human coronary and carotid atherosclerotic lesions: PON1 esterase and peroxidase-like activities. Circulation 2000;101:2510–2517.

205. Shih DM, Gu L, Hama S, et al. Genetic-dietary regulation of serum paraoxonase expression and its role in atherogenesis in a mouse model. J Clin Invest 2003;97:1630–1639.

206. Herdick CC, Hassan K, Hough GP, et al. Short-term feeding of atherogenic diet to mice results in reduction of HDL and paraoxonase that may be mediated by an immune mechanism. Arterioscl Thromb Vasc Biol 2000;20:1946–1952.

207. Sutherland WHF, Walker RJ, de Jong SA, van Rij AM, Phillips V, Walker HL. Reduced postprandial serum paraoxonase activity after a meal rich in used cooking fat. Arterioscl Thromb Vasc Biol 1999;19:1340–1347.

208. Paragh G, Balogh Z, Seres I, Harangi M, Boda J, Kovacs P. Effect of gemfibrozil on HDL-associated serum paraoxonase activity and lipoprien profile in patients with hyperlipidemia. Clin Drug Invest 2000;19:277–282.

209. Tomas M, Senti M, Garcia-Faria F, Vila J, Torrents A, Covas M, Effect of simvastatin therapy on paraoxonase activity and related lipoproteins in familial hypercholesterolemic patients. Arterioscl Thromb Vasc Biol 2000;20:2113–2119.

210. Aviram M, Rosenblat M, Bisgaier CL, Newton RS. Atorvastatin and gemfibrozil metabolites, but not the parent drugs are potent antioxidants against lipoprotein oxidation. Atherosclerosis 1998;138:271–280.

211. Durrington PN, Mackness MI, Bhatnagar D, et al. Effects of two different fibric acid derivatives on lipoproteins, cholesteryl ester transfer, fibrinogen, plasminogen activator inhibitor and paraoxonase activity in type IIb hyperlipoproteinemia. Atherosclerosis 1998;138:217–225.

212. Cushing SD, Berliner JA, Valente AJ. Minimally modified LDL induces monocyte chemotactic protein 1 in human endothelial cells and smooth muscle cells. Proc Natl Acad Sci USA 1990;87:5134–5138.

213. Kugiyama K, Kerns SA, Morrisett JD, Roberts R, Henry PD. Impairment of endothelium-dependent arterial relaxation by lysolecithin in modified lipoproteins. Nature 1990;344: 160–162.

214. Avogaro P, Bittolo Bon G, Cazzolato G. Presence of a modified LDL in humans. Arteriosclerosis 1988;8:79–87.

215. Haberland ME, Fong D, Cheng L. Malondialdehyde-altered protein occurs in atheroma of WHHL rabbits. Science 1988; 241:215–218.

216. Palinski W, Rosenfeld ME, Yla-Herttuala S, et al. LDL undergoes oxidative modification in vivo. Proc Natl Acad Sci USA 1989;86:1372–1376.

217. Holvoet P, Perez G, Zhao Z, et al. MDA-modified LDL in patients with atheroscleotic disease. J Clin Invest 1995;95:2611–2619.

218. Itabe H, Yamamoto H, Imanaka T, et al. Sensitive detection of oxidatively modified LDL using a monoclonal antibody. J Lipid Res 1996;37:45–53.

219. Palinski W, Horkko S, Miller E, et al. Cloning of MAb to epitopes of oxidized lipoproteins from apoE-deficient mice. Demonstration of epitopes of oxidized LDL in human plasma. J Clin Invest 1996;98:800–814.

220. Parthasarathy S, Wieland E, Steinberg D. A role of endothelial cell lipoxygenase in the oxidative modification of LDL. Proc Natl Acad Sci USA 1989;86:1046–1050.

221. Jessup W, Rankin SM, DeWhalley CV, et al. Alpha-tocopherol consumption during LDL oxidation. Biochem J 1990;265:390–105.

222. Esterbauer H, Gebicki J, Puhl H, Jurgens G. The role of lipid peroxidation and antioxidants in oxidative modification of LDL. Free Radical Biol Med 1992;13:341–390.

223. Hoff HF, Gaubatz JW. Isolation, purification and characterization of a lipoprotein containing apoB from the human aorta. Atherosclerosis 1982;42:273–297.

224. Yla-Herttuala S, Palinski W, Butler SW, Picard S, Steinberg D, Witztum JL. Rabbit and human atherosclerotic lesions contain IgG that recognizes epitopes of oxidized LDL. Arterioscl Thromb 1994;14:32–40.

225. Tertov VV, Orkhov AN, Kacharava AG. LDL-containing circulating immune complexes and coronary atherosclerosis. Exp Mol Pathol 1990;52:300–308.

226. Chumburidze T, Li X, Sung K, Le NA, Pitt B, Brown WV. Levels of autoantibodies against MDA-LDL are not increased in patients with documented CAD. J Invest Med 1997; 45:216A.

227. van de Vijver LPL, Steyger R, van Poppel G, et al. Autoantibodies against MDA-LDL in subjects with severe and minor atherosclerosis and healthy population controls. Atherosclerosis 1996;122:245–253.

228. Salonen JT, Yla-Herttuala S, Yamamoto R. Autoantibody against LDL and progression of carotid atherosclerosis. Lancet 1992;339:883–887.

229. Maggi E, Finardi G, Poli G. Specificity of autoantibodies against oxLDL predicting myocardial infarction. Cor Artery Dis 2001;4:1119–1122.

230. Palinski W, Miller E, Witztum JL. Immunization of LDL receptor-deficient rabbits with homologous malondialdehyde-modified LDL reduces atherosclerosis. Proc Natl Acad Sci USA 1995;92:821–825.

231. Ameli S, Hultgardh-Nilsson A, Rengstrom J, et al. Effect of immunization with homologous LDL and oxidized LDL on early atherosclerosis in hypercholesterolemic rabbits. Arterioscler Thromb Vasc Biol 1996;16:1074–1079.

232. Babior BM. Oxygen-dependent microbial killing by phagocytes. N Engl J Med 1978;298:659–668.

233. Uhlinger DJ, Burnham DN, Mullins RE, Lambeth D, Merrill A. Functional differences in human neutrophils isolated pre- and post-prandially. FEBS Letters 1991;286:28–32.

234. Ji LL. Oxidative stress during exercise: implication of antioxidant nutrients. Free Rad Biol Med 1995;18:1079–1086.

235. Le NA, Li X, Kyung S, Brown WV. Evidence for the in vivo generation of oxidatively modified epitopes in patients with documented CAD. Metabolism 2000;49:1271–1277.

236. Gradek Q, Harris M, Yahia N, Davis WW, Le N-A, Brown WV. Polyunsaturated fatty acids acutely suppress antibodies to malondialdehyde-modified lipoproteins in patients with vascular disease Am J Cardiol 2004;93:881-885.

237. Wilson PWF, d'Agostino RB, Levy D, Belanger AM, Silbershatz H, Kannel WB. Prediction of coronary heart disease using risk factor categories. Circulation 1998;97:1837–1847.

238. Wilson PWF, Kannel WB, Silbershatz H, d'Agostino RB. Clustering of metabolic factors and coronary heart disease. Arch Inter Med 1999;159:1104–1109.

239. Lakka H-M, Laaksonen DE, Lakka TA, et al. The metabolic syndrome and total and cardiovascular disease mortality in middle-aged men. JAMA 2002;288:2709–2716.

240. Steinmetz A, Fenselau S, Schrezenmeir J. Treatment of dyslipoproteinemia in the metabolic syndrome. Exp Clin Endocrinol Diabetes 2001;109:S548–S559.

241. Lichstenstein AH, Ausman LM, Jalpert SM, Schaefer EJ. Effects of different forms of dietary hydrogenated fats on serum lipoprotein cholesterol levels. N Engl J Med 1999;340: 1933–1940.

242. Lichstenstein AH. Trans fatty acid and cardiovascular disease risk. Curr Opinion Lipidol 2000;11:37–42.

243. Stone NJ. Fish consumption, fish oil, lipids, and coronary heart disease. Circulation 1996;94:2337–2340.

244. Angere P, von Schacky C. n-3 polyunsaturated fatty acids and the cardiovascular system. Curr Opinion Lipidol 2000;11:57–63.

245. Rimm EB, Klatsky A, Grobbee D, Stampfer MJ. Review of moderate alcohol consumption and reduced risk of coronary heart disease: is the effect due to beer, wine or spirits. Br Med J 1996;23:731.

246. Hjermann I, Holme I, Velve Byre K, Leren P. Effect of diet and smoking intervention on the incidence of coronary heart disease: Report from the Oslo Study group of a randomised trial in healthy men. Lancet 1981;2:1303–1310.

247. de leogeril M, Salen P, Paillard F, Laporte F, Boucher F, de Leiris J. Mediterranean diet and the French paradox: two distinct biogeographoc concepts for one consolidated scientific theory on the role of nutrition in coronary heart disease. Cardiovasc Res 2002;54:503–515.

248. Hallikainen MA, Uusitupa MI. The effect of two low-fat stanol ester-containing margerines on serum cholesterol concentrations as part of a low-fat diet in hypercholesterolemic subjects. Am J Clin Nutr 1999;69:403–410.

249. Nguyen TT, Dale LC, von Bergmann K, Croghan IT. Cholesterol-lowering effect of stanol ester in a US population of mildly hypercholesterolemic men and women: A randomized controlled trial. Mayo Clin Proc 1999;74:1198–1206.

250. Schwartz GG, Olson AG, Eskowitz MD, et al. Effects of atorvastatin on early recurrent ischemic events in acute coronary syndromes: the MIRACL study. A randomized controlled trial. JAMA 2001;285:1711–1718.

251. Stamler J. The Coronary Drug Project: Findings with regard to estrogen, dextrothyroxine;clofibrate and niacin. Adv Exp Med Biol 1977;82:52–75.

252. Canner PL, Berger KG, Wenger NK, et al. Fifteen year mortality in Coronary Drug Project patients: long-term benefit with niacin. J Am Coll Cardiol 1986;8:1245–1255.

253. Oliver MF, Heady JA, Morris JN, Cooper J. A cooperative trial in the primary prevention of ischaemic heart disease using clofibrtate: Report from the Committee of Principal Investigators. Br Heart J 1978;40:1069–1118.

254. Manninen V, Elo O, Haapa K, et al. Lipid alterations and decline in the incidence of coronary heart disease in the Helsinki Heart Study. JAMA 1988;260:641–651.

255. Carlson LA, Rosenhamer G. Reduction of mortality in the Stockholm Ischaemic Heart Disease Secondary Prevention

Study by combined treatment with clofibrate and nicotinic acid. Acta Med Scand 1988;223:405–418.

256. Kjekshus J, Pederson TR, for the 4S Group. Reducing the risk of coronary events: Evidence from the Scandinavian Simvastatin Survival Study (4S). Am J Cardiol 1995;76:64C–68C.

257. Sacks FM, Pfeffer MA, Moye LA, et al. The effect of pravastatin on coronary events after myocardial infarction in patients with average cholesterol levels: Cholesterol and Recurrent Events. N Engl J Med 1996;335:1001–1009.

258. The Long-term Intervention with Pravastatin in Ischaemic Disease. Prevention of cardiovascular events and death with pravastatin in patients with coronary heart disease and a borad range of initial cholesterol levels. N Engl J Med 1998;339:1349–1357.

259. Heart Protection Study Collaborative Group. MRC/BHF Heart Protection Study of cholesterol-lowering with simvastatin in 20,536 high-risk individuals: a randomised placebo-controlled trial. Lancet 2002;360:7–22.

260. Downs JR, Clearfield M, Weis S, et al. Primary prevention of acute coronary events with lovastatin in men and women with average cholesterol levels: Results of the AFCAPS/TexCAPS. JAMA 1998;279:1615–1622.

261. Shepherd J, Blauw GJ, Murphy MB, et al. Pravastatin in elderly individuals at risk of vascular disease (PROSPER): A randomised controlled trial. Lancet 2002;360:1623–1630.

262. Knopp RH. Drug treatment of lipid disorders. N Engl J Med 1999;341:498–551.

263. Andrews TC, Ballantyne CM, Hsia JA, Kramer JH. Achieving and maintaining NCEP LDL-cholesterol goal with five statins. Am J Med 2001;111:185–191.

264. Istvan ES, Deisenhofer J. Structural mechanism for statin inhibition of HMGCoA reductase. Science 2001;292: 1160–1164.

265. Wang SL, Du EZ, Martin TD, Davis RA. Coordinate regulation of lipogenesis, the assembly and secretion of apoB-containing lipoproteins by SRBP-1. J Biol Chem 1997;272:19351–19358.

266. Laufs U, La Fata V, Plutzky J, Liao JK. Upregulation of endothelial nitric oxide synthase by HMG CoA reductase inhibitors. Circulation 1998;97:1129–1135.

267. Beaird SL. HMG-CoA reductase inhibitors: Assessing differences in drug interactions and safety profiles. J Am Pharm Assoc 2000;40:637–644.

268. Herman RJ. Drug interactions and the statins. Can Med Assoc J 1999;161:1281–1286.

269. Corsini A, Bellosta S, Baetta R, Fumagalli R, Paoletti R, Bernini F. New insights into the pharmacodynamic and pharmacokinetic properties of statins. PharmacolTher 1999;84:413–428.

270. Bottorff M, Hansten P. Long-term safety of hepatic HMG-CoA reductase inhibitors. Arch Inter Med 2000;160:2273–2280.

271. Pasternak RC, Smith SC, Bairey-Merz CN, Grundy SM, Cleeman JI, Lenfant C. ACC/AHA/NHLBI clinical advisory on the use and safety of statins. Circulation 2002;106: 1024–1028.

272. Grunden JW, Fisher KA. Lovastatin-induced rhabdomyolysis potentially associated with clarithromycin and azithromycin. Ann Pharmacother 1997;31:859–863.

273. Maltz HC, Balog DL, Cheigh JS. Rhabdomyolysis associated with concomitant use of atorvastatin and cyclosporine. Ann Pharmacother 1999;33:1176–1179.

274. Fears R, Brown R, Ferres H, Grenier F, Tyrell AW. Effect of novel bile salts on cholesterol metabolism in rats and guinea pigs. Biochem Pharmacol 1990;40:2029–2037.

275. Higaki J, Hara S, Takasu N, et al. Inhibition of ileal Na+/bile acid cotransporter by S-8921 reduces serum cholesterol and prevents atherosclerosis in rabbits. Arterioscl Thromb Vasc Biol 1998;18:1304–1311.

276. Davidson MH, Dillon MA, Gordon B, et al. Colesevelam hydrochloride (Cholestagel): a new potent bile acid sequestrant associated with a low incidence of gastrointestinal side effects. Arch Inter Med 1999;159:1893–1900.

277. Blankenhorn DH, Nessim SA, Johnson RL, Sanmarco ME, AzenSP, Cahin-Hemphill L. Beneficial effects of combined colestipol-niacin therapy on coronary atherosclerosis and coronary venous bypass grafts. JAMA 1987;257:3233–3240.

278. Brown G, Albers JJ, Fisher LD, et al. Regression of CAD as a result of intensive lipid-lowering therapy in men with high levels of apoB. N Engl J Med 1990;323:1289–1298.

279. Kane JP, Malloy MJ, Ports TA, Phillips NR, Diehl JC, Havel RJ. Regression of coroanry atherosclerosis during treatment of familial hypercholesterolemia with combined drug regimens. JAMA 1990;264:3007–3012.

280. Cashin-Hemphill L, Mack WJ, Pogoda JM, Sanmarco ME, Azen SP, Blankenhorn DH. Beneficial effects of colestipol-niacin on coronary atherosclerosis. A 4-year follow-up. JAMA 1990;264:3013–3017.

281. Altschul R, Hoffer A, Stephen JD. Influence of nicotinic acid on cholesterol in man. Arch Biochem 1955;54:558–559.

282. Crouse JR. New developments in the use of niacin for treatment of hyperlipidemia: New considerations in the use of an old drug. Cor Artery Dis 1996;7:321–326.

283. Guyton JR. Effect of niacin on atherosclerotic cardiovascular disease. Am J Cardiol 1998;82:18U–23U.

284. Grundy SM, Mok HYI, Zech L, Berman M. Influence of nicotinic acid on metabolism of cholesterol and triglycerides in man. J Lipid Res 1981;22:24–36.

285. Carlson LA, Hamsten A, Asplund A. Pronounced lowering of serum level of Lp(a) in hyperlipidemic subjects treated with nicotinic acid. J Internal Med 1989;226:271–276.

286. Morgan JM, Capuzzi DM, Guyton JR, et al. Treatment effect of Niaspan, a controlled-release niacin in patients with hypercholesterolemia: a placebo-controlled trial. J cardiovasc Pharmacol Ther 1996;1:195–202.

287. Morgan JM, Capuzzi DM, Guyton JR. A new extended-release niacin (Niaspan): Efficacy, tolerability, and safety in hypercholesterolemic patients. Am J Cardiol 1998;82:29U–34U.

288. Morrow JD, Parsons WG, Roberts LJ. Release of markedly increased quantities of prostaglandins D2in vivo in humans following the administration of nicotinic acid. Prostaglandins 1989;38:263–274.

289. Knopp RH. Clinical profiles of plain versus sustained-release niacin and the physiologic rationale for nighttime dosing. Am J Cardiol 1998;82:35U–38U.

290. Jay RH, Dickson AC, Betteridge DJ. Effects of aspirin upon the flushing reaction induced by niceritrol. Br J Clin Pharm 1990;29:120–122.

291. Goldberg A, Alagona P, Capuzzi DM, et al. Multiple-dose efficacy and safety of an extended-release form of niacin in the management of hyperlipidemia. Am J Cardiol 2000;85:1100–1105.

292. Brown WV. Niacin for lipid disorders. Postgrad Medicine 1995;98:185–196.

293. Grundy SM, Vega GL, McGovern ME, et al. Efficacy, safety and tolerability of once-daily niacin for the treatment of dyslipidemia associated with type 2 diabetes: Results of the

assessment of diabetes control and evaluation of the efficacy of niaspan trial. Arch Inter Med 2002;162:1568–1576.

294. Grundy SM, Gibbons LW, Gonzalez V, Gordon N. The prevalence of side-effects with regular and sustained-release nicotinic acid. Am J Med 1995;99:378–385.

295. Grundy SM, Ahrens EH, Salen G, Schreibman PH, Nestel PJ. Mechanisms of action of clofibrate on cholesterol metabolism in patients with hyperlipidemia. J Lipid Res 1972;13:531–551.

296. Brown WV. Fenofibrate: a third-generation fibric acid derivative. Am J Med 1987;83:1–89.

297. Grundy SM, Vega GL. Fibric acids: effects on lipids and lipoprotein metabolism. Am J Med 1987;83:9–20.

298. Staels B, Dallongeville J, Auwerx J, Schoonjans K, Leitersdorf E, Fruchart JC. Mechanism of action of fibrates on lipid and lipoprotein metabolism. Circulation 1998;98:2088–2093.

299. Schoonjans K, Staels B, Auwerx J. Role of the peroxisome proliferator-activated receptor (PPAR) in mediating the effects of fibrates and fatty acids on gene expression. J Lipid Res 1996;37:907–925.

300. Gervois P, Chopin-Delannoy S, Fadel A, et al. Fibrates increase human REV-ERBalpha expresion in liver via a novel peroxisome proliferator-activated receptor response element. Mol Endocrinol 1999;13:400–409.

301. Staels B, Schoonjans K, Fruchart JC, Auwerx J. The effects of fibrates and thiazolidinediones on plasma triglyceride metabolism are mediated by distinct peroxisome proliferator activated receptors (PPARs). Biochimie 1997;79:95–99.

302. Haubenwallner S, Essenburg AD, Barnett BC, et al. Hypolipidemic activity of select fibrates correlates to changes in hepatic apolipoprotein C-III expression: a potential physiologic basis for their mode of action. J Lipid Res 1995;36:2541–2551.

303. Goto D, Okimoto T, Ono M, et al. Upregulation of LDL receptor by gemfibrozil, a hypolipidemic agent, in human hepatoma cells through stabilization of mRNA transcripts. Arterioscl Thromb Vasc Biol 1997;17:2707–2712.

304. Hunt MC, Yang Y-Z, Eggertsen G, et al. The PPAR alpha regulates bile acid synthesis. J Biol Chem 2000;275:28947–28953.

305. Post SM, Duez H, Gervois P, Staels B, Kuipers F, Princen HMG. Fibrates suppress bile acid synthesis via PPAR alpha mediated downregulation of cholesterol 7alpha-hydrolase and sterol 27-hydrolase expression. Arterioscl Thromb Vasc Biol 2001;21:1840–1845.

306. Plat J, Kerckhoffs DAJM, Mensink RP. Therapeutic potential of plant sterols and stanols. Curr Opinion Lipidol 2000;11:571–576.

307. Lees AM, Mok HYI, Lees RS, McCluskey MA, Grundy SM. Plant sterols as cholesterol-lowering agents: clinical trials in patients with hypercholesterolemia and studies of sterol balance. Atherosclerosis 1977;28:325–338.

308. Miettinen TA, Puska P, Gylling H, Vanhanen H, Vartiainen E. Serum cholesterol lowering by sitostanol ester margerine in a mildly hypercholesterolemic random population. N Engl J Med 1995;333:1308–1312.

309. Bhattacharyya AK, Connor WE. Beta-sitosterolemia and xanthomatosis. J Clin Invest 1974;53:1033–1043.

310. Salen G, Shefer S, Nguyen L. Sitosterolemia. J Lipid Res 1992;33:945–955.

311. van Heek M, France CF, Compton DS, et al. In vivo metabolism-based discovery of a potent cholesterol absorption inhibitor, SCH58235, in the rat and rhesus monkey through the identification of the active metabolites of SCH48461. J Pharmacol Exp Ther 1997;283:157–163.

312. van Heek M, Farley C, Compton D, Hoos L, Davis HR. Ezetimibe selectively inhibits intestinal cholesterol absorption in rodents in the absence and presence of exocirne pancreatic function. Br J Pharmacol 2001;134:409–417.

313. Dujovne CA, Ettinger MP, McNeer JF, et al. Efficacy and safety of a potent new cholesterol absorption inhibitor, ezetimibe, in patients with primary hypercholesterolemia. Am J Cardiol 2002;90:1092–1097.

314. van Heek M, Farley C, Compton D, et al. The potent cholesterol absorption inhibitor, ezetimibe, is glucurodinated in the intestine, localizes to the intestine, and circulates enterohepatically. Atherosclerosis 2000;151:155(Abstr).

315. van Heek M, Farley C, Compton DS, et al. Comparison of the activity and disposition of the novel cholesterol absorption inhibitor SCH58235, and its glucoronide, SCH60663. Br J Pharmacol 2000;129:1748–1754.

316. Gagne C, Bays HE, Weiss SR, et al. Efficacy and safety of ezetimibe added to ongoing statin therapy of patients with primary hypercholesterolemia. Am J Cardiol 2002;90:1084–1091.

317. Davidson MH, McGarry T, Bettis R, et al. Ezetimibe coadministered with simvastatin in patients with primary hypercholesterolemia. J Am Call Cardiol 2002;40:2125–2134.

318. Cagne C, Gaudet D, Bruckert E, for the Ezetimibe Study Group. Efficacy and safety of ezetimibe coadministered with atorvastatin or simvastatin in patients with homozygous familial hypercholesterolemia. Circulation 2002;105:2469–2475.

319. Kosoglou T, Guillame M, Sun S, et al. Pharmacodynamic interactions betweeen fenofibrate and the cholesterol absorption inhibitor ezetimibe. Atherosclerosis 2001;2:38(Abstract).

320. Reyderman, Kosoglou T, Statkevich P, et al. Assessment of a multiple dose drug interaction between ezetimibe and gemfibrozil. Drugs Affecting Lipid Metabolism XIV Symposium, Dordrecht, The Netherlands: Kluwer Academic Publishers; 2001.

321. Yokohama S, Hayashi R, Satani M, Yamamoto A. Selective removal of LDL by plasmapheresis in familial hypercholesterolemia. Arteriosclerosis 1985;5:613–622.

322. Gordon BR, Stein E, Jones P, Illingworth DR. Indications for LDL apheresis. Am J Cardiol 1994;74:1109–1113.

323. Gordon BR, Kelsey SF, Dau PC, Gotto AM, Liposorber Study Group. Long-term effects of LDL apheresis using an automated dextran sulfate cellulose adsorption system. Am J Cardiol 1998;81:407–411.

324. Kroon AA, Aengevaeren WRM, van der Werf T, et al. LDL Atherosclerosis Regression Study: Effect of aggressive versus conventional lipid lowering treatment on coronary atherosclerosis. Circulation 1996;93:1826–1835.

325. Nishimura S, Sekiguchi M, Kano T, et al. Effects of intensive lipid-lowering by LDL apheresis on regression of coronary atherosclerosis in patients with familial hypercholesterolemia: Japan LDL-apheresis Coronary Atherosclerosis Prospective Study. Atherosclerosis 1998;144:409–417.

326. Tatami R, Inoue N, Itoh H, et al. Regression of coronary atherosclerosis by combined LDL-apheresis and lipid-lowering drug therapy in patients with familial hypercholesterolemia: a multicenter study. Atherosclerosis 1992;95:1–13.

29 Vascular Aging

From Molecular to Clinical Cardiology

Samer S. Najjar, MD and Edward G. Lakatta, MD

CONTENTS

INTRODUCTION

Advancing age is the most powerful predictor of cardiovascular morbidity, mortality, and disability. Age has traditionally been ignored as a risk factor for cardiovascular disease because it is considered a non-modifiable risk. However, close examination of the age-associated changes in cardiovascular structure and function may help explain why aging is such a strong predictor of adverse events. Findings from recent clinical studies have shown that the age-associated changes in vascular structure and function, previously not defined as clinical or subclinical diseases, are themselves risk factors for cardiovascular diseases. These novel risk factors, including intimal medial thickness, vascular stiffness, and endothelial dysfunction, alter the substrate upon which the cardiovascular diseases are superimposed; therefore, they affect the development, manifestation, severity, and prognosis of these diseases. The risk factors directly and indirectly modulate disease states, but,

in turn, these diseases affect the risk factors. Thus, age-associated changes in vascular structure and function cannot be ignored and cannot be viewed as simply part of normative aging. Instead, the clinical implications and the profound impact of aging on cardiovascular diseases need to be recognized, and acted upon accordingly, by those who shape medical policy and by those who set research priorities.

We propose a research agenda that would (1) establish a framework for future studies aimed at defining the underlying mechanisms and pathophysiologic correlates and the clinical sequelae associated with these new risk factors and (2) catalyze interest in developing efficacious, cost-effective, and practical guidelines for screening, preventing, and treating these age-associated risk factors for cardiovascular diseases. Successful implementation of this formidable research agenda will require the close collaboration of cardiovascular researchers with expertise in diverse areas, including molecular cardiologists, cardiovascular physiologists, and clinical trialists.

From: *Contemporary Cardiology: Principles of Molecular Cardiology*
Edited by: M. S. Runge and C. Patterson © Humana Press Inc., Totowa, NJ

AGING AS A CARDIOVASCULAR RISK FACTOR

The world population in both industrialized and developing countries is aging. For example, in the United States 35 million people are over the age of 65 yr, and the number of older Americans is expected to double by the year 2030. The clinical and economic implications of this demographic shift are staggering because age is the most powerful risk factor for cardiovascular diseases. The incidence and prevalence of hypertension *(1)* (Fig. 1A), coronary artery disease *(2)*, congestive heart failure *(3)* (Fig. 1B), and stroke *(4)* increase exponentially with age.

Although epidemiologic studies indicate that several risk factors, such as hypertension, hypercholesterolemia, diabetes mellitus, smoking, sedentary lifestyle, and genetic factors, contribute to the development of coronary artery disease, age is the most potent individual risk factor for coronary atherosclerosis, especially in individuals over the age of 50 *(5)*. In older community-dwelling healthy volunteers, the incidence of silent coronary atherosclerosis, assessed by combined electrocardiographic treadmill stress testing and thallium perfusion imaging, increases dramatically with age *(6)*. Age influences not only the incidence and prevalence of coronary atherosclerosis but also the severity and prognosis of this disease. In survivors of a myocardial infarction, age is an independent predictor of short- and long-term morbidity, mortality, and disability, even after adjusting for infarct size and location, the number of diseased vessels, and the extent of coronary artery disease *(7–9)*. Similar considerations pertain to the effects of age on other cardiovascular diseases, such as hypertension, congestive heart failure, and stroke.

Traditional Perspectives

Because of the dominant effect of age on cardiovascular diseases, aging has often been considered synonymous with disease. However, this view has been discredited by clinical data showing that many individuals can achieve old age without evidence of cardiovascular diseases. This pattern of aging, called "successful" *(10)* cardiovascular aging, is the *El Dorado* of cardiovascular gerontologists.

Despite the plethora of compelling epidemiological evidence indicating age is a potent risk factor for cardiovascular diseases, the "risky" components of aging have not been identified, in part because age has traditionally been viewed as a homogeneous chronological process. The heterogeneous pathophysiological implications of aging have been overlooked, and age has been considered an unmodifiable—and hence unpreventable or

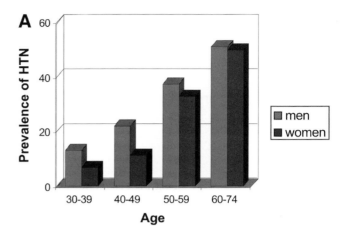

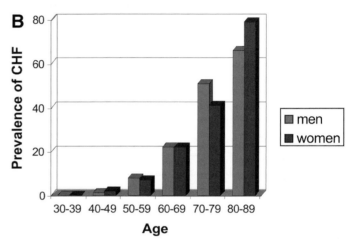

Fig. 1. The prevalence of cardiovascular diseases increases with advancing age. **(A)** Prevalence of hypertension (HTN), defined as having systolic blood pressure greater than 140 mm Hg or diastolic blood pressure greater than 90 mm Hg or currently using medication to treat elevated blood pressure. Data are based on the National Health and Nutrition Examination Surveys III (1988–1991). From Burt et al. *(1)*, with permission. **(B)** Prevalence of congestive heart failure (CHF) (per 1000 subjects) in the Framingham Heart Study. Reprinted with permission from *(3)*.

untreatable—process. Thus, age is a recognized cardiovascular risk factor that has been largely ignored from an interventional or therapeutic standpoint. The risky components of aging have been attributed to an increased time of exposure to other more traditional cardiovascular risk factors *(11)*, which, in turn, may vary in number and severity with increasing age. Many investigators have focused their efforts on searching for novel "subclinical" cardiovascular risk factors *(12)*, which would explain the increased age-associated risk that is not accounted for by the traditional risk markers. However, this view neglects the fact that a cardiovascular aging process accompanies chronologic aging and that this cardiovascular aging process is independent of cardiovascular diseases *(13)*.

This aging process has been described in humans and in several animal models of aging *(14)*.

Contemporary Perspectives

A new generation of cardiovascular gerontologists has acknowledged that although the aging process is independent of cardiovascular diseases, the observed cardiovascular phenotype is a result of the interaction between the aging process and these disease states *(15)*. In other words, cardiovascular diseases can alter the natural history of the cardiovascular aging process, and, for a given time at risk, the cardiovascular aging process itself can affect the threshold, manifestation, severity, and prognosis of these diseases by altering the substrate upon which these pathophysiologic mechanisms are superimposed. Thus, aging and cardiovascular diseases are interdependent, and the independent effects of aging can be best evaluated in the absence of disease (or unhealthy lifestyle).

A very important corollary is that the age-associated changes in vascular structure and function may help define the role of aging as a potent risk factor for cardiovascular diseases. Quantitative information on these age-related changes is available because traditional gerontologists have painstakingly described the age-associated changes in cardiovascular structure and function in community-dwelling individuals who did not have (or had not yet experienced) clinical disease *(13)*. The new generation of cardiovascular gerontologists, having gained an appreciation for the interaction between the aging process and cardiovascular diseases, expanded on this database by grouping individuals by age categories and stratifying them according to the magnitude or level of a given vascular variable. Each variable is classified as beneficial or deleterious, based on epidemiologic and clinical studies of its clinical and prognostic significance. Individuals with extreme measures of vascular variables are then considered to be aging successfully or unsuccessfully. Because patients with defined overt or occult clinical disease were excluded, unsuccessful aging does not mean having clinical or subclinical disease. Instead, unsuccessful aging should be defined as being at risk for future clinical cardiovascular disease because of a high measurement for a deleterious variable. Identifying and characterizing potentially detrimental vascular variables will help define why aging is associated with high risk for cardiovascular diseases.

A comprehensive description of the partnership between the aging process and cardiovascular diseases requires a thorough understanding of the interplay of complex genetic traits. Although our knowledge of the underlying genetic determinants is minimal, breakthroughs are imminent, heralded by the recent advances

Table 1
Age-Associated Changes in Human Arterial Structure and Function

Increases with Age

　Lumen size

　Intimal–medial thickness

　Collagen content and cross-linking

　Vessel wall stiffness

　Systolic blood pressure

　Pulse pressure

　Elastin fragmentation

Decreases with Age

　Elastin content

　Endothelial function

in genomics and proteomics, including the sequencing of the human genome and the availability of high-throughput genotyping to detect single nucleotide polymorphisms and allelic variations on a population-wide basis.

During the past two decades, the effects of aging on multiple aspects of cardiovascular structure and function were characterized in participants from the Baltimore Longitudinal Study on Aging (BLSA). These community-dwelling volunteers are rigorously screened to detect both clinical and occult cardiovascular disease, and lifestyle habits (e.g., diet and exercise) of participants are well characterized. Findings from these studies and from studies in other aging populations and in animal models of aging are reviewed here in light of recent epidemiologic studies of the deleterious (or beneficial) potential of age-associated vascular changes.

AGE-ASSOCIATED CHANGES IN VASCULAR STRUCTURE AND FUNCTION

Human Studies

Many age-associated changes are seen in the large arteries of humans (Table 1). Cross-sectional studies show that central elastic arteries dilate with age, leading to an increase in lumen size *(16)*. In addition, post mortem studies have indicated an age-associated increase in arterial wall thickening, which is caused mainly by an increase in intimal thickening *(17)*. In cross-sectional studies, carotid intimal–medial thickening increases nearly threefold between the ages of 20 and 90 yr *(18)* (Fig. 2A). The range of values for intimal–medial thickness in Fig. 2A is much greater in older individuals than in younger ones. The increase in arterial wall thickening is accompanied by an increase in vascular stiffening (reduction in vascular compliance) *(19)* (Fig. 2B), which is due to several structural

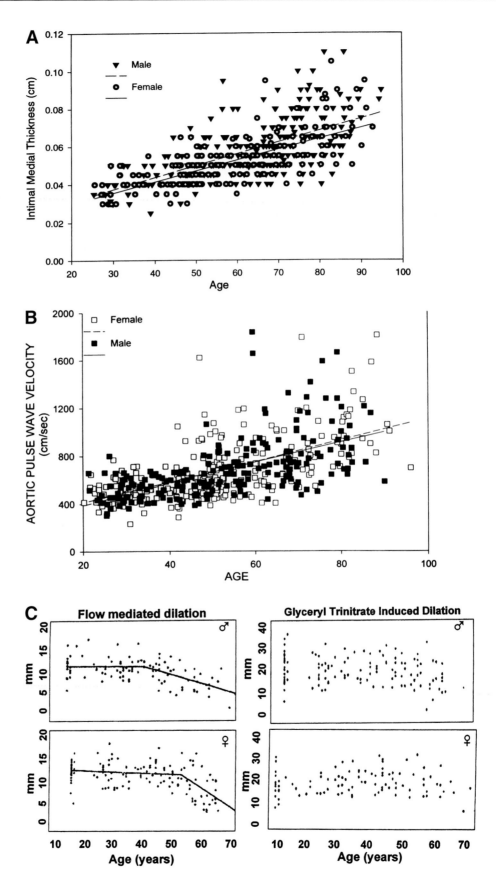

changes in the arterial wall *(14)*. These changes include an increase in collagen content, cross-linking of adjacent collagen molecules to form advanced glycosylation end products *(20)*, fraying of elastin, and a decrease in the amount of elastin. In addition to structural changes, functional alterations include an age-associated deterioration in vascular endothelial vasoreactivity *(21,22)* (Fig. 2C).

Animal Studies

Age-associated morphologic changes in the vascular walls of rodents (Table 2) and nonhuman primates, which are similar changes to those seen in age-related arterial remodeling in humans, include luminal dilation *(23)*, intimal and medial thickening *(24–26)*, vascular stiffening *(23,26)*, and endothelial dysfunction *(27,28)*. Animal models of aging can be used to study the molecular mechanisms that underlie macroscopic vascular changes.

INTIMAL CHANGES

The thickened intima in older rats comprises matrix molecules, including collagen, fibronectin, and proteoglycans, and vascular smooth muscle cells (SMCs). SMCs are usually not seen in the intima of young rats *(24)*. The thickened intima of older arteries has significantly higher levels of transforming growth factor beta (TGF-β) and intercellular adhesion molecules (ICAM-1) than younger vessels *(24)*. In addition, levels of the zinc-dependent endopeptidase type 2 matrix metalloproteinase (MMP-2) *(24)* and its activator membrane type 1 matrix metalloproteinase (MT1-MMP) are significantly higher in the thickened intima of older rats than in younger rats, whereas levels of the endogenous tissue inhibitor of metalloproteinase 2 (TIMP-2) are similar between the two groups *(29)* (Table 3). MMP-2 promotes protein degradation and accumulates in the aged aortae in areas surrounding SMCs that are located near breaks in the internal elastic lamina and along the elastic lamina throughout the media. This finding suggests that MMP-2 may be involved in the age-associated increase in fragmentation of the elastic lamina *(24)*.

SMOOTH MUSCLE CELLS

Because vascular SMCs are not terminally differentiated, their phenotype can be modulated, and they can change to a proliferative, secretory, or migratory mode.

Activated SMCs help repair vascular damage and contribute to the vascular pathologies seen in hypertension and atherosclerosis. The intimal growth that occurs during aging in rodents and nonhuman primates in the absence of experimental injury, resembles, in some ways, the neointimal formation seen after vascular injury induced by arterial catheter balloon inflation *(30–33)* or after aortocoronary saphenous vein graft implantation *(34)*. The neointimal growth in response to endothelial injury is markedly higher in older rats than in younger ones. This growth response is caused by factors intrinsic to the vessel wall, because excessive intimal hyperplasia is seen when aortae from old animals are transplanted into younger ones *(35)*. SMCs play an important role in this growth response *(36)*. After balloon injury to the rat carotid artery, medial SMCs are activated and begin to proliferate (Fig. 3A). Then, they migrate to the intimal layer and invade the complex extracellular matrix of the vessel wall through discontinuities in the internal elastic lamina. In addition, hematopoietic stem cells that originate in the bone marrow may contribute to the neointimal proliferation after arterial injury by migrating into the subendothelial layer from the luminal side of the vascular wall and differentiating into vascular SMCs *(37)*.

MATRIX METALLOPROTEASE (TYPE II)

The dissolution of the basement membrane that enables the migration of SMCs may result from the action of elastases and gelatinases (such as MMP-2) *(24)* that are secreted by activated SMCs (see below). However, the excessive intimal hyperplasia and the increased SMC invasiveness seen after carotid arterial injury are attenuated by the overexpression of TIMP-2, an endogenous inhibitor of MMP-2 *(38)*. Thus, the MMPs are important in the remodeling of blood vessels after experimental injury. In addition, nitric oxide may modulate this process; nitric oxide has antiproliferative actions on vascular cells *(39)*, and chronic inhibition of nitric oxide synthesis accelerates neointimal formation in cholesterol-fed rabbits *(40)*.

Studies of cultured vascular SMCs have shown that the chemotactic invasion of a reconstituted basement membrane requires MMP-2 activity *(41)*. MMP-2, in turn, is potentially derived from cytokine-stimulated vascular SMCs. When stimulated with the cytokines interleukin-1α,

---

Fig. 2. Age-associated changes in vascular structure and function in humans. **(A)** The common carotid intimal–medial thickness in healthy BLSA volunteer subjects, as a function of age and gender. Note that the values for intimal–medial thickness are much greater in older individuals than in younger ones. **(B)** Aortic pulse wave velocity in healthy BLSA volunteer subjects, as a function of age and gender. Pulse wave velocity is an index of arterial stiffness. **(C)** Endothelial-flow mediated and non-endothelial (glyceryl trinitrate) induced arterial dilatation in apparently healthy individuals. Note that the marked age-associated accelerated decline in endothelial-mediated dilatation occurs about a decade later in women than in men. Reprinted with permission from *(21)*.

Table 2
Age-Associated Changes in Rodent Aortae

Increased vessel diameter *(23)*
Increased wall stiffness *(23,26)*
Increased wall thickness
   Intima
      Increased thickness (smooth muscle cells and matrix) *(24–26)*
      Increased TGB-β *(24)* with decreased antiproliferative effects *(49)*
      Increased MMP-2 *(24,29)*
      Increased expression of adhesion molecules *(24)*
      Increased nitrite and nitrate levels *(55)*
      Decreased eNOS activity *(53,55)*
      Increased ACE activity *(53)*
   Media
      Increased thickness *(23,29)*
      Increase in size but decrease in number of smooth muscle cells *(23)*
   Matrix
      Increased collagen content *(23,29)*
      Increased collagen cross-linking (nonenzymatic glycation) *(242)*
      Increased fibronectin *(50)*
      Decreased elastin: calcification and fragmentation *(23,29)*
      Increased glycosaminoglycans *(24,243)*
Endothelial dysfunction
   Decreased vasoreactivity *(27,146)*
   Increased expression of adhesion molecules *(24)*
   Increased permeability *(152)*
   Decreased angiogenesis (in rabbits) *(169)*
   Decreased VEGF (in rabbits) *(169)*
Exaggerated wound repair response *(31,33,35,36)*

TGF-β, transforming growth factor beta; MMP-2, type 2 matrix metalloproteinase; eNOS, endothelial nitric oxide synthase; ACE, angiotensin converting enzyme; VEGF, vascular endothelial growth factor.

Table 3
Primary Antibody Staining of Rat Aortic Intimal and Medial Tissue

	Intima			*Media*	
	Young (2 mo)	*Old (30 mo)*		*Young (2 mo)*	*Old (30 mo)*
MMP-2	1.0 ± 0.0	$4.0 \pm 0.0^*$		1.0 ± 0.0	$2.5 \pm 0.6^*$
TIMP-2	4.0 ± 0.0	4.0 ± 0.0		3.0 ± 0.8	$1.0 \pm 0.0^*$
MTI-MMP	1.5 ± 0.6	$3.5 \pm 0.6^*$		1.5 ± 0.6	2.0 ± 0.8

Data are means ± standard error of percent staining.
$^*p < 0.05$ versus young group. MMP-2, type 2 matrix metalloprotease; TIMP-2, tissue inhibitor of MMP-2; MTI-MMP, membrane bound tissue activator of MMP-2.

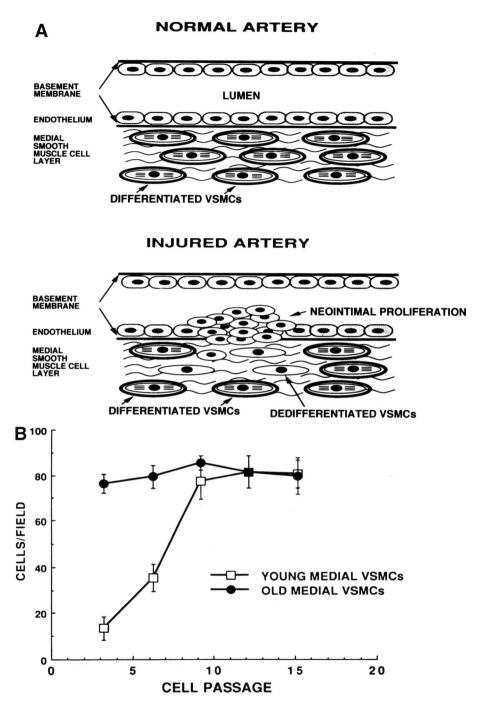

Fig. 3. (A) After injury to the artery, vascular smooth muscle cells (VSMCs) dedifferentiate, proliferate, and migrate to the intimal layer, contributing to neointimal proliferation. **(B)** Chemotactic response of young and old medial VSMCs.

tumor necrosis factor-α, and TGF-β *(24)*, early passage vascular SMCs from aged aortae secrete more MMP-2 than those from young aortae. This finding suggests that increased levels of MMP-2 in the thickened intima of aortae from aged rats may reflect a chronically increased level of cytokine stimulation in vivo. In addition, early passage aortic vascular SMCs of old rats have an exaggerated chemotactic response to platelet-derived growth factor (PDGF), whereas cells from young aortae require several additional passages in culture to generate an equivalent response *(42)* (Fig. 3B). The exaggerated response of old vessels to experimental injury in vivo *(36)* may be attributable, in part, to increased SMC chemotaxis or proliferation in response to growth factors such as PDGF *(43)*.

The excessive neointimal formation seen after balloon injury to the rat carotid artery can be prevented by cleaving the mRNA of the early growth response gene, Egr-1, a zinc-finger transcription factor that modulates several stress-responsive genes (including PDGF and TGF-β) (44). Furthermore, Egr-1 levels are increased in human atherosclerotic plaques (45). In contrast, studies in human fibroblasts indicate that the expression and activity of Egr-1 are decreased in senescent cells (46).

TRANSFORMING GROWTH FACTOR-β

The thickened intima of older aortae contains high levels of TGF-β, which is a member of the superfamily of cytokines that are important in vascular remodeling. TGF-β regulates cellular proliferation, migration, and apoptosis. In addition, it suppresses proteases, activates tissue inhibitors of MMP, and stimulates synthesis of extracellular matrix proteins; therefore, an increase in TGF-β can lead to excessive fibrosis (47). The cellular effects of TGF-β are mediated through at least three types of cell surface receptors. The intracellular signaling downstream from TGF-β involves a recently described family of intracellular signaling proteins, the Smad proteins, which interact with the conserved nuclear transcriptional coactivator CREB binding protein (48). The antiproliferative actions of TGF-β decrease with aging (49). Aortic SMCs from young and old rats produce similar amounts of TGF-β1 and equivalent levels of its mRNA. However, old SMCs are refractory to the inhibitory effects of TGF-β1 on proliferation, whereas young SMCs are significantly inhibited by low levels of TGF-β1. This loss of inhibition is caused by a reduced binding capacity of TGF-β1 to old SMCs, which, in turn, results from an age-related reduction in the expression of the type II receptor (48). Thus, proliferation of SMCs is increased in older animals because they do not respond to the autocrine growth inhibitory effects of TGF-β1.

TGF-β and MMP-2 accumulate in the same intimal regions of aged rats, which may account for the concomitant increase in fibronectin (24,50). Fibronectin and TGF-β expression are both regulated by angiotensin II (51). Chronic administration of angiotensin-converting enzyme (ACE) inhibitors significantly delays many of the age-associated intimal and matrix changes in normotensive and hypertensive rats (23,52). This finding suggests that the age-associated changes in the local vascular angiotensin system may modulate the age-associated vascular remodeling process. An age-associated increase in aortic intimal–medial angiotensin II has been described in rats (53) and in nonhuman primates, where angiotensin II co-localized with both ACE and MMP-2 (54).

NITRIC OXIDE

The vasoconstrictor response to angiotensin II is reduced in aging rats, and the inhibition of nitric oxide synthesis returns this reduced response to normal levels (55). Aging rats have increased plasma levels of nitrite and nitrate (55). Conflicting results have been reported in studies of age-associated changes in aortic levels of cGMP and age-associated changes in aortic expression of endothelial constitutive nitric oxide synthase (eNOS) and inducible nitric oxide synthase (iNOS) (53,55). However, activity of the eNOS isoform is markedly reduced in aging rats (55) and in aging rabbits (56). These findings suggest a mechanism of age-associated impairment in endothelial vasoreactivity because vasoreactivity depends on NO generated by eNOS.

INTIMAL–MEDIAL THICKNESS

Studies of morphologic, cellular, enzymatic, and biochemical changes in animal models have increased our understanding of age-associated arterial remodeling in humans. For example, the age-associated intimal–medial thickening seen in humans is often ascribed to "subclinical" atherosclerosis (57–60). This idea has become so well accepted that intimal thickening is used as a surrogate measure of atherosclerosis (61,62). However, intimal–medial thickening is only weakly associated with the extent and severity of coronary artery disease (63). Furthermore, findings in rodent (24) and nonhuman primate (28) models of aging clearly indicate that intimal–medial thickening is an age-related process that is separate from atherosclerosis because atherosclerosis is absent in both of these animal models. The use of poor terminology may have helped blur the boundaries between the aging and the atherosclerotic processes. Referring to intimal–medial thickening as subclinical atherosclerosis gives the false impression that the atherosclerotic process is already present in the arterial wall, whereas intimal–medial thickening clearly occurs in the absence of atherosclerosis. In summary, excessive intimal–medial thickening is not necessarily synonymous with early or subclinical atherosclerosis (64).

Nonetheless, an association (not a correlation) between intimal–medial thickening and carotid (65–67), aortic (68), and coronary (62) atherosclerosis has been documented in humans. In individuals rigorously screened for the absence of cardiovascular disease, excessive intimal–medial thickening at a given age predicts silent coronary artery disease (18) (Fig. 4A), which, in turn, progresses to clinical ischemic heart disease. In the Atherosclerosis Risk In Communities (ARIC) study, which comprised middle-aged adults, intimal–medial thickening was associated with a greater prevalence of cardiovascular diseases (69) and was an independent predictor of stroke (70). In the Cardiovascular Health Study (CHS), which comprised individuals over the age of 65, intimal–medial thickening was an independent predictor of future myocardial infarction and stroke (71) (Fig. 4B). In the CHS study, subjects were grouped according to quintiles of intimal–medial thickening, and the results indicated a non-linear gradation in risk, with higher quintiles conferring a greater risk for cardiovascular diseases (59) (Fig. 4B). In fact, the strength of intimal–medial thickening as a risk factor for cardiovascular diseases equals or exceeds that of most other traditional risk factors (Fig. 4C).

Thus, intimal–medial thickening is not a manifestation of atherosclerosis but is associated with it. Intimal–medial thickening is an aging-related process that is separate from the pathophysiologic process of atherosclerosis, yet intimal thickening is a risk factor for atherosclerosis. Intimal–medial thickening has previously been classified in the same disease category as atherosclerosis, but should be correctly reclassified as a marker of arterial aging. When intimal–medial thickening is accelerated, or when the extent of thickening exceeds the value in age- and gender-matched controls, it is a risk factor associated with adverse cardiovascular outcomes, and it should be recognized as a subclinical or clinical vascular disease. The threshold and cut-off values for considering intimal–medial thickening as a clinical or subclinical vascular disease have not been defined, but some investigators are beginning to address these issues (72).

Intimal–Medial Thickening and Atherosclerosis

Animal models of aging have contributed significantly to our understanding of the pathophysiologic mechanisms that underlie the association of intimal–medial thickening with atherosclerosis. The age-associated cellular, enzymatic, and molecular mechanisms that underlie the phenotypic appearance of intimal–medial thickening include the migration of activated vascular SMCs into the intima and increased levels of MMP-2, MT1-MMP, TGF-β, and ICAM-1 (24). These age-associated changes create a metabolically active environment that induces, contributes to, or is a result of endothelial dysfunction (27,28,73) and permeability (74). These same metabolic, enzymatic, cellular, and endothelial alterations are important in developing and promoting atherosclerosis, vascular inflammation, vascular remodeling, and oxidant stress (73,75–78). In other words, many of the same factors that underlie the age-associated structural and functional intimal and medial alterations contribute to the pathogenesis of clinical cardiovascular diseases. These changes could help explain the risky component of aging.

Because atherosclerosis is localized to the intima–lumen interface (54,79) (at least in early and mid stages), it is affected by age-associated alterations in the intimal and medial environments. In pathologic studies in humans, atherosclerosis was present in arteries as early as the second decade of life, manifesting as innocuous fatty streaks (80). Thus, atherosclerosis may precede the age-associated structural and functional vascular alterations. However, once the changes appear, they may contribute to, or catalyze, the activation of fatty streaks, which then transform and mature into potentially significant clinical plaques. This interaction is supported by results from studies in which feeding rabbits (56) or nonhuman primates (81) an atherogenic diet caused markedly more severe atherosclerotic lesions in older animals than in younger animals, despite both groups having similar increases in plasma lipid levels (Fig. 5). In the rabbits, older animals had a higher percentage of myocytes, lymphocytes, proliferating cells, and apoptotic cells in the atherosclerotic lesions than younger animals (56). The atherosclerotic process, through its structural invasion and destruction of the inner layers of the vascular wall and its metabolic and cellular activity, should modulate intimal–medial thickening. Although this concept has not been directly tested, supporting indirect evidence comes from observational studies in which patients with carotid atherosclerotic plaques have more intimal–medial thickening than age- and risk factor-matched subjects who do not have carotid plaques (64).

The purported crosstalk between the atherosclerotic plaque and the vascular wall in which it is embedded is the molecular counterpart of the vascular aging and cardiovascular disease partnership that is observed clinically. These interactions, both at the molecular and phenotypic levels, are affected by risk factors such as hypertension, smoking, dyslipidemia, diabetes, diet, and genetic factors. In this context, atherosclerosis can be viewed as a physiologic process in humans (i.e., initially manifesting as innocuous fatty streaks). This process can be potentially accelerated and exacerbated by interactions with several factors, including intrinsic features related to vascular aging; traditional atherosclerotic, inflammatory, oxidative, and other unidentified risk factors; and complex genetic determinants. Further research is needed to delineate the components of the purported crosstalk between the atherosclerotic plaque and the vascular wall, to define the initiator signals and the modulators of this communication, and to study the effects of aging on this process.

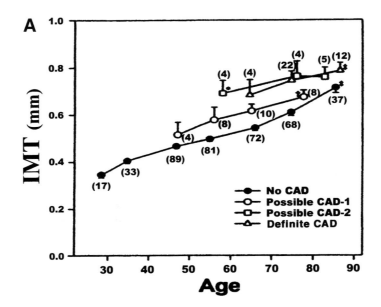

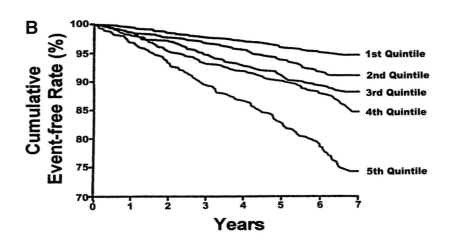

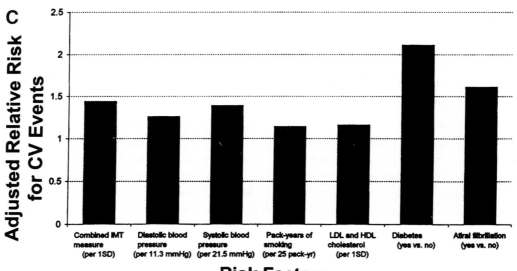

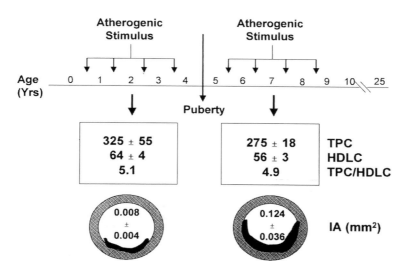

Fig. 5. Effects of age on the susceptibility of cynomolgus monkeys to diet-induced coronary artery atherosclerosis. Older monkeys developed greater atherosclerosis than younger monkeys even though both groups had similar diet-induced atherogenic stimuli and elevated cholesterol levels. TPC, total plasma cholesterol; HDLC, high density lipoprotein cholesterol; IA, intimal atherosclerosis. Reprinted with permission from (81).

VASCULAR STIFFNESS

Similar considerations to those discussed with intimal–medial thickening pertain to the age-associated increase in vascular stiffening, which has been seen in humans (19,82–84) and in animal models of aging (23,26). Studies in animals have shown several structural changes in the vascular wall, such as increased collagen content, reduced elastin content, and calcification and fragmentation of elastin, and result in alterations in smooth muscle tone and endothelial function, which underlie the observed phenotypic compliance changes (14). Strictly speaking, stiffness and its inverse, distensibility, depend on intrinsic structural properties of the blood vessel wall that relate pressure with a corresponding change in volume. However, in this chapter, the terms stiffness and compliance will be used in a broader sense to denote the overall lumped stiffness and compliance, which include the additional effects of vascular tone, blood pressure, and other modulating factors.

Pulse Wave Velocity

With each systolic contraction of the ventricle, a propagation wave that is generated in the arterial wall travels centrifugally down the arterial tree. This propagation wave accompanies (and slightly precedes) the luminal flow wave generated during systole. The velocity of propagation of this wave is proportional to the stiffness of the arterial wall. This situation is analogous to the flow of a wave on a string; as the string is stretched, it becomes less compliant, and the velocity of the flow wave increases. The velocity of the pulse wave in vivo is determined not only by the intrinsic stress/strain relationship (stiffness) of the vascular wall, but also by the smooth muscle tone, which is reflected by the mean arterial pressure (85).

The availability of noninvasive measures of the velocity of this pulse wave allows for large-scale epidemiological studies. Pulse wave velocity was assessed in BLSA participants who were rigorously screened for the

Fig. 4. Carotid intimal–medial thickness and cardiovascular diseases. **(A)** Common carotid intimal–medial thickness (CCA IMT) as a function of age, stratified by coronary artery disease (CAD) classification, in Baltimore Longitudinal Study on Aging subjects. CAD-1 denotes a subset with positive exercise electrocardiogram (ECG) but negative thallium scans; CAD-2 represents a subset with concordant positive exercise ECG and thallium scans. **(B)** Common carotid intimal–medial thickness as a predictor of future cardiovascular events in the Cardiovascular Health Study (CHS). Note the non-linear increase in the risk for cardiovascular event rates with increasing quintiles. From O'Leary et al. *(71)*, with permission. **(C)** Comparisons of the associations of age- and sex-adjusted cardiovascular risk factors with the combined events of stroke or myocardial infarction in the CHS study, using Cox proportional hazards models. Note that intimal–medial thickness is a potent risk factor for future cardiovascular events. Adapted with permission from *(71)*.

absence of overt or silent cardiovascular disease *(19)* and in other populations with varying degrees of prevalence of cardiovascular disease *(82,83,86–89)*. In all these studies, a significant age-associated increase in pulse wave velocity has been observed in both men and women.

Elegant experiments in canines have shown several detrimental hemodynamic effects when the heart is switched from ejecting into a compliant vessel to ejecting into a stiff conduit, especially in the setting of myocardial ischemia *(90)*. In support of these animal studies, several clinical studies have recently shown the adverse cardiovascular effects of accelerated vascular stiffening. In the ARIC study, several vascular compliance indices were predictors of hypertension *(91)* (Fig. 6A). In hypertensive patients, pulse wave velocity was a marker of cardiovascular risk *(92)* and coronary events *(93)* (Fig. 6B) and was an independent predictor of mortality *(94)*. Pulse wave velocity was also an independent predictor of mortality in subjects over 70 yr of age *(95)* and in patients with end-stage renal disease *(96)*. Other noninvasive indices of vascular compliance, including stroke volume divided by pulse pressure *(97)* (Fig. 6C) and the incremental modulus of elasticity *(98)*, were independent predictors of adverse outcomes. Thus, vascular stiffening, like intimal–medial thickening, should be viewed as another marker of aging, which, when accelerated, also becomes a risk factor for cardiovascular diseases.

The interaction between vascular wall stiffening and cardiovascular diseases may set in motion a vicious cycle. Pulse wave velocity is determined, in part, by SMC tone, which, in turn, is partially regulated by endothelial cells. Moreover, endothelial dysfunction is seen early in several cardiovascular disorders including atherosclerosis *(77)*, diabetes *(99)*, and hypertension *(100)*. Thus, in this cycle, alterations in the mechanical properties of the vessel wall contribute to endothelial cell dysfunction and, ultimately, vascular stiffening.

Reflected Waves

In addition to the forward pulse wave, each cardiac cycle generates a reflected wave, which travels back up the arterial tree toward the central aorta. This reflected wave, which originates in the smaller arteries and arterioles, alters the arterial pressure waveform *(101)* and is modulated, in part, by nitric oxide *(102)*. The velocity of the reflected flow wave is proportional to the stiffness of the arterial wall *(85)*. Thus, in young individuals whose vascular wall is compliant, the reflected wave does not reach the large elastic arteries until diastole. With advancing age and increasing vascular stiffening, the

velocity of the reflected wave increases, and the wave reaches the central circulation earlier in the cardiac cycle, during the systolic phase. This reflected wave can be noninvasively assessed from recordings of the carotid *(103,104)* or radial *(103,105,106)* arterial pulse waveforms by arterial applanation tonometry and high-fidelity micromanometer probes. Inspection of the recorded arterial pulse wave contour shows an inflection point, which heralds the arrival of the reflected wave *(107)* (Fig. 7A). The distance from the inflection point to the peak of the arterial waveform is the pressure pulse augmentation that is due to the early arrival of the reflected wave. Dividing this augmentation by the distance from the peak to the trough of the arterial waveform (corresponding to the pulse pressure) yields the augmentation index *(107)*. The augmentation index, like the pulse wave velocity, increases with age *(19,101,103,106,108)* (Fig. 7B).

Because reflected waves originate in small arteries and arterioles, the age-associated changes in this index are probably determined, in part, by the age-associated changes in the structure and function of distal vessels and by the age-associated alterations in the structure and function of large elastic arteries. Although attention has been focused on the transmission velocity of reflected waves as an index of arterial stiffness, evaluation of the pulse wave contour may provide valuable insight into the characteristics and the pathology of more distal vessels, where reflected waves originate *(109)*.

The pressure pulse augmentation provided by the early return of the reflected wave is an added load against which the ventricle must contract *(110)*. Furthermore, the loss of the diastolic augmentation seen in compliant vessels caused by the late return of the reflected waves decreases diastolic blood pressure and thus has the potential to reduce coronary blood flow because most coronary flow occurs during diastole *(110)*. These considerations suggest that excessively early return of the reflected waves, which can be assessed with the augmentation index, may be detrimental to the cardiovascular system. In fact, the augmentation index is a predictor of adverse events in end-stage renal disease patients *(111)* (Fig. 7C). Thus, this index is another marker of vascular aging that is a risk factor for cardiovascular diseases.

Pulse Pressure

As blood vessels stiffen, their diameter increases, which decreases wall strain. Moreover, the combination of arterial wall stiffening and early return of the reflected waves widens the pulse pressure *(112)*. Indeed, a high

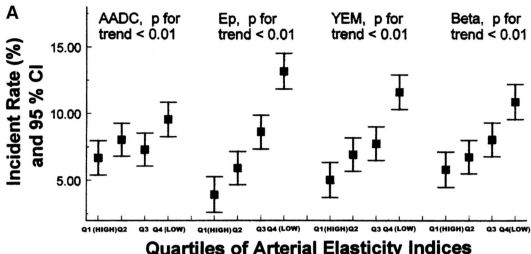

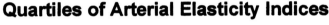

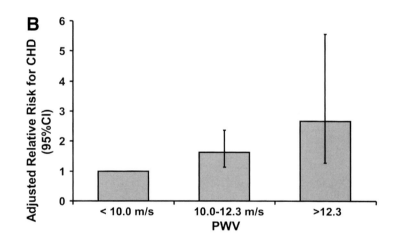

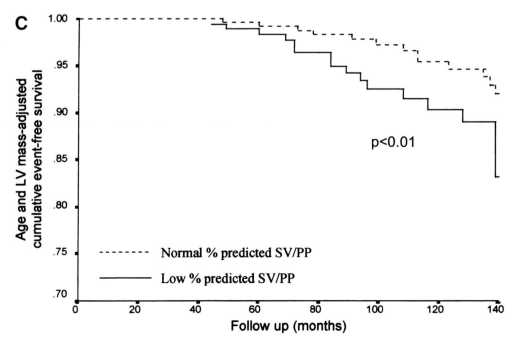

systolic blood pressure generates a similar distention of hardened capacitance vessels, while a lower diastolic blood pressure results, in part, from the loss of diastolic augmentation. Thus, pulse pressure is a useful hemodynamic marker of the vascular stiffness of conduit arteries. Clinical and epidemiological studies in several different populations with varying prevalences of cardiovascular diseases have confirmed the prognostic importance of pulse pressure *(113–127)*. Furthermore, in several studies, pulse pressure was a stronger predictor of outcomes than systolic or diastolic blood pressures.

As clinical studies have shown the deleterious effects of hypertension, recommendations for the treatment of elevated blood pressures have been adjusted accordingly. The emphasis was initially on treating increases in diastolic blood pressure. However, the finding that systolic hypertension is a predictor of adverse events prompted the use of increased systolic blood pressure as an indication for treatment. Although the initial cut-off value for normal systolic pressure was 160 mm Hg, the value was adjusted downward when studies showed that pressures between 140 and 160 mm Hg conferred added risk. The systolic value was recently pushed further down to 130 mm Hg for patients with diabetes mellitus *(128)*. The finding that pulse pressure may be a stronger predictor of outcomes than systolic or diastolic blood pressures indicates the need for studies to evaluate whether pulse pressure should replace systolic or diastolic pressures as a screening criterion or as a therapeutic endpoint in the treatment of hypertension.

Isolated Systolic Hypertension

Both systolic and pulse pressures increase with age in all adults, whereas diastolic blood pressure increases until the fifth decade and then levels off before decreasing after 60 yr of age *(83,129)* (Fig. 8A–D). These age-dependent changes in systolic, diastolic, and pulse pressures are consistent with the idea that in younger people, blood pressure is determined largely by peripheral vascular resistance, whereas in older people blood pressure is determined mainly by the stiffness of central

conduit vessels *(83)*. Isolated systolic hypertension is defined as a systolic blood pressure >140 mm Hg and a diastolic blood pressure <90 mm Hg (i.e., a widened pulse pressure). The most common form of hypertension in older individuals, isolated systolic hypertension, could be described as a disease related, in part, to arterial stiffening *(130)*. Even mild isolated systolic hypertension (stage 1) is associated with an appreciable increase in cardiovascular disease risk *(131,132)*.

Hypertension

Recent studies showing that increased vascular stiffness may precede the development of hypertension have underscored the relationship between hypertension and arterial wall stiffening *(91)*. This concept has been overshadowed by the notion that an increase in mean arterial pressure (or peripheral resistance) is the predominant cause of increased stiffness of large arteries. The increase in mean blood pressure that occurs with hypertension can lead to a secondary increase in large-artery stiffness; however, the primary age-associated increase in large-artery stiffness can lead to an increase in arterial pressures. Thus, hypertension can be defined as a disease that is, in part, determined or modulated by properties of the arterial wall. An even broader view recognizes hypertension as a syndrome *(133)*, with blood pressure increases representing only one (albeit late) manifestation.

Recognizing the independence of arterial wall stiffening from hypertension has important clinical implications. In a study of patients with end-stage renal disease who required dialysis, Guerin et al. *(134)* reported that treatment of hypertension had differing effects on pulse wave velocity, despite having similar blood pressure–lowering effects in patients *(134)* (Fig. 9). Mortality was higher in the group in which pulse wave velocity increased in spite of therapy, and progression of vascular stiffening was an independent predictor of mortality. These observations suggest that treating increases in blood pressure is necessary but not sufficient therapy for the syndrome of hypertension.

Fig. 6. Vascular stiffness and cardiovascular outcomes. **(A)** Reduced arterial elasticity and incidence of hypertension in the Atherosclerosis Research In Communities (ARIC) study. Values 1–4 denote the highest to lowest quartiles. Note that for all indices, decreased elasticity is associated with an increased incidence of hypertension ($p < 0.01$). CI, confidence interval; AADC, adjusted arterial diameter change; EP, Peterson's elastic modulus; YEM, Young's elastic modulus; BETA, β stiffness index. Reprinted with permission from *(91)*. **(B)** Relative risk for coronary heart disease (CHD) events, adjusted for age, sex, blood pressure, heart rate, diabetes mellitus, smoking, and previous antihypertensive treatment, by tertiles of pulse wave velocity (PWV). CI, confidence interval. Adapted with permission from *(93)*. **(C)** Cumulative event-free survival, adjusted for age and left ventricular mass, relative to total arterial compliance indexed as stroke volume (SV)/pulse pressure (PP). Note that reduced arterial compliance is a predictor of cardiovascular events. Reprinted with permission from *(97)*.

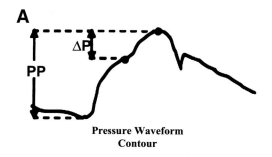

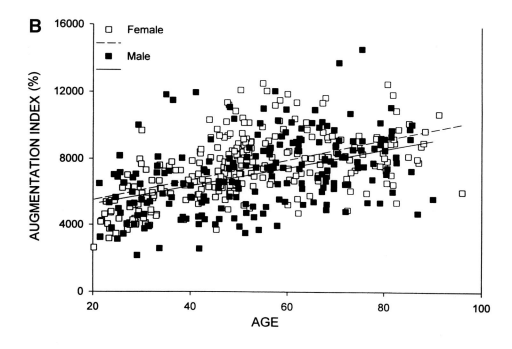

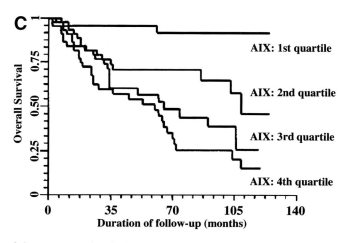

Fig. 7. (A) Graphic representation of the augmentation index, which is defined as the ratio of the distance from the inflection point to the peak of the arterial waveform (ΔP), over the pulse pressure (PP). **(B)** The augmentation index in healthy Baltimore Longitudinal Study on Aging volunteer subjects, as a function of age and gender. **(C)** Probability of overall survival in patients with end-stage renal failure, stratified by quartiles of augmentation index (AIX). Reprinted with permission from *(111)*.

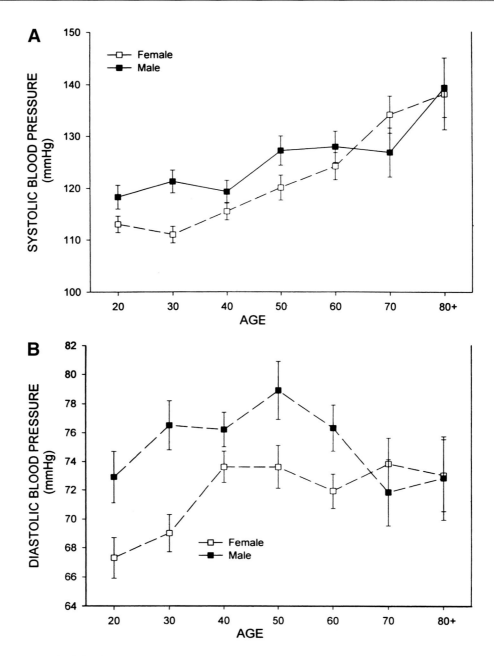

Fig. 8. (**A–C**) Average systolic (**A**), diastolic (**B**), and pulse (**C**) pressures and age, in Baltimore Longitudinal Study on Aging participants stratified by gender. Values are mean ± SEM. (**D**) Scatterplot of pulse pressure versus age in Baltimore Longitudinal Study on Aging participants stratified by gender. In addition to an overall age-associated effect, within a particular age-group there is a greater range of values in older as compared with younger individuals.

Studying the relationship between primary age-associated vascular wall remodeling and cardiovascular diseases has led researchers to search for new phenotypic manifestations of arterial remodeling to explore their clinical and prognostic significance. For example, the various carotid geometric patterns that are derived by combining the measurements of vascular mass with wall-to-lumen ratio were recently associated with unique

functional and hemodynamic profiles that are largely independent of age and hypertension *(135)*.

Diabetes Mellitus

Several studies have documented a robust association between diabetes mellitus and increased vascular stiffening *(136–139)*. Increased levels of hemoglobin A1c *(86)* and fasting glucose *(136)* are associated with greater arterial

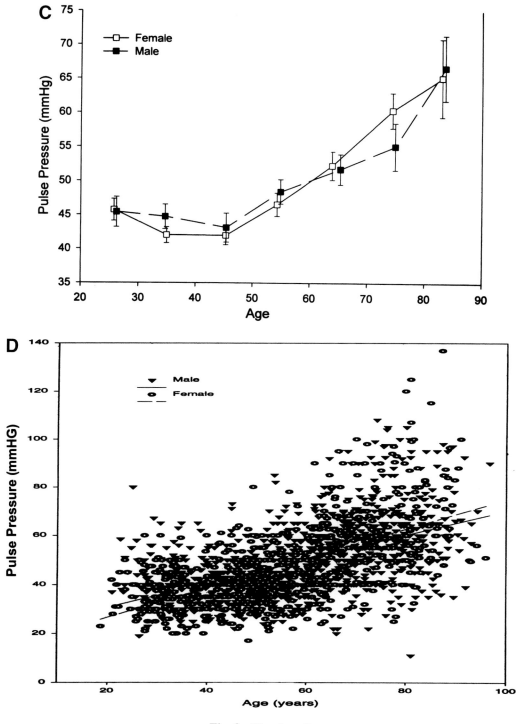

Fig. 8. *(Continued)*

stiffness, even in nondiabetic subjects. This association may be due to the increased glycosylation of long-lived matrix proteins (such as collagen) in the vascular wall during hyperglycemia and the subsequent irreversible covalent cross-linking of these proteins to form advanced glycation end products *(20)*.

The metabolic syndrome, which includes insulin resistance, obesity (particularly abdominal adiposity), hypertension, and dyslipidemia (increased triglycerides with low HDL), is associated with a markedly increased incidence of cardiovascular diseases. Furthermore, greater waist circumference *(86)* and levels of insulin *(86,88,136)*,

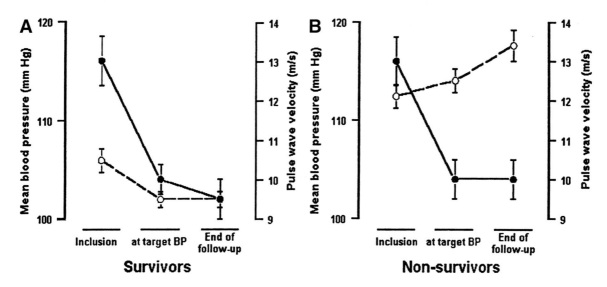

Fig. 9. Changes in mean blood pressure (solid circles) and aortic pulse wave velocity (open circles) in survivor and nonsurvivor patients with end-stage renal failure. Follow-up occurred at a mean of 51 ± 38 mo. Values are means ± standard error. Reprinted with permission from *(134).*

triglycerides *(86,136)*, and visceral adiposity *(88)* are all associated with arterial stiffening. Thus, the deleterious effects of the metabolic syndrome may be mediated via acceleration of vascular stiffening.

ENDOTHELIAL FUNCTION

Age-Associated Endothelial Dysfunction

Endothelial cells are extremely important and powerful regulators of the vasculature. Several cardiovascular conditions and risk factors are associated with endothelial dysfunction, including hypercholesterolemia, insulin resistance, cigaret smoking, and heart failure *(140)*. Endothelial cells contribute to the pathogenesis of hypertension *(100)* and atherosclerosis *(77,141)*. In addition, endothelial cells play a pivotal role in regulating vascular tone, vascular permeability, and the response to inflammation *(141–143)*. Several features of these arterial properties undergo age-associated alterations in function.

VASOREACTIVITY

With advancing age, nitric oxide–dependent mechanical and agonist-mediated endothelial vasodilatation is reduced in humans *(21,22,144,145)* (Fig. 2C) and animals *(28,146)*. This vasoreactivity depends on nitric oxide generated by eNOS. In aging rats *(55)* and rabbits *(56)*, activity of the eNOS isoform is markedly reduced.

INFLAMMATION

Aging is associated with increased expression of adhesion molecules in rats *(24)* and increased adherence of

monocytes to the endothelial surface in rabbits *(56)*. Adhesion molecules on the luminal surface of endothelial cells mediate leukocyte binding to endothelial cells and subendothelial migration *(75)*. This process is probably facilitated by the actions of MMPs *(147–149)*. Serum levels of adhesion molecules show age-associated alterations in humans *(150,151)*. In patients with hypercholesterolemia and ischemic heart disease, serum levels of soluble vascular cell adhesion molecule-1, but not soluble ICAM-1, are positively associated with aging *(151)*.

PERMEABILITY

In rat aortae, aging is associated with increased permeability to albumin *(152)*. Moreover, glycosaminoglycans *(56)*, which help regulate several arterial properties including vascular permeability *(153)*, accumulate in greater number in the intima of older rabbits. Within hours of an acute arterial balloon injury to the rabbit carotid artery, the pericellular distribution of glycosaminoglycans is significantly reduced in the arterial wall, and this loss is associated with a significant expansion of the extracellular space. The glycosaminoglycans were rapidly replaced by SMCs in the media but not in the developing neointima *(154)*.

VASCULAR-WALL SHEAR STRESS

Vascular-wall shear stress is important in modulating endothelial morphology and function *(141,143,155)*. The identities of the mechanoreceptors that transduce the frictional forces of blood, the various effector systems and component molecules that are activated, and the disparate second-messenger signaling systems involved have not been well defined. Nonetheless, changes in vascular-wall shear stress result in acute and chronic alterations in the synthetic and metabolic activities of endothelial cells (143,155). Arterial regions with low shear stress are particularly vulnerable to the development of atherosclerosis (155).

NONINVASIVE ASSESSMENT OF ENDOTHELIAL FUNCTION

Studying endothelial function is severely hindered by technical and methodological constraints, including the lack of noninvasive, easy-to-perform, reproducible, and widely applicable measurements. The most widely used noninvasive method relies on ultrasonographic assessment of changes in brachial artery diameter in response to mechanical or pharmacological maneuvers. Although this technique has traditionally had technical and interpretive limitations, its reproducibility has been steadily improving (156), and it has been used in large-scale epidemiological studies (156). However, surrogate markers of endothelial function are needed, and techniques that can easily, reliably, and reproducibly assess alterations in endothelial function are being studied. Recent studies of contrast magnetic resonance imaging to evaluate vascular reactivity (157,158) and local vascular-wall shear stress forces (159,160) show promise.

Endothelial Dysfunction and Cellular Senescence

Telomeres, which are DNA–protein complexes that form the ends of chromosomes, and telomerase, a unique enzyme that regulates telomere length, may be important in cellular senescence (161). Because telomeres shorten with each replicative cell division (162), they may be good indicators of biologic aging. Telomere length is a marker of cellular turnover in human vascular tissue (163), where it is inversely associated with age (164) and with atherosclerotic grade (165). In a study of Danish twins, telomere length of chromosomes in white blood cells was negatively associated with pulse pressure (166). In a normotensive French cohort, telomere length of chromosomes in white blood cells was longer in women than in men but contributed significantly to variations in pulse pressure and pulse wave velocity only in men (167). Loss of telomere function induces endothelial dysfunction in vascular endothelial cells, whereas inhibition of telomere shortening suppresses age-associated dysfunction in these cells (168).

Endothelial Dysfunction and Angiogenesis

Endothelial cells play a pivotal role in angiogenesis in which new vessels grow from the existing microvasculature. Studies in animal models of aging indicate that angiogenesis is impaired with advancing age (169). Angiogenesis requires the migration and proliferation of endothelial cells in response to cytokines. Migration of endothelial cells, in turn, requires an optimal level of adhesion to matrix proteins, which is regulated by matrix-degrading metalloproteases such as MMP-1. In microvascular endothelial cells from aged mice, expression of MMP-1 is decreased, whereas expression of its inhibitor TIMP1 is increased (170). Furthermore, in these aged animals, expression of the growth factor TGF-β1 and the matrix protein type 1 collagen is decreased (171). Recent evidence suggests that the expression of growth factors is modulated by advanced glycosylation end products (172). Thus, the age-associated impairment in angiogenesis is due, in part, to changes in the levels of extracellular enzymes, matrix proteins, and growth factors, which affect endothelial cell migration.

AN INTEGRATED VIEW OF VASCULAR AGING

An integrated and comprehensive conceptualization of arterial aging requires improved methods for studying endothelial function and an understanding of as yet unrecognized genetic and polymorphic components of arterial structure and function. Furthermore, interactions among traditional vascular variables need to be defined. These vascular variables have been studied separately, and the emphasis has been placed on their relationships to cardiovascular diseases, not on their relationships with each other. In addition to being intimately involved with cardiovascular diseases, these traditional vascular factors are interrelated and interdependent. For example, in a longitudinal study of a large population of relatively aged subjects, increased baseline levels of pulse pressure were associated with progression of intimal–medial thickening, and baseline intimal–medial thickening, in turn, was associated with greater widening of the pulse pressure (173). After all the components of arterial aging are identified, a comprehensive vascular aging profile may be developed for each individual that represents the integrated sum of all the vascular processes.

TREATMENT OF VASCULAR AGING

We have reviewed the evidence indicating that several age-associated structural and functional vascular changes, including intimal–medial thickening, dilation and stiffening of conduit arteries, and endothelial dysfunction, formerly thought to be part of the normal aging process, precede clinical disease and predict a higher risk for developing clinical disease. In other words, aging blood

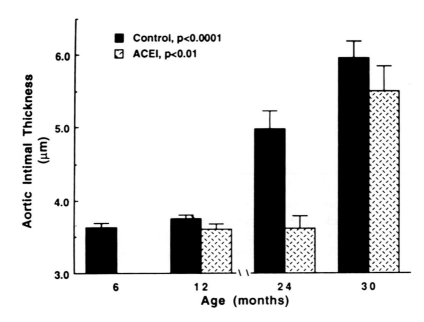

Fig. 10. Effects of aging and angiotensin-converting enzyme inhibitors (ACE-I) on intimal thickness in rodent aortae. ACE-I significantly reduced the age-associated increase in intimal thickening. Adapted with permission from *(23)*.

vessels provide an excellent environment for the development of cardiovascular diseases.

Many of these age-related structural and functional vascular changes should be regarded as risk factors for diseases. Furthermore, when extreme, these changes could be viewed as subclinical or clinical vascular diseases. Cut-off values have been established for LDL cholesterol above which pharmacological interventions are recommended even in a primary preventive setting *(174)*. These cut-off values are lowered when the diagnosis of atherosclerosis is established (in secondary prevention) *(174)*. Similar considerations may eventually be applied to these age-related vascular changes because the dynamic definition of disease used in clinical medicine recognizes the importance of other risk factors in defining the threshold for disease. For example, recommendations of the sixth report of the Joint National Committee on prevention, detection, evaluation, and treatment of high blood pressure (JNC 6) *(128)* established a systolic blood pressure of 140 mm Hg as a cut-off for the diagnosis of hypertension and initiation of interventions in nondiabetics, whereas the systolic blood pressure cut-off value for diabetics is lower at 130 mm Hg. Furthermore, a systolic blood pressure of 130–139 mm Hg in nondiabetics was considered high normal, an indirect reference to subclinical disease, which requires lifestyle changes and close follow-up and monitoring.

No cut-off values for age-associated changes have been established that define thresholds for subclinical or clinical

disease. Age-associated changes have not yet been recognized or accepted as risk factors or diseases by the clinical community; therefore, no screening or prevention guidelines exist to address these newly recognized vascular risk factors, and no treatment strategies that directly target them have been approved. Recognizing the importance and the potential pathophysiologic implications of these new cardiovascular risk factors and vascular disease entities is essential in shaping new medical policy and prioritizing resource allocations.

Pharmacological Interventions

INTIMAL–MEDIAL THICKNESS

The treatment of intimal–medial thickening has been the most extensively studied of the vascular variables associated with aging because intimal–medial thickness has traditionally been regarded as a marker of subclinical atherosclerosis. Medications that were used to treat atherosclerosis were tested for their effects on intimal–medial thickening. The cholesterol-lowering combination of colestipol and niacin reduced the progression of intimal–medial thickening *(175)*. Statins significantly inhibited the progression of intimal–medial thickening in patients with coronary artery disease *(58,176)* and in hypercholesterolemic subjects *(57,177,178)*. Many of the beneficial cardiovascular effects of statins may be due to non–lipid-related mechanisms *(179,180,181)*, including favorable effects on endothelial function, plaque architecture and stability, inflammation, and the inhibition of cellular proliferation. Because of these pleiotropic effects on the arterial wall, and because intimal–medial thickening is not synonymous with atherosclerosis, statins should be further tested as modulators of vascular aging.

Chronic administration of ACE inhibitors can markedly delay the age-associated intimal thickening in rodents (23) (Fig. 10). In humans, administration of ACE inhibitors significantly reduces the progression of intimal–medial thickening in patients at high risk for coronary artery disease (182) and in diabetic patients with hypertension (183). Similarly, treatment with beta-blockers reduces the rate of intimal–medial thickening in hypercholesterolemic patients (184) and in asymptomatic patients with carotid plaque (185). In addition, administration of the calcium channel blocker amlodipine significantly reduces intimal–medial thickening in subjects with untreated hypertension (186) and in diabetic patients with hypertension (187). The calcium channel blockers nifedipine and verapamil (188,189), but not isradipine (190), have stronger salutary effects on intimal–medial thickening than diuretics. The antioxidant probucol reduces the progression of intimal–medial thickening in asymptomatic hypercholesterolemia patients significantly more than placebo (191).

Because many of the molecular changes seen in intimal–medial thickening associated with aging contribute to the pathogenesis of atherosclerosis, therapies for atherosclerosis, not surprisingly, attenuate age-associated intimal–medial thickening. Developing more selective therapies for age-associated intimal–medial thickening requires a better understanding of the biochemical and cellular changes associated with this process. These therapies may, in turn, be efficacious in treating atherosclerosis.

Vascular Stiffness

The effects of traditional cardiovascular medications on vascular stiffness have been assessed. ACE inhibitors reduce vascular stiffening in humans, as assessed by arterial wall hypertrophy (192), vascular distensibility (192), pulse wave velocity (193,194), and arterial wave reflections (193–196). The effects of angiotensin receptor blockers on vascular stiffness have been assessed in only a few studies. Klemsdal et al. (197) administered losartan for 4 wk to 16 hypertensive individuals and noted improvement in vascular compliance as assessed by finger plethysmography. In contrast, Benetos et al. (198) reported that an 8-wk regimen of irbesartan in hypertensive patients did not affect carotid distensibility. Mahmud and Feely (199) added valsartan to a regimen of ACE inhibitors for 2 wk in 18

hypertensive patients and noted a significant decrease in the augmentation pressure. However, these studies were small and of short duration.

Acute (195) and chronic administration of beta-blockers reduces vascular stiffness as assessed by pulse wave velocity (200,201) and augmentation index (195,201). Similarly, studies of pulse wave velocity and augmentation index have shown that acute (195) and chronic administration of calcium channel blockers reduces vascular stiffness (193).

Few studies have evaluated the effects of statins on vascular stiffness. Smilde et al. (202) reported that 1 yr of therapy with statins significantly improved the distensibility and compliance of the femoral artery, but not the common carotid artery, in 45 middle-aged hypercholesterolemic patients. Ferrier et al. (203) reported that 3 mo of therapy with high-dose atorvastatin significantly increased arterial compliance in patients with isolated systolic hypertension. However, Ubels et al. (204) found that intensifying statin therapy in hypercholesterolemic patients did not significantly reduce vascular stiffness. This observation suggests that the beneficial effects of statins on the vascular wall may be related to non–lipid-related mechanisms of action (179–181).

Vascular stiffness can be modulated by strategies that interfere with the synthesis or availability of nitric oxide. In healthy young men, inhibition of constitutive nitric oxide synthesis with N^G-monomethyl-L-arginine (L-NMMA) (205) or with N^G-nitro-L-arginine methyl ester (L-NAME) (102) decreases arterial compliance (102,205) and increases pulse wave velocity (205). These vascular alterations are reversed with the administration of the nitric oxide precursor L-arginine, but not with the infusion of its stereoisomer D-arginine, which is not a substrate for the enzyme nitric oxide synthase. Furthermore, administering nitroglycerine, which is a nitric oxide donor, increases vascular compliance and decreases pulse wave velocity (205). Administering sodium nitroprusside, also a nitric oxide donor, significantly decreases the augmentation index but not the pulse wave velocity (206).

An emerging concept in the treatment of hypertension is that progressive vascular damage can occur even when arterial pressure is controlled. For example, in a cohort of hypertensive patients who were followed for 20 yr, total peripheral vascular resistance and arterial rigidity increased despite treatment of diastolic blood pressure with diuretics or beta-blockers (207). Moreover, in a subgroup of hypertensive patients with end-stage renal disease, pulse wave velocity progressed even when blood pressure was controlled with antihypertensive medications *(134)*; increased vascular stiffening in this cohort was an independent predictor of mortality *(134)*. These findings underscore the need to change the current approach to and evaluation of antihypertensive therapies *(208)*. In addition to lowering blood pressure, antihypertensive agents may inhibit or reverse the age-associated remodeling and stiffening of the vascular wall, which may be an important determinant of their efficacy.

This concept, if supported by clinical studies, has immediate clinical implications. For example, the effects of traditional antihypertensive therapies on pulse pressure need to be examined because pulse pressure is a better predictor of cardiovascular outcomes than systolic or diastolic blood pressures. Current guidelines for the treatment of hypertension *(128)* overlook the prognostic importance of pulse pressure and emphasize the use of systolic or diastolic blood pressures as targets to monitor efficacy of therapy.

Although we have focused on properties of the vasculature, cardiac factors are also important determinants of blood pressure in normotensive and hypertensive individuals *(209)*. The contributions of each cardiac factor to hypertension depend, in part, on the patterns of left-ventricular remodeling *(210)*. Furthermore, age-associated arterial stiffening is matched by an age-associated ventricular systolic stiffening *(211)*. Thus, a comprehensive assessment of interventions aimed at modifying blood pressure or vascular stiffness should include an evaluation of their effects on cardiac remodeling and hypertrophy *(14)*.

ENDOTHELIAL FUNCTION

During the past decade, several studies have shown that endothelial function can be improved by several traditional pharmacological agents. Statins *(212–214)*, the combination of statins with probucol or cholestyramine *(215)*, ACE inhibitors *(216,217)*, angiotensin receptor blockers *(218,219)*, and hormone replacement therapy *(220,221)* increase endothelium-dependent vasodilatation. Similarly, administration of vitamin C *(222)* and parenteral *(144,223)*, but not oral *(224)*, L-arginine improve endothelial function.

Angiogenesis, which is impaired with aging, can be affected by the administration of angiogenic growth factors such as vascular endothelial growth factor (VEGF). Expression of VEGF decreases with aging *(169)*, a process attributed to lower transcriptional activity under hypoxic conditions. This lower transcriptional activity, in turn, is due to an age-associated reduction in hypoxia inducible factor 1 activity *(225)*.

New Pharmacotherapies

Most pharmacologic therapies evaluated for treating vascular aging rely heavily on traditional cardiovascular therapies such as angiotensin antagonists, beta-blockers, and calcium channel blockers. Although these agents predominantly affect vascular tone, load, or function, the recently identified class of thiazolium compounds appears to directly target structural glycoproteins in the vascular wall *(226)* and cleaves the covalent cross-links of advanced glycosylation end products that form between adjacent proteins. These advanced glycosylation end products, which increase with age and increase markedly with diabetes, may contribute to the age- and disease-related increases in large artery stiffening *(20)*. Thiazolium agents reduce indices of arterial stiffening in rodents *(227)*, nonhuman primates *(228)* (Fig. 11A), and humans *(229)* (Fig. 11B).

As the molecular mechanisms that underlie age-associated vascular alterations are identified, new therapies can be developed that will specifically target these pathways.

Lifestyle Interventions

Lack of vigorous exercise, which is a lifestyle risk factor, increases dramatically with age in healthy persons *(230)*. Older persons who are physically conditioned have lower pulse pressure, pulse wave velocity, and carotid augmentation index *(19,231)* and better baroreceptor reflex function *(232)* and endothelial vasoreactivity *(233)* than sedentary controls. The effects of exercise training on vascular stiffness are not fully defined. Cameron and Dart *(234)* reported that a 4-wk exercise training program improved arterial compliance in healthy sedentary individuals, whereas Ferrier et al. *(235)* found that an 8-wk exercise training program did not significantly reduce arterial compliance in hypertensive patients.

Studies evaluating the effects of lifestyle interventions on intimal–medial thickening have been published. Tanaka et al. *(236)* observed that a 3-month endurance-training program did not reduce intimal–medial thickening in healthy sedentary subjects. However, Mavri et al. *(237)* showed a beneficial effect of weight loss on intimal–medial progression in obese premenopausal women. Nonpharmacologic dietary and lifestyle modification programs in other populations have yielded conflicting results *(59,238)*.

Dietary interventions can affect vascular properties. High-fat meals adversely affect vascular compliance *(239)* and endothelial function *(240)*. Diets low in sodium are associated with reduced arterial stiffening with aging, independent of the effect of lowering blood pressure *(241)*.

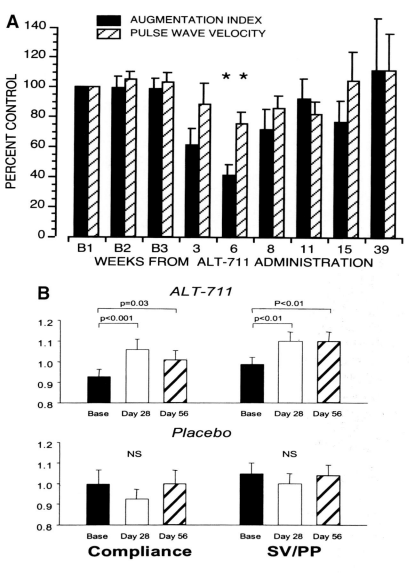

Fig. 11. (A) Measures of vascular stiffness after administering the thiazolium derivative ALT-711 (a synthetic compound that breaks cross-links between glycosylation end products) to nonhuman primates. ALT-711 was administered for 3 wk, but the peak effects on pulse wave velocity and augmentation index were observed at 6 wk ($p < 0.05$). B1, B2, B3 denote the baseline measurements performed before initiation of study medication. (B) The effects of ALT-711 versus placebo on indices of total arterial compliance in hypertensive subjects with elevated vascular stiffness. SV, stroke volume; PP, pulse pressure.

The effect of pharmacological or lifestyle interventions in preventing or inhibiting unsuccessful aging of the vasculature in younger middle-aged individuals with excessive subclinical evidence of unsuccessful aging is unknown.

RESEARCH AGENDA

Although vascular aging is becoming recognized as an important cardiovascular risk factor, many issues are poorly understood. We believe future studies should focus on defining the underlying mechanisms of these new risk factors and identifying their pathophysiologic correlates and clinical sequelae. Priority areas of study in the field of vascular aging are listed in (Table 4). Several of these age-associated risk factors are being studied with an emphasis on their relationship to atherosclerosis rather than on their relationship to aging.

We hope this research agenda will galvanize investigators to develop efficacious, cost-effective, and practical guidelines for screening, preventing, and treating newly recognized age-associated vascular risk factors. To be successful, this plan will require the close collaboration of a consortium of researchers that includes molecular cardiologists, cardiovascular physiologists, and clinical trialists.

Table 4
Research Agenda for Vascular Aging

Animal Models of Aging

- Describe the cellular, molecular, and enzymatic changes that are associated with age-related changes in vascular structure and function.
- Identify the signals that modulate age-related changes and the alterations that lead to the deleterious vascular phenotypes.
- Characterize the relationships among the elements of the vascular wall.
- Identify therapeutic strategies that selectively target the changes that accelerate age-associated vascular changes.
- Study the contribution of the surrounding environment, including rheological factors and vessel-wall shear stress, on age-associated changes in vascular structure and function.
- Identify the molecular processes involved in cellular senescence, including the role of telomeres and telomerases.
- Evaluate the role of the endothelial layer in the pathophysiology of age-associated cardiovascular diseases.

Clinical Studies

- Define "normative" vascular aging for each age-associated vascular variable in the context of successful and accelerated aging.
- Assess the impact of age-associated vascular changes on the risk, development, expression, manifestation, and progression of cardiovascular diseases and on the response to therapy and prognosis.
- Identify phenotypic changes or biomarkers of age-associated changes in vascular structure and function that are of clinical and prognostic value.
- Define the genomic and proteomic principles that control structural and functional vascular aging.
- Characterize the complex genetic traits that determine the qualitative and quantitative responses to aging-related stimuli.
- Construct and validate a vascular aging scoring system that accurately reflects biologic vascular aging.
- Establish guidelines for cost-effective screening for vascular aging.
- Develop effective primary and secondary preventive strategies for accelerated vascular aging based on cardiovascular risk profiles.
- Define, for each age-associated vascular risk variable, normal levels and levels associated with subclinical and clinical disease.
- Study pharmacological and nonpharmacological (lifestyle) measures for treating age-associated vascular risk factors, and establish dose-response curves for each measure.
- Improve current noninvasive techniques for quantifying and characterizing the phenotypic and molecular age-associated structural and functional vascular changes.
- Develop and validate simple and reproducible noninvasive tools for assessing these vascular properties that can be used in population studies.
- Search for easily identifiable and measurable surrogate markers for age-associated endothelial dysfunction.

ACKNOWLEDGMENTS

We would like to thank Christina Link and Denise Dunaway for their expert secretarial assistance.

REFERENCES

1. Burt VL, Cutler JA, Higgins M, et al. Trends in the prevalence, awareness, treatment, and control of hypertension in the adult US population. Data from the health examination surveys, 1960 to 1991. Hypertension 1995;26:60–69.
2. Wilson PW, Castelli WP, Kannel WB. Coronary risk prediction in adults (the Framingham Heart Study). Am J Cardiol 1987;59:91G–94G.
3. Ho KK, Pinsky JL, Kannel WB, Levy D. The epidemiology of heart failure: the Framingham Study. J Am Coll Cardiol 1993;22:6A–13A.
4. Wolf PA, D'Agostino RB, O'Neal MA, et al. Secular trends in stroke incidence and mortality. The Framingham Study. Stroke 1992;23:1551–1555.
5. Wilson PW, D'Agostino RB, Levy D, et al. Prediction of coronary heart disease using risk factor categories. Circulation 1998;97:1837–1847.
6. Fleg JL, Gerstenblith G, Zonderman AB, et al. Prevalence and prognostic significance of exercise-induced silent myocardial ischemia detected by thallium scintigraphy and electrocardiography in asymptomatic volunteers. Circulation 1990;81:428–436.
7. White HD, Barbash GI, Califf RM, et al. Age and outcome with contemporary thrombolytic therapy. Results from the GUSTO-I trial. Global Utilization of Streptokinase and TPA for Occluded coronary arteries trial. Circulation 1996;94:1826–1833.
8. Aguirre FV, McMahon RP, Mueller H, et al. Impact of age on clinical outcome and postlytic management strategies in

patients treated with intravenous thrombolytic therapy. Results from the TIMI II Study. TIMI II Investigators. Circulation 1994;90:78–86.

9. Maggioni AP, Maseri A, Fresco C, et al. Age-related increase in mortality among patients with first myocardial infarctions treated with thrombolysis. The Investigators of the Gruppo Italiano per lo Studio della Sopravvivenza nell'Infarto Miocardico (GISSI-2). N Engl J Med 1993;329:1442–1448.

10. Rowe JW, Kahn RL. Successful aging. Gerontologist 1997;37: 433–440.

11. Grundy SM. Age as a risk factor: you are as old as your arteries. Am J Cardiol 1999;83:1455–1457, A7.

12. Grundy SM. Coronary plaque as a replacement for age as a risk factor in global risk assessment. Am J Cardiol 2001;88:8E–11E.

13. Lakatta EG. Cardiovascular aging in health. Clin Geriatr Med 2000;16:419–444.

14. Lakatta EG. Cardiovascular regulatory mechanisms in advanced age. Physiol Rev 1993;73:413–467.

15. Lakatta EG. Age-associated cardiovascular changes in health: impact on cardiovascular disease in older persons. Heart Fail Rev 2002;7:29–49.

16. Gerstenblith G, Frederiksen J, Yin FC, et al. Echocardiographic assessment of a normal adult aging population. Circulation 1977;56:273–278.

17. Virmani R, Avolio AP, Mergner WJ, et al. Effect of aging on aortic morphology in populations with high and low prevalence of hypertension and atherosclerosis. Comparison between occidental and Chinese communities. Am J Pathol 1991;139:1119–1129.

18. Nagai Y, Metter EJ, Earley CJ, et al. Increased carotid artery intimal-medial thickness in asymptomatic older subjects with exercise-induced myocardial ischemia. Circulation 1998;98: 1504–1509.

19. Vaitkevicius PV, Fleg JL, Engel JH, et al. Effects of age and aerobic capacity on arterial stiffness in healthy adults. Circulation 1993;88:1456–1462.

20. Brownlee M, Cerami A, Vlassara H. Advanced glycosylation end products in tissue and the biochemical basis of diabetic complications. N Engl J Med 1988;318:1315–1321.

21. Celermajer DS, Sorensen KE, Spiegelhalter DJ, et al. Aging is associated with endothelial dysfunction in healthy men years before the age-related decline in women. J Am Coll Cardiol 1994;24:471–476.

22. Gerhard M, Roddy MA, Creager SJ, Creager MA. Aging progressively impairs endothelium-dependent vasodilation in forearm resistance vessels of humans. Hypertension 1996;27:849–853.

23. Michel JB, Heudes D, Michel O, et al. Effect of chronic ANG I-converting enzyme inhibition on aging processes. II. Large arteries. Am J Physiol 1994;267:R124–135.

24. Li Z, Froehlich J, Galis ZS, Lakatta EG. Increased expression of matrix metalloproteinase-2 in the thickened intima of aged rats. Hypertension 1999;33:116–123.

25. Guyton JR, Lindsay KL, Dao DT. Comparison of aortic intima and inner media in young adult versus aging rats. Stereology in a polarized system. Am J Pathol 1983;111:234–246.

26. Fornieri C, Quaglino D, Jr., Mori G. Role of the extracellular matrix in age-related modifications of the rat aorta. Ultrastructural, morphometric, and enzymatic evaluations. Arterioscler Thromb 1992;12:1008–1016.

27. Haudenschild CC, Prescott MF, Chobanian AV. Aortic endothelial and subendothelial cells in experimental hypertension and aging. Hypertension 1981;3:I148–I153.

28. Asai K, Kudej RK, Shen YT, et al. Peripheral vascular endothelial dysfunction and apoptosis in old monkeys. Arterioscler Thromb Vasc Biol 2000;20:1493–1499.

29. Wang M, Lakatta EG. Altered regulation of matrix metalloproteinase-2 in aortic remodeling during aging. Hypertension 2002;39:865–873.

30. Zalewski A, Shi Y. Vascular myofibroblasts. Lessons from coronary repair and remodeling. Arterioscler Thromb Vasc Biol 1997;17:417–422.

31. Jenkins GM, Crow MT, Bilato C, et al. Increased expression of membrane-type matrix metalloproteinase and preferential localization of matrix metalloproteinase-2 to the neointima of balloon-injured rat carotid arteries. Circulation 1998;97: 82–90.

32. Galis ZS, Sukhova GK, Libby P. Microscopic localization of active proteases by in situ zymography: detection of matrix metalloproteinase activity in vascular tissue. Faseb J 1995;9:974–980.

33. Majesky MW, Lindner V, Twardzik DR, Schwartz SM, Reidy MA. Production of transforming growth factor beta 1 during repair of arterial injury. J Clin Invest 1991;88:904–910.

34. Motwani JG, Topol EJ. Aortocoronary saphenous vein graft disease: pathogenesis, predisposition, and prevention. Circulation 1998;97:916–931.

35. Hariri RJ, Alonso DR, Hajjar DP, Coletti D, Weksler ME. Aging and arteriosclerosis. I. Development of myointimal hyperplasia after endothelial injury. J Exp Med 1986;164:1171–1178.

36. Stemerman MB, Weinstein R, Rowe JW, et al. Vascular smooth muscle cell growth kinetics in vivo in aged rats. Proc Natl Acad Sci U S A 1982;79:3863–3866.

37. Sata M, Saiura A, Kunisato A, et al. Hematopoietic stem cells differentiate into vascular cells that participate in the pathogenesis of atherosclerosis. Nat Med 2002;8:403–409.

38. Cheng L, Mantile G, Pauly R, et al. Adenovirus-Mediated Gene Transfer of the Human Tissue Inhibitor of Metalloproteinase-2 Blocks Vascular Smooth Muscle Cell Invasiveness In Vitro and Modulates Neointimal Development In Vivo. Circulation 1998;98:2195–2201.

39. Garg UC, Hassid A. Nitric oxide-generating vasodilators and 8-bromo-cyclic guanosine monophosphate inhibit mitogenesis and proliferation of cultured rat vascular smooth muscle cells. J Clin Invest 1989;83:1774–1777.

40. Cayatte AJ, Palacino JJ, Horten K, Cohen RA. Chronic inhibition of nitric oxide production accelerates neointima formation and impairs endothelial function in hypercholesterolemic rabbits. Arterioscler Thromb 1994;14:753–759.

41. Pauly RR, Passaniti A, Bilato C, et al. Migration of cultured vascular smooth muscle cells through a basement membrane barrier requires type IV collagenase activity and is inhibited by cellular differentiation. Circ Res 1994;75:41–54.

42. Pauly RR, Passaniti A, Crow M, et al. Experimental models which mimic the differentiation and dedifferentiation of vascular cells. Circulation 1992;86(suppl 6): III-68–III-73.

43. McCaffrey TA, Nicholson AC, Szabo PE, Weksler ME, Weksler BB. Aging and arteriosclerosis. The increased proliferation of arterial smooth muscle cells isolated from old rats is associated with increased platelet-derived growth factor-like activity. J Exp Med 1988;167:163–174.

44. Santiago FS, Lowe HC, Kavurma MM, et al. New DNA enzyme targeting Egr-1 mRNA inhibits vascular smooth muscle proliferation and regrowth after injury. Nat Med 1999;5:1264–1269.

45. McCaffrey TA, Fu C, Du B, et al. High-level expression of Egr-1 and Egr-1-inducible genes in mouse and human atherosclerosis. J Clin Invest 2000;105:653–662.

46. Meyyappan M, Wheaton K, Riabowol KT. Decreased expression and activity of the immediate-early growth response (Egr-1) gene product during cellular senescence. J Cell Physiol 1999;179:29–39.

47. Border WA, Ruoslahti E. Transforming growth factor-beta in disease: the dark side of tissue repair. J Clin Invest 1992;90:1–7.

48. Topper JN, DiChiara MR, Brown JD, et al. CREB binding protein is a required coactivator for Smad-dependent, transforming growth factor beta transcriptional responses in endothelial cells. Proc Natl Acad Sci 1998;95:9506–9511.

49. McCaffrey TA, Falcone DJ. Evidence for an age-related dysfunction in the antiproliferative response to transforming growth factor-beta in vascular smooth muscle cells. Mol Biol Cell 1993;4:315–322.

50. Takasaki I, Chobanian AV, Sarzani R, Brecher P. Effect of hypertension on fibronectin expression in the rat aorta. J Biol Chem 1990;265:21935–21939.

51. Crawford DC, Chobanian AV, Brecher P. Angiotensin II induces fibronectin expression associated with cardiac fibrosis in the rat. Circ Res 1994;74:727–739.

52. Levy BI, Michel JB, Salzmann JL, Devissaguet M, Safar ME. Remodeling of heart and arteries by chronic converting enzyme inhibition in spontaneously hypertensive rats. Am J Hypertens 1991;4:240S–245S.

53. Challah M, Nadaud S, Philippe M, et al. Circulating and cellular markers of endothelial dysfunction with aging in rats. Am J Physiol 1997;273(4 Pt 2):H1941–H1948.

54. Wang M, Takagi G, Asai K, et al. Discoordinate regulation of matrix metalloprotease-2 in the thickened aortic intima of older non-human primates. Arterioscler Thromb Vasc Biol 2002 supplement.

55. Cernadas MR, Sanchez de Miguel L, Garcia-Duran M, et al. Expression of constitutive and inducible nitric oxide synthases in the vascular wall of young and aging rats. Circulation Research 1998;83:279–286.

56. Orlandi A, Marcellini M, Spagnoli LG. Aging influences development and progression of early aortic atherosclerotic lesions in cholesterol-fed rabbits. Arterioscler Thromb Vasc Biol 2000;20:1123–1136.

57. Salonen R, Nyssonen K, Porkkala-Sarataho E, Salonen JT. The Kuopio Atherosclerosis Prevention Study (KAPS): effect of pravastatin treatment on lipids, oxidation resistance of lipoproteins, and atherosclerotic progression. Am J Cardiol 1995;76:34C–39C.

58. Hodis HN, Mack WJ, LaBree L, et al. Reduction in carotid arterial wall thickness using lovastatin and dietary therapy: a randomized controlled clinical trial. Ann Intern Med 1996;124:548–556.

59. Markus RA, Mack WJ, Azen SP, Hodis HN. Influence of lifestyle modification on atherosclerotic progression determined by ultrasonographic change in the common carotid intima-media thickness. Am J Clin Nutr 1997;65:1000–1004.

60. Woo KS, Chook P, Raitakari OT, et al. Westernization of Chinese adults and increased subclinical atherosclerosis. Arterioscler Thromb Vasc Biol 1999;19:2487–2493.

61. Crouse JR, 3rd, Byington RP, Bond MG, et al. Pravastatin, Lipids, and Atherosclerosis in the Carotid Arteries (PLAC-II). Am J Cardiol 1995;75:455–459.

62. Barth JD. An update on carotid ultrasound measurement of intima-media thickness. Am J Cardiol 2002;89:32B–38B; discussion 38B–39B.

63. Adams MR, Nakagomi A, Keech A, et al. Carotid intima-media thickness is only weakly correlated with the extent and severity of coronary artery disease. Circulation 1995;92:2127–2134.

64. Homma S, Hirose N, Ishida H, Ishii T, Araki G. Carotid plaque and intima-media thickness assessed by b-mode ultrasonography in subjects ranging from young adults to centenarians. Stroke 2001;32:830–835.

65. Wendelhag I, Wiklund O, Wikstrand J. On quantifying plaque size and intima-media thickness in carotid and femoral arteries. Comments on results from a prospective ultrasound study in patients with familial hypercholesterolemia. Arterioscler Thromb Vasc Biol 1996;16:843–850.

66. Rosfors S, Hallerstam S, Jensen-Urstad K, Zetterling M, Carlstrom C. Relationship between intima-media thickness in the common carotid artery and atherosclerosis in the carotid bifurcation. Stroke 1998;29:1378–1382.

67. Zureik M, Ducimetiere P, Touboul PJ, et al. Common carotid intima-media thickness predicts occurrence of carotid atherosclerotic plaques: longitudinal results from the Aging Vascular Study (EVA) study. Arterioscler Thromb Vasc Biol 2000;20:1622–1629.

68. Kallikazaros IE, Tsioufis CP, Stefanadis CI, Pitsavos CE, Toutouzas PK. Closed relation between carotid and ascending aortic atherosclerosis in cardiac patients. Circulation 2000;102:III263–III268.

69. Burke GL, Evans GW, Riley WA, et al. Arterial wall thickness is associated with prevalent cardiovascular disease in middle-aged adults. The Atherosclerosis Risk in Communities (ARIC) Study. Stroke 1995;26:386–391.

70. Chambless LE, Folsom AR, Clegg LX, et al. Carotid wall thickness is predictive of incident clinical stroke: the Atherosclerosis Risk in Communities (ARIC) study. Am J Epidemiol 2000;151:478–487.

71. O'Leary DH, Polak JF, Kronmal RA, et al. Carotid-artery intima and media thickness as a risk factor for myocardial infarction and stroke in older adults. Cardiovascular Health Study Collaborative Research Group. N Engl J Med 1999;340:14–22.

72. Aminbakhsh A, Mancini GB. Carotid intima-media thickness measurements: what defines an abnormality? A systematic review. Clin Invest Med 1999;22:149–157.

73. Galis ZS, Khatri JJ. Matrix metalloproteinases in vascular remodeling and atherogenesis: the good, the bad, and the ugly. Circ Res 2002;90:251–262.

74. Nguyen M, Arkell J, Jackson CJ. Human endothelial gelatinases and angiogenesis. Int J Biochem Cell Biol 2001;33:960–970.

75. Ross R. Atherosclerosis—an inflammatory disease. N Engl J Med. 1999;340:115–126.

76. Libby P, Ridker PM, Maseri A. Inflammation and atherosclerosis. Circulation 2002;105:1135–1143.

77. Shimokawa H. Primary endothelial dysfunction: atherosclerosis. J Mol Cell Cardiol 1999;31:23–37.

78. Lum H, Roebuck KA. Oxidant stress and endothelial cell dysfunction. Am J Physiol Cell Physiol 2001;280:C719–C741.

79. Guyton JR, Klemp KF. Development of the lipid-rich core in human atherosclerosis. Arterioscler Thromb Vasc Biol 1996;16:4–11.

80. Stary HC. Evolution and progression of atherosclerotic lesions in coronary arteries of children and young adults. Arteriosclerosis 1989;9:I19–I32.

81. Clarkson TB. Nonhuman primate models of atherosclerosis. Lab Anim Sci 1998;48:569–572.

82. Avolio AP, Chen SG, Wang RP, et al. Effects of aging on changing arterial compliance and left ventricular load in a northern Chinese urban community. Circulation 1983;68:50–58.

83. Franklin SS, Gustin Wt, Wong ND, et al. Hemodynamic patterns of age-related changes in blood pressure. The Framingham Heart Study. Circulation 1997;96:308–315.

84. Smulyan H, Asmar RG, Rudnicki A, London GM, Safar ME. Comparative effects of aging in men and women on the properties of the arterial tree. J Am Coll Cardiol 2001;37:1374–1380.

85. Nichols WW, O'Rourke MF. Aging. In: Nichols WW, O'Rourke MF, eds. McDonald's Blood Flow in Arteries. London: Edward Arnold; 1998.

86. Sutton-Tyrrell K, Newman A, Simonsick EM, et al. Aortic stiffness is associated with visceral adiposity in older adults enrolled in the study of health, aging, and body composition. Hypertension 2001;38:429–433.

87. Asmar R, Rudnichi A, Blacher J, London GM, Safar ME. Pulse pressure and aortic pulse wave are markers of cardiovascular risk in hypertensive populations. Am J Hypertens 2001;14:91–97.

88. Mackey RH, Sutton-Tyrrell K, Vaitkevicius PV, et al. Correlates of aortic stiffness in elderly individuals: a subgroup of the Cardiovascular Health Study. Am J Hypertens. 2002;15:16–23.

89. Safar ME, Blacher J, Pannier B, et al. Central pulse pressure and mortality in end-stage renal disease. Hypertension 2002;39:735–738.

90. Saeki A, Recchia F, Kass DA. systolic flow augmentation in hearts ejecting into a model of stiff aging vasculature. Influence on myocardial perfusion-demand balance. Circ Res 1995;76:132–141.

91. Liao D, Arnett DK, Tyroler HA, et al. Arterial stiffness and the development of hypertension. The ARIC study. Hypertension 1999;34:201–206.

92. Blacher J, Pannier B, Guerin AP, et al. Carotid arterial stiffness as a predictor of cardiovascular and all- cause mortality in end-stage renal disease. Hypertension 1998;32:570–574.

93. Boutouyrie P, Tropeano AI, Asmar R, et al. Aortic stiffness is an independent predictor of primary coronary events in hypertensive patients: a longitudinal study. Hypertension 2002;39:10–15.

94. Laurent S, Boutouyrie P, Asmar R, et al. Aortic stiffness is an independent predictor of all-cause and cardiovascular mortality in hypertensive patients. Hypertension 2001;37:1236–1241.

95. Meaume S, Benetos A, Henry OF, Rudnichi A, Safar ME. Aortic pulse wave velocity predicts cardiovascular mortality in subjects >70 yr of age. Arterioscler Thromb Vasc Biol 2001;21:2046–2050.

96. Blacher J, Guerin AP, Pannier B, et al. Impact of aortic stiffness on survival in end-stage renal disease. Circulation 1999;99:2434–2439.

97. de Simone G, Roman MJ, Koren MJ, et al. Stroke volume/pulse pressure ratio and cardiovascular risk in arterial hypertension. Hypertension 1999;33:800–805.

98. Blacher J, Asmar R, Djane S, London GM, Safar ME. Aortic pulse wave velocity as a marker of cardiovascular risk in hypertensive patients. Hypertension 1999;33:1111–1117.

99. Goligorsky MS, Chen J, Brodsky S. Workshop: endothelial cell dysfunction leading to diabetic nephropathy : focus on nitric oxide. Hypertension 2001;37:744–748.

100. Boulanger CM. Secondary endothelial dysfunction: hypertension and heart failure. J Mol Cell Cardiol 1999;31:39–49.

101. McVeigh GE, Bratteli CW, Morgan DJ, et al Age-related abnormalities in arterial compliance identified by pressure pulse contour analysis: aging and arterial compliance. Hypertension 1999;33:1392–1398.

102. McVeigh GE, Allen PB, Morgan DR, Hanratty CG, Silke B. Nitric oxide modulation of blood vessel tone identified by arterial waveform analysis. Clin Sci (Lond) 2001;100:387–393.

103. Kelly R, Hayward C, Avolio A, O'Rourke M. Noninvasive determination of age-related changes in the human arterial pulse. Circulation 1989;80:1652–1659.

104. Chen CH, Nevo E, Fetics B, et al. Estimation of central aortic pressure waveform by mathematical transformation of radial tonometry pressure. Validation of generalized transfer function. Circulation 1997;95:1827–1836.

105. Chen CH, Ting CT, Nussbacher A, et al. Validation of carotid artery tonometry as a means of estimating augmentation index of ascending aortic pressure. Hypertension 1996;27:168–175.

106. Cameron JD, McGrath BP, Dart AM. Use of radial artery applanation tonometry and a generalized transfer function to determine aortic pressure augmentation in subjects with treated hypertension. J Am Coll Cardiol 1998;32:1214–1220.

107. Murgo JP, Westerhof N, Giolma JP, Altobelli SA. Aortic input impedance in normal man: relationship to pressure wave forms. Circulation 1980;62:105–116.

108. Wilkinson IB, Prasad K, Hall IR, et al. Increased central pulse pressure and augmentation index in subjects with hypercholesterolemia. J Am Coll Cardiol 2002;39:1005–1011.

109. McVeigh GE, Hamilton PK, Morgan DR. Evaluation of mechanical arterial properties: clinical, experimental and therapeutic aspects. Clin Sci (Lond) 2002;102:51–67.

110. O'Rourke MF. Towards optimization of wave reflection: therapeutic goal for tomorrow? Clin Exp Pharmacol Physiol 1996;23:S11–S15.

111. London GM, Blacher J, Pannier B, et al. Arterial wave reflections and survival in end-stage renal failure. Hypertension 2001;38:434–438.

112. Dart AM, Kingwell BA. Pulse pressure—a review of mechanisms and clinical relevance. J Am Coll Cardiol 2001;37:975–984.

113. Darne B, Girerd X, Safar M, Cambien F, Guize L. Pulsatile versus steady component of blood pressure: a cross-sectional analysis and a prospective analysis on cardiovascular mortality. Hypertension 1989;13:392–400.

114. Madhavan S, Ooi WL, Cohen H, Alderman MH. Relation of pulse pressure and blood pressure reduction to the incidence of myocardial infarction. Hypertension 1994;23:395–401.

115. Mitchell GF, Moye LA, Braunwald E, et al. Sphygmomanometrically determined pulse pressure is a powerful independent predictor of recurrent events after myocardial infarction in patients with impaired left ventricular function. SAVE investigators. Survival and Ventricular Enlargement. Circulation 1997;96:4254–4260.

116. Chae CU, Pfeffer MA, Glynn RJ, et al. Increased pulse pressure and risk of heart failure in the elderly. JAMA 1999;281:634–639.

117. Domanski MJ, Sutton-Tyrrell K, Mitchell GF, et al. Determinants and prognostic information provided by pulse pressure in patients with coronary artery disease undergoing revascularization. The Balloon Angioplasty Revascularization Investigation (BARI). Am J Cardiol 2001;87:675–679.

118. Franklin SS, Khan SA, Wong ND, Larson MG, Levy D. Is pulse pressure useful in predicting risk for coronary heart Disease? The Framingham heart study. Circulation 1999;100:354–360.

119. Millar JA, Lever AF, Burke V. Pulse pressure as a risk factor for cardiovascular events in the MRC Mild Hypertension Trial. J Hypertens 1999;17:1065–1072.

120. Domanski MJ, Davis BR, Pfeffer MA, Kastantin M, Mitchell GF. Isolated systolic hypertension : prognostic information provided by pulse pressure. Hypertension 1999;34:375–380.

121. Benetos A, Gautier S, Lafleche A, et al. Blockade of angiotensin II type 1 receptors: effect on carotid and radial artery structure and function in hypertensive humans. J Vasc Res 2000;37:8–15; Discussion 68–70.

122. Glynn RJ, Chae CU, Guralnik JM, Taylor JO, Hennekens CH. Pulse pressure and mortality in older people. Arch Intern Med 2000;160:2765–2772.

123. Sesso HD, Stampfer MJ, Rosner B, et al. Systolic and Diastolic Blood Pressure, Pulse Pressure, and Mean Arterial Pressure as Predictors of Cardiovascular Disease Risk in Men. Hypertension 2000;36:801–807.

124. Fang J, Madhavan S, Alderman MH. Pulse pressure: a predictor of cardiovascular mortality among young normotensive subjects. Blood Press 2000;9:260–266.

125. Domanski M, Norman J, Wolz M, Mitchell G, Pfeffer M. Cardiovascular risk assessment using pulse pressure in the first national health and nutrition examination survey (NHANES I). Hypertension 2001;38:793–797.

126. Fagard RH, Pardaens K, Staessen JA, Thijs L. The pulse pressure-to-stroke index ratio predicts cardiovascular events and death in uncomplicated hypertension. J Am Coll Cardiol 2001; 38:227–231.

127. Domanski MJ, Mitchell GF, Norman JE, et al. Independent prognostic information provided by sphygmomanometrically determined pulse pressure and mean arterial pressure in patients with left ventricular dysfunction. J Am Coll Cardiol 1999;33:951–958.

128. The sixth report of the Joint National Committee on prevention, detection, evaluation, and treatment of high blood pressure. Arch Intern Med 1997;157:2413–2446.

129. Burt VL, Whelton P, Roccella EJ, et al. Prevalence of hypertension in the US adult population. Results from the Third National Health and Nutrition Examination Survey, 1988-1991. Hypertension 1995;25:305–313.

130. Franklin SS. Is there a preferred antihypertensive therapy for isolated systolic hypertension and reduced arterial compliance? Curr Hypertens Rep 2000;2:253–259.

131. Sagie A, Larson MG, Levy D. The natural history of borderline isolated systolic hypertension. N Engl J Med 1993;329: 1912–1917.

132. Kannel WB. Elevated systolic blood pressure as a cardiovascular risk factor. Am J Cardiol 2000;85:251–255.

133. Neutel JM. Beyond the sphygmomanometric numbers: hypertension as a syndrome. Am J Hypertens 2001;14:250S–257S.

134. Guerin AP, Blacher J, Pannier B, et al. Impact of aortic stiffness attenuation on survival of patients in end-stage renal failure. Circulation 2001;103:987–992.

135. Scuteri A, Chen CH, Yin FC, et al. Functional correlates of central arterial geometric phenotypes. Hypertension 2001;38:1471–1475.

136. Salomaa V, Riley W, Kark JD, Nardo C, Folsom AR. Non-insulin-dependent diabetes mellitus and fasting glucose and insulin concentrations are associated with arterial stiffness indexes. The ARIC Study. Atherosclerosis Risk in Communities Study. Circulation 1995 ;91:1432–1443.

137. Lambert J, Smulders RA, Aarsen M, Donker AJ, Stehouwer CD. Carotid artery stiffness is increased in microalbuminuric IDDM patients. Diabetes Care 1998;21:99–103.

138. Aoun S, Blacher J, Safar ME, Mourad JJ.Diabetes mellitus and renal failure: effects on large artery stiffness. J Hum Hypertens 2001;15:693–700.

139. Bella JN, Devereux RB, Roman MJ, et al. Separate and joint effects of systemic hypertension and diabetes mellitus on left ventricular structure and function in American Indians (the Strong Heart Study). Am J Cardiol 2001 ;87:1260–1265.

140. Anderson TJ. Assessment and treatment of endothelial dysfunction in humans. J Am Coll Cardiol 1999;34:631–638.

141. Toborek M, Kaiser S. Endothelial cell functions. Relationship to atherogenesis. Basic Res Cardiol 1999;94:295–314.

142. Vane JR, Anggard EE, Botting RM. Regulatory functions of the vascular endothelium. N Engl J Med 1990;323:27–36.

143. Gimbrone MA. Vascular endothelium, hemodynamic forces, and atherogenesis. AJP 1999;155:1–5.

144. Chauhan A, More RS, Mullins PA, et al. Aging-associated endothelial dysfunction in humans is reversed by L-arginine. J Am Coll Cardiol 1996;28:1796–1804.

145. Taddei S, Virdis A, Mattei P, et al. Aging and endothelial function in normotensive subjects and patients with essential hypertension. Circulation 1995;91:1981–1987.

146. Hongo K, Nakagomi T, Kassell NF, et al. Effects of aging and hypertension on endothelium-dependent vascular relaxation in rat carotid artery. Stroke 1988;19:892–897.

147. Romanic AM, Madri JA. T cell adhesion to endothelial cells and extracellular matrix is modulated upon transendothelial cell migration. Lab Invest 1997;76:11–23.

148. Amorino GP, Hoover RL. Interactions of monocytic cells with human endothelial cells stimulate monocytic metalloproteinase production. Am J Pathol 1998;152:199–207.

149. Rosenberg GA, Estrada EY, Dencoff JE. Matrix metalloproteinases and TIMPs are associated with blood-brain barrier opening after reperfusion in rat brain. Stroke 1998;29:2189–2195.

150. Blann AD, Daly RJ, Amiral J. The influence of age, gender and ABO blood group on soluble endothelial cell markers and adhesion molecules. Br J Haematol 1996;92:498–500.

151. Morisaki N, Saito I, Tamura K, et al. New indices of ischemic heart disease and aging: studies on the serum levels of soluble intercellular adhesion molecule-1 (ICAM-1) and soluble vascular cell adhesion molecule-1 (VCAM-1) in patients with hypercholesterolemia and ischemic heart disease. Atherosclerosis 1997;131:43–48.

152. Belmin J, Corman B, Merval R, Tedgui A. Age-related changes in endothelial permeability and distribution volume of albumin in rat aorta. Am J Physiol 1993;264(3 Pt 2):H679–H685.

153. Wight TN. Cell biology of arterial proteoglycans. Arteriosclerosis 1989;9:1–20.

154. Bingley JA, Hayward IP, Campbell GR, Campbell JH. Relationship of glycosaminoglycan and matrix changes to vascular smooth muscle cell phenotype modulation in rabbit arteries after acute injury. J Vasc Surg 2001;33:155–164.

155. Malek AM, Alper SL, Izumo S. Hemodynamic shear stress and its role in atherosclerosis. JAMA 1999;282:2035–2042.

156. Corretti MC, Anderson TJ, Benjamin EJ, et al. Guidelines for the ultrasound assessment of endothelial-dependent flow-mediated vasodilation of the brachial artery: a report of the International Brachial Artery Reactivity Task Force. J Am Coll Cardiol 2002;39:257–265.

157. Silber HA, Bluemke DA, Ouyang P, et al. The relationship between vascular wall shear stress and flow-mediated dilation: endothelial function assessed by phase-contrast magnetic resonance angiography. J Am Coll Cardiol 2001;38:1859–1865.

158. Alexander MR, Kitzman DW, Khaliq S, et al. Determination of femoral artery endothelial function by phase contrast magnetic resonance imaging. Am J Cardiol 2001;88:1070–1074.

159. Stokholm R, Oyre S, Ringgaard S, et al. Determination of wall shear rate in the human carotid artery by magnetic resonance techniques. Eur J Vasc Endovasc Surg 2000;20: 427–433.

160. Kohler U, Marshall I, Robertson MB, et al.MRI measurement of wall shear stress vectors in bifurcation models and comparison with CFD predictions. J Magn Reson Imaging 2001;14:563–573.

161. Weng NP, Hodes RJ. The role of telomerase expression and telomere length maintenance in human and mouse. J Clin Immunol 2000;20:257–267.

162. Harley CB, Futcher AB, Greider CW. Telomeres shorten during ageing of human fibroblasts. Nature 1990;345:458–460.

163. Chang E, Harley CB. Telomere length and replicative aging in human vascular tissues. Proc Natl Acad Sci U S A 1995;92: 11190–11194.

164. Aviv H, Khan MY, Skurnick J, et al. Age dependent aneuploidy and telomere length of the human vascular endothelium. Atherosclerosis 2001;159:281–287.

165. Okuda K, Khan MY, Skurnick J, et al. Telomere attrition of the human abdominal aorta: relationships with age and atherosclerosis. Atherosclerosis 2000;152:391–398.

166. Jeanclos E, Schork NJ, Kyvik KO, et al. Telomere length inversely correlates with pulse pressure and is highly familial. Hypertension 2000;36:195–200.

167. Benetos A, Okuda K, Lajemi M, et al. Telomere length as an indicator of biological aging: the gender effect and relation with pulse pressure and pulse wave velocity. Hypertension 2001;37: 381–385.

168. Minamino T, Miyauchi H, Yoshida T, et al. Endothelial cell senescence in human atherosclerosis: role of telomere in endothelial dysfunction. Circulation 2002;105:1541–1544.

169. Rivard A, Fabre JE, Silver M, et al. Age-dependent impairment of angiogenesis. Circulation 1999;99:111–120.

170. Reed MJ, Corsa AC, Kudravi SA, McCormick RS, Arthur WT. A deficit in collagenase activity contributes to impaired migration of aged microvascular endothelial cells. J Cell Biochem 2000;77:116–126.

171. Reed MJ, Corsa A, Pendergrass W, et al. Neovascularization in aged mice: delayed angiogenesis is coincident with decreased levels of transforming growth factor beta1 and type I collagen. Am J Pathol 1998;152:113–123.

172. Treins C, Giorgetti-Peraldi S, Murdaca J, Van Obberghen E. Regulation of vascular endothelial growth factor expression by advanced glycation end products. J Biol Chem 2001;276: 43836–43841.

173. Zureik M, Touboul PJ, Bonithon-Kopp C, et al. Cross-sectional and 4-year longitudinal associations between brachial pulse pressure and common carotid intima-media thickness in a general population. The EVA study. Stroke 1999;30:550–555.

174. Executive Summary of The Third Report of The National Cholesterol Education Program (NCEP) Expert Panel on Detection, Evaluation, And Treatment of High Blood Cholesterol In Adults (Adult Treatment Panel III). JAMA 2001;285:2486–2497.

175. Blankenhorn DH, Selzer RH, Crawford DW, et al. Beneficial effects of colestipol-niacin therapy on the common carotid artery. Two- and four-year reduction of intima-media thickness measured by ultrasound. Circulation 1993;88:20–28.

176. Crouse JR, 3rd. Predictive value of carotid 2-dimensional ultrasound. Am J Cardiol 2001;88:27E–30E.

177. Furberg CD, Adams HP, Jr., Applegate WB, et al. Effect of lovastatin on early carotid atherosclerosis and cardiovascular events. Asymptomatic Carotid Artery Progression Study (ACAPS) Research Group. Circulation 1994;90:1679–1687.

178. Mercuri M, Bond MG, Sirtori CR, et al. Pravastatin reduces carotid intima-media thickness progression in an asymptomatic hypercholesterolemic mediterranean population: the Carotid Atherosclerosis Italian Ultrasound Study. Am J Med 1996;101: 627–634.

179. Maron DJ, Fazio S, Linton MF. Current perspectives on statins. Circulation 2000;101:207–213.

180. Koh KK. Effects of statins on vascular wall: vasomotor function, inflammation, and plaque stability. Cardiovasc Res 2000; 47:648–657.

181. Faggiotto A, Paoletti R. State-of-the-Art lecture. Statins and blockers of the renin-angiotensin system: vascular protection beyond their primary mode of action. Hypertension 1999;34:987–996.

182. Lonn E, Yusuf S, Dzavik V, et al. Effects of ramipril and vitamin E on atherosclerosis: the study to evaluate carotid ultrasound changes in patients treated with ramipril and vitamin E (SECURE). Circulation 2001;103:919–925.

183. Migdalis IN, Gerolimou B, Kozanidou G, Hatzigakis SM, Karmaniolas KD. Effect of fosinopril sodium on early carotid atherosclerosis in diabetic patients with hypertension. J Med 1997;28:371–380.

184. Wiklund O, Hulthe J, Wikstrand J, et al. Effect of controlled release/extended release metoprolol on carotid intima-media thickness in patients with hypercholesterolemia: a 3-year randomized study. Stroke 2002;33:572–577.

185. Hedblad B, Wikstrand J, Janzon L, Wedel H, Berglund G. Low-dose metoprolol CR/XL and fluvastatin slow progression of carotid intima-media thickness: Main results from the Beta-Blocker Cholesterol-Lowering Asymptomatic Plaque Study (BCAPS). Circulation 2001;103:1721–1726.

186. Stanton AV, Chapman JN, Mayet J, et al, Thom SA. Effects of blood pressure lowering with amlodipine or lisinopril on vascular structure of the common carotid artery. Clin Sci (Lond) 2001;101:455–464.

187. Koshiyama H, Tanaka S, Minamikawa J. Effect of calcium channel blocker amlodipine on the intimal-medial thickness of carotid arterial wall in type 2 diabetes. J Cardiovasc Pharmacol 1999;33:894–896.

188. Simon A, Gariepy J, Moyse D, Levenson J. Differential effects of nifedipine and co-amilozide on the progression of early carotid wall changes. Circulation 2001;103:2949–2954.

189. Zanchetti A, Rosei EA, Dal Palu C, et al. The Verapamil in Hypertension and Atherosclerosis Study (VHAS): results of long-term randomized treatment with either verapamil or chlorthalidone on carotid intima-media thickness. J Hypertens 1998;16:1667–1676.

190. Borhani NO, Mercuri M, Borhani PA, et al. Final outcome results of the Multicenter Isradipine Diuretic Atherosclerosis Study (MIDAS). A randomized controlled trial. JAMA 1996;276:785–791.

191. Sawayama Y, Shimizu C, Maeda N, et al. Effects of probucol and pravastatin on common carotid atherosclerosis in patients with asymptomatic hypercholesterolemia. Fukuoka Atherosclerosis Trial (FAST). J Am Coll Cardiol 2002;39:610–616.

192. Girerd X, Giannattasio C, Moulin C, et al. Regression of radial artery wall hypertrophy and improvement of carotid artery compliance after long-term antihypertensive treatment in elderly patients. J Am Coll Cardiol 1998;31:1064–1073.

193. London GM, Pannier B, Guerin AP, et al. Cardiac hypertrophy, aortic compliance, peripheral resistance, and wave reflection in

end-stage renal disease. Comparative effects of ACE inhibition and calcium channel blockade. Circulation 1994;90:2786–2796.

194. Asmar R, Topouchian J, Pannier B, Benetos A, Safar M. Pulse wave velocity as endpoint in large-scale intervention trial. The Complior study. Scientific, Quality Control, Coordination and Investigation Committees of the Complior Study. J Hypertens 2001;19:813–818.

195. Ting CT, Chen CH, Chang MS, Yin FC. Short- and long-term effects of antihypertensive drugs on arterial reflections, compliance, and impedance. Hypertension 1995;26:524–530.

196. Dart AM, Reid CM, McGrath B. Effects of ACE inhibitor therapy on derived central arterial waveforms in hypertension. Am J Hypertens 2001;14:804–810.

197. Klemsdal TO, Moan A, Kjeldsen SE. Effects of selective angiotensin II type 1 receptor blockade with losartan on arterial compliance in patients with mild essential hypertension. Blood Press 1999;8:214–219.

198. Benetos A, Zureik M, Morcet J, et al. A decrease in diastolic blood pressure combined with an increase in systolic blood pressure is associated with a higher cardiovascular mortality in men. J Am Coll Cardiol 2000;35:673–680.

199. Mahmud A, Feely J. Favourable effects on arterial wave reflection and pulse pressure amplification of adding angiotensin II receptor blockade in resistant hypertension. J Hum Hypertens 2000;14:541–546.

200. Kahonen M, Ylitalo R, Koobi T, Turjanmaa V, Ylitalo P. Influences of nonselective, beta(1)-selective and vasodilatory beta(1)-selective beta-blockers on arterial pulse wave velocity in normotensive subjects. Gen Pharmacol 2000;35:219–224.

201. Asmar RG, London GM, O'Rourke ME, Safar ME. Improvement in blood pressure, arterial stiffness and wave reflections with a very-low-dose perindopril/indapamide combination in hypertensive patient: a comparison with atenolol. Hypertension 2001;38:922–926.

202. Smilde TJ, van den Berkmortel FW, Wollersheim H, et al. The effect of cholesterol lowering on carotid and femoral artery wall stiffness and thickness in patients with familial hypercholesterolaemia. Eur J Clin Invest 2000;30:473–480.

203. Ferrier KE, Waddell TK, Gatzka CD, et al. Aerobic exercise training does not modify large-artery compliance in isolated systolic hypertension. Hypertension 2001;38:222–226.

204. Ubels FL, Muntinga JH, van Doormaal JJ, Reitsma WD, Smit AJ. Effects of initial and long-term lipid-lowering therapy on vascular wall characteristics. Atherosclerosis 2001;154:155–161.

205. Kinlay S, Creager MA, Fukumoto M, et al. Endothelium-derived nitric oxide regulates arterial elasticity in human arteries in vivo. Hypertension 2001;38:1049–1053.

206. Nussbacher A, Gerstenblith G, O'Connor FC, et al. Hemodynamic effects of unloading the old heart. Am J Physiol 1999;277:H1863–1871.

207. Lund-Johansen P. Twenty-year follow-up of hemodynamics in essential hypertension during rest and exercise. Hypertension 1991;18(5 Suppl):III54–III61.

208. Safar ME, Rudnichi A, Asmar R. Drug treatment of hypertension: the reduction of pulse pressure does not necessarily parallel that of systolic and diastolic blood pressure. J Hypertens 2000;18:1159–1163.

209. Ganau A, Devereux RB, Roman MJ, et al. Patterns of left ventricular hypertrophy and geometric remodeling in essential hypertension. J Am Coll Cardiol 1992;19:1550–1558.

210. Segers P, Stergiopulos N, Westerhof N. Quantification of the contribution of cardiac and arterial remodeling to hypertension. Hypertension 2000;36:760–765.

211. Chen CH, Nakayama M, Nevo E, et al. Coupled systolic-ventricular and vascular stiffening with age: implications for pressure regulation and cardiac reserve in the elderly. J Am Coll Cardiol 1998;32:1221–1227.

212. O'Driscoll G, Green D, Taylor RR. Simvastatin, an HMG-coenzyme A reductase inhibitor, improves endothelial function within 1 month. Circulation 1997;95:1126–1131.

213. Jarvisalo MJ, Toikka JO, Vasankari T, et al. HMG CoA reductase inhibitors are related to improved systemic endothelial function in coronary artery disease. Atherosclerosis 1999;147:237–242.

214. Holm T, Andreassen AK, Ueland T, et al. Effect of pravastatin on plasma markers of inflammation and peripheral endothelial function in male heart transplant recipients. Am J Cardiol 2001;87:815–818, A9.

215. Anderson TJ, Meredith IT, Yeung AC, et al. The effect of cholesterol-lowering and antioxidant therapy on endothelium-dependent coronary vasomotion. N Engl J Med 1995;332:488–493.

216. Antony I, Lerebours G, Nitenberg A. Angiotensin-converting enzyme inhibition restores flow-dependent and cold pressor test-induced dilations in coronary arteries of hypertensive patients. Circulation 1996;94:3115–3122.

217. Higashi Y, Sasaki S, Nakagawa K, et al. A comparison of angiotensin-converting enzyme inhibitors, calcium antagonists, beta-blockers and diuretic agents on reactive hyperemia in patients with essential hypertension: a multicenter study. J Am Coll Cardiol 2000;35:284–291.

218. Cheetham C, Collis J, O'Driscoll G, et al. Losartan, an angiotensin type 1 receptor antagonist, improves endothelial function in non-insulin-dependent diabetes. J Am Coll Cardiol 2000;36:1461–1466.

219. Rajagopalan S, Brook R, Mehta RH, Supiano M, Pitt B. Effect of losartan in aging-related endothelial impairment. Am J Cardiol 2002;89:562–566.

220. Gerhard M, Walsh BW, Tawakol A, et al. Estradiol therapy combined with progesterone and endothelium-dependent vasodilation in postmenopausal women. Circulation 1998;98:1158–1163.

221. Higashi Y, Sanada M, Sasaki S, et al. Effect of estrogen replacement therapy on endothelial function in peripheral resistance arteries in normotensive and hypertensive postmenopausal women. Hypertension 2001;37:651–657.

222. Ting HH, Timimi FK, Haley EA, et al. Vitamin C improves endothelium-dependent vasodilation in forearm resistance vessels of humans with hypercholesterolemia. Circulation 1997;95:2617–2622.

223. Quyyumi AA, Dakak N, Diodati JG, et al. Effect of L-arginine on human coronary endothelium-dependent and physiologic vasodilation. J Am Coll Cardiol 1997;30:1220–1227.

224. Blum A, Hathaway L, Mincemoyer R, et al. Oral L-arginine in patients with coronary artery disease on medical management. Circulation 2000;101:2160–2164.

225. Rivard A, Berthou-Soulie L, Principe N, et al. Age-dependent defect in vascular endothelial growth factor expression is associated with reduced hypoxia-inducible factor 1 activity. J Biol Chem 2000 ;275:29643–29647.

226. Vasan S, Zhang X, Kapurniotu A, et al An agent cleaving glucose-derived protein crosslinks in vitro and in vivo. Nature 1996;382:275–278.

227. Wolffenbuttel BH, Boulanger CM, Crijns FR, et al. Breakers of advanced glycation end products restore large artery properties in experimental diabetes. Proc Natl Acad Sci U S A 1998;95:4630–4634.

228. Vaitkevicius PV, Lane M, Spurgeon H, et al. A cross-link breaker has sustained effects on arterial and ventricular properties in older rhesus monkeys. Proc Natl Acad Sci U S A 2001;98:1171–1175.

229. Kass DA, Shapiro EP, Kawaguchi M, et al Improved arterial compliance by a novel advanced glycation end-product crosslink breaker. Circulation 2001;104:1464–1470.

230. Talbot LA, Metter EJ, Fleg JL. Leisure-time physical activities and their relationship to cardiorespiratory fitness in healthy men and women 18-95 yr old. Med Sci Sports Exerc 2000;32:417–425.

231. Tanaka H, DeSouza CA, Seals DR. Absence of age-related increase in central arterial stiffness in physically active women. Arterioscler Thromb Vasc Biol 1998;18:127–132.

232. Hunt BE, Farquhar WB, Taylor JA. Does reduced vascular stiffening fully explain preserved cardiovagal baroreflex function in older, physically active men? Circulation 2001;103:2424–2427.

233. Rywik TM, Blackman MR, Yataco AR, et al. Enhanced endothelial vasoreactivity in endurance-trained older men. J Appl Physiol 1999;87:2136–2142.

234. Cameron JD, Dart AM. Exercise training increases total systemic arterial compliance in humans. Am J Physiol 1994;266: H693–H701.

235. Ferrier KE, Muhlmann MH, Baguet JP, et al. Intensive cholesterol reduction lowers blood pressure and large artery stiffness in isolated systolic hypertension. J Am Coll Cardiol 2002;39: 1020–1025.

236. Tanaka H, Seals DR, Monahan KD, et al. Regular aerobic exercise and the age-related increase in carotid artery intima-media thickness in healthy men. J Appl Physiol 2002;92:1458–1464.

237. Mavri A, Stegnar M, Sentocnik JT, Videcnik V. Impact of weight reduction on early carotid atherosclerosis in obese premenopausal women. Obes Res 2001;9:511–516.

238. Agewall S, Fagerberg B, Berglund G, et al. Multiple risk intervention trial in high risk hypertensive men: comparison of ultrasound intima-media thickness and clinical outcome during 6 yr of follow-up. J Intern Med 2001;249:305–314.

239. Nestel PJ, Shige H, Pomeroy S, Cehun M, Chin-Dusting J. Post-prandial remnant lipids impair arterial compliance. J Am Coll Cardiol 2001;37:1929–1935.

240. Brown AA, Hu FB. Dietary modulation of endothelial function: implications for cardiovascular disease. Am J Clin Nutr 2001;73:673–686.

241. Avolio AP, Clyde KM, Beard TC, et al. Improved arterial distensibility in normotensive subjects on a low salt diet. Arteriosclerosis 1986;6:166–169.

242. Cantini C, Kieffer P, Corman B, et al. Aminoguanidine and aortic wall mechanics, structure, and composition in aged rats. Hypertension 2001;38:943–948.

243. Chajara A, Delpech B, Courel MN, et al. Effect of aging on neointima formation and hyaluronan, hyaluronidase and hyaluronectin production in injured rat aorta. Atherosclerosis 1998;138:53–64.

30 Oxidative Stress

Nageswara R. Madamanchi, PhD and Marschall S. Runge, MD, PhD

CONTENTS

PATHOGENESIS OF ATHEROSCLEROSIS

Atherosclerosis is a chronic inflammatory disease resulting from the interaction of multiple regulatory factors with cells. An important initiating event for atherosclerosis is the interaction of oxidized lipoproteins with the cellular constituents of the arterial wall. The inflammatory reactions and oxidation-mediated signals that follow this event perpetuate the formation of atherosclerotic lesions. Lesion formation begins with the development of fatty streaks in the arterial wall beneath the endothelial cells. The initial event in the development of the fatty streak may be the transport of low-density lipoproteins (LDL) into the arterial wall *(1,2)*. Fatty streaks may develop in response to oxidized phospholipids present in the LDL.

Animal models have shown that LDL rapidly crosses the endothelium and becomes trapped in a network of fibers and fibrils secreted by the cells of the arterial wall into the subendothelial space *(3)*. Although the mechanism of oxidation of phospholipids in LDL trapped in the arterial wall is not known, evidence suggests that endothelial cells, smooth muscle cells, and macrophages are the source of oxidants for the oxidative modification of the phospholipids. Oxidized lipids induce the expression of adhesive molecules, such as P-selectin *(4)*, and monocyte-activating proteins, such as monocyte chemoattractant protein-1 *(5)* and macrophage colony stimulating factor *(6)*, which leads to the activation and attachment of monocytes and T lymphocytes to the endothelial cells *(7)*. Growth factors and chemoattractants secreted by endothelial cells, leukocytes, and smooth muscle cells induce the migration of monocytes and leukocytes into the subendothelial space *(8)*. In the subendothelial space, monocytes mature into macrophages that generate reactive oxygen species (ROS), which convert oxidized LDL into highly oxidized LDL. Scavenger and oxidized LDL receptors take up the highly oxidized LDL in an unregulated process, which leads to intracellular cholesterol accumulation and the formation of "foam cells." Lymphocytes together with the foam cells become the fatty streak. Another hypothesis of the initial event in fatty streak formation is that the migration of monocytes, macrophages, and leukocytes into the vessel wall results from other forces, including alterations in fluid shear stress at areas of flow disruption, such as vessel branching points *(9,10)*.

Whatever the initiating event, formation of fatty streaks clearly involves recruitment of circulating cells to the subendothelial area at discrete locations in the

From: *Contemporary Cardiology: Principles of Molecular Cardiology*
Edited by: M. S. Runge and C. Patterson © Humana Press Inc., Totowa, NJ

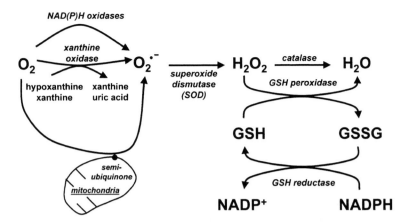

Fig. 1. Pathways of ROS production and clearance. GSH, glutathione; GSSG, glutathione disulfide. Reprinted, with permission *(71)*.

vasculature. In addition, smooth muscle cells are recruited to these lesions, and large numbers of intimal smooth muscle cells often surround fatty streaks *(11)*. With continued influx and proliferation of monocytes and macrophages, fatty streaks progress to more advanced lesions and, ultimately, to a fibrous plaque that protrudes into the arterial lumen. Coronary angiography, although not able to detect fatty streaks, can identify fibrous plaques. Fibrous plaques that only modestly impinge on the vessel lumen (<50% stenosis) are unlikely to cause symptoms of ischemia; however, they can rupture and initiate thrombus formation that results in vessel occlusion and end-organ damage. In the coronary vasculature, this sequence of events leads to myocardial infarction and even sudden cardiac death *(12)*. However, a fatty streak does not have to inevitably progress to myocardial infarction and cardiac death. Recent studies have shown that lifestyle changes and pharmacological therapies, such as 3-hydroxy-3-methylglutaryl coenzyme A (HMG Co-A) reductase inhibitors (statins) or angiotensin-converting enzyme (ACE) inhibitors, can dramatically reduce risk, even in patients with severe coronary atherosclerosis. Although statins and ACE inhibitors were developed for other purposes, an important effect of these drugs may be the ability to block growth signals for vascular cells.

OXIDATIVE STRESS

Oxidative stress is a general term used to describe a shift in the normal cellular balance between ROS production and antioxidant capacity. Oxidants are usually produced in eukaryotic cells during metabolic respiration or phagocytosis or in response to the action of various growth factors and cytokines. Oxidative stress occurs when the cumulative action of oxidative species damages the lipids, membranes, proteins, and DNA of the cell beyond repair.

Reactive Oxygen Species

Oxygen, an abundant molecule in biological systems, is invariably associated with aerobic existence. The most biologically relevant ROS, superoxide ($O_2^{.-}$), peroxide (O_2^{2-}), and hydroxyl radical (OH·), are produced in vivo through partial reduction of triplet-state molecular oxygen in normal metabolic processes. Univalent reduction of ground state triplet oxygen leads to the formation of superoxide radical anion. Superoxide anion is dismutated enzymatically to hydrogen peroxide (H_2O_2) by the action of superoxide dismutases (SOD) *(13,14)* (Fig. 1). In addition, superoxide can be converted nonenzymatically to H_2O_2 and singlet oxygen ($^1O_2$) in biological tissues *(15)*. H_2O_2 reacts with reduced transition metals such as Fe^{2+} to produce highly reactive hydroxyl radicals by the Fenton reaction. Initially, oxidation of superoxide by Fe^{3+} generates molecular oxygen and Fe^{2+}. The resultant Fe^{2+} initiates the Fenton reaction and regenerates Fe^{3+} to propagate the reaction *(16)*. The oxidative potential of H_2O_2 can be amplified by myeloperoxidase, a heme protein secreted by phagocytes *(17)*. Hypochlorus acid (HOCl) is the major oxidant generated by the myeloperoxidase-H_2O_2-Cl^- system at physiological concentrations of Cl^- *(18)*. HOCl can react with $O^{.-}$ to produce OH· *(19)*.

Additional pathways of ROS generation include mitochondrial electron transport, peroxisomal fatty acid metabolism, and cytochrome P450 reactions *(20)*. Mitochondria consume approx 90% of the oxygen, and about 1–2% of the oxygen metabolized by mitochondria is converted to $O_2^{.-}$ at several sites in the respiratory chain and matrix *(21)* (Fig. 1).

Reactive Nitrogen Species

Studies on reactive nitrogen species often focus on nitric oxide, but reactive nitrogen species include several other reactive moieties that are important in modulating cellular oxidative stress. Reactive nitrogen species are derived from the oxidation of the guanido nitrogen of L-arginine. Production of the nitric oxide (NO) radical (NO$\cdot$) is catalyzed by a family of NO synthases, which includes constitutively expressed isoforms (neuronal and endothelial NO synthases) and an inducible form *(22)*. NO$\cdot$ has a wide range of biological roles, including regulation of vascular tone, memory formation, and inflammation *(23)*. However, other important functions of NO$\cdot$ are phagocytosis and mediation of cellular injury in pathological processes such as reperfusion injury and rheumatoid arthritis *(24–26)*. NO$\cdot$ can react with $O_2^{\cdot-}$ at near diffusion-limited rates (10^9 M^{-1} s^{-1}) to form peroxynitrite *(27)*, which is a stronger oxidant than either NO$\cdot$ or $O_2^{\cdot-}$ *(28)*. Nitration of protein tyrosines is increased in human atherosclerotic lesions *(29)*, and the balance between NO$\cdot$ and $O_2^{\cdot-}$ within the vasculature may determine whether the net outcome is injury resolution and repair or chronic inflammation *(30)*.

MOLECULAR EVENTS THAT REGULATE OXIDANT PRODUCTION

Reactive Oxygen Species Production by Phagocytic NADPH Oxidase

ROS production by phagocytic cells, neutrophils, monocytes, and macrophages is an essential mechanism by which these cells kill invading pathogens. In phagocytic cells, engulfment of bacteria or other pathogens initiates ROS generation that is associated with an abrupt but transient increase in oxygen consumption and a robust release of $O_2^{\cdot-}$. This metabolic event is called the "respiratory burst." NADPH oxidase is a membrane-associated enzyme that generates $O_2^{\cdot-}$ in these cells by catalyzing the one-electron reduction of oxygen to $O_2^{\cdot-}$ by using NADPH as the electron donor *(31)*. The key role of NADPH oxidase in the defense against pathogens was elucidated in studies on patients with chronic granulomatous disease (CGD). CGD is an inherited disorder in which NADPH oxidase activity is absent or near absent because of a mutation in one of the subunits of the enzyme. In patients with CGD, phagocytic cells can endocytose bacteria but cannot kill the bacteria because of the absence of the oxidative burst. CGD patients are predisposed to bacterial infections *(32)* and the formation

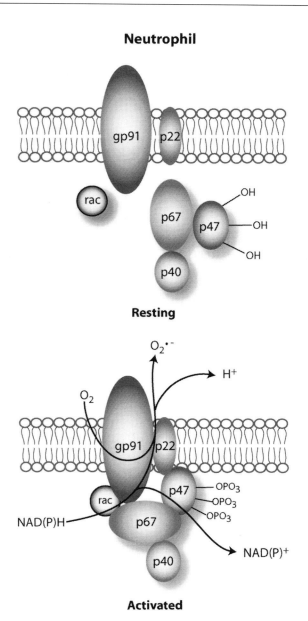

Fig. 2. Activation of the neutrophil NAD(P)H oxidase. gp91^{phox} and p22^{phox} form the electron transfer component of the oxidase, and p47^{phox}, p40^{phox}, p67^{phox}, and rac are the cytosolic components. When the cell is activated, p47^{phox} undergoes phosphorylation and the cytosolic components migrate to the gp91^{phox} and p22^{phox} complex in the membrane to form a functional oxidase. Reprinted, with permission *(42)*.

of inflammatory, "granulomatous" lesions at sites of infection.

The molecular constituents of the NADPH oxidase are a membrane-bound cytochrome, b558, comprising gp91^{phox} and p22^{phox}, and three cytosolic proteins: p47^{phox}; p67^{phox}; and a G protein, rac1 or rac2 *(33)* (Fig. 2). A recently described component, p40^{phox}, is probably a subunit of

NADPH oxidase in many settings. Together with p22[phox], gp91[phox], which contains binding sites for heme, FAD, and NADPH *(34,35)*, supports the flow of electrons from NADPH to O_2 *(34)*. p40[phox] was recently identified as part of the cytosolic complex of p67[phox] and p47[phox] in human neutrophils *(36,37)*. The likelihood that p40[phox] is important for NAD(P)H oxidase activity is based on the following observations. First, p40[phox] has significant sequence homology with p47[phox] and p67[phox], and p40[phox] expression is markedly reduced in the cell cytosol of CGD patients with p67[phox] deficiency. Finally, p40[phox] is phosphorylated and translocated to the plasma membrane in a manner similar to that of p47[phox] during neutrophil activation. p40[phox] increases NAD(P)H oxidase activity by increasing the affinity of p47[phox] for the enzyme *(38)*. p67[phox] may be the bridging molecule that connects p40[phox] and p47[phox] *(39)*.

The activity of the phagocytic NADPH oxidase is tightly regulated because uncontrolled production of ROS would lead to phagocyte dysfunction and inflammatory reactions in the surrounding tissues *(32,33)*. Initial activation of the phagocytic NADPH oxidase occurs upon phosphorylation of p47[phox] *(40)* and translocation of cytosolic p47[phox], p67[phox], and rac to the membrane-bound cytochrome b_{558} (Fig. 2). The enzyme is activated by bacterial lipopolysaccharides, lipoproteins, or cytokines such as interferon-γ, interleukin-1β, or interleukin-8 *(41)*.

Reactive Oxygen Species Production by Nonphagocytic NAD(P)H Oxidases

Multiple cell types in the blood vessel wall generate ROS *(42)* by using, at least in part, an oxidase analogous to the phagocytic NADPH oxidase. ROS generation by endothelial cells, vascular smooth muscle cells (VSMC), and adventitial fibroblasts is mediated by membrane-associated isoforms of NAD(P)H oxidase that can use either NADPH or NADH *(43)*. Superoxide production in vascular cells differs from that in phagocytic cells because of differences in the function of superoxide in the two cell types. Endothelial cells and fibroblasts release $O_2^{.-}$ extracellularly, whereas ROS production in smooth muscle cells is mainly intracellular *(42)*. In contrast to those in neutrophils, nonphagocytic NAD(P)H oxidases are active even during normal metabolic events, and a sustained activation of the enzyme occurs in response to agonists. However, the overall production of superoxide in vascular cells is approximately 10- to 20-fold lower than that of neutrophils *(42)*. Vascular oxidases are induced in response to hormones such as angiotensin II *(43)*, proteases such as thrombin *(44)*, growth factors such as platelet-derived growth factor (PDGF) *(45)*, cytokines

Vascular Smooth Muscle Cell

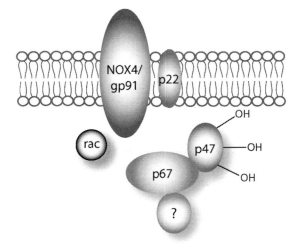

Resting

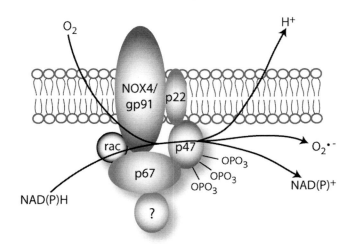

Activated

Fig. 3. Vascular smooth muscle cell NAD(P)H oxidase. gp91[phox] and/or a homologue, Nox4, complex with p22[phox] to make up the membrane component of the oxidase. Phosphorylation of p47[phox] is accompanied by NAD(P)H oxidase activation as in neutrophils. In vitro reconstitution studies of the functional NAD(P)H oxidase were not performed because of the low concentrations of the components in the vascular cells. Adapted from *(42)*.

such as tumor necrosis factor-α *(46)*, and hemodynamic forces such as shear stress *(47)*. In vascular cells, changes in superoxide levels may initiate intracellular signaling, and NAD(P)H oxidases may be essential in these cells for growth, migration, and modification of the extracellular matrix.

Vascular NAD(P)H oxidases are similar but not identical in structure to neutrophil oxidases (Fig. 3), and subtle differences may be seen in NAD(P)H oxidase function among various vascular cell types. Vascular endothelial cells *(48–50)* and fibroblasts *(51)* express gp91^{phox}, whereas a homolog, Nox4, may be the functional component of smooth muscle cell NAD(P)H oxidase *(52)*. In addition, a Nox4-based NAD(P)H oxidase has been described in human embryonic kidney 293 cells *(53)*. Expression of Nox1 and Nox4 increases ROS levels in fibroblasts, suggesting that these proteins contribute to vascular NAD(P)H oxidase function *(54,55)*. Another gp91^{phox} homolog, tox-1, is the main catalytic component of the thyroid NADPH oxidase *(56)*. p22^{phox} and p47^{phox} are expressed in endothelial cells *(48,49,57)*, VSMC *(44,48,58,59)*, and fibroblasts *(51)*. Expression of p67^{phox} is reported in endothelial cells *(49,50)* and fibroblasts *(51,60)* but not in VSMC *(44)*. However, the presence of both gp91^{phox} and p67^{phox} in human VSMC was recently reported *(61)*. Participation of small G protein rac in the activation of vascular NAD(P)H oxidase is well documented *(44,62–64)*.

Unlike the components of neutrophil NADPH oxidase, whose function in enzyme activity is shown by genetic *(65)* and biochemical reconstitution assays *(66)*, the role of the vascular NAD(P)H oxidase components in oxidase activity has been inferred from loss of function or correlational studies. The lack of confirmation is due, in large part, to the lower expression levels in vascular cells than in phagocytic cells.

Decreased intracellular superoxide production was observed in agonist-treated VSMC from p47$^{phox-/-}$ mice *(59,67)*. The requirement for p47^{phox} in oxidase activity was shown independently by the abolition of superoxide generation in angiotensin II-treated rat VSMC depleted of p47^{phox} *(68)*. Similarly, an essential role for p47^{phox} in endothelial cell superoxide production in response to agonists was recently reported *(57)*. A positive correlation between superoxide production and expression and translocation of p47^{phox} and rac was seen in human smooth muscle cells treated with thrombin, suggesting that these components participate in the active enzyme complex *(44)*. Furthermore, the requirement for p67^{phox} activity in vascular NAD(P)H oxidase function was shown in analogous studies. Immunodepletion of p67^{phox} decreased superoxide production in fibroblasts treated with angiotensin II *(51)*. In addition, rac1 is necessary for superoxide production in fibroblasts *(45)*. Studies with p22^{phox} antisense cDNA suggest that p22^{phox} is a critical component of induced rat VSMC NAD(P)H oxidase activity *(69)*. However, the components that make up the functional oxidases in different vascular cell types and the molecular rearrangements that occur during activation and assembly of these enzymes have not been completely

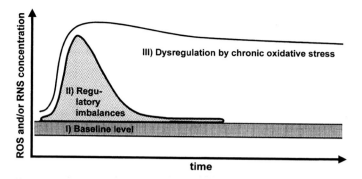

Fig. 4. Regulatory events and their dysregulation depend on the magnitude and duration of the change in the concentration of reactive oxygen species or reactive nitrogen species. Adapted from *(171)*.

defined. Subsequent studies will focus on the organization of the NAD(P)H oxidase in different vascular cell types and the mechanisms by which its function can be modulated in the vasculature.

ANTIOXIDANT DEFENSE MECHANISMS

Enzymatic and nonenzymatic defense mechanisms have evolved in aerobic organisms to minimize the cellular damage resulting from interactions between cellular constituents and ROS *(70)*. Under normal conditions, a balance is maintained between the rates of ROS production and clearance by antioxidant defense mechansims in the cell. This balanced state is called redox homeostasis (Fig. 4; I, baseline level). Under conditions of oxidative stress, redox homeostasis is perturbed because of excess production of ROS and reactive nitrogen species. In response to oxidative stress, genes involved in antioxidant defense mechanisms are expressed, and the excess oxidants produced are scavenged. Thus, the physiological response to increased oxidative stress restores the redox homeostasis (Fig. 4; II, regulatory imbalances). However, during chronic oxidative stress, the antioxidant defense capacity of the cell is overwhelmed, which results in the dysregulation of cellular redox homeostasis (Fig. 4; III, chronic oxidative stress) and alterations in the redox-sensitive signaling pathways. Dysregulation of redox homeostasis is often associated with many pathlogical conditions, including atherosclerosis *(71)*.

Antioxidants compete with oxidizable substrates at relatively low concentrations and, thus, significantly delay or inhibit the oxidation of these substrates *(72)*. The numerous antioxidant systems in vascular cells are probably targeted at modulating oxidative stress under different circumstances. Enzymatic antioxidants include various forms of SOD, catalase, glutathione peroxidase, enzymes involved in glutathione redox homeostasis such as glutathione reductase, and glucose 6-phosphate dehydrogenase, which is involved in the generation of NADPH in the pentose phosphate pathway (70).

SOD catalyzes diffusion-limited degradation of O_2^- into H_2O_2 and O_2. Three different forms of SOD are found in vascular cells. The copper–zinc SOD (SOD1) is primarily expressed in the cytosol, whereas manganese SOD (SOD2) is located in the mitochondrial matrix (73). A third SOD, extracellular SOD (ecSOD), is found in intravascular and extracellular fluids (74) and makes up about 50% of the total SOD in the vessel wall (75,76). Because of its site of expression, SOD2 may play a more critical role than other SOD isoforms in antioxidant defense under normal physiologic conditions. A vascular cell not stressed by agonists or physical changes in its environment probably generates the majority of superoxide as a byproduct of oxidative phosphorylation, and this production is balanced by SOD2 activity. In addition, SOD2 is important under conditions that lead to increased oxidative phosphorylation, including pathogenic stimuli such as lipopolysaccharides, growth factors, cytokines (77), ionizing radiation (78), phorbol esters (79), and redox-cycling drugs (80). Studies in knockout mice have shown the importance of SODs in protection against oxidative stress. SOD2$^{-/-}$ mice develop severe dilated cardiomyopathy and die within 10 d after birth (81). Atherosclerosis is accelerated in hybrid hypercholesterolemic mice deficient in SOD2. Increased expression of ecSOD in atherosclerotic vessels and in foam cells suggests that ecSOD is induced in response to the oxidative environment of the atherosclerotic vessel and macrophages (82). Overexpression of ecSOD improves endothelial function in stroke-prone spontaneously hypertensive rats (83).

Thus, cells respond to maintain a critical balance in superoxide generation and degradation. Indeed, overexpression of SODs could lead to ROS generation and toxicity because SODs can also act as peroxidases and oxidases leading to oxidative injury (84,85). An increase in fatty streak formation occurs in mice overexpressing SOD1 and consuming a high-fat diet (86).

Glutathione peroxidase catalyzes the reduction of H_2O_2 and various hydroperoxides by using glutathione as a reducing agent to form water and corresponding alcohols, respectively (70). At least four major isoforms of this selenium-dependent enzyme are found in mammalian cells. Knocking out glutathione peroxidase enzyme renders mice susceptible to acute paraquat toxicity, myocardial ischemia-reperfusion injury (70), virus-induced myocarditis (87), and neurotoxicity (88). Catalase is a heme-containing peroxidase that catalyzes

the decomposition of H_2O_2 either by catalysis or by peroxidation; the catalytic reaction is favored under high concentrations of H_2O_2 (89). Catalase activity is usually low in the heart and brain, perhaps reflecting the high sensitivity of these organs to oxidative stress (90); however, the reason for low catalase activity in metabolically active organs is unknown. Transgenic mice overexpressing human catalase have significantly lower levels of LDL oxidation in aortic segments and smooth muscle cells than wild-type mice (91). In addition, overexpression of catalase protects against doxorubicin (92), H_2O_2 (93), and ischemia-reperfusion injury (94). These findings suggest that catalase may be important in protecting against oxidative stress.

Nonenzymatic antioxidants include ascorbate (vitamin C), β-carotene, α-tocopherol (vitamin E), glutathione, and NADPH. Ascorbate may inhibit free radical chain propagation reactions by scavenging alkoxy radicals (72). Ascorbate reduces the cytotoxic effects of oxidized LDL (95) and protects against glutathione depletion and DNA and protein damage induced by hypochlorous acid (96). β-Carotene, a carotenoid pigment obtained from fruits and vegetables, circulates in human plasma, predominantly in LDL (97). Enrichment of LDL with β-carotene inhibits endothelial cell–mediated oxidation of LDL (98). β-carotene may inhibit lipid peroxidation by scavenging lipid hydroperoxyl radical generated during the propagation stage (99). In addition to its antioxidant properties, β-carotene and another carotenoid, lycopene, inhibit smooth musclFe cell proliferation (100).

Vitamin E (primarily α-tocopherol), the major lipid-soluble antioxidant in LDL (101), scavenges the highly reactive lipid peroxyl and alkoxyl radicals, which would otherwise propagate the chain reaction of lipid peroxidation (102). However, the resistance of LDL to oxidation does not correlate with its vitamin E content (103,104). α-Tocopherol oxidation is limited to advanced human atherosclerotic lesions, and studies on vitamin E have failed to show complete inhibition of LDL oxidation in the arterial wall (105). In fact, vitamin E can also act as pro-oxidant in LDL, via α-tocopheroxyl radical-mediated formation of lipid radicals (104,106). In the presence of other antioxidants such as ascorbate (107) and ubiquinol-10 (93), α-tocopherol can be converted in the vasculature from an oxidant to an antioxidant (101,108,109). The actions of vitamin E may depend on its interactions with other antioxidants, which may explain why foods containing small amounts of vitamin E provide greater benefits than larger doses of vitamin E alone (110).

Glutathione provides antioxidant protection in multiple ways. Glutathione may prevent lipid peroxidation from entering the propagation stage by scavenging the lipid alkyl or lipoxyl radicals formed during the initiation stage (111). By slowing the oxidation of α-tocopherol (112), glutathione facilitates vitamin E's antioxidant activity. In addition, glutathione stabilizes cellular enzymes from inactivation because the thiol-group of glutathione is preferentially oxidized over other enzymes (113). Exogenous addition of glutathione protects monocyte-macrophages in vitro against oxidized LDL (114), and induction of glutathione along with other antioxidants protects smooth muscle cells against oxidants (115). Thiol supplementation with glutathione improves endothelial dysfunction by increasing NO activity in patients with atherosclerosis or its risk factors (116). NAD(P)H has recently been proposed as a major antioxidant for mitochondria-generated ROS (117). NAD(P)H traps trioxocarbonate ($CO_3{}^{\cdot-}$) and nitrogen dioxide ($NO_2{}^{\cdot-}$) radicals derived from peroxynitrite, in addition to supporting glutathione regeneration and its antioxidative action.

Although inhibiting the production of ROS with antioxidant vitamins and reducing agents is easy in cultured cells or organ baths, results from large clinical trials regarding the use of antioxidants (e.g., vitamin E) for prevention of atherosclerosis have been mixed and, most recently (118–122), disappointing. Large prospective trials with clinical end points have limitations, and the use of surrogate markers of subclinical atherosclerosis, such as intimal–medial thickness (123,124), for evaluating antioxidants has been proposed. In the SECURE trial (Study to Evaluate Carotid Ultrasound changes in patients treated with Ramipril and vitamin E), which was a substudy of the HOPE (Heart Outcomes Prevention Evaluation) trial, administration of 400 IU/d did not affect atherosclerosis progression (125). Furthermore, the Perth Carotid Ultrasound Disease Assessment Study (CUDAS) showed little support for an association between antioxidant intake and/or plasma levels and early carotid atherosclerosis (126). The most notable exception is the report from the Antioxidant Supplementation in Atherosclerosis Prevention (ASAP) study, wherein vitamin E and slow-release vitamin C retarded the progression of carotid atherosclerosis in a small subgroup of hypercholestrolemic men who smoked (127).

However, most data fail to show clear evidence that antioxidant vitamin supplements reduce the risk of atherosclerosis. The reason why results in human studies differ markedly from those of preclinical animal studies is unclear. Several possibilities may account for these differences. First, the vitamin formulations used may have resulted in suboptimal dosing. Second, subcellular localization of ROS generation may preclude adequate

inhibition by the antioxidants used. Finally, the lack of an adequate method to identify those who would most benefit from antioxidant therapy may make positive results more difficult to obtain in large populations. These potential limitations will be addressed in recently designed clinical trials so that the role of antioxidant vitamins can be clearly established.

OXIDATIVE STRESS AND STATINS

Data from numerous large clinical trials have shown that statins decrease the incidence of coronary heart disease in patients with hypercholesterolemia and atherosclerosis (128–131). Statins lower LDL levels by interfering with L-mevalonic acid synthesis via inhibition of HMG Co-A reductase. In addition to their effect on LDL levels, statins increase HDL cholesterol levels and decrease triglyceride levels. Subgroup analysis of trials suggests that statins might have beneficial effects independent of their effects on plasma cholesterol levels (132). One of the cholesterol-independent pleiotropic effects of statins is their antioxidant function. Statins decrease vascular oxidative stress by their inhibitory effect on lipid synthesis (133,134). In addition, statins directly inhibit production of ROS such as $O_2{}^{\cdot-}$ and $OH^{\cdot}$ (135). The mechanism involved in the antioxidant effect of statins has been studied in VSMC; statin-mediated inhibition of rac1 decreases NAD(P)H oxidase activity (136, our unpublished results).

OXIDATIVE STRESS AND ATHEROGENIC RISK FACTORS

In addition to hyperlipidemia, many pathophysiological processes such as hyperglycemia, hypertension, homocysteinemia, and local hemodynamic stresses are risk factors for atherosclerosis (137,138). Genetic determinants (139,140), aging (141), smoking (142), and obesity (143) are other important risk factors for the disease (Fig. 5). Many investigators have proposed that oxidative stress is a unifying mechanism of these risk factors in atherogenesis. For example, vascular dysfunction in diabetes-associated hyperglycemia is probably caused by increased oxidative stress and can be reversed with antioxidants (144). Exposure of VSMC to high glucose activates intracellular signals responsible for proliferation, and ROS generated by high glucose may prime these signaling networks (145). In endothelial cells, high levels of glucose generate ROS and induce LDL peroxidation (146). Moreover, oxidative stress induced by triglycerides and free fatty acids causes insulin resistance and hyperinsulinemia. Obesity is associated with insulin

Risk factors for atherosclerosis: Oxidative stress is a potential unifying mechanism

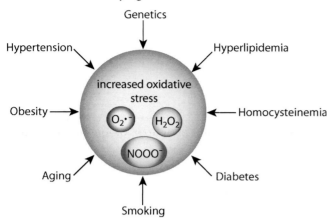

Fig. 5. Oxidative stress is a potential unifying mechanism of various risk factors for atherosclerosis.

resistance and hyperinsulinemia, and oxidative stress inherent in obesity may also involve these common mechanisms *(147)*.

Hypertension predisposes to and accelerates atherosclerosis at least in part by exerting oxidative stress on the arterial wall *(148)*. Recent studies have indicated that much of the oxidative stress in hypertension results from angiotensin II–mediated activation of the smooth muscle cell NAD(P)H oxidase *(42)*. The increased risk for atherosclerotic complications seen in patients with increased homocysteine levels may relate, in part, to oxidative mechanisms. The sulfhydryl group of homocysteine reacts catalytically with ferric or cupric ions in a mixed function oxidase system to generate H_2O_2, oxygen radicals, and homocysteine radicals *(149)*. Homocysteine-induced H_2O_2 toxicity has been attributed to endothelial cell damage *(150)*.

Age is an independent risk factor for atherosclerosis, and adults over age 70 are four times more likely to suffer from cardiovascular disease than younger adults *(141)*. Oxidants generated by mitochondria may be important in the generation of the atherosclerotic lesions that accumulate with age *(151)*. The oxidative hypothesis of aging is supported by increased levels of cellular oxidative stress as measured by increased peroxide levels *(152)* and oxidized proteins *(153)* in aged animals models.

OXIDATIVE STRESS AND VASCULAR SMOOTH MUSCLE CELL GROWTH

Oxidative stress, in addition to the mechanisms described above, modulates important signal transduction pathways that regulate vascular cell function. ROS can

stimulate tyrosine and serine/threonine phosphorylation of protein kinases and initiate activation of transcription factors that control gene regulation. For example, lipid peroxidation products, linoleic acid and its metabolites, initiate mitogen–activated protein kinase (MAPK) activation and protooncogene mRNA expression and stimulate VSMC proliferation *(150)*. Similarly, 4-hydroxy-2-nonenal, another important lipid peroxidation product, induces VSMC growth through MAPK activation, redox-sensitive mechanisms, and growth factor expression *(154)*. Janus kinase (JAK) activation and STAT (signal transducers and activators of transcription) tyrosine phosphorylation in thrombin-treated VSMC are mediated via ROS, and JAK-STAT pathway activation is necessary for thrombin-induced growth *(155)*. The observation that oxidative stress induces growth is further supported by H_2O_2-induced JAK-STAT activation and growth of VSMC *(156)* and fibroblasts *(157)*. The finding that ROS are mitogenic for smooth muscle cells supports the hypothesis that oxidative stress induces VSMC growth *(158)*. Data from our laboratory focus on the role of thrombin as an activator of the smooth muscle cell NAD(P)H oxidase, but other agonists such as angiotensin II and PDGF cause similar effects.

In addition to stimulating cell growth, ROS act as second messengers for signal transduction and cell growth *(44,71,159,160)*. AP-1 and NF-κB are the most studied redox-sensitive transcription factors *(161)*, and most ROS-induced vascular cell signals are mediated by either AP-1 or NF-κB. Activation of AP-1 and generation of ROS are inhibited by treatment with antioxidants such as DPI, *N*-acetyl-cysteine, whereas angiotensin II-induced cardiac myocyte hypertrophy is mediated through NF-κB activation via the generation of ROS *(162)*. These data support the hypothesis that ROS-mediated VSMC growth and migration is one important mechanism by which oxidative stress contributes to atherosclerosis.

OXIDATIVE STRESS AND ATHEROSCLEROSIS: ANIMAL MODELS

The importance of specific proteins and pathways can be studied in genetically altered mouse models. To gain a better understanding of the role of ROS in atherosclerosis and smooth muscle cell function in our laboratory, we have studied atherosclerosis in vivo in mouse models and VSMC signaling in vitro in cells isolated from these mice. VSMC from mice genetically deficient in the NAD(P)H component p47^phox−/− have decreased responsiveness to serum and thrombin as measured by ROS generation and proliferation *(59)*. The importance of this in vitro finding was confirmed by in vivo studies showing that ROS production was less in p47$^{phox-/-}$ aortas than in wild-type aortas. To determine the role of NAD(P)H oxidase–mediated ROS generation in atherosclerosis, we compared lesion formation in mice deficient in ApoE (atherosclerosis prone) (162) with lesions in mice deficient in both ApoE and p47^{phox}. ApoE$^{-/-}$/p47$^{phox-/-}$ mice formed significantly fewer and smaller atherosclerotic lesions than ApoE$^{-/-}$/p47$^{phox+/+}$ mice. Together, these findings support the hypothesis that NAD(P)H oxidase is important in cellular ROS generation and that NAD(P)H-generated ROS are important in atherogenesis.

Another strategy for genetic manipulation of oxidative stress involves targeted disruption of SOD1 and SOD2 genes. The cellular specificity of these enzymes allows for the discrimination between cytosolic and mitochondrial oxidative stress in the development of cardiovascular disease. SOD1$^{-/-}$, SOD1$^{+/-}$ mouse hearts are more susceptible to ischemic reperfusion injury than wild-type mouse hearts, suggesting that SOD1 is a critical antioxidant defense mechanism in the heart (163). Similarly, SOD2 may be important for myocardial function. On some backgrounds, SOD2 deficiency (SOD2$^{+/-}$) produces dilated cardiomyopathy in the absence of an injury. Complete deficiency of SOD2 is lethal at or shortly after birth. At least part of this effect involves increased oxidative damage to mitochondrial protein and DNA (164).

We have recently shown a feedback mechanism involving mitochondria that perpetuates initial oxidative damage. When vascular cells are exposed to ROS, mitochondrial DNA is less protected than nuclear DNA and other cellular constituents. This decreased protection is due in part to the lack of associated proteins (histones protect nuclear DNA from damage) and to the less robust repair mechanisms for mitochondrial DNA than for nuclear DNA. Mitochondrial DNA damage, in addition to being a sensitive marker for oxidative stress, decreases oxidative energetic capacity via impaired oxidative phosphorylation and increases ROS generation (165–167). Thus, oxidative stress–induced mitochondrial damage leads to continued mitochondrial ROS generation and VSMC dysfunction. To test the hypothesis that mitochondrial DNA damage is a cause rather than an effect of atherosclerosis, we examined the relation between mitochondrial DNA damage and atherosclerotic lesion progression in human arterial specimens and in genetically modified (ApoE$^{-/-}$ and ApoE$^{-/-}$/SOD2$^{+/-}$) mice (168). Mitochondrial DNA damage was significantly higher in human atherosclerotic aorta than in nonatherosclerotic aorta, suggesting that increased mitochondrial DNA damage correlates with atherosclerosis. Furthermore, mitochondrial DNA damage

preceded atherosclerotic lesion development in ApoE$^{-/-}$ mice compared with age-matched control animals. ApoE$^{-/-}$/SOD2$^{+/-}$ mice had increased mitochondrial DNA damage and atherosclerotic lesions compared with age-matched ApoE$^{-/-}$ mice, indicating that the ApoE$^{-/-}$/SOD2$^{+/-}$ phenotype is the result of an interaction between a proatherogenic lipid milieu of ApoE$^{-/-}$ background and an increased oxidative milieu of SOD2$^{+/-}$ background. Findings in these mouse models suggest a role for mitochondrial oxidative stress in the development of atherosclerosis.

To investigate other possible mechanisms by which oxidative stress can affect atherosclerotic phenotype, we cultured VSMC from age-matched wild-type (C57BL/6) mice and SOD1$^{+/-}$ and SOD2$^{+/-}$ mice with C57BL/6 background. SOD1$^{+/-}$ and SOD2$^{+/-}$ VSMC have greater constitutive and agonist-induced proliferation capacity than control VSMC, and increased proliferation correlated with increased ROS generation (our unpublished results). Increased cytosolic oxidative stress in SOD1$^{+/-}$ VSMC leads to enhanced constitutive and thrombin-induced MAPK activation, whereas increased mitochondrial oxidative stress increased STAT3 phosphorylation. These findings suggest that oxidative stress in different subcellular compartments affects VSMC proliferation, and hence atherosclerotic phenotype, via different signaling cascades.

The oxidative hypothesis of aging suggests that chronic or abnormal ROS generation may contribute to the age-associated incidence of atherosclerosis in humans (141). To assess the effect of age on atherosclerosis, we have studied VSMC isolated from aortas of young (4 mo old) and old (16 mo old) mice (169). The constitutive and agonist-induced proliferation rate in VSMC is lower in aged mice than in young mice, but aged mice produce higher levels of ROS and have constitutively higher MAPK activity in VSMC than younger mice. The increase in chronic oxidative stress in VSMC from older mice was associated with increased lipid peroxidation and mitochondrial DNA damage. Increased ROS levels in older mice may indicate impaired antioxidant capacity because SOD2 expression and activity and glutathione levels are reduced. This seemingly contradictory observation of inverse correlation between ROS generation and cell proliferation in VSMC from older mice is due to dysregulation of cell cycle–associated proteins. In VSMC from older mice, upregulation of G1 phase-associated cyclin D1 was decreased, and Cdk inhibitor p27Kip1 was not efficiently depleted in response to growth factor stimulation. Paradoxically, the decreased proliferation of VSMC with age can contribute to atherosclerosis because smooth muscle cells protect the integrity of the unstable fibrous cap of athersclerotic plaques, and loss of smooth muscle cell proliferation can result in plaque destabilization *(169,170)*.

SUMMARY

In the search for common underlying mechanisms for the multifaceted disease of atherosclerosis, many investigators have focused on oxidative stress and inflammation. The slightest perturbation of the delicate balance between oxidants and antioxidants can alter cellular function and lead to an increased risk for diseases such as atherosclerosis. While this general concept is widely accepted, the specifics of cellular compartmentalization of ROS and ROS-scavenging enzymes, susceptibility to ROS, and the lack of an effect of antioxidant vitamins in clinical trials leave more questions unanswered than answered. As investigators continue their efforts towards a comprehensive understanding of the relation between clinical disease and oxidative stress, general approaches of proven efficacy become clear. Caloric restriction, moderate exercise, and consumption of fruits and vegetables rich in antioxidant vitamins are approaches to be considered. For patients with known cardiovascular risk factors, therapies such as the use of ACE inhibitors for hypertension and statins for hypercholesterolemia reduce coronary risk. Future research will focus on the development of reliable markers for oxidative phenotype and the use of antioxidants, statins, and other therapies for the treatment of the oxidative subset of atherosclerosis patients.

ACKNOWLEDGMENT

We thank Chris Horaist for assistance in the preparation of the manuscript.

REFERENCES

1. Navab M, Berliner JA, Watson AD, et al. The yin and yang of oxidation in the development of the fatty streak. Arterioscler Thromb Vasc Biol 1996;16:831–842.
2. Young SG, Parthasarathy S. Why are low density lipoproteins atherogenic? West J Med 1994;160:153–164.
3. Nievelstein PF, Fogelman AM, Mottino G, Frank JS. Lipid accumulation in rabbit aortic intima 2 hours after bolus infusion of low-density lipoprotein: a deep-etch and immunolocalization study of rapidly frozen tissue. Arterioscler Thromb 1991;11:1795–1805.
4. Vora DK, Fang ZT, Liva SM, et al. Induction of P-selectin by oxidized lipoproteins. Separate effects on synthesis and surface expression. Circ Res 1997;80:810–818.
5. Cushing SD, Berliner JA, Valente AJ. Minimally modified LDL-induces monocyte chemotactic protein-1 in human endothelial and smooth muscle cells. Proc Natl Acad Sci USA 1990;87:5134–5138.
6. Rajavashisth TB, Andalibi A, Territo MC, et al. Induction of endothelial cell expression of granulocyte and macrophage-colony stimulating factors by modified low density lipoproteins. Nature 1990;344:254–257.
7. McEver RP. Leukocyte-endothelial interactions. Curr Opin Cell Biol 1992;4:840–849.
8. Ross R. The pathogenesis of atherosclerosis: a perspective for the 1990s. Nature 1993;362:801–809.
9. Caro CG, Fitz-Gerald JM, Schroter RC. Arterial wall shear and distribution of early atheroma in man. Science 1969;223:1159–1161.
10. Gimbrone MA Jr. Vascular endothelium, hemodynamic forces, and atherogenesis. Am J Pathol 1999;155:1–5.
11. Thomas WA, Lee KT, Kim DN. Cell population kinetics in atherogenesis. Cell births and losses in intimal cell mass-derived lesions in the abdominal aorta of swine. Ann N Y Acad Sci 1985;454:305–315.
12. Ross R. Cellular and molecular studies of atherogenesis. Atherosclerosis 1997;131:S3–S4.
13. Fridovich I. The biology of oxygen radicals. Science 1978;201:875–880.
14. Deby C, Goutier R. New perspectives on the biochemistry of superoxide anion and the efficiency of superoxide dismutases. Biochem Pharmacol 1990;39:399–405.
15. Steinbeck MJ, Khan AU, Karnovsky MJ. Extracellular production of singlet oxygen by stimulated macrophages quantified using 9, 10-dipheylanthracene and perylene in a polystyrene film. J Biol Chem 1993;268:15649–15654.
16. Kehrer JP. The Haber-Weiss reaction and mechanisms of toxicity. Toxicology 2000;149:43–50.
17. Schraufstatter IU, Browne K, Harris A, et al. Mechanisms of hypochlorite injury of target cells. J Clin Invest 1990;85:554–562.
18. Foote CS, Goyne TE, Lehrer RI. Assessment of chlorination by human neutrophils. Nature 1983;301:715–716.
19. Herdener M, Heigold S, Saran M, Bauer G. Target cell–derived superoxide anions cause efficiency and selectivity of intercellular induction of apoptosis. Free Radic Biol Med 2000;29:1260–1271.
20. Ames BN, Shigenaga MK, Hagen TM. Oxidants, antioxidants, and the degenerative disease of aging. Proc Natl Acad Sci USA 1993;90:7915–7922.
21. Chance B, Sies H, Boveris A. Hydroperoxide metabolism in mammalian organs. Physiol Rev 1979;59:527–605.
22. Clancey RM, Amin AR, Abramson SB. The role of nitric oxide in inflammation and immunity. Arthritis Rheum 1998;41:1141–1151.
23. Moncada S, Higgs A. The L-arginine-nitric oxide pathway. N Engl J Med 1993,329:2002–2012.
24. Murrant CL, Reid M. Detection of reactive oxygen and reactive nitrogen species in skeletal muscle. Microsc Res Tech 2001;55:236–248.
25. Hibbs JB, Taintor RR, Vavrin Z, et al. Synthesis of nitric oxide from a terminal guanidino nitrogen atom of L-arginine: a molecular mechanism regulating cellular proliferation that targets intracellular iron. In: Moncada S, Higgs EA, eds. Nitric oxide from L-arginine: a bioregulatory system. Amsterdam: Elsevier; 1990:189–223.
26. Mazzetti I, Grigolo B, Pulsatelli L, et al. Differential roles of nitric oxide and oxygen radicals in chondrocytes affected by osteoarthritis and rheumatoid arthritis. Clin Sci 2001;101:593–599.
27. Kissner R, Nauser T, Bugnon P, Lye PG, Loppenol WH. Formation and properties of peroxynitrite as studied by laser flash photolysis, high-pressure stopped-flow technique, and pulse radiolysis. Chem Res Toxicol 1997;10:1285–1292.

28. Beckman JS, Koppenol WH. Nitric oxide, superoxide, and peroxynitrite: the good, the bad, and the ugly. Am J Physiol 1996; 271:C1424–C1437.

29. Beckmann JS, Ye YZ, Anderson PG, et al. Extensive nitration of protein tyrosines in human atherosclerosis detected by immunohistochemistry. Biol Chem Hoppe Seyler 1994;375:81–88.

30. Darley-Usmar V, Wiseman H, Halliwell B. Nitric oxide and oxygen radicals: a question of balance. FEBS Lett 1995;369: 131–135.

31. Babior BM, Curnutte JT, McMurrich BJ. The particulate superoxide-forming system from human neutrophils. Properties of the system and evidence supporting its participation in the respiratory burst. J Clin Invest 1976;58:989–996.

32. Smith RM, Curnutte JT. Molecular basis of chronic granulomatous disease. Blood 1991;77:673–686.

33. Babior BM. NADPH oxidase: an update. Blood 1999;93: 1464–1476.

34. Yu L, Quinn MT, Cross AR, Dinauer MC. Gp91(phox) is the heme binding subunit of the superoxide-generating NADPH oxidase. Proc Natl Acad Sci USA 1998;95:7993–7998.

35. Segal AW, West I, Wientjes F, et al. Cytochrome b-245 is a flavocytochrome containing FAD and the NADPH-binding site of the microbicidal oxidase of phagocytes. Biochem J 1992;284:781–788.

36. Someya A, Nagoka I, Nunoi H, Yamashita T. Translocation of guinea pig p40phox during activation of NADPH oxidase. Biochim Biophys Acta 1996;1277:217–225.

37. Wientjes FB, Panayotou G, Reeves E, Segal W. Interactions between cytosolic components of the NADPH oxidase: p40phox interacts with both p67phox and p47phox. Biochem J 1996;317:919–924.

38. Cross AR. p40phox participates in the activation of NADPH oxidase by increasing the affinity of p47phox for flavocytochrome b_{558}. Biochem J 2000;349:113–117.

39. Lapouge K, Smith SJ, Groemping Y, Rittinger K. Architecture of the p40-p47-p67phox complex in the resting state of the NADPH oxidase. A central role for p67phox. J Biol Chem 2002;277:10121–10128.

40. Johnson JL, Park JW, Benna JE, Faust LP, Inanami O, Babior BM. Activation of p47(PHOX), a cytosolic subunit of the leukocyte NADPH oxidase. Phosphorylation of ser-359 or ser-370 precedes phosphorylation at other sites and is required for activity. J Biol Chem 1998;273:35147–35152.

41. Bonizzi G, Piette J, Merville MP, Bours V. Cell-type specific role for reactive oxygen species in nuclear factor (B activation by interleukin-1. Biochem Pharmacol 2000;59:7–11.

42. Griendling KK, Sorescu D, Ushio-Fukai M. NAD(P)H oxidase: role in cardiovascular biology and disease. Circ Res 2000;86: 494–501.

43. Griendling KK, Minieri CA, Ollerenshaw JD, Alexander RW. Angiotensin II stimulates NADH and NADPH oxidase activity in cultured vascular smooth muscle cells. Circ Res 1994;74:1141–1148.

44. Patterson C, Ruef J, Madamanchi NR, et al. Stimulation of vascular smooth muscle cell NAD(P)H oxidase by thrombin. Evidence that p47(phox) may participate in forming this oxidase in vitro and in vivo. J Biol Chem 1999;274:19814–19822.

45. Irani K, Xia Y, Zweier JL, et al. Mitogenic signaling mediated by oxidants in ras-transformed fibroblasts. Science 1997;275: 1649–1652.

46. De Keulenaer GW, Alexander RW, Ushio-Fukai M, Ishizaka N, Griendling KK. Tumor necrosis factor-α activates a p22phox-based NADH oxidase in vascular smooth muscle cells. Biochem J 1998;329:653–657.

47. Yeh LH, Kinsey AM, Chatterjee S, Alevriadou BR. Lactosylceramide mediates shear-induced endothelial superoxide production and intercellular adhesion molecule-1 expression. J Vasc Res 2001;38:551–559.

48. Gorlach A, Brandes RP, Nguyen K, Amidi M, Dehghani F, Busse R. A gp91phox containing NADPH oxidase selectively expressed in endothelial cells is a major source of oxygen radical generation in the arterial wall. Circ Res 2000;87:26–32.

49. Jones SA, O'Donnell VB, Wood JD, Broughton JP, Hughes EJ, Jones OT. Expression of phagocyte NAD(P)H oxidase components in human endothelial cells. Am J Physiol 1996; 271:H1626–H1634.

50. Bayraktutan U, Draper N, Lang D, Shah AM. Expression of functional neutrophil-type NADPH oxidase in cultured rat coronary microvascular endothelial cells. Cardiovasc Res 1998; 38:256–262.

51. Pagano PJ, Clark JK, Cifuentes-Pagano ME, Clark SM, Callis GM, Quinn MT. Localization of a constitutively active , phagocyte-like NADPH oxidase in rabbit aortic adventitia: enhancement by angiotensin II. Proc Natl Acad USA 1997;94: 14483–14488.

52. Sorescu D, Weiss MD, Lasségue B, et al. Superoxide production and expression of Nox family proteins in human atherosclerosis. Circulation 2002;105:1429–1435.

53. Shiose A, Kuroda J, Tsuruya K, et al. A novel superoxide-producing NAD(P)H oxidase in kidney. J Biol Chem 2001;276: 1417–1423.

54. Suh Y, Arnold RS, Lasségue B, et al. Cell transformation by the superoxide-generating oxidase mox1. Nature 1999;401:79–82.

55. Geiszt M, Kopp JB, Varnai P, Leto TL. Identification of renox, an NAD(P)H oxidase in kidney. Proc Natl Acad Sci USA 2000;97:8010–8014.

56. Dupuy C, Ohayon R, Valent A, Noel-Hudson MS, Déme D, Virion A. Purification of a novel flavoprotein involved in the thyroid NADPH oxidase. J Biol Chem 1999;274:37265–37269.

57. Li JM, Mullen AM, Yun S, et al. Essential role of the NADPH oxidase subunit p47phox in endothelial cell superoxide production in response to phorbol ester and tumor necrosis factor-α. Circ Res 2002;90:143–150.

58. Fukui T, Lasségue B, Kai H, Alexander RW, Griendling KK. cDNA cloning and mRNA expression of cytochrome b_{558} α-subunit in rat vascular smooth muscle cells. Biochim Biophys Acta 1995;1231:215–219.

59. Barry-Lane PA, Patterson C, van der Merwe M, et al. p47phox is required for atherosclerotic lesion progression in ApoE(−/−) mice. J Clin Invest 2001;108:1513–1522.

60. Pagano PJ, Chanock SJ, Siwik DA, Colucci WS, Clark JK. Angiotensin II induces p67phox mRNA expression and NADPH oxidase superoxide generation in rabbit aortic adventitial fibroblasts. Hypertension 1998;32:331–337.

61. Toyuz RM, Chen X, Tabet F, et al. Expression of a functionally active gp91phox-containing neutrophil-type NAD(P)H oxidase in smooth muscle cells from human resistance arteries. Regulation by angiotensin II. Circ Res 2002;90:1205–1213.

62. Sohn HY, Keller M, Gloe T, Morawietz H, Rueckschloss U, Pohl U. The small G-protein Rac mediates depolarization-induced superoxide formation in human endothelial cells. J Biol Chem 2000;275:18745–18750.

63. Wagner AH, Kohler T, Ruckschloss U, Just I, Hecker M. Improvement of nitric oxide-dependent vasodilatation by

HMG-CoA reductase inhibitors through attenuation of endothelial superoxide anion formation. Arterioscler Thromb Vasc Biol 2000;20:61–69.

64. Wung BS, Cheng JJ, Shyue SK, Wang DL. NO modulates monocyte chemotactic protein-1 expression in endothelial cells under cyclic strain. Arterioscler Thromb Vasc Biol 2001;21:1941–1947.

65. Price MO, McPhail LC, Lambeth JD, Han CH, Knaus UG, Dinauer MC. Creation of a genetic system for analysis of the phagocyte respiratory burst: high-level reconstitution of the NADPH oxidase in a nonhematopoietic system. Blood 2002;99:2653–2661.

66. Ebisu K, Nagasawa T, Watanabe K, Kakinuma K, Miyano K, Tamura M. Fused p47phox and p67phox truncations efficiently reconstitute NADPH oxidase with higher activity and stability than the individual components. J Biol Chem 2001;276:24498–24505.

67. Lavigne MC, Malech HL, Holland SM, Leto TL.Genetic disruption of p47phox-dependent superoxide anion production in murine vascular smooth muscle cells. Circulation 2001;104:79–84.

68. Schieffer B, Luchtefeld M, Braun S, Hilfiker A, Hilfiker-Kleiner D, Drexler H. Role of NAD(P)H oxidase in angiotensin II-induced JAK/STAT signaling and cytokine induction. Circ Res 2000;87:1195–11201.

69. Ushio-Fukai M, Zafari AM, Fukui T, Ishizaka N, Griendling KK. p22phox is a critical component of the superoxide-generating NADH/NADPH oxidase system and regulates angiotensin II-induced hypertrophy in vascular smooth muscle cells. J Biol Chem 1996;271:23317–23321.

70. Ho YS, Magnenat JL, Gargano M, Cao J. The nature of antioxidant defense mechanisms: a lesson from transgenic studies. Environ Health Perspect 1998;106:1219–1228.

71. Dröge W. Free radicals in the physiological control of cell function. Physiol Rev 2002;82:47–95

72. Halliwell B, Gutteridge JMC. Free Radicals in Biology and Medicine. 2nd ed. Oxford, England: Clarendon; 1989.

73. Weisiger RA, Fridovich I. Superoxide dismutase: organelle specificity. J Biol Chem 1973;248:3582–3592.

74. Marklund SL, Holme E, Hellner L. Superoxide dismutase in extracellular fluids. Clin Chim Acta 1982;126:41–51.

75. Stralin P, Karlsson K, Johansson BO, Marklund SL. The interstitium of the human arterial wall contains very large amounts of extracellular superoxide dismutase. Arterioscler Thromb Vasc Biol 1995;15:2032–2036.

76. Oury TD, Day BJ, Crapo JD. Extracellular superoxide dismutase in vessels and airways of humans and baboons. Free Radic Biol Med 1996;20:957–965.

77. Visner GA, Dougall WC, Wilson JM, Burr IA, Nick HS. Regulation of manganese superoxide dismutase by lipopolysaccharide, interleukin-1, and tumor necrosis factor. Role in the acute inflammatory response. J Biol Chem 1990;265:2856–2864.

78. Poswig A, Wenk J, Brenneisen P, et al. Adaptive antioxidant response of manganese-superoxide dismutase following repetitive UVA irradiation. J Invest Dermatol 1999;112:13–18.

79. Fujii J, Taniguchi N. Phorbol ester induces manganese-superoxide dismutase in tumor necrosis factor-resistant cells. J Biol Chem 1991;266:23142–23146.

80. Kumar S, Millis AJ, Baglioni C. Expression of interleukin 1-inducible genes and production of interleukin 1 by aging human fibroblasts. Proc Natl Acad Sci USA 1992;89:4683–4687.

81. Li Y, Huang TT, Carlson EJ, et al. Dilated cardiomyopathy and neonatal lethality in mutant mice lacking manganese superoxide dismutase. Nat Genet 1995;11:376–381.

82. Fukai T, Galis ZS, Meng XP, Parthasarathy S, Harrison DJ. Vascular expression of extracellular superoxide dismutase in atherosclerosis. J Clin Invest 1998;101:2101–2111.

83. Fennel JP, Brosnan MJ, Frater AJ, et al. Adenovirus-mediated overexpression of extracellular superoxide dismutase improves endothelial dysfunction in a rat model of hypertension. Gene Ther 2002;9:110–117.

84. Yim MB, Chock PB, Stadtman ER. Enzyme function of copper, zinc superoxide dismutase as a free radical generator. J Biol Chem 1993;268:4099–4105.

85. Liochev SI, Fridovich I. Copper- and zinc-containing superoxide dismutase can act as a superoxide reductase and a superoxide oxidase. J Biol Chem 2000;275:38482–38485.

86. Tribble DL, Gong EL, Leeuwenburgh C, et al. Fatty streak formation in fat-fed mice expressing human copper-zinc superoxide dismutase. Circ Res 1997;17:1734–1740.

87. Beck MA, Esworthy RS, Ho YS, Chu FF. Glutathione peroxidase protects mice from viral-induced myocarditis. FASEB J 1998;12:1143–1149.

88. Kilvenyi P, Andreassen OA, Ferrante RJ, et al. Mice deficient in cellular glutathione peroxidase show increased vulnerability to malonate, 3-nitropropionic acid, and 1-methyl-4-phenyl-1,2,5,6-tetrahydropyridine. J Neurosci 2000;20:1–7.

89. Winston GW. Physiological basis for free radical formation in cells: production and defenses. In: Alscher RG, Cumming JR, eds. Stress Responses in Plants: Adaptation and Acclimation Mechanisms. New York: John Wiley & Sons; 1990:57–86.

90. Kang YJ, Chen Y, Epstein PN. Suppression of doxorubicin cardiotoxicity by overexpression of catalase in the heart of transgenic mice. J Biol Chem 1996;271:12610–12616.

91. Guo Z, Van Remmen H, Yang H, et al. Changes in expression of antioxidant enzymes affect cell-mediated LDL oxidation and oxidized LDL-induced apoptosis in mouse aortic cells. Arterioscler Thromb Vasc Biol 2001;21:1131–1138.

92. Kang YJ, Sun X, Chen Y, Zhou Z. Inhibition of doxorubicin chronic toxicity in catalase-overexpressing transgenic mouse hearts. Chem Res Toxicol 2002;15:1–6.

93. Xu B, Moritz JT, Epstein P. Overexpression of catalase provides partial protection to transgenic mouse beta cells. Free Radic Biol Med 1999;27:830–837.

94. Li G, Chen Y, Saari JT, Kang YJ. Catalase-overexpressing transgenic mouse heart is resistant to ischemia-reperfusion injury. Am J Physiol 1997;273:H1090–H1095.

95. Siow RC, Richards JP, Pedley KC, Leake DS, Mann GE. Ascorbate protects human vascular smooth muscle cells against apoptosis induced by moderately oxidized LDL containing high levels of lipid hydroperoxides. Arterioscler Thromb Vasc Biol 1999;19:2387–2394.

96. Jenner AM, Ruiz JE, Dunster C, Halliwell B, Mann GE, Siow RC. Vitamin C protects against hypochlorous acid–induced glutathione depletion and DNA base and protein damage in human vascular smooth muscle cells. Arterioscler Thromb Vasc Biol 2002;22:574–580.

97. Romanchik J, Morel D, Harrison E. Distribution of carotenoids and α-tocopherol among lipoproteins does not change when human plasma is incubated in vitro. J Nutr 1995;125:2610–2617.

98. Dugas T, More DW, Harrison EH. Impact of LDL carotenoid and α-tocopherol content on LDL oxidation by endothelial cells in culture. J Lipid Res 1998;39:999–1007.

99. Burton CW, Ingold KU. β-carotene: An unusual type of lipid antioxidant. Science 1984;224:569–573.

100. Carpenter KL, Hardwick SJ, Albarani V, Mitchinson MJ. Carotenoids inhibit DNA synthesis in human aortic smooth muscle cells. FEBS Lett 1999;447:17–20.

101. Stocker R, Bowry VW, Frei B. Ubiquinol-10 protects human low density lipoprotein more efficiently against lipid peroxidation than does α-tocopherol. Proc Natl Acad Sci USA 1991;88:1646–1650.

102. Niki E, Saito T, Kawakami A, Kamiya Y. Inhibition of oxidation of methyl linoleate in solution by vitamin E and vitamin C. J Biol Chem 1984;259:4177–4182.

103. Diaz MN, Frei B, Vita JA, Keaney JF. Antioxidants and atherosclerotic heart disease. N Engl J Med 1997;337:408–416.

104. Neuzil J, Thomas SR, Stocker R. Requirement for, promotion, or inhibition by α-tocopherol of radical-induced initiation of plasma lipoprotein lipid peroxidation. Free Radic Biol Med 1997;22:57–71.

105. Terentis AC, Thomas SR, Burr JA, Liebler DC, Stocker R. Vitamin E oxidation in human atherosclerotic lesions. Circ Res 2002;90:333–339.

106. Bowry VW, Ingold KU, Stocker R. Vitamin E in human low-density lipoprotein. When and how this antioxidant becomes a pro-oxidant. Biochem J 1992;288:341–344.

107. Suarna C, Dean RT, May J, Stocker R. Human atherosclerotic plaque contains both oxidized lipids and relatively large amounts of α-tocopherol and ascorbate. Arterioscler Thromb Vasc Biol 1995;15:1616–1624.

108. Frei B, England L, Ames BN. Ascorbate is an outstanding antioxidant in human blood plasma. Proc Natl Acad Sci USA 1989;86:6377–6381.

109. Carr AC, Zhu BZ, Frei B. Potential antiatherogenic mechanisms of ascorbate (vitamin C) and α-tocopherol (vitamin E). Circ Res 2000;87:349–354.

110. Herrera E, Barbas C. Vitamin E: action, metabolism and perspectives. J Physiol Biochem 2001;57:43–56.

111. Liebler DC, Kling DS, Reed DJ. Antioxidant protection of phospholipid bilayers by α-tocopherol. Control of α-tocopherol status and lipid peroxidation by ascorbic acid and glutathione. J Biol Chem 1986;261:12114–12119.

112. Hill KE, Burk RF. Influence of vitamin E and selenium on glutathione-dependent protection against microsomal lipid peroxidation. Biochem Pharmacol 1984;33:1065–1068.

113. Halliwell B. Chloroplast Metabolism. Oxford, England: Clarendon Press; 1984.

114. Hardwick SJ, Carpenter KL, Allen EA, Mitchinson MJ. Glutathione (GSH) and the toxicity of oxidized low-density lipoprotein to human monocyte-macrophages. Free Radic Res 1999;30:11–19.

115. Cao Z, Li Y. Chemical induction of cellular antioxidants affords marked protection against oxidative injury in vascular smooth muscle cells. Biochem Biophys Res Commun 2002;22:50–57.

116. Prasad A, Andrews NP, Padder FA, Husain M, Quyyumi AA. Glutathione reverses endothelial dysfunction and improves nitric oxide bioavailability. J Am Coll Cardiol 1999;34:507–514.

117. Kirsch M, Groot HD. NAD(P)H, a directly operating antioxidant? FASEB J 2001;15:1569–1574.

118. Yusuf S, Dagenais G, Pogue J, Bosch J, Sleight P. Vitamin E supplementation and cardiovascular events in high-risk patients. N Engl J Med 2000;342:154–160.

119. GISSI-Prevenzione Investigators. Dietary supplementation with n-3 polyunsaturated fatty acids and vitamin E after myocardial infarction: results of the GISSI-Prevenzione trial. Lancet 1999;354:447–455.

120. Rapola JM, Virtamo J, Ripatti S, et al. Randomised trial of α-tocopherol and β-carotene supplements on incidence of major coronary events in men with previous myocardial infarction. Lancet 1997;349:1715–1720.

121. Stephens NG, Parsons A, Schofield PM, Kelly F, Cheeseman K, Mitchinson MJ. Randomised control trial of vitamin E in patients with coronary artery disease: Cambridge Heart Antioxidant Study (CHAOS). Lancet 1996;347:781–786.

122. Patterson C, Madamanchi NR, Runge MS. The oxidative paradox: another piece in the puzzle. Circ Res 2000;87:1074–1076.

123. Steinberg D, Parthasarathy S, Carew TE, Khoo JC, Witztum JL. Beyond cholestrol: modifications of low-density lipoprotein that increase its atherogenicity. N Engl J Med 1989;320:915–924.

124. Lonn E. Modifying the natural history of atherosclerosis: the SECURE trial. Int J Clin Pract Suppl 2001;117:13–18.

125. Lonn E, Yusuf S, Dzavik V, et al. Effects of ramipril and vitamin E on atherosclerosis. The Study to Evaluate Carotid Ultrasound changes in patients treated with Ramipril and vitamin E (SECURE). Circulation 2001;103:919–925.

126. McQuillan BM, Hung J, Beilby JP, Nidorf M, Thompson PL. Antioxidant vitamins and the risk of carotid atherosclerosis. J Am Coll Cardiol 2001;38:1788–1794.

127. Salonen JT, Nyyssonen K, Salonen R, et al. Antioxidant Supplementation in Atherosclerosis Prevention (ASAP) study: a randomized trial of the effect of vitamins E and C on 3-year progression of carotid atherosclerosis. J Intern Med 2000; 248:377–386.

128. Prevention of cardiovascular events and death with pravastatin in patients with coronary heart disease and a broad range of initial cholesterol levels: the Long-Term Intervention With Pravastatin in Ischaemic Disease (LIPID) Study Group. N Engl J Med 1998;339:1349–1357.

129. Sacks FM, Pfeffer MA, Moye LA, et al. The effect of pravastatin on coronary events after myocardial infarction in patients with average cholesterol levels: Cholesterol and Recurrent Events Trial Investigators. N Eng J Med 1996;335: 1001–1009.

130. Shepherd J, Cobbe SM, Ford I, et al. Prevention of coronary heart disease with pravastatin in men with hypercholesterolemia: West Of Scotland Coronary Prevention Study Group. N Engl J Med 1995;333:1301–1307.

131. Downs JR, Clearfield M, Weis S, et al. Primary prevention of acute coronary events with lovastatin in men and women with average cholesterol levels: results of AFCAPS/TexCAPS: Air Force/Texas Coronary Atherosclerosis Prevention Study. JAMA 1998;279:1615–1622.

132. Takemoto M, Liao JK. Pleiotropic effects of 3-hydroxy-3-methylglutaryl coenzyme A reductase inhibitors. Arterioscler Thromb Vasc Biol 2001;21:1712–1719.

133. Cai H, Harrison DG. Endothelial dysfunction in cardiovascular diseases: the role of oxidant stress. Circ Res 2000;87:840–844.

134. Landmesser U, Hornig B, Drexler H. Endothelial dysfunction in hypercholestrolemia: mechanisms, pathophysiological importance, and therapeutic interventions. Semin Thromb Hemost 2000;26:529–537.

135. Rikitake Y, Kawashima S, Takeshita S, et al. Anti-oxidative properties of fluvastatin, an HMG-CoA reductase inhibitor, contribute to prevention of atherosclerosis in cholesterol-fed rabbits. Atherosclerosis 2001;154:87–96.

136. Wassman S, Laufs U, Baumer AT, et al. Inhibition of geranylgeranylation reduces angiotensin II-mediated free radical production in vascular smooth muscle cells; involvement of

angiotensin AT1 receptor expression and Rac1 GTPase. Mol Pharmacol 2001;59:646–654.

137. Prasad K. Homocysteine, a risk factor for cardiovascular disease. Int J Angiol 1999;8:76–86.

138. Kunsch C, Medford RM. Oxidative stress as a regulator of gene expression in the vasculature. Circ Res 1999;85:753–766.

139. Lange LA, Bowden DW, Langefeld CD, et al. Heritability of carotid artery intima-medial thickness in type 2 diabetes. Stroke 2002;33:1876–1881.

140. Broeckel U, Hengstenberg C, Mayer B, et al. A comprehensive linkage analysis for myocardial infarction and its related risk factors. Nat Genet 2002;30:210–214.

141. Patterson C. Things have changed: cell cycle dysregulation and smooth muscle cell dysfunction in atherogenesis. Aging Res Rev 2002;1:167–179.

142. Glantz SA, Parmley WW. Even a little second hand smoke is dangerous. JAMA 2001;286:462–463.

143. Perticone F, Ceravolo R, Candigliota M, et al. Obesity and body fat distribution induce endothelial dysfunction by oxidative stress: protective effect of vitamin C. Diabetes 2001;50:159–165.

144. Baynes JW. Role of oxidative stress in development of complications in diabetes. Diabetes 1991;40:405–412.

145. Srivastava AK. High glucose-induced activation of protein kinase signaling pathways in vascular smooth muscle cells: a potential role in the pathogenesis of vascular dysfunction in diabetes. Int J Mol Med 2002;9:85–89.

146. Graier WF, Simecek S, Kukovetz WR, Kostner JM. High-D-glucose-induced change in endothelial Ca^{2+}/EDRF signaling are due to generation of superoxide anions. Diabetes 1996;45:1386–1395.

147. Sanchez-Margalet V, Valle M, Ruz FJ, Gascon F, Mateo J, Goberna R. Elevated plasma total homocysteine levels in hyperinsulinemic obese subjects. J Nutr Biochem 2002;13:75–79.

148. Alexander RW. Theodore Cooper Memorial Lecture. Hypertension and the pathogenesis of atherosclerosis: oxidative stress and the mediation of arterial inflammatory response: a new perspective. Hypertension 1995;25:155–161.

149. Olszewski AJ, McCully KS. Homocysteine metabolism and the oxidative modification of proteins and lipids. Free Radic Biol Med 1993;14:683–693.

150. Blundell G, Jones BG, Rose FA, Tudball N. Homocysteine mediated endothelial cell toxicity and its amelioration. Atherosclerosis 1996;122:163–172.

151. Shigenaga MK, Hagen TM, Ames BN. Oxidative damage and mitochondrial decay in aging. Proc Natl Acad Sci USA 1994;91:10771–10778.

152. Spencer NF, Poynter ME, Im SY, Daynes RA. Constitutive activation of NF-kappa B in an animal model of aging. Int Immunol 1997;9:1581–1588.

153. Berlett BS, Stadtman ER. Protein oxidation in aging, disease, and oxidative stress. J Biol Chem 1997;272:20313–20316.

154. Rao GN, Alexander RW, Runge MS. Linoleic acid and its metabolites, hydroperoxyoctadecadienoic acids, stimulate c-FOS, c-Jun, and c-Myc mRNA expression, mitogen-activated protein kinase activation, and growth in rat aortic smooth muscle cells. J Clin Invest 1995;96:842–847.

155. Ruef J, Rao GN, Li F, et al. Induction of rat aortic smooth muscle cell growth by the lipid peroxidation product 4-hydroxy-2-nonenal. Circulation 1998;97:1071–1078.

156. Madamanchi NR, Li S, Patterson C, Runge MS. Thrombin regulates vascular smooth muscle cell growth and heat shock proteins via the JAK-STAT pathway. J Biol Chem 2001;276:18915–18924.

157. Madamanchi NR, Li S, Patterson C, Runge MS. Reactive oxygen species regulate heat-shock protein 70 via the JAK/STAT pathway. Arterioscler Thromb Vasc Biol 2001;21:321–326.

158. Abe J, Berk BC. Fyn and JAK2 mediate ras activation by reactive oxygen species. J Biol Chem 1999;274:21003–21010.

159. Suzuki YJ, Forman HJ, Sevanian A. Oxidants as stimulators of signal transduction. Free Radic Biol Med 1997;22:269–285.

160. Sundaresan M, Yu ZX, Ferrans VJ, Irani K, Finkel T. Requirement for generation of HO for platelet-derived growth factor signal transduction. Science 1995;270:296–299.

161. Hirotani S, Otsu K, Nishida K, et al. Involvement of nuclear factor–kB and apoptosis signal-regulating kinase 1 in G-protein-coupled receptor agonist-induced cardiomyocyte hypertrophy. Circulation 2002;105:509–515.

162. Zhang SH, Reddick RL, Piedrahita JA, Maeda N. Spontaneous hypercholesterolemia and arterial lesions in mice lacking apolipoprotein E. Science 1992;258:468–471.

163. Yoshida T, Maulik N, Engelman RM, Ho YS, Das DK. Targeted disruption of the mouse SOD1 gene makes the hearts vulnerable to ischemic reperfusion injury. Circ Res 2000;86:264–269.

164. Williams MD, Remmen HV, Conrad CC, Huang TT, Epstein CJ, Richardson A. Increased oxidative damage is correlated to altered mitochondrial function in heterozygous manganese superoxide dismutase knockout mice. J Biol Chem 1998;273:28510–28515.

165. Ballinger SW, Patterson C, Yan CN, et al. Hydrogen peroxide- and peroxynitrite-induced mitochondrial DNA damage and dysfunction in vascular endothelial and smooth muscle cells. Circ Res 2000;86:960–966.

166. Ferrari R. The role of mitochondria in ischemic heart disease. J Cardiovasc Pharmacol 1996;28:S1–S10.

167. Ide T, Tsutsui H, Kinugawa S, et al. Direct evidence for increased hydroxyl radicals originating from superoxide in the failing myocardium. Circ Res 2002;86:152–157.

168. Ballinger SW, Patterson C, Knight-Lozano CA, et al. Mitochondrial integrity and function in atherogenesis. Circulation 2002;106:544–549.

169. Moon SK, Thompson LJ, Madamanchi N, et al. Aging, oxidative responses, and proliferative capacity in cultured mouse aortic smooth muscle cells. Am J Physiol Heart Circ Physiol 2001;280:H2779–H2788.

170. Newby AC, Zaltsman AB. Fibrous cap formation or destruction—the critical importance of vascular smooth muscle cell proliferation, migration and matrix formation. Cardiovasc Res 1999;41:345–360.

31 Diabetes Mellitus

An Important Cardiovascular Risk Factor

David R. Clemmons, MD

CONTENTS

INTRODUCTION

Diabetes is associated with a significant increase in the risk of coronary heart disease, peripheral vascular disease, and stroke. The relative risk ratio for coronary heart disease for both men and women with diabetes is increased. Most epidemiologic studies in which relative risk has been assessed have been conducted in patients with type 2 diabetes; however, patients with type 1 diabetes, particularly those with renal failure, are at increased risk. Comorbidity factors associated with diabetes include hyperlipidemia, hypertension, and insulin resistance.

In a large study in England, the incidence of myocardial infarction over a 7-yr period in patients with no history of infarction was 18.8% in diabetics and 3.5% in nondiabetics. In patients with a history of infarction, the relative risks were 45% in diabetics and 20% in nondiabetics *(1)*. These findings indicate that the likelihood of infarction in a diabetic patient with no history of infarction is equal to that of a nondiabetic patient who has had a previous infarction. In addition, patients with diabetes have a high fatality rate after myocardial infarction. At 1 yr after infarction, the case fatality rate is 45% for diabetic men, 38% for nondiabetic men, 39% for diabetic women, and 25% for nondiabetic women. Macrovascular disease, which accounts for 59% to 70% of the deaths in patients with type 2 diabetes, is the most important long-term complication of this disease. The relative risk of stroke is two- to threefold higher in diabetic individuals with type 2 diabetes than in nondiabetic individuals. Identifying the major factors that underlie the pathogenesis of vascular disease in diabetes is critical in constructing rational treatment regimens.

ETIOLOGY AND PATHOGENESIS

The prevalence of type 1 diabetes is lower than that of type 2 diabetes. Among patients younger than 30 yr, the

From: *Contemporary Cardiology: Principles of Molecular Cardiology*
Edited by: M. S. Runge and C. Patterson © Humana Press Inc., Totowa, NJ

prevalence of type 1 diabetes is approx 0.3%, whereas the prevalence of type 2 diabetes may be as high as 3% in those over age 60 yr.

Although type 1 diabetes is an autoimmune disease, no single etiologic agent that triggers this autoimmune response has been identified. Both viral and chemical agents have been indicated as etiologic agents. Certain human leukocyte antigen (HLA) haplotypes are associated with a tendency to produce islet cell autoantibodies that may contribute to the pathogenesis of diabetes. On chromosome 6, the HLA haplotypes that are the most likely to result in diabetes include DQB*10302-A1 0*301-DRB104 and DQB1*0201-A10501-DRB*103 (2). HLA haplotypes that protect against the development of diabetes, such as DQB1*0602, have been identified (3). HLA phenotype can account for 60% of the genetic risk. The genetic inheritance pattern is complex and involves the interaction of multiple polymorphisms. Epidemiologic studies support the role of viral interactions with genetic factors; however, identifying one virus in the etiology of diabetes is difficult because of the complexity of the genetic markers with which they interact at a pathophysiologic level (4). An inciting agent such as viral infection in a patient with a predisposing HLA haplotype results in an autoimmune inflammatory response that produces high titers of anti-islet cell antibodies, which may cause long-term β cell destruction. Clinically significant diabetes does not always develop in these patients, but insulin secretion is usually significantly impaired. Anti-islet cell antibodies may remain for several years after diagnosis, which indicates the potential for ongoing β cell destruction. When β cell reserve is reduced to less than 5% of normal levels, patients usually develop symptoms associated with increased plasma levels of glucose, including polyuria, polydipsia, and polyphagia with weight loss. Diabetes is strictly defined as a glucose level of 200 mg/dL 2 h after eating or a fasting glucose level greater than 126 mg/dL (5). The peak incidence in type 1 diabetes occurs between 11 and 12 yr of age, but the disease may present in older patients because of prolonged autoimmune destruction.

Type 2 diabetes is more prevalent than type 1 and is therefore a more common cause of vascular disease. Like type 1 diabetes, type 2 has a significant genetic component. For example, in identical twins, the concordance rate is 91% (6). The prevalence of type 2 diabetes varies between ethnic groups. Type 2 diabetes develops in 35% of Pima Indians (and in as much as 80% in Pima Indians when both parents have diabetes), which is 10–20 times more frequent than in Caucasian populations (7). Modifying factors such as obesity, hypertension, sedentary lifestyle, and increasing age strongly predispose to the development of type 2 diabetes in genetically susceptible individuals. These factors increase the incidence of insulin resistance in the general nondiabetic population. If β cell function is normal, insulin resistance leads to chronic hyperinsulinemia, which allows those individuals to maintain relatively normal glucose tolerance. However, if insulin secretion becomes impaired, then impaired glucose tolerance develops, followed by overt diabetes. The development of type 2 diabetes in insulin-resistant adults depends on ethnicity and genetic factors. In Caucasians, the rate of progression from impaired glucose tolerance (e.g., fasting glucose >110 mg/dL) to type 2 diabetes is 2% to 6% per year over a 10-year period (8). The loss of the ability to secrete adequate insulin to compensate during this period is caused by acquired β cell toxicity, which results from increased glucose concentrations (9), and by genetic abnormalities (10).

PATHOPHYSIOLOGY

The pathophysiology of type 2 diabetes involves the development of insulin resistance. Factors that predispose individuals to the development of insulin resistance include genetics, obesity, hypertension, stress, and medications. In these patients, the three major sites of glucose metabolism—the liver, fatty tissue, and skeletal muscle—become resistant to the actions of insulin. The liver is the major site of glucose production, and muscle and fat are sites of glucose disposal. When these sites become resistant to the actions of insulin, normal concentrations of glucose cannot be maintained in the bloodstream. Because insulin resistance develops slowly over time, hyperinsulinemia exists for several years before type 2 diabetes develops in most patients. These patients usually develop reduced glucose tolerance manifested by fasting glucose concentrations between 110 and 126 mg/dL and an impaired insulin response to glucose administration; therefore, they secrete less insulin at any given glucose level than normoglycemic subjects (11).

The molecular pathogenesis of insulin resistance is not well defined. Although mutations in the insulin receptor have been described, they are rare (< 0.5% of patients). In addition, anti-insulin and anti-insulin receptor antibodies have rarely been associated with insulin resistance. More than 80% of patients with type 2 diabetes have no defined molecular etiology.

Metabolic abnormalities, such as an increase in free fatty acids, may mediate the progressive loss of insulin sensitivity. The release of free fatty acids increases with the development of obesity. The use of free fatty acids as a source of energy in skeletal muscle impairs glucose use in response to insulin (12). In addition, free fatty acids reduce the ability of insulin to suppress hepatoglucose output. Increased levels of cytokines, seen during sepsis, cirrhosis, and severe illness, can briefly and severely worsen insulin resistance (13).

Most studies indicate that the uptake of insulin from blood vessels and the transport of insulin to peripheral tissues are normal in patients with type 2 diabetes. Furthermore, the binding of insulin is normal in most tissues, which indicates the defect is at a postreceptor level. Many intermediary signaling molecules are activated after the insulin receptor is activated. These intermediary molecules include the insulin receptor substrate (IRS) family of proteins and members of the phosphoinositol (PI)-3 kinase signal transduction family that are necessary for activation of Glut-4, the primary glucose transporter in skeletal muscle and adipose tissue. Genetic defects in several of these proteins have been described as rare causes of type 2 diabetes, but their frequency is low and they do not contribute to etiology in most patients with type 2 diabetes. Skeletal muscle accounts for 80–85% of insulin-mediated uptake of glucose, and studies have shown that this response is markedly impaired in patients with type 2 diabetes (14). Although the uptake of glucose into fat cells is also impaired, insulin resistance in fat contributes much less to the total impairment in peripheral glucose uptake.

A second major site of impaired insulin action is the liver. Glucose output in the liver is usually reduced to levels between 30% and 60% of normal (15). Because the liver is a major source for maintaining nighttime glucose levels, early morning fasting glucose measurements are often significantly increased. In addition, glycogen synthesis in muscle is reduced because of the decreased glucose transport and impaired glucose phosphorylation (16). Free fatty acid levels are increased, which further aggravates insulin resistance in the liver and skeletal muscle. This increase in insulin resistance increases fasting and postprandial plasma insulin concentrations. Chronic elevation of insulin concentrations leads to a rightward shift of the insulin dose–response curve and a reduction in the number of insulin receptors; therefore, higher insulin concentrations are required to maximally stimulate glucose transport in patients with diabetes (17). Secondary causes of insulin insensitivity such as glucocorticoid therapy and acromegaly will result in hyperinsulinemia and a reduction in insulin receptor number. Weight loss in patients with type 2 diabetes improves the ability of insulin to stimulate tyrosine kinase activity of the insulin receptor and partially reverses some of the changes associated with insulin resistance. Although 50 mutations have been identified in the insulin receptor, many are functionally insignificant and they account for less than 1% of all cases

of type 2 diabetes. Levels of the glucose transport protein Glut-4 are reduced in adipose tissue in type 2 diabetics. Glut-4 levels are normal in skeletal muscle, but the ability of insulin to stimulate translocation of Glut-4 to the plasma membrane, which is required for normal muscle glucose transport, is impaired (18). This translocation defect occurs in obesity with insulin resistance before the development of diabetes.

Mutations in Glut-4 are rare causes of type 2 diabetes. The reason for the functional defect in Glut-4 translocation in skeletal muscle has not been determined. Changes in levels of IRS-1 (which regulates Glut-4-dependent translocation) cannot explain this defect because IRS-1 levels are reduced in adipose tissue but not in skeletal muscle. The defect that accounts for resistance to insulin suppression of hepatic glucose output has not been defined. The overproduction in glucose is secondary to increased gluconeogenesis, but the inability of insulin to suppress this process has not been defined at the molecular level. In the postprandial state, the defect in skeletal muscle glucose uptake accounts for most of the increase in plasma glucose (19); 60% to 90% of ingested carbohydrate bypasses the liver, and failure to incorporate this glucose into muscle accounts for the marked increase in blood glucose that occurs after a meal in diabetic individuals (20). Therefore, postprandial hyperglycemia is due primarily to insulin resistance in skeletal muscle (19), whereas in the fasting state suppression of hepatoglucose output is the primary determinant of abnormal glucose levels in type 2 diabetes (21).

Therapy for type 1 diabetes, which involves administration of insulin, is straightforward; however, therapy for type 2 diabetes is difficult because of the lack of drugs that can counteract insulin resistance. Three classes of drugs other than insulin are used: secretogogues, biguanides, and thiazolidinediones. Insulin secretogogues stimulate increased insulin production by β cells. Because insulin production by β cells is usually decreased in patients with type 2 diabetes, secretogogues can help patients maintain glycemic control. Sulfonylureas, the main drug in the secretogogue class, partially reverse the effect of glucotoxicity and the suppression of islet cell function. These drugs are effective in early stages of type 2 diabetes because improving glucose concentrations by increasing insulin secretion may further improve insulin secretion by partially reversing glucose toxicity. The second category of drugs, the biguanides, act primarily at the level of the liver to reverse insulin resistance. The final class, the thiazolidinediones, act on the peroxisome proliferator activated receptor (PPAR) γ receptors to increase insulin sensitivity. The thiazolidinediones lower insulin resistance not only in liver but also in fat and skeletal muscle.

PATHOPHYSIOLOGY OF VASCULAR DISEASE IN DIABETES

Several variables interact to accelerate the development of vascular disease in patients with type 1 and type 2 diabetes. These variables have been studied primarily in patients with type 2 diabetes. The most common secondary abnormality in type 2 diabetes is an altered lipoprotein profile. Although lipoprotein abnormalities confer no greater risk for vascular disease in diabetics than in nondiabetics, the prevalence of lipoprotein abnormalities is much higher in patients with type 2 diabetes than in the general population. At least 80% of diabetics will develop some form of dyslipidemia (8).

Similarly, hypertension, although conferring no greater risk in diabetics than in nondiabetics, is found more frequently in patients with diabetes. Diabetic patients who develop renal failure are almost always hypertensive, and aggressive control of blood pressure in these patients significantly reduces the rate of progression of vascular disease. In addition, hypertension exacerbates insulin resistance and, if present before the development of type 2 diabetes, accelerates disease progression.

High blood glucose levels are epidemiologically linked to the development of vascular disease in diabetics but do not contribute further risk to the effect of insulin resistance. High glucose levels can lead to secondary abnormalities such as glycosylation of lipoproteins, which increases their atherogenic potential. In contrast, insulin resistance as a primary abnormality is a major predisposing factor to the development of vascular disease. The risk is increased in nondiabetic, insulin resistant patients, as well as in diabetic patients.

Platelet and blood coagulation abnormalities are associated with diabetes. Defects in platelet aggregation and adhesion in diabetes increase the predisposition to myocardial infarction. Plasma fibrinogen levels and plasminogen activator inhibitor-I (PAI-1) levels are high in diabetic patients, which can lead to a hypercoagulable state. Finally, diabetic patients, particularly those with renal disease, have increased levels of plasma homocysteine, which can accelerate atherosclerosis.

LIPOPROTEIN ABNORMALITIES

Insulin resistance is usually associated with increased plasma levels of triglycerides and apoplipoprotein-B 100 and decreased levels of high-density lipoprotein (HDL) (22). In addition, evidence indicates an increased formation of small, dense low-density lipoprotein (LDL) particles that carry greater risk for the development of vascular disease

Table 1
Pathophysiological Abnormalities in Diabetes

Lipoprotein Abnormalities*
  Increased triglycerides
  Increased apolipoprotein B-100
  Decreased high-density lipoprotein
  Increased lipoprotein[a]
  Increased small dense low-density lipoprotein
  Glycation of low-density lipoprotein

Abnormalities of Blood Vessel Function
  Decreased release of nitric oxide
  Decreased vasodilatation mediated by nitric oxide
  Increased contractility of arterioles
  Increased vascular response to angiotensin II
  Increased inactivation of nitric oxide

Coagulation Abnormalities
  Increased platelet aggregation
  Increased fibrinogen
  Increased factor VII
  Decreased antithrombin III
  Decreased protein C
  Increased plasminogen activator inhibitor-1

*Seen mainly in type 2 diabetes.

than an increase in the total plasma LDL concentration (23). The development of dyslipidemia in patients with type 1 diabetes is often related to the development of nephropathy. Nephropathy may be associated with increased plasma levels of lipoprotein [a] (Lp[a]), which is an independent risk factor for coronary artery disease (24). The kidneys are involved in the catabolism of Lp[a]; therefore, the clearance of Lp[a] in patients with nephropathy is decreased and plasma concentrations are increased.

Microalbuminuria, an early manifestation of nephropathy, correlates strongly with the presence of vascular disease in diabetics (24). Familial combined hyperlipidemia is often inherited in a manner that is similar to inheritance of the predisposition to type 1 diabetes, and therefore these two diseases often coexist (25).

Type 2 diabetic patients often present with HDL levels that are below 35 mg/dL and triglyceride levels above 200 mg/dL (Table 1). Diabetics are twice as likely to have these changes as the general population. These alterations in lipid levels often occur before the development of hyperglycemia; therefore, the period of exposure to abnormal lipoprotein concentrations is longer than the duration of diabetes. In one study, 14% of middle-aged men with these abnormal lipid concentrations and who had not yet developed diabetes had a coronary event within 8 yr of having abnormal lipid profiles (26). This syndrome, called the metabolic syndrome or syndrome X, is usually accompanied by a waist-to-hip ratio greater than 1.0 in men and greater than 0.85 in women. Factors that induce insulin resistance in these patients are increased release of free fatty acids from adipose tissue and hypersecretion of very low density lipoproteins (VLDL) by the liver (27). Insulin normally stimulates adipocytes to secrete lipoprotein lipase, which hydrolyzes the triglycerides in VLDL and in chylomicrons; therefore, in patients with insulin resistance, hydrolysis is impaired and VLDL levels are increased. In addition, the transfer of cholesterol ester from HDL to VLDL is increased, which affects LDL composition in diabetics. In one theory, the LDL comprises two subfractions: one that contains large particles and one that contains small particles. The small particles are metabolized rapidly by lipoprotein lipase to intermediate-density lipoprotein and then to LDL, whereas the large particles are metabolized directly to small dense LDL, primarily in the liver (28). VLDL apolipoprotein B production is significantly increased in diabetes, and the metabolism of intermediate-density lipoprotein to LDL is decreased; therefore, the concentration of small dense LDL is increased.

Small, dense LDL may be more atherogenic than LDL because of its ability to cross endothelial barriers and deposit in the subendothelial space of medium and small arteries (29). In diabetes, the major abnormality in LDL is its increased oxidation rate. Another important modification is glycation of LDL (30). Abnormally high chronic glucose levels lead to nonenzymatic glycation of LDL, which increases monocyte chemoattraction into the subendothelial space and thus contributes to the progression of atherogenesis (31,32). Finally, sialation of LDL increases its binding to proteoglycans, and, therefore, its atherogenecity. Sialic acid levels in plasma are increased in diabetes, possibly because of the abnormal rates of desylation of LDL. Plasma sailic acid concentrations may predict progression of vascular disease in diabetic patients (33).

Although mean triglyceride levels are higher in diabetics, most patients are not hypertriglyceridemic (33). The prevalence of hypertriglyceridemia is 19% in diabetic men and 17% in diabetic women, whereas the prevalence in nondiabetics is 8% in men and 9% in women (34). The prevalence of low HDL levels is increased in diabetics; low HDL levels are seen in 21% of diabetic men and 25% of diabetic women, whereas only 9% of nondiabetic men and 10% of nondiabetic women have low HDL levels (34). The increased levels

of hepatic lipase seen in diabetics may contribute to the suppression of HDL. Treatment of type 2 diabetes often lowers triglyceride levels and increases HDL concentrations. These benefits can occur even in the presence of weight gain and increased body fat content (35). However, HDL levels may increase with weight loss. Even when hyperglycemia is controlled, low HDL and high triglyceride levels may persist in cases of chronic diabetes; therefore, the abnormal lipid profile may relate more to insulin resistance than the absolute level of glucose.

Conflicting results have been reported in epidemiologic studies of the relative risk of high triglyceride levels for predicting vascular disease. In the Paris prospective study, hypertriglyceridemia predicted increased mortality associated with coronary artery disease in patients with impaired glucose tolerance or diabetes (36). In the Finnish study of patients with diabetes, LDL triglyceride levels correlated positively with the development of coronary artery disease over a 7-year period, and HDL cholesterol was inversely associated with risk for CAD (37). In diabetics, both HDL and triglyceride levels were better predictors of risk for CAD than LDL cholesterol levels. In contrast, in the United Kingdom Progressive Diabetes Study (UKPDS), LDL cholesterol was a better predictor than HDL and triglyceride levels; low HDL was a good predictor, whereas triglycerides were only a weak predictor (38).

Total cholesterol levels are usually normal in diabetics, except in patients with an inherited disorder of LDL catabolism (39). Treatment that improves LDL catabolism increases HDL levels. The increase in LDL that occurs in patients with diabetes is mainly caused by increases in levels of intermediate-density lipoprotein that result from an abnormally high rate of VLDL metabolism (39,40). In this situation, small dense LDL increases (41). LDL particle size is inversely related to hemoglobin A_1C levels in diabetics (39). In addition, increased activity of hepatic lipase contributes to the increase in small dense LDL because remnant VLDL particles are preferentially processed to small dense LDL by hepatic lipase (42).

Lp[a] comprises an LDL linked by a disulfide bond, apolipoprotein a. Lp[a] has increased atherogenic properties and is thrombogenic. Lp[a] levels are increased in type 1 diabetes, but controlling glycemic levels improves Lp[a] concentration (43). The presence of microalbuminuria in patients with type 1 diabetes predicts high Lp[a] levels. Nephropathy accelerates Lp[a] abnormality in patients with diabetes (44). Diabetic patients with microalbuminuria have higher triglyceride and apolipoprotein B levels than diabetic patients without microalbuminuria. The development of macroproteinuria further increases LDL levels and reduces HDL cholesterol *(45)*. The use of prednisone for immunosuppression after renal transplant may accelerate the progression of lipoprotein abnormalities in all transplant patients.

METABOLIC SYNDROME

Increased insulin resistance is the first manifestation of type 2 diabetes. Patients with the metabolic syndrome present with fasting hyperinsulinemia and increased waist-to-hip ratios and also have increased levels of free fatty acids, triglycerides, and small dense LDL, and decreased levels of HDL. In addition, sodium retention and sympathetic nervous system activity are increased, levels of PAI-I and fibrinogen are increased, and hypertension is present *(46)*. VLDL synthesis is markedly increased. The metabolic abnormalities are worsened in the postprandial state, and the increase in triglyceride-rich lipoproteins is exaggerated *(47)*. This increase in triglycerides correlates with the increase in insulin and small dense LDL. These defects exist for several years in patients with metabolic syndrome before diabetes develops and places patients at increased risk for coronary artery disease once diabetes develops. The activation of the sympathetic nervous system in patients with metabolic syndrome leads to an increased heart rate in normotensive patients once diabetes develops *(48)*. Sodium retention is increased in individuals with insulin resistance. The prevalence of hyperinsulinemia, a consequence of insulin resistance, is higher in hypertensive populations with or without diabetes; hypertension is seen in 45% of patients with a fasting insulin level greater than 80 uU/mL but only in 10% of normoinsulinemic subjects *(49)*. Insulin resistance is found in first-degree relatives of hypertensive patients with normotensive siblings, which suggests that insulin resistance and hypertension may be causally related. Many of the abnormalities of the metabolic syndrome that aggravate vascular disease in patients with diabetes are found during the insulin resistant hyperglycemic phase of the disease.

HYPERTENSION

Diabetic patients are twice as likely as nondiabetic patients to develop hypertension, and the chance of developing macrovascular complications is significantly increased in diabetics if systolic blood pressure is high *(50)*. Each 10 mm increase in mean arterial blood pressure is associated with a 15% risk of cardiovascular death for patients with diabetes *(51)*. In type 1 diabetes, nephropathy is often the basis for hypertension. In type 2 diabetes,

vascular expansion occurs and sodium retention increases before a change in renal function occurs. Hyperinsulinemia is associated with a reduction in vascular wall nitric oxide (NO), and loss of NO-mediated vasodilatation increases vascular sensitivity to the effects of sodium *(52)* (Table 1). Interventions that target insulin resistance, such as weight loss, can reduce these vascular abnormalities. Insulin usually increases vascular NO production and sodium pump activity; however, in patients with insulin resistance, both these actions are impaired. Furthermore, mobilization of free calcium by arterial smooth muscle is defective in insulin-resistant patients, which increases contractility and angiotensin II activation. These changes interfere with insulin-mediated PI-3 kinase activation, and insulin resistance worsens *(53)*. Oxidized LDL reduces endothelium-dependent vascular relaxation, and transient postprandial hyperglycemia can increase vascular activity while reducing NO synthesis *(54)*. In addition, glycation of LDL may inactivate NO, and diets rich in oleic acid will improve endothelial dependent vasodilatation in patients with diabetes *(55)*. These findings suggest multiple interactions between hypertension and aggravation of insulin resistance.

GLYCEMIA

Epidemiologic studies indicate a relation between glycemia and the development of myocardial infarction or stroke, irrespective of insulin levels. The UKPDS showed a correlation between hemoglobin A_1C and the development of myocardial infarction and stroke. For each 1% increase in glycosylated hemoglobin, death from myocardial infarction increased by 21%, the rate of myocardial infarction increased by 14%, and stroke increased by 12% *(56)*. However, insulin resistance and hyperglycemia were not differentiated in this study. Other studies have shown a relation between the 2-hour postprandial glucose level and coronary artery disease that is stronger than the relation between fasting glucose and coronary artery disease. These findings suggest the presence of an effect by blood glucose levels that is additional to the effect of insulin levels *(57)*.

The mechanisms that have been proposed to account for the effects of hyperglycemia include endothelial dysfunction, oxidative stress, and glycation of several proteins, including the lipoproteins. High glucose concentrations reduce endothelium-dependent vasodilatation and increase vasoconstriction *(54,58)*. Glycation of LDL increases its ability to penetrate the subendothelial space and induce macrophage infiltration *(59)*. In addition, high glucose levels directly interfere with the ability of endothelium to generate NO. LDL is more likely to become oxidized and therefore more atherogenic in the setting of hyperglycemia. In a large study, a 1% increase in glycated hemoglobin was associated with only a 10% increase in the incidence of coronary artery disease, although the correlation between hemoglobin (HB)A$_1$C and vasculopathy is much weaker than the correlation between HBA$_1$C and the development of retinopathy or nephropathy (60). In UKPDS, increased HBA$_1$C was more reliable for predicting the development of retinopathy than for predicting the development of macrovascular disease (38). None of these studies accounted for the effect of insulin resistance independent of glycemia; therefore, assessing whether glucose had an independent effect on the development of coronary artery disease or on mortality is difficult.

Interest has recently developed in receptor for advanced glycation end products (RAGE), which is a receptor for glycated proteins that is important in removing products of oxidative stress such as oxidized hemoglobin and oxidized LDL (61). Activation of RAGE by advanced glycation end products (AGE) can increase macrophage secretion of inflammatory mediators that accelerate atherogenesis. RAGE is found on cells of the vessel wall, for example, smooth muscle cells, macrophages, and endothelial cells. Therefore, this receptor can modify the pathogenesis of lesion formation and the ability of vessels to respond to normal changes in blood flow and blood pressure (62). In animal models of atherosclerosis, blockade of RAGE suppresses the development of atherogenesis in diabetic and nondiabetic animals. In summary, glycemia is a modest risk factor for atherogenesis.

COAGULATION DISORDERS

Platelet activation and aggregation are increased in patients with diabetes (Table 1). Platelet activity is altered by multiple factors in diabetes, including an increase in the mobilization of platelet calcium and a high turnover of phosphoinositide (63). Some of these changes result from glycation of platelet membrane proteins and decreased NO production by cells of the vessel wall and by platelets. In addition, blood coagulation is increased in diabetics because of increased concentrations of fibrinogen, PAI-I, factor VII, and von Willebrand factor (64). Antithrombotic factors such as antithrombin III and protein C are decreased in hyperglycemic patients. This increased propensity for the development of thrombosis mitigates against the use of hormonal replacement therapy in postmenopausal diabetic women (65). An increase in factor VII is an independent risk factor for cardiovascular disease. Postprandial hyperglycemia and hypertriglyceridemia

seen in diabetics increases the activation of factor VII (66). These changes occur concomitantly with increases in PAI-I, which is one of the first proteins to be increased in the serum of insulin resistant patients. Abnormalities in many of the proteins involved in coagulation often correlate with a higher fatality rate associated with myocardial infarction in diabetics (67). Finally, fibrinogen levels are increased in patients with overt diabetes mellitus. Although fibrinogen is increased in patients with insulin resistance, the correlation between high fibrinogen levels and the development of acute coronary thrombosis is not nearly as strong as the correlation between PAI-1 and thrombosis, which suggests that fibrinogen may be a less important variable (68).

HOMOCYSTEINE

Increased plasma levels of homocysteine may be associated with coronary disease. The prevalence of hyperhomocysteinemia is two to four times higher in diabetics (69). Furthermore, hyperhomocysteinemia is almost always seen in diabetic patients with impaired renal function and may lead to further endothelial damage and loss of NO release (70). In diabetic patients, the increase in homocysteine levels is usually proportionate to the degree of loss of renal function. One large study showed that the odds ratio for development of coronary artery disease in diabetic patients with hyperhomocysteinemia was 6.6, and plasma homocysteine was an independent predictor of coronary artery disease in diabetics but not in nondiabetic patients (71). These findings suggest an interaction between homocysteine and other risk factors for coronary artery disease that are specific for diabetes. Other studies have reported that diabetics, even those without nephropathy, have significantly higher homocysteine levels than nondiabetics. Thus, epidemiologic evidence suggests an interaction between increased homocysteine levels in the presence of diabetes and the prediction of risk for coronary artery disease. However, these data have been obtained in case control studies; large prospective controlled trials or interventional trials are necessary to assess whether lowering homocysteine levels will affect the incidence of coronary artery disease in diabetics.

MECHANISMS OF LESION DEVELOPMENT IN DIABETES

No single molecular mechanism for lesion development in patients with diabetes has been identified; however, several variables that accentuate the underlying inflammatory process in the vessel walls of nondiabetics are also present in diabetics. After the deposition of oxidized

LDL in vessel walls, macrophages infiltrate into the subendothelial space. In patients with diabetes, macrophage activation may be increased because of glycation of LDL and abnormal oxidation rates of LDL (72). Accelerated macrophage activation may result in increased lipid and lipoprotein deposition with excessive release of biologic response modifiers (73). Furthermore, an increase in macrophage expression of scavenger receptors such as CD36 may result in greater oxidized LDL binding and expression of tumor necrosis factor α and interleukin-1β. Proper metabolism of LDL depends on cyclooxygenase-2 induction in macrophages. In diabetes, cyclooxygenase 2 (Cox)-2 is downregulated and this may be another mechanism for prolonging the half-life of oxidized LDL within the vessel wall (74). Oxidized LDL aggravates plaque instability and stimulates metalloproteinase secretion by endothelial cells, which contributes to plaque instability and thrombus formation (75). In addition, oxidized LDL can increase macrophage expression of CCR2, which is a receptor for monocyte chemotactic protein-1 (MCP-1). This increased binding of MCP-1 will increase macrophage penetration into the subendothelial space (76). Furthermore, PPAR γ agonists regulate proinflammatory cytokine gene expression by activated macrophages, which may be one mechanism by which these drugs retard vascular disease progression in diabetes.

Oxidized and glycated LDL forms penetrate the subendothelial space and stimulate the release of multiple cytokines that stimulate recruitment of macrophages and migration of smooth muscle cells. The stimulated macrophages secrete mitogens into the neointima, which causes growth of smooth muscle cells. In addition, AGE-activated monocytes secrete growth factors that stimulate lesion growth. Glycated LDL stimulates mitogen secretion, and chronic hyperglycemia results in increased expression of growth factors such as platelet-derived growth factor, heparin-binding epidermal growth factor, and insulin-like growth factor-1 (77). Moreover, high glucose concentrations increase transcriptional activation of β fibroblast growth factor and transforming growth factor-α in aortic smooth muscle cells (78,79). A glucose response element in the promotor of these genes suggests a direct correlation between increased gene expression and increased glucose levels. In addition, high glucose levels result in increased secretion of vascular endothelial growth factor. Hyperglycemia and hyperinsulinemia increase the synthesis of extracellular matrix components that are deposited into blood vessel walls such as fibronectin and PAI-1 (80). Increased deposition of type IV collagen and heparan-sulfate containing glycosaminoglycans, both of which activate smooth muscle cells, is seen in patients with hyperglycemia and hyperinsulinemia (81). Macrophage growth responses to colony stimulating factor-1 are accentuated in hyperglycemia. Hyperinsulinemia increases sodium potassium exchange, calcium exchange, and sodium potassium ATPase activity in smooth muscle cells (82). Glycation of fibronectin, heparan sulfate proteoglycans, and type I collagen may lead to changes in smooth muscle cell function. Similarly, glycation of MCP-1 and intercellular adhesion molecules may increase monocyte adhesion (83). All of these changes result in stimulation of smooth muscle cell growth and lesion development. Increased inflammatory cell deposition alone may be a risk factor because they contribute to plaque instability and rupture.

IMPLICATIONS FOR THERAPY

Therapy for type 1 diabetes, which involves administration of insulin, is straightforward; however, therapy for type 2 diabetes is difficult because of the lack of drugs that can counteract insulin resistance. Three classes of drugs other than insulin are used: secretogogues, biguanides, and thiazolidinediones. Insulin secretogogues stimulate increased insulin production by β cells. Because insulin production by β cells is usually decreased in patients with type 2 diabetes, secretogogues can help patients maintain glycemic control. Sulfonylureas, the main drug in the secretogogue class, partially reverse the effect of glucotoxicity and the suppression of islet cell function. These drugs are effective in early stages of type 2 diabetes because improving glucose concentrations by increasing insulin secretion may further improve insulin secretion by partially reversing glucose toxicity. The second category of drugs, the biguanides, act primarily at the level of the liver to reverse insulin resistance. The final class, the thiazolidinediones, act on the PPAR γ receptors to increase insulin sensitivity. The thiazolidinediones lower insulin resistance not only in liver but also in fat and skeletal muscle.

Insulin Resistance

Most of the pathophysiologic processes discussed in this chapter are seen in nondiabetic patients; however, some aspects of diabetic pathophysiology merit special consideration in planning a treatment regimen designed to reduce risk factors in diabetic patients. Treatment should focus on reduction of insulin resistance. Specifically, patients should be started on a weight loss and exercise program designed to decrease waist-to-hip ratios, body fat content, and free fatty acid levels (84,85).

Each of these interventions will improve insulin sensitivity and lower the risk of vascular disease. In patients who do not improve on this regimen, the use of insulin sensitizing agents, such as biguanides and peroxisome proliferator activated receptor (PPAR) γ agonists, may be necessary. The efficacy of these drugs in nondiabetic patients with impaired glucose tolerance or insulin resistance is unknown, but patients with overt diabetes will benefit from the addition of these agents. Although PPAR γ agonists are associated with weight gain and increased body fat content, these disadvantages are offset by the beneficial effects of improved insulin sensitivity and reduced monocyte activation (86).

Hyperglycemia

In addition to treating insulin resistance, improving hyperglycemia is important because of the strong association of hemoglobin A_1C with coronary disease outcome. Although difficult to achieve, target values for hemoglobin A_1C in patients with abnormal lipid profiles should be less than 7%. New insulin-sensitizing drugs may be helpful in reaching this goal. However, many patients will require intensive therapy with insulin which may result in weight gain and worsening of lipoprotein profiles in some patients; therefore, the benefits and disadvantages of intensive insulin therapy should be carefully considered (87). Whether the high insulin levels required to achieve glycemic control are a primary risk factor for coronary artery disease has not been determined.

Lipoprotein Abnormalities

The goal in treating lipoprotein abnormalities is to reduce triglyerides, increase HDL levels, and lower LDL levels. Because of the increased risk of coronary disease associated with the interaction between diabetes and high LDL cholesterol, statins are important in drug therapy. Although LDL cholesterol is greater than120 μg/dL in only a small percentage of patients, the five large studies that have assessed the benefit of lowering LDL cholesterol in diabetics have found a beneficial effect (88–92). The American Heart Association (AHA) and the American Diabetes Association (ADA) recommendations are based on results from these trials, and both agencies recommend LDL cholesterol levels of less than 100 mg/dL for primary prevention therapy (93,94). Targeting LDL levels is recommended as the first priority probably because of the lack of availability of drugs other than fibrates that increase HDL cholesterol and lower trigylcerides. Because of these recommendations statins will be used as a first line therapy in most patients.

Triglyceride levels are increased and HDL levels are reduced in most diabetics; therefore, physicians should consider combination therapy with fibrates rather than statins only, particularly in patients with a fasting HDL below 30 mg/dL. Fibrates moderately increase HDL cholesterol and lower LDL cholesterol and triglycerides (95). The effect of fenofibrate on coronary artery progression was recently studied in a large trial of 731 patients with type 2 diabetes who were assigned to treatment with 200 mg/day of fenofibrate or placebo (96). Angiographic findings showed that stenosis associated with coronary artery disease was significantly smaller in the fenofibrate group than in the placebo group. In addition, HDL cholesterol was increased 8% in fenofibrate patients and only 0.5% in placebo patients, whereas total cholesterol was reduced 10% in fenofibrate patients and was unchanged in the placebo group. Triglycerides were reduced by 30% in the treatment group. Although clinical endpoints were not examined, the trial clearly showed that treatment with fenofibrate substantially improved HDL cholesterol levels and reduced progression of atherosclerotic lesions. The authors concluded that patients with type 2 diabetes should be treated with fenofibrate even if only minimal abnormalities in lipoproteins are found on baseline evaluation. Fibrates remain the best therapeutic choice under these circumstances. The ADA recommends treatment of patients with HDL levels less than 35 mg/dL, and the AHA recommends treatment of patients with HDL levels less than 45 mg/dL.

Nicotinic acid is another treatment option that increases HDL levels. However, nicotinic acid can worsen carbohydrate intolerance, and patients with diabetes, even mild diabetes, should be monitored because the underlying disease may be significantly exacerbated by treatment with nicotinic acid. The major problem with using fibric acid derivatives in conjunction with statins is myositis, drug-induced muscle inflammation, which may occur in as many as 5% of patients taking lovastatin and gemfibrozil (97). However, the risk of myositis is probably lower than 5% in patients without renal failure. Patients with renal disease should not be treated with this drug combination. Muscle enzymes should be monitored at frequent intervals during the first six months of therapy in patients in whom combination therapy is used. The treatment of hypertriglyceridemia alone has not been adequately studied. Triglyceride levels can be lowered with weight loss, decreased alcohol consumption, and increased physical exercise. In addition, patients with triglyceride levels greater than 500 mg/dL should restrict dietary fat to less than 10% of total calories to reduce the risk of pancreatitis. However, primary drug treatment in patients with triglyceride levels between 200 and 500 mg/dL to lower the risk for vascular disease has not proved to be beneficial. Statins may help lower triglyceride levels, particularly in patients with significantly high levels. Patients with triglyceride levels from 200–500 mg/dL range will benefit from fibrate therapy, and if HDL levels are low in patients with very high triglyceride levels, fibrate therapy should be considered as the primary form of therapy.

Hypertension

Lowering blood pressure, particularly systolic pressure, is beneficial in patients with diabetes and hypertension. In UKPDS, by adding either the ACE inhibitor captopril or the β blocker atenolol, the incidence of stroke was reduced by 44% (38). Death was reduced by 32% by both drugs. Although both drugs were equally effective, ACE inhibitors may be considered as the primary therapy because of previously mentioned theoretical reasons. In the Heart Outcomes Prevention Evaluation (HOPE) study, treatment with ramapril reduced the risk of myocardial infarction by 22% and the incidence of stroke by 33% in all patients, even though mean arterial pressure was lowered by only 2.4 mm (98). Because of their nephroprotective effect, ACE inhibitors should be the drug of choice for treating hypertension in patients with microalbuminuria. In addition, ACE inhibitors have the theoretical benefit of improving insulin resistance because angiotension II induces resistance by inhibiting the ability of insulin to activate the PI-3 kinase pathway as outlined previously (99). Furthermore, ACE inhibitors improve blood flow to muscle and lower triglyceride and free fatty acid levels, and all three of these actions improve insulin sensitivity. By counteracting some of the effect of insulin resistance on endothelial NO production and action and by reducing oxidative stress, ACE inhibitors reduce the levels of oxidized LDL. In summary, ACE inhibitors are the drug of choice in patients with microalbuminuria and should be strongly considered as first-line therapy for hypertension in diabetic patients without microalbuminuria.

Hypertension often develops early in patients with type 1 diabetes, and the onset of microalbuminuria often precedes the development of hypertension. Most physicians recommend treating microalbuminuria with an ACE inhibitor independently of an increase in blood pressure (100). Aggressive therapy with ACE inhibitors should be initiated as soon as hypertension develops in patients with microalbuminuria. In patients with advancing nephropathy (e.g., creatinine >2.0 mg/dL), three- and four-drug therapy is often required to reduce blood pressure;

aggressive therapy is warranted to attenuate the decline in renal function and the development of vascular abnormalities. In patients with labile hypertension, β blockers are important in maintaining normal blood pressure; however, β blockers can alter autonomic responses that alert patients to the hypoglycemic state and should be used with caution in patients who are treated with insulin. In patients treated with oral agents, β blockers are an important second-line drug after the initiation of ACE inhibitors to control blood pressure.

Homocysteinemia

The identification of hyperhomocysteinemia as an important problem, particularly in type 1 diabetics with nephropathy, has led to a resurgence in the use of folate to control homocysteine levels (101). Prospective trials assessing the efficacy of folate in reducing vascular events have not been completed; however, the excellent safety profile and the low cost of therapy warrants consideration of the use of folate in all patients.

Platelet Abnormalities

Although specific antithrombotic therapies are not recommended, the daily ingestion of aspirin in patients with longstanding diabetes, particularly diabetes with nephropathy, is important. Aspirin is clearly beneficial in preventing myocardial infarction in patients with established diabetes (1). No specific therapy is recommended to treat increased procoagulant activity; however, postmenopausal women with type 2 diabetes should avoid hormone replacement therapy (65). Hormone replacement therapy can be considered if levels of protein C, antithrombin-III, and factor-VIII are normal; estrogen therapy should be avoided in patients with abnormal levels of any of these factors.

ACKNOWLEDGMENTS

The author wishes to thank Ms. Laura Lindsey for her help in preparing the manuscript.

This work was supported by grants from the National Institutes of Health HL56850 and HL 69067.

REFERENCES

1. Haffner SM, Lehto S, Ronnemaa T, Pyorala K, Laakso M. Mortality from coronary heart disease in subjects with type 2 diabetes and in nondiabetic patients with and without prior myocardial infarction. N Engl J Med 1998;339:229–234.
2. Schranz D, Lernmark A. Immunology in diabetes: an update. Diabetes Metab Rev 1998;14:3–29.
3. Nepom GT, Kwok WW. Molecular basis for HLA-DQ associations with IDDM. Diabetes 1998;47:1177–1184.

4. Yoon JW, Austin M, Onodera T, Notkins AL. Isolation of a virus from the pancreas of a child with diabetic ketoacidosis. N Engl J Med 1979;300:1173–1179.

5. Report of the Expert Committee on the Diagnosis and Classification of Diabetes Mellitus. Diabetes Care 1997;20: 1183–1197.

6. Barnett AH, Eff C, Leslie RD, Pyke DA. Diabetes in identifical twins: A study of 200 pairs. Diabetologia 1981;20:87–93.

7. Knowler WC, Bennett PH, Pettit D, Pettitt DJ, Savage PJ, Bennett PH. Diabetes incidence in Pima indians: contributions of obesity and parental diabetes. Am J Epidemol 1981; 113:144–156.

8. Alberti KG. The clinical implications of impaired glucose intolerance. Diabet Med 1996;13:927:937.

9. Leahy JL, Bonner-Weir S, Weir GC. Beta-cell dysfunction induced by chronic hyperglycemia. Current ideas on mechanism of impaired glucose-induced insulin secretion. Diabetes Care 1992;15:442–455.

10. Pimenta W, Korytkowski M, Mitrakou A, et al. Pancreatic beta-cell dysfunction as the primary genetic lesion in NIDDM. Evidence from studies in normal glucose-tolerant individuals with a first-degree NIDDM relative. JAMA 1995;273:1855–1861.

11. Polonsky KS, Sturis J, Bell GI. Seminars in Medicine of the Beth Israel Hospital, Boston. Non-insulin dependent diabetes mellitus — a genetically programmed failure of the beta cell to compensate for insulin resistance. N Engl J Med 1996;34: 777–783.

12. Rebrin K, Steil GM, Getty L, Bergman RN. Free fatty acid as a link in the regulation of hepatic glucose output by peripheral insulin. Diabetes 1995;44:1038–1045.

13. Lang CH, Dobrescu C, Bagby GJ. Tumour necrosis factor impairs insulin action on peripheral glucose disposal and hepatic glucose output. Endocrinology 1992;130:43–52.

14. Edelman SV, Laakso M, Wallace P, Brechtel G, Olefsky JM, Baron AD. Kinetics of insulin-mediated and non-insulin-mediated glucose uptake in humans. Diabetes 1990;39:955–964.

15. Dinneen S, Gerich J, Rizza R. Carbohydrate metabolism in non-insulin-dependent diabetes mellitus. N Engl J Med 1992; 327:707–713.

16. Kelley DE, Mokan M, Mandarino LJ. Intracellular defects in glucose metabolism in obese patients with NIDDM. Diabetes 1992;41:698–706.

17. Thies RS, Molina JM, Ciaraldi TP, Freidenberg GR, Olefsky JM. Insulin receptor autophosphorylation and endogenous substrate phosphorylation in human adipocytes from control, obese, and NIDDM subjects. Diabetes 1990;39:250–259.

18. Kelley DE, Mintun MA, Watkins SC, et al. The effect of non-insulin-dependent diabetes mellitus and obesity on glucose transport and phosphorylation in skeletal muscle. J Clin Invest 1996;97:2705–2713.

19. DeFronzo RA, Jacot E, Jequier E, Maeder E, Wahren J, Felber JP. The effect of insulin on the disposal of intravenous glucose. Results from indirect calorimetry and hepatic and femoral venous catheterization. Diabetes 1981;30:1000–1007.

20. Huang SW, Haedt LH, Rich S, Barbosa J. Prevalence of antibodies to nucleic acids in insulin-dependent diabetes and their relatives. Diabetes 1981;30:873–874.

21. Consoli A, Nurjhan N, Reilly JJ, Bier DM, Gerich JE. Mechanism of increase gluconeogenesis in noninsulin-dependent diabetes mellitus. Role of alterations in systemic, hepatic, and muscle lactate and alanine metabolism. J Clin Invest 1990;86:2038–2045.

22. Wilson PW, Kannel WB, Anderson KM. Lipids, glucose intolerance and vascular disease: the Framingham Study. Monogr Atheroscler 1985;13:1–11.

23. Barakat HA, Carpenter JW, McLendon VD, et al. Influence of obesity, impaired glucose tolerance, and NIDDM on LDL structure and composition. Possible link between hyperinsulinemia and atherosclerosis. Diabetes 1990;39:1527–1533.

24. McKenna K, Thompson C. Microalbuminuria: a marker to increased renal and cardiovascular risk in diabetes mellitus. Scott Med J 1997;42:99–104.

25. Abbate SL, Brunzell JD. Pathophysiology of hyperlipidemia in diabetes mellitus. J Cardiovasc Pharmacol 1990;16:S1–S7.

26. Stamler J, Vaccaro O, Neaton JD, Wentworth D. Diabetes, other risk factors, and 12-yr cardiovascular mortality for men screened in the Multiple Risk Factor Intervention Trial. Diabetes Care 1993;16:434–444.

27. Reaven GM. Banting lecture 1988. Role of insulin resistance in human disease. Diabetes 1988;37:1595–1607.

28. Brunzell JD, Hokanson JE. Low-density and high-density lipoprotein subspecies and risk for premature coronary artery disease. Am J Med 1999;107:16S–18S.

29. Anber V, Griffin BA, McConnell M, Packard CJ, Shepherd J. Influence of plasma lipid and LDL-subfraction profile on the interaction between low density lipoprotein with human arterial wall proteoglycans. Atherosclerosis 1996;124:261–271.

30. Bowie A, Owens D, Collins P, Johnson A, Tomkin GH. Glycosylated low density lipoprotein is more sensitive to oxidation: implications for the diabetic patient? Atherosclerosis 1993;102:63–67.

31. Rajavashisth TB, Liso JK, Galis ZS, et al. Inflammatory cytokines and oxidized low density lipoproteins increase endothelial cell expression of membrane type 1-matrix metalloproteinase. J Biol Chem 1999;274:11924–11929.

32. Xu XP, Meisel SR, Ong JM, et al. Oxidized low-density lipoprotein regulates matrix metalloproteinase-9 and its tissue inhibitor in human monocyte-derived macrophages. Circulation 1999;99:993–998.

33. Crook MA, Pickup JC, Lumb PJ, et al. Relationships between plasma sialic acid concentration and microvascular and macrovascular complications in type 1 diabetes. Diabetes Care. 2001;24:316–22.

34. Miettinen H, Lehto S, Salomaa V, et al. Impact of diabetes on mortality after the first myocardial infarction. The FINMONICA Myocardial Infarction Register Study Group. Diabetes Care 1998;21:69–75.

35. Haffner SM. Management of dyslipidemia in adults with diabetes. Diabetes Care 1998;21:160–178.

36. Fontbonne A, Eschwege E, Cambien F, et al. Hypertriglyceridemia as a risk factor of coronary heart disease mortality in subjects with impaired glucose tolerance or diabetes. Diabetologia 1989;32:300–304.

37. Laakso M, Lehto S, Penttila I, Pyorala K. Lipids and lipoproteins predicting coronary heart disease mortality and morbidity in patients with non-insulin-dependent diabetes. Circulation 1993;99:1421–1430.

38. Turner RC, Millns H, Neil HA, et al. Risk factors for coronary artery disease in non-insulin dependent diabetes mellitus: United Kingdom Prospective Diabetes Study (UKPDS: 23), B M J 1998;316:823–828.

39. Okumura K, Matsui H, Kawakami K, et al. Low density lipoprotein particle size is associated with glycosylated hemoglobin levels regardless of plasma lipid levels. Intern Med 1998;37:273–279.

40. Siegel RD, Cupples A, Schaefer EJ, Wilson PW. Lipoproteins, apolipoproteins, and low-density lipoprotein size among diabetics in the Framingham offspring study. Metabolism 1996;45:1267–1272.

41. Feingold KR, Grunfeld C, Pang M, Doerrler W, Krauss RM. LDL subclass phenotypes and triglyceride metabolism in non-insulin-dependent diabetes. Arterioscler Thromb 1992; 12:1496–1502.

42. Taskinen MR. Lipoprotein lipase in diabetes. Diabetes Metab Rev 1987;3:551–570.

43. Haffner SM. Lipoprotein(a) and diabetes. An update. Diabetes Care 1993;16:835–840.

44. Jenkins AJ, Steele JS, Janus ED, Best JD. Increased plasma apoliporotein (a) levels in IDDM patients with microalbuminuria. Diabetes 1991;40:787–790.

45. Joven J, Villabona C, Vilella E. Pattern of hyperlipoproteinemia in human nephrotic syndrome: influence of renal failure and diabetes mellitus. Nephron 1993;64:565–569.

46. Haffner SM, Valdez RA, Hazuda HP, Mitchell BD, Morales PA, Stern MP. Prospective analysis of the insulin-resistance syndrome (syndrome X). Diabetes 1992;41:715–722.

47. Kuusisto J, Mykkanen L, Pyorala K, Laakso M. NIDDM and its metabolic control predict coronary heart disease in elderly subjects. Diabetes 1994;43:960–967.

48. Reaven GM, Lithell H, Landsberg L. Hypertension and associated metabolic abnormalities—the role of insulin resistance and the sympathoadrenal system. N Engl J Med 1996;334:374–381.

49. Zavaroni I, Mazza S, Dall'Aglio E, Gasparini P, Passeri M, Reaven GM. Prevalence of hyperinsulinaemia in patients with high blood pressure. J Intern Med 1992;231:235–240.

50. Gress, TW, Nieto FJ, Shahar E, Wofford MR, Brancati FL. Hypertension and antihypertensive therapy as risk factors for type 2 diabetes mellitus. Atherosclerosis Risk in Communities Study. N Engl J Med 2000;342:905–912.

51. Adler, AI, Stratton IM, Neil HA, et al. Association of systolic blood pressure with macrovascular and microvascular complications of type 2 diabetes (UKPDS 36): prospective observational study. B M J 2000;321:412–419.

52. Sowers JR, Draznin B. Insulin, cation metabolism and insulin resistance. J Basic Clin Physiol Pharmacol 1998;9:223–233.

53. Zeng G, Quon MJ. Insulin-stimulated production of nitric oxide is inhibited by wortmannin. Direct measurement in vascular endothelial cells. J Clin Invest 1996;98:894–898.

54. Williams SB, Goldfine AB, Timimi FK, et al. Acute hyperglycemia attenuates endothelium-dependent vasodilation in humans in vivo. Circulation 1998;97:1695–1701.

55. Hogan M, Cerami A, Bucala R. Advanced glycosylation endproducts block the antiproliferative effects of nitric oxide. Role in the vascular and renal complications of diabetes mellitus. J Clin Invest 1992;90:1110–1115.

56. Stratton IM, Adler AI, Neil HA, et al. Association of glycaemia with macrovascular and microvascular complications of type 2 diabetes (UKPDS 35): prospective observational study. B M J 2000;321:405–412.

57. de Vegt F, Dekker JM, Ruhe HG, et al. Hyperglycaemia is associated with all-cause and cardiovascular mortality in the Hoorn population: the Hoorn Study. Diabetologi 1999;42:926–931.

58. Chan NN, Vallance P, Colhoun HM. Nitric oxide and vascular responses in Type 1 diabetes. Diabetologi 2000;43:137–147.

59. Witztum JL, Mahoney EM, Branks MJ, Fisher M, Elam R, Steinberg D. Nonezymatic glycosylation of low-density lipoprotein alters its biologic activity. Diabetes 1982;31:283–291.

60. Klein R. Hyperglycemia and microvascular and macrovascular disease in diabetes. Diabetes Care 1995;18:258–268.

61. Schmidt AM, Stern DM. RAGE: a new target for the prevention and treatment of the vascular and inflammatory complications of diabetes. Trends Endocrinol Metab 2000;11:368–375.

62. Vlassara H. The AGE-receptor in the pathogenesis of diabetic complications. Diabetes Metab Res Rev 2001;17:436–443.

63. Schaeffer G, Wascher TC, Kostner GM, Graier WF. Alterations in platelet Ca2+ signalling in diabetic patients is due to increased formation of superoxide anions and reduced nitric oxide production. Diabetologia 1999;42:167–176.

64. Sowers JR, Lester MA. Diabetes and cardiovascular disease. Diabetes Care 1999;22:C14–C20.

65. Sowers JR. Diabetes mellitus and cardiovascular disease in women. Arch Intern Med 1998;158:617–621.

66. Junker R, Heinrich J, Schulte H, van de Loo J, Assmann G. Coagulation factor VII and the risk of coronary heart disease in healthy men. Arterioscler Thromb Vasc Biol 1997;17:1539–1544.

67. Hamsten A, de Faire U, Walldius G, et al. Plasminogen activator inhibitor in plasma: risk factor for recurrent myocardial infarction. Lancet 1987;2:3–9.

68. Landin K, Tengborn L, Smith U. Elevated fibrinogen and plasminogen activator (PAI-1) in hypertension are related to metabolic risk factors for cardiovascular disease. J Intern Med 1990;227:273–278.

69. Smulders YM, Rakic M, Slaats EH, et al. Fasting and postmethionine homocysteine levels in NIDDM. Determinants and correlations with retinopathy, albuminuria, and cardiovascular disease. Diabetes Care 1999;22:125–132.

70. Hofmann MA, Kohl B, Zumbach MS, et al. Hyperhomocyst(e)inemia and endothelial dysfunction in IDDM. Diabetes Care 1998;21:841–848.

71. Hoogeveen EK, Kostense PJ, Jakobs C, et al. Hyperhomocysteinemia increases risk of death, especially in type 2 diabetes: 5-year follow up of the Hoorn study. Circulation 2000;101:1506–1511.

72. Tribe RM, Poston L. Oxidative stress and lipids in diabetes: a role in endothelium vasodilator dysfunction? Vasc Med 1996;1:195–206.

73. Feener EP, King GL. Vascular dysfunction in diabetes mellitus. Lancet 1997;350:SI9–SI13.

74. Kol A, Sukhova GK, Lichtman AH, Libby P. Chlamydial heat shock protein 60 localizes in human atheroma and regulates macrophage tumor necrosis factor-alpha and matrix mellatoproteinase expression. Circulation 1998;98:300–307.

75. Huang Y, Mironova M, Lopes-Virella MF. Oxidized LDL stimulates matrix metalloproteinase-1 expression in human vascular endothelial cells. Arterioscler Thromb Vasc Biol 1999;19:2640–2647.

76. Han KH, Tangirala RK, Green SR, Quehenberger O. Chemokine receptor CCR2 expression and monocyte chemoattractant protein-1 mediated chemotaxis in human monocytes. A regulatory role for plasma LDL. Arterioscler Thromb Vasc Biol 1998;18:1983–1991.

77. Kirstein M, Aston C, Hintz R, Vlassara H. Receptor-specific induction of insulin-like growth factor I in human monocytes by advanced glycosylation end product-modified proteins. J Clin Invest 1992;90:439–446.

78. McClain DA, Patterson AJ, Roos MD, Wei X, Kudlow JE. Glucose and glucosamine regulate growth factor gene expression in vascular smooth muscle cells. Proc Natl Acad Sci USA 1992;89:8150–8154.

79. Murphy PR, Sato Y, Sato R, Friesen HG. Regulation of multiple basic fibroblast growth factor messenger ribonucleic acid transcripts by protein kinase C activators. Mol Endocrinol 1988;2:1196–1201.

80. Nordt TK, Sawa H, Fujii S, Sobel BE. Induction of plasminogen activator inhibitor type-1 (PAI-1) by proinsulin and insulin in vivo. Circulation 1995;91:764–770.

81. Heickendorff L, Ledet T, Rasmussen LM. Glycosaminoglycans in the human aorta in diabetes mellitus: a study of tunica media from areas with and without atherosclerotic plaque. Diabetologia 1994;37:286–292.

82. Sowers JR. Effects of insulin and IGF-I on vascular smooth muscle glucose and cation metabolism. Diabetes 1996;45:S47–S51.

83. O'Brien KD, Allen MD, McDonald TO, et al. Vascular cell adhesion molecule-1 is expressed in human coronary atherosclerotic plaques. Implications for the mode of progression of advanced coronary atherosclerosis. J Clin Invest 1993;92:945–951.

84. American Diabetes Association. Nutrition recommendations and principles for people with diabetes mellitus. Diabetes Care 2000;23:S43–S46.

85. Mayer-Davis EJ, D'Agostino RJ, Karter AJ et al. Intensity and amount of physical activity in relation to insulin sensitivity: the Insulin Resistance Atherosclerotic Study. JAMA 1998;279:669–674.

86. Olefsky JM, Saltiel AR. PPAR and the treatment of insulin resistance. Trends Endocrinol Metab 2000;11:362–368.

87. Henry RR, Gumbiner B, Ditzler T, Wallace P, Lyon R, Glauber HS. Intensive conventional insulin therapy for type II diabetes. Metabolic effects during a 6-mo outpatient trial. Diabetes Care 1993;16:21–31.

88. Pyorala K, Pedersen TR, Kjekshus J, Faergeman O, Olsson AG, Thorgeirsson G. Cholesterol lowering with simvastatin improves prognosis of diabetic patients with coronary heart disease. A subgroup analysis of the Scandinavian Simvastatin Survival Study (4S). Diabetes Care 1997;20:614–620.

89. Haffner S, Alexander CM, Cook TJ, et al. Reduced coronary events in simvastatin-treated patients with coronary heart disease and diabetes or impaired fasting glucose levels: subgroup analyses in the Scandinavian Simvastatin Survival Study. Arch Intern Med 1999;159:2661–2667.

90. Goldberg RB, Mellies MJ, Sacks FM, et al. Cardiovascular events and their reduction with pravastatin in diabetic and glucose-intolerant myocardial infarction survivors with average cholsterol levels: subgroup analyses in the cholesterol and recurrent events (CARE) trial. The Care Investigators. Circulation 1998;98:2513–2519.

91. Prevention of cardiovascular events and death with pravastatin in patients with coronary heart disease and a broad range of initial cholesterol levels. The Long-Term Intervention with Pravastatin in Ischaemic Disease (LIPID) Study Group. N Engl J Med 1998;339:1349–1357.

92. Downs JR, Clearfield M, Weis S et al. Primary prevention of acute coronary events with lovastatin in men and women with average cholesterol levels: results of AFCAPS/TexCAPS. Air Force/Texas Coronary Atherosclerosis Prevention Study. JAMA 1998;279:1615–1622.

93. Grundy SM, Benjamin IJ, Burke GL, et al. Diabetes and cardiovascular disease: a statement for healthcare professionals from the American Heart Association. Circulation 1999;100: 1134–1146.

94. American Diabetes Association. Management of dyslipidemia in adults with diabetes. Diabetes Care 2000;23:S57–S60.

95. Koskinen P, Manttari M, Manninen V, Huttunen JK, Heinonen OP, Frick MH. Coronary heart disease incidence in NIDDM patients in the Helsinki Heart Study. Diabetes Care 1992;15:820–825.

96. Effect of fenofibrate on progression of coronary-artery disease in type 2 diabetes: the Diabetes Atherosclerotic Intervention Study, a randomised study. Lancet 2001;357:905–910.

97. Pierce LR, Wysowski DK, Gross TP. Myopathy and rhabdomyolosis associated with lovastatin-gemfibrozil combination therapy. JAMA 1990;264:71–75.

98. The Heart Outcomes Prevention Evaluation Study Investigators. Effects of an angiotensin-converting-enzyme inhibitor, ramipril, on cardiovascular events in high-risk patients. N Engl J Med 2000;342:145–153.

99. McFarlane SI, Banerji M. Sowers JR. Insulin resistance and cardiovascular disease. J Clin Endocrinol Metab 2001;96:713–718.

100. Lewis EJ, Hunsicker LG, Bain RP, Rohde RD. The effect of angiotensin-converting enzyme inhibition on diabetic nephropathy. The Collaborative Study Group. N Engl J Med 1993;329:1456–1462.

101. Jacques PF, Selhub J, Bostom AG, Wilson PW, Rosenberg IH. The effect of folic acid fortification on plasma folate and total homocysteine concentrations. N Engl J Med 1999;340: 1449–1454.

32   Vascular Inflammation as a Cardiovascular Risk Factor

Allan R. Brasier, MD, Adrian Recinos III, PhD, and Mohsen S. Eledrisi, MDS

CONTENTS

INTRODUCTION

Basic and epidemiologic studies indicate that vascular inflammation is an independent risk factor for the development of atherosclerosis. Otherwise healthy patients with chronic increases in circulating interleukin-6 (IL-6) or its biomarkers, the hepatic acute-phase reactants, are at increased risk for the development and progression of atherosclerosis. Epidemiologic studies indicate that vascular inflammation is a risk independent of those produced by conventional factors including serum lipids, smoking, family history, or hypertension. This finding suggests that vascular inflammation may have a separate mechanistic role in atherogenesis. In fact, the basic process underlying atherosclerosis is inflammatory and depends on continuous recruitment of circulating monocytes into the vessel wall in response to cytokines released by the atherosclerotic plaque. In the absence of other inflammatory processes, the detection of increased circulating IL-6 or its biomarkers can indicate subclinical vascular inflammation. The primary underlying causes of increased vascular IL-6 secretion are probably multifactorial and are incompletely characterized.

Vascular inflammation can result from various processes such as endovascular infection, direct injury through deposition of oxidized lipoproteins, increased reactive oxygen species (ROS) formation through local actions of angiotensin II or thrombin, or a combination of these. Regardless of the underlying initiating event, vascular wall-produced IL-6 has important local and systemic cardiovascular actions that increase the atherosclerotic process. IL-6 induces the hepatic synthesis of acute-phase reactant proteins, which have pro-atherogenic properties.

In this chapter, we will review the mechanisms of vascular inflammation and the vascular cytokine cascade. We will examine the local and systemic actions of IL-6 and how it induces expression of important cardioregulatory molecules including C-reactive protein (CRP), serum amyloid A (SAA), fibrinogen, and angiotensinogen (AGT). In addition, we will discuss epidemiological evidence linking each acute-phase reactant to atherosclerotic risk and the current clinical methods for measuring vascular inflammation. Finally, we will describe therapeutic agents used to reduce vascular inflammation.

From: *Contemporary Cardiology: Principles of Molecular Cardiology*
Edited by: M. S. Runge and C. Patterson © Humana Press Inc., Totowa, NJ

THE INFLAMMATORY PROCESS OF ATHEROSCLEROSIS

Ross initially proposed that atherosclerosis is initiated as a result of injury (denudation) to the vascular endothelial lining (1). This "response to injury hypothesis" has recently been modified to state that the initiating event in atherosclerosis produces endothelial "dysfunction" in which pre-atherosclerotic vessels undergo a paradoxical vasoconstrictive response to exogenously administered acetylcholine. This response probably reflects abnormalities in nitric oxide tone (2). Endothelial dysfunction/atherosclerosis can be induced by several agents including endovascular infection (with the β herpes virus, cytomegalovirus, *Helicobacter pylori*, or the obligate intracellular parasite, *Chlamydia trachomatis*), vascular toxicity initiated by smoking, increased low density lipoprotein (LDL) cholesterol, hypertension, or increased plasma homocysteine (2,3). LDL cholesterol, identified as a major cause of injury to the endothelium, is the focus of multiple therapeutic interventions (2,4).

Although initial endothelial injury is required to initiate the process of atherosclerosis, atherosclerosis also involves a series of coordinated cellular and molecular events characteristic of inflammation (Fig. 1). The first pathological manifestation of atherosclerosis, the fatty streak, is an inflammatory reaction that comprises lipid, monocytes, and T lymphocytes that have been recruited into the subendothelial space. In hypercholesterolemia, mononuclear cells are recruited into the vessel wall to phagocytose LDL. Lipid-laden macrophages become foam cells, a hallmark of the early atherosclerotic lesion. Oxidized LDL particles, preferentially internalized by macrophages and further oxidized into lipid peroxides, become potent signaling compounds that attract additional monocytes. In fatty streaks destined to become atherosclerotic plaques, the continuous recruitment of monocytes and T cells and the proliferation of smooth muscle cells in response to increased production of ROS give rise to established fibro-fatty plaques.

Mononuclear cell recruitment into the vascular lesion depends on the endothelial cell surface and gradients of chemotactic cytokines produced by cells of the vessel wall. Endothelial cells overlying active vascular lesions are activated in response to cytokines and the effects of local ROS production related to LDL oxidation. These activated endothelial cells express receptors such as E-selectin and vascular cell adhesion molecules (VCAMs). Circulating monocytes interacting with these cell surface adhesion molecules are induced to roll along the endothelium. Leukocytes extravasate when this low affinity, selectin-mediated interaction is converted into high affinity, integrin-mediated interactions via chemotactic cytokine (chemokine) gradients released from monocytes and smooth muscle cells residing within the vessel wall.

In addition to mononuclear cell recruitment, a prominent pathological feature of atherosclerosis is vascular smooth muscle cell (VSMC) proliferation at the site of the lesion (1). Local production of ROS and growth factors, including angiotensin II and thrombin, induce migration and proliferation of smooth muscle cells and formation of fibrous tissue. In established plaques, resident inflammatory mononuclear leukocytes and activated smooth muscle cells express several peptide molecules, including IL-6, monocyte chemotactic protein-1 (MCP-1), macrophage-derived chemokine, and fractalkine, and growth factors, such as platelet derived growth factor (PDGF), insulin-like growth factor (IGF), and fibroblast growth factor (2). Local (paracrine) actions of this environment enriched with cytokines, growth factors and ROS lead to the formation of the advanced "complicated" lesion. These large fibro-fatty plaques eventually become unstable and rupture, producing thrombosis or aneurysmal dilatation. Plaque rupture primarily occurs at the edge of the fibrous cap in areas of accumulated inflammatory cells, macrophages, T lymphocytes, and mast cells. Activated inflammatory cells may stimulate the erosion of extracellular matrix through the release of proteases or the induction of critical structural cells (5,6). Because the atherosclerotic lesion is initiated and maintained through an orchestrated inflammatory cellular response involving chemotactic cytokines and growth factors, atherosclerosis is clearly a form of chronic inflammation.

THE VASCULAR CYTOKINE CASCADE

Cytokines produced during atherogenesis have important local (paracrine) and systemic (endocrine) actions. Local actions include the induction of leukocyte chemotaxis and activation and differentiation of monocytes, vascular smooth muscle cells, and endothelial cells. The cytokines, interleukin-1 (IL-1), tumor necrosis factor (TNF), and interferon-γ are activating peptides and are released mainly by activated immune and mononuclear cells. These cytokines induce adhesion molecule, cytokine, and chemokine expression by resident non-immune cells; these downstream peptides coordinate the cellular response to injury and are responsible for recruiting leukocyte subsets into the vessel wall. Activating cytokines induce expression of the leukocyte adhesion molecules, VCAM-1, intercellular adhesion molecule-1 (ICAM-1), and E-selectin by adjacent endothelial cells and VSMCs. Many downstream chemokines and cytokines are

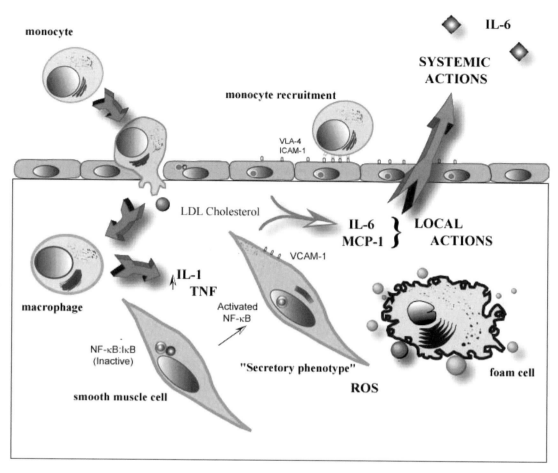

Fig. 1. Cytokine cascade in atherosclerosis. Schematic diagram of the activation of the cytokine cascade in the pre-atherosclerotic blood vessel. Circulating monocytes are the source for tissue-resident macrophages. In response to reactive oxygen species generated by LDL oxidation or endovascular infections with CMV, *Helicobacter pylori*, or *Chlamydia trachomatis*, the activating cytokines IL-1 and TNF are secreted. These cytokines signal inactive cytoplasmic NF-κB to enter the nucleus in smooth muscle cells, endothelial cells, and fibroblasts to induce expression of downstream cytokines, including MCP-1, IL-6, and others (see text). These cytokines work on local (paracrine) targets to increase monocyte recruitment and LDL oxidation and on systemic (endocrine) targets to induce expression of hepatic acute-phase reactants. ICAM-1, intercellular adhesion molecule-1; IκB, protein inhibitor of κB; ILκ1, interleukin-1; IL-6, interleukin-6; LDL, low density lipoprotein; MCP-1, monocyte chemoattractant protein-1; NF-κB, nuclear factor-κB; ROS, reactive oxygen species; TNF, tumor necrosis factor; VCAM-1, vascular cell adhesion molecule-1; VLA-4, very late antigen-4.

expressed in the vessel wall *(2,7–9)*. Of these, MCP-1 *(10,11)*, IL-8 *(12)*, RANTES *(13)*, macrophage inflammatory protein-1α (MIP-1α) *(14)*, growth related oncogene-α *(15)*, and cytokine-induced neutrophil chemoattractant (KC) *(16)* are largely responsible for monocyte recruitment, which is an important initial step in atherosclerotic progression. MCP-1 is a small 8–10 kDa β (CC-type) chemokine that specifically attracts monocytes and memory T lymphocytes expressing the CCR2 receptor, both of which are found in all stages of the atherosclerotic lesion. MCP-1/CCR2 interactions are important in atherosclerosis because hyperlipidemic-atherosclerotic prone mice made genetically deficient in MCP-1 *(17)* or CCR2 *(18)* have

reduced numbers of vascular macrophages and develop fewer atherosclerotic lesions than controls. Macrophage colony stimulating factor (MCSF), a cytokine produced locally in the vascular wall by smooth muscle cells and macrophages, stimulates proliferation, differentiation, and LDL uptake by macrophages through the scavenger receptor *(19,20)*. As with MCP-1 deficiency, hyperlipidemic MCSF-deficient animals have smaller atherosclerotic lesions because of decreased monocyte recruitment into the vessel wall *(8,20)*. Although initially described as a plasma cell growth factor, IL-6, abundantly secreted by activated monocytes and VSMCs *(21,22)*, is a 26 kDa cytokine that promotes smooth muscle cell proliferation through a paracrine mechanism involving the local production of PDGF (23). IL-6 is significant because it induces systemic responses to vascular inflammation through the hepatic acute-phase response. Finally, the insulin-like growth factors (IGFs), single chain polypeptides with significant homology to insulin, and their receptor are produced by endothelial cells and VSMCs within the atherosclerotic plaque (24). IGF-1 plays an important role in stimulating the phenotypic switch of the smooth muscle cell from the contractile to the secretory state, inducing smooth muscle cell proliferation and migration, accumulating extracelluar matrix, and forming the fibrous cap in the advanced lesion. These findings suggest that local expression of chemokines by the injured vascular wall coordinates multicellular responses required for the recruitment and differentiation of monocytes and the migration and proliferation of smooth muscle cells to develop the advanced complicated lesion.

Mechanisms for the Vascular Cytokine Cascade

The cytokine cascade is an important upstream regulator of the cellular responses to atherosclerosis and is a possible target for therapeutic intervention; therefore, the mechanisms controlling the cytokine cascade in the vessel wall have been intensively studied. The ubiquitous cytoplasmic transcription factor, nuclear factor-κB (NF-κB), is central in controlling the expression of inflammatory immune response and cellular survival genes (25–27). NF-κB is a family of highly inducible DNA binding proteins that is regulated by a family of cytoplasmic inhibitors, IκBs, that bind and specifically inactivate NF-κB members. The nuclear localization sequence of NF-κB is masked by IκBs, and nuclear entry is prevented (28–30). NF-κB activation is a sequential process that results in nuclear translocation of sequestered cytoplasmic NF-κB complexes through targeted proteolysis of the IκB inhibitors. Intracellular NF-κB activating signals converge on the multiprotein cytoplasmic IκB kinase complex (IKK), which phosphorylates IκB on two serine residues (Ser^{32} and Ser^{36}) in its NH$_2$-regulatory domain (26). PhosphoIκB is then ubiquitinated and proteolyzed through the proteasome (26,31,32) and calpain pathways (33,34). After IκB proteolysis, liberated NF-κB enters the nucleus to activate target gene transcription.

Activated NF-κB has been identified in smooth muscle cells, macrophages, and endothelial cells in human atherosclerotic plaques in situ (35). In addition, gene regulation studies have shown that the inducible adhesion molecules (ICAM, VCAM, E-selectin), cytokines (MCSF, IL-6), and chemokines (MCP-1) that are expressed within the atherosclerotic lesion contain NF-κB binding sites. Together, these findings indicate that NF-κB plays an

upstream central role in initiating the cytokine cascade required for atherosclerotic development (22,36–38). In monocytes and endothelial cells, IL-1, TNFα, and oxidized LDL induce NF-κB to increase the expression of adhesion molecules and chemotactic cytokines (38,39). In VSMCs, the vasoactive peptide angiotensin II induces the activation and translocation of NF-κB through an ROS-dependent mechanism (22,37,40,41). The finding that angiotensin II is a pro-inflammatory molecule due to its ability to activate NF-κB provides a potential mechanistic link for why hypertension accelerates the development of atherosclerosis (30) and how inhibitors of the renin-angiotensin system may reduce atherosclerotic complications (discussed below). In addition, the sensitivity of NF-κB to the effects of antioxidants may provide a mechanistic linkage for manners in which antioxidants reduce vascular atherosclerosis and inflammation. Thus, NF-κB is a central regulator of inflammatory cytokine production in the vessel wall and is an attractive target for inhibition by anti-atherogenic drugs.

Systemic Actions of Vascular Cytokines

Significant changes in the composition of the blood stream can be detected in patients with acute illness (42). Many of these changes, reflected in blood sedimentation properties, are the result of a genetic switch in plasma protein synthesis by the inflamed liver, a process called the hepatic acute-phase response. The hepatic acute-phase response can be activated to various degrees in response to systemic microbial infections, collagen-vascular diseases, myocardial ischemia/infarction, systemic malignancy, burns, and vascular injury after angioplasty or in response to the atherosclerotic process (43). Complete activation of the hepatic acute-phase response is characterized by systemic fever, malaise, leukocytosis, alterations in endocrine regulators (glucagon, ACTH, cortisol, catecholamines), and metabolic changes (increased protein catabolism, negative nitrogen balance) (44). Although cytokines produced by atherosclerotic vessels do not produce obvious systemic manifestations in healthy patients, their biochemical detection with sensitive immunodetection methods is of prognostic value for the presence of clinically significant atherosclerosis.

Hepatic acute-phase reactants are defined as proteins with plasma concentrations that change by 25% or more during systemic inflammation (44). Many acute-phase reactants have significant cardiovascular actions. In humans, the complement factors (C3, C4, C9, Factor B), coagulant/fibrinolytic factors (fibrinogen, plasminogen, tissue plasminogen activator), antiproteases (α1 antitrypsin), components of the innate immune system

(CRP), apolipoproteins (SAA), and the vasoactive precursor AGT are acute-phase reactants *(30,43)*. Because of their wide range of biological roles, acute-phase reactants may be important in restoring homeostasis after an inflammatory injury by promoting clearance of infectious agents, facilitating wound repair, and ensuring adequate blood pressure and salt homeostasis *(43)*. Of the acute-phase reactants, CRP, SAA, fibrinogen, and AGT have particular cardiovascular significance.

Induction of Hepatic Acute-Phase Reactants

Hepatic acute-phase reactants have been subclassified by their responsiveness to the major cytokines and steroids that are involved in their upregulation. Although many cytokines induce hepatic acute-phase synthesis *(43,45–47)*, IL-6 is the primary mediator in humans. Class 1 acute-phase reactant genes are induced mainly by IL-1, alone or combined with IL-6, or by IL-1 and IL-6 in combination with glucocorticoids, whereas class 2 genes are induced by IL-6 alone. For example, IL-6 in combination with cortisol synergistically stimulates AGT and fibrinogen synthesis *(48,49)*. In the presence of IL-1, IL-6 synergistically upregulates CRP and SAA synthesis *(43)* but downregulates fibrinogen expression *(48)*. These broad generalizations, however, do not reflect the complex and subtle variation in the manners in which subsets of these classes and specific acute-phase reactants are regulated. The complex interplay between circulating cytokines allows for heterogeneity in plasma protein synthesis in response to different inflammatory stimuli.

Because IL-6 is the major hormonal mediator of the hepatic acute-phase reaction, the mechanisms by which IL-6 signals in the hepatocyte have been extensively studied. IL-6 induces acute-phase reactant synthesis by two distinct signaling pathways initiated through the IL-6 receptor. Type I IL-6 signaling is mediated through a tyrosine kinase pathway involving the janus kinase (JAK)-signal transducer and activator of transcription (STAT) pathway, whereas type II IL-6 signaling is mediated through a Ras/mitogen-activated protein (MAP) kinase/nuclear factor-IL6 (NF-IL6) pathway *(50)*. Gene transfer studies and genetic knockout experiments both indicate that the type I (JAK-STAT) pathway is the major pathway responsible for acute-phase reactant synthesis *(51,52)* **(Fig. 2)**. IL-6 activates the JAK-STAT pathway in hepatocytes by binding on its target cells to a high-affinity membrane protein receptor called the IL-6R alpha chain (IL-6Rα), which lacks intrinsic kinase activity. Two molecules of the liganded IL-6-IL–6Rα complex then associate with two molecules of transducin (gp130), forming the active hexameric signaling complex.

Oligomerization of this large receptor complex brings gp130-associated tyrosine kinases, JAK-1 and JAK-2, and Tyk 2 kinases close enough to phosphorylate gp130 on specific tyrosine residues. Tyrosine-phosphorylated gp130 is a docking site for cytoplasmic transcription factors, STAT1 and STAT3, to bind gp130 via src homology-2 (SH2) domains. These inactive STATs are tyrosine phosphorylated, which allows them to associate (dimerize) and translocate into the nucleus where they bind to target acute-phase response genes *(53)*. STATs 1 and 3 bind to response elements containing the sequence $TTCN_3GAA$ in the promoters of target genes. Upon binding to their cognate response elements, STATs recruit bridging coactivators, such as p300/CBP (Creb-binding protein), which serve as molecular bridges to communicate with RNA polymerase, and through histone acetylase activity, p300/CBP modifies the chromatin structure of its target genes *(49,54,55)*. Although IL-6 induces tyrosine phosphorylation, nuclear translocation, and DNA binding of both STAT 1 and 3 subunits, only STAT3 is predominantly responsible for mediating synthesis of acute-phase reactants *(51,52)*. These observations indicate that the role of STAT depends on the cell type and hormonal stimulus.

IL-6–MEDIATED INFLAMMATION AND ATHEROSCLEROTIC RISK

Several studies have linked increased IL-6 levels with myocardial ischemia and atherosclerosis. In patients with acute coronary syndromes, high concentrations of IL-6 within 48 h of hospitalization indicated increased cardiac events in patients with unstable angina *(56)*; therefore, IL-6 may be a marker for plaque instability in patients with active ischemia *(57)*. Furthermore, patients with unstable coronary artery disease who had increased plasma levels of IL-6 had the highest mortality rates after adjustment for other risk factors. Early revascularization significantly reduced mortality rates among those with increased IL-6 levels, whereas mortality was not reduced among patients without increased IL-6 concentrations *(58)*. These findings suggest that the presence of vascular inflammation may be used to identify a subgroup of patients who would benefit from more aggressive therapy.

In healthy populations, prospective observational studies have shown that plasma levels of IL-6 in the upper quartile of the normal range are independently predictive of an increased risk of all-cause and cardiovascular mortality *(59)* and future myocardial infarction (MI) *(60)*. In the Physicians' Health Study, a prospective case-control study of healthy men, IL-6 levels in 202 participants who

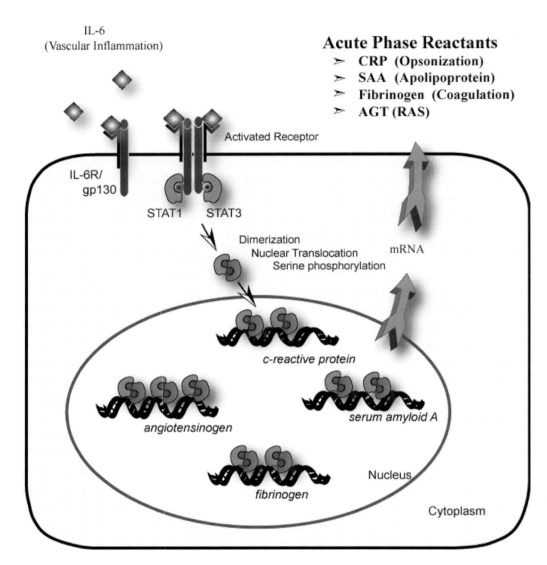

Fig. 2. Mechanisms for the induction of the hepatic acute-phase response by vascular inflammation through the IL-6 Type I (JAK-STAT) signaling pathway. Circulating IL-6 derived from vascular sources induces hepatic signaling by binding the high-affinity IL-6Rα, a process that initiates receptor oligomerization. The active signaling complex is a hexamer of 2 molecules of IL-6, 2 molecules of IL-6Rα, and 2 molecules of gp130. Cytoplasmic transcription factors, STAT1 and STAT3, bind tyrosine phosphorylated gp130 through their SH2 domains. STAT1 and STAT3, in molecular contact with the janus kinases, are tyrosine phosphorylated, which allows these molecules to self-associate and enter the nucleus. Target genes for STAT-dependent activation include CRP, SAA, fibrinogen, and angiotensinogen. These acute-phase reactants are translated and secreted through the constitutive protein synthesis pathway to affect pathways important in wound repair, lipid transport, coagulation, and blood pressure control. AGT, angiotensinogen; CRP, c-reactive protein; IL-6, interleukin-6; IL-6R, interleukin-6 receptor; mRNA, messenger ribonucleic acid; RAS, renin-angiotensin system; SAA, serum amyloid A; STAT, signal transducer and activator of transcription.

subsequently developed MI were compared with those in 202 individuals, matched for age and smoking status, who did not develop vascular disease during a 6-year follow-up *(60)*. Median concentrations of IL-6 at baseline were higher among those who subsequently had an MI than those who did not. The risk of future MI increased with increasing quartiles of baseline IL-6 levels; the relative risk was 2.3 times higher for men in the highest quartile at entry than for those in the lowest quartile, and the risk increased 38% for each quartile increase in IL-6. This relationship was significant after adjustment for other cardiovascular risk factors, was stable over the study period, and was seen in all low-risk groups including nonsmokers.

These epidemiologic studies indicate the strong link between IL-6 and atherosclerotic risk but do not define the biological mechanism. IL-6 is an important inducer of hepatic acute-phase reactant proteins, which have significant cardiovascular actions.

HEPATIC ACUTE-PHASE REACTANTS

C-reactive Protein

After the first observation in 1930 that the sera of patients with acute fever could be uniquely precipitated with an extract (Fraction C) of pneumococcus, this "C-precipitin" protein, later called CRP, was not found in the blood of healthy persons (61,62). CRP is induced during the acute phase of a variety of states, febrile and non-febrile, infectious and noninfectious, and after MI and surgery (61,62). Purified as a lipid- and carbohydrate-free protein, CRP comprises five identical 2-kDa noncovalently linked subunits that aggregate as a cyclic pentamer (63,64). Partial amino acid sequences of CRP indicated that it was one of a structural group of evolutionarily conserved calcium-binding proteins called pentraxins whose members participate in the acute-phase responses of different species (64). The binding of CRP to the cell wall of *Streptococcus pneumoniae* is a calcium-dependent association that requires phosphocholine substrates found on many bacteria, yeast, and fungal pathogens. After CRP binds to cell walls on pathogens, or on damaged or necrotic host cells, it then binds to the high-affinity IgG receptors on phagocytic cells (FcγR1 and FCγRII) and increases phagocytic uptake. Exogenous CRP administration increases survival from lethal *S. pneumoniae* infection (65). This property underlies one of the putative primary biological activities of CRP as a nonspecific opsonin. Other potential biological functions of CRP include activation of the classic complement pathway through association with C1q and inhibition of the alternative complement pathway to increase host immune defenses during the acute-phase response.

REGULATION OF C-REACTIVE PROTEIN BY INFLAMMATION

CRP, erythrocyte sedimentation rate (ESR), and other markers of the acute-phase response have been used as indices of inflammation and necrosis. Of the circulating markers found in vertebrates, CRP and SAA are the major acute-phase proteins in humans. Their plasma concentrations increase rapidly after the onset of inflammation and return to basal levels upon removal of inflammatory stimuli, which makes them useful as markers of inflammation. CRP, produced in the liver in response to IL-6, is the best studied acute-phase reactant in relation to vascular disease and has been most consistently associated with cardiovascular risk in clinical settings. Healthy individuals have trace blood levels of CRP that can increase (sometimes more than a 1000-fold) to concentrations greater than 30 mg/dL in severe infection (66). The regulation of CRP expression occurs mainly at the transcriptional level in the liver as shown by human CRP-expressing transgenic mice after stimulation with bacterial lipopolysaccharide (LPS) and analysis by nuclear run-on experiments (67).

In vitro and in vivo studies with DNase I-hypersensitivity footprinting and analysis of transfected CRP promoter constructs have identified two closely spaced sequences in the CRP promoter called acute-phase response elements (APREs) (61,66,68). These elements map in the proximal 137 bp of the 5′-flanking region of the CRP gene and appear to act independently of each other. Removal of the downstream APRE (nucleotides -94 to -46) does not affect LPS inducibility and reflects a redundancy unique to the CRP promoter among other acute-phase response genes. This redundancy probably contributes to its capacity for massive stimulation of expression levels (66). IL-6 activates transcription of CRP, and IL-1β, with no effect of its own, synergistically increases IL-6–induced CRP promoter activity (69–72). In vitro studies have shown that 157 bp of upstream CRP sequence was sufficient to confer these activities in CRP transcription reporter constructs. In addition, several genetic cis-elements and protein transcription factors and transactivators are required for the transcription of CRP in response to treatment with IL-6 or cytokines present in monocyte conditioned cell culture medium. IL-6–inducible C/EBP (CCAAT/enhancer binding protein) family members bind two C/EBP binding sites in the proximal CRP promoter (73), and binding sites for hepatic nuclear factor-1 (HNF-1) are adjacent to these C/EBP sites and are required for CRP transcription (74). Although one of these HNF-1 sites is necessary and sufficient for IL-6–inducible CRP transcription, the presence of both sites markedly increases expression levels, which suggests synergistic promoter transactivation by two HNF-1 molecules bound simultaneously at two distinct sites. STAT3 is another signaling protein that has recently been added to the list of molecules that participate in the transcriptional activation of CRP in response to IL-6. The STAT3-specific binding motif $TT(N)_4AA$ (75) was identified at position −112 in the 5′-flanking CRP sequence and was shown via mutation analysis to be required for optimal IL-6 induction in liver cells transfected with reporter constructs driven by the −157 to + 3 CRP promoter region (72,76). Overexpression of STAT3 and treatment of these transfected liver cells with IL-6 was sufficient to induce reporter gene expression containing two copies of the STAT3 binding motif and a minimal thymidine kinase promoter from which the inherent C/EBP site had been removed. These findings indicate that STAT3, or a closely related molecule, is involved in the IL-6 stimulation of human CRP (hCRP) transcription.

In vitro studies in cultured hepatocytes are a solid first step in characterizing the regulation of CRP gene expression, but animal studies indicate that control of this acute-phase reactant is very complex. Regulatory factors that confer inducible CRP expression with reporter constructs in cell lines are insufficient for induction in transgenic mice expressing hCRP (77). The degree of participation of the pentraxins in the acute-phase response is usually species-specific. In the acute-phase response of the mouse, serum amyloid proteins (e.g., serum amyloid P component [SAP]) are highly upregulated (78,79), whereas CRP remains almost at basal levels (80); however, a 31 kb genomic hCRP construct expressed in transgenic mice was regulated the same as in humans (67). Studies in transgenic mice with various deletion constructs of the parent 31 kb hCRP fragment have shown that constructs lacking sequence regions surrounding the poly (A) site were not expressed with or without LPS induction. These studies also showed that liver specific but constitutive expression required at least 540 and 1200 bases, respectively, of upstream and downstream hCRP gene-flanking sequence. Furthermore, extended 5′ and 3′ flanking regions were required to silence expression before induction of the acute-phase response (77). These findings and peak levels and timing of CRP expression after stimulation were independent of copy number and integration site for each of the various hCRP transgenes. Overall, these results indicate that the minimal cis-regulatory CRP gene sequences previously shown to confer LPS-inducible expression in hepatocyte cell lines are insufficient in transgenic mice and that the capacity to generate necessary transactivating factors (which interact with distal genetic elements both 5′ and 3′ to the hCRP gene) is conserved from mouse to human (77,81).

Plasma levels of CRP are rapidly increased with the onset of inflammation and subsequently reduced to basal levels upon withdrawal of inflammatory stimuli (e.g., infection). Genomic signaling networks must be efficient to silence and upregulate CRP expression, and the proper balance of these factors may be missed in in vitro studies with gene expression constructs. Moreover, the extensive intricate web of powerful paracrine and endocrine effects can be elicited completely only in animal models. The use of transgenic mouse techniques, in which CRP and other molecules are expressed or not expressed in their native context, have helped tremendously in applying these studies to cardiovascular disease.

Early studies in transgenic mice showed that CRP expression was sex dependent. Both constitutive and LPS-induced serum concentrations of CRP were significantly higher in transgenic males than in females, and these increased levels were directly attributed to testosterone (81). Another unexpected observation in transgenic mice was that IL-6, a potent inducer of CRP in humans, did not upregulate the hCRP transgene in these mice but did induce endogenous mouse SAA (81). The involvement of IL-6 in the LPS-stimulation of the hCRP transgene was studied in female mice with double genetic modifications that expressed the 31kb hCRP transgene and were deficient for IL-6 (82,83). In these mice, hCRP stimulation by LPS was eliminated and could not be reinstated by treatment with IL-6; however, a combination of LPS and IL-6 did rescue the response, which indicates that IL-6 is necessary but not sufficient for the induction of the hCRP transgene. To clarify this issue and discrepancies from human cell culture experiments in which IL-6 could independently induce CRP expression, several cytokines were screened in hCRP transgenic mice that were both IL-6$^{+/+}$ and IL-6$^{-/-}$. IL-1β, oncostatin M, and leukemia inhibitory factor (LIF) could induce hCRP in both genetic backgrounds, suggesting the presence of both IL-6–independent and IL-6–dependent mechanisms for regulating hCRP (84). Oncostatin M and LIF both activate STAT signaling through the same gp130 transducing receptor used by IL-6. The mechanism involved in the activation of CRP expression by oncostatin M and LIF has not been determined, but may be related to ligand-dependent differences in gp130-mediated signaling pathways.

The above results were studied further in independently produced, but phenotypically identical, doubly modified 31 kb hCRP transgenic/IL-6$^{-/-}$ mice (85) by carefully tracking sex and CRP and endogenous SAP (another pentraxin) expression and by administering various cytokines with and without testosterone (86). Three major findings were reported in this mouse model. First, testosterone was required for basal hCRP expression but not for endogenous SAP, which is a major acute-phase reactant in mice. Second, IL-6 was necessary and sufficient for induction of hCRP in male mice, but hCRP induction in females required IL-6 plus a second signal that could be initiated either by LPS or testosterone. Finally, IL-1, which did not seem to significantly affect hCRP induction, was required along with IL-6 for full induction of mouse SAP (86). In addition, the authors noted that these and previous findings indicate that partial release of one of the two strong negative control elements in the distal 5′ and 3′ flanking regions of the hCRP gene is necessary for constitutive expression of the hCRP gene. In transgenic mice, this expression is mediated by testosterone through a subsequent downstream mediator(s) such as growth hormone (87). Humans do not have sexually dimorphic patterns of CRP expression, and this mediator(s) is probably not under androgen control. The other negative control element is relieved by an LPS-induced mediator(s). Acute-phase induction by LPS occurs when at least one of the negative controls is significantly relieved and requires only IL-6 (81). Pronounced acute-phase induction of CRP amplification might then occur through release of negative control at both flanking elements.

To a lesser extent, CRP is regulated in the acute-phase response by post-transcriptional mechanisms. CRP is normally synthesized slowly, which corresponds to its trace plasma levels, but with transcript upregulation, hepatocyte secretion of CRP becomes more efficient. During upregulation, the half-time for exit from the endoplasmic reticulum is reduced from 18 h to 75 min because of altered interactions of CRP with two carboxylesterases in the endoplasmic reticulum (88–90). Nevertheless, the major mode of CRP upregulation during the acute-phase is a STAT-mediated transcriptional activation.

C-REACTIVE PROTEIN AND ATHEROSCLEROSIS

Increased CRP levels were noted in patients with acute ischemia as early as the 1940s; this increase was considered part of the "acute-phase response." Since then, a several 100-fold increase in CRP levels has been noted in response to acute injury, infection, and other inflammatory stimuli that is maintained over long periods in the absence of new stimuli, depending on the rate of hepatic production (78,91). As laboratory and clinical data indicating the role of inflammation in atherosclerosis accumulated, investigators hypothesized that CRP may be an adjunct for assessment of cardiovascular risk. Moreover, CRP levels in the low-normal range were noted to have a predictive value for patients presenting with acute coronary ischemia (92–94). Overall however, interpretations of increased CRP levels in settings of acute ischemia remained unclear. CRP testing as a predictor of coronary heart disease risk needed to be evaluated in large-scale prospective studies of healthy individuals in which baseline levels of CRP could be related to future risk of cardiovascular events. Highly sensitive and fully automated CRP assays were used in these studies (95,96).

Epidemiological studies have strengthened the role of plasma levels of CRP as an independent predictor of risk of future MI, stroke, peripheral vascular disease and vascular mortality among individuals with no known cardiovascular disease. In a population-based cross-sectional study from general practice registries in the United Kingdom, the prevalence of coronary heart disease among 388 men aged 50 to 69 years was noted to increase 1.5-fold for each doubling of CRP concentration (97). In this study, increased levels of CRP were associated with increased age, smoking, body mass index and exposure to certain infectious agents. These latter confounding effects could not be adequately controlled, and the authors could not conclude whether the relation between CRP and symptomatic coronary heart disease was due to cause or effect. In a series of prospective epidemiologic studies, increased baseline levels of CRP correlated with future cardiovascular morbidity and mortality among individuals with no clinical evidence of vascular disease even after adjustment for many of those potential confounding factors (59,98–107). For example, in a cohort of 22,000 middle-aged healthy men, for those with baseline CRP levels in the highest quartile, the risk of MI increased threefold, the risk of stroke increased twofold, and the risk of peripheral vascular disease increased fourfold (100,103). These effects were independent of cardiovascular disease risk factors, including total and high density lipoprotein cholesterol, triglycerides, fibrinogen, and lipoprotein [a], and were not modified by smoking status. Further analysis of these data showed that risk stratification that included both CRP and lipid parameters was superior to that based on lipids alone and that high CRP levels predicted a higher risk of MI for men at low and high risk for coronary heart disease as indicated by lipid values (108).

CRP measurement is a predictor of cardiovascular events in healthy postmenopausal women (98,102). For example, in a prospective nested case-control study of 22,263 postmenopausal women, 12 markers of coronary heart disease, including several lipid and lipoprotein variables, CRP, homocysteine levels, and others, were measured at baseline with a mean follow-up period of 3 years (98). CRP measurement was the strongest predictor of cardiovascular events; the relative risk of events for women in the highest as compared with the lowest quartile was 4.4 (more than a fourfold increase). Moreover, levels of CRP were significant predictors of cardiac risk even in the subgroup of women who had normal LDL cholesterol. In addition, high CRP levels increased the risk for cardiovascular disease in patients with chronic renal insufficiency on maintenance hemodialysis (109).

These data suggest that serum concentration of CRP is a risk factor for cardiovascular disease in patients with acute coronary ischemia, stable angina pectoris, or a history of MI *(92–94,97,108,109)*. In a case-control analysis of patients who had a MI in the Cholesterol and Recurrent Events (CARE) trial, CRP values were predictive of higher risk for recurrent nonfatal MI or coronary death with a 75% higher relative risk in the highest versus lowest quintile group *(110)*. Similarly, a European study found that among 2,121 patients with angina pectoris, each standard deviation increase in baseline CRP was associated with a 45% increase in the relative risk of nonfatal MI or sudden cardiac death *(97)*.

Increased serum CRP concentrations at admission are a predictor for short- and long-term adverse outcomes in patients with unstable angina *(92–94,111–113)*. In a study of 276 patients in which CRP levels were determined before coronary artery stenting, the incidence of restenosis, repeat intervention of the stented vessel, MI, and cardiac death at 6 months was greater in those with CRP values in the highest quintile *(114)*. High CRP levels are predictive of graft failure in patients undergoing cardiac transplantation *(115)*. The association between acute coronary syndromes and CRP suggests that chronic inflammation of the coronary arterial wall may be important in these pathophysiologic events. The increase in CRP levels is not the cause of plaque rupture; rather, the acute-phase response appears to be a marker of hyperresponsiveness of the inflammatory system *(113,116)*.

For clinical applications, high sensitivity-CRP (HSCRP) values are divided into population-based quintiles. Risk estimates derived from studies of healthy American men and women are available (Table 1). These data are adjusted for age, smoking status, hypertension, family history of premature coronary artery disease, diabetes, dyslipidemia, exercise level, and body mass index. For each quintile increase in HSCRP, the adjusted relative risk of having a future cardiovascular event increased 26% for men and 33% for women *(117)*.

C-REACTIVE PROTEIN AND ATHEROGENESIS

The strong epidemiological link between CRP and atherosclerotic risk suggests that CRP may play a direct mechanistic role in atherogenesis rather than being an epiphenomenon that indirectly reflects the extent of tissue damage or ischemia associated with the acute-phase reaction *(118)*. However, the cause and effect relationship has not been established for some of the associations of CRP with cardiovascular disease. For example, chronic infection (outside of the cardiovascular system) is associated with increased risk for vascular disease, possibly caused by the increase in CRP that coincides with the acute-phase response *(119)*. However, CRP is not selectively induced by the acute-phase response, and CRP could be a marker for another inflammatory product that increases cardiovascular risk.

The biological actions of CRP may provide clues for its role in atherogenesis. CRP was discovered and named based on its binding specificity for phosphocholine, which is a component of many bacterial and fungal polysaccharides, most biological membranes, and apolipoprotein B-containing lipoproteins (LDL and very low density lipoproteins [VLDL]) *(61,120)*. In addition, CRP binds nuclear constituents such as histones and small ribonucleoproteins *(121)*. Ligand-complexed CRP is recognized by complement component C1q, which activates the classical complement cascade *(122)*. mRNA for CRP and complement components C1 to C9 have been detected in normal arterial and plaque tissue *(123)*. When levels of CRP and complement components were compared in plaque tissue, normal artery, and liver, the levels were highest in plaque tissue, followed by normal artery, and then liver. Furthermore, some key inhibitors of the classical cascade that might be expected to be upregulated in plaque were not *(124)*.

Other studies have indicated a direct pro-inflammatory role for CRP in initiating or exacerbating vascular disease because of its action as an opsonin for several biological particles, such as modified LDL (oxidized or acetylated) that is important to early atherosclerotic lesion development. Phagocytosis of CRP-opsonized zymosan in mice proceeds through the FcγRI macrophage IgG receptor *(125)*. The CRP-mediated macrophage uptake of native LDL occurs via the related low-affinity receptor FCγRIIα (CD32) *(120)*. These findings suggest that CRP plays an important role in foam cell formation. In addition, CRP directly interacts with the vessel wall by inducing the expression of monocyte- and lymphocyte-recruiting adhesion molecules on human endothelial cells *(126,127)*, and this is important in promoting the local inflammatory response within atherosclerotic plaques. Expression of vascular adhesion molecules ICAM-1 and E-selectin is upregulated in the presence of CRP and human serum. This serum factor may be activated complement because upregulation of ICAM-1 in rats required both cytokines and complement; ICAM-1 upregulation in human infarcted myocardium always co-localizes with complement *(128,129)*. Finally, the direct role of CRP in vascular inflammation is supported by the recent finding that CRP increases the secretion of MCP-1 by cultured human endothelial cells sevenfold *(126)*. Taken together, these results suggest that

Table 1
Hepatic Acute-Phase Reactants

Acute-phase reactant	Assay	Normal values (SI units)	Increase in acute-phase reactant	Comments
Interleukin-6	ELISA	Limit of detection depends on assay (<5 ng/L)	Variable (levels to 400 ng/L)	Short half life, impractical for routine clinical assays
C-reactive protein	Latex agglutination immunonephelometry	0–12 mg/L	1000-fold	Influenced by obesity smoking, diabetes; Quartiles predict cardiovascular risk
ESR	Westergren method	0–15 mm/h in males 0–20 mm/h in females	Variable	Influenced by age and many diseases; Indirect measurement of fibrinogen
Serum amyloid A	ELISA	0.5–10 mg/L	100–1000-fold	Values usually <3, higher in elderly; Limit of detection varies by assay
Fibrinogen	Automated clotting	1.75–4.0 µmol/L	2–4-fold	Influenced by smoking, age, lipids, blood pressure, obesity
Angiotensinogen	Radioimmunoassay	1293 ± 277 ng AI/ml in males 1344 ± 292 ng AI/ml in females	1.5–2.0-fold	Influenced by genotype, steroid hormone prescription; For research applications

Values for nonsmoking men; must adjust for smoking status and gender.
ELISA, enzyme-linked immunosorbent assay; ESR, erythrocyte sedimentation rate.

CRP, in addition to being a significant and predictive marker of inflammation, may contribute mechanistically to the development and progression of atherosclerosis.

Serum Amyloid A

SAA was first recognized in the early 1970s as a plasma protein that was antigenically related to the main fibrillar compound in deposits of reactive AA amyloid (130–134). The amyloid A protein deposit, and its precursor SAA, are part of a large group of heterogenous proteins. Disorders of the proteins (amyloidoses) involve folding anomalies and deposition. The A proteins are usually involved in the pathophysiology of immunity and inflammation, producing deposits chiefly in the liver, kidney, and spleen (135,136). Early studies showed that, like CRP, SAA levels increased in inflammatory conditions, particularly those characterized by high neutrophil counts (137). Subsequent early studies focused on the fractionation of immune cell extracts that mediated induction of SAA synthesis and the characterization of SAA and proteins structurally associated with it (138). When mRNA was isolated and translated from LPS-stimulated mouse liver, a major protein product was identified at 13-14 kDa that immunoprecipitated with anti-mouse AA, and the production of monoclonal antibodies facilitated detection of heterogeneous human SAA proteins that had

similar molecular weights but different solubility and isoelectric charge properties (139). SAA was further identified as an apolipoprotein associated with apoAI and apoAII mainly in the high density lipoprotein 3 (HDL) subfraction of HDL (140). In humans, the SAA gene family comprises four closely clustered members on chromosome 11 that are divided into two classes, the acute-phase and constitutive SAAs (139,141). The acute-phase SAAs, SAA1 and SAA2, are highly inducible with inflammation (up to 1000-fold), whereas the constitutive SAA4 is induced only slightly (SAA3 is a pseudogene and not expressed) (142,143). Most acute-phase SAA originates in the liver but can be induced in other tissues by inflammatory cytokines such as IL-1, IL-6, and TNFα (144–147). All SAA protein isoforms are expressed in atherosclerotic lesions in humans.

Like CRP, SAA has multiple functions. Recombinant acute-phase SAA binds cholesterol with high affinity and increases cholesterol uptake by cultured hepatocytes (148). Antibody mapping and peptide competition experiments showed that the amino-terminal region of acute-phase, but not constitutive, SAA specifically bound cholesterol and increased its transport into aortic smooth muscle cells and hepatocytes (149). Because SAA associates with HDL, the constitutive SAA4 may be involved in normal HDL function, and the acute-phase SAAs may function differently or may contribute to the markedly altered lipoprotein profiles seen during the acute-phase response and chronic inflammation (150,151). Studies in which SAAs were overexpressed in transgenic mice have not clarified these issues. SAAs alone, expressed at levels equivalent to those seen in systemic inflammation, are insufficient to alter HDL cholesterol or apoAI levels (152). However, very high levels of the constitutive SAA4 protein increased VLDL and triglyceride levels through unknown mechanisms.

SAA interferes with platelet function; acute-phase SAA isolated and purified from the sera of trauma patients inhibited thrombin-induced platelet aggregation at physiological concentrations, but did not perturb the clotting or amidolytic activities of thrombin. These findings suggest a thrombin-specific protective role for SAA in thromboembolic disease (153). Earlier studies suggested that SAA may have immunosuppressive effects on macrophage-T cell interactions (154), but more recent studies have shown that SAA is strongly chemotactic for monocytes, neutrophils, and T lymphocytes, both in cell culture and in recruiting infiltration to injection sites in mice (155,156). These observations suggest a pleiotropic role for SAA in lipoprotein metabolism, neutrophil recruitment, and possibly platelet function in inflamed vessels.

Analyses of the SAA1 gene promoter have shown that 304 bp of 5′-flanking sequence in CAT reporter constructs are sufficient for its hepatocyte-specific expression and its 15- to 20-fold induction by conditioned medium from mixed lymphocyte cultures, IL-1, or the phorbol ester, 12-O-tetradecanoylphorbol-13-acetate (157). Further deletion analyses identified a 65 bp DNA fragment (−135 to −71) that conferred cytokine responsiveness onto a heterologous thymidine kinase promoter in both liver and non-liver cells. Binding sites for NF-κB and C/EBP identified within this region had synergistic effects on induced SAA1 expression. A third transcription factor, YY1, interacts between the NF-κB and C/EBP sites in a repressive manner by inhibiting NF-κB binding (158). Disruption of YY1 binding increased basal and induced promoter activity, and overexpression of YY1 transrepressed this activity. This YY1 repression may contribute to the transient nature of SAA expression after inflammation (158). Detailed transfection analyses identified a 29 bp tissue-specific repressor (TSR) element distal to the cytokine response region. This element inhibited SAA reporter expression (in an orientation- and distance-independent manner) and formed specific protein-DNA complexes with nuclear proteins in several nonliver cell lines and placenta (159). The authors concluded that liver-specific expression of SAA1 may be

regulated by both positive and negative regulatory elements. Surprisingly, purification of the TSR protein from HeLa cells, with amino acid sequencing and antibody supershift experiments, identified it as transcription factor AP-2, showing a new function. Furthermore, this function could be derepressed in HeLa cells by mutation of the AP-2 DNA binding site or by introduction of a dominant negative AP-2 expression construct (160). This same group recently reported that the repressive effects of AP-2 on the expression of transfected and endogenous hepatocyte genes indicate that AP-2 may also function as a negative regulator of some liver genes in non-hepatic cells. In addition, heterologous AP-2 expression in a hepatocyte background can repress inducible and constitutive liver-specific genes but has no effect on the expression of genes that are also natively expressed in non-hepatocytes.

SAA levels are a significant predictor of the risk of cardiovascular events in healthy individuals. In a prospective, case-control study involving 28,263 participants in the Women's Health Study, the relative risk for cardiovascular events was three times higher in healthy women in the highest quartile than in those in the lowest quartile (98). The levels of SAA were significant predictors of cardiovascular risk even in the subgroup of women with normal LDL cholesterol. In addition, SAA concentrations predicted the risk of recurrent coronary events in patients with established ischemic heart disease; the relative risk was 1.74 times higher in patients with SAA levels in the highest quintile than in those with levels in the lowest quintile (110).

Fibrinogen

Fibrinogen, long recognized to be important in thrombotic processes, has integral functions in platelet aggregation and controls cellular and enzymatic processes that affect the vascular wall (161,162). In addition, fibrinogen contributes significantly to changes in blood viscosity during inflammation as an acute-phase reactant. Abundantly secreted by the liver into the plasma, fibrinogen is a glycoprotein composed of a 340 kDa dimer with each half made up of three different polypeptide subunits, Aα, Bβ, and γ, interconnected by five symmetrical disulfide bridges (163). The amino-terminal region of each Aα chain contains a sequence that is proteolyzed by thrombin at the site of local vessel injury. This cleavage initiates fibrin assembly through the exposure of a polymerization site which, in turn, via complementary binding stoichiometries, forms double-stranded twisting fibrils that reassociate and branch in the complex fiber network required for thrombosis. This thrombin-induced biochemical cascade exposes specific binding sites for extrinsic proenzymes, clotting factors, and cell receptors (163). Fibrinogen–fibrin molecules have many biological roles, including blood coagulation, cellular and matrix interactions, inflammation, and wound repair. The important role of fibrinogen in atherosclerosis is supported by its ability to promote adenosine diphosphate-dependent platelet aggregation, induce vascular smooth muscle proliferation, bind LDL, and facilitate monocyte adherence to the vascular endothelium (164,165).

FIBRINOGEN REGULATION BY INFLAMMATION

The three fibrinogen subunits are encoded by separate genes that are closely linked within 65 kb of each other on chromosome 4. Coordinate expression of the fibrinogen subunits ensures that the correct stoichiometry is maintained for their assembly into the mature fibrinogen molecule. Although Aα, Bβ, and γ fibrinogen subunits are constitutively expressed, the fibrinogen locus is inducibly and coordinately regulated by systemic inflammation. Like CRP and SAA, the three human fibrinogen genes and those of the rat contain cis-regulatory elements that specify liver expression and cytokine response (163,166–169). The liver specific factors include HNF-1 and NF-IL6/C/EBPβ, a protein that binds in the proximal promoter of Aα, Bβ, and γ fibrinogen genes (48). The transcriptional control mechanisms for inducible fibrinogen synthesis have been extensively studied. IL-6 is the major acute-phase mediator of fibrinogen expression; IL-6 activates the Aα, Bβ, and γ fibrinogen genes through the cis-regulatory motifs containing the sequence CTGGGAAA that bind the IL-6–inducible STAT3 transcription factor (48). Typical of a class I acute-phase reactant, cortisol markedly increases the effect of IL-6 on fibrinogen synthesis, which is a glucocorticoid receptor-dependent phenomenon that either increases recruitment of the coactivator p300/CBP to the fibrinogen promoter or increases expression of the IL-6 signaling pathway (48,170). Basal and IL-6–induced fibrinogen expression are negatively regulated by fibric acid (fibrate) derivatives, drugs used to treat hypertryglyceridemia, by activating the nuclear receptor peroxisome proliferator activated receptor α (PPARα). PPARα may compete for coactivator binding with the liver specific protein NF-IL6/C/EBPβ (171), thereby reducing fibrinogen expression.

FIBRINOGEN AND ATHEROSCLEROSIS

An increase in circulating levels of fibrinogen is a well-established risk factor for the development of coronary events and for stroke in men and women with established coronary artery disease (164,165,172–175). More than 20 yr ago, in the Northwick Park Heart study of 1,510 white men aged 40–64 yr, a significant association between death from cardiovascular disease and initial fibrinogen values was discovered (176). In this and subsequent studies, the association of fibrinogen and cardiac events was stronger than that of cholesterol and cardiac events. In the Gothenborg study of 792 men followed for 13.5 years, univariate analysis identified cholesterol and fibrinogen as predictors of MI and blood pressure and fibrinogen as predictors of stroke. Patients hospitalized with unstable angina pectoris who had fibrinogen levels in the highest quartile had a 3.5-fold increased risk for cardiac death and future coronary events over those in the lowest quartile (173). Similar observations linking fibrinogen levels to the risk of coronary artery disease were seen in studies that included non-Western populations such as Chinese, Japanese, and Indian groups (177–179). The Bezafibrate Infarction Prevention (BIP) study showed that baseline levels of plasma fibrinogen independently predicted cardiovascular events in patients with coronary artery disease and that the incidence of cardiac death and ischemic stroke was reduced in patients who had high baseline fibrinogen values (180). Although the –455G/A polymorphism of the beta-fibrinogen gene affects levels of plasma fibrinogen, the results of studies evaluating its role as a predictive factor in the development of coronary artery disease have been inconsistent (181–183).

The role of plasma fibrinogen in cardiovascular disease risk is less evident and, in fact, absent in some studies of individuals with no clinically apparent coronary artery disease (184,185). One study found that fibrinogen levels predicted the development of coronary artery disease among patients with diabetes who had no history of coronary heart disease (186). Fibrinogen values correlated with the quantity of coronary artery calcification, a marker for preclinical coronary atherosclerosis, determined by electron beam computed tomography in middle-aged women without cardiovascular disease (187). Although fibrinogen may be causally related to atherosclerosis, no direct clinical evidence supports this relationship. Fibrinogen levels have not been selectively lowered in a study with agents that did not also have hypolipidemic effects—a problem also seen with CRP and SAA.

Angiotensinogen

Angiotensinogen (AGT) is a glycoprotein hormone secreted by the liver and is the only known precursor of the angiotensin peptides, generated by activity of the renin-angiotensin system (RAS). The RAS is an endocrine system involved in acute homeostatic control of peripheral vascular resistance and electrolyte homeostasis *(188,189)*. In the intravascular compartment, physiologic regulators of blood pressure and fluid balance induce the production of the potent vasoactive angiotensin peptides as a consequence of sequential proteolysis of the AGT prohormone, catalyzed initially by the aspartyl protease renin. Renin release from storage granules in specialized endocrine cells in the kidney (juxtaglomerular apparatus) is stimulated by changes in renal perfusion pressure, sympathetic outflow, and sodium load. In the presence of renin, the amino-terminus of the AGT precursor is cleaved into the decapeptide angiotensin I (AI). AI, in turn, is rapidly processed into the octapeptide angiotensin II through angiotensin-converting enzyme (ACE) appearing ubiquitously on the vascular endothelium. After formation of the angiotensin peptides, blood pressure and extracellular fluid volume are restored to normal levels *(188–190)*. Data support an expanded role of the RAS in the long-term control of blood pressure *(191)*, the pathobiology of diabetic nephropathy *(192)*, the edema of congestive heart failure *(193)*, and the control of the development (or progression) of atherosclerosis *(194,195)*.

Several studies indicate that circulating AGT concentration is an important factor controlling RAS tone. Under normal conditions, AGT circulates at concentrations less than the Km of renin *(1 μmol/L)*, and AGT abundance is rate-limiting for maximal velocity of AI formation *(189)*. Changes in AGT concentration, therefore, can affect RAS tone. Several physiologic observations support this critical relationship between AGT synthesis and RAS tone: (1) AGT concentrations correlate positively with blood pressure in ambulatory patients *(196)*; (2) pharmacologic manipulations (such as steroid administration) increase AGT and blood pressure in humans *(197)*; (3) gene dosage studies in mice show a linear 8 mm Hg increase in blood pressure with AGT copy number *(198)*; (4) transgenic mice overexpressing human AGT and renin genes are severely hypertensive *(199)*; and (5) human genetic linkage studies have associated polymorphisms of certain AGT alleles with hypertensive disease states, including essential hypertension *(191,200)*, preeclampsia *(201,202)*, and an intermediate phenotype of hypertension characterized by a blunted renal vascular response to angiotensin II (nonmodulators) *(203)*. In hypertensive individuals, changes in circulating plasma AGT of twofold or less are associated with significant differences in blood pressure and RAS tone. Although not systematically studied, changes in circulating AGT levels may significantly affect local RASs, such as the vascular RAS, which have independent angiotensin II–generating systems

free of the feedback regulatory mechanisms that normally control renin release.

Angiotensinogen Regulation by Inflammation

AGT is a member of the serine protease inhibitor (serpin) family, a family of acute-phase inducible genes that includes α1 antitrypsin, antithrombin, and ovalbumin. These serpins have evolved from a common ancestral gene *(204)*. In rodents, systemic inflammation is a well-established inducer of AGT expression. For example, 8 hours after stimulation, a single dose of bacterial endotoxin upregulates steady state AGT mRNA levels fivefold *(205)* and circulating AGT threefold *(206)*. This upregulation is mediated through TNF and IL-1–dependent activation of the NF-κB transcription factor *(30)*. Although human AGT has the same overall genomic organization as that of the rodent gene, detailed study of the sequence and organization of the *cis* control elements has shown significant divergence, indicating species-specific differences in AGT regulation *(207)*. The authors recently showed that human AGT (hAGT) is as not strongly upregulated by IL-1 or TNF as it is in the rodent gene. Instead, inducible hepatic hAGT expression is primarily mediated by IL-6 at the transcriptional level *(51)*. Like CRP, the acute-phase regulation of AGT shows species specificity. The mechanism for IL-6–mediated upregulation of hAGT is similar to that described for the other acute-phase reactants, CRP, SAA, and fibrinogen. IL-6 induces an increase in steady state AGT mRNA at the transcriptional level mediated by three reiterated TTCTGGGAA (STAT) binding motifs located in the first 300 nucleotides of the human proximal promoter *(51)*. Expression of dominant negative isoforms of STAT1 and STAT3 showed that STAT3 was the only major STAT transactivating form of AGT expression. These studies were independently confirmed in mice by tissue specific knock-out studies of STAT3 in the liver with the use of Cre-recombinase technology *(52)*; expression of acute-phase reactants was significantly inhibited in these animals deficient in hepatic STAT3. Finally, the authors have demonstrated a role for STAT3–dependent chromatin remodeling through recruitment of histone acetyltransferase activity of the p300/CBP coactivator to the AGT promoter *(49)*. Histone acetyltransferase activity is important in chromatin (nucleosomal) remodeling in the process of gene activation *(37,54)*. Together, these studies suggest a molecular mechanism for how vascular wall inflammation might affect RAS activity. Although the vascular wall releases mediators that upregulate the expression of hAGT, reciprocally circulating AGT may have important pro-atherogenic actions in the vessel wall by supplying increased substrate to the local vascular RAS.

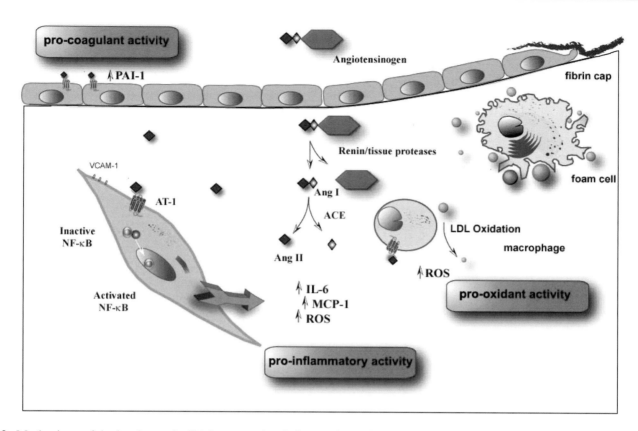

Fig. 3. Mechanisms of the local vascular RAS to potentiate inflammation and atherosclerosis. Schematic diagram of a complex atherosclerotic plaque and processing enzymes for local angiotensin II production from circulating angiotensinogen. Circulating angiotensinogen can be cleaved into the decapeptide angiotensin I by the action of renin or several tissue proteases. Angiotensin I is rapidly converted into the vasoactive octapeptide angiotensin II by the action of angiotensin-converting enzyme produced by activated mononuclear cells in the atherosclerotic plaque. Angiotensin II binds to a 7-transmembrane spanning domain receptor expressed by vascular smooth muscle cells, endothelial cells, and macrophages. Note that the actions of angiotensin II are similar to those of the activating cytokines in the vascular cytokine cascade (see Fig. 1) by increasing expression of monocytic chemokines (IL-6 and MCP-1) and stimulating formation of reactive oxygen species. Angiotensin II affects coagulation cascades through its potent effects on plasminogen activator inhibitor-1 expression by endothelial cells. ACE, angiotensin-converting enzyme; Ang, angiotensin; AT-1, angiotensin type 1 receptor; IL-6, interleukin-6; LDL, low density lipoprotein; MCP-1, monocyte chemoattractant protein-1; NF-κB, nuclear factor-κB; PAI-1, plasminogen activator inhibitor-1; ROS, reactive oxygen species; VCAM-1, vascular cell adhesion molecule-1.

ATHEROSLCEROTIC PLAQUE AS A LOCAL GENERATOR OF ANGIOTENSIN II

RAS has been divided into two categories: the circulating intravascular RAS and the local tissue RASs, which are important in controlling organ function. Local RASs are assumed to operate in tissues that have the ability to express the necessary components for local angiotensin II generation. Local RASs have been described for brain, kidney, heart, and adipose tissue *(207,208)*, with evidence for a vascular RAS. The detailed in situ hybridization work of Campbell and Habener *(209,210)* has shown that the vessel wall is not a significant source of AGT expression. However, the circulating plasma provides a constant source of AGT, derived mainly from hepatic secretion, to the vessel wall *(30,211)*. In the case

of the vessel wall, local angiotensin II can be generated by the expression of processing enzymes that would convert circulating AGT into angiotensin peptides (Fig. 3). Renin and several renin-like enzymes that release AI from AGT, including cathepsin D, aspartyl proteases, have been identified in vascular tissue *(208,212)*. In addition, atherosclerotic plaques are rich in the converting enzymes that process AI into angiotensin II, including classical ACE expressed by activated monocyte/macrophages in the vascular wall *(213)*. Moreover, cells in atherosclerotic lesions make other ACE-like enzymes that produce active angiotensin II. Some of these enzymes include cathepsin G (expressed by neutrophils) *(214)* and chymase (a component of mast cells) *(215)*. Atherosclerotic plaques are not surprisingly positive for angiotensin II by immunohistochemical staining *(216)*. These findings strongly suggest that the atherosclerotic plaque has a local tissue angiotensin II–generating mechanism that can use circulating AGT substrate, but this mechanism escapes the negative feedback controls that normally regulate activity of the intravascular RAS (30).

Pro-atherogenic Actions of Angiotensin II

Angiotensin II affects the atherosclerotic vessel by binding a high affinity G-protein–coupled 7-transmembrane receptor expressed on endothelial cells, VSMCs, and monocytes (37,217,218). Several vascular actions of angiotensin II are pro-inflammatory and pro-atherogenic. On endothelial cells, angiotensin II upregulates the expression of the endothelial oxidized LDL receptor, the lectin-like oxLDL receptor-1 (219). Angiotensin II increases production of ROS and catabolism of nitric oxide and contributes to early endothelial dysfunction. In response to ROS, endothelial cells upregulate expression of adhesion molecules such as VCAM (220), which in turn increase monocyte recruitment. By increasing IL-6 production, angiotensin II stimulates monocytes to increase LDL uptake and catabolism, which results in foam cell formation (221). Angiotensin II may alter the balance between the fibrinolytic and coagulation systems by increasing expression of plasminogen activator inhibitor-1 (222), a process that promotes thrombogenesis on the unstable atherosclerotic plaque.

The effects of angiotensin II on the VSMCs have been studied intensively. As with endothelial cells, angiotensin I induces adhesion molecule upregulation on VSMCs. In addition, angiotensin II induces oxidative stress through an NADH/NADPH oxidase system, which has some components common to the macrophage NADPH oxidase (223–225). ROS production is a key intracellular signal and is linked to activation of tyrosine kinase–coupled receptors, including the epithelial growth factor receptor, which activates p38 mitogen-activated protein kinase (MAPK), extracellular signal–related kinase (ERK), c-fos expression, and vascular hypertrophy (37,218,226). As a consequence of activation of MAP, ERK, and the jun amino-terminal kinases, angiotensin II upregulates inflammatory cytokine expression by VSMCs. Of these cytokines, IL-6 and MCP are well established targets for angiotensin II signaling (22,41,227). These chemokines act locally to induce monocyte migration into the plaque, promote monocyte maturation, and initiate the hepatic acute-phase response.

Renin–Angiotensin System Activity and Atherosclerosis

The finding that ACE inhibitors profoundly reduce ischemic vascular events in clinical trials suggests an important relation between the RAS and atherogenesis. In the Studies of Left Ventricular Dysfunction (SOLVD) trial, a prospective double-blind trial examining the development of MI or unstable angina in 6,800 patients with low ejection fraction, enalapril reduced the incidence of recurrent MI by 23% (228). A 25% reduction in recurrent MI was seen in the Survival and Ventricular Enlargment (SAVE) trial in patients with left ventricular dysfunction after MI (229). The Heart Outcomes Prevention Evaluation (HOPE) study, involving 9,297 high-risk patients with vascular disease, provided further evidence of the beneficial effects of ACE inhibitors on cardiovascular events (230). In contrast with earlier trials of patients with severe left ventricular dysfunction, patients in the HOPE study had normal left ventricular function; the study was terminated early (after 5 yr) because of the statistically significant 22% reduction in MI, cerebrovascular accidents, or death from cardiovascular causes seen in the group given ramipril (230). ACE inhibitor therapy was significant after 2 yr of treatment. The authors suggested that that the effect of lowering blood pressure was modest and could not account completely for the risk reduction observed in the study. Although these results strongly suggest that blocking angiotensin II formation may reduce cardiovascular mortality, the actions of the ACE inhibitor may have been due, in part, to non-angiotensin II actions (e.g., inhibition of bradykinin breakdown). Although similar clinical studies are needed to clarify the mechanism, data support a central role for angiotensin II in the vascular pathobiology of atherosclerosis.

Angiotensin II Enhancement of Atherosclerosis and Vascular Inflammation

Several observations have suggested mechanisms for manners in which angiotensin II may synergize with hyperlipidemia to accelerate atherosclerosis. As in human studies, ACE inhibitors reduce the development of atherosclerosis in experimental animals including the Watanabe hypercholesterolemic rabbit (231), the apolipoprotein E deficient mouse (232), minipigs (233), and hyperlipidemic hamsters (234). Losartan (Dup 753), a selective angiotensin II receptor antagonist, recently reversed the increase in ROS formation and endothelial dysfunction in the early atherosclerotic lesion; this study supports an early role for angiotensin II in the atherogenic process (223). In addition, losartan reduced lesion size in the cholesterol-fed cynomologous monkey, indicating a role for angiotensin II in LDL-induced atherosclerosis (235). In contrast, transgenic mice with constitutively high levels of circulating angiotensin II, caused by transgenic co-expression of the human renin and AGT genes, develop extensive aortic root lesions in response to a high-fat diet *(236)*. Two groups recently evaluated the effects of a 4- to 8-wk subcutaneous angiotensin II infusion in the atherosclerosis-susceptible apolipoprotein E–deficient (apoE$^{-/-}$) mouse, which lacks the ability to clear LDL cholesterol and is deficient in HDL reverse cholesterol transport from tissue to plasma *(237)*. Chronic angiotensin II infusion dramatically accelerated the generation of atherosclerotic aortic lesions from 4% surface area involvement in control mice to 70% in angiotensin II–treated apoE$^{-/-}$ mice *(238)* and increased the formation of aortic aneurysms and macrophage recruitment to the underlying adventitia *(239)*. In control experiments, angiotensin II infusion in control (apoE$^{+/+}$) mice did not detectably induce aneurysms or atherosclerosis *(239)*. The combined effect of the angiotensin II infusion with hyperlipidemia may have a synergistic effect on angiotensin II action and LDL oxidation to increase ROS production in the vessel wall *(195,223,224)*. Together, these data strongly suggest that angiotensin II potentiates the development of atherosclerosis in experimental models of hyperlipidemia and may account for the cardioprotective actions of ACE inhibitors seen in human trials.

BIOCHEMICAL ASSESSMENT OF VASCULAR INFLAMMATION

The hepatic acute-phase response is a nonspecific response to the presence of inflammation from infectious agents, rheumatologic conditions, and the presence of systemic malignancy. These conditions must be excluded before sensitive biochemical measurements of inflammation can be interpreted. In the absence of these other inflammatory processes, the detection of increased circulating IL-6 or CRP is an indicator of subclinical vascular inflammation, a process underlying atherogenesis. Although it is seemingly the most direct method, measuring circulating IL-6 in patients with suspected vascular disease is problematic. In nonstressed conditions, IL-6 circulates at such low concentrations (<5 ng/L) that it is not normally detectable by conventional enzyme-linked immunosorbent assay (ELISA). Because of rapid in vivo turnover, uncomplexed IL-6 has an estimated serum half life of about 2 min, which necessitates the use of sequential sampling to determine steady state IL-6 concentrations *(240)*. More important, IL-6 is bound in plasma by the soluble (s) forms of the high-affinity IL-6 receptor, sIL-6R, and transducin, sgp130 *(241)*. The IL-6:sIL-6R complex extends the biologic half life of IL-6 and activates IL-6 signaling in cells expressing gp130 (but otherwise lacking the IL-6R). Under normal conditions, sIL-6R circulates at concentrations of 30 to 70 ng/mL, which

are significant relative to the concentration of IL-6, and is itself regulated by infectious processes *(242)*. In contrast, sgp130, which selectively complexes with IL-6:sIL-6R and inhibits its activity, acts as a sink for the cytokine and determines the biologically active fraction of IL-6. sgp130 circulates at concentrations of up to 400 ng/L, and the effect of inflammation on sgp130 levels is not understood. Therefore, assays for detecting the biologically active form of IL-6 are not routinely used in clinical settings.

C-reactive Protein Measurement—A Sensitive Biomarker of IL-6 Production

Because of the difficulties in measuring IL-6 directly, measurements of CRP, the biological target of IL-6, are used as a marker for subclinical vascular inflammation. CRP levels are stable and reflect the biologic activity of IL-6. The original standard clinical assays for CRP measurements, developed with immunoturbidimetric and immunophelometric techniques, were used primarily to detect active inflammation and infection. The dynamic range of these assays extends from a detection level of 3 mg/L, which corresponds to the 90th percentile of the general population, to over 200 mg/L. However, these assays lack sensitivity within the low–normal range and therefore are not effective for determining the risk of cardiovascular disease in healthy individuals.

To improve the sensitivity and reproducibility of CRP measurements, high sensitivity CRP (HSCRP) assays were developed. In early studies, an ELISA method with polyclonal antibodies was used in the HSCRP assays *(243)*. A commercially available automated latex-enhanced technique has been used recently *(91,244–246)*. In comparison assays, results of these two HSCRP methods were similar *(244)*. Current HSCRP assays can detect concentrations as low as 0.15 mg/L (<2.5th percentile of the general population); however, these assays may have different sensitivities, especially at lower limits of quantification, which may result in significant discrepancies between different commercial kits *(243,245,247)*. These discrepancies may lead to misclassification of cardiovascular risk and inappropriate management of patients, suggesting the need for standardization of current HSCRP assays. The most effective method is to have a single HSCRP assay in the clinical laboratory that can measure concentrations at both low and high ends, or physicians should request HSCRP assays specifically performed for cardiovascular risk prediction *(248)*.

Because HSCRP levels increase with acute infection and trauma *(249)*, testing is not recommended in patients who have had an acute illness such as an upper respiratory tract infection until recovery is complete. HSCRP testing may be of limited value in patients with inflammatory conditions such as rheumatoid arthritis or lupus because CRP levels are usually high in these patients. Large-scale survey studies indicate that less than 2% of the population screened have HSCRP values that are greater than 1.5 mg/dL, a level considered to be indicative of a clinically relevant inflammatory condition *(117)*. When above 1.5 mg/dL, the HSCRP measure should be repeated in 2–3 wk to exclude the possibility of a recent infection. If the CRP level is high a second time, the patient should be evaluated for a previously unsuspected inflammatory condition.

HSCRP levels do not show circadian variation *(250)*; thus, testing can be performed at any time of day. The within-person biologic variability of HSCRP is low over an extended period of time, which indicates the biologic stability of the molecule in the absence of active infection *(251)*.

For assessing the risk of future cardiovascular events, HSCRP values are divided into five population-based quintiles based on studies in healthy American men and women *(117)*. The ranges of these values are 0.01–0.069 (low relative risk), 0.07–0.11 (mild relative risk), 0.12–0.19 (moderate relative risk), 0.20–0.38 (high relative risk), and >0.38 mg/dL (highest relative risk) *(117)*.

Serum Amyloid A Assay

The various methods for measuring SAA include radioimmunoassay (RIA), radial immunodiffusion, latex-enhanced immunonephelometry, and ELISA. The commercially available ELISA assay is the most sensitive method and has a lower limit of detection of 100 ng/L *(146)*. The normal range of SAA is 0.5–10 mg/L; most healthy subjects have values less than 3 mg/L, and the value is slightly higher in the elderly *(252)*. Levels of SAA dramatically increase in inflammatory conditions, depending on the severity. For example, in acute MI, levels of SAA usually increase to 100–1000 mg/L.

Erythrocyte Sedimentation Rate

The ESR has been widely used for more than 50 years to detect the acute-phase reaction. In the Westergren method for measuring ESR, a calibrated tube of standard diameter with anticoagulated whole blood is used to measure the rate of red blood cell (RBC) sedimentation after 1 h. When the RBCs settle toward the bottom of the tube they leave an increasingly large zone of clear plasma which is the area measured. Most changes in sedimentation rate are caused by alterations in plasma proteins, mainly fibrinogen, with a much smaller contribution

from immunoglobulins. Many disease states such as acute and chronic inflammation, tissue injury, malignancy, and collagen vascular disease may result in increased levels of ESR, which reflects its poor specificity. Studies of the association of ESR and the risk of coronary heart disease are few and the results are conflicting. A meta-analysis comparing ESR values in individuals in the upper third of the normal distribution with those in the lower third showed a risk ratio of 1.3 *(253)*. However, ESR failed to predict subsequent MI in American men and women *(254)* and Swedish women *(255)*. In a large prospective European study of 2014 healthy men aged 40 to 60 years who were followed for 23 yr, ESR correlated with coronary heart disease mortality, but did not predict the development of nonfatal MI *(256)*. The study was limited by the absence of adjustment for serum fibrinogen, albumin, and immunoglobulins. The value of measuring ESR for the prediction of coronary heart disease has not been established *(257)*.

Fibrinogen

Clinical laboratories measure plasma fibrinogen by an automated clotting assay *(258)*. Although plasma levels of fibrinogen are high in the unstressed state (2.5–3.0 mg/mL), changes in circulating levels of fibrinogen, such as those induced by inflammation, may affect the extent of thrombosis *(259)*. Circulating levels of fibrinogen are strongly affected by age, smoking, gender, and many pharmaceuticals *(164)*. For example, smokers have levels that are about 0.3 g/L higher than those of nonsmokers, and high levels persist for up to 20 years after smoking cessation. In addition, women tend to have fibrinogen levels that are 0.1 g/L higher than those of men. When these factors are controlled for, circulating fibrinogen concentration is upregulated in the hepatic acute-phase reaction, but only three- to fourfold within the first 24 h of the inflammatory stimulus *(260)*.

Renin–Angiotensin System Activity

RAS components are usually measured in the laboratory by indirect assays because the plasma concentrations of angiotensin II are extremely labile due to its rapid half life. The most widely used indirect assay is the plasma renin activity (PRA) test, which measures angiotensin release from endogenous substrate by incubation in vitro *(261)*. The PRA is sensitive to volume status, ambulatory state, and hypertensive treatment (especially diuretics). Although qualitative measurements of AGT concentrations have been estimated by rocket immunoelectrophoresis *(262)*, indirect assays have been most widely used. In the indirect technique, a plasma sample is extensively digested by active renin in the presence of converting enzyme inhibitors, and the amount of AI formation is then determined by radioimmunoassay *(191)*. Normal circulating levels of AGT depend on genotype, gender, drugs (progestins, estrogens, and cortisol increase its expression), and inflammation (Table 1). In one study, circulating AGT levels were increased twofold in 70% of patients with severe infection *(262)*. Although numerically small, this change is biologically significant and is similar to the twofold increase in circulating AGT seen in patients with autosomal-dominant (angiotensin II–dependent) hypertension *(191)*. Because of its difficulty and numerous confounding factors, measurement of RAS activity is used only for specific research applications.

MANAGEMENT OF VASCULAR INFLAMMATION IN ATHEROSCLEROSIS

Markers of vascular inflammation would be clinically useful in two groups: patients with acute ischemia and healthy individuals for whom atherosclerotic risk is being detected. First, increased IL-6 or CRP secretion is of prognostic value for short- and intermediate-term outcome in patients with unstable angina. However, whether the presence of inflammation can be used to identify a subgroup of patients that may be responsive to particular therapies is unknown. In a recent Scandanavian prospective study of 3489 patients with unstable angina randomized to two treatment regimens (invasive or noninvasive), early invasive treatment substantially reduced 12-month mortality among those with increased IL-6 levels *(58)*. Furthermore, mortality was reduced more in patients with increased IL-6 levels who were placed on low molecular weight heparin than in patients on heparin therapy without increased IL-6. These findings need to be replicated before formal recommendations can be made for patient management; however, inflammation in patients with acute ischemia may be useful in identifying subgroups that are responsive to particular therapies.

The relation of increased IL-6 or acute-phase reactants with atherosclerotic risk raises the question as to whether these factors could be used to identify a subgroup of patients that should be treated with anti-inflammatory therapy. Few studies have addressed this question. In the Physicians' Health Study, aspirin therapy reduced the risk of MI by 55.7% in healthy individuals with baseline levels of CRP in the highest quartile *(100)*. However, aspirin reduced risk by only 13.9%, a nonsignificant effect, in patients with CRP levels in the lowest quartiles. These findings suggest that the efficacy of aspirin

in cardiovascular disease prevention could be due in part to its anti-inflammatory effect, in addition to its effects on platelet aggregation. Aspirin reduces vascular NF-κB activation, which may contribute to its beneficial effects in clinical studies *(263)*.

Several other established anti-atherogenic therapies have anti-inflammatory actions in the vessel wall. For example, baseline levels of CRP are modified by treatment with 3-hydroxy-3-methylglutaryl coenzyme A (HMG-CoA) reductase inhibitors, or statins. Statin therapy reduces serum CRP levels in patients treated with statins for primary hypercholesterolemia *(264,265)* and in patients being treated for secondary prevention of coronary artery events *(110,265,266)*. The lowering of CRP levels was independent of the changes in plasma lipid values in response to HMG-CoA reductase inhibitors *(110,265,266)*. These observations suggest that, in addition to their ability to reduce LDL cholesterol, statins may favorably modify the atherosclerotic process by inhibiting inflammatory and possibly noninflammatory mechanisms that induce the acute-phase response *(267–269)*. Statins reduce the in vitro secretion of IL-6 and inducible nitric oxide synthase by VSMCs and improve endothelial function *(270)*. The biochemical mechanism of an inflammatory effect has not been shown, but suggested mechanisms include depletion of cholesterol in the membranes of inflammatory cells and reduced isoprenylation of signaling proteins in these membranes *(267)*. Reports on the effect of statins on other acute-phase proteins such as fibrinogen and plasminogen-activator inhibitor-I have been inconsistent *(271,272)*, suggesting that statins may effect expression of certain acute-phase reactants more than others. Postmenopausal women on hormone replacement therapy have higher levels of serum CRP than those not on hormone replacement *(273–275)*; this difference was not affected by the hormone used in such therapy. The clinical signficance of these findings has not been determined. Finally, fibric acid derivatives, a class of hypolipidemic drugs used to treat hypertrigyceridemia, antagonize cytokine signaling in VSMCs *(276)*. In addition, fibrates reduce circulating fibrinogen levels through transcriptional inhibition of fibrinogen expression mediated by the nuclear hormone receptor peroxisome proliferator-α *(171,277)*. In fact, plasma fibrinogen levels were significantly reduced in patients with coronary artery disease and mixed hyperlipidemia (increased LDL cholesterol and triglycerides) after 6 months of therapy with combined treatment with fluvastatin and bezafibrate or with bezafibrate alone. Data on coronary events or mortality have not been reported

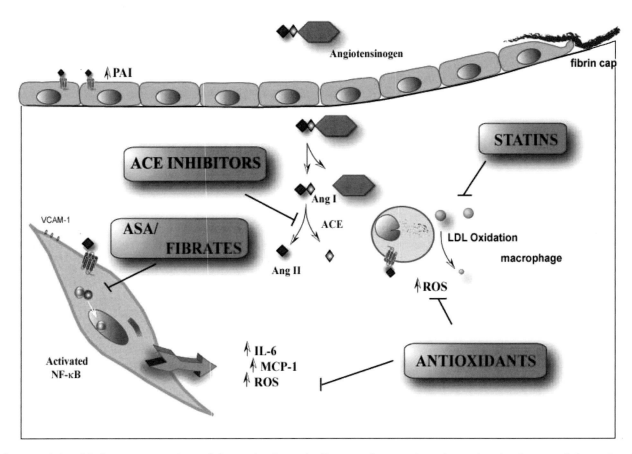

Fig. 4. Potential anti-inflammatory actions of drugs. A schematic diagram of a complex atherosclerotic plaque and the major sites of drug actions that affect local vascular inflammation. The anti-inflammatory actions of ACE inhibitors and antioxidants have not been shown clinically. ACE, angiotensin-converting enzyme; Ang, angiotensin; ASA, acetylsalicylic acid; IL-6, interleukin-6; LDL, low density lipoprotein; MCP-1, monocyte chemoattractant protein-1; NF-κB, nuclear factor-κB; PAI, plasminogen activator inhibitor; ROS, reactive oxygen species; VCAM-1, vascular cell adhesion molecule-1.

(172). These findings suggest that some of the benefits of fibrate action may be mediated by anti-inflammatory actions locally at the vessel wall and systemically via reduction in fibrinogen. Figure 4 shows the major sites of action of conventional anti-inflammatory agents on the vessel wall.

The effects of anti-inflammatory therapy intended to reduce acute-phase reactant markers of atherosclerosis have not been assessed in clinical trials without ancillary platelet or lipid-lowering effects. CRP reduction, per se, has not yet been shown to reduce cardiovascular events.

Future Directions

Although epidemiological studies have produced strong evidence supporting the relation between vascular inflammation and atherosclerosis, these studies do not address the mechanisms by which chronic inflammation is produced or by which it increases cardiovascular risk. For example, is activation of the acute-phase reaction only a measure of the severity of vascular inflammation or does it play a role in the pathobiology of atherosclerosis? Which products of the acute-phase response, if any, participate in the atherogenic process? When in the process of atherosclerosis is inflammation seen? Does inflammation play a role at the fatty streak stage or after an established atherosclerotic plaque is formed? Do combinations of acute-phase reactants contribute independently to cardiovascular risk? Should the presence of inflammation be clinically addressed? Should these patients be more aggressively managed, and should anti-inflammatory therapy be initiated when an increased HSCRP value is measured? What is the best agent(s) to treat patients with vascular inflammation? These questions need to be addressed by basic and clinical research with specific pharmacologic tools that interfere with the action or expression of individual acute-phase reactants.

REFERENCES

1. Ross R, Glomset JA. Atherosclerosis and the arterial smooth muscle cell: Proliferation of smooth muscle is a key event in the genesis of the lesions of atherosclerosis. Science 1973;180:1332–1339.
2. Ross R. Atherosclerosis—an inflammatory disease. N Engl J Med 1999;340:115–126.
3. Kullo KJ, Gau G, Tajik AJ. Novel risk factors for atherosclerosis. Mayo Clinic Proc 2000;75:369–380.
4. Griendling KK, Alexander RW. Oxidative stress and cardiovascular disease. Circulation 1997;96:3264–3265.
5. Libby P. Molecular base of the acute coronary syndrome. Circulation 1995;21:2844–2850.
6. Galis ZS, Muszynski M, Sukhova GK, et al. Cytokine-stimulated smooth muscle cells synthesize a complement of enzymes required for extracellular matrix digestion. Circ Res 1994;75:181–189.
7. Ross R. Growth regulatory mechanisms and formation of the lesions of atherosclerosis. Ann N Y Acad Sci 1995;748:1–6.
8. Lusis AJ. Atherosclerosis. Nature 2000;407:233–241.
9. Knowles JW, Maeda N. Genetic modifiers of atherosclerosis in mice. Arterioscler Thromb Vasc Biol 2000;20:2336–2345.
10. Takeya M, Yoshimura T, Leonard EJ, Takahashi K. Detection of monocyte chemoattractant protein-1 in human atherosclerotic lesions by an anti-monocyte chemoattrantant protein-1 monoclonal antibody. Hum Pathol 1993;24:534–539.
11. Gerszten RE, Garcia-Zepeda EA, Lim YC, et al. MCP-1 and IL-8 trigger firm adhesion of monocytes to vascular endothelium under flow conditions. Nature 1999;398:718–723.
12. Koch AE, Kunkel SL, Pearce WH, et al. Enhanced production of the chemotactic cytokines interleukin-8 and monocyte chemoattractant protein-1 in human abdominal aortic aneurysms. Am J Pathol 1993;142:1423–1431.
13. Pattison JM, Nelson PJ, Huie P, Sibley RK, Krensky AM. RANTES chemokine expression in transplant-associated accelerated atherosclerosis. J Heart Lung Transplant 1996;15:1194–1199.
14. Wilcox JN, Nelken NA, Coughlin SR, Gordon D, Schall TJ. Local expression of inflammatory cytokines in human atherosclerotic plaques. J Atheroscler Thromb 1994;1:S10–S13.
15. Weber KS, von Hundelshausen P, Clark-Lewis I, Weber PC, Weber C. Differential immobilization and hierarchical involvement of chemokines in monocyte arrest and transmigration on inflamed endothelium in shear flow. Eur J Immunol 1999;29:700–712.
16. Huo Y, Weber C, Forlow SB, et al. The chemokine KC, but not monocyte chemoattractant protein-1, triggers monocyte arrest on early atherosclerotic endothelium. J Clin Invest 2001;108:1307–1314.
17. Gu L, Okada Y, Clinton SK, et al. Absence of monocyte chemoattractant protein-1 reduces atherosclerosis in low density lipoprotein receptor-deficient mice. Mol Cell 1998;2: 275–281.
18. Boring L, Gosling J, Cleary M, Charo IF. Decreased lesion formation in CCR2–/– mice reveals a role for chemokines in the initiation of atherosclerosis. Nature 1998;394:894–897.
19. Clinton SK, Underwood R, Hayes L, Sherman ML, Kufe DW, Libby P. Macrophage colony-stimulating factor gene expression in vascular cells and in experimental and human atherosclerosis. Am J Pathol 1992;140:301–316.
20. Smith JD, Trogan E, Ginsberg M, Grigaux C, Tian J, Miyata M. Decreased atherosclerosis in mice deficient in both macrophage

21. colony-stimulating factor (op) and apolipoprotein E. Proc Natl Acad Sci USA 1995;92:8264–8268.
21. Loppnow H, Libby P. Proliferating or interleukin-1 activated human vascular smooth muscle cells secrete copious interleukin-6. J Clin Invest 1990;85:731–738.
22. Han Y, Runge MS, Brasier AR. Angiotensin II induces interleukin-6 transcription in vascular smooth muscle cells through pleiotropic activation of nuclear factor-kappa B transcription factors. Circ Res 1999;84:695–703.
23. Ikeda U, Ikeda M, Oohara T, et al. Interleukin-6 stimulates growth of vascular smooth muscle cells in a PDGF-dependent manner. Am J Physiol 1991;260:H1713–H1717.
24. Bayes-Genis A, Conover CA, Schwartz RS. The insulin-like growth factor axis: A review of atherosclerosis and restenosis. Circ Res 2000;86:125–130.
25. Barnes PJ, Karin M. Nuclear factor-kappaB: a pivotal transcription factor in chronic inflammatory diseases. N Engl J Med 1997;336:1066–1071.
26. Karin M. The beginning of the end: IkappaB kinase (IKK) and NF-kappaB activation. J Biol Chem 1999;274:27339–27342.
27. Garofalo R, Sabry M, Jamaluddin M, et al. Transcriptional activation of the interleukin-8 gene by respiratory syncytial virus infection in alveolar epithelial cells: nuclear translocation of the RelA transcription factor as a mechanism producing airway mucosal inflammation. J Virol 1996;70:8773–8781.
28. Han Y, Brasier AR. Mechanism for biphasic rel A. NF-kappaB1 nuclear translocation in tumor necrosis factor alpha-stimulated hepatocytes. J Biol Chem 1997;272:9825–9832.
29. Henkel T, Machleidt T, Alkalay I, Kronke M, Ben-Neriah Y, Baeuerle PA. Rapid proteolysis of I kappa B-alpha is necessary for activation of transcription factor NF-kappa B. Nature 1993;365:182–185.
30. Brasier AR, Li J. Mechanisms for inducible control of angiotensinogen gene transcription. Hypertension 1996;27: 465–475.
31. Brown K, Gerstberger S, Carlson L, Franzoso G, Siebenlist U. Control of Ikappa B-alpha proteolysis by site-specific, signal-induced phosphorylation. Science 1995;267:1485–1488.
32. Karin M, Ben Neriah Y. Phosphorylation meets ubiquitination: the control of NF-[kappa]B activity. Annu Rev Immunol 2000;18:621–663.
33. Jamaluddin M, Casola A, Garofalo RP, et al. The major component of IkappaBalpha proteolysis occurs independently of the proteasome pathway in respiratory syncytial virus-infected pulmonary epithelial cells. J Virol 1998;72:4849–4857.
34. Han Y, Weinman S, Boldogh I, Walker PK, Brasier AR. Tumor necrosis factor-alpha-inducible IkappaBalpha proteolysis mediated by cytosolic m-calpain. A mechanism parallel to the ubiqiuitin-proteasome pathway for nuclear factor-kappaB activation. Biol Chem 1999;274:787–794.
35. Brand K, Page S, Rogler G, et al. Activated transcription factor nuclear factor-kappaB is present in the atherosclerotic lesion. J Clin Invest 1996;97:1715–1722.
36. Li J, Brasier AR. Angiotensinogen gene activation by angiotensin II is mediated by the rel A (nuclear factor-kappaB p65) transcription factor: one mechanism for the renin angiotensin system positive feedback loop in hepatocytes. Mol Endocrinol 1996;10:252–264.
37. Brasier AR, Jamaluddin M, Han Y, Patterson C, Runge MS. Angiotensin II induces gene transcription through cell-type dependent effects on the nuclear factor-kB (NF-kappaB) transcription factor. Mol Cell Biochem 2000;212:155–169.

38. Collins T, Cybulsky MI. NF-kappaB: pivotal mediator or innocent bystander in atherogenesis? J Clin Invest 2001;107:255–264.

39. Vlahopoulos S, Boldogh I, Casola A, Brasier AR. Nuclear factor-kappaB-dependent induction of interleukin-8 gene expression by tumor necrosis factor alpha: evidence for an antioxidant sensitive activating pathway distinct from nuclear translocation. Blood 1999;94:1878–1889.

40. Bourcier T, Sukhova G, Libby P. The nuclear factor kappa-B signaling pathway participates in dysregulation of vascular smooth muscle cells in vitro and in human atherosclerosis. J Biol Chem 1997;272:15817–15824.

41. Kranzhofer R, Schmidt J, Pfeiffer CA, Hagl S, Libby P, Kubler W. Angiotensin induces inflammatory activation of human vascular smooth muscle cells. Arterioscler Thromb Vasc Biol 1999;19:1623–1629.

42. Fahraeus R. The suspension stability of the blood. Acta Med Scand 1921;55:1.

43. Gabay C, Kushner I. Acute-phase proteins and other systemic responses to inflammation. N Engl J Med 1999;340:448–454.

44. Kushner I. The phenomenon of the acute phase response. Ann N Y Acad Sci 1982;389:39–48.

45. Metz R, Ziff E. cAMP stimulates the C/EBP-related transcription factor rNFIL-6 to trans-locate to the nucleus and induce c-fos transcription. Genes Dev 1991;5:1754–1766.

46. O'Neil KT, Shuman JD, Ampe C, DeGrado WF. DNA-induced increase in the alpha-helical content of C/EBP and GCN4. Biochemistry 1991;30:9030–9034.

47. Steel DM, Whitehead AS. The major acute phase reactants: C-reactive protein, serum amyloid P component and serum amyloid A protein. Immunol Today 1994;15:81–88.

48. Fuller GM, Zhang Z. Transcriptional control mechanism of fibrinogen gene expression. Ann N Y Acad Sci 2001;936:469–479.

49. Ray S, Sherman C, Lu M, Brasier AR. Angiotensinogen gene expression is dependent on signal transducer and activator of transcription 3-mediated p300/cAMP response element binding protein-binding protein coactivator recruitment and histone acetyltransferase activity. Mol Endocrinol 2002;16: 824–836.

50. Akira S, Nishio Y, Tanaka T, et al. Transcription factors NF-IL6 and APRF involved in gp130-mediated signaling pathway. Ann N Y Acad Sci 1995;762:15–28.

51. Sherman CT, Brasier AR. Role of signal transducers and activators of transcription 1 and -3 in inducible regulation of the human angiotensinogen gene by interleukin-6. Mol Endocrinol 2001;15:441–457.

52. Alonzi T, Maritano D, Gorgoni B, Rizzuto G, Libert C, Poli V. Essential role of STAT3 in the control of the acute-phase response as revealed by inducible gene inactivation [correction of activation] in the liver. Mol Cell Biol 2001;21:1621–1632.

53. Ihle J. STATs: signal transducers and activators of transcription. Cell 1996;84:331–334.

54. Shikama N, Lyon J, LaThangue NB. The p300/CBP family: integrating signals with transcription factors and chromatin. Trends Cell Biol 1997:7:230–236.

55. Bannister AJ, Kouzarides T. The CBP co-activator is a histone acetyltransferase. Nature 1996;384:641–643.

56. Miyao Y, Yasue H, Ogawa H, et al. Elevated plasma interleukin-6 levels in patients with acute myocardial infarction. Am Heart J 1993;126:1299–1304.

57. Biasucci LM, Liuzzo G, Fantuzzi G, et al. Increasing levels of interleukin (IL)-1Ra and IL-6 during the first 2 days of hospitalization in unstable angina are associated with increased risk of in-hospital coronary events. Circulation 1999;99:2079–2084.

58. Lindmark E, Diderholm E, Wallentin L, Siegbahn A. Relationship between interleukin 6 and mortality in patients with unstable coronary artery disease: effects of an early invasive or noninvasive strategy. JAMA 2001;286:2107–2113.

59. Harris TB, Ferrucci L, Tracy RP, et al. Associations of elevated interleukin-6 and C-reactive protein levels with mortality in the elderly. Am J Med 1999;106:506–512.

60. Ridker PM, Rifai N, Stampfer MJ, Hennekens CH. Plasma concentration of interleukin-6 and the risk of future myocardial infarction among apparently healthy men. Circulation 2000;101:1767–1772.

61. Volanakis JE. Human C-reactive protein: expression, structure, and function. Mol Immunol 2001;38:189–197.

62. Gewurz H, Mold C, Siegel J, Fiedel B. C-reactive protein and the acute phase response. Adv Internal Med 1982;27:345–372.

63. Oliveira EB, Gotschlich C, Liu TY. Primary structure of human C-reactive protein. J Biol Chem 1979;254:489–502.

64. Osmand AP, Friedenson B, Gewurz H, Painter RH, Hofmann T, Shelton E. Characterization of C-reactive protein and the complement subcomponent C1t as homologus proteins displaying cyclic pentameric symmetry (pentraxins). Proc Natl Acad Sci USA 1997;74:739–743.

65. Szalai AJ, Briles DE, Volanakis JE. Human C-reactive protein is protective against fatal Streptococcus pneumoniae infection in transgenic mice. J Immunol 1995;155:2557–2563.

66. Toniatti C, Arcone R, Majello B, Ganter U, Arpaia G, Ciliberto G. Regulation of the human C-reactive protein gene, a major marker of inflammation and cancer. Mol Biol Med 1990;7:199–212.

67. Ciliberto G, Arcone R, Wagner EF, Ruther U. Inducible and tissue–specific expression of human C-reactive protein in transgenic mice. EMBO J 1987;6:4017–4022.

68. Arcone R, Gualandi G, Ciliberto G. Identification of sequences responsible for acute-phase induction of human C-reactive protein. Nucleic Acids Res 1988;16:3195–3207.

69. Ganter U, Arcone R, Toniatti C, Morrone G, Ciliberto G. Dual control of C-reactive protein gene expression by interleukin-1 and interleukin-6. EMBO J 1989;8:3773–3779.

70. Majello B, Arcone R, Toniatti C, Ciliberto G. Constitutive and IL-6-induced nuclear factors that interact with the human C-reactive protein promoter. EMBO J 1990;9:457–465.

71. Zhang D, Jiang SL, Rzewnicki D, Samols D, Kushner I. The effect of interleukin-1 on C-reactive protein expression in Hep3B cells is exerted at the transcriptional level. Biochem J 1995;310:143–148.

72. Zhang D, Sun M, Samols D, Kushner I. STAT3 participates in transcriptional activation of the C-reactive protein gene by interleukin-6. J Biol Chem 1996;271:9503–9509.

73. Ramji DP, Vitelli A, Tronche F, Cortese R, Ciliberto G. The two C/EBP isoforms, IL-6DBP/NF-IL6 and C/EBP delta/NF-IL6 beta, are induced by IL-6 to promote acute phase gene transcription via different mechanisms. Nucleic Acids Res 1993;21:289–294.

74. Toniatti C, Demartis A, Monaci P, Nicosia A, Ciliberto G. Synergistic trans-activation of the human C-reactive protein promoter by transcription factor HNF-1 binding at two distinct sites. EMBO J 1990;9:4467–4475.

75. Seidel HM, Milocco LH, Lamb P, Darnell JE Jr, Stein RB, Rosen J. Spacing of palindromic half sites as a determinant of selective STAT (signal transducers and activators of transcription) DNA binding and transcriptional activity. Proc Natl Acad Sci USA 1995;92:3041–3045.

76. Johnson PF. Identification of C/EBP basic region residues involved in DNA sequence recognition and half-site spacing preference. Mol Cell Biol 1993;13:6919–6930.

77. Murphy C, Beckers J, Ruther U. Regulation of the human C-reactive protein gene in transgenic mice. J Biol Chem 1995;270:704–708.

78. Pepys MB, Baltz ML. Acute phase proteins with special reference to C-reactive protein and related proteins (pentaxins) and serum amyloid A protein. Adv Immunol 1983;34: 141–212.

79. Grange T, Roux J, Rigaud G, Pictet R. Cell-type specific activity of two glucocorticoid responsive units of rat tyrosine aminotransferase gene is associated with multiple binding sites for C/EBP and a novel liver-specific nuclear factor. Nucleic Acids Res 1991;19:131–139.

80. Whitehead AS, Zahedi K, Rits M, Mortensen RF, Lelias JM. Mouse C-reactive protein. Generation of cDNA clones, structural analysis, and induction of mRNA during inflammation. Biochem J 1990;266:283–290.

81. Szalai AJ, van Ginkel FW, Dalrymple SA, Murray R, McGhee JR, Volanakis JE. Testosterone and IL-6 requirements for human C-reactive protein gene expression in transgenic mice. J Immunol 1998;160:5294–5299.

82. Weinhold B, Bader A, Poli V, Ruther U. Interleukin-6 is necessary, but not sufficient, for induction of the human C-reactive protein gene in vivo. Biochem J 1997;325:617–621.

83. Poli V, Balena R, Fattori E, et al. Interleukin-6 deficient mice are protected from bone loss caused by estrogen depletion. EMBO J 1994;13:1189–1196.

84. Weinhold B, Ruther U. Interleukin-6-dependent and -independent regulation of the human C-reactive protein gene in vivo. Biochem J 1997;327:425–429.

85. Dalrymple SA, Lucian LA, Slattery R, et al. Interleukin-6-deficient mice are highly susceptible to Listeria monocytogenes infection: correlation with inefficient neutrophilia. Infect Immun 1995;63:2262–2268.

86. Szalai AJ, van Ginkel FW, Dalrymple SA, Murray R, McGhee JR, Volanakis JE. Testosterone and IL-6 requirements for human C-reactive protein gene expression in transgenic mice. J Immunol 1998;160:5294–5299.

87. Georgatsou E, Bourgarel P, Meo T. Male-specific expression of mouse sex-limited protein requires growth hormone, not testosterone. Proc Natl Acad Sci USA 1993;90:3626–3630.

88. Macintyre SS, Kushner I, Samols D. Secretion of C-reactive protein becomes more efficient during the course of the acute phase response. J Biol Chem 1985;260:4169–4173.

89. Macintyre S, Samols D, Dailey P. Two carboxylesterases bind C-reactive protein within the endoplasmic reticulum and regulate its secretion during the acute phase response. J Biol Chem 1994;269:24496–24503.

90. Yue CC, Muller-Greven J, Dailey P, Lozanski G, Anderson V, Macintyre S. Identification of a C-reactive protein binding site in two hepatic carboxylesterases capable of retaining C-reactive protein within the endoplasmic reticulum. J Biol Chem 1996;271:22245–22250.

91. Macy EM, Hayes TE, Tracy RP. Variability in the measurement of C-reactive protein in healthy adults: implications for reference intervals and epidemiological applications. Clin Chem 1997;43:52–58.

92. Liuzzo G, Biasucci LM, Gallimore JR, et al. The prognostic value of C-reactive protein and serum amyloid a protein in severe unstable angina. N Engl J Med 1994;331:417–424.

93. Morrow DA, Rifai N, Antman EM, et al. C-reactive protein is a potent predictor of mortality independently and in combination with troponin T in acute coronary syndromes: a TIMI 11A substudy. Thrombolysis in Myocardial Infarction. J Am Coll Cardiol 1998;31:1460–1465.

94. Biasucci LM, Liuzzo G, Grillo RL, et al. Elevated levels of C-reactive protein at discharge in patients with unstable angina predict recurrent instability. Circulation 1999;99:855–860.

95. Hynes RO, Wagner DD. Genetic manipulation of vascular adhesion molecules in mice. J Clin Invest 1996;98:2193–2195.

96. Wilkins J, Gallimore JR, Moore EG, Pepys MB. Rapid automated high sensitivity enzyme immunoassay of C-reactive protein. Clin Chem 1998;44:1358–1361.

97. Haverkate F, Thompson SG, Pyke SD, Gallimore JR, Pepys MB. Production of C-reactive protein and risk of coronary events in stable and unstable angina. European Concerted Action on Thrombosis and Disabilities Angina Pectoris Study Group. Lancet 1997;349:462–466.

98. Ridker PM, Hennekens CH, Buring JE, Rifai N. C-reactive protein and other markers of inflammation in the prediction of cardiovascular disease in women. N Engl J Med 2000;342:836–843.

99. Kuller LH, Tracy RP, Shaten J, Meilahn EN. Relation of C-relative protein and coronary heart disease in the MRFIT nested case-control study. Multiple Risk Factor Intervention Trial. Am J Epidemiol 1996;143:1107–1115.

100. Ridker PM, Cushman M, Stampfer MJ, Tracy RP, Henneken CH. Inflammation, aspirin, and the risk of cardiovascular disease in apparently healthy men. N Engl J Med 1997;336:973–979.

101. Tracy RP, Lemaitre RN, Psaty BM, et al. Relationship of C-reactive protein to risk of cardiovascular disease in the elderly. Results from the Cardiovascular Health Study and the Rural Health Promotion Project. Arterioscler Thromb Vasc Biol 1997;17:1121–1127.

102. Ridker PM, Buring JE, Shih J, Matias M, Hennekens CH. Prospective study of C-reactive protein and the risk of future cardiovascular events among apparently healthy women. Circulation 1998;98:731–733.

103. Ridker PM, Cushman M, Stampfer MJ, Tracy RP, Hennekens CH. Plasma concentration of C-reactive protein and risk of developing peripheral vascular disease. Circulation 1998;97:425–428.

104. Koenig W, Sund M, Frohlich M, et al. C-reactive protein, a sensitive marker of inflammation, predicts future risk of coronary heart disease in initially health middle-aged men: results from the MONICA (Monitoring Trends and Determinants in Cardiovascular Disease) Augsberg Cohort Study, 1984 to 1992. Circulation 1999;99:237–242.

105. Roivainen M, Viik-Kajander M, Palosuo T, et al. Infections, inflammation, and the risk of coronary heart disease. Circulation 2000;101:252–257.

106. Danesh J, Whincup P, Walker M, et al. Low grade inflammation and coronary heart disease: prospective study and updated meta-analyses. Br Med J 2000;321:199–204.

107. Mendall MA, Strachan DP, Butland BK, et al. C-reactive protein: relation to total mortality, cardiovascular mortality and cardiovascular risk factors in men. Eur Heart J 2000;21: 1584–1590.

108. Ridker PM, Glynn RJ, Hennekens CH. C-reactive protein adds to the predictive value of total and HDL-cholesterol in determining risk of first myocardial infarction. Circulation 1998;97:2007–2011.

109. Zimmermann J, Herrlinger S, Pruy A, Metzger T, Wanner C. Inflammation enhances cardiovascular risk and mortality in hemodialysis patients. Kidney Int 1999;55:648–658.

110. Ridker PM, Rifai N, Pfeffer M, et al. Inflammation, pravastatin, and the risk of coronary events after myocardial infarction in patients with average cholesterol levels. Circulation 1998;98:839–844.

111. Heeschen C, Hamm CW, Bruemmer J, Simoons ML. Predictive value of C-reactive protein and troponin T in patients with unstable angina: a comparative analysis. CAPTURE Investigators. Chimeric c7E3 Antiplatelet Therapy in Unstable angina REfractory to standard treatment trial. J Am Coll Cardiol 2000;35:1535–1542.

112. Toss H, Lindahl B, Siegbahn A, Wallentin L. Prognostic influence of increased fibrinogen and C-reactive protein levels in unstable coronary artery disease. FRISC Study Group. Fragmin during Instability in Coronary Artery Disease. Circulation 1997;96:4204–4210.

113. Liuzzo G, Buffon A, Biasucci LM, et al. Enhanced inflammatory response to coronary angioplasty in patients with severe unstable angina. Circulation 1998;98:2370–2376.

114. Walter DH, Fichtlscherer S, Sellwig M, Auch-Schwelk W, Schachinger V, Zeiher AM. Preprocedural C-reactive protein levels and cardiovascular events after coronary stent implantation. J Am Coll Cardiol 2001;37:839–846.

115. Eisenberg MS, Chan HJ, Warshofsky MK, et al. Elevated levels of plasma C-reactive protein are associated with decreased graft survival in cardiac transplant recipients. Circulation 2000;102:2100–2104.

116. Liuzzo G, Biasucci LM, Gallimore JR, et al. Enhanced inflammatory response in patients with preinfarction unstable angina. J Am Coll Cardiol 1999;34:1696–1703.

117. Ridker PM. High-sensitivity C-reactive protein: potential adjunct for global risk assessment in the primary prevention of cardiovascular disease. Circulation 2001;103:1813–1818.

118. Lagrand WK, Visser CA, Hermens WT, et al. C-reactive protein as a cardiovascular risk factor: more than an epiphenomenon? Circulation 1999;100:96–102.

119. Malik I, Danesh J, Whincup P, et al. Soluble adhesion molecules and prediction of coronary heart disease: a prospective study and meta-analysis. Lancet 2001;358:971–976.

120. Zwaka TP, Hombach V, Torzewski J. C-reactive protein-mediated low density lipoprotein uptake by macrophages: implications for atherosclerosis. Circulation 2001;103:1194–1197.

121. Pepys MB, Booth SE, Tennent GA, Butler PJ, Williams DG. Binding of pentraxins to different nuclear structures: C-reactive protein binds to small nuclear ribonucleoprotein particles, serum amyloid P component binds to chromatin and nucleoli. Clin Exp Immunol 1994;97:152–157.

122. Volanakis JE. Complement activation by C-reactive protein complexes. Ann N Y Acad Sci 1982;389:235–250.

123. Yasojima K, Schwab C, McGeer EG, McGeer PL. Generation of C-reactive protein and complement components in atherosclerotic plaques. Am J Pathol 2001;158:1039–1051.

124. Yasojima K, Schwab C, McGeer EG, McGeer PL. Complement components, but not complement inhibitors, are upregulated in atherosclerotic plaques. Arterioscler Thromb Vasc Biol 2001; 21:1214–1219.

125. Mold C, Gresham HD, Du Clos TW. Serum amyloid P component and C-reactive protein mediate phagocytosis through murine Fc gamma Rs. J Immunol 2001;166:1200–1205.

126. Pasceri V, Chang JS, Willerson JT, Yeh ET, Chang J. Modulation of C-reactive protein-mediated monocyte chemoattractant protein-1 induction in human endothelial cells by anti-atherosclerosis drugs. Circulation 2001;103:2531–2534.

127. Patel SS, Thiagarajan R, Willerson JT, Yeh ET. Inhibition of alpha4 integrin and ICAM-1 markedly attenuate macrophage homing to atherosclerotic plaques in apoE-deficient mice. Circulation 1998;97:75–81.

128. Pasceri V, Willerson JT, Yeh ET. Direct proinflammatory effect of C-reactive protein on human endothelial cells. Circulation 2000;102:2165–2168.

129. Lagrand WK, Niessen HW, Nijmeijer R, Hack CE. Role for complement as an intermediate between C-reactive protein and intercellular adhesion molecule-1 expression? Circulation 2001;104:E46.

130. Benditt EP, Eriksen N. Chemical classes of amyloid substance. Am J Pathol 1971;65:231–252.

131. Benditt EP, Eriksen N. Chemical characteristics of the substance of typical amyloidosis in monkeys. Acta Pathol Microbiol Scand 1972;233:103–108.

132. Hermodson MA, Kuhn RW, Walsh KA, Neurath H, Eriksen N, Benditt EP. Amino acid sequence of monkey amyloid protein A. Biochemistry 1972;11:2934–2938.

133. Levin M, Pras M, Franklin EC. Immunologic studies of the major nonimmunoglobulin protein of amyloid. I. Identification and partial characterization of a related serum component. J Exp Med 1973;138:373–380.

134. Husby G, Natvig JB. A serum component related to nonimmunoglobulin amyloid protein AS, a possible precursor of the fibrils. J Clin Invest 1974;53:1054–1061.

135. Sipe JD, Cohen AS. Review: history of the amyloid fibril. J Struct Biol 2000;130:88–98.

136. Sipe JD. Amyloidosis. Annu Rev Biochem 1992;61:947–975.

137. McAdam KP, Anders RF, Smith SR, Russell DA, Price MA. Association of amyloidosis with erythema nodosum leprosum reactions and recurrent neutrophil leucocytosis in leprosy. Lancet 1975;2:572–573.

138. McAdam KP, Li J, Knowles J, et al. The biology of SAA: identification of the inducer, in vitro synthesis, and heterogeneity demonstrated with monoclonal antibodies. Ann N Y Acad Sci 1982;389:126–136.

139. Sellar GC, Oghene K, Boyle S, Bickmore WA, Whitehead AS. Organization of the region encompassing the human serum amyloid A (SAA) gene family on chromosome 11p15.1. Genomics 1994;23:492–495.

140. Benditt EP, Eriksen N. Amyloid protein SAA is associated with high density lipoprotein from human serum. Proc Natl Acad Sci USA 1977;74:4025–4028.

141. Kumon Y, Loose LD, Birbara CA, Sipe JD. Rheumatoid arthritis exhibits reduced acute phase and enhanced constitutive serum amyloid A protein in synovial fluid relative to serum. A comparison with C-reactive protein. J Rheumatol 1997;24: 14–19.

142. Meek RL, Urieli-Shoval S, Benditt EP. Expression of apolipoprotein serum amyloid A mRNA in human atherosclerotic lesions and cultured vascular cells: implications for serum amyloid A function. Proc Natl Acad Sci USA 1994;91:3186–3190.

143. Sellar GC, Whitehead AS. The putative fifth human serum amyloid A protein (SAA)-related gene "SAA5" is defined by SAA3. Biochem Biophys Res Comm 1994;200:202–205.

144. Kushner I. The acute phase response: an overview. Methods Enzymol 1988;163:373–383.

145. Edbrooke MR, Foldi J, Cheshire JK, Li F, Faulkes DJ, Woo P. Constitutive and NF-kappa B-like proteins in the regulation of the serum amyloid A gene by interleukin 1. Cytokine 1991;3:380–388.

146. Yamada T. Serum amyloid A (SAA): a concise review of biology, assay methods and clinical usefulness. Clin Chem Lab Med 1999;37:381–388.

147. Baumann H, Gauldie J. The acute phase response. Immunol Today 1994;15:74–80.

148. Liang JS, Sipe JD. Recombinant human serum amyloid A (apoSAAp) binds cholesterol and modulates cholesterol flux. J Lipid Res 1995;36:37–46.

149. Liang JS, Schreiber BM, Salmona M, et al. Amino terminal region of acute phase, but not constitutive, serum amyloid A (apoSAA) specifically binds and transports cholesterol into aortic smooth muscle and HepG2 cells. J Lipid Res 1996;37:2109–2116.

150. Bausserman LL, Bernier DN, McAdam KP, Herbert PN. Serum amyloid A and high density lipoproteins during the acute phase response. Eur J Clin Invest 1988;18:619–626.

151. Malle E, Steinmetz A, Raynes JG. Serum amyloid A (SAA): an acute phase protein and apolipoprotein. Atherosclerosis 1993;102:131–146.

152. Kindy MS, de Beer MC, Yu J, de Beer FC. Expression of mouse acute-phase (SAA1.1) and constitutive (SAA4) serum amyloid A isotypes: influence on lipoprotein profiles. Arterioscler Thromb Vasc Biol 2000;20:1543–1550.

153. Zimlichman S, Danon A, Nathan I, Mozes G, Shainkin-Kestenbaum R. Serum amyloid A, an acute phase protein, inhibits platelet activation. J Lab Clin Med 1990;116:180–186.

154. Aldo-Benson MA, Benson MD. SAA suppression of immune response in vitro: evidence for an effect on T cell-macrophage interaction. J Immunol 1982;128:2390–2392.

155. Badolato R, Wang JM, Murphy WJ, et al. Serum amyloid A is a chemoattractant: induction of migration, adhesion, and tissue infiltration of monocytes and polymorphonuclear leukocytes. J Exp Med 1994;180:203–209.

156. Xu L, Badolato R, Murphy WJ, et al. A novel biologic function of serum amyloid A. Induction of T lymphocyte migration and adhesion. J Immunol 1995;155:1184–1190.

157. Li XX, Liao WS. Expression of rat serum amyloid A1 gene involves both C/EBP-like and NF kappa B-like transcription factors. J Biol Chem 1991;266:15192–15201.

158. Lu SY, Rodriguez M, Liao WS. YY1 represses rat serum amyloid A1 gene transcription and is antagonized by NF-kappa B during acute-phase response. Mol Cell Biol 1994;14:6253–6263.

159. Li L, Liao WS. An upstream repressor element that contributes to hepatocyte-specific expression of the rat serum amyloid A1 gene. Biochem Biophys Res Comm 1999;264:395–403.

160. Ren Y, Reddy SA, Liao WS. Purification and identification of a tissue-specific repressor involved in serum amyloid A1 gene expression. J Biol Chem 1999;274:37154–37160.

161. Dang CV, Bell WR, Shuman M. The normal and morbid biology of fibrinogen. Am J Med 1989;87:567–576.

162. Williams MS, Bray PF. Genetics of arterial prothrombotic risk states. Exp Biol Med 2001;226:409–419.

163. Mosesson MW, Siebenlist KR, Meh DA. The structure and biological features of fibrinogen and fibrin. Ann N Y Acad Sci 2001;936:11–30.

164. Montalescot G, Collet JP, Choussat R, Thomas D. Fibrinogen as a risk factor for coronary heart disease. Eur Heart J 1998;19:H11–H17.

165. Ernst E. Fibrinogen as a cardiovascular risk factor-interrelationship with infections and inflammation. Eur Heart J 1993;14:82–87.

166. Mizuguchi J, Hu CH, Cao Z, Loeb KR, Chung DW, Davie EW. Characterization of the 5'-flanking region of the gene for the gamma chain of human fibrinogen. J Biol Chem 1995;270:28350–28356.

167. Hu CH, Harris JE, Davie EW, Chung DW. Characterization of the 5'-flanking region of the gene for the alpha chain of human fibrinogen. J Biol Chem 1995;270:28342–28349.

168. Zhang Z, Fuentes NL, Fuller GM. Characterization of the IL-6 responsive elements in the gamma fibrinogen gene promoter. J Biol Chem 1995;270:24287–24291.

169. Anderson GM, Shaw AR, Shafer JA. Functional characterization of promoter elements involved in regulation of human B beta-fibrinogen expression. Evidence for binding of novel activator and repressor proteins. J Biol Chem 1993;268:22650–22655.

170. Fischer CP, Bode BP, Takahashi K, Tanabe KK, Souba WW. Glucocorticoid-dependent induction of interleukin-6 receptor expression in human hepatocytes facilitates interleukin-6 stimulation of amino acid transport. Ann Surg 1996;223:610–618.

171. Gervois P, Vu-Dac N, Kleemann R, et al. Negative regulation of human fibrinogen gene expression by peroxisome proliferator-activated receptor alpha agonists via inhibition of CCAAT box/enhancer-binding protein beta. J Biol Chem 2001;276:33471–33477.

172. Jousilahti P, Salomaa V, Rasi V, Vahtera E, Palosuo T. The association of c-reactive protein, serum amyloid a and fibrinogen with prevalent coronary heart disease—baseline findings of the PAIS project. Atherosclerosis 2001;156:451–456.

173. Koukkunen H, Penttila K, Kemppainen A, et al. C-reactive protein, fibrinogen, interleukin-6 and tumor necrosis factor-alpha in the prognostic classification of unstable angina pectoris. Ann Med 2001;33:37–47.

174. Eriksson M, Egberg N, Wamala S, Orth-Gomer K, Mittleman MA, Schenck-Gustafsson K. Relationship between plasma fibrinogen and coronary heart disease in women. Arterioscler Thromb Vasc Biol 1999;19:67–72.

175. Koenig W. Fibrinogen and coronary risk. Curr Cardiol Rep 1999;1:112–118.

176. Meade TW, North WR, Chakrabarti R, et al. Haemostatic function and cardiovascular death: early results of a prospective study. Lancet 1980;1:1050–1054.

177. Lam T, Liu LJ, Janus ED, Lau CP, Hedley AJ. Fibrinogen, angina and coronary heart disease in a Chinese population. Atherosclerosis 2000;149:443–449.

178. Sato S, Nakamura M, Iida M, et al. Plasma fibrinogen and coronary heart disease in urban Japanese. Am J Epidemiol 2000;152:420–423.

179. Gheye S, Lakshmi AV, Krishna TP, Krishnaswamy K. Fibrinogen and homocysteine levels in coronary artery disease. Indian Heart J 1999;51:499–502.

180. Secondary prevention by raising HDL cholesterol and reducing triglycerides in patients with coronary artery disease: the Bezafibrate Infarction Prevention (BIP) study. Circulation 2000;102:21–27.

181. Folsom AR, Aleksic N, Ahn C, Boerwinkle E, Wu KK. Beta-fibrinogen gene -455G/A polymorphism and coronary heart disease incidence: the Atherosclerosis Risk in Communities (ARIC) Study. Ann Epidemiol 2001;11:166–170.

182. Weng X, Cloutier G, Genest J Jr. Contribution of the -455 G/A polymorphism at the beta-fibrinogen gene to erythrocyte aggregation in patients with coronary artery disease. Thromb Haemost 1999;82:1406–1411.

183. Carter AM, Mansfield MW, Stickland MH, Grant PJ. Beta-fibrinogen gene -455G/A polymorphism and fibrinogen levels. Risk factors for coronary artery disease in subjects with NIDDM. Diabetes Care 1996;19:1265–1268.

184. Cooper JA, Miller GJ, Bauer KA, et al. Comparison of novel hemostatic factors and conventional risk factors for prediction of coronary heart disease. Circulation 2000;102:2816–2822.

185. Breddin HK, Lippold R, Bittner M, Kirchmaier CM, Krzywanek HJ, Michaelis J. Spontaneous platelet aggregation as a predictive risk factor for vascular occlusions in health volunteers? Results of the HAPARG Study. Hemaostatic parameters as risk factors in healthy volunteers. Atherosclerosis 1999;144:211–219.

186. Saito I, Folsom AR, Brancati FL, Duncan BB, Chambless LE, McGovern PG. Nontraditional risk factors for coronary heart disease incidence among persons with diabetes: the Artherosclerosis Risk in Communities (ARIC) Study. Ann Intern Med 2000;133:81–91.

187. Bielak LF, Klee GG, Sheedy PF 2nd, Turner ST, Schwartz RS, Peyser PA. Association of fibrinogen with quantity of coronary artery calcification measured by electron beam computed tomography. Arterioscler Thromb Vasc Biol 2000;20:2167–2171.

188. Peach MJ. Renin-angiotensin system: biochemistry and mechanisms of action. Physiol Rev 1977;57:313–370.

189. Reid IA, Morris BJ, Ganong WF. The renin-angiotensin system. Annu Rev Physiol 1978;40:377–410.

190. Tigerstedt R, Bergman P. Niere and Kreislauf. Scand Arch Physiol 1898;8:223–271.

191. Jeunemaitre X, Soubrier F, Kotelevtsev YV, et al. Molecular basis of human hypertension: role of angiotensinogen. Cell 1992;71:169–180.

192. Burns KD. Angiotensin II and its receptors in the diabetic kidney. Am J Kidney Dis 2000;36:449–467.

193. Schrier RW, Abraham WT. Hormones and hemodynamics in heart failure. N Engl J Med 1999;341:577–585.

194. Dzau VJ. Theodore Cooper Lecture: Tissue angiotensin and pathobiology of vascular disease: a unifying hypothesis. Hypertension 2001;37:1047–1052.

195. Weiss D, Sorescu D, Taylor WR. Angiotensin II and atherosclerosis. Am J Cardiol 2001;87:25C–32C.

196. Walker WG, Whelton PK, Saito H, Russel RP, Hermann J. Relation between blood pressure and renin, renin substrate, angiotensin II, aldosterone and urinary sodium and potassium in 574 ambulatory subjects. Hypertension 1979;1:287–291.

197. Krakoff LR. Measurement of plasma-renin substrate by radioimmunoassay of angiotensin I. Concentration in syndromes associated with steroid excess. J Clin Endocrinol Metab 1973;37:110–117.

198. Kim HS, Krege JH, Kluckman KD, et al. Genetic control of blood pressure and the angiotensinogen locus. Proc Natl Acad Sci USA 1995;92:2735–2739.

199. Fukamizu A, Sugimura K, Takimoto E, et al. Chimeric renin-angiotensin system demonstrates sustained increase in blood pressure of transgenic mice carrying both human renin and human angiotensinogen genes. J Biol Chem 1993;268:11617–11621.

200. Caulfield M, Lavender P, Farrall M, et al. Linkage of the angiotensinogen gene to essential hypertension. N Engl J Med 1994;330:1629–1633.

201. Morgan T, Craven C, Nelson L, Lalouel JM, Ward K. Angiotensinogen T235 expression is elevated in decidual spiral arteries. J Clin Invest 1997;100:1406–1415.

202. Ward K, Hata A, Jeunemaitre X, et al. A molecular variant of angiotensinogen associated with preeclampsia. Nat Genet 1993;4:59–61.

203. Hopkins PN, Lifton RP, Hollenberg NK, et al. Blunted renal vascular response to angiotensin II is associated with a common variant of the angiotensinogen gene and obesity. J Hypertens 1996;14:199–207.

204. Doolittle RF. Angiotensinogen is related to the antitrypsin-antithrombin-ovalbumin family. Science 1983;222:417–419.

205. Ron D, Brasier AR, Wright KA, Tate JE, Habener JF. An inducible 50-kilodalton NF kappa B-like protein and a constitutive protein both bind the acute-phase response element of the angiotensinogen gene. Mol Cell Biol 1990;10:1023–1032.

206. Okamoto H, Hatta A, Itoh N, Ohashi Y, Arakawa K, Nakanishi S. Acute phase responses of plasma angiotensinogen and T-kininogen in rats. Biochem Pharmacol 1987;36:3069–3073.

207. Brasier AR, Han Y, Sherman CT. Transcriptional regulation of angiotensinogen gene expression. Vitam Horm 1999;57: 217–247.

208. Campbell DJ. Circulating and tissue angiotensin systems. J Clin Invest 1987;79:1–6.

209. Campbell DJ, Habener JF. Angiotensinogen gene is expressed and differentially regulated in multiple tissues of the rat. J Clin Invest 1986;78:31–39.

210. Campbell DJ, Habener JF. Cellular localization of angiotensinogen gene expression in brown adipose tissue and mesentery: quantification of messenger ribonucleic acid abundance using hybridization in situ. Endocrinology 1987;121:1616–1626.

211. Bouhnik J, Cassio D, Coezy E, Corvol P, Weiss MC. Angiotensinogen production by rat hepatoma cells in culture and analysis of its regulation by techniques of somatic cell genetics. J Cell Biol 1983;97:549–555.

212. Lilly LS, Pratt RE, Alexander RW, et al. Renin expression by vascular endothelial cells. Circ Res 1985;57:312–318.

213. Diet F, Pratt RE, Berry GJ, Momose N, Gibbons GH, Dzau VJ. Increased accumulation of tissue ACE in human atherosclerotic coronary artery disease. Circulation 1996;94:2756–2767.

214. Snyder RA, Kaempfer CE, Wintroub BU. Chemistry of a human monocyte-derived cell line (U937): identification of the angiotensin I-converting activity as leukocyte cathepsin G. Blood 1985;65:176–182.

215. Kinoshita A, Urata H, Bumpus FM, Husain A. Multiple determinants for the high substrate specificity of an angiotensin II-forming chymase from the human heart. J Biol Chem 1991;266:19192–19197.

216. Schieffer B, Schieffer E, Hilfiker-Kleiner D, et al. Expression of angiotensin II and interleukin 6 in human coronary atherosclerotic plaques: potential implications for inflammation and plaque instability. Circulation 2000;101:1372–1378.

217. Murphy TJ, Alexander RW, Griendling KK, Runge MS, Bernstein KE. Isolation of a cDNA encoding the vascular type-1 angiotensin II receptor. Nature 1991;351:233–236.

218. Griendling KK, Ushio-Fukai M, Lassegue B, Alexander RW. Angiotensin II signaling in vascular smooth muscle. New concepts. Hypertension 1997;29:366–373.

219. Morawietz H, Rueckschloss U, Niemann B, et al. Angiotensin II induces LOX-1, the human endothelial receptor of oxidized low-density lipoprotein. Circulation 1999;100:899–902.

220. Pueyo ME, Gonzalez W, Nicoletti A, Savoie F, Arnal JF, Michel JB. Angiotensin II stimulates endothelial vascular cell adhesion molecule-1 via nuclear factor-kappaB activation induced by intracellular oxidative stress. Arterioscler Thromb Vasc Biol 2000;20:645–651.

221. Keidar S, Heinrich R, Kaplan M, Hayek T, Aviram M. Angiotensin II administration to atherosclerotic mice increases macrophage uptake of oxidized ldll: a possible role for interleukin-6. Arterioscler Thromb Vasc Biol 2001;21: 1464–1469.

222. Vaughan DE, Lazos SA, Tong K. Angiotensin II regulates the expression of plasminogen activator inhibitor-1 in cultured endothelial cells. A potential link between the renin-angiotensin system and thrombosis. J Clin Invest 1995;95:995–1001.

223. Warnholtz A, Nickenig G, Schulz E, et al. Increased NADH-oxidase mediated superoxide production in the early stages of

atherosclerosis: evidence for involvement of the renin-angiotensin system. Circulation 1999;99:2027–2033.

224. Griendling KK, Minieri CA, Ollerenshaw JD, Alexander RW. Angiotensin II stimulates NADH and NADPH oxidase activity in cultured vascular smooth muscle cells. Circ Res 1994;74:1141–1148.

225. Patterson C, Ruef J, Madamanchi NR, et al. Stimulation of a vascular smooth muscle cell NAD(P)H oxidase by thrombin. Evidence that p47(phox) may participate in forming this oxidase in vitro and in vivo. J Biol Chem 1999;274: 19814–19822.

226. Frank GD, Eguchi S, Yamakawa T, Tanaka S, Inagami T, Motley ED. Involvement of reactive oxygen species in the activation of tyrosine kinase and extracellular signal-regulated kinase by angiotensin II. Endocrinology 2000;141: 3120–3126.

227. Hernandez-Presa M, Bustos C, Ortego M, et al. Angiotensin-converting enzyme inhibition prevents arterial nuclear factor-kappa B activation, monocyte chemoattractant protein-1 expression, and macrophage infiltration in a rabbit model of early accelerated atherosclerosis. Circulation 1997;95:1532–1541.

228. Yusuf S, Pepine C, Garces C, et al. Effect of enalapril on myocardial infarction and unstable angina in patients with low ejection fractions. Lancet 1992;340:1173–1178.

229. Rutherford JD, Pfeffer MA, Moye LA, et al. Effects of captopril on ischemic events after myocardial infarction. Results of the Survival and Ventricular Enlargment trial. SAVE Investigators. Circulation 1994;90:1731–1738.

230. Yusef S, Sleight P, Pogue J, Bosch J, Davies R, Dagenais G. Effects of an angiotensin-converting-enzyme inhibitor, ramipril, on cardiovascular events in high-risk patients. The Heart Outcomes. N Engl J Med 2000;342:145–153.

231. Chobanian AV, Haudenschild CC, Nickerson C, Drago R. Antiatherogenic effect of captopril in the Watanabe heritable hyperlipidemic rabbit. Hypertension 1990;15:327–331.

232. Hayek T, Attias J, Smith J, Breslow JL, Keidar S. Antiatherosclerotic and antioxidative effects of captopril in apolipoprotein E-deficient mice. J Cardiovasc Pharmacol 1998; 31:540–544.

233. Charpiot P, Rolland PH, Friggi A, et al. ACE inhibition with perindopril and atherogenesis-induced structural and functional changes in minipig arteries. Arterioscler Thromb Vasc Biol 1993;13:1125–1138.

234. Kowala MC, Recce R, Beyer S, Aberg G. Regression of early atherosclerosis in hyperlipidemic hamsters induced by fosinopril and captopril. J Cardiovasc Pharmacol 1995;25:179–186.

235. Strawn WB, Chappell MC, Dean RH, Kivlighn S, Ferrario CM. Inhibition of early atherogenesis by losartan in monkeys with diet-induced hypercholesterolemia. Circulation 2000; 101:1586–1593.

236. Sugiyama F, Haraoka S, Watanabe T, et al. Acceleration of atherosclerotic lesions in transgenic mice with hypertension by the activated renin-angiotensin system. Lab Invest 1997; 76:835–842.

237. Breslow JL. Mouse models of atherosclerosis. Science 1996 ;272:685–688.

238. Weiss D, Kools JJ, Taylor WR. Angiotensin II-induced hypertension accelerates the development of atherosclerosis in apoE-deficient mice. Circulation 2001;103:448–454.

239. Daugherty A, Manning MW, Cassis LA. Angiotensin II promotes atherosclerotic lesions and aneurysms in apolipoprotein E-deficient mice. J Clin Invest 2000;105:1605–1612.

240. Castell JV, Geiger T, Gross V, et al. Plasma clearance, organ distribution and target cells of interleukin-6/hepatocyte-stimulating factor in the rat. Eur J Biochem 1988;177: 357–361.

241. Jones SA, Horiuchi S, Topley N, Yamamoto N, Fuller GM. The soluble interleukin 6 receptor: mechanisms of production and implications in disease. FASEB J 2001;15:43–58.

242. Honda M, Yamamoto S, Cheng M, et al. Human soluble IL-6 receptor: its detection and enhanced release by HIV infection. J Immunol 1992;148:2175–2180.

243. Ledue TB, Weiner DL, Sipe JD, Poulin SE, Collins MF, Rifai N. Analytical evaluation of particle-enhanced immunonephelometric assays for C-reactive protein, serum amyloid A and mannose-binding protein in human serum. Ann Clin Biochem 1998;35:745–753.

244. Rifai N, Tracy RP, Ridker PM. Clinical efficacy of an automated high-sensitivity C-reactive protein assay. Clin Chem 1999;45:2136–2141.

245. Roberts WL, Sedrick R, Moulton L, Spencer A, Rifai N. Evaluation of four automated high-sensitivity C-reactive protein methods: implications for clinical and epidemiological applications. Clin Chem 2000;46:461–468.

246. Roberts WL, Moulton L, Law TC, et al. Evaluation of nine automated high-sensitivity C-reactive protein methods: implications for clinical and epidemiological applications. Part 2. Clin Chem 2001;47:418–425.

247. Johnson AM, Sampson EJ, Blirup-Jensen S, Svendsen PJ. Recommendations for the selection and use of protocols for assignment of values to reference materials. Eur J Clin Chem Clin Biochem 1996;34:279–285.

248. Rifai N, Ridker PM. High-sensitivity C-reactive protein: a novel and promising marker of coronary heart disease. Clin Chem 2001;47:403–411.

249. Pepys MG. The acute phase response and C-reactive protein. In: Weatherall D, Ledingham J, Warrell D, eds. Oxford Textbook of Medicine. 3rd ed. Oxford, England: Oxford University Press; 1995:1527–1533.

250. Meier-Ewert HK, Ridker PM, Rifai N, Price N, Dinges DF, Mullington JM. Absence of diurnal variation of C-reactive protein concentrations in healthy human subjects. Clin Chem 2001;47:426–430.

251. Ridker PM, Rifai N, Pfeffer M, Sacks F, Braunwald E. Long-term effects of pravastatin on plasma concentration of C-reactive protein. Circulation 1999;100:230–235.

252. Yamada T, Uchiyama K, Yakata M, Gejyo F. Sandwich enzyme immunoassay for serum amyloid A protein (SAA). Clin Chim Acta 1989;178:169–175.

253. Danesh J, Collins R, Peto R, Lowe GD. Haematocrit, viscosity, erythrocyte sedimentation rate: meta-analyses of prospective studies of coronary heart disease. Eur Heart J 2000;21: 515–520.

254. Rafnsson V, Bengtsson C. Erythrocyte sedimentation rate and cardiovascular disease. Results from a population study of women in Goteborg, Sweden. Atherosclerosis 1982;42: 97–107.

255. Gillum RF, Mussolino ME, Makuc DM. Erythrocyte sedimentation rate and coronary heart disease: the NHANES I Epidemiologic Follow-up Study. J Clin Epidemiol 1995;48: 353–361.

256. Erikssen G, Liestol K, Bjornholt JV, Stormorken H, Thaulow E, Erikssen J. Erythrocyte sedimentation rate: a possible marker of atherosclerosis and a strong predictor of coronary heart disease mortality. Eur Heart J 2000;21:1614–1620.

257. Rapaport E. Erythrocyte sedimentation rate: is it a useful marker for coronary heart disease? Eur Heart J 2000;21:1567–1569.

258. Kratz A, Lewandrowski KB. Case records of the Massachusetts General Hospital. Weekly clinicopathological exercises. Normal reference laboratory values. N Engl J Med 1998;339:1063–1072.

259. Chooi CC, Gallus AS. Acute phase reaction, fibrinogen level and thrombus size. Thromb Res 1989;53:493–501.

260. Aronsen KF, Ekelund G, Kindmart CO, Laurell CB. Sequential changes of plasma proteins after surgical trauma. Scand J Clin Lab Invest Suppl 1972;124:127–136.

261. Oparil S. Theoretical approaches to estimation of plasma renin activity: a review and some original observations. Clin Chem 1976;22:583–593.

262. Hoj Nielsen A, Knudsen F. Angiotensinogen is an acute-phase protein in man. Scand J Clin Lab Invest 1987;47:175–178.

263. Muller DN, Heissmeyer V, Dechend R, et al. Aspirin inhibits NF-kappaB and protects from angiotensin II-induced organ damage. FASEB J 2001;15:1822–1824.

264. Ridker PM, Rifai N, Lowenthal SP. Rapid reduction in C-reactive protein with cerivastatin among 785 patients with primary hypercholesterolemia. Circulation 2001;103:1191–1193.

265. Albert MA, Danielson E, Rifai N, Ridker PM; PRINCE Investigators. Effect of statin therapy on C-reactive protein levels: the pravastatin inflammation/CRP evaluation (PRINCE): a randomized trial and cohort study. JAMA 2001; 286:64–70.

266. Ridker PM, Rifai N, Clearfield M, et al. Measurement of C-reactive protein for the targeting of statin therapy in the primary prevention of acute coronary events. N Engl J Med 2001;344: 1959–1965.

267. Sparrow CP, Burton CA, Hernandez M, et al. Simvastatin has anti-inflammatory and antiatherosclerotic activities independent of plasma cholesterol lowering. Arterioscler Thromb Vasc Biol 2001;21:115–121.

268. Ferro D, Parrotto S, Basili S, Alessandri C, Violi F. Simvastatin inhibits the monocyte expression of proinflammatory cytokines in patients with hypercholesterolemia. J Am Coll Cardiol 2000;36:427–431.

269. Munford RS. Statins and the acute-phase response. N Engl J Med 2001;344:2016–2018.

270. Chen H, Ikeda U, Shimpo M, Shimada K. Direct effects of statins on cells primarily involved in atherosclerosis. Hypertens Res 2000;23:187–192.

271. Jialal I, Stein D, Balis D, Grundy SM, Adams-Huet B, Devaraj S. Effect of hydroxymethyl glutaryl coenzyme a reductase inhibitor therapy on high sensitive C-reactive protein levels. Circulation 2001;103:1933–1935.

272. Rosenson RS, Tangney C. Antiatherothrombotic properties of statins: implications for cardiovascular event reduction. JAMA 1998;279:1643–1650.

273. Garcia-Moll X, Zouridakis E, Cole D, Kaski JC. C-reactive protein in patients with chronic stable angina: differences in baseline serum concentration between women and men. Eur Heart J 2000;21:1598–1606.

274. Cushman M, Legault C, Barrett-Connor E, et al. Effect of post-menopausal hormones on inflammation-sensitive proteins: the Postmenopausal Estrogen/Progestin Interventions (PEPI) Study. Circulation 1999;100:717–722.

275. Ridker PM, Hennekens CH, Rifai N, Buring JE, Manson JE. Hormone replacement therapy and increased plasma concentration of C-reactive protein. Circulation 1999;100:713–716.

276. Staels B, Koenig W, Habib A, et al. Activation of human aortic smooth-muscle cells is inhibited by PPARalpha but not by PPARgamma activators. Nature 1998;393:790–793.

277. Kockx M, Gervois PP, Poulain P, et al. Fibrates suppress fibrinogen expression in rodents via activation of the peroxisome proliferator-activated receptor-alpha. Blood 1999;93:2991–2998.

INDEX